Fifth Edition

Cowell and Tyler's
Diagnostic Cytology and Hematology
of the Dog and Cat

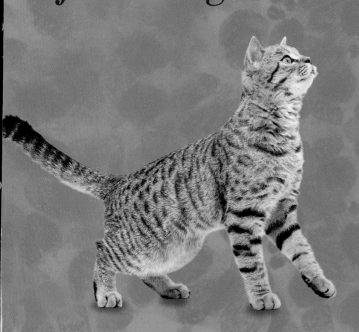
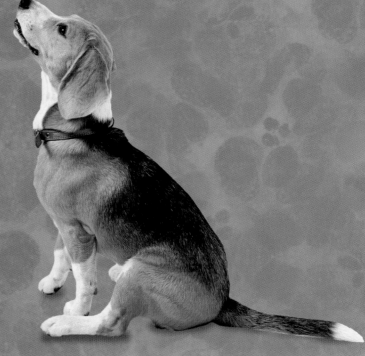

AMY C. VALENCIANO, DVM, MS, DACVP
Veterinary Clinical Pathologist
IDEXX Laboratories, Inc.
Dallas, Texas

RICK L. COWELL, DVM, MS, DACVP
Veterinary Clinical Pathologist
Stillwater, Oklahoma

ELSEVIER

Senior Content Strategist: Jennifer Catando
Senior Content Development Manager: Ellen Wurm-Cutter
Content Development Specialist: Laura Klein
Publishing Services Manager: Julie Eddy
Book Production Specialist: Clay S. Broeker
Design Direction: Brian Salisbury

Printed in China

Last digit is the print number: 9   8   7   6   5   4   3   2   1

ELSEVIER

3251 Riverport Lane
St. Louis, Missouri 63043

Working together
to grow libraries in
developing countries

www.elsevier.com • www.bookaid.org

To Dr. Rick Cowell, an inspiration and excellent pathologist and mentor. Thank you for sharing your projects, insights, and laughter and for entrusting *Diagnostic Cytology and Hematology of the Dog and Cat* to me. I can only hope to chase your footsteps. I dedicate my efforts to God and my family: Daniel (husband), Avery (daughter), Ty (son), Bonny (twin), and my dear parents (Norman and Mary Ann). I thank my wonderful mentors, especially Drs. Dave Fisher, Sonjia Shelly, Carol Grindem, Jan Andrews, Mary Jo Burkhard, Gregg Dean, Christine Stanton, and Lon Rich.

Amy C. Valenciano

To my parents who taught me the value of honesty and instilled in me a work ethic that has served me well through the years.

To my wife (Annette) and daughter (Anne) who have continually given support, meaning, and inspiration to my life.

To my daughter (Rebecca) who showed me the face of true courage and taught me to laugh and love even in the worst of times. While she lost her battle with cancer at the age of 11, her memories and life lessons will forever be remembered.

To the many outstanding veterinary clinical pathologists I have had the opportunity to learn from, especially Drs. Ronald D. Tyler, James Meinkoth, and Dennis DeNicola.

To the many veterinary practitioners, residents, and students who taught me much more than I could ever have hoped to teach them and have become colleagues and friends.

To Dr. Dean Cornwell for his support and encouragement.

To Dr. Amy Valenciano for being willing to assume editorial responsibilities; I have great faith in her ability and knowledge.

Rick L. Cowell

CONTRIBUTORS

Robin W. Allison, DVM, PhD, DACVP
Associate Professor
Department of Veterinary Pathobiology
Center for Veterinary Health Sciences
Oklahoma State University
Stillwater, Oklahoma
Subcutaneous Glandular Tissue: Mammary, Salivary, Thyroid, and Parathyroid
Female Reproductive Tract

Anne M. Barger, DVM, MS, DACVP
Clinical Associate Professor
Department of Pathobiology
College of Veterinary Medicine
University of Illinois
Urbana, Illinois
Immunocytochemistry

Regan R. W. Bell, DVM, MS, DACVP
Clinical Pathologist
IDEXX Laboratories, Inc.
Portland, Oregon
The Pancreas

Deborah C. Bernreuter, DVM, MS
Veterinary Clinical Pathologist
Department of Clinical Pathology
IDEXX Laboratories, Inc.
Irvine, California
Oropharynx and Tonsils

Melissa Blauvelt, DVM, MS, DACVP
Doctor
Clinical Pathology
IDEXX Laboratories, Inc.
Worthington, Ohio
The Lymph Nodes

Dori L. Borjesson, DVM, PhD, DACVP
Professor
Department of Pathology, Microbiology, and Immunology
School of Veterinary Medicine
University of California
Davis, California
The Pancreas

Melinda S. Camus, DVM, DACVP
Associate Professor
Department of Pathology
University of Georgia
Athens, Georgia
Female Reproductive Tract
Immunocytochemistry

Janice Cruz Cardona, DVM, DACVP
Clinical Pathologist
IDEXX Laboratories, Inc.
Houston, Texas
The Spleen

Sabrina D. Clark, DVM, DACVP
Assistant Lecturer/Graduate Student
Department of Veterinary Pathobiology
College of Veterinary Medicine and Biomedical Science
Texas A&M University
College Station, Texas
Male Reproductive Tract: Prostate. Testes, Penis, and Semen

Jennifer R. Cook, DVM, MS, DACVP
Clinical Pathologist
IDEXX Laboratories, Inc.
Detroit, Michigan
Cerebrospinal Fluid and Central Nervous System Cytology

Stephanie C. Corn, DVM, DACVP
Clinical Pathologist
IDEXX Laboratories, Inc.
Worthington, Ohio
Special Tests: Flow Cytometry

Dean Cornwell, DVM, PhD
Regional Head
Department of Clinical Pathology
IDEXX Laboratories, Inc.
Dallas, Texas
Molecular Methods in Lymphoid Malignancies

Rick L. Cowell, DVM, MS, DACVP
Clinical Pathologist
Stillwater, Oklahoma
Sample Collection and Preparation
Cell Types and Criteria of Malignancy
Selected Infectious Agents
Transtracheal and Bronchoalveolar Washes
The Kidneys

Heather L. DeHeer, DVM, DACVP
Regional Manager of Clinical Pathology North US
Department of Pathology
IDEXX Laboratories, Inc.
Newark, Delaware
The External Ear Canal

Dennis B. DeNicola, DVM, PhD, DACVP
Medical Affairs Fellow
Department of Hematology/Urinalysis Research and Development
IDEXX Laboratories, Inc.
Westbrook, Maine
Adjunct Full Professor of Veterinary Clinical Pathology
Department of Veterinary Pathobiology
College of Veterinary Medicine
Purdue University
West Lafayette, Indiana
Round Cells

Roberta Di Terlizzi, DVM, MRCVS, DACVP
Veterinary Clinical Pathologist
Clinical Pathology Lab
IDEXX Laboratories, Inc.
North Grafton, Massachusetts
Transtracheal and Bronchoalveolar Washes

Kate English, BSc, BVetMed, FRCPath, MRCVS
Lecturer
Veterinary Clinical Pathology
Department of Pathology and Pathogen Biology
Royal Veterinary College
North Mymms
Hatfield, United Kingdom
Transtracheal and Bronchoalveolar Washes

Patty J. Ewing, DVM, MS, DACVP
Director
Clinical Laboratory
Department of Pathology
Angell Animal Medical Center
Boston, Massachusetts
The Kidneys

Peter J. Fernandes, DVM, DACVP
Veterinary Clinical Pathologist
IDEXX Laboratories, Inc.
Irvine, California
Synovial Fluid Analysis

Susan E. Fielder, DVM, MS, DACVP
Clinical Pathologist
Texas A&M Veterinary Medical Diagnostic Laboratory
College Station, Texas
The Musculoskeletal System

David J. Fisher, DVM, DACVP
Veterinary Clinical Pathologist
IDEXX Laboratories, Inc.
West Sacramento, California
Cutaneous and Subcutaneous Lesions

Michael M. Fry, DVM, MS, DACVP
Associate Professor
Department of Biomedical and Diagnostic Sciences
College of Veterinary Medicine
University of Tennessee
Knoxville, Tennessee
The Lung and Intrathoracic Structures

Carolyn N. Grimes, DVM, DACVP
Regional Clinical Laboratory Director
Ethos Diagnostic Science
Ethos Veterinary Health
San Diego, California
The Lung and Intrathoracic Structures

Carol B. Grindem, DVM, PhD
Professor Emeritus
Department of Population Health and Pathobiology
College of Veterinary Medicine
North Carolina State University
Raleigh, North Carolina
Bone Marrow

Jamie L. Haddad, VMD, DACVP
Veterinary Anatomic and Clinical Pathologist
Animal Medical Center
IDEXX Laboratories, Inc.
New York, New York
The Gastrointestinal Tract
Bone Marrow

Gary J. Haldorson, DVM, PhD, DACVP
Assistant Professor
Department of Veterinary Microbiology and Pathology
College of Veterinary Medicine
Washington State University
Pullman, Washington
The Adrenal Gland

Silke Hecht, DVM, DACVR, DECVDI
Professor in Radiology
Department of Small Animal Clinical Sciences
College of Veterinary Medicine
University of Tennessee
Knoxville, Tennessee
The Lung and Intrathoracic Structures

Natalie Hoepp, DVM, MS, DACVP
Veterinary Clinical Pathologist
Pathobiology
University of Pennsylvania
Philadelphia, Pennsylvania
Round Cells

Kathryn Jacocks, DVM, DACVP
Doctor
Clinical Pathology
IDEXX Laboratories, Inc.
Dallas, Texas
Round Cells

Jocelyn D. Johnsrude, DVM, MS, DACVP
Clinical Pathologist
Department of Clinical Pathology
IDEXX Laboratories, Inc.
West Sacramento, California
The Spleen

Lisa S. Kelly, DVM, PhD
Clinical Pathologist
Department of Clinical Pathology
Antech Diagnostics
Atlanta, Georgia
Immunocytochemistry

Laura V. Lane, DVM, DACVP
Veterinary Clinical Pathologist
Department of Pathology
IDEXX Laboratories, Inc.
Irvine, California
Selected Infectious Agents

Jean-Sébastien Latouche, BSc, DVM, DES
Veterinary Clinical Pathologist
IDEXX Laboratories, Inc.
Portland, Oregon
The Pancreas

Casey J. LeBlanc, DVM, PhD, DACVP
Clinical Pathologist and Chief Executive Office
Eastern VetPath, LLC
Bethesda, Maryland
The Lung and Intrathoracic Structures

Christian M. Leutenegger, DVM, PhD, FVH
Regional Head of Molecular Diagnostics
IDEXX Laboratories, Inc.
Sacramento, California
Molecular Methods in Lymphoid Malignancies

Gwendolyn J. Levine, BS, DVM, DACVP
Clinical Assistant Professor
Department of Veterinary Pathobiology
College of Veterinary Medicine and Biomedical Sciences
Texas A&M University
College Station, Texas
Cerebrospinal Fluid and Central Nervous System Cytology

Elizabeth K. Little, BA, VMD
Doctor
Clinical Pathology
IDEXX Laboratories, Inc.
North Grafton, Massachusetts
The Adrenal Gland

Peter S. MacWilliams, DVM, PhD, DACVP
Chief of Staff
Diagnostic Services
Professor of Clinical Pathology
Department of Pathobiological Sciences
School of Veterinary Medicine
University of Wisconsin
Madison, Wisconsin
The Spleen

Patricia M. McManus, VMD, PhD, DACVP
Veterinary Clinical Pathologist
IDEXX Laboratories, Inc.
Portland, Oregon
The Spleen

James H. Meinkoth, DVM, PhD, DACVP
Professor
Department of Veterinary Pathobiology
College of Veterinary Medicine
Oklahoma State University
Stillwater, Oklahoma,
Sample Collection and Preparation,
Cell Types and Criteria of Malignancy,
Transtracheal and Bronchoalveolar Washes,
The Kidneys

Joanne B. Messick, VMD, PhD, DACVP
Associate Professor
Department of Comparative Pathobiology
College of Veterinary Medicine
Purdue University
West Lafayette, Indiana
The Lymph Nodes

Doris Miller, DVM, PhD
Professor
Athens Veterinary Diagnostic Lab
College of Veterinary Medicine
University of Georgia
Athens, Georgia
Female Reproductive Tract

Peter F. Moore, BVSc, PhD
Professor
Department of Veterinary Medicine Pathology, Microbiology,
    and Immunology
School of Veterinary Medicine
University of California
Davis, California
Molecular Methods in Lymphoid Malignancies

Rebecca J. Morton, BS, MS, DVM, PhD
Professor Emeritus
Department of Veterinary Pathobiology
Center for Veterinary Health Sciences
Oklahoma State University
Stillwater, Oklahoma
Sample Collection and Preparation

Mary B. Nabity, DVM, PhD, DACVP
Assistant Professor
Department of Veterinary Pathobiology
College of Veterinary Medicine and Biomedical Sciences
Texas A&M University
College Station, Texas
Male Reproductive Tract: Prostrate, Testes, Penis, and Semen

Jennifer A. Neel, DVM
Associate Professor
Clinical Pathology
Department of Population Health and Pathobiology
College of Veterinary Medicine
North Carolina State
Raleigh, North Carolina
The Gastrointestinal Tract

Reema T. Patel, DVM, DACVP
Clinical Pathologist
VCA ANTECH Diagnostics
Mars Petcare
Fairfax, Virginia
The External Ear Canal

M. Judith Radin, DVM, PhD, DACVP
Professor Emertius
Department of Veterinary Biosciences
Ohio State University
Columbus, Ohio
Nasal Exudates and Masses

Theresa E. Rizzi, DVM, DACVP
Clinical Associate Professor
Department of Veterinary Pathobiology
Center for Veterinary Health Sciences
Oklahoma State University
Stillwater, Oklahoma
Abdominal, Thoracic, and Pericardial Effusions

Sarah C. Roode, DVM, PhD
Resident
Veterinary Clinical Pathology
Department of Population Health and Pathobiology
College of Veterinary Medicine
North Carolina State University
Raleigh, North Carolina
Bone Marrow

Deanna M. W. Schaefer, DVM, MS, MT (ASCP), DACVP
Assistant Professor
Veterinary Clinical Pathology
Department of Biomedical and Diagnostic Sciences
University of Tennessee
Knoxville, Tennessee
Special Tests: Flow Cytometry

Andrea Siegel, DVM, ACVP
Clinical Pathologist
Department of Pathology
IDEXX Laboratories, Inc.
New York, New York
The Liver

Devorah A. Marks Stowe, DVM
Clinical Assistant Professor
Clinical Pathology
Department of Population Health and Pathobiology
College of Veterinary Medicine
North Carolina State University
Raleigh, North Carolina
The Gastrointestinal Tract

Leandro B. C. Teixeira, DVM, MSc, DACVP
Assistant Professor
Department of Pathobiological Sciences
University of Wisconsin, Madison
Madison, Wisconsin
Eyes and Associated Structures

Ronald D. Tyler, BS, DVM, PhD
Distinguished Research Fellow
Department of Comparative Biology and Safety Sciences
Amgen Inc.
Harlingen, Texas
Sample Collection and Preparation
Cell Types and Criteria of Malignancy
Transtracheal and Bronchoalveolar Washes
The Kidneys

Amy C. Valenciano, DVM, MS, DACVP
Veterinary Clinical Pathologist
IDEXX Laboratories, Inc.
Dallas, Texas
Abdominal, Thoracic, and Pericardial Effusions

William Vernau, BSc, BVMS, DVSc, PhD
Professor
Department of Veterinary Medical Pathology, Microbiology,
    and Immunology
University of California, Davis
Davis, California
Molecular Methods in Lymphoid Malignancies

Dana B. Walker, DVM, MS, PhD, DACVP
Team Lead
Global Pharmacovigilance and Epidemiology
Bristol-Myers Squibb
Wallingford, Connecticut
Peripheral Blood Smears

Koranda A. Walsh, VMD, DACVIM (SAIM), DACVP
Assistant Professor
Department of Pathobiology
University of Pennsylvania
Philadelphia, Pennsylvania
The External Ear Canal

Raquel M. Walton, VMD, MS, PhD
Clinical Pathologist
Center for Animal Referral and Emergency Services
IDEXX Laboratories, Inc.
Langhorne, Pennsylvania
*Subcutaneous Glandular Tissue: Mammary, Salivary, Thyroid,
    and Parathyroid*

Heather L. Wamsley, BS, DVM, PhD, DACVP
Veterinary Clinical Pathologist
VCA ANTECH Diagnostics
Mars Petcare
Tampa, Florida
Examination of the Urine Sediment

Maxey L. Wellman, MS, DVM, PhD, DACVP
Professor
Department of Veterinary Biosciences
Ohio State University
Columbus, Ohio
Nasal Exudates and Masses

Tamara B. Wills, DVM, MS, DACVP
Regional Head of Clinical Pathology
IDEXX Laboratories, Inc.
Pullman, Washington
The Adrenal Gland

Michael D. Wiseman, DVM, MS, DACVP
Veterinary Clinical Pathologist
IDEXX Laboratories, Inc.
New York, New York
The Liver

Pi Jie Yang, BVSc, DACVP
Clinical Pathologist
Department of Clinical Pathology
IDEXX Laboratories, Inc.
Irvine, California
Selected Infectious Agents

Karen M. Young, VMD, PhD
Professor of Clinical Pathology
Department of Pathobiological Sciences
School of Veterinary Medicine
University of Wisconsin, Madison
Madison, Wisconsin
Eyes and Associated Structures

Shanon M. Zabolotzky, DVM, DACVP
Veterinary Clinical Pathologist
Reference Laboratory
IDEXX Laboratories, Inc.
Elmhurst, Illinois
Peripheral Blood Smears

Cytologic evaluation of blood, fluid, and tissue specimens is an especially valuable diagnostic aid in veterinary medicine. Reliable, confident interpretation of carefully obtained, well-preserved, representative cellular samples is essential for accurate diagnosis, prognosis, and treatment. *Cowell and Tyler's Diagnostic Cytology and Hematology of the Dog and Cat,* fifth edition, is a comprehensive yet practical reference designed to help the reader develop and enhance the necessary clinical laboratory and interpretive skills for a wide variety of pathologic conditions seen in everyday practice, along with those less frequently encountered.

The goal of this reference text is to provide small-animal veterinary clinicians and cytology students with the knowledge and skills required to apply cytodiagnostic techniques to sample collection, preparation, microscopic assessment, and interpretation. It is intended to be a familiar and trusted bench-top reference and guide alongside the microscope. The numerous tables and flowcharts that accompany the text assist the reader in both the development of a cytological opinion and in correlation of the cytological findings with clinical signs and history, physical examination, diagnostic imaging, and other clinical laboratory findings to achieve the most accurate and specific diagnosis possible, while still being rapid and efficient.

Written in a logical, highly visual manner, we believe we have provided a resource that will establish and maintain a secure clinical foundation for the technical as well as interpretive aspects of cytological diagnostic screening. The straightforward text is organized for quick information retrieval. Over 1000 high-resolution, full-color photomicrographs illustrate pertinent features of lesions; aid in the identification of many bacterial, fungal, and protozoal organisms and in the differentiation of normal cells from abnormal cells; and demonstrate the variability of patterns seen in certain conditions. Helpful and easy-to-follow algorithms and tables are distributed throughout the text to facilitate rapid and efficient progression through the diagnostic process. As inappropriate sample collection and poor slide preparation are often the major impediments to sample quality, we have included valuable information on collection and preparation techniques. This not only facilitates accurate on-site diagnosis but also permits the practitioner to confidently submit diagnostic-quality samples to a cytopathologist for interpretation.

The fifth edition maintains the practical diagnostic approach of its predecessors. All chapters from the previous edition have been substantially updated to include recently recognized conditions, new terminology, new procedures, and numerous new photomicrographs. Histopathology photomicrographs of both normal morphology and selected pathologic conditions have been added to enhance knowledge of tissue architecture in relation to cytology. In addition, five chapters in particular—Round Cells, The Spleen, The Liver, Female Reproductive Tract, and Bone Marrow—offer more expanded coverage and have been reorganized to integrate relevant information for better understanding.

The authors hope that you will truly find this one of the most used references in your clinical library. We also believe that, with the knowledge and skills you glean from use of this resource, you will reduce your clinical time and frustrations and, most importantly, improve the quality of the care you deliver to your patients and their people.

Amy C. Valenciano
Rick L. Cowell

ACKNOWLEDGMENTS

We thank our families for their support and understanding. Many other people deserve acknowledgment and sincere thanks also. These include Elsevier's excellent editors and staff and the many veterinary pathologists who sent slides or pictures for use in the text.

It was an honor and privilege to work with each of the authors. They are exceptional veterinarians, scientists, and teachers. We thank them for sharing their time, talent, and expertise, and we thank their families for sharing them.

Amy C. Valenciano
Rick L. Cowell

CONTENTS

Sample Collection and Preparation

James H. Meinkoth, Rick L. Cowell, Ronald D. Tyler, and Rebecca J. Morton

Evaluation of cytological samples has become well established as a method of obtaining a diagnosis of lesions in a wide variety of tissues. Cytology and histopathology will likely always remain complementary diagnostic procedures, reflecting a trade-off between the lower cost, reduced invasiveness of sample collection, and more rapid turnaround time with cytology and the increased amount of information available from the ability to evaluate tissue architecture with histopathology. However, the ever-increasing availability of advanced imaging techniques has resulted in an increased reliance on cytopathology to evaluate focal lesions of internal organs, which previously could not be reliably sampled. As clinicians have increased their use of this diagnostic modality and cytopathologists have become more experienced with the wider variety of lesions and tissues sampled, the spectrum of disease processes that can be identified by cytology and the reliability and precision of the diagnoses for lesions of many tissues have increased.

Other than the experience of the cytopathologist evaluating the samples, one of the major factors determining the diagnostic value of cytological specimens is the quality of the sample. The diagnostic yield of cytology is noticeably higher in the hands of clinicians who have a great deal of experience with obtaining cytological specimens. With histological specimens, once the tissue sample is collected and placed in an appropriate amount of formalin, laboratory technicians handle the remainder of sample preparation. With cytology, the clinician is faced with the responsibility of not only collecting an adequately representative specimen but also preparing the slides that are to be examined and, often, staining of the slides as well. Because the cells to be examined are not grossly visible during sample collection and slide preparation, it is often difficult to tell whether an adequate specimen has been obtained at the time of the sampling procedure.

Collection and preparation of cytological specimens is definitely a skill gained only through experience and refinement of technique based on the results obtained. Many clinicians (and owners) are understandably frustrated when a sample submitted is determined to be nondiagnostic. Fortunately, an understanding of some basic principles of sample collection and familiarity with some of the more common pitfalls related to cytological sample preparation can increase the odds of a diagnostic result.[1-5]

METHODS OF SAMPLE COLLECTION

Several methods of collecting samples for cytological analysis exist. The indications for each are outlined in Table 1.1.

Fine-Needle Biopsy

Fine-needle biopsy (FNB) can be performed by using a standard syringe and needle with or without aspiration (as described later). This is the best overall method for sampling any cutaneous mass or proliferative lesion.[1] FNB allows for collection of cells from deep within the lesion, avoiding surface contamination with inflammatory cells and organisms that often plague impression smears, swabs, or scrapings. Surface cells are often poorly preserved and may show artifacts related to cellular aging and exposure to secondary inflammation responses, especially with ulcerated masses. These changes can make evaluation of the significance of cellular atypia more difficult. A classic example of this is masses of the urinary bladder. Samples collected by traumatic catheterization often contain cells that show significant degeneration and artifact from aging and prolonged exposure to urine (Fig. 1.1). Conversely, samples collected via FNB from deep within the lesion are typically well preserved and easier to evaluate (see Fig. 1.1, A). FNB is also the only practical technique for sampling of subcutaneous or internal organs or masses.

Selection of Syringe and Needle

FNB specimens are collected with a 22- to 25-gauge needle and a 3- to 20-mL syringe. The softer the tissue, the smaller are the needle and syringe used. It is seldom necessary to use a needle larger than 22-gauge for aspiration, even for firm tissues. When needles larger than 22-gauge are used, tissue cores tend to be aspirated, resulting in a poor yield of free cells. Also, larger needles tend to cause greater blood contamination. For aspirating lesions deep within body cavities, longer needles may be needed, but the diameter should remain the same. Whenever aspirating lesions within body cavities, the needle may pass through, and collect cells from, nontarget organs. Serosal mesothelial cells are particularly common. Using a needle with a stylet in place and removing the stylet only when the lesion is entered can help reduce inadvertent collection of nontarget tissue.

The size of the syringe is not critical when the samples are collected by using the nonaspiration technique. If using the aspiration technique, the size of syringe used is influenced by the consistency of the tissue being aspirated. Softer tissues, such as lymph nodes, often can be aspirated with a 3-mL syringe. Firm tissues, such as fibromas and squamous cell carcinomas, require a larger syringe to maintain adequate negative pressure (suction) for collection of a sufficient number of cells. A 12-mL syringe is a good choice if the texture of the tissue is unknown.

Preparation of the Site for Aspiration

If microbiological tests are to be performed on a portion of the sample collected or a body cavity (peritoneal and thoracic cavities, joints, etc.) is to be penetrated, the area of aspiration is surgically prepped. Otherwise, skin preparation is essentially that required for vaccination or venipuncture. An alcohol swab can be used to clean the area. If the samples are being collected under ultrasound guidance, it is important to avoid the use of ultrasound gel, substituting alcohol as a

TABLE 1.1	Indications for Various Methods of Sample Collection	
Collection Method	**Indications for Uses**	**Comments**
Fine-needle biopsy (aspiration or nonaspiration method)	Masses (surface or internal)	Best method for cutaneous or subcutaneous masses because it avoids surface contamination
	Lymph nodes	
	Internal organs	Best method for minimally invasive sampling of internal organs or masses
	Fluid collection	
Impression smear	Exudative cutaneous lesions	Most useful for identification of infectious organisms
		May yield only surface cells and contamination (problem with ulcerated tumors)
	Preparation of cytology samples from biopsy specimens	With biopsy specimens, it is imperative to blot excess blood from sample
		Impression smears of biopsy specimens must be made before exposure of biopsy sample to formalin
Scraping	Used with flat cutaneous lesions that are not amenable to fine-needle biopsy	With dry cutaneous lesions (e.g., ringworm), it is important to scrape sufficiently to obtain some blood or serum to help cells stick to slide
	Preparation of cytology samples from poorly exfoliative biopsy specimens	
Swab		Generally used only when anatomical location not amenable to collection by other means
	Vaginal smears	
	Fistulous tracts	With fistulous tracts, most useful in classifying type of inflammatory response and identifying infectious organisms

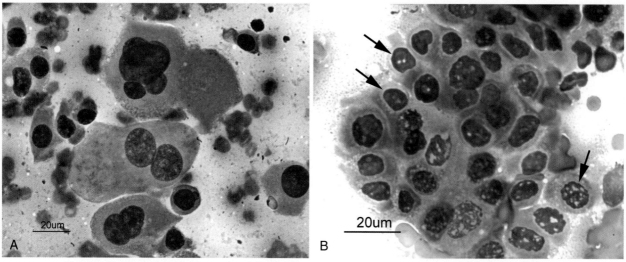

Fig. 1.1 Photomicrograph of samples collected from transitional cell carcinoma. (A) Sample collected by fine-needle biopsy of the mass. The cells are well preserved, allowing for examination of nuclear and cytoplasmic detail. (B) Sample collected by traumatic catheterization. These samples typically collect superficial cells that show marked changes resulting from cellular aging and exposure to urine. Nuclear degeneration is noted as a homogeneous light pink-purple color as well as fragmentation with numerous clear spaces evident *(arrows)*. (Courtesy Oklahoma State University teaching files.)

contact agent instead. Ultrasound gel stains pink with commonly used cytology stains. Even a small amount of ultrasound gel picked up as a contaminant when the needle passes through the skin is enough to completely obscure the cells and render a slide nondiagnostic.

Nonaspiration Procedure (Capillary Technique, Stab Technique)

Currently, most clinicians prefer to collect FNB specimens without the application of negative pressure. This technique yields samples of equal or better quality compared with those obtained with the older aspiration technique.[4-6] The nonaspiration technique works well for most masses, especially those that are highly vascular.[1] The procedure is performed by using a small-gauge needle on a 3- to 12-mL syringe. The barrel of the syringe is filled with air before the collection attempt to allow for rapid expulsion of material onto a glass slide. The syringe is grasped at or near the needle hub with the thumb and forefinger (much like holding a dart) to allow for maximal control (Fig. 1.2). The mass to be aspirated is stabilized with a free hand, and the needle is

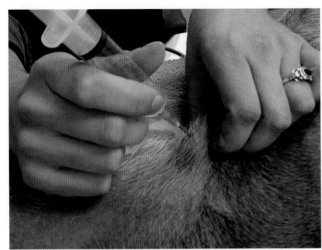

Fig. 1.2 Nonaspiration technique of fine-needle biopsy. The syringe is held at or near the needle hub with the thumb and forefinger. Note that the syringe is prefilled with air. The free hand is used to stabilize the mass. This technique allows greater control over movement of the needle. (Courtesy Oklahoma State University teaching files.)

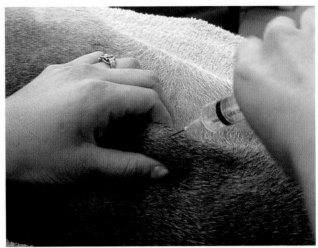

Fig. 1.3 Aspiration technique of fine-needle biopsy. The mass is stabilized with one hand while the needle is introduced into the center of the mass. The hand holding the syringe is used to pull back on the plunger, creating negative pressure. (Courtesy Oklahoma State University teaching files.)

inserted into the mass. The needle is rapidly moved back and forth in a stabbing motion in an attempt to stay along the same tract, similar to the action of a sewing machine. This allows for collection of cells by cutting and tissue pressure. Care must be taken to keep the needle tip within the mass to prevent contamination with surrounding tissue. The needle is then withdrawn, the material in the needle is rapidly expelled onto a clean glass slide, and a smear is made by using one of the techniques listed later in this chapter (see "Preparation of Slides").

Having the syringe prefilled with air allows the sample to be expelled onto a slide more quickly, and this helps avoid desiccation (drying out) of the collected cells and coagulation of the sample.[6]

Some perform the nonaspiration technique with a needle only, with no syringe attached. This may allow for even greater control of the placement and movement of the needle, although the syringe must then be attached after sample collection to expel the material from the needle. Another variation that has been recommended for ultrasound-guided collection is to have an intravenous fluid extension set placed between the needle and the syringe.[6] This allows freedom of movement of the needle with one hand during the collection procedure. The syringe can be hung over the shoulder during collection, and then the other hand can be used to quickly expel the material onto the slide.

Aspiration Procedure

With the older aspiration method of FNB, the mass is stabilized with one hand while the needle, with syringe attached, is introduced into the center of the mass (Fig. 1.3). Strong negative pressure is applied by withdrawing the plunger to about three-fourths the volume of the syringe (Fig. 1.4). If the mass is sufficiently large and the patient sufficiently restrained, negative pressure can be maintained while the needle is moved back and forth repeatedly, passing through about two-thirds of the diameter of the mass. With large masses, the needle can be redirected to several areas within the mass to increase the amount of tissue sampled. Alternatively, several different areas of the mass can be sampled with separate collection attempts. Care should be taken to not allow the needle to exit the mass while negative pressure is being applied because this can result in either aspiration of the sample into the barrel of the syringe (where it may not be retrievable) or contamination of the sample with tissue surrounding the mass.

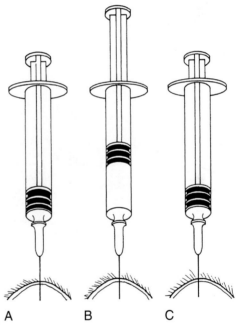

A   B   C

Fig. 1.4 Fine-needle aspiration from a solid mass. After the needle is within the mass (A), negative pressure is placed on the syringe by rapidly withdrawing the plunger (B), usually one-half to three-fourths the volume of the syringe barrel. The needle is redirected several times while negative pressure is maintained, if this can be accomplished without the needle's point leaving the mass. Before the needle is removed from the mass, the plunger is released, relieving negative pressure on the syringe (C).

The negative pressure should not be applied for more than a few seconds in any one area. Often, no material will be visible in the syringe or in the hub of the needle, even though an adequate sample has been obtained. With excessive force or prolonged application of negative pressure, disruption of blood vessels will eventually occur, and the sample will be contaminated with peripheral blood, diluting the tissue cells and rendering the sample nondiagnostic.

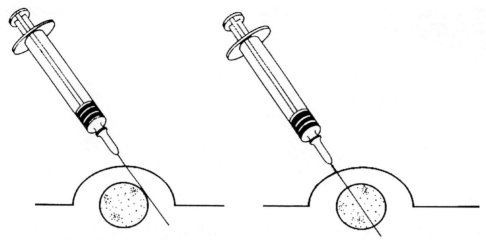

Fig. 1.5 Geographical miss. Sometimes, the needle is not in the area containing representative tissue of the lesion during sample collection. This is common in obese animals where the lesion may be surrounded by abundant subcutaneous fat. (Courtesy Oklahoma State University teaching files.)

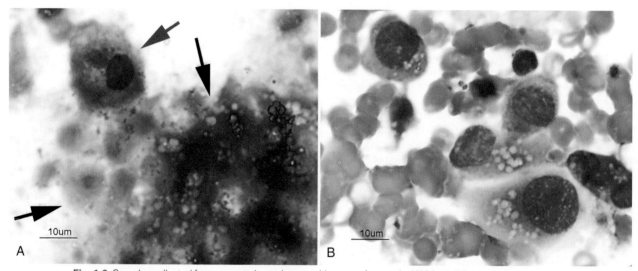

Fig. 1.6 Samples collected from a prostatic carcinoma with areas of necrosis. (A) Most slides were from aspirates of necrotic areas and contain predominantly necrotic cellular debris *(black arrows)*. A single partially intact cell is present *(blue arrow)*. These slides would be nondiagnostic. (B) One of the aspiration attempts sampled a nonnecrotic area, and the resulting slides contained numerous intact cells, allowing a diagnosis to be made. This demonstrates the importance of sampling multiple sites of a mass. (Courtesy Oklahoma State University teaching files.)

After several areas are sampled, the negative pressure is released, and the needle is removed from the mass and skin. The needle is removed from the syringe, and air is drawn into the syringe. The needle is replaced onto the syringe, and some of the tissue in the barrel and hub of the needle is expelled onto one end of a glass microscope slide by rapidly depressing the plunger. When possible, several preparations should be made, as described later in this chapter (see "Preparation of Slides").

If possible, it is optimal to perform multiple collection attempts at various sites within the mass to increase the chance of obtaining diagnostic material and to ensure a representative sampling of the lesion.

Collection Tips

Make and submit multiple slides. This is likely the single most important thing that can be done to increase the diagnostic yield. Small-gauge needles are used for collecting cytological specimens, and the procedure is usually relatively painless. It takes less time to

perform several collection attempts and prepare multiple slides when the animal is first presented than to repeat a procedure after finding the specimen to be nondiagnostic, often after the animal has already been discharged from the hospital. This is particularly important if sedation or anesthesia is required for collection. It is optimal to stain and briefly examine one or two slides to ensure that they are adequately cellular while the patient is still in the hospital (or before animal has recovered, if anesthesia or sedation is required). If the slides stained are not cellular, additional collection attempts can be performed immediately.

There are many possible reasons for any one slide being nondiagnostic. The slide may not have any diagnostic cells because the needle missed the lesion during collection (geographical miss) (Fig. 1.5) or may have been in a nonrepresentative portion of the lesion (e.g., an area of inflammation or necrosis within a neoplasm (Fig. 1.6). In addition, some lesions simply do not exfoliate cells well. Even if adequate cells were collected, many times the cells do not spread out well and the slides are too thick to be evaluated (especially common in the case

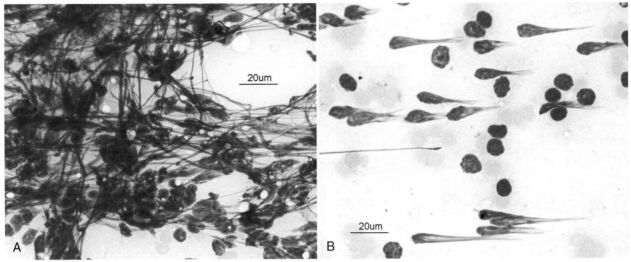

Fig. 1.7 Images from an aspirate of a reactive lymph node. This sample was nondiagnostic because all of the cells have been ruptured as a result of excessive downward pressure being applied during sample preparation. (A) The linear streaks of material represent nuclear chromatin of ruptured cells. (B) Ruptured cells often appear to have "comet tails" all going the same direction. (Courtesy Oklahoma State University teaching files.)

of lymph node aspirates), or all of the cells are ruptured during smear preparation (Fig. 1.7). Even in the hands of clinicians who are highly experienced in sample collection, it is not unusual to have multiple slides from a single lesion and all but one of the slides being nondiagnostic for one reason or another.

If possible, a minimum of four to five slides, representing collection attempts from several sites within the lesion, should be submitted from any lesion. If some of the samples appear to be excessively thick or if little to no material is apparent on the slides, additional slides should be made. With multiple slides, the chances of at least one of them being of diagnostic quality are increased.

If multiple masses are sampled, a new needle and syringe should be used with each mass. If this is not done, slides from one mass may be contaminated with cells left in the needle from previous collection attempts. Each slide should be clearly labeled as to the anatomical site sampled.

Avoid blood dilution. Blood contamination (hemodilution) is another common cause of nondiagnostic slides. FNB with aspiration will collect the tissue of least resistance. If blood vessels within the lesion have been ruptured, the tissue of least resistance will be peripheral blood. Once significant blood contamination has occurred, it is difficult to salvage the sample. Additional collection attempts should be made using a clean syringe and a clean needle.

The two major causes of blood contamination are the use of too large a needle (<22-gauge) and prolonged aspiration. Larger-bore needles do not usually collect more cells but are more likely to rupture small blood vessels. As mentioned before, material is often not visible in the syringe during sample collection despite adequate numbers of cells being present within the needle. Any time material is visible in the hub of the needle, the collection procedure should be stopped and slides made immediately.

Some lesions are highly vascular, making it difficult to avoid blood contamination, even with good collection technique. In these cases, use of a nonaspiration technique may result in less blood contamination and more tissue cells for evaluation.

Do not be timid. Other reasons for poor cellularity of a sample are inadequate negative pressure (aspiration technique) and slow or shallow needle passages (nonaspiration technique). When using the

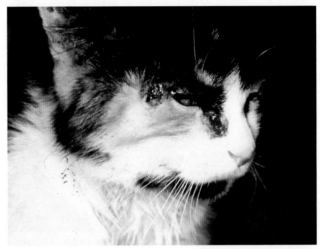

Fig. 1.8 Ulcerative, exudative lesions on the face of a cat. This lesion is well suited for impression smears. Slides from these lesions revealed inflammatory cells and many *Sporothrix* organisms. (Courtesy Oklahoma State University teaching files.)

nonaspiration technique, the clinician is relying on the cutting action of the needle going through the tissue to create a slurry of cells and tissue fluid, which will enter the needle by capillary action. Needle passages should be quick and of sufficient length (although the size of the mass may limit the length of the needle pass).

Impression Smears

Impression smears can be made from ulcerated or exudative superficial lesions (Fig. 1.8) or tissue samples collected at surgery or necropsy (Fig. 1.9). Impression smears from superficial lesions often yield only inflammatory cells, even if the inflammation is a secondary process; neoplastic cells may not exfoliate in exudates or impression smears of ulcerated masses. If possible, FNB of tissue under the ulcerated or exudative area should be collected in addition to the impression smears. Inserting the needle at a nonulcerated area will help reduce contamination during collection. Impression smears of exudates or ulcers are

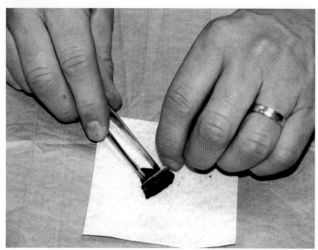

Fig. 1.9 Impression smear of tissue removed at surgery. The tissue is trimmed so that a fresh surface is created for making the impression smear. If normal tissue surrounding a mass has been excised, it is important to be sure that the tissue is cut through the area of interest. (Courtesy Oklahoma State University teaching files.)

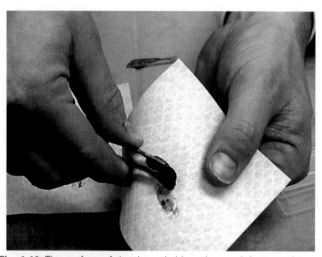

Fig. 1.10 The surface of the tissue is blotted several times against an absorbent material to remove excess blood and tissue fluid. This is extremely important to avoid slides that contain only peripheral blood. (Courtesy Oklahoma State University teaching files.)

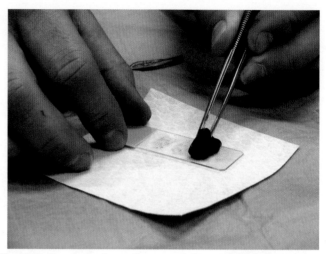

Fig. 1.11 The tissue is gently pressed (not smeared) several times against the surface of a clean glass slide. (Courtesy Oklahoma State University teaching files.)

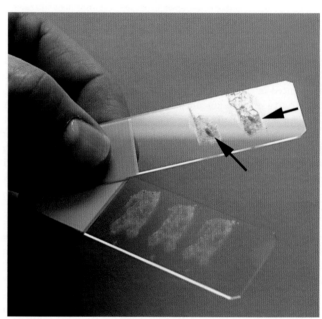

Fig. 1.12 The resulting slides from an impression smear. The slide on the bottom is properly made and has several slightly opaque areas where the tissue has been touched to the slide indicating cells have probably been transferred to the slide. The slide on top has excessive peripheral blood *(arrows)*, indicating that the tissue was not properly blotted against absorbent material before making the impression smear. This slide will likely contain only peripheral blood, or if cells are present, they may not be well spread out. (Courtesy Oklahoma State University teaching files.)

most beneficial for determining whether bacterial or fungal organisms are present. Keep in mind that bacteria may reflect only a secondary bacterial infection.

Ulcerated areas should be imprinted before they are cleaned. The lesion should then be cleaned with a saline-moistened surgical sponge and reimprinted or scraped.

To collect impression smears from tissues collected during surgery or necropsy, the tissue should first be cut so that a fresh surface for imprinting is created (see Fig. 1.9). Next, the excess blood and tissue fluid should be removed from the surface of the lesion being imprinted by blotting with a clean absorbent material (Fig. 1.10). Excessive blood and tissue fluids inhibit tissue cells from adhering to the glass slide, producing a poorly cellular preparation. Also, excessive fluid inhibits cells from spreading and assuming the size and shape they usually have in air-dried smears. After excess blood and tissue fluids have been blotted from the surface of the lesion, the surface of the lesion is touched (pressed) against the middle of a clean glass microscope slide and lifted

directly up (Fig. 1.11). This should be repeated several times so that several tissue imprints are present on the slide. If the excess blood has been adequately removed, the tissue will stick somewhat to the slide and will appear to peel off the slide, if removed slowly. Properly made slides will have slightly opaque areas at the areas of the impressions but should not have excessively thick areas of blood (Fig. 1.12).

No further smearing of the material is necessary. The tissue should not be allowed to slide around on the glass surface, as this causes cells to rupture. When possible, several slides should be imprinted so that a few can be retained in case special stains are necessary. After making

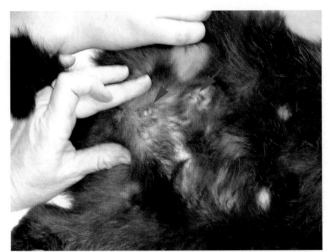

Fig. 1.13 Multiple plaquelike and raised lesions on the ventrum of a cat with eosinophilic granuloma lesions. The lesions were not thick enough to obtain good aspirates but yielded diagnostic cells via scraping. The ulcerated lesions are those that have already been scraped *(arrows)*. Scraping to the point of obtaining a small amount of blood or serum helps the cells adhere to the slides and also increases the chance of bypassing surface contamination and obtaining representative cells. (Courtesy Oklahoma State University teaching files.)

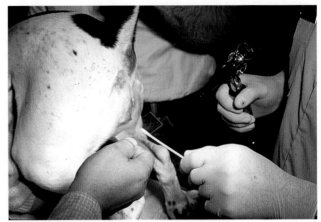

Fig. 1.14 Preparation of a vaginal swab from a dog. The swab containing the sample is gently rolled along the slide. Sliding or smearing the swab across the slide will result in excessive rupturing of the cells. (Courtesy Oklahoma State University teaching files.)

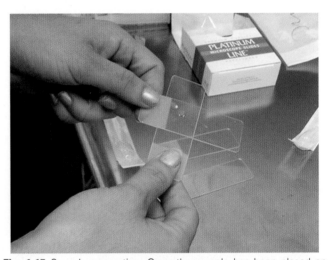

Fig. 1.15 Squash preparation. Once the sample has been placed on a clean glass slide, a second slide is placed on top of the sample and is used to spread out the sample. It is important that no downward pressure be applied on the top slide during spreading of the sample. (Courtesy Oklahoma State University teaching files.)

sufficient impression smears, the tissue used should be placed in an appropriate amount of formalin so that it may be submitted for histological evaluation, if necessary.

Scrapings

Scrapings can be made from external lesions or tissue obtained from surgery or necropsy. Generally, scrapings will result in more cellular slides than will impression smears; however, like impression smears, scrapings may contain mostly surface contamination or inflammation if made from the surface of ulcerated cutaneous lesions. Generally, scrapings are not as valuable for diagnosing neoplasia as slides made from FNB. Scrapings are valuable in collecting samples from cutaneous lesions that are flat and dry and thus not amenable to FNB or impression and from samples collected at surgery or necropsy (Fig. 1.13).[1] Two examples of lesions in which scrapings are beneficial are feline eosinophilic granuloma complex lesions and dermatophytosis.[7] Scrapings are prepared by holding a scalpel blade perpendicular to the lesion's surface and pulling the blade toward oneself several times. When scraping dry, nonulcerated lesions, such as dermatophyte lesions, scrapings should be sufficiently deep to cause exudation of serum or blood. This proteinaceous and fibrin-rich fluid will help the collected cells (and hairs when looking for dermatophytes) adhere to the slide and prevent them from being washed off during staining. The material collected on the blade is transferred to the middle of a glass microscope slide and spread either by smearing gently with the scalpel blade or by one of the techniques described later for preparation of smears from aspirates of solid masses.

Swabs

Generally, swabs are used only when other collection methods are not practical, as when obtaining samples from the vagina or the external ear or from within fistulous tracts. Swabs from the external ear canal and fistulous tracts are most useful for identifying infectious organisms. Specimens are collected from the site by using a sterile cotton swab. If the lesion is moist, the cotton swab need not be moistened. However, if the lesion is not very moist, moistening the swab with sterile saline is suggested because this helps minimize disruption of the cells that might occur during collection

and sample preparation. Use of lubricant gels (e.g., K-Y Jelly) should be avoided when collecting swabs because they can coat the sample and interfere with staining of the cells, rendering the slide uninterpretable. Once the sample has been collected, the swab is gently rolled across the surface of a clean glass slide. It is important to not swipe the swab across the slide because this will often result in rupture of all the cells (Fig. 1.14).

PREPARATION OF SLIDES: SOLID TISSUE ASPIRATES

Slide-Over-Slide Smears ("Squash Preps")

When used properly, this is generally the best method for preparing slides from FNB or scrapings of solid tissue lesions. The goal is to prepare a thin film in which the cells are spread out into a single layer, without rupturing the cells. The material collected from the FNB procedure is expelled near one end (approximately one-half inch) of a clean glass slide (sample slide). A second glass slide (spreader slide) is placed on top of and perpendicular to the slide containing the sample directly over the specimen (Fig. 1.15). The specimen will usually spread out between the two slides because of the weight of the spreader slide alone. If the sample is thick or granular and does not spread out well, light momentary downward pressure may be applied to the spreader slide and then released. The spreader slide is then lightly drawn out across the length of the bottom slide, spreading the sample (Fig. 1.16). Despite the (poorly worded) name "squash prep," it is important that no downward pressure be applied to the spreader slide while smearing the sample because this usually results in rupturing the majority of the cells.

If done properly, the smear should have a "flame shape" that does not extend to the edge of the slide. This is important because, as with a blood smear, often it is only at the edges of the sample where the cells are spread out sufficiently thin to be evaluated. Smears that extend off the edge of the slides are usually too thick to be evaluated. Also, many automated slide stainers do not stain the entire slide but leave an unstained area approximately one-quarter to one-half inch wide on either end of the slide. Cells in these areas will not be stained and therefore cannot be evaluated. Even when using dip-staining methods

that stain the entire slide, material at the very edges of a slide may be impossible to view on some microscopes.

When done correctly, this technique does a good job of spreading out the cells, even those in clusters, so that cellular detail can be adequately evaluated. The main disadvantage of this method, particularly in inexperienced hands, is excessive cell rupturing. Lymphoid cells are particularly fragile and will often rupture if even moderate pressure is used when preparing slides with this technique.

Blood Smear Technique

With many samples, especially lymph node aspirates, the material expelled from the syringe onto the slide will have enough tissue fluid, blood, or both so that the sample can be smeared out as if making a blood smear (Fig. 1.17).[1] This technique will result in less cell rupturing, especially with fragile cell populations, and generally produces thin smears with intact cells that are well spread out.

As with the slide-over-slide technique, the sample is expelled from the syringe near one end of the sample slide. The long edge of the

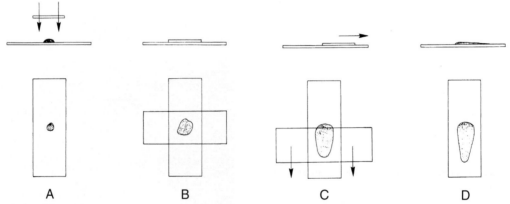

Fig. 1.16 Squash preparation. (A) A portion of the aspirate is expelled onto a glass microscope slide, and another slide is placed over the sample. (B) This spreads the sample. If the sample does not spread well, gentle digital pressure can be applied to the top slide. Care must be taken not to place excessive pressure on the slide, causing the cells to rupture. (C) The slides are smoothly slid apart. (D) This usually produces well-spread smears but may result in excessive cell rupture.

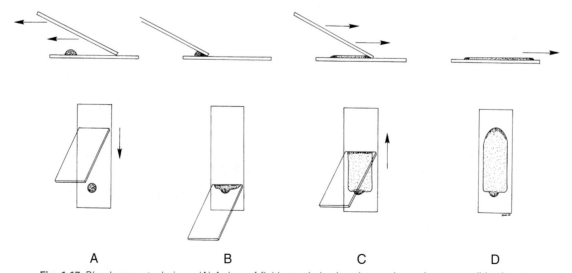

Fig. 1.17 Blood smear technique. (A) A drop of fluid sample is placed on a glass microscope slide close to one end, then another slide is slid backward to contact the front of the drop. (B) When the drop is contacted, it rapidly spreads along the juncture between the two slides. (C) and (D) The spreader slide is then smoothly and rapidly slid forward the length of the slide, producing a smear with a feathered edge.

spreader slide is placed onto the flat surface of the sample slide in front of the sample. The spreader slide is tilted to a 45-degree angle with respect to the sample slide and pulled backward about a third of the way into the aspirated material. The spreader slide is then smoothly and rapidly slid forward, as if making a blood smear. The smear should end in a feathered edge at least 0.5 inch from the opposite end of the spreader slide. If the sample smear extends all the way to the edge of a slide, additional slides should be made, and a smaller amount of sample should be put on the slide.

"Starfish" Preps

This is another technique used by some people, but generally is not the preferred technique because it may not produce good-quality smears. In this method, the aspirated material is dragged peripherally in several directions with the point of a syringe needle, producing a starfish shape (Figs. 1.18 and 1.19). This technique tends to avoid damaging fragile cells but allows a thick layer of tissue fluid to remain around the cells. Often, the thick layer of fluid prevents the cells from spreading well, and there may be few or no areas of the slides adequate for evaluation. Overall, a gentle slide-over-slide is recommended, but this technique can be considered if excessive cell rupturing is a problem.

Preparation Tips
Do Not Let the Sample Dry or Clot

If the sample clots or dries out on the slide before smears can be made, the cells may not spread out sufficiently to be evaluated. Also, the cells will often be distorted or not stain well because they are incorporated in a clot. Several clean slides should be laid out in an easily accessible area before the collection procedure to reduce the time between collections and final smear preparation.

One common mistake is to spray the sample from the needle onto the slide from a distance. This results in the sample being spread out in many small drops over the slide, much like a shotgun blast (Fig. 1.20). The problem is that these small drops tend to dry before the operator has time to make a smear. When viewed under the microscope, small clusters of cells appear poorly spread out (Fig. 1.21), and it is usually impossible to adequately visualize the morphology of the cells. When transferring the sample to the slide, the edge of the needle should be held very close to the slide, and the sample should be sprayed in one

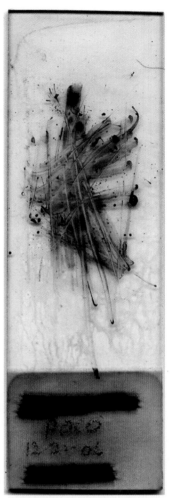

Fig. 1.19 Slide prepared using starfish or needle spread technique depicted in Fig. 1.18. Blue streaks indicating cellular areas are seen where the needle was dragged repeatedly across the slide and through the sample. (Courtesy Oklahoma State University teaching files.)

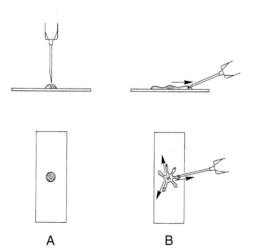

Fig. 1.18 Needle spread or "starfish" preparation. (A) A portion of the aspirate is expelled onto a glass microscope slide. (B) The tip of a needle is placed in the aspirate and moved peripherally, pulling a trail of the sample with it. This procedure is repeated in several directions, resulting in a preparation with multiple projections.

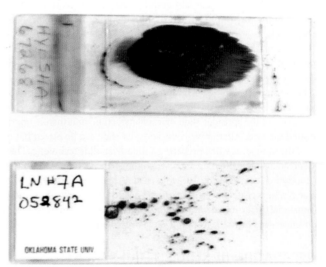

Fig. 1.20 Example of a poorly smeared sample. The slide on top is well made. However, the bottom slide shows what happens when a sample is sprayed onto the slide from a distance resulting in a shotgun blast–like arrangement of small drops. These drops dry quickly and then cannot be spread out. (Courtesy Oklahoma State University teaching files.)

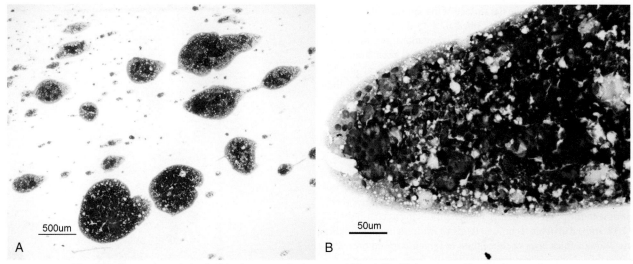

Fig. 1.21 Photomicrograph of slide shown on the bottom of Fig. 1.20. (A) Low-magnification image shows that the cells are all present in thick drops where the sample landed and that they were not spread out before the sample dried. (B) Higher-magnification image of one of the drops shows that the individual cells cannot be seen, resulting in a nondiagnostic sample. (Courtesy Oklahoma State University teaching files.)

drop, if possible. The sample should then be immediately smeared by using one of the techniques described previously. If sufficient sample is obtained to put on more than one slide, it is important to make all smears quickly before the sample dries. When using the nonaspiration technique, prefilling the syringe with air will shorten the time between sample collection and smear preparation and will reduce the likelihood of the sample clotting before smears can be made.

Avoid Making Too Thick a Smear

When smears are too thick, the cells will not spread out adequately, making it impossible to evaluate them. Samples that yield thick smears are those that are contaminated with excessive amounts of peripheral blood or samples collected from tissues that easily exfoliate large numbers of cells (e.g., lymph node aspirates). Ideally, only a small drop of sample should be applied to a slide (about the size of drop used in making a blood smear). If a large amount of sample is applied to a single smear, the smear generally ends up being too thick. If the sample extends all the way to the far end of the slide, the smear will probably be too thick.

Generally, the amount of sample being applied to the slide can be controlled when the material is expelled from the syringe. If too large a drop is applied to a slide, a thin smear can still be obtained by using the blood smear technique. The spreader slide is drawn back just to the point that it barely contacts the sample, which will begin to spread across the surface of the spreader slide by capillary action, and then is rapidly smeared forward. Alternatively, the spreader slide can be placed flat on top of the sample, as when preparing a slide-over-slide technique. Then, the spreader slide is lifted up and used to transfer a portion of the sample to another clean glass slide, on which a smear can be made. This technique can be repeated more than once, if needed, and finally the remaining material on the initial sample slide is smeared out. In this way, several thin smears can be made from one large drop of sample.

PREPARATION OF SLIDES: FLUID SAMPLES

A fluid sample can be obtained when sampling body cavities (e.g., thoracocentesis, joint tap), when performing washings (e.g., transtracheal wash), or when aspirating a cystic lesion (e.g., benign cyst, cystic tumor, sialocele). Proper handling of fluid samples is essential to obtaining diagnostic information. The two main considerations are preserving cell morphology during transit of the sample and preparing smears that are sufficiently cellular to allow for adequate evaluation.

Any fluid sample on which cytological evaluation is going to be performed should be placed in an appropriate amount of ethylenediaminetetraacetic acid (EDTA). EDTA will prevent coagulation of the sample (which can alter cell counts obtained from the specimen) and help preserve cell morphology during transport to the laboratory. This is especially important if the sample will be mailed. Usually, but not always, EDTA will adequately preserve cell morphology overnight and possibly longer. Refrigeration of the sample will extend the length of time that readable smears can be made from the sample. If culture of the fluid is anticipated, a portion of the sample should be placed separately into an appropriate transport medium or other sterile tube. It is important that a sufficient amount of sample fluid be added to the EDTA tube. EDTA has a very high refractive index, and if only a small amount of sample is added to a large EDTA tube, the total protein estimation determined by a refractometer will be artifactually elevated.

Even when fluid samples are placed in EDTA tubes and refrigerated or kept cool with ice packs, cells will undergo aging changes and eventually become too degenerate to be evaluated. Depending on the cellularity, type of cells present, and physical composition of the fluid (i.e., protein concentration), significant morphological changes may occur within 24 hours. The best way to preserve cell morphology is to send premade, air-dried smears. Once smears are made, cell morphology will be preserved for several days, even without fixation of the slides. If possible, premade smears should always be made and sent along with the fluid sample itself. Glass slides should never be placed in the refrigerator because condensation forming on the slide can result in lysis of the cells.

Fluid samples can vary from virtually acellular (cerebrospinal fluid) to extremely cellular (septic exudate). Depending on the nature of the sample, different techniques can be used to produce slides of adequate cellularity. Smears can be prepared directly from fresh, well-mixed fluid or from the sediment of a centrifuged sample using blood smear (direct smears) (see Fig. 1.17), line smear (Figs. 1.22 and 1.23), and squash prep (see Fig. 1.16) techniques. Table 1.2 outlines the samples to be prepared and submitted from fluid samples based on the characteristics of the specimen.

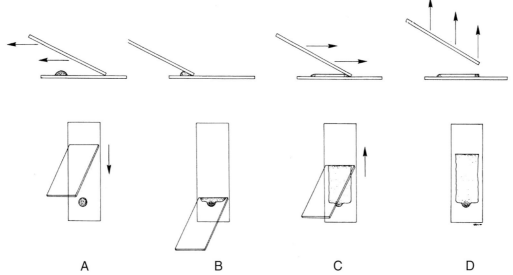

Fig. 1.22 Line smear concentration technique. (A) A drop of fluid sample is placed onto a glass microscope slide close to one end, and another slide is slid backward to contact the front of the drop. (B) When the drop is contacted, it rapidly spreads along the juncture between the two slides. (C) The spreader slide is then slid forward smoothly and rapidly. (D) After the spreader slide has been advanced about two-thirds to three-fourths of the distance required to make a smear with a feathered edge, the spreader slide is raised directly upward. This produces a smear with a line of concentrated cells at its end, instead of a feathered edge.

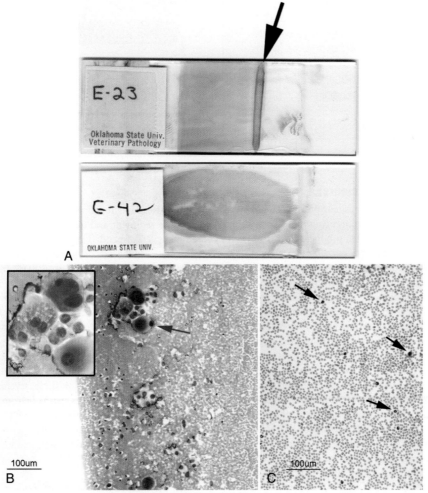

Fig. 1.23 Line smear made from fluid sample. (A) The slide on the bottom was made using a standard blood smear technique. Toward the right, the sample forms a typical feathered edge. The slide on the top was made using a line smear technique. Toward the right, the smear ends abruptly, forming a thick line with a higher concentration of large nucleated cells *(arrow)*. (B) and (C) Images taken from the line smear of a fluid sample. The main portion of the smear (C: right) is of low cellularity, consisting mostly of blood but with low numbers of nucleated cells *(black arrows)*. These relatively small cells are neutrophils and macrophages. At the line edge (B: left), there are increased numbers of nucleated cells, especially clusters of large neoplastic epithelial cells. Inset shows higher magnification of cell cluster indicated by the red arrow. (A, Courtesy Oklahoma State University teaching files.)

TABLE 1.2 Methods of Preparing Cytology Slides From Fluid Samples

Types or Characteristics of Fluid	Samples to Prepare or Submit
Peripheral blood for cytology	Make several air-dried direct smears (blood smear method).
	Submit remainder in EDTA.
Clear, transparent fluids (e.g., abdominal fluid)	Make one to two direct smears (can be used to estimate cellularity) and line smears.
	Centrifuge a portion of the sample and make smears from sediment.
	Submit a portion of fluid in EDTA.
	Submit a portion of fluid in sterile container if culture is desired.
Turbid or opaque fluids	Make one to two direct smears.
	Submit a portion of the fluid in EDTA.
	Submit a portion of the fluid in sterile container if culture is desired.
Clear fluid with flecks or mucous strands (e.g., transtracheal wash fluid, bone marrow samples in EDTA)	Make several direct smears from fluid.
	Make "squash preps" (slide-over-slide preps) of particles or mucous strands removed from the fluid using either a pipette, needle, or capillary tube.
	Submit a portion of the fluid in EDTA.
	Submit a portion of the fluid in sterile container if culture is desired.

EDTA, ethylenediaminetetraacetic acid.

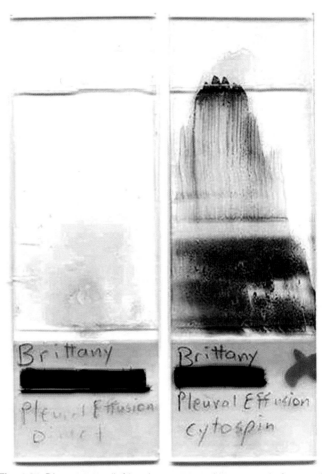

Fig. 1.24 Direct smear *(left)* and concentrated smear made from sediment *(right)* of pleural effusion from a dog. The dark color on the concentrated smear is the result of markedly increased cellularity. (Courtesy Oklahoma State University teaching files.)

Blood Smear Technique (Direct Smears)

The blood smear technique (direct smear) usually produces well-spread smears of sufficient cellularity from homogeneous fluids containing 5000 cells per microliter (cells/μL) but often produces smears of insufficient cellularity from fluids containing less than 5000 cells/μL. The line smear technique can be used to concentrate fluids of low cellularity but often does not sufficiently spread cells from highly cellular fluids. In general, translucent fluids are of low to moderate cellularity, whereas opaque fluids are usually highly cellular. Therefore translucent fluids often require concentration, either by centrifugation or by the line smear technique. When possible, concentration by centrifugation is preferred. The "squash prep" technique often spreads viscous samples (e.g., transtracheal wash [TTW]) and samples with flecks of particulate material better compared with the blood smear and line smear techniques.

To prepare a smear by the blood smear technique, place a small drop of the fluid on a glass slide about 0.5 inch from the end. Slide another slide backward at a 30- to 40-degree angle until it contacts the drop. When the fluid flows sideways along the crease between the slides, slide the second slide forward quickly and smoothly until the fluid has all drained away from the second slide. This makes a smear with a feathered edge.

Sediment Preps (Centrifugation Preps)

To concentrate fluids by centrifugation, the fluid is centrifuged for 5 minutes at 165 to 360 × g (gravitational force). This is achieved by operating a centrifuge with a radial arm length of 14.6 centimeters (cm) (the arm length of most urine centrifuges) at 1000 to 1500 revolutions per minute

(rpm). After centrifugation, the majority of the supernatant is separated from the sediment and analyzed for total protein concentration. The sediment is resuspended in a few drops of supernatant left in the tube by gently tapping the side of the tube. A drop of the resuspended sediment is placed on a slide, and a smear is made by the blood smear or squash prep technique (Fig. 1.24). Alternatively, a plastic pipette can be placed through the supernatant and used to remove the pellet of cells from the bottom of the tube and transfer it to a glass slide and make smears using a slide-over-slide technique. An absorbent tissue may be used to wick away excess supernatant before smear preparation, if needed.

Sediment-concentrated slides can produce highly cellular smears even from fluids of low cellularity and help identify cells present in low numbers (Fig. 1.25). When possible, several smears should be made by each technique. When slides are made from the sediment of a fluid sample, it is not possible to estimate the cellularity of the sample from the slides. Therefore it is imperative to either retain a portion of sample for cell counts or to make direct smears in addition to the sediment preps.

Line Smears

When the fluid cannot be concentrated by centrifugation or the centrifuged sample is of low cellularity, the line smear technique (see Fig. 1.22) can be used to concentrate cells in the smear. A drop of fluid is placed on a clean glass slide, and the blood smear technique is used, but the spreading slide is stopped and raised directly upward about three fourths of the way through the smear. This will result in a line containing a much higher concentration of cells than the rest of the slide (see

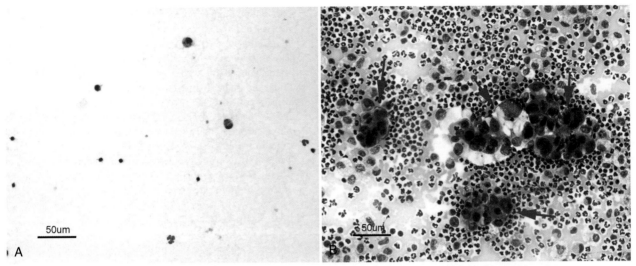

Fig. 1.25 Photomicrographs taken from slides shown in Fig. 1.24. (A) Low-magnification image taken from direct smear of pleural fluid shows relatively sparse cellularity consisting mostly of nondegenerate neutrophils and macrophages. This image is representative of the slide. (B) Low-magnification image taken from the concentrated sediment preparation of the same fluid sample. The slide is highly cellular. In addition to the neutrophils and macrophages seen on the direct smear, clusters of neoplastic epithelial cells (arrows) are easily found.

Fig. 1.23). Unfortunately, the cells that are present in the line may not be well spread out, making evaluation difficult.

Fluid is sometimes obtained when sampling a mass or other proliferative lesion. When this occurs, as much fluid as possible should be drained from the lesion and handled as described above. The lesion should then be reevaluated. If a solid tissue component still remains, that component should be sampled by using FNB with either the aspiration or the nonaspiration technique. Many times, cystic neoplasia will not exfoliate overtly neoplastic cells into the cystic fluid. The material obtained from direct FNB may have a completely different cell population compared with that present in the fluid itself.

STAINING CYTOLOGICAL PREPARATIONS

To Stain or Not to Stain?

If you intend to send the slides to a laboratory for evaluation, it is not necessary to stain the slides or do any special fixation at all. Air-dried smears will hold up quite well over the length of time necessary for transport to an outside laboratory. In fact, if the slides are to be submitted for analysis, unstained slides are preferable. This will allow the cytologist to stain the smears with the type of stain he or she is used to viewing. However, it is usually advisable to stain at least one slide to ensure that an adequately cellular sample was obtained before paying for interpretation of the smears. All slides collected from the lesion, both stained and unstained, should be submitted for evaluation, in case not all slides were adequately cellular.

Types of Stain

Several types of stains have been used for cytological preparations.[8] The two general types most commonly used are (1) the Romanowsky-type stains (Wright stain, Giemsa stain, Diff-Quik stain) and Papanicolaou stain and its derivatives, such as Sano's trichrome. Papanicolaou stains and their derivatives require the specimen to be wet fixed (i.e., the smear must be fixed before the cells have dried). Usually, this is achieved by spraying the smear with a cytological fixative or placing it in ethanol immediately after preparation. Such procedures are not necessary and are actually undesirable if the samples are to be stained with Romanowsky-type stains. Papanicolaou-type stains give excellent nuclear detail and are routinely used in human

cytopathology.[8] However, these stains require multiple staining steps, do not stain many organisms or cell cytoplasm well, and are not practical for use in most clinics. They are rarely used in veterinary cytology. The remainder of this chapter (and text) deals with Romanowsky-type stains.

Romanowsky-type stains are inexpensive, readily available to the practicing veterinarian, and easy to prepare, maintain, and use. They stain organisms and the cytoplasm of cells excellently. Although the nuclear and nucleolar details cannot be perceived as well with Romanowsky-type stains as with Papanicolaou-type stains, the nuclear and nucleolar details are sufficient for differentiating neoplasia and inflammation and for evaluating neoplastic cells for cytological evidence of malignant potential (criteria of malignancy). Smears to be stained with Romanowsky-type stains are first air-dried. Air-drying partially preserves (fixes) the cells and causes them to adhere to the slide so that they do not fall off during the staining procedure.

Romanowsky stains may be either aqueous based or methanol based.[9] Wright and Giemsa stains are examples of methanol-based stains. Diff-Quik and Hema 3 are commonly used aqueous-based Romanowsky stains, but others exist. Most, if not all, Romanowsky stains are acceptable for staining cytological preparations. Aqueous-based stains are often used in private-practice settings because of ease of use and rapid staining times. However, the aqueous-based stains may fail to stain the granules of mast cells, basophils, and large granular lymphocytes.[9] When mast cell granules do not stain, the mast cells may be misclassified as macrophages or plasma cells. This can lead to confusion in examination of some mast cell tumors. Similarly, basophils may appear as neutrophils if their granules do not stain. Although uncommonly encountered, distemper inclusions stain more prominently with aqueous-based stains than with alcohol-based stains.[9]

Each stain usually has its own recommended staining protocol. These procedures should be followed in general but adapted to the type and thickness of smear being stained and to the evaluator's preference. The thinner the smear and the lower the total protein concentration of the fluid, the less is the time needed in the stain. The thicker the smear and the greater the total protein concentration of the fluid, the more is the time needed in the stain. As a result, fluid smears with low protein and low cellularity, such as some abdominal fluid samples, may stain better using half or less of the recommended time. Thick smears, such as smears of neoplastic lymph nodes, may need to be stained twice the recommended time or longer.

Each person tends to have a specific technique that he or she prefers. By trying variations in the recommended time intervals for stains, the evaluator can establish which times produce the preferred staining characteristics.

Poor staining quality is a common problem for a variety of reasons. It can be confusing to the novice when trying to examine his or her own slides because the cells may appear completely unrecognizable. Most staining problems can be avoided by applying the following precautions:

- *Use only new, clean slides.* Attempts to reuse slides are usually doomed to failure. Even if they are cleaned and dried, the samples often do not spread out well or do not stain properly because the surface properties of the glass have been altered.
- *Use fresh, well-filtered (if periodic filtering is required) stains.* Over time, with repeated use, stains will "fatigue," form excessive precipitate, or may become contaminated with organisms or cell debris from previous slides.
- *Make sure that the slides are completely air-dried before staining.* This is particularly important when examining blood smears. Some water will remain even after slides appear grossly to have dried. Slides should be air-dried for 5 to 10 minutes or dried briefly with a hair dryer before staining.
- *Do not touch the surface of the slide or smear at any time.* Likewise, make sure the slide is not contaminated with ultrasound gel or other lubricant gels (e.g., K-Y Jelly).

Table 1.3 lists some problems that can occur with Romanowsky-type stains and some proposed solutions to these problems. One of the most commonly encountered problems simply is understaining of

TABLE 1.3   Some Possible Solutions to Problems Seen with Common Romanowsky-Type Stains

Problem	Solution
Excessive Blue Staining (red blood cells may be blue-green)	
Prolonged stain contact	Decrease staining time.
Inadequate wash	Wash for longer time.
Specimen too thick	Make thinner smears, if possible.
Stain, diluent, buffer, or wash water too alkaline	Check with pH paper and correct pH.
Exposure to formalin vapors	Store and ship cytological preps separate from formalin containers.
Wet fixation in ethanol or formalin	Air-dry smears before fixation.
Delayed fixation	Fix smears sooner, if possible.
Surface of the slide being alkaline	Use new slides.
Excessive Pink Staining	
Insufficient staining time	Increase staining time.
Prolonged washing	Decrease duration of wash.
Stain or diluent too acidic	Check with pH paper and correct pH; fresh methanol may be needed.
Excessive time in red stain solution	Decrease time in red solution.
Inadequate time in blue stain solution	Increase time in blue stain solution.
Mounting coverslip before preparation is dry	Allow preparation to dry completely before mounting coverslip.
Weak Staining	
Insufficient contact with one or more of the stain solutions	Increase staining time.
Fatigued (old) stains	Change stains.
Another slide covered specimen during staining	Keep slides separate.
Uneven Staining	
Variation of pH in different areas of slide surface (may be from slide surface being touched or slide being poorly cleaned)	Use new slides and avoid touching them before and after preparation.
Water allowed to stand on some areas of the slide after staining and washing	Tilt slides close to vertical to drain water from the surface, or dry with a fan.
Inadequate mixing of stain and buffer	Mix stain and buffer thoroughly.
Precipitate on preparation	
Inadequate stain filtration	Filter or change the stain(s).
Inadequate washing of slide after staining	Rinse slides well after staining.
Dirty slides used	Use clean new slides.
Stain solution drying during staining	Use sufficient stain, and do not leave it on slide too long.
Miscellaneous	
Overstained preparations	Destain with 95% methanol and restain; Diff-Quik–stained smears may have to be destained in the red Diff-Quik stain solution to remove the blue color; however, this damages the red stain solution.
Refractile artifact red blood cells with Diff-Quik stain (usually as a result of moisture in fixative)	Change the fixative.

slides. Slides are often understained when they are highly cellular or stained with old stains. With well-stained smears, the nucleus of most cells should be a dark purple, and clear demarcation of the nucleus and cytoplasm should be present (see Chapter 2). When slides are understained, cells and nuclei may appear pink, it may be difficult to distinguish the boundary between the nucleus and the cytoplasm, or the cells may just appear excessively faded or "muted." It may be difficult for the beginning cytologist to recognize understaining if he or she is not familiar with what the cells should look like. However, most cytology preparations will contain some neutrophils or other peripheral blood cells whose morphology is more likely to be familiar to the observer. These cells can be used as an internal control for staining quality. If the slides appear understained, they can simply be placed in the stains for an additional period. However, restaining should optimally be done before immersion oil is placed on the slides.

SUBMISSION OF SAMPLES TO THE LABORATORY

If the clinician is not going to evaluate the slides in-house, the final step in processing of cytological samples is ensuring that they arrive at the laboratory intact. Many well-made, potentially diagnostic slides have met their doom at the hands of various postal services. Thin cardboard slide mailers (Fig. 1.26) do not offer adequate protection for slides being mailed to outside laboratories and often result in broken, unreadable

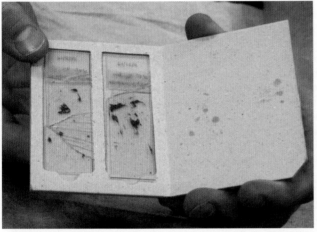

Fig. 1.26 Cardboard containers do not offer sufficient protection for mailing slides. If the slides are not put in additional protective packaging, they often become broken in transit. (Courtesy Oklahoma State University teaching files.)

slides. Rigid plastic or polystyrene foam mailers (Fig. 1.27) are excellent for mailing slides and generally prevent breakage. Often, even if the polystyrene foam box has been severely damaged in transport, the slides inside remain unbroken (Fig. 1.28). If these are not available, slides should be wrapped in protective material (e.g., paper towel) and mailed in a small, sturdy box. Alternatively, slides can be placed in a large plastic pill bottle and then placed in a mailing envelope.

If samples of body fluids are submitted along with slides, small EDTA tubes will fit inside standard polystyrene foam slide mailers or can be placed inside a larger cardboard box. Most overnight mailing services require that body fluids be double-sealed and placed in specially designed plastic envelopes, which are provided by these services.

Slides mailed to an outside laboratory should be labeled with the names of the patient and the owner and the body location from which the sample was collected. Microscope slides used for cytology (or hematology) should have frosted or colored edges that can be written on with a pencil. It is difficult to permanently label slides without frosted edges, and this can lead to samples being mixed up. The ink from most marking pens (even "permanent" markers) is soluble in cytological stains and will wash off during the staining procedure, leaving the slides unidentifiable. In contrast, pencil markings on frosted slides will not get erased during staining. Many slides without frosted ends arrive at laboratories with patient identification written on small pieces of white bandage tapes affixed to the edge of the slide. With many types of automatic slide stainers, these labels must be removed before the slides can be stained, and this, again, may result in potential misidentification of the sample.

As a final note, unstained cytology slides should never be mailed with, or even stored near, samples in formalin. Formalin fumes will penetrate most packaging, even biopsy samples in plastic jars with screw-top lids that are sealed in plastic zip-top bags. Formalin fumes partially fix the cells on air-dried smears and markedly interfere with subsequent staining (Fig. 1.29), often making the slides totally uninterpretable.

SUBMISSION OF SAMPLES FOR CULTURE

Although this text deals primarily with cytological evaluation of samples, with many samples (particularly fluids) submitted for cytology, culture is also indicated. Culture results are strongly influenced by sample collection, preparation, and transport. The following procedures are suggested to optimize success in culturing lesions and fluids:
- Call the laboratory before collecting the sample.
- Collect the sample as aseptically as possible.
- Submit fresh samples for culture.

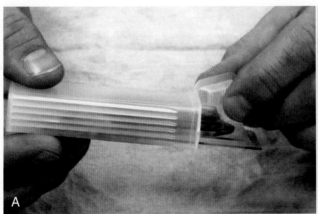
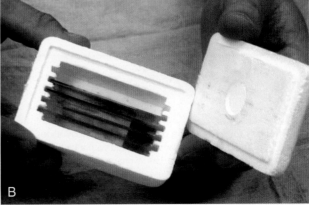

Fig. 1.27 Rigid plastic (A) and polystyrene foam mailers (B), shown here, do a good job of protecting slides for mailing. Slides in these types of containers can usually be put directly in mailing envelopes with no additional protective packaging. (Courtesy Oklahoma State University teaching files.)

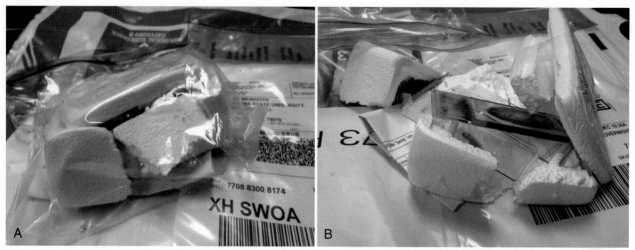

Fig. 1.28 (A) Cytology sample as received from overnight courier. The polystyerene mailer was severely damaged. (B) Upon opening the bag, the mailer was broken into several pieces. Despite this, the enclosed slides remained unbroken. These holders do an excellent job of protecting the enclosed slides. (Courtesy Oklahoma State University teaching files.)

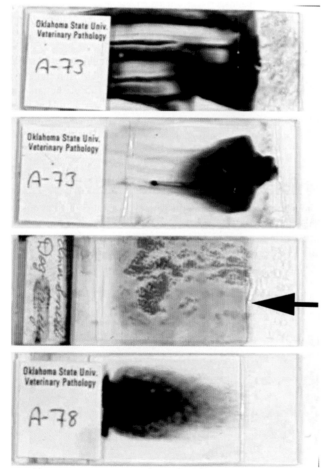

Fig. 1.29 Effect of formalin fumes on unstained cytology slides. The slide second from the bottom *(arrow)* was mailed with a biopsy sample in formalin. After staining, the slide has a characteristic color that is different from the other slides that were not exposed to formalin. This partial fixation alters the staining of the cells and often makes it impossible to interpret the sample.

- Use proper methods for collection and transport of the sample.
- Use a timely transportation service.

Call the Laboratory Before Collecting the Sample

Techniques, media, days when cultures are read or subcultures are performed, and so forth, often vary from laboratory to laboratory. By contacting the laboratory to which the sample will be submitted, such matters as the optimal sample type, transport medium, day of the week to submit the sample, and so on can be discussed. Also, some laboratories furnish culture supplies. Supplies that are expensive, quickly outdated, or both (e.g., blood culture tubes) may be ordered from the laboratory on an as-needed basis. Early communication with the laboratory also allows the laboratory to prepare for the sample and ensure that any special media required are available.

Collect Samples as Aseptically as Possible

All samples should be collected as aseptically as possible. Even samples collected from lesions that naturally are exposed to secondary contamination (e.g., cutaneous ulcers) should be protected from further contamination. When samples are collected from more than one lesion, care should be taken not to cross-contaminate the samples. Finding the same organism in several different lesions is strong evidence that the organism is involved in the development of the lesions. Therefore cross-contamination of samples from different lesions can lead to misinterpretation of culture results. When fluids are collected, anticoagulant and serum tubes should not be presumed to be sterile. Serum tubes generally are identified as sterile or non-sterile on the label of the tube. Also, EDTA, because of its effect on bacterial cell walls, can be bacteriostatic or bactericidal and should therefore be avoided.

Submit Fresh Samples

Samples should be submitted as soon as possible after collection. Fluid aspiration, resection of lesions to be cultured, exploratory surgeries during which culture is anticipated, and other procedures that may produce samples to be cultured should be scheduled to allow for immediate transportation of samples to the laboratory. During transport, samples should be kept cool but not frozen.

Use Proper Methods for Collection and Transport of Samples

Tissue and fluid samples usually are more rewarding than swab samples for isolation of a causative agent. Individual tissue samples submitted for culture should be about 4 cm^2 or larger. Whirl-Pak bags, which are sterile and sealable, are excellent for submitting samples for culture. If the interior of the tissue is to be cultured by the laboratory, clean and sealable plastic bags are sufficient. To avoid cross-contamination, all tissues should be packaged separately. To prevent drying during transport, small biopsies, such as punch biopsies of skin lesions, should be placed in a transport system with maintenance medium. Shipping biopsies in sterile saline should be avoided because this may result in false-negative culture results.

Culture of subcutaneous or internal tissues can be collected in a minimally invasive manner by performing a fine-needle aspiration procedure into a syringe that has been prefilled with an appropriate liquid culture medium, such as from blood culture bottles. Following the aspiration procedure, the culture medium in the syringe is expelled, through the needle containing the collected tissue, into a sterile tube.[10]

Fluid samples (i.e., urine, milk, joint fluid, thoracic fluid, abdominal fluid, abscess aspirates) to be cultured should be placed in containers that are sterile and leak-proof, such as sterile Vacutainer tubes or sterile disposable syringes.

For collection of samples for which swabs must be used (epithelial surfaces, fistulous tracts), the swabs should be placed in a maintenance medium that allows for preservation with little to no replication of microbes so that the quantity and quality of the microbial flora of the swab remain as intact as possible. Transport tubes containing maintenance media for optimal transport of swabs for isolating bacteria, chlamydia, or viruses are commercially available (Culturette, Transwab, Transtube, and CultureSwab). The bacterial media systems usually support a wide variety of bacteria for up to 72 hours at 20°C to 25°C. Swabs without media can dry out during transport, resulting in false-negative results, whereas in swabs submitted in broth culture medium, often there is overgrowth of contaminants. Separate swabs should be submitted if additional cultures for fungi, viruses, or both are desired.

Samples for anaerobic culturing require special handling and transport. The main objective is to limit, as much as possible, the exposure of the sample to oxygen and, thus, to air. Swabs are the least desirable means for specimen collection for anaerobes because of the difficulty of limiting the exposure of the sample to air. Fluids for anaerobic culturing should be collected in syringes, with air excluded. The needle is then plugged with a sterile rubber stopper or bent double to prevent intake of air and transported immediately to the laboratory for culture. If samples for anaerobic culturing cannot reach the laboratory within 2 hours, the sample must be placed into some type of anaerobic transport system. Several commercial systems are now available for transporting all types of specimens for anaerobic culture. Port-A-Cul systems contain a prereduced transport medium in a soft agar with reducing agents to maintain anaerobiosis and offer vials for fluid specimens, jars for small tissues and swabs, and tubes for swabs. Self-contained, gas-generating systems are also available, and these systems provide their own anaerobic atmosphere once the sample is placed in the container and the system sealed. Such systems are available for swabs (Anaerobic Culturette; Becton Dickinson Microbiology Systems) and as sealable plastic bags (Bio-Bag, Gas-Pak Pouch). The bags can be used for transporting large tissue specimens, fluids contained within syringes, and aerobic swab systems for anaerobic culturing.

In general, samples submitted for fungal culture should be collected and transported in the same manner as samples for bacterial culture, with the exception of dermatophyte cultures.

Scrapings and hair plucked from the periphery of suspected dermatophyte lesions should be submitted in clean containers that remain dry during transit. Bacterial overgrowth of dermatophyte cultures is a common problem and can be eliminated by disinfecting suspect dermatophyte lesions with alcohol before obtaining samples. Vacutainer tubes and similar tightly sealable containers are to be avoided because condensate tends to form within them, allowing overgrowth of contaminants. Clean paper envelopes are suitable specimen containers. For transport, the envelope should be packaged within a more durable wrapper. Swabs are the least preferred samples for fungal cultures and should never be used for dermatophyte isolation.

Use a Timely Transportation Service

Care in collection of samples would be futile if the samples were not received in the laboratory in a timely manner, generally within 48 hours or less. Most microbiology laboratories deal with various carriers on a daily basis and can recommend what carrier to use. Packaging specimens to guard against breakage and leakage not only protects against specimen loss but also protects package handlers against potential infection. The clinician must be aware of special requirements to be taken when shipping biohazardous materials, including some clinical specimens. If in doubt regarding how to package specimens for transport, the microbiology laboratory to which the specimens will be sent should be contacted for instructions.

REFERENCES

1. Meinkoth JH, Cowell RL. Sample collection and preparation in cytology: increasing diagnostic yield. *Vet Clin North Am.* 2002;32:1187–1207.
2. Meyer DJ, Connolly SL, Heng HG. The acquisition and management of cytology specimens. In: Raskin RE, Meyer DJ, eds. *Atlas of Canine and Feline Cytology.* 2nd ed. Philadelphia: Saunders; 2010:1–14.
3. Lumsden JH, Baker R. Cytopathology techniques and interpretation. In: Baker R, Lumsden JH, eds. *Color Atlas of Cytology of the Dog and Cat.* St. Louis, MO: Mosby; 2000:7–20.
4. Menard M, Papageorges M. Fine-needle biopsies: how to increase diagnostic yield. *Comp Cont Ed Pract Vet.* 1997;19:738–740.
5. DeMay RM. *The Art and Science of Cytopathology.* Chicago, IL: ASCP; 1996:464–483.
6. Menard M, Papageorges M. Technique for ultrasound-guided fine needle biopsies. *Vet Rad Ult.* 1995;36:137–138.
7. Caruso K, Cowell RL, Cowell AK, et al. Skin scraping from a cat. *Vet Clin Path.* 2002;31(1):13–15.
8. Jörundsson E, Lumsden JH, Jacobs RM. Rapid staining techniques in cytopathology: a review and comparison of modified protocols for hematoxylin and eosin, Papanicolaou and Romanowsky stains. *Vet Clin Path.* 1999;28:100–108.
9. Allison RW, Velguth KE. Appearance of granulated cells in blood films stained by automated aqueous versus methanolic Romanowsky methods. *Vet Clin Path.* 2009;39:99–104.
10. Meinkoth KR, Morton RJ, Meinkoth JH. Naturally occurring tularemia in a dog. *J Am Vet Med Assoc.* 2004;225:545–547.

2

Cell Types and Criteria of Malignancy

James H. Meinkoth, Rick L. Cowell, and Ronald D. Tyler

Examining cytological preparations often presents a potentially confusing array of different cell types and a potentially endless variety of cell debris and contaminants. With experience, most of the common lesions are recognized quickly. In case of a lesion or sample site not previously encountered, it is helpful to keep in mind certain fundamental questions that need to be considered when evaluating a sample. Cells can usually be classified into one of a few basic categories, based on common features shared by different cells in that category.[1-4] Recognizing the common features of the different basic cell types sometimes makes it possible to classify cells that are not obvious at first.

An orderly approach to examining slides and answering certain questions in a logical order will reduce the chances of missing important information or misdiagnosing or overdiagnosing the sample.

ARE SUFFICIENT NUMBERS OF WELL-STAINED, WELL-PRESERVED, INTACT CELLS PRESENT TO BE EVALUATED?

A basic premise of cytology is that interpretations are generally based on entire populations of cells, not on low numbers of individual cells. Any one cell or few cells from a lesion may show features that are atypical or unusual. This is especially true if cells are coming from a tissue in which the cells are not well preserved or exposed to injurious stimuli. Cells coming from inflammatory reactions or areas of tissue repair often show cellular atypia that is the result of dysplasia.

In addition to atypia seen with inflammation and tissue repair, cells that undergo aging changes may be difficult to interpret. Cells present in fluid samples (e.g., thoracocentesis, abdominocentesis) may undergo morphological changes over time if slides are not made immediately after collection. These changes can range from subtle alterations, such as cellular or nuclear swelling and altered staining characteristics, to overt pyknosis or lysis. Even if slides are prepared immediately after collection, cells may have undergone in vivo aging. Cells from the fluid portion of cystic lesions (e.g., some mammary tumors) or cells that have been in prolonged contact with urine (e.g., urine sediment preparations or urethral or bladder samples collected by traumatic catheterization) often have significant artifacts that must not be misinterpreted as criteria of malignancy.

Interpretations based on inadequately cellular specimens that may not contain a representative sample of the lesion could give a false impression of normalcy or, even worse, may result in a false impression of malignancy that is not really present. Although no easily defined limit to the question "How many cells are enough?" exists, slides should have many cells per field across a large portion of the slide. It has been said that if the question "Is the specimen adequately cellular or not?" even comes to mind when looking at the slide, it probably is not.[3] When a large lesion is being evaluated, several smears of

good cellularity collected from different areas of the lesion should be evaluated to assess any variability that may be present within different parts of the lesion. Large neoplasms may have areas of inflammation or necrosis that will yield markedly different cell populations compared with adjacent areas. It is common to collect 5 to 10 slides representing multiple attempts to aspirate from a lesion, sometimes more when evaluating some organs, such as the liver or spleen, where there may be a mixture of normal and abnormal appearing tissue.

The cellularity of the smear is often evident the moment the slides are stained. A slide containing high numbers of nucleated cells is visibly blue after staining. Slides that are perfectly clear after staining probably have low numbers of nucleated cells, although sufficient cells may still be present for a diagnosis. Therefore cellularity must be confirmed by looking at the slide under the microscope. Even for practitioners who do not have the time or desire to evaluate cytology preparations themselves, it is beneficial to stain one or two smears and determine that an adequately cellular specimen is being sent off for evaluation.

When examined microscopically, the slides should first be scanned using low power (10× to 20×) to assess the cellularity of the slide and find the area(s) containing the highest number of well-stained, well-spread-out, intact cells for evaluation (Fig. 2.1). Cells are often unevenly distributed across the slides, especially with impression smears or aspirates of solid tissue lesions. Even with slides made from fluid samples, large cells may all be pulled out to the feathered edge, where they can be easily overlooked if the whole slide is not scanned first (Fig. 2.2).

After locating the cellular areas of the slides, it is important to determine whether the cells are sufficiently spread out for evaluation, intact, and well stained. This can usually also be done on low power (10× to 20×), which will allow a greater portion of the slide to be evaluated in a short time. Inexperienced cytologists often frustrate themselves by spending an inordinate amount of time trying to identify cells that cannot be interpreted because they are not spread out, are poorly stained, or are ruptured. Intact, well-stained, well-spread cells should have a clearly evident demarcation between the nucleus and the cytoplasm (Fig. 2.3). The nucleus may be irregularly shaped (particularly in neoplastic cells), but the nuclear outline should be smooth and distinct. A fuzzy, irregular or indistinct appearance around the outline of the nucleus generally indicates that the cell has been minimally traumatized during sample collection, preparation, or both. More significant cell trauma can result in the nucleus appearing fragmented or full of holes (see Fig. 2.3). Severely traumatized cells will often appear only as strands of light pink nuclear chromatin (Fig. 2.4). Some traumatized or ruptured cells will be present in virtually any cytological specimen. The sample is usually still interpretable if the majority of the cells are intact; however, the traumatized cells are not evaluated. This is particularly important when determining criteria of malignancy because

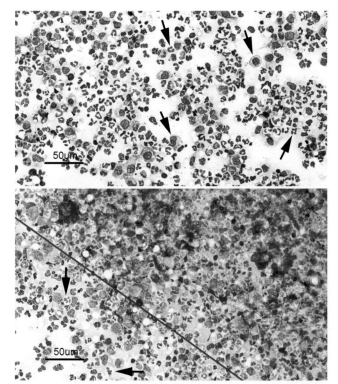

Fig. 2.1 Low-power image of different areas of a slide. The top image shows an area that, although highly cellular, is well spread out and the cells are well stained. The cell details are difficult to evaluate at this magnification, but it is possible to see the characteristic nuclear shape of some well-spread-out neutrophils and to differentiate the nucleus and cytoplasm of mononuclear cells *(arrows)*. The lower image shows another area from the same slide where the cells are not well spread out and thus have not stained well. Most of the area above and to the right of the red line is too thick to evaluate. A few well-spread-out cells are seen in the lower left *(arrows)*.

nuclei may appear enlarged and nucleoli may appear more prominent in traumatized cells. If the majority of the cells are traumatized or ruptured, additional samples usually need to be collected.

Cells that are not well spread out often stain diffusely dark, and it is difficult to recognize the line of demarcation and color distinction between the cytoplasm and the nucleus (Fig. 2.5). Usually, the contrast between the blue cytoplasm and the purple (or pink-purple) nucleus can be seen at relatively low magnification if the cells are well spread out. Poorly spread, poorly stained cells often appear only as different shades of blue. This allows the observer to scan large areas of the slide quickly at low magnification to find areas of the slide worth examining at higher magnification.

Nucleoli will often be more prominent than usual in understained cells, and this can result in a false impression of malignancy if this artifact is not recognized. The nuclei of well-stained cells are usually dark purple, generally more intensely and deeply stained compared with the surrounding cytoplasm. Some variation between cell types will exist in the intensity and pattern of nuclear staining. In case of uncertainty as to whether light staining of nuclei is a characteristic of the cell or the result of understaining, it may be helpful to evaluate the staining of more familiar cells. Usually, some neutrophils will be present as a result of peripheral blood contamination or inflammation within the lesion and make a good reference to evaluate how well cells are stained (and spread out).

In most specimens, significant variation in cellularity, degree of cell spreading, and, hence, staining quality from area to area on the slide will exist. This is particularly true of highly cellular specimens, such as lymph node aspirates, which may have areas that are of diagnostic quality, even if the majority of the slide is thick and understained. Diligent scanning of the slides on low power is necessary to find these areas before attempting to evaluate the cells at higher magnification. With overly thick smears, a thin rim of well-spread, well-stained cells can sometimes be found at either the feathered edge or the sides of the slides. If the entire slide is found to be understained, restaining the slide before immersion oil is added may improve the staining quality and result in a diagnostic sample.

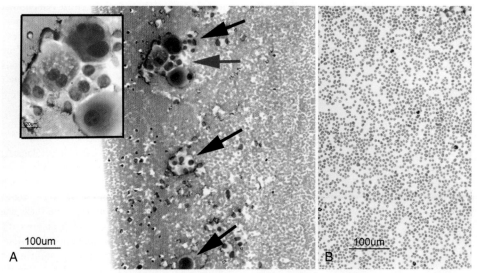

Fig. 2.2 Images from a slide made from hemorrhagic pleural effusion showing uneven distribution of cells on the slide. (A) Numerous large clusters of cells *(arrows)* have all been pulled out to the edge of the smear. Some of these show marked atypia allowing for a diagnosis of neoplastic effusion (carcinoma). Inset shows higher magnification of atypical cell cluster indicated by the red arrow. (B) The majority of the smear contained predominantly erythrocytes with a few small nuclei (neutrophils and macrophages) visible. Scanning on low power quickly allowed the atypical cells to be found at the edge of the smear. These could have easily been overlooked if the observer started out at high magnification in the body of the smear.

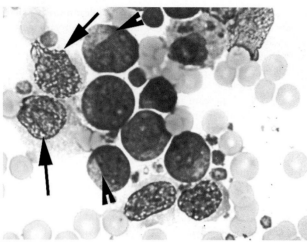

Fig. 2.3 Lymph node aspirate from a dog showing well-spread-out cells. A clear distinction can be seen between the nucleus and the cytoplasm *(arrowheads)*. Several traumatized cells are also present. Note that their nuclear chromatin appears excessively fragmented *(arrows)*.

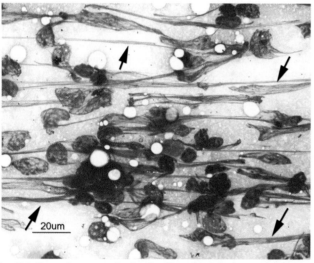

Fig. 2.4 Severely traumatized cells. The streaks of material *(arrows)* represent smeared-out nuclear chromatin from ruptured cells.

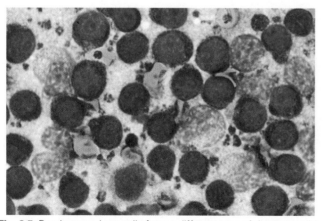

Fig. 2.5 Poorly spread-out cells from a different area of the same slide shown in Fig 2.3. The cells are diffusely dark with the nuclei and cytoplasm staining different shades of blue. Compare this with the purple color of the well-spread-out nuclei in Fig 2.3. Also, it is difficult to discern the demarcation between the nucleus and the cytoplasm.

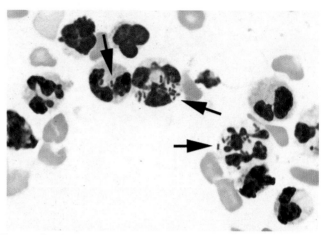

Fig. 2.6 Septic neutrophilic inflammation. Many neutrophils are present, some of which contain phagocytized bacterial rods *(arrows)*.

ARE ALL OF THE CELLS ON THE SMEAR INFLAMMATORY CELLS?

A good initial decision, particularly for the beginning cytologist, is to determine whether the smear is composed entirely of inflammatory cells. In many primary care practices, inflammatory lesions are more commonly sampled compared with neoplastic lesions. Also, most clinicians initially feel more comfortable recognizing inflammatory cells because they are more familiar with the morphology of these cells, having viewed them many times in peripheral blood smears. Many clinicians choose to screen their cytology specimens, interpreting inflammatory lesions in-house and submitting those composed of tissue cells to an outside laboratory. Although inflammatory cells in tissues often look the same as they do in peripheral blood, some may appear different because of morphological changes induced by their presence in a focus of inflammation or simply because they are not well spread out. It is important to remember that it may not be possible to identify every cell present on a slide, or even on any given field, and that the interpretation is based on the entire cell population present.

If a lesion is found to be composed entirely of inflammatory cells, the relative percentages of the various types of inflammatory cells should be noted because this may provide clues as to the etiology of the inflammation. Finally, a search for infectious agents should be conducted. A discussion of the various inflammatory patterns and morphology of common infectious agents will be covered more completely in Chapters 3 and 5 of this text.

Neutrophils

Neutrophils are commonly found in cytological specimens. Their morphology is often similar to that observed in peripheral blood smears (Fig. 2.6). Normal neutrophil nuclei stain dark purple and contain one to multiple distinct segments or lobes. The neutrophil cytoplasm is typically clear. Neutrophils are phagocytic cells and typically are the cells that phagocytize pathogenic bacteria, if present (see Fig. 2.6). Although neutrophils contain intracytoplasmic granules, in most domestic animals these generally do not stain prominently with cytological stains. Sometimes, however, these granules will be discernible as elongated, faintly eosinophilic structures, and they must not be confused with bacteria or lightly staining eosinophil granules.

In thick preparations or in viscous fluids, such as synovial fluid, neutrophils may not spread out well, and the segmented nature of their nucleus may be less evident. Sometimes, the nucleus will appear essentially round as a result of being poorly spread out and, thus, mimic

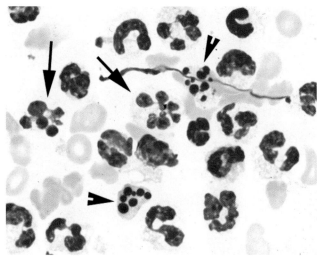

Fig. 2.7 Sample from a nonseptic inflammatory lesion. Many of the neutrophils show nuclear hypersegmentation *(arrows)*, an aging artifact. This will ultimately lead to pyknotic change *(arrowheads)*, where the nuclear chromatin condenses and fragments into several discrete, dense spheres.

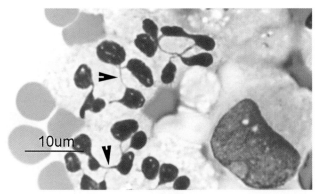

Fig. 2.8 Hypersegmentation of neutrophils in which elongated thin filaments connect the nuclear lobes *(arrowheads)*. This is a common manifestation of aged neutrophils in fluid samples prepared by cytocentrifugation.

that of a lymphocyte, but the cell can still be identified as a neutrophil by the lobulated outline of the nucleus. More normal neutrophil morphology can be observed in the thinner areas (often along the edges) of the smear.

Neutrophils may undergo several morphological changes in tissues. Aging change is a commonly encountered phenomenon. The initial change seen is hypersegmentation of the nucleus (Fig. 2.7). Sometimes, an elongated thin strand of nuclear material (Fig. 2.8) connects the nuclear lobes of aged neutrophils. This is commonly seen in cytocentrifuged preparations from fluids. The end result of aging change is pyknosis of the nucleus. *Pyknosis* is condensation of the nuclear chromatin into one or more small discrete, densely staining spheres lacking any nuclear chromatin pattern (see Fig. 2.7). Aging artifact simply represents neutrophils dying of "old age" and must not be confused with degenerative change.

Degenerative change occurs when neutrophils are present in an environment that is damaging to the cell. It is commonly seen in neutrophils from lesions in which endotoxin-producing bacteria are present. The presence of a predominance of neutrophils with marked degenerative change should prompt a diligent search for bacteria. Degenerative change is an acquired change and is distinct from the toxic changes

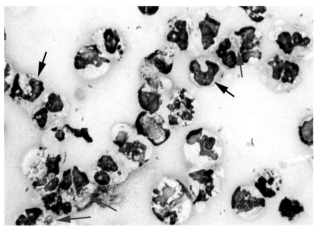

Fig. 2.9 Neutrophils showing degenerative change. Degenerative change is evidenced by nuclear swelling *(black arrows)*, which leads to loss of distinct segmentation. As the nucleus swells the neutrophils may appear band shaped, or in more severe change, the nucleus may appear round or overtly lytic. Degenerative change is commonly associated with the presence of endotoxin-producing-bacteria. Many bacterial rods *(red arrows)* were present on this slide.

noted in peripheral blood neutrophils. Degenerative change occurs when the neutrophil is unable to control water homeostasis and undergoes hydropic degeneration. The hallmark of degenerative change is nuclear swelling (Fig. 2.9). The nucleus of the cell swells and appears thicker, stains a lighter eosinophilic color, and loses nuclear lobation. Degenerative neutrophils often resemble large band cells. Any markedly inflamed lesion is likely to have some neutrophils undergoing degenerative change. Also, aged neutrophils, such as those in fluids samples that have sat for prolonged periods before slides are made, may sometimes undergo lysis rather than pyknosis and mimic degenerative change. Ultimately, although degenerative neutrophils may prompt suspicion of a septic process, sepsis can be definitively confirmed only by findings organisms on the slides or by culture if bacterial numbers are low.

Macrophages

Macrophages in inflammatory lesions are derived from peripheral blood monocytes. Many tissues have low numbers of fixed tissue macrophages as normal resident cells (e.g., Kupffer cells in the liver). Macrophages may display extremely variable morphology in tissues, which can be somewhat confusing. Initially, they may resemble peripheral blood monocytes (Fig. 2.10). With time, the nucleus becomes round, and the cell enlarges as the cytoplasm becomes greatly expanded and, sometimes, extremely vacuolated. Macrophages are also phagocytic cells, typically phagocytizing larger structures, such as fungal organisms and other cells. Many times, the cytoplasm of macrophages will contain partially phagocytized debris that cannot be identified but must not be misinterpreted as an infectious agent.

Binucleate or multinucleate macrophages are commonly encountered in longstanding inflammatory lesions (Fig. 2.11). Multinucleate macrophages can get very large and are referred to as *inflammatory giant cells*. In some chronic inflammatory lesions, *epithelioid macrophages* may be encountered (Fig. 2.12). This term is applied to macrophages that are enlarged with expansive cytoplasm that stains uniformly basophilic, giving the cell the look of an epithelial cell. Because these macrophages can also show variation in size and multinucleation, they could potentially be misinterpreted as neoplastic epithelial cells. Extreme caution should be exercised when diagnosing malignancy in the face of inflammation because of the potential of macrophages displaying atypical criteria.

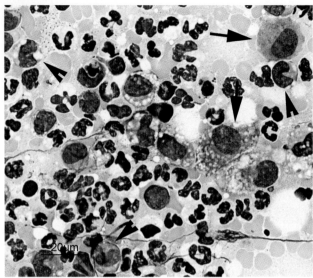

Fig. 2.10 Pyogranulomatous inflammatory response demonstrating many macrophages. Some macrophages resemble peripheral blood monocytes *(arrowheads)*. Other macrophages are variably increased in size resulting from increased amounts of cytoplasm that is sometimes vacuolated *(arrows)*.

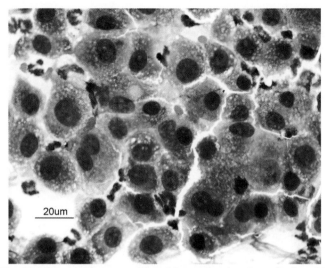

Fig. 2.12 Impression smear of a nodule on pleural surface of a dog with pyothorax caused by *Actinomyces* spp. infection. Numerous large epithelioid macrophages are present. These cells have abundant basophilic cytoplasm that may be nonvacuolated to minimally vacuolated. They may also occur in large aggregates resembling epithelial cell clusters.

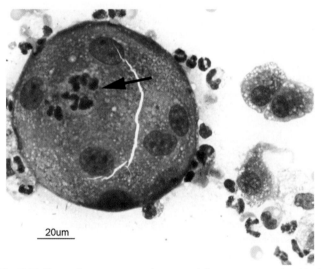

Fig. 2.11 Smear from a pyogranulomatous inflammatory reaction (*Actinomyces* infection). An extremely large, multinucleate macrophage is present. The macrophage has phagocytized several neutrophils.

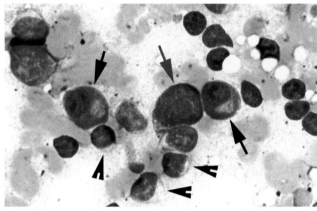

Fig. 2.13 Smear made from an aspirate of a reactive lymph node. Many small lymphocytes are present *(arrowheads)*. These cells have scant amounts of cytoplasm that do not appear to encircle the nucleus. Two plasma cells *(arrows)* are also present. One large lymphoid cell (large lymphocyte) is present *(red arrow)*. Note that the large lymphocyte and plasma cells are similar in size. However, the large lymphocyte has a larger nucleus, whereas the nucleus of the plasma cell is similar in size to a small lymphocyte.

Lymphocytes (Small, Medium, and Large)

Small lymphocytes are smaller than neutrophils with rounded nuclei and scant basophilic cytoplasm (Fig. 2.13). The nucleus is small (often about the diameter of a red blood cell [RBC] or slightly larger) and is generally not perfectly round but will have a flattened or indented area on one side. The nuclear chromatin has a smudged appearance and is usually *condensed*, having a dark purple appearance. Nucleoli are not visible; however, darker areas (heterochromatin) and lighter areas (euchromatin) are often visible. Generally, the cytoplasm is not visible completely around the circumference of the nucleus but is visible only on one side of the nucleus.

Medium-sized lymphocytes have nuclei that are somewhat larger, with lighter pink-purple chromatin and may have nucleoli visible. They have moderately increased amounts of cytoplasm often visible approximately halfway or more around the nuclear perimeter.

Large lymphocytes are large cells (often bigger than a neutrophils) with enlarged nuclei (often 2× the diameter of RBCs or greater) and *dispersed* chromatin that stains a lighter pink-purple than that of small lymphocytes (Fig. 2.14). Cytoplasm is more abundant, is often visible around the complete circumference of the nucleus, and is typically deeply basophilic. Distinct nucleoli are often visible, and multiple nucleoli may be observed. Large lymphocytes are commonly encountered in aspirates of lymphoid tissue and lymphoid neoplasms and may also be present in low numbers in inflammatory lesions.

A note on terminology regarding these cells is important. Large lymphocytes are sometimes alternatively referred to as either *lymphoblasts* or *immature lymphoid cells*, although both these terms are problematic. The term *lymphoblast* refers to a very specific morphological form of cell in the human classification of lymphoma, rather than being a general term for large lymphoid cells, as has been previously used in veterinary medicine. Also, because lymphocytes are not

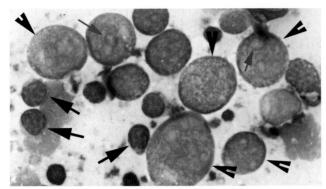

Fig. 2.14 Image of a fine-needle aspirate smear of a lymph node from a dog with lymphoma containing numerous large lymphocytes *(arrowheads)* and lymphocytes *(arrows)*. The large lymphocytes are larger and have more abundant cytoplasm. Nuclei are large with light staining, dispersed chromatin and often show prominent nucleoli *(red arrows)*.

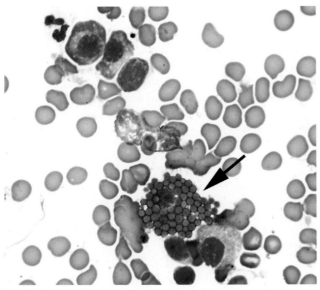

Fig. 2.15 Image from a lymph node aspirate demonstrates small lymphocytes, plasma cells, and one Mott cell with numerous Russell bodies *(arrow)*. The Russell bodies may range from appearing as clear vacuoles to being somewhat basophilic as in this image. (Courtesy Dr. Robin Allison, Oklahoma State University.)

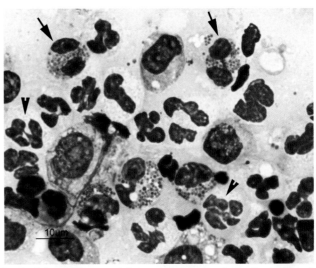

Fig. 2.16 Image from an inflammatory reaction in the intestines of a dog containing a mixture of neutrophils, eosinophils, and macrophages. The nuclei of the eosinophils are typically less lobulated *(arrows)* compared with those of the neutrophils *(arrowheads)*.

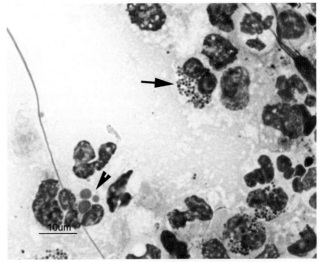

Fig. 2.17 Image from the same slide as Fig 2.16. In the dog, eosinophils have numerous small granules *(arrow)* or just a few large granules *(arrowhead)*.

terminally differentiated cells but can be stimulated to repeatedly replicate, small lymphocytes are not necessarily more "mature" than large lymphocytes, as is true with most other leukocytes. Nonetheless, any of these terms may be seen in reports and should not cause confusion for the reader.

Reactive lymphocytes are those responding to antigenic stimulation. They have moderately increased amounts of basophilic cytoplasm. Plasma cells are differentiated B-lymphocytes stimulated to produce antibodies. Plasma cells have a round, eccentrically placed nucleus, moderate amounts of deeply basophilic cytoplasm, and usually a distinct clear area located next to the nucleus (see Fig. 2.13). This clear area represents the Golgi apparatus and is often located between the nucleus and the greatest volume of cytoplasm. Plasma cells and large lymphocytes are both larger than small lymphocytes, but in plasma cells most of the increase in size is caused by more abundant cytoplasm, whereas in the large lymphocyte the nucleus has enlarged (see Fig. 2.13). Some plasma cells (termed *Mott cells*) have numerous large clear to basophilic vacuoles (termed *Russell bodies*) filling their cytoplasm (Fig. 2.15). These vacuoles represent retained immunoglobulin.

Eosinophils

Eosinophils are slightly larger than neutrophils. Their nuclei are segmented but are commonly less lobated than those of neutrophils and often divided into only two distinct lobes (Fig. 2.16). Rarely, eosinophils with perfectly round nuclei will be identified in cytological specimens, most often from the respiratory tract. The cytoplasm of eosinophils contains prominent orange-to-pink granules. In dogs, eosinophil granules are round and vary widely in size and number (Fig. 2.17). Eosinophil granules are numerous, small, and rod shaped in cats (Fig. 2.18). The delicate, densely packed granules of feline eosinophils are often less obvious than those of the dog, particularly in thick specimens (e.g., transtracheal washes) that may not stain well. Also, neutrophils in exudates will occasionally have mild eosinophilic stippling. Care must be taken not to confuse neutrophils and poorly stained eosinophils when trying to differentiate eosinophilic from neutrophilic inflammatory reactions in cats. The slightly larger and minimal nuclear lobation can help make the distinction. Often, it is easier to identify feline eosinophils that have been traumatized during slide preparation as their granules spread out and become more obvious. If many eosinophils have been ruptured during sample collection (e.g., with scraping of feline eosinophilic granuloma complex lesions), high numbers of eosinophil granules will be present throughout the background of the smear and may be identified before intact cells are seen.

Occasionally, eosinophil granules will not stain well with Diff-Quik stain (similar to what sometimes occurs with mast cells) yet stain prominently with Wright stain or Wright-Giemsa stain.

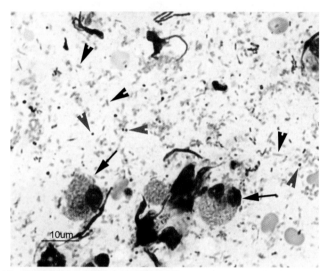

Fig. 2.18 Scraping from an eosinophilic granuloma complex lesion in a cat. Cat eosinophils *(arrows)* have densely packed granules, often making it difficult to see the individual granules in intact cells. Numerous free granules *(black arrowheads)* released from ruptured cells are present and demonstrate the slender rod shape typical of feline eosinophil granules. Numerous bacteria *(red arrowheads)* are also present free in the background.

IF A SMEAR IS COMPOSED OF TISSUE CELLS RATHER THAN INFLAMMATORY CELLS, WHAT TYPE OF CELLS ARE PRESENT?

A wide variety of specific cells may be encountered from the various normal tissues and tumors sampled cytologically. With experience, most of these cells can be easily recognized, particularly with the knowledge of what structure is being sampled. However, even if the cells are not immediately recognizable, they can generally be classified into one of three major categories on the basis of certain common cytological features (Table 2.1):

1. Discrete cells (or round cells)
2. Epithelial cells
3. Mesenchymal cells

Categorization of cells according to the major group they belong to helps the evaluator identify the specific cell type present. Even if precise identification cannot be made, relevant information, such as the presence of a cell type abnormal for the tissue sampled (e.g., epithelial cells in a lymph node aspirate), may be gained.

Discrete Cells (Round Cells)

Discrete cells are a group of cells that share certain cytological features because they are present individually in tissues, not adhered to other cells or a connective tissue matrix. The majority of these cells are of hematogenous origin. Aspirates of normal lymphoid tissue, such as the spleen and lymph nodes, yield cell populations that have a discrete cell pattern. Other than normal lymphoid tissue, a discrete cell pattern usually indicates the presence of one of a group of tumors termed *discrete cell tumors* (or *round cell tumors*). Recognition of discrete cell tumors is important because these are some of the more common neoplasms encountered in small animal practice. Also, cells of most discrete cell tumors have cytological characteristics that are sufficiently distinct to allow for a specific diagnosis.

TABLE 2.1	General Cytological Characteristics of Different Tissue Cell Types		
	Round Cells	**Epithelial Cells**	**Mesenchymal Cells**
Cellularity of slides	High cellularity	High cellularity	Low to high cellularity
			Normal mesenchymal cells and many tumors are of low cellularity because of adherence of cell in matrix
			Malignant tumors may yield high numbers of cells
Cell distribution	Evenly distributed across slide	Typically present in clusters	Discretely oriented or adhered in aggregates by extracellular matrix
		Malignant cells may lose cohesion	
Cell size and shape	Small to medium	Small to large, depending on tissue samples	Often fusiform or "spindle shaped"
	Generally round with distinct cell borders	Cuboidal to columnar to round, depending on specific tissue	Some cells may be plump or round (particularly cells from bone or bone tumors)
		Generally distinct cell borders when cells are individually oriented or at the edges of cell clusters	Often have indistinct cytoplasmic borders
Other features suggestive of this cell type	Distinctive morphology or select individual cell types	Formation of acini or tubules	Production of eosinophilic extracellular matrix
		Extremely large cells with abundant cytoplasm	
		Squamous differentiation	

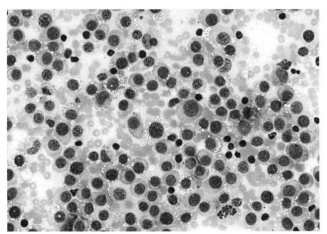

Fig. 2.19 This slide, made from an aspirate of a transmissible venereal tumor, shows a typical discrete cell pattern. The slide is highly cellular and the cells are evenly spread out throughout the smear. This pattern can usually be recognized from low-power magnification.

General Cytological Characteristics of Discrete Cell Populations

Because discrete cells are not adhered to other structures within the tissues, they generally exfoliate very readily during fine-needle biopsy (FNB). Hence, the cellularity of the resulting smears is usually very high. In addition, the individual cells are usually evenly spread throughout the smear (Fig. 2.19). Cell clusters or aggregates are not present; however, the extremely high cellularity of the smears may result in cells being piled on top of each other in thicker areas of the smears, and this may be misinterpreted as cell adhesion (or cell clustering). In the thinner areas of the smears, the cells can be seen to be individually oriented.

The individual cells tend to be of small to medium size and round. If the cells have not been traumatized during sample preparation, they typically have distinct cytoplasmic borders (i.e., the boundary of the cell is well defined).

Specific Discrete Cell Tumors

The discrete cell tumors are mast cell tumor, lymphoma (formerly termed *lymphosarcoma*), canine cutaneous histiocytoma, histiocytic sarcoma, plasmacytoma, and transmissible venereal tumor. In addition, melanocytic tumor can be a great imitator, yielding cell populations that may appear discrete, epithelial, or mesenchymal.

Mast cell tumor. Mast cell tumors are the only lesions that will yield highly cellular smears consisting entirely or predominantly of mast cells. Mast cells are recognized by their distinctive small, red-purple intracytoplasmic granules (Fig. 2.20). The number of granules in mast cells varies tremendously, even within cells from the same tumor (Fig. 2.21). Most mast cell tumors yield cells that contain a sufficient number of granules to be easily recognized as mast cells. Sometimes, the cells are so densely packed with granules that the cytoplasm will appear diffusely dark purple and the individual granules difficult or impossible to discern. In this situation, the granules will be evident in cells that have been ruptured. Because mast cell granules have such a high affinity for most cytological stains, the nucleus of a heavily granulated mast cell may appear pale or even totally unstained, giving the cell the look of a photographic negative with dark cytoplasm and a pale nucleus (Fig. 2.22). Some of the components of mast cell granules are chemotactic for eosinophils. The number of eosinophils present in smears from a mast cell tumor varies from very few to many. Occasionally, an aspirate from a mast cell tumor

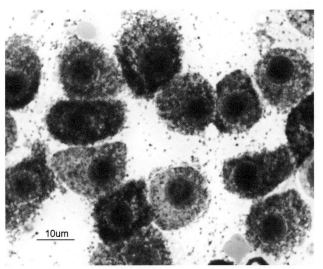

Fig. 2.20 Smear made from a mast cell tumor has a pure population of heavily granulated mast cells. The nuclei of these cells are often obscured by the granulation. Numerous free granules are present in the background.

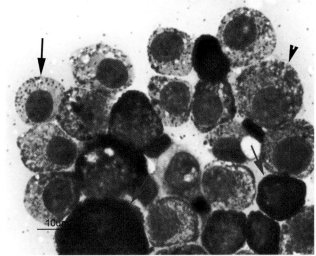

Fig. 2.21 Image from a mast cell tumor. Some cells are sparsely granulated and the individual granules are easy to see *(black arrow)*. In some heavily granulated cells, the cytoplasm appears diffusely pink-purple, but some individual granules can be seen and the outline of the nucleus can still be visualized *(black arrowhead)*. Some cells are so densely packed with granules that neither individual granules nor the nucleus can be seen, making the cell appear as a dark purple mass *(red arrows)*.

will yield predominantly eosinophils with fewer mast cells (Fig. 2.23). In this case, it can be difficult to differentiate a mast cell tumor from a hypersensitivity response. Generally, if there are areas on the slides containing large "sheets" where mast cells are present to the exclusion of other cells, mast cell tumor is most likely.

Cells from some mast cell tumors contain relatively few granules. If a mast cell tumor had degranulated during or before aspiration, a percentage of the cells may have relatively few granules. Generally, some granules will still be evident in most cells, and some cells will remain heavily granulated. In addition, high numbers of free granules may be present in the background of the slides. Aspirates of degranulated mast cell tumors may be of lower than normal cellularity because of resultant tissue edema. Anaplastic (poorly differentiated) mast cell tumors may yield cells virtually devoid of granules because the cells have not

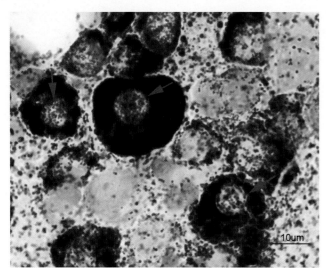

Fig. 2.22 Image from a mast cell tumor. The densely packed granules in the cytoplasm have a high affinity for the stain and the nuclei of many cells are understained, giving the cells the look of a photographic negative.

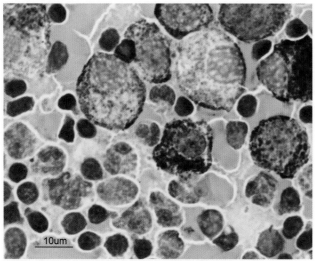

Fig. 2.23 Mast cell tumor metastasis to a lymph node. Many mast cells are present, but greater numbers of eosinophils are attracted by constituents of mast cell granules. In some cases, the number of eosinophils can be greater than the number of mast cells in an aspirate from a mast cell tumor.

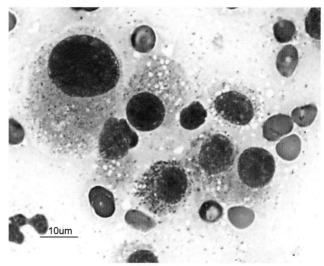

Fig. 2.24 Aspirate from a poorly differentiated (grade III) mast cell tumor. The poorly differentiated cells contain relatively few granules. The individual cells show marked atypia including significant variation of cell size, nuclear size, and nuclear-to-cytoplasmic ratio.

differentiated sufficiently to produce them (Fig. 2.24). In this case, the cells generally display marked atypia (see the section "Do the Tissue Cells Present Display Significant Criteria of Malignancy?"). Finally, Diff-Quik stain sometimes fails to stain the granules of mast cell tumors. Slides from the same tumor stained with the Wright stain may be heavily granulated (Fig. 2.25). This is an inconsistent event, occurring only in some mast cell tumors and not others. When it occurs, mast cells may resemble plasma cells or macrophages. A diligent search of the slides will usually reveal low numbers of identifiable, although poorly stained, granules in some cells. A person routinely using the Diff-Quik stain should always consider this possibility when evaluating a discrete cell population.

Cells from mast cell tumors should be evaluated for criteria of malignancy, as described later in this chapter. Although cytology cannot help evaluate tissue invasion by neoplastic cells, a newly proposed two-tier histological grading scheme for canine cutaneous mast cell tumors relies on nuclear atypia rather than depth of invasion.[5]

The majority of tumors composed of poorly granulated cells that display marked cytological atypia will have an aggressive biological behavior. A small percentage of tumors composed of heavily granulated, well-differentiated cells will be behaviorally malignant, and thus all mast cell tumors should be removed with wide surgical excision, if possible, and submitted for histology to grade the neoplasm and evaluate completeness of excision.

Examination of peripheral blood smears or buffy coat preparations, bone marrow aspirates, and aspirates of any enlarged lymph nodes or abdominal organs (particularly liver and spleen) can be useful in detecting systemic spread of the mast cell tumor.

Lymphoma (Lymphosarcoma). Most cases of lymphoma in dogs and cats are high-grade tumors composed predominantly of large blastic lymphocytes (Fig. 2.26). If large, blastic lymphocytes constitute greater than 50% of the cells in a highly cellular smear from lymphoid tissue containing mostly intact cells, a diagnosis of lymphoma can reliably be made. Large lymphocytes can usually be differentiated from the cells of other discrete cell tumors, on the basis of their higher nuclear-to-cytoplasmic (N:C) ratio and the intensely basophilic cytoplasm. Also, in aspirates from lymphoma, usually, numerous small but different-sized basophilic fragments of cytoplasm (lymphoglandular bodies) are scattered among the cells (see Fig. 2.26). Lymphoid cells, particularly large lymphocytes, are fragile cells and easily ruptured during slide preparation. If an overwhelming majority of the cells on the smears is ruptured, one cannot be confident that the remaining cells accurately represent the cell population in the lymph node. In this situation, additional samples must be collected for a diagnosis. Submission of multiple slides from different lymph nodes will increased chances of a diagnostic slide.

Sometimes, lymphoma is well differentiated and composed of small- to medium-sized lymphocytes rather than large, blastic cells. Such tumors can be difficult to differentiate from normal or reactive lymphoid tissue solely on the basis of cytology, and confirmation may be required either through molecular techniques such as polymerase chain reaction for antigen receptor rearrangement (PARR) or flow cytometry (see Chapters 30 and 31) or may require histological examination of a surgically removed lymph node, which can demonstrate architectural effacement and capsular invasion.

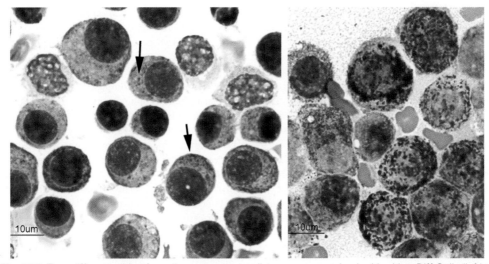

Fig. 2.25 Two different slides from the same mast cell tumor were stained with either Diff-Quik *(left)* or Wright-Giemsa *(right)* stain. Although the sample stained with Wright-Giemsa stain shows that the cells are heavily granulated, Diff-Quik stain did not stain the granules of the cells well in this tumor. Some granules can be seen in the Diff-Quik–stained specimen *(arrows)*.

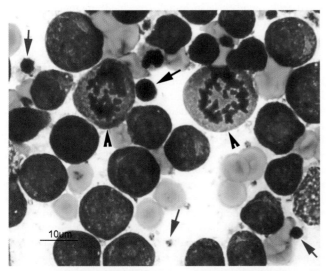

Fig. 2.26 Aspirate of the lymph nodes of a dog with lymphoma. The slide consists almost entirely of large blastic lymphoid cells. One poorly spread-out small lymphocyte is present *(black arrow)*. Two mitotic figures are present *(arrowheads)* and numerous cytoplasmic fragments of lymphoid cells (lymphoglandular bodies) are present in the background *(red arrows)*.

Canine cutaneous histiocytoma. Canine cutaneous histiocytoma is a benign tumor of dendritic cell origin and occurs commonly in young dogs (Fig. 2.27). Tumor cells are medium sized, slightly larger than neutrophils. Nuclei are generally round to oval but may be indented to irregular in shape. The nucleus has finely stippled chromatin and may have indistinct nucleoli. They have a moderate amount of light blue-gray cytoplasm. If a significant amount of protein-rich tissue fluid is present between cells, the cytoplasm of the cells may appear lighter than the background (Fig. 2.28), or the cell borders may be indistinct.

Histiocytomas usually regress spontaneously within a few weeks to months. Regression is associated with an infiltration of small lymphocytes into the tumor. Therefore aspirates from these tumors will sometimes contain a mixture of tumor cells and small lymphocytes (see Fig. 2.28). The presence of small lymphocytes among the larger tumor cells must not lead to misidentification of histiocytoma cells as

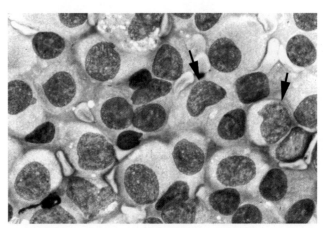

Fig. 2.27 Smear made from a histiocytoma. Histiocytoma cells have moderate amounts of light-colored cytoplasm. Nuclei are usually round to oval but may be indented, kidney shaped, or irregular *(arrows)*.

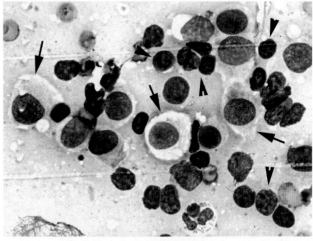

Fig. 2.28 Smear made from a histiocytoma. Regression of a histiocytoma is associated with an infiltration of small lymphocytes *(arrowheads)*, which may be more numerous than the histiocytoma cells *(arrows)*.

large lymphocytes. The irregular shape of the nuclei, the light color and greater volume of the cytoplasm, and the lack of lymphoglandular bodies help differentiate histiocytoma cells from lymphoid cells.

Histiocytic sarcoma complex. These tumors result from proliferation of either dendritic cells or macrophages of bone marrow origin.[6,7] Older publications may refer to this tumor as "malignant histiocytosis." Cytology alone may not be able to differentiate these diseases from each other or from inflammatory proliferations of macrophages (granulomatous inflammation) when the cells are of macrophage rather than dendritic cell origin.

Cytological appearance of histiocytic sarcoma varies from a population of cells resembling relatively well-differentiated macrophages to histiocytic cells with marked atypia (Figs. 2.29, 2.30, and 2.31).[7] Common features include large discrete cells with abundant vacuolated cytoplasm, prominent cytophagia, and multinucleation (see Fig. 2.30, B). With tumors of dendritic cell origin, the cytoplasmic vacuoles are often small and of uniform size and may lack the presence

of phagocytic debris common in macrophages seen in inflammatory lesions (see Fig. 2.29). The cells may demonstrate marked anisocytosis, anisokaryosis, and variation of the N:C ratio (see Fig. 2.31, A). Macrocytosis, karyomegaly, and the presence of large multinucleate cells are common (see Fig. 2.31, B).

When masses are composed of histiocytic cells showing marked atypia, a diagnosis of histiocytic sarcoma can be made. However, when the cells consist of macrophages that appear relatively bland, definitive diagnosis may not be possible solely on the basis of cytology. It should be noted that many of these lesions with relatively bland cytological appearance may have an aggressive biological behavior.

Plasmacytoma. Tumors of plasma cell origin include multiple myeloma (plasma cell myeloma), a systemic tumor arising primarily in bone marrow, and extramedullary plasmacytomas. Extramedullary plasmacytomas are commonly cutaneous tumors but have been described as occurring in other sites, including the gastrointestinal (GI) tract. Cutaneous plasmacytomas are typically benign.[8] It has been suggested that a greater likelihood of aggressive biological behavior exists with plasmacytomas arising from the GI tract other than the oral areas.[9]

Well-differentiated plasmacytomas yield cells that resemble normal plasma cells (Fig. 2.32, A). Distinguishing features include eccentrically placed small, round nuclei surrounded by a moderate amount of deeply basophilic cytoplasm with or without the characteristic distinct paranuclear clear zone. In some well-differentiated plasma cell tumors, the paranuclear clear zone will not be evident, even though the cells otherwise resemble well-differentiated plasma cells. Poorly differentiated plasmacytomas may yield a less distinct population of discrete cells that demonstrate significant cytological atypia. Anisocytosis, anisokaryosis, and variation of the N:C ratio can be prominent. Binucleate and multinucleate cells are common in both well-differentiated and poorly differentiated tumors (see Fig. 2.32, B). This, together with a lack of lymphoglandular bodies, helps differentiate these tumors from lymphoma. Cytological atypia often does not correlate with an aggressive biological behavior. Many neoplasms effacing bone marrow or the spleen comprise uniform, well-differentiated plasma cells, whereas benign cutaneous tumors may show significant pleomorphism.

Some plasma cells have a distinct red color to the periphery of their cytoplasm and are referred to as *flame cells* (Fig. 2.33). Rarely, an eosinophilic extracellular matrix representing amyloid (composed of immunoglobulin light chain) is seen among the neoplastic cells.

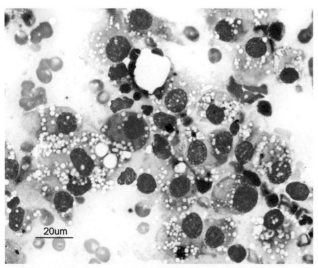

Fig. 2.29 Splenic aspirate from a dog with histiocytic sarcoma. The spleen was markedly enlarged and consisted almost entirely of a population of discretely oriented, heavily vacuolated histiocytic cells. Many of the cells were fairly uniform, although other cells showed significant atypia.

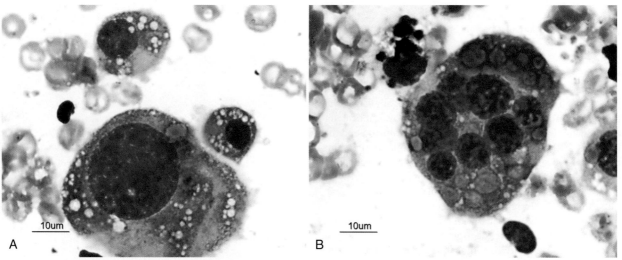

A   B

Fig. 2.30 Same slide as in Fig 2.29. (A) Some macrocytic, karyomegalic cells were also present. Note the phagocytosis of several red blood cells. (B) Large multinucleate cell showing erythrophagia.

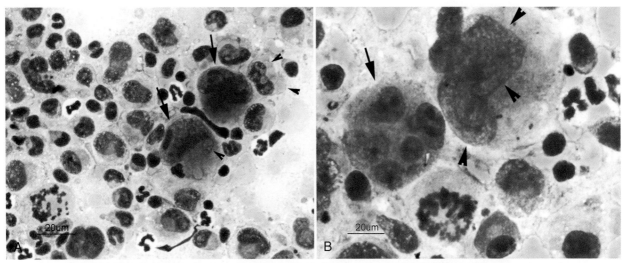

Fig. 2.31 Splenic aspirate from another dog with histiocytic sarcoma. (A) Cells from this tumor showed marked atypia including anisocytosis, anisokaryosis, and nuclear pleomorphism. Large, karyomegalic cells with large, prominent, irregularly shaped nucleoli are present *(arrows)*. Many of the cells in this tumor demonstrated erythrophagia *(arrowheads)*. (B) Both large multinucleate cells and large cells with a single, pleomorphic, karyomegalic nucleus *(arrowheads)* are common in this tumor.

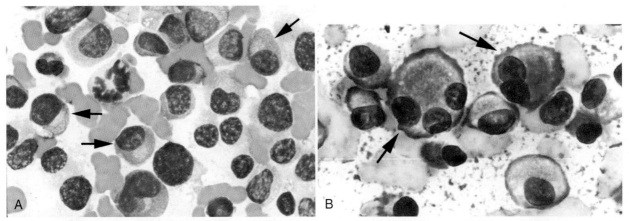

Fig. 2.32 Smears made from an extramedullary plasmacytoma. (A) Cells show a typical discrete cell pattern. Many cells resemble mature plasma cells having eccentric nuclei and distinct perinuclear clear areas *(arrows)*. (B) Binucleate and multinucleate cells *(arrows)* are common in tumors of plasma cell origin.

Transmissible venereal tumor. Except in certain geographical areas, transmissible venereal tumors (TVTs) are less commonly encountered compared with other discrete cell tumors. TVTs are often present on the external genitalia but may occur in other locations as well.

The cells from a TVT are typically more pleomorphic compared with those from most other discrete cell tumors (Fig. 2.34). They have moderate amounts of smoky to light blue cytoplasm with sharply defined cytoplasmic boundaries. A prominent characteristic of TVT cells that helps distinguish them from other discrete cell tumors is the presence of numerous, distinctly walled, cytoplasmic vacuoles (see Fig. 2.34). These vacuoles can also be found extracellularly, appearing as clear areas against a proteinaceous background of tissue fluid. Nuclei show moderate to marked anisokaryosis and have a coarse nuclear chromatin pattern. Nucleoli may be prominent, and mitotic figures, often atypical, are common.

Melanocytic tumors. Tumors of melanocytic origin are great imitators; cells may show features of discrete cells, epithelial cells, or mesenchymal cells. Often, a mixture of all three of these morphological appearances will be present within an aspirate from a single tumor. Sometimes, however, aspirates will consist entirely of discretely oriented, round cells giving the appearance of a "round cell tumor." Melanocytic tumors are usually easily recognized by their pigmentation. Individual melanin granules are rod-shaped granules that typically stain dark green to black. When these granules are densely packed within cells, they appear black. The appearance of the cells from a melanoma may range from heavily pigmented to sparsely pigmented, depending on the degree of differentiation of the tumor.

With heavily pigmented tumors, the cells often appear simply as dark black, circular to spherical objects (Fig. 2.35). Visualization of cell detail is often completely obscured by the pigmentation. Nuclei may be seen in cells that are traumatized, and often a background containing numerous free melanin granules is present (see Fig. 2.35).

In poorly differentiated tumors, pigmentation may be sparse (Fig. 2.36) to absent, requiring a lengthy search to find any pigment granules at all. These cells typically show marked criteria of malignancy (see subsequent section in this chapter) (see Fig. 2.36).

Most poorly pigmented tumors with marked cytological atypia have a malignant biological behavior. It is difficult to assess the malignant potential of heavily pigmented tumors because individual cells cannot

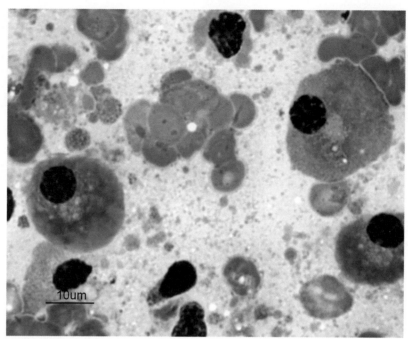

Fig. 2.33 Smear made of a spleen aspirate from a dog with a plasma cell tumor. Plasma cells show a distinct red color at the periphery of their cytoplasm and are termed *flame cells*.

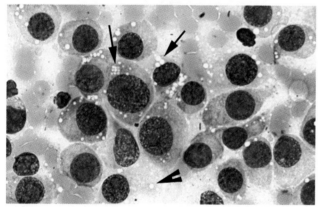

Fig. 2.34 Smear made from a transmissible venereal tumor (TVT). Cells from a TVT are characterized by numerous clear vacuoles within the cytoplasm of the cells *(arrows)* and free in the background *(arrowhead)*. Many of the cells have coarse nuclear chromatin and large nucleoli.

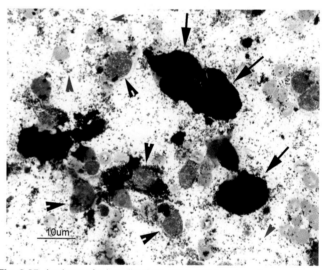

Fig. 2.35 Aspirate of a heavily pigmented cutaneous melanoma from a dog. In most of the intact cells *(arrows)*, the cellular detail is completely obscured by the pigmentation, preventing evaluation of these cells. Nuclei can be seen in some cells *(arrowheads)* that appear partially ruptured. Numerous free melanin granules *(red arrowheads)* are present in the background of the smear.

be evaluated. Although many heavily pigmented tumors are benign, some of these may also demonstrate aggressive biological behavior. The anatomical location of the tumor greatly affects the likelihood of malignancy in dogs, with tumors of the oral cavity, mucocutaneous junctions, and nail bed carrying a greater likelihood of malignant behavior.

A note on terminology is important because it has changed over the years. Currently, the term *melanocytoma* is typically used to refer to a benign tumor and *melanoma* to indicate a malignant tumor or a tumor with higher potential for malignant behavior. Many years ago, the term *melanoma* was more widely used with benign tumors, whereas the term *malignant melanoma* was used when criteria of malignancy were clear. The potential for malignancy is also hard to determine because invasion of the lymphatics and vessels cannot be evaluated via cytology and because cellular morphology may be obscured by the pigment; therefore, the more general term *melanocytic neoplasia* may be used to denote the cell of origin without restricting to either a benign or

malignant process. The most important thing is that the clinician is clear about the intent of the terms used by the pathologist; if there is any uncertainty, a phone call can help clarify the intent.

Epithelial Cells

Normal epithelial cells are commonly encountered in many cytological preparations. Surface epithelium will be present in most surface scrapings or swabs (e.g., squamous cells from skin scrapings and nasal or vaginal swabs), in washings (e.g., columnar cells from transtracheal washes), and as the result of normal exfoliation (e.g., transitional cells from urine sediments). In addition, epithelial cells will be the major cellular component of smears made from FNB of many parenchymal

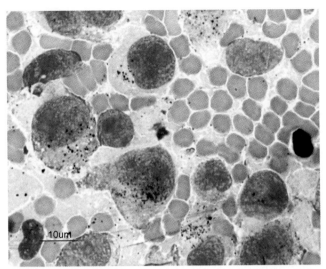

Fig. 2.36 Aspirate from a poorly pigmented malignant melanoma from the oral cavity of a dog. The slide consists of large, pleomorphic cells with a high nuclear-to-cytoplasmic ratio and large prominent nucleoli. Most cells have a few cytoplasmic melanin granules that are easily recognizable.

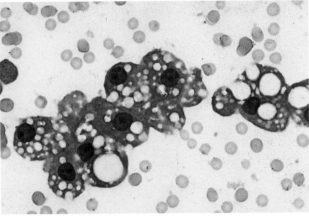

Fig. 2.37 Smear made from an aspirate of a feline kidney. Numerous renal tubular epithelial cells are present. Epithelial cells tend to form cell clusters. Feline renal tubular cells may have numerous lipid vacuoles within their cytoplasm.

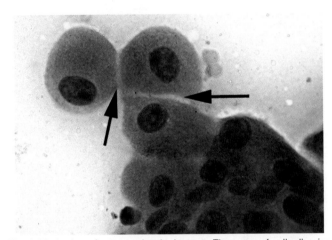

Fig. 2.38 Aspirate from a perianal adenoma. The areas of cell adhesion can be seen in some cells *(arrows)*.

organs (e.g., hepatocytes and bile duct epithelium from liver aspirates, renal tubular cells from kidney aspirates) and glandular aspirates (e.g., mammary, prostate).

Epithelial cells may also originate from a hyperplastic proliferation or neoplasm. Cells from benign epithelial tumors may be difficult to impossible to differentiate from their normal, or hyperplastic, counterparts solely on the basis of cytology. However, combining clinical and cytological findings can often allow one to make the diagnosis of a benign epithelial proliferation. For example, a discrete wartlike mass on an older dog that yields numerous clusters of normal-appearing sebaceous epithelial cells suggests a sebaceous adenoma or sebaceous gland hyperplasia.

Epithelial cells that display sufficient cytological criteria of malignancy indicate the presence of a carcinoma or adenocarcinoma. A specific diagnosis of cell type may or may not be possible solely on the basis of cytology and depends on how well differentiated and characteristic the cells are. Histopathology may be required for a more specific diagnosis of cell type. However, the ability to confirm the presence of a malignant epithelial tumor by cytology is often sufficient to guide clinical management of a case.

General Cytological Characteristics of Epithelial Cell Populations

A main feature of epithelial cells is cell-to-cell adhesion (Fig. 2.37). Normal epithelial cells are typically present in different-sized sheets or clusters. Sometimes, the area of adhesion between individual cells can be seen (Fig. 2.38). True cell clustering from cell-to-cell adhesion must be differentiated from crowding of cells in highly cellular aspirates of any cell type. This can usually be accomplished by looking at thinner areas of the smear. In thin areas, if the cells are still present in clusters but are separated by acellular areas, cell-to-cell adhesion is documented.

Mesenchymal cells are sometimes held together by an extracellular matrix, resulting in large aggregates of cells, which resembles cell adhesion. Often, this extracellular matrix is apparent as a brightly eosinophilic, homogeneous material between the cells and can be used to identify the type of cell present.

Normal epithelial cells vary in size from small (e.g., basal cells) to large, depending on the specific type and stage of maturation. They may be round, polygonal, columnar, or caudate in shape and typically have distinct, sharply defined cytoplasmic borders. Cytoplasmic borders within cell clusters may be difficult to discern; however, the outer edges of the cells in the clusters typically are clearly demarcated. Nuclei of epithelial cells are generally round to somewhat oval in shape. A single, small, round nucleolus may be visible in certain types of epithelial cells, such as hepatocytes and renal tubular epithelium (see Fig. 2.37).

Epithelial Criteria Specific to Certain Cell Types

Mature squamous epithelial cells are often found in samples collected from surface swabs or scrapings. These tend to be more individually oriented and may not show prominent cell clustering (Fig. 2.39). Fully mature (cornified or keratinized) squamous cells have abundant cytoplasm with angular cytoplasmic borders. Their nuclei become small and pyknotic, and eventually the cell becomes anucleate (see Fig. 2.39). Less differentiated squamous cells, often present in swabs or scrapings along with mature cells, are more cohesive, and have a greater tendency to be in clusters (Fig. 2.40). These cells are round and have variable amounts of cytoplasm, increasing as the cell matures. Nuclei of these cells are large and round with functional (nonpyknotic) chromatin (see Fig. 2.40). Because of the potential to have a mixture of cells at different stages of maturation, squamous cell populations may normally show significant variation in cell size and nuclear size.

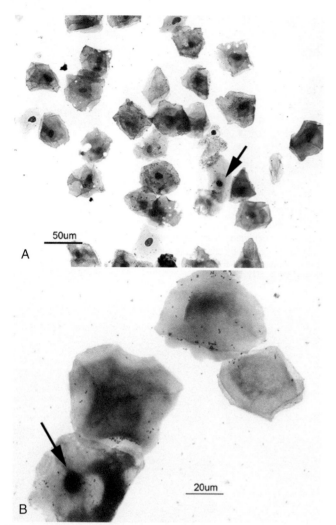

Fig. 2.39 Mature, cornified cells from a canine vaginal swab. (A) Low-magnification image shows that these cells tend to exfoliate individually rather than in cohesive clusters. Individual cells show angular cytoplasmic borders. Nuclei become pyknotic *(arrow)* and eventually disappear, leaving anucleate cells. (B) High-magnification image showing three anucleate squamous cells and one mature squamous cell with a condensed pyknotic nucleus *(arrow)*.

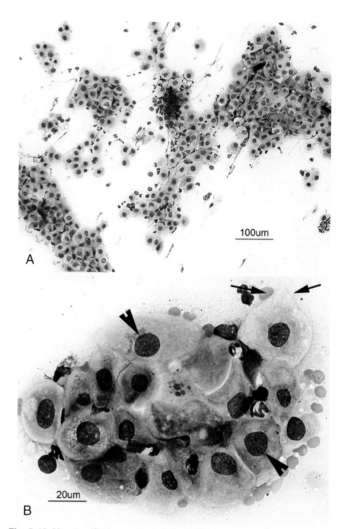

Fig. 2.40 Noncornified squamous cells from a canine vaginal swab. These cells are less differentiated than those shown in Fig 2.39. These cells can be seen in surface swabs and scraping and may be intermixed with fully keratinized cells. (A) Low-magnification image shows that these cells tend to demonstrate cell-to-cell adhesion, being present in cohesive clusters. (B) High magnification of one cluster of noncornified squamous cells. The cells tend to be round, although some cells are beginning to develop angular borders. Amount of cytoplasm is variable, depending on stage of maturation. Cells have functional, nonpyknotic nuclei *(arrowheads)*.

Epithelial cells from the respiratory and GI tract are distinctly columnar. Cell clusters may show long rows of cells, with nuclei lined up at the basal end of the cell (Fig. 2.41). Often, cilia can be seen at the apical surface of samples from the respiratory tract (Fig. 2.42). Normal epithelial cells from the GI tract are often present in large, pavemented clusters, often with clear cytoplasm, suggesting their secretory nature (Fig. 2.43). The columnar nature of the cells may be evident only at the sides of the clusters, where the cells have arranged on their sides (rather than a "top down" view seen in the middle of the clusters) (Fig. 2.44).

Although most tissue architecture is lost during fine-needle aspiration, some architectural arrangements may endure. Epithelial cells of glandular origin may show evidence of tubular or acinar formation (Figs. 2.45 and 2.46). Papillary or trabecular patterns may also be retained in some epithelial tumors.

Tumors of endocrine epithelial cells (e.g., thyroid carcinoma) and neuroendocrine cells (e.g., pheochromocytoma, chemodectoma) often yield cell populations with characteristic features (Fig. 2.47). The slides are highly cellular and consist of loosely cohesive types. In addition, these cells tend to be fragile, and smears typically contain many bare nuclei admixed

with the loosely cohesive intact cells. Bare nuclei of fragile cell populations must be differentiated from bare nuclei occurring from cell rupturing caused by poor smearing technique (i.e., excessive pressure during smearing). Bare nuclei from endocrine or neuroendocrine populations often have relatively intact nuclear outlines, as opposed to the traumatized, irregular appearance often seen with poor smearing technique.

Mesenchymal Cells
Origin of Mesenchymal Cells in Cytological Samples
Mesenchymal cells are cells that form connective tissue, blood vessels, and lymphatics. Because blood is considered a connective tissue, hematopoietic cells (including many of the cells described in the section on discrete cells) are technically classified as mesenchymal cells. However, because these hematopoietic cells have a cytological appearance (i.e., discrete cell appearance) that is highly distinct from the other connective tissues, they are typically considered a separate classification. Most often, the discussion of mesenchymal cells in cytology texts implies stromal connective tissue cells.

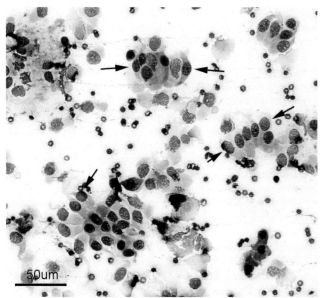

Fig. 2.41 Smear of a bronchial brushing from a dog. Low-magnification image shows numerous clusters of columnar epithelial cells. In some of the well-spread-out cells, the columnar nature is evident, and the nuclei can be seen lining up on what was the basal surface of the cell.

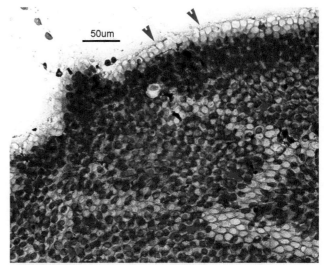

Fig. 2.43 Aspirate of intestinal epithelial cells from a cat. Low magnification shows large, tightly cohesive clusters of cells in a pavemented monolayer. The secretory nature of the cells is evident by the clear nature of the cytoplasm of many of the cells *(red arrows)*. The columnar nature of the cells is evident only at the edges of the cluster *(red arrowheads)*.

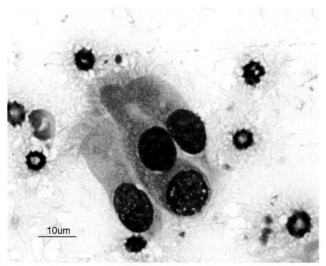

Fig. 2.42 Higher magnification of slide from Fig 2.41. Cilia can be seen on the apical surface of the columnar epithelial cells.

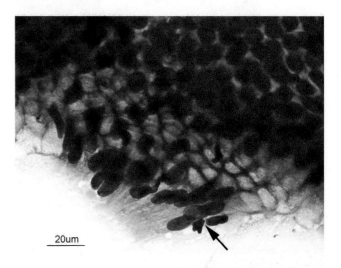

Fig. 2.44 Higher magnification of intestinal epithelial cells shown in Fig 2.43. The columnar nature of the cells and palisading nuclear arrangement can be seen on the edge of the cluster *(arrow)*. Again, many of the cells have clear, distended cytoplasm typical of secretory cells.

Most normal connective tissues exfoliate very few, if any, cells when sampled by FNB. Sometimes, small fragments of mature muscle will be seen in samples as inadvertent sampling of muscle surrounding a lesion (Fig. 2.48). Muscle fragments appear as basophilic, irregularly shaped structures from low magnification. At high magnification, regularly spaced, ovoid nuclei may be noted, and striations may be seen in the cytoplasm by focusing up and down on the tissue fragment. Fibroblasts and fibrocytes are the one nonneoplastic mesenchymal cell type that is commonly encountered in cytological specimens. Clusters of normal stromal cells can be seen in aspirates of internal organs, particularly the spleen. Scattered individual fibroblasts may be seen in aspirates from virtually any tissue. Reactive fibroblasts may be present in significant numbers in aspirates from areas of inflammation or tissue repair (e.g., surgical scars). Reactive fibroblasts (fibroplasia) may show many of the cytological criteria of malignancy, so caution should be exercised in evaluating mesenchymal cells when a significant inflammatory response is present. Reactive fibroblasts should be suspected when scattered mesenchymal cells are present along with a population of inflammatory cells (Fig. 2.49).

Mesenchymal neoplasia is the other main consideration for a cytological specimen containing mesenchymal cells. Highly cellular smears containing a pure population of mesenchymal cells that show cytological atypia are likely to indicate mesenchymal neoplasia. Malignant tumors of mesenchymal origin are by definition sarcomas, although the names of some tumors do not follow the standard nomenclature (e.g., *malignant fibrous histiocytoma, hemangiopericytoma*).

General Cytological Characteristics of Mesenchymal Cell Populations

As previously mentioned, aspirates of normal mesenchymal tissue are usually sparsely cellular because of the tightly cohesive nature of

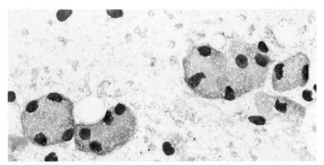

Fig. 2.45 Smear from an aspirate of a normal salivary gland (accidentally aspirated instead of the submandibular lymph node). The cells are arranged in an acinar pattern with nuclei at the periphery of the acinus. Individual cells are relatively small with small, round nuclei showing mature chromatin and abundant cytoplasm yielding a low nuclear-to-cytoplasmic ratio.

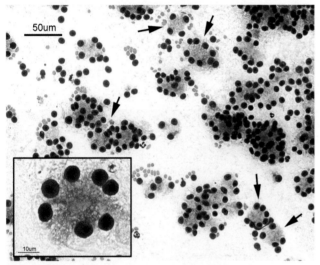

Fig. 2.46 Smear of a pancreatic aspirate from a cat. Uniform epithelial cells are in clusters and show acinus formation (arrows) indicating a glandular origin. Inset, Higher magnification of a single acinus with evidence of secretory material (slightly pink) in the center of the acinus.

connective tissue. Benign mesenchymal tumors tend to exfoliate very few cells, and samples of diagnostic quality may be difficult to obtain. In contrast, malignant mesenchymal tumors may yield highly cellular aspirates (Fig. 2.50). The cells are usually individually oriented, although large aggregates may be present, particularly if held together by an extracellular matrix (see below).

Mesenchymal cells are often fusiform cells with cytoplasm that tapers in one or more directions (Fig. 2.51). These are commonly referred to as *spindle cells*. Mesenchymal cells may range from extremely elongated, fusiform cells with thin, rod-shaped nuclei (Fig. 2.52) to cells that are plump and minimally tapered and have round nuclei (Fig. 2.53). Aspirates from malignant mesenchymal tumors often show a mixture of cells of various shapes, so the entire population must be examined to determine the cell type (see Fig. 2.50). Depending on the histological subtype, cells from primary bone tumors (e.g., osteosarcoma, chondrosarcoma) may show virtually no spindling and may have well-defined cytoplasmic borders mimicking discrete cells or epithelial cells (see Fig. 2.53). Usually, these are identified as being mesenchymal in nature on the basis of clinical suspicion (i.e., lytic bone lesion), the presence of extracellular matrix, the presence of osteoclasts (Fig. 2.54), and the characteristic appearance of the cells (see Fig. 2.53).

In contrast to other cell types (discrete and epithelial), the cytoplasmic borders of mesenchymal cells are often indistinct (Fig. 2.55). The cytoplasm may blend imperceptibly with the background, making it nearly impossible to distinguish the limits of the cell membrane. Ruptured cells may also have indistinct cytoplasmic borders. In these traumatized cells, the nuclear membrane is usually also disrupted, whereas the nuclear outline of intact mesenchymal cells is well defined. Another characteristic of mesenchymal cells is production of an extracellular matrix (Fig. 2.56). This is seen as a variably eosinophilic material present between cells, often holding them in large aggregates.

These descriptions outline general characteristics. The entire cell population present should be carefully evaluated because no single criterion will definitively identify a cell population. Sometimes, particularly with poorly differentiated malignant tumors, the cells will show criteria of more than one category. In these cases, it may be impossible to accurately classify the type of cell present. If cell type cannot be categorized, the cells should be evaluated for criteria of malignancy because identification of a malignant tumor may be sufficient information to direct management of the case. Surgical biopsy and histopathology may be able to provide a more specific diagnosis as to tissue of origin, if needed.

DO THE TISSUE CELLS PRESENT DISPLAY SIGNIFICANT CRITERIA OF MALIGNANCY?

Tissue cells should be evaluated for cytological atypia (criteria of malignancy). If sufficient criteria are present, a diagnosis of malignant neoplasia can be made. Cells from normal tissue, hyperplastic tissue, and benign neoplasia generally do not contain significant criteria of malignancy.

Cytological Criteria of Malignancy

Although some assessment of the arrangement of cells within cell clusters can be made, cytological samples often lack the architectural information that is available on histological sections. Therefore, some factors, such as disruption of normal architecture and invasion of suspect cells into adjacent normal tissue or lymphatics, usually cannot be determined. Evaluation of malignant potential in cytology specimens involves evaluating cell populations for lack of differentiation and cellular atypia. In general, benign lesions yield morphologically uniform populations of well-differentiated cells, whereas malignant tumors are characterized by variability of cell features. Cytological criteria are divided into general criteria of malignancy and nuclear criteria of malignancy (Table 2.2). Nuclear criteria of malignancy are more reliable because they are less likely to be induced by nonneoplastic processes, such as inflammation-induced dysplasia. No single criterion indicates the presence of malignancy, and any of the features described below may be seen in certain cells or cell populations.

General Criteria of Malignancy

Anisocytosis and macrocytosis. Anisocytosis (Fig. 2.57) refers to variation in cell size, whereas *macrocytosis* (Fig. 2.58) refers to exceptionally large cells. Macrocytic cells are most commonly observed in tumors of epithelial origin. Both are atypical findings in most cell populations, although exceptions do exist. In samples of normal or reactive lymphoid tissue, variation in cell size is an expected finding because of the variety of different cell types present (i.e., small lymphocytes, large lymphocytes, plasma cells). In contrast, lymphoid malignancy yields a uniform, monomorphic population of large lymphocytes. In scrapings from skin surfaces and some vaginal swabs, moderate to marked anisocytosis of the squamous epithelial cells may exist. This relates to the fact that such samples can collect squamous cells

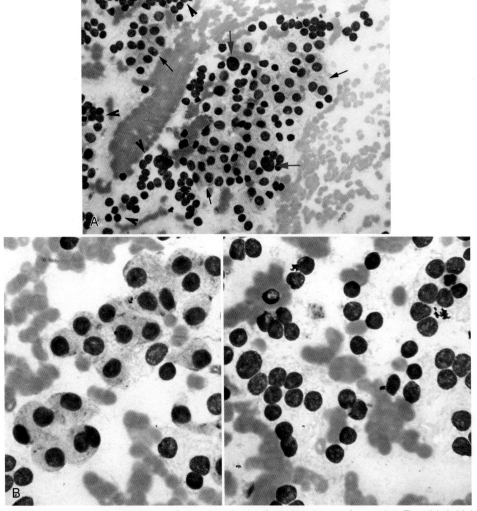

Fig. 2.47 (A) Low-magnification image of a neuroendocrine (heart base) tumor from a dog. The slide is highly cellular and consists of a mixture of loosely cohesive intact cells *(black arrows)* and bare nuclei of ruptured cells *(black arrowheads)*. The cells are fairly uniform, although some karyomegalic cells are seen *(red arrows)*. (B) Higher magnification of same slide as in image A. On the left, the intact cells appear fairly uniform and have small nuclei with mature, condensed chromatin and moderate amounts of lightly basophilic cytoplasm. On the right, a different field shows many bare nuclei suggesting the fragile nature of the cells. Note that although the cells are ruptured, the bare nuclei appear intact rather than the nuclear streaming often seen when cells are ruptured from excessive pressure during slide preparation.

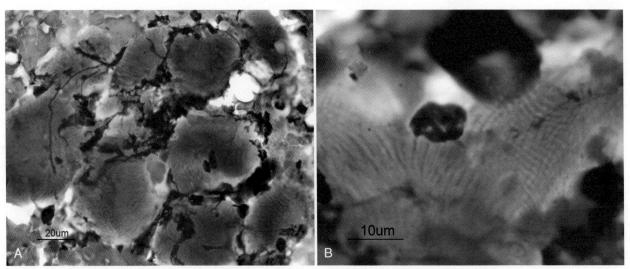

Fig. 2.48 Aspirate of a perianal gland tumor from a dog. (A) Numerous circular to oval, basophilic structures represent fragments of normal striated muscle. (B) Higher magnification of another area from the same slide shows distinct striations within the cytoplasm.

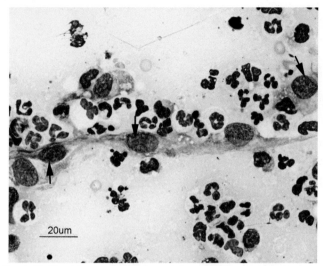

Fig. 2.49 Fibroblasts present in an inflammatory reaction. Note that the fibroblasts have prominent nucleoli *(arrows)*. In many cases, reactive fibroblasts will show other atypical features often associated with malignancy, such as marked anisocytosis and anisokaryosis. When large numbers of inflammatory cells are present, as in this case, reactive fibroblasts should be suspected, and great caution exercised before diagnosis of mesenchymal neoplasia (i.e., biopsy).

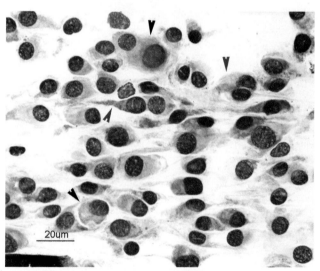

Fig. 2.50 Aspirate from a tumor of mesenchymal origin. The slide is highly cellular and the population of mesenchymal cells has a mixture of tapered cells *(red arrowheads)* to cells that are essentially round *(black arrowheads)*, demonstrating the need to evaluate the entire cell population to determine the cell type present. Contrast this with the appearance of the cells in Fig 2.51.

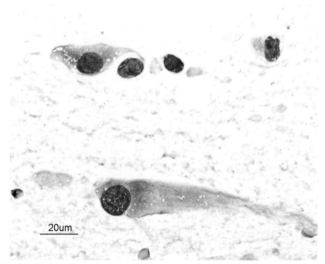

Fig. 2.51 Spindle cells from a malignant tumor of mesenchymal origin (myxosarcoma). Note the elongated appearance of the cells with cytoplasm that tapers in one or more directions.

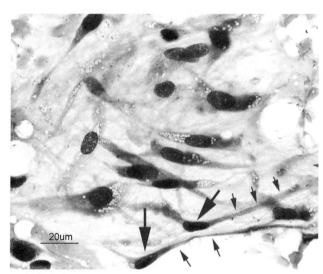

Fig. 2.52 Cells from a malignant mesenchymal tumor (fibrosarcoma). Note that most cells are extremely elongated with thin, tapered cytoplasm *(red arrows)*. The majority of the nuclei are also fusiform *(blue arrows)*.

of varying degrees of maturation, ranging from small, immature basal or parabasal cells to mature, fully keratinized, superficial squamous cells. Transitional epithelial cells also show moderate anisocytosis as a normal feature of that cell type. Finally, macrophages in inflammatory reactions can show marked variation in size (see Figs. 2.10 and 2.11) and many other atypical features.

Some degree of anisocytosis is normal in any cell population. The tendency of many beginning cytologists is to overinterpret normal variability in cell size rather than to ignore significant variation when it is present; therefore, caution is warranted in evaluating subjective parameters. Significant variation in cell size is when one cell is multiple times (e.g., 2×, 3×) the size of other cells from the same population. No easily defined objective criteria of macrocytosis exist, although this usually indicates cells that are decidedly larger than what is normal for the cell population. Obviously, this requires having sufficient experience to recognize the limits of normal. If normal cells from the tissue in question are present along with neoplastic cells, this can give a valuable reference point from which to judge the degree of variability (Fig. 2.59).

Hypercellularity. Malignant tumors tend to exfoliate high numbers of cells, even when arising from tissues that would not normally exfoliate any cells. A classic example of this is primary bone tumors, such as osteosarcoma and chondrosarcoma. Normal bone will obviously exfoliate very few, if any, cells. However, aspirates from primary bone tumors are often highly cellular (Fig. 2.60). Cells in malignant tumors are often anaplastic and have not differentiated to the point where they develop cell receptors or produce the extracellular matrix that makes them adhesive to other tissues in the body. Therefore these cells will exfoliate very well by FNB. Similarly, these cells will often demonstrate loss of cohesion, if epithelial in origin. Highly malignant epithelial tumors may yield cells that distribute in more of a discrete cell pattern, with fewer cell clusters (Fig. 2.61).

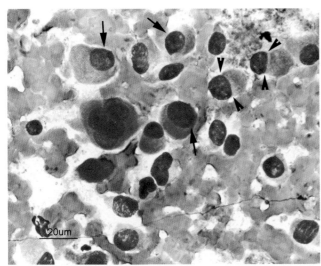

Fig. 2.53 Cells from a canine osteosarcoma. The osteoblasts show little to no spindling and have distinct cytoplasmic borders. Note that most of the cells have eccentrically placed nuclei *(arrows)*. Often, the nuclei appear to be partially outside the cytoplasmic borders *(arrowheads)*. The mesenchymal nature of these cells is suggested by the presence of an extracellular matrix.

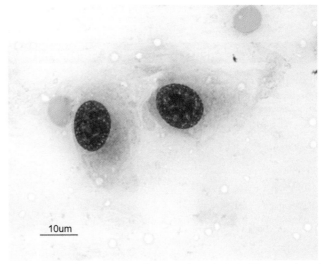

Fig. 2.55 Cells from a tumor of mesenchymal origin. The cytoplasmic boundary of these cells is extremely indistinct; the cytoplasm seems to fade gradually into the background. This is another common feature of cells of mesenchymal origin.

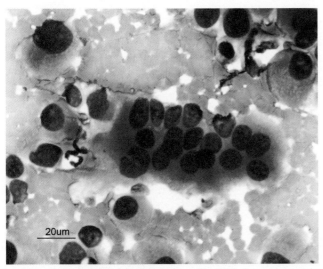

Fig. 2.54 High magnification of slide from Fig 2.53. A large osteoclast is present in the center, surrounded by osteoblasts. Osteoclasts often have 10 to 20 nuclei or more.

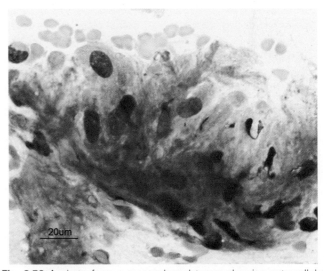

Fig. 2.56 Aspirate from a mesenchymal tumor showing extracellular matrix production. Numerous mesenchymal cells are present, which appear to be embedded in a brightly eosinophilic extracellular matrix.

Obviously, hypercellularity as a criterion of malignancy must be viewed in terms of the tissue sampled. Inflammatory lesions (see Fig. 2.1), lymphoid tissue, and some other tissues normally yield high numbers of cells. In these instances, hypercellularity cannot be considered a criterion of malignancy. However, highly cellular slides containing a single population of mesenchymal cells is not a normal finding (see Fig. 2.50). Hypercellularity is also important because the sample is more likely to be representative of the lesion than if relatively few cells are present. A definitive diagnosis of malignancy should be made with extreme caution if the sample is of low cellularity.

Pleomorphism. Pleomorphism, which refers to variability in the shape of cells, may be normal if more than one cell type is present on a smear. Also, pleomorphism among cells of a single cell type is seen in some normal tissue, such as transitional cells from the urinary tract, and in samples containing squamous cells of varying degrees of maturation (skin scrapings and vaginal smears).

Nuclear Criteria of Malignancy

Anisokaryosis and macrokaryosis (karyomegaly). Anisokaryosis and *macrokaryosis* (karyomegaly) are terms that refer to variation in nuclear size (see Fig. 2.57) and excessively large nuclei (see Fig. 2.58), respectively. Nuclei that are multiple times the size of those in other cells within the same population represent significant anisokaryosis. In some malignant tumors, particularly carcinomas, macronuclei, which may be larger than some entire cells of the same population, may be present.

Anisokaryosis is a normal finding in samples containing squamous epithelial cells. As squamous cells mature, the nucleus becomes small and pyknotic, eventually disappearing from the cell.

Multinucleation. Cells with multiple nuclei may be seen in malignant tumors of any cell type. Multinucleation is particularly important when anisokaryosis is present among nuclei within a single

TABLE 2.2   Easily Recognized General and Nuclear Criteria of Malignancy

Criteria	Description	Schematic Representation
General Criteria		
Anisocytosis and macrocytosis	Variation in cell size, with some cells ≥2 times larger than normal	
Hypercellularity	Increased cell exfoliation caused by decreased cell adherence	Not depicted
Pleomorphism (except in lymphoid tissue)	Variable size and shape in cell of the same type	
Nuclear Criteria		
Macrokaryosis	Increased nuclear size; cell with nuclei larger than 20 micrometers (µm) in diameter suggest malignancy	RBC
Increased nuclear-to-cytoplasmic ratio (N:C)	Normal nonlymphoid cells usually have a N:C of 1:3–1:8, depending on the tissue; increased ratio (1:2,1:1, etc.) suggests malignancy	See "macrokaryosis"
Anisokaryosis	Variation in nuclear size; especially important if the nuclei of multinucleate cells vary in size.	
Multinucleation	Multiple nuclei in a cell; especially important if the nuclei vary in size	
Increased mitotic figures	Mitosis is rare in normal tissue	normal abnormal
Abnormal mitosis	Improper alignment of chromosomes	See "increased mitotic figures"
Coarse chromatin pattern	The chromatin pattern is coarser than normal; may appear ropy or cordlike	
Nuclear molding	Deformation of nuclei by other nuclei within the same cell or adjacent cells	
Macronucleoli	Nucleoli are increased in size; nucleoli ≥5 µm strongly suggest malignancy. For reference, RBCs are 5–6 µm in the cat and 7–8 µm in the dog.	RBC
Angular nucleoli	Nucleoli are fusiform or have other angular shapes instead of their normal round to slightly oval shape	
Anisonucleoliosis	Variation in nucleolar shape or size (especially important if the variation is within the same nucleus)	See "angular nucleoli"

RBC, red blood cell.

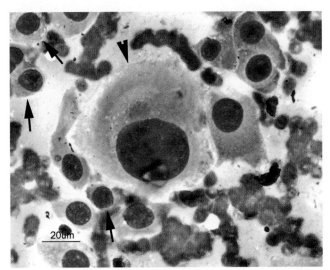

Fig. 2.57 Aspirate from a transitional cell carcinoma. The cells show significant anisocytosis and anisokaryosis. Some cells *(arrowhead)* are several times larger than other cells in the population *(arrows)*.

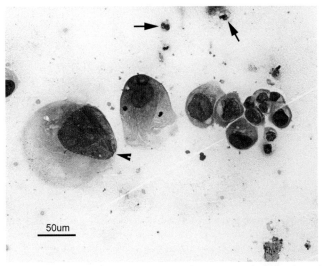

Fig. 2.58 Low-power photomicrograph of smears made from thoracic fluid of a cat with a metastatic carcinoma. Atypically macrocytic cells almost 100 micrometers (μm) in diameter with macronuclei (karyomegaly) greater than 50 μm are present. Macrophages *(arrows)* are present for size comparison.

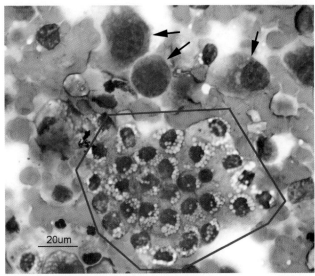

Fig. 2.59 Aspirate of a carcinoma from the prostate of a dog. In this case the presence of relatively normal, uniform prostatic cells in the middle *(surrounded by the red boundary)* allows for easier recognition of the surrounding abnormal larger cells with larger nuclei and prominent nucleoli.

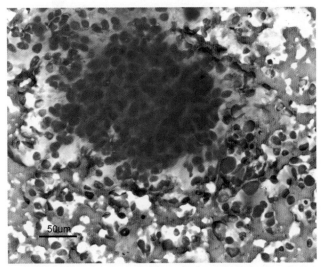

Fig. 2.60 Aspirate from a canine osteosarcoma demonstrating the hypercellularity that may be seen with malignant tumors. Normal bone would exfoliate no cells, whereas an osteosarcoma often yields highly cellular slides.

cell (Fig. 2.62). Multinucleation in neoplastic cells results from nuclear division without cell division. Usually, in multinucleate cells, even numbers of nuclei are present. Odd numbers of nuclei indicate atypical nuclear division and are an important finding (Fig. 2.63).

Multinucleation can also be seen in nonneoplastic lesions. Inflammatory lesions may have macrophages that are multinucleate (multinucleate inflammatory giant cells) (see Fig. 2.11). Osteoclasts are also normally multinucleate (see Fig. 2.54). Megakaryocytes, which are commonly present in the spleen as a reflection of extramedullary hematopoiesis, may have multiple nuclear lobes (Fig. 2.64) and may appear to be multinucleate. Binucleate cells are commonly found in aspirates of epithelial tissue undergoing hyperplasia or regeneration (e.g., hepatic nodular hyperplasia). Also, some benign tumors, such as cutaneous plasmacytomas, may have many binucleate and multinucleate cells (see Fig. 2.33).

Abnormal nuclear-to-cytoplasmic ratio (N:C ratio). The term *N:C ratio* refers to the relative areas occupied by the nucleus and cytoplasm of the cell. A low N:C ratio indicates a cell with a relatively small nucleus and vast amounts of cytoplasm (Fig. 2.65). In contrast, cells with only scant amounts of cytoplasm have a high N:C ratio (Fig. 2.66). Epithelial and mesenchymal cells having a high N:C ratio are suggestive of malignancy. A high N:C ratio is a particularly important finding in very large cells because some small cells (e.g., mature lymphocytes, basal epithelial cells) normally have a high N:C ratio. A high N:C ratio in a large cell generally indicates a poorly differentiated cell. As a rule of thumb, if two nuclei would not fit in the cytoplasmic borders of a medium to large cell, it has a high N:C ratio.

Marked variation in the N:C ratio of cells within a single population is also an abnormal finding (Fig. 2.67). Again, exceptions exist. Slides of normal lymphoid tissue and scrapings containing normal squamous cells of varying stages of maturation will demonstrate variation in the N:C ratio.

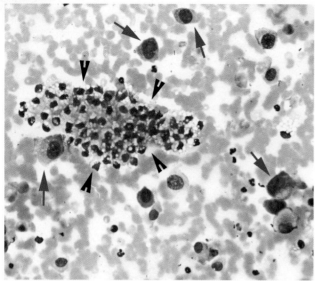

Fig. 2.61 Aspirate from a carcinoma in the prostate of a dog. Note that the smaller, uniform cells representing normal prostatic epithelium *(black arrowheads)* are in a tightly cohesive cluster, whereas the larger, neoplastic cells are largely individually oriented because of loss of cellular cohesion *(red arrows)*.

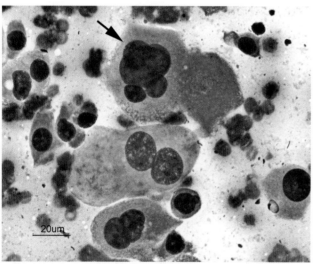

Fig. 2.62 Aspirate of a transitional cell carcinoma from a dog. Two binucleate cells are present with equally sized nuclei. However, one multinucleate cell *(arrow)* shows significant variation in nuclear size.

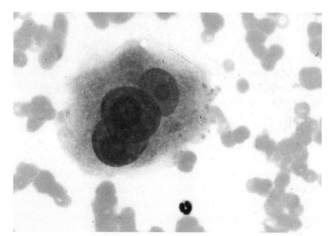

Fig. 2.63 A multinucleate cell with an odd number of nuclei. Prominent, large nucleoli of varying size are also present. The erythrocytes and neutrophil can be used for size comparison.

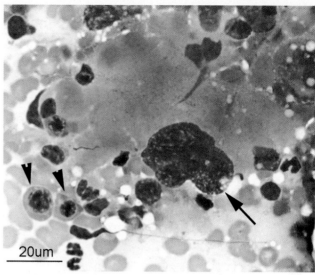

Fig. 2.64 Splenic aspirate from a dog with extramedullary hematopoiesis. A single megakaryocyte is present. This large cell has expansive cytoplasm and a single, multilobulated nucleus and can resemble a multinucleate cell.

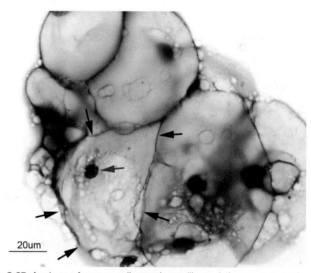

Fig. 2.65 Aspirate of mature adipose tissue (lipoma) demonstrates a low nuclear-to-cytoplasmic ratio. The cells are extremely large *(black arrows outline the cytoplasmic boundaries of a single adipocyte)* yet have very small nuclei *(red arrow)*.

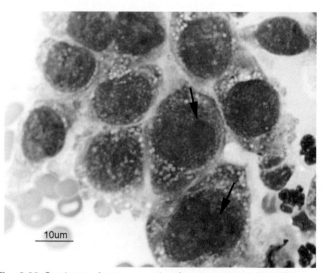

Fig. 2.66 Carcinoma from a sample of canine pleural fluid. The neoplastic cells demonstrate a high nuclear-to-cytoplasmic (N:C) ratio. Note that the nucleus takes up well over half of the volume of the entire cell. Some cells have only scant amounts of visible cytoplasm. A high N:C ratio is normal in some cells, such as lymphocytes and basal epithelial cells, but in large cells, such as this, it generally indicates undifferentiated cells. Also, note the large nucleoli *(arrows)*.

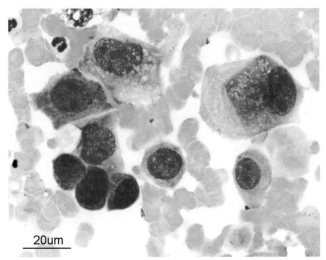

Fig. 2.67 Aspirate from a carcinoma. Note the variation in nuclear-to-cytoplasmic ratio.

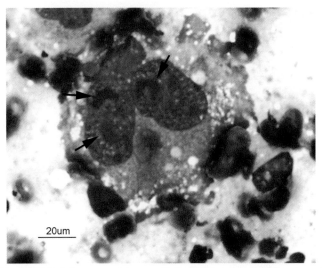

Fig. 2.68 Cell from a carcinoma. Note the large, irregularly shaped nucleoli *(arrows)*.

Abnormal nucleoli. Nucleoli are areas within the nucleus that are responsible for production of ribosomal ribonucleic acid (RNA). All cells have nucleoli, but they are usually small and often not readily visible. Nucleoli that are abnormally large (macronucleoli), that are atypically shaped (angular), or that vary in size are strong indicators of malignancy. Nucleoli in normal cells are small, approximately 1 to 2 micrometers (μm) in diameter. Nucleoli greater than 5 μm in diameter are suggestive of malignancy (see Fig. 2.66). Erythrocytes can be used as a reference for evaluating the size of nucleoli. Canine erythrocytes are 7 to 8 μm, whereas feline erythrocytes are approximately 5 to 6 μm in diameter, if well spread out.

Normal cells have round nucleoli. Fusiform, pleomorphic, or angular nucleoli are indicative of malignancy (Fig. 2.68). Diff-Quik stain often stains nucleoli more prominently compared with other cytological stains, so this must be considered when evaluating cells for malignant potential. Also, nucleoli may be more prominent than normal in cells that are either ruptured or understained.

Abnormal mitosis. Mitotic figures are rare in samples from most normal tissue cell populations. Exceptions are lymphoid tissue and bone marrow, where mitoses may be common. Also, macrophages can divide in tissues, and so mitotic figures are frequently seen in inflammatory responses with numerous macrophages (Fig. 2.69). Increased numbers of mitoses in other tissues or mitotic figures showing abnormal alignment of chromosomes are suggestive of malignancy (Figs. 2.70, 2.71, and 2.72).

Coarse or immature nuclear chromatin. Nuclear chromatin patterns are not as distinctive and evident in cells stained with Romanowsky-type stains as they are when cells are wet fixed and stained with Papanicolaou-type stains. Still, an abnormally coarse nuclear chromatin pattern is often visible in malignant cells. Also, mature cells tend to have nuclear chromatin that is condensed and thus stains a dark purple. Immature cells may have light staining chromatin lacking aggregates of heterochromatin often described as "dispersed" or "open" (see Fig. 2.14).

Abnormal nuclear arrangement. Although the majority of tissue architecture is lost when performing fine-needle aspiration, some cellular structure is still evident in cell clusters. Normal cell clusters tend to have a very uniform arrangement of the nuclei, giving them a honeycomb appearance (Fig. 2.73). Because mature cells typically have a lower N:C ratio, the nuclei often appear evenly spaced and not touching each other (see Fig. 2.73). In contrast, clusters of neoplastic

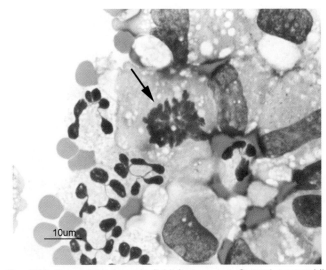

Fig. 2.69 Transtracheal wash fluid from a cat. Several neutrophils and macrophages are shown. One macrophage is undergoing mitosis *(arrow)*.

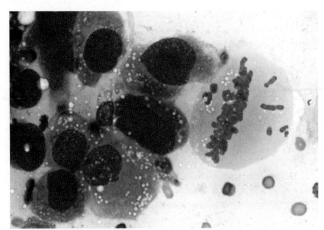

Fig. 2.70 Smear from a malignant tumor in the lung of a cat. One abnormal mitotic figure is present, which demonstrates some lagging chromosomes.

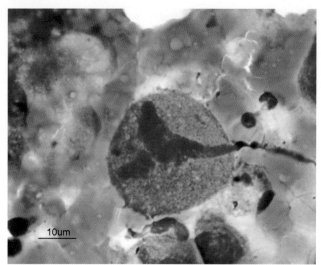

Fig. 2.71 Abnormal mitotic figure in a sample of a malignant tumor from a dog. The nuclear material has formed a "Y" shape rather than forming a straight line.

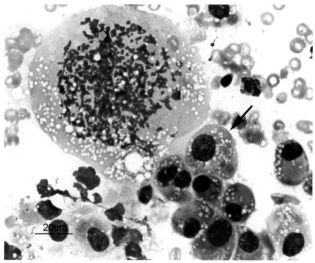

Fig. 2.72 Extremely large, bizarre mitotic figure from a spleen aspirate of a dog with histiocytic sarcoma. Several other histiocytic cells are present, one of which shows erythrophagocytosis *(arrow)*.

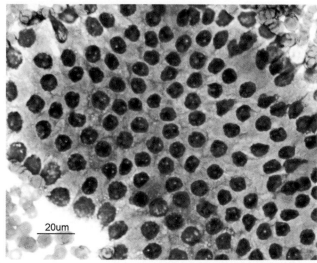

Fig. 2.73 Prostatic aspirate from a dog with benign prostatic hyperplasia. The slide consists of mature, well-differentiated prostatic epithelial cells. Note the uniform and even spacing of the nuclei in the center of this cell cluster. The nuclei are round and have densely stained, mature chromatin. Around the edges of the cell cluster, some of the cells have been traumatized, resulting in lighter staining nuclei with irregular outlines.

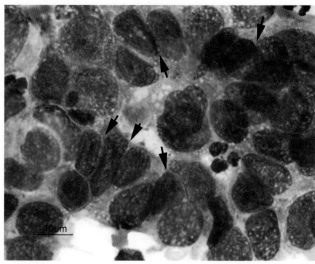

Fig. 2.74 Aspirate of a carcinoma from a dog. The cells lack the regular arrangement of benign well-differentiated cells. Nuclei are crowded together and pile on top of each other. The cells have a high nuclear-to-cytoplasmic ratio and many have prominent nucleoli.

cells often show irregular arrangement (Fig. 2.74). Lack of normal contact inhibition can result in nuclei that are crowded together and piled on top of each other (see Fig. 2.74).

Sometimes, the nucleus of one cell can be seen to deform around the nucleus of another cell (or another nucleus within a multinucleate cell). This is referred to as *nuclear molding* and indicates rapid growth and loss of contact inhibition (Fig. 2.75).

General Cautions Regarding Evaluating Cytological Criteria of Malignancy

No single cellular feature clearly distinguishes malignant cells from benign cells. A reliable diagnosis of malignancy can usually be made if three or more nuclear criteria of malignancy are present in a majority of the cells present in the smear. If cytological features of malignancy are not unambiguous, the diagnosis should be confirmed with a biopsy and histological evaluation. It is imperative that a representative sample (highly cellular) is available and that only intact (nontraumatized), well-spread-out, well-stained cells are evaluated. Nucleoli are often more distinct in understained cells present in thick areas of the smears.

When cells are partially ruptured, the nuclear chromatin spreads out and uncoils. This results in the nucleus appearing larger than it really is and also makes the nucleoli, normally obscured by the condensed chromatin, more visible.

Caution should be exercised in diagnosing neoplasia in the face of inflammation. Inflammation can induce dysplastic changes in tissue cells that can mimic neoplasia. Inflammatory lesions may also contain large, epithelioid macrophages and proliferating fibroblasts, both of which may have some features that are similar to malignant cells.

Conversely, not every malignant tumor shows marked cellular atypia and variability. Some tumors may yield relatively uniform populations of cells yet exhibit aggressive biological behavior. This finding is frequently encountered in endocrine tumors. The majority of thyroid tumors in dogs is malignant, yet samples from some thyroid carcinomas contain relatively uniform cells without marked criteria of

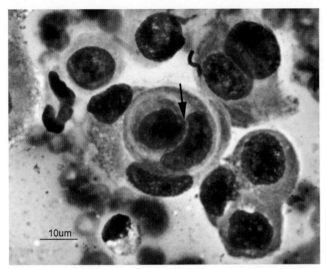

Fig. 2.75 Cells from a transitional cell carcinoma from a dog. Nuclear molding is seen in the center, where the nucleus of one cell is wrapping around that of another.

malignancy. The same situation is described in other tumors of endocrine and neuroendocrine origins. Many other well-differentiated carcinomas (e.g., perianal gland tumors) are difficult to distinguish from a benign proliferation solely on the basis of cytological examination findings. In some cases, this differentiation is also difficult to make on histological examination. Thus, although an understanding of general features of cellular atypia is helpful, experience with the peculiarities of each individual tumor type is needed for correct interpretation of many samples.

REFERENCES

1. Meinkoth JH, Cowell RL. Recognition of basic cell types and criteria of malignancy. *Vet Clin North Am.* 2002;32:1209–1235.
2. Raskin R. General categories of cytologic interpretation. In: Raskin RE, Meyer DJ, eds. *Atlas of Canine and Feline Cytology.* 2nd ed. Philadelphia, PA: Saunders; 2010:5–25.
3. McKinley ET. General cytologic principles. In: Atkinson BF, ed. *Atlas of Diagnostic Cytopathology.* 2nd ed. Philadelphia, PA: Saunders; 2004:1–30.
4. Kocjan G. *Fine Needle Aspiration Cytology: Diagnostic Principles and Dilemmas.* New York: Springer; 2006:35–58.
5. Kiupel M, Webster JD, Bailey KL, et al. Proposal of a 2-tier histologic grading system for canine cutaneous mast cell tumor to more accurately predict biological behavior. *Vet Pathol.* 2011;48:147–155.
6. Affolter VK, Moore PF. Localized and disseminated histiocytic sarcoma of dendritic cell origin in dogs. *Vet Pathol.* 2002;39:74–83.
7. Moore PF, Affolter VK, Vernau W. Canine hemophagocytic histiocytic sarcoma: a proliferative disorder of CD11d+ macrophages. *Vet Pathol.* 2006;43:632–645.
8. Clark GN, Berg J, Engler SJ, et al. Extramedullary plasmacytomas in dogs: results of surgical excision in 131 cases. *J Am Anim Hosp Assoc.* 1992;28:105–111.
9. Vail DM. Plasma cell neoplasms. In: Withrow SJ, Vail DM, eds. *Small Animal Clinical Oncology.* 4th ed. St. Louis, MO: Saunders; 2007:769–794.

3

Selected Infectious Agents

Laura V. Lane, Pi Jie Yang, and Rick L. Cowell

Microorganisms are often encountered when evaluating cytological samples and can be primary etiological agents, opportunistic secondary overgrowths, part of the normal flora, or contaminants. This chapter is intended to aid recognition of the more commonly encountered infectious agents in canine and feline cytopathology. Discussions of pathological changes and conditions associated with these organisms are found in the following relevant chapters. Sample collection, staining, and culture submission were previously covered in Chapter 1.

IDENTIFICATION OF ORGANISMS

Size, shape, and staining characteristics are important in the cytological identification of organisms. The staining characteristics described in this chapter are for commonly available Romanowsky-type stains such as Wright, modified Wright, Wright-Giemsa, Diff-Quik, or Dip-Stat stains, unless otherwise stated.

BACTERIA

Most gram-positive or gram-negative bacteria stain blue to purple with routine Romanowsky-type stains. Once bacteria have been identified, Gram stains can be used to differentiate between gram-positive and gram-negative bacteria. However, Gram stains often do not give reproducible, accurate results in exudates because cells, exudative proteins, and bacteria all tend to stain red.

Bacteria may not be readily detected if present in low numbers. In addition, the presence of proteinaceous or cellular debris can limit sensitivity of microscopy for the detection of bacteria. Hence, failure to detect bacteria in an inflammatory lesion does not exclude an underlying bacterial infection, and aerobic and anaerobic cultures are still recommended.

Intracellular bacteria indicate an active infection (primary or secondary), whereas extracellular bacteria may represent an active infection, normal microflora, or contamination. A monomorphic bacterial population (only one bacterial type) suggests infection, whereas a pleomorphic population (mixture of different sized rods and/or cocci) may be seen with contamination, normal microflora, or a mixed bacterial infection. Mixed bacterial infections may be associated with conditions such as gastrointestinal (GI) infections, bite wounds, and foreign bodies.

Bacterial Cocci

Pathogenic bacterial cocci (Fig. 3.1) are usually gram positive and of the genera *Staphylococcus*, *Streptococcus*, or *Peptostreptococcus*. *Staphylococcus* spp. usually occur in clusters, whereas *Streptococcus* and *Peptostreptococcus* spp. tend to occur in chains. *Staphylococcus* and *Streptococcus* spp. are facultative anaerobes (can grow in aerobic and anaerobic conditions), and *Peptostreptococcus* spp. is anaerobic. Aerobic and anaerobic cultures and sensitivity testing are needed to identify the organism(s) and to guide optimal antibiotic therapy. If treatment is deemed necessary before culture results are available, antibiotics effective against gram-positive organisms should be considered.

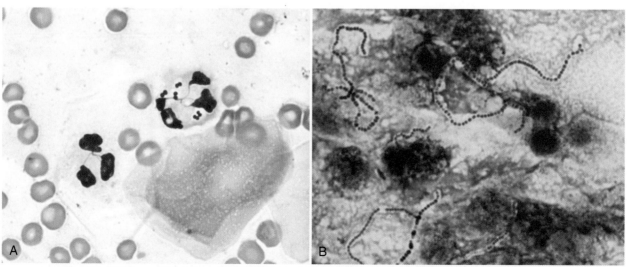

Fig. 3.1 (A) Neutrophilic inflammation with intracellular bacterial cocci in pairs (Wright stain). (B) Bacterial cocci arranged in chains (Wright stain).

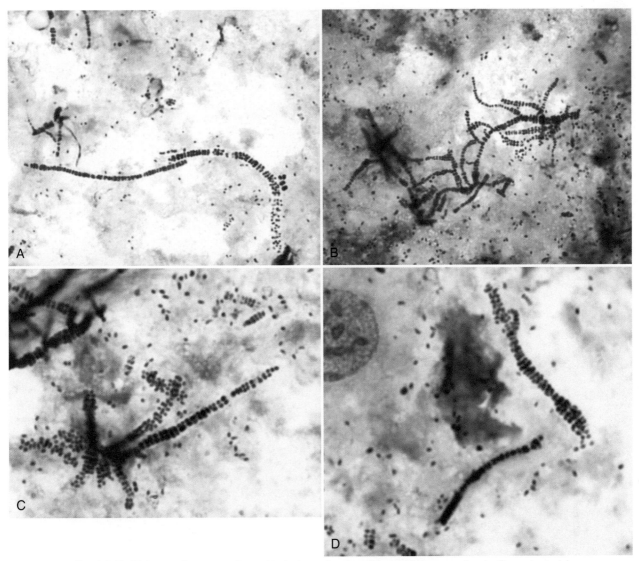

Fig. 3.2 (A–D) Impression smear from skin lesions showing *Dermatophilus congolensis.* These bacterial cocci replicate by transverse and longitudinal division, producing long chains of cocci in paired rows that resemble small, blue railroad tracks (Wright stain).

Dermatophilus congolensis replicate by transverse and longitudinal divisions to form elongated branching structures of cocci arranged in paired rows, resembling railroad tracks (Fig. 3.2). In dogs, these organisms infect the epidermis, causing crusty lesions, and samples from the undersurface of scabs are most rewarding in demonstrating organisms. Cats more often develop deeper abscesses in muscles, lymph nodes, and subcutaneous tissues. On cytological preparations, the organisms can be scattered in the background or embedded within aggregates of neutrophils.

Small Bacterial Rods

Most small bacterial rods are gram negative (e.g., *Escherichia coli*, *Pasteurella* spp., *Pseudomonas* spp.). Some bacterial rods, such as *Pasteurella* and *Yersinia* spp., exhibit bipolar staining (Fig. 3.3). Aerobic and anaerobic cultures and sensitivity testing are needed to identify the organism(s) and to guide optimal antibiotic therapy. If treatment is deemed necessary before culture results are available, antibiotics effective against gram-negative organisms should be considered.

Filamentous Rods

Pathogenic filamentous rods are typically *Nocardia* or *Actinomyces* spp. Rarely, *Fusobacterium* spp. can also appear filamentous. These fine filamentous bacterial rods are typically light blue with intermittent, small, pink-to-purple areas creating a distinctive "beaded" appearance (Fig. 3.4). Samples may contain macroscopic white or tan tissue granules (i.e., sulfur granules), which are seen microscopically as dense bacterial mats. If sulfur granules are noted during sample collection, they should be gently squashed on a slide for evaluation. Aerobic and anaerobic cultures are required for identification and to guide optimal antibiotic therapy. The laboratory should be alerted to the presence of filamentous bacteria because culture of these organisms can take longer than that for most common bacteria.

Mycobacterium spp.

Mycobacteriosis in dogs and cats can be caused by many different *Mycobacterium* spp. and can result in different clinical presentations. Lesions may be localized to cutaneous or subcutaneous tissue (e.g., canine leproid granuloma, feline leprosy), or they can be disseminated with systemic involvement (e.g., *M. bovis, M. avium complex*).[1]

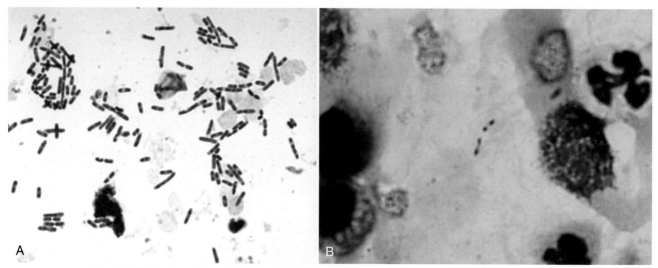

Fig. 3.3 (A) Bipolar rods in cat (Wright stain). (B) Higher magnification of bipolar rods (Wright stain).

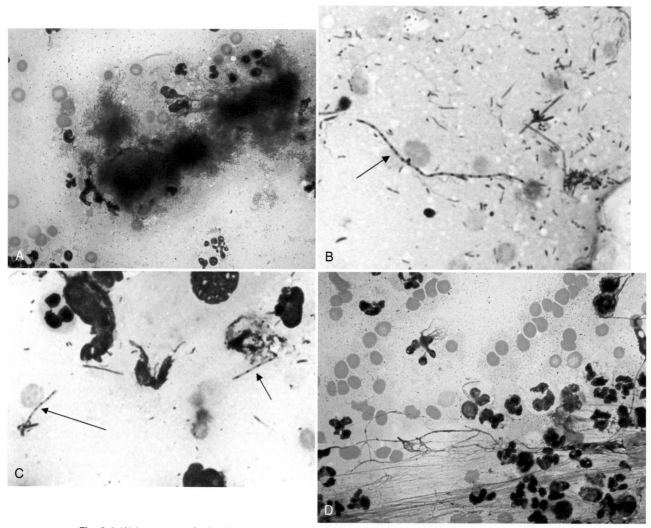

Fig. 3.4 (A) Large mat of mixed bacteria with filamentous rods (Wright stain). (B and C) Filamentous rods *(arrows)* typical of *Actinomyces* or *Nocardia* spp. (Wright stain). (D) Filamentous rod noted within a disrupted neutrophil (Wright stain).

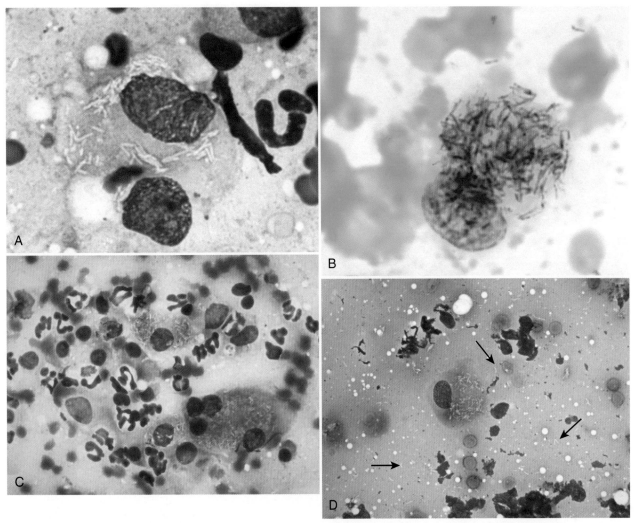

Fig. 3.5 (A) Cat liver aspirate. Macrophage contain nonstaining bacterial rods indicative of *Mycobacterium* infection (Wright stain). (B) Cat liver *Mycobacterium* (acid-fast stain). (C) Dog ear mass, leproid granuloma, nonstaining bacterial rods also in multinucleated giant cell (Wright stain). (D) Dog ear mass, leproid granuloma. Note nonstaining bacterial rods free in the background *(arrows)* (Wright stain).

The cell walls of *Mycobacterium* spp. have high lipid content, resulting in negative staining rods with Romanowsky-type stains (Fig. 3.5).[1] They can be seen in macrophages, other inflammatory cells, or in the background. Macrophages in these lesions can appear epithelioid, as characterized by increased cytoplasmic basophilia, minimal vacuolation, and tendency to occur in groups. If a sample contains epithelioid macrophages, a careful search for negative staining rods should be made.

Mycobacterium spp. stain bright pink with acid-fast stains, which can be performed to aid detection of these organisms (see Fig. 3.5, B). Mycobacterial culture is typically needed for confirmation and further characterization. Growth characteristics in culture can be slow or fast, and some organisms are difficult to cultivate, requiring polymerase chain reaction (PCR) for identification.

Clostridium spp.

Clostridium spp. can infect cutaneous and subcutaneous tissue after penetrating injury, resulting in severe pain, edema, and swelling. Gas production from these organisms can result in cutaneous/subcutaneous crepitus. *Clostridium* spp. are large anaerobic bacterial rods that are usually gram positive.[1] These organisms can form clear, round to oval subterminal endospores under anaerobic conditions, which

can sometimes be observed cytologically (Fig. 3.6). Bacterial culture is needed for definitive identification. Although *Clostridium* spp. are anaerobic bacteria, both aerobic and anaerobic cultures are recommended to exclude concurrent infection with other bacteria.

Oral Bacteria

The oral cavity of clinically healthy dogs and cats hosts a myriad of aerobic and anaerobic bacteria, some of which have distinctive morphology on cytology.

Simonsiella spp. are large, nonpathogenic bacterial rods that divide lengthwise and are arranged in parallel rows, resulting in a structure resembling a large stack of coins or a large foot print (Fig. 3.7, A and B). The presence of these organisms in cytology samples can reflect oropharyngeal contamination or underlying pathology. For example, the presence of *Simonsiella* spp. in transtracheal fluid or bronchoalveolar lavage fluid suggest contamination from the oropharynx (passage of endotracheal tube) or inhalation of oropharyngeal material in coughing or dyspneic animals. Similarly, the presence of *Simonsiella* spp. in a nasal flush may reflect contamination or presence of an oronasal fistula. The appearance of these organisms adhered to squamous epithelial cells in an aspirate from a cutaneous or subcutaneous lesion suggest licking by the animal.

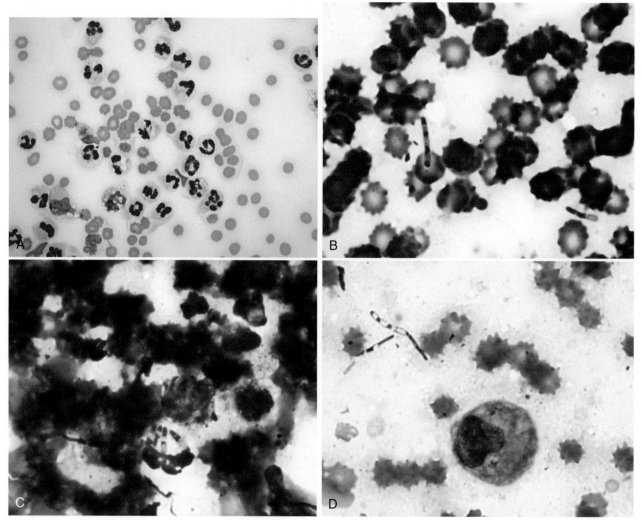

Fig. 3.6 (A) Spore-forming bacterial rod in a neutrophil (Wright stain). (B) Scattered red blood cells (RBCs) and two large extracellular spore-forming bacterial rods typical of *Clostridium* spp. (Wright stain). (C) Multiple phagocytized spore-forming bacterial rods (Wright stain). (D) *Clostridium* organisms from mass on dog (Wright stain).

Other bacteria that can be associated with oral microflora are fine thread-like spirochetes (see Fig. 3.7, C and D), which can be pathogens. Spirochetes in a subcutaneous inflammatory lesion can be seen with bite wounds or lesions that communicate with the oral cavity (e.g., tooth root abscess, penetrating injury from within the oral cavity).

FUNGUS

Fungal organisms that cause disease in dogs and cats are often seen in yeast and/or hyphal forms. Although some organisms exhibit distinctive morphological features that allows for identification on cytology (Table 3.1), others require additional tests, such as fungal culture, molecular tests, and serology.

Fungal infections (mycoses) are typically associated with pyogranulomatous (mixture of neutrophils, macrophages, lymphocytes, and/or plasma cells) to granulomatous (macrophage predominant) inflammatory response. However, a neutrophilic or eosinophilic response can also be seen.

Many pathogenic fungi are saprophytic, but some also have zoonotic potential, especially for humans who are immunocompromised. Hence, caution is warranted when handling patients and samples from cases of suspected mycoses.

Sporothrix schenckii

Sporothrix schenckii is a thermal dimorphic fungus that is often found in yeast form at body temperature (37°C), although hyphal forms have been described.[2] It often causes proliferative or ulcerative cutaneous lesions, although mucosal, lymphatic, and respiratory infections can occur. Transmission is typically via direct inoculation (scratches or bites) and, less commonly, via inhalation.

The organisms are widespread in nature and often isolated from aging or dead vegetation. They are also often found on the skin, teeth, and claws of many animals, although cats are the only proven reservoir for the organism. Cutaneous sporotrichosis in humans is known as "rose gardeners' disease," as it usually results from contact with infected plant material. Sporotrichosis is a zoonotic disease and can be transmitted via animal bites or scratches.

The inflammatory response seen with sporotrichosis is typically pyogranulomatous to granulomatous. Numerous yeasts are often found in samples from cats, but they may be hard to find in samples from dogs.[1] Organisms can be found intra- and extracellularly, are round to oval to fusiform ("cigar shape"), measure approximately 1 to 3 μm wide and 3 to 9 μm long, contain light blue cytoplasm, an eccentrically located pink-to-purple nucleus, and a thin clear cell wall (Fig. 3.8).

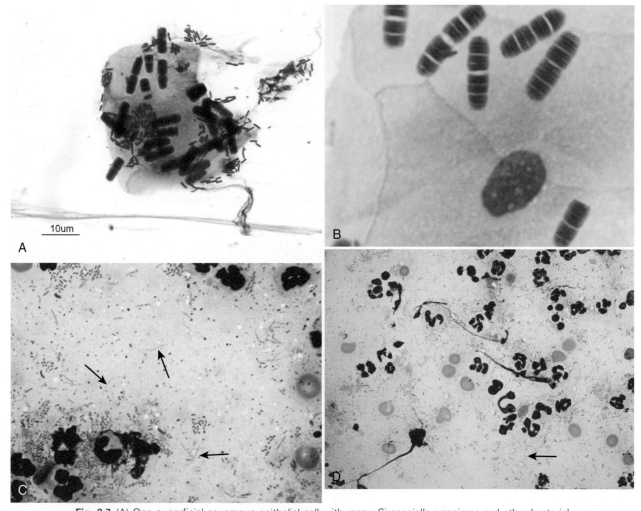

Fig. 3.7 (A) One superficial squamous epithelial cell with many *Simonsiella* organisms and other bacterial rods (Wright stain). (B) Higher magnification, showing *Simonsiella* organisms as large rods arranged in parallel rows, resembling a stack of coins or footprint (Wright stain). (C and D) Large number of spirochetes *(arrows)* (Wright stain).

Narrow-based budding may be observed. The round to oval forms are morphologically similar to *Histoplasma capsulatum*, but the presence of fusiform yeasts is only seen with *S. schenckii*.

Skin biopsy for fungal culture or histopathology with the aid of immunohistochemical stains can be used for confirmation

Histoplasma capsulatum

Histoplasma capsulatum is a dimorphic fungus that is found throughout the world and is endemic in temperate and subtropical regions of the United States. *H. capsulatum* grows in soil and material contaminated with bird or bat droppings (guano), and infection in people and animals is likely caused by inhalation of spores from the mycelial phase.

Infections can be localized or disseminated, and symptoms are dependent on the tissue affected. Organisms can be found in skin, lymph nodes, internal organs, joints, bone marrow, peripheral blood, or, rarely, cerebrospinal fluid (CSF). The inflammatory response is pyogranulomatous to granulomatous, and infected tissues usually yield abundant organisms that are generally in macrophages and occasionally neutrophils. *Histoplasma* organisms (Fig. 3.9) are usually seen as small yeasts, 2 to 4 μm in diameter and round to oval in shape, with an eccentric crescent-shaped pink-to-purple nucleus, light to

medium blue cytoplasm, and a thin clear cell wall. Narrow-based budding may be seen. The lack of fusiform shapes differentiates this yeast from *S. schenckii*. Rarely, hyphal forms of *H. capsulatum* have been reported.[3]

Additional tests for confirmation or to enhance detection include PCR, serology, and biopsy for histopathology with fungal stains. Urine antigen detection can be used to monitor response to treatment.[4] Culture is not recommended because of the risk for infection.

Blastomyces dermatitidis

Blastomyces dermatitidis is a dimorphic fungus that is found primarily in the midwestern and northern United States and Canada. Most cases of blastomycosis are acquired by inhalation of spores of the mycelial phase. The organism cannot be transmitted via aerosols between animals and humans; however, direct inoculation can produce infections in humans.[1]

Blastomycosis in dogs and cats can disseminate to involve any body system, and lesions in the lung, eye, skin, and bone are common. Cutaneous lesions are commonly found on the nose and extremities and are usually ulcerated and draining. The inflammatory response is typically pyogranulomatous, and the number of organisms is variable. The organisms are often surrounded by a ring of neutrophils, and

TABLE 3.1 Common Dimorphic Fungi That Form Yeasts in Tissue

Yeast	Distinguishing Characteristics
Small Yeasts	
Sporothrix schenckii	• Round to oval to fusiform (cigar-shaped) • 1–3 μm wide × 3–9 μm long • Light blue cytoplasm, eccentric pink-to-purple nucleus, thin clear cell wall • Narrow-based budding
Histoplasma capsulatum	• Round to oval, NOT fusiform • 2–4 μm in diameter • Light to medium blue cytoplasm; eccentric crescent-shaped, pink-to-purple nucleus; thin clear cell wall • Narrow-based budding • Rare hyphal forms in tissue
Medium-Sized Yeasts	
Blastomyces dermatitidis	• Spherical • 8–20 μm in diameter • Deeply blue, with thick, refractile double wall • Broad-based budding • Rare hyphal forms in tissue
Cryptococcus spp.	• Round to oval to elongated • 4–15 μm diameter without capsule; 8–40 μm diameter with capsule • Pink to purple and granular with thick, colorless to light pink capsule; rough coated forms lack the capsule • Narrow-based budding • Rare hyphal forms
Large Yeasts	
Coccidioides spp.	Spherules: • Round • 10–200 μm diameter • Blue, often folded or crumpled protoplasm • Endosporulation Endospores: • Round to ovoid • 2–5 μm in diameter • Clear to light blue cytoplasm, dark blue to purple eccentric nuclei, thin clear cell wall

rarely organisms may be in macrophages. *B. dermatitidis* (Fig. 3.10) are medium sized, spherical, 8 to 20 μm in diameter, deeply basophilic with a thick, refractile double wall and occasional broad-based budding. Rarely, hyphating forms have been reported.[5] The presence of broad-based budding differentiates *B. dermatitidis* from pollen and smaller *Coccidioides* spherules.

Additional tests for confirmation or to enhance detection include PCR, serology, and biopsy for histopathology with fungal stains. Urine antigen detection can be used to monitor response to treatment.[6] Culture is not recommended because of the risk for infection.

Cryptococcus spp.

The two most common pathogenic species of *Cryptococcus* are *C. neoformans* and *C. gattii*.[1] These are dimorphic fungi found in yeast form at 37°C, although hyphal forms have been rarely reported.[7] *C. neoformans*

is found worldwide, whereas *C. gattii* is mostly found in tropical and subtropical regions. More recently, *C. gattii* has been reported in the Pacific Northwest of the United States and southwestern Canada.[1]

Upper respiratory infection is most common in cats, forming a nasal mass or swelling that may involve the frontal sinus. Otitis media, mandibular lymphadenopathy, oral lesions, cutaneous lesions, and central nervous system (CNS), ocular, and systemic involvement can occur. Dogs often develop severe disseminated disease, with involvement of the CNS, eyes, urinary system, and nasal cavity.

Organisms may be seen in aspirates of mass lesions and in CSF when there is neurological involvement. Few inflammatory cells that may be present are often macrophages, admixed with fewer lymphocytes and neutrophils. Eosinophils may predominate in CSF. The yeasts often contain a thick nonstaining or light pink polysaccharide capsule, although nonencapsulated ("rough coated") forms can occur. The yeasts are round to oval to elongated, measure approximately 4 to 15 μm without capsule, or 8 to 40 μm with capsule, stain pink to purple, and occasionally show internal granularity (Fig. 3.11). Narrow-based budding may be observed.

Serum and CSF can be used for capsular antigen detection via latex agglutination, and serum antigen titer is also useful for monitoring response to treatment. PCR is sensitive and specific; however, fungal culture is needed to differentiate between *C. neoformans* and *C. gattii*.

Coccidioides spp.

Coccidioidomycosis is caused by *Coccidioides immitis* or *C. posadasii*. These are dimorphic fungi that form spherules at 37°C, which internally divide to form endospores. The organism is found in soil from desert regions of southwestern United States, Mexico, and Central and South Americas.[1]

Pulmonary disease is common in dogs and can disseminate systemically to involve the bones, eyes, heart and pericardium, CNS, spleen, liver, and kidneys. Draining skin lesions in dogs are often associated with underlying bone lesions. Cutaneous involvement without underlying bone involvement is most common in cats. Bone lesions are rare in cats.

Needle aspirate of mass lesions, enlarged lymph nodes, and impression smears of draining tracts typically reveal pyogranulomatous inflammation and may contain very few organisms. Spherules are blue, round structures that measure approximately 10 to 200 μm in diameter, are double walled, and contain finely granular protoplasm or appear folded or crumpled (Fig. 3.12). Endospores may be visualized within spherules, phagocytized by neutrophils or macrophages, and scattered in the background. The endospores (see Fig. 3.12, D) are small, round to ovoid, approximately 2 to 5 μm in diameter, contain a thin clear cell wall, clear to light blue cytosol, and dark blue to purple eccentrically located nuclei.[8]

Small- to medium-sized spherules can morphologically resemble *B. dermatitidis*. However, the lack of budding, the tremendous variation in size of the spherules, and the presence of endospores help identify *Coccidioides* spp.

Cokeromyces recurvatus may be another consideration when spherule-like structures are observed in samples with GI material, as it is morphologically similar to *Coccidioides* spp.[9]

If organisms are not readily identified on cytology or histopathology, diagnosis of coccidioidomycosis can be based on history, clinical findings, and serological test results. PCR is also available.

Direct transmission from animals to humans is rarely reported, but precaution should still be taken when coccidioidomycosis is suspected. Fungal culture is not recommended because of the risk for infection.

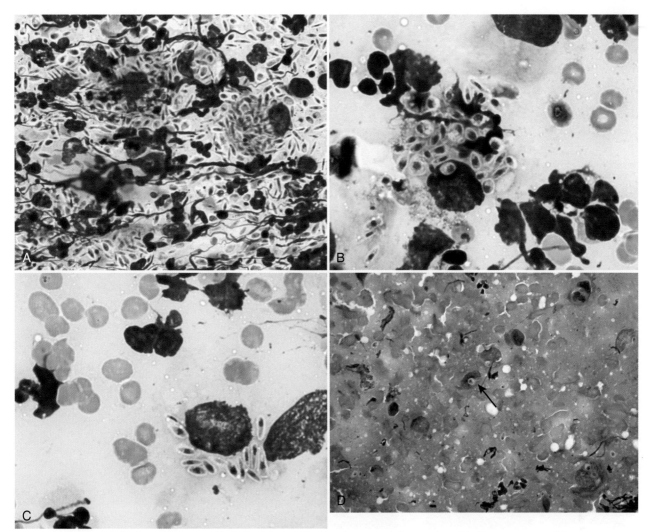

Fig. 3.8 (A) Scraping from a skin lesion in a cat. Pyogranulomatous inflammation with disrupted neutrophils, macrophages, and numerous intracellular and extracellular *Sporothrix* organisms (Wright stain). (B) Macrophage containing round, oval, and fusiform *Sporothrix* organisms (Wright stain). (C) A ruptured cell that contained fusiform *Sporothrix* organisms (Wright stain). (D) Dog, skin lesion. Note narrow-based budding *(arrow)* (Wright stain).

Malassezia spp.

Malassezia spp. are a group of lipophilic nonmycelioid yeasts, of which *M. pachydermatis* is a common skin commensal and opportunistic pathogen in dogs and cats. Warm and moist skin environments, such as ears, chin, axilla, groin, and feet, are often affected in dogs.

These yeasts are small, gram positive, typically peanut or footprint shaped, but may be globose or ellipsoidal, and exhibit broad-based budding (Fig. 3.13). Tape preparation, swab rolled onto a slide, or impression smears are the preferred samples for cytology. Culture may be performed for confirmation.

Dermatophytes

Microsporum and *Trichophyton* spp. are keratinophilic fungi that commonly cause dermatophytosis (ringworm) in dogs and cats. Dermatophytosis is zoonotic, and similar lesions can be noted in humans who come in close contact with affected animals.

The lesions are often crusty, focal, scaly, and alopecic and occur on the head, feet, and tail of the animals. Scrapings from the edge of active lesions are best for visualizing dermatophytes. They can be identified on unstained oil immersion preparations (with or without 10%

potassium hydroxide treatment), in wet-mount preparations from dermatophyte test medium (DTM) culture colonies stained with new methylene blue, or air-dried smears stained with routine cytological stains.

Pyogranulomatous inflammation may be present, and fungal mycelia and arthrospores are found adhered to the surface of epithelial cells, free in the background, within hair shafts (*Trichophyton* spp.) or on the hair shaft surface (*Microsporum* spp.). The mycelia and spores stain medium to dark blue with a thin, clear cell wall (Fig. 3.14). Silver staining (e.g., Gomori methenamine silver) or periodic acid–Schiff reaction can be used to highlight spores. Fungal culture or PCR is needed for definitive identification.

HYPHATING FUNGI AND FUNGAL-LIKE ORGANISMS

Many fungi and fungal-like organisms that infect dogs and cats can form hyphae in tissue (Fig. 3.15). These include opportunistic pathogens (e.g., *Aspergillus fumigatus*), commensal microflora (e.g., *Candida albicans*), aquatic oomycetes (e.g., *Pythium insidiosum*, *Lagenidium* spp.),

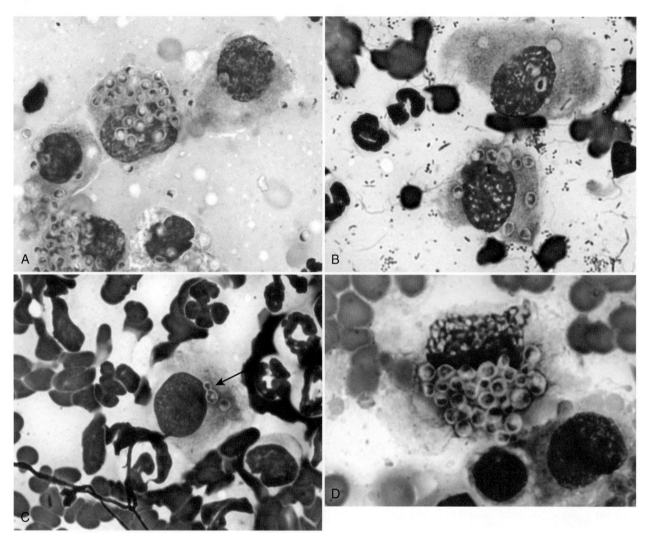

Fig. 3.9 (A) Lung aspirate showing macrophages containing many *Histoplasma* organisms (Wright stain). (B) Scraping from an ulcerated mass in the mouth of a cat. Several *Histoplasma* organisms are observed within macrophages. Moderate numbers of mixed bacteria, blood, and few neutrophils are present in the background (Wright stain). (C) Pyogranulomatous inflammation with a *Histoplasma* organism showing narrow-based budding *(arrow)* (Wright stain). (D) *Histoplasma* organisms from intraabdominal aspirate (Wright stain).

and saprophytic fungi causing zygomycosis, hyalohyphomycoses, and phaeohyphomycoses.[1] Fungal organisms often induce a pyogranulomatous to granulomatous inflammatory response, and many eosinophils may be present. Although hyphal characteristics such as width, branching, septae, pseudohyphae formation, staining, and negative images (see Fig. 3.15) may suggest a specific organism, definitive diagnosis requires culture and histopathological evidence of tissue invasion. PCR, serology, and immunohistochemical staining may also be available, depending on the organism.

Pneumocystis spp.

Pneumocystis spp. is phylogenetically characterized as a fungus but has both fungal and protozoal characteristics.[1] This organism is an opportunistic pulmonary (alveolar) pathogen with suspected airborne transmission. Several species, most notably *P. carinii*, affect animals and humans, and a compromised immune system is the greatest risk factor for clinical and, rarely, disseminated disease. Bronchoalveolar and transtracheal

washes, fine-needle aspirates, and impression smears from biopsy samples may contain 5- to 10-μm diameter cysts with up to eight purple intracystic bodies (Fig. 3.16) and small 1- to 2-μm trophozoites. Biopsy with histopathology and PCR of respiratory washes can be used for confirmation.

Rhinosporidium seeberi

Rhinosporidium seeberi is a eukaryotic pathogen in a class between fungi and animals.[1] It is generally found in tropical regions and is associated with aquatic environments. Rhinosporidiosis in dogs and cats[10-12] is characterized by polypoid nasal growths with a granular surface that can resemble neoplastic lesions. It is diagnosed by finding round to oval endospores in nasal exudates or tissue imprints. Mature endospores are approximately 7 to 15 μm in diameter, stain bright pink, have internal eosinophilic globules, and are surrounded by bilamellar cell walls (Fig. 3.17). Large 100- to 450-μm sporangia, which produce many immature endospores, may be occasionally observed. Biopsy with histopathology and PCR are available for confirmation.

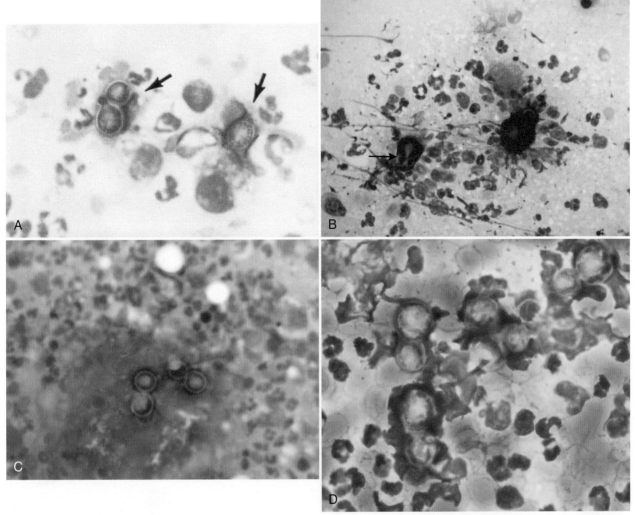

Fig. 3.10 (A) *Blastomyces dermatitidis* is a deeply basophilic, spherical, double-walled, fungal organism *(arrows)* that measure approximately 8 to 20 μm in diameter (Wright stain). (B) *Blastomyces* organism with broad-based budding *(arrow)* (Wright stain). (C and D) *Blastomyces* organisms (Wright stain).

ALGAE

Prototheca zopfii and *P. wickerhami* are achlorophilic unicellular algae, which are ubiquitous in soil and water in warm humid environments worldwide but only sporadically cause disease. In dogs, prototitecosis is often disseminated, with GI, CNS, ocular, and, occasionally, cutaneous manifestations. Lesions in cats are localized cutaneous or subcutaneous masses. Cytological preparations from rectal scrapes, mass and lymph node aspirates, CSF, and urine sediment reveal pyogranulomatous to granulomatous inflammation, and many eosinophils may be present. Organisms may be few or many and are generally extracellular. *Prototheca* are oval to kidney bean shaped, are 1 to 14 μm wide and 1 to 16 μm long, and have granular basophilic cytoplasm and a thin clear cell wall (Fig. 3.18). Mature organisms contain a small nucleus that stain pink to deep purple. A single alga may consist of two to four or more endospores, and occasional empty casings (theca) may be seen.[13] Culture is required for definitive diagnosis.

PROTOZOA

Leishmania spp.

Dogs are the main reservoir for *Leishmania infantum* (*chagasi*), which causes human visceral leishmaniasis. It is endemic in the Mediterranean basin, Middle East, and South America. Cases in North America are sporadic, but outbreaks have been reported in foxhounds.[14] Feline leishmaniosis occurs only sporadically in endemic regions.

Sandflies are the main vector for transmission in endemic areas, and only a small percentage of infected dogs develop clinical disease. Organisms can be found in any tissue or body fluid. Cutaneous lesions are common, and lymphadenomegaly and splenomegaly are often present.

The amastigotes of *Leishmania* spp. may be seen in impression smears of ulcerative lesions, aspirates of nodules, lymph node, spleen, or bone marrow, which often have pyogranulomatous or granulomatous inflammation. The amastigotes are ovoid, approximately 2.5 to 5 μm long and 1.5 to 2 μm wide, and contain an oval, pink-to-purple nucleus and a small, dark blue–to–purple, rod-shaped kinetoplast (Fig. 3.19).

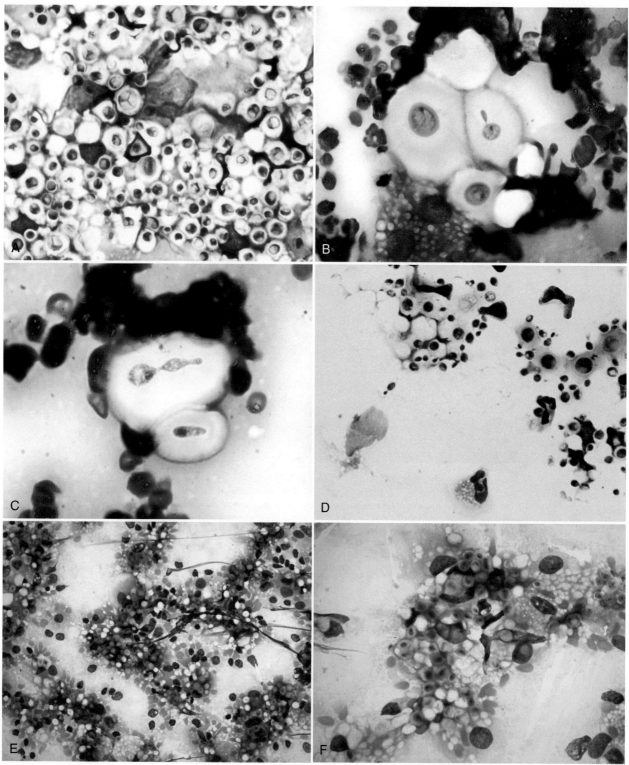

Fig. 3.11 (A) Low-power view of numerous *Cryptococcus* organisms with clear capsules. Note the lack of an inflammatory response (Wright stain). (B) *Cryptococcus* organisms with thick clear capsules and narrow-based budding (Wright stain). (C) *Cryptococcus* organisms showing narrow-based budding (Wright stain). (D) *Cryptococcus* organisms found in cerebrospinal fluid, with rare eosinophils present in the background (Wright stain). (E and F) Rough-coated *Cryptococcus* organisms. Note the lack of clear capsules (Wright stain).

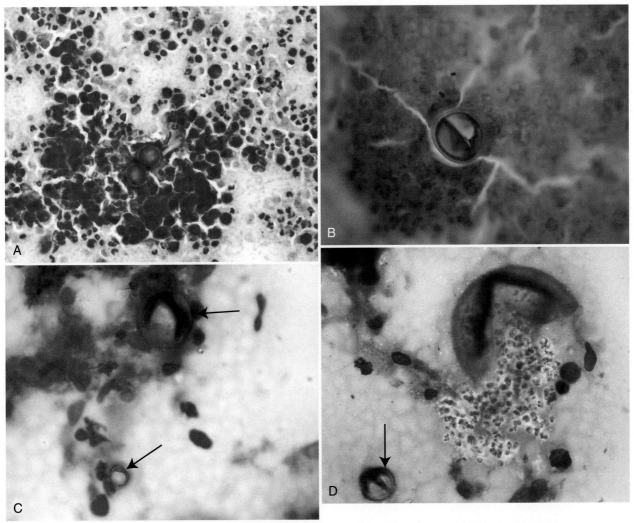

Fig. 3.12 (A) Low-power view showing pyogranulomatous inflammation and two large *Coccidioides* organisms (Wright stain). (B) Large *Coccidioides* spherule with a distinct fold (Wright stain). (C) Two *Coccidioides* organisms *(arrows)* showing the marked variation in size that can occur with the organisms (Wright stain). (D) Large ruptured *Coccidioides* organism releasing endospores, and a smaller *Coccidioides* organism *(arrow)* (Wright stain).

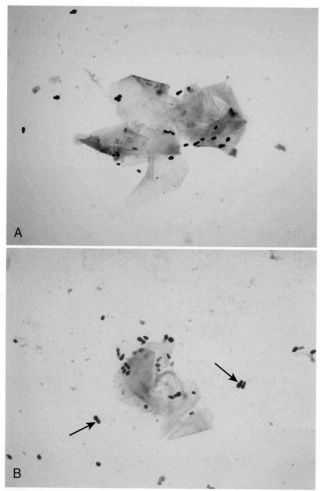

Fig. 3.13 (A and B) Canine ear swab showing numerous *Malassezia* organisms adhered to squamous epithelial cells and free in the background. Note some yeasts show broad-based budding *(arrows)* (Wright stain).

The presence of a kinetoplast distinguishes this organism from *Toxoplasma* spp. and small fungal yeasts, such as *Histoplasma* spp. The amastigote of *Trypanosoma* spp. can appear morphologically similar to *Leishmania* spp.[15] PCR is recommended for confirmation.

Toxoplasma gondii, *Neospora caninum*, and *Hammondia* spp.

The definitive hosts for *Toxoplasma gondii* are domestic cats and other felids. Severe toxoplasmosis in cats is most commonly seen in kittens and immunocompromised cats. Toxoplasmosis can affect all warm-blooded animals, including dogs and humans.

The domestic dog and some canids are definitive hosts for *Neospora caninum*. Severe and disseminated neosporosis is usually seen in puppies less than 6 months old. Immunosuppression in adult dogs can lead to reactivation of previous infection. Natural cases of neosporosis have not been reported in cats or humans.

Both coccidia form cysts in extraintestinal tissue of the intermediate host and the low numbers of definitive hosts that succumb to clinical disease. Disseminated toxoplasmosis in cats can affect the lungs, CNS, liver, pancreas, and eyes. Toxoplasmosis in young dogs is often disseminated, whereas older dogs tend to develop neurological and muscular signs. Neosporosis in dogs can involve many tissues, but CNS and muscular involvement predominate. Immunosuppression in dogs can lead to cutaneous neosporosis.

Tachyzoites of *T. gondii* and *N. caninum* are morphologically indistinguishable on light microscopy and can be found in pleural or peritoneal fluid, blood, CSF, tissue aspirates, and bronchoalveolar lavage fluid during the acute phase of the disease. The tachyzoites are ovoid to crescent shaped, are approximately 5 to 7 μm long and 2 μm wide, and contain light blue cytoplasm and one to two pink-to-purple nuclei (Fig. 3.20).

The zoites of *Hammondia hammondi* (in cats) and *H. heydorni* (in dogs) are also morphologically similar and can be encountered in duodenal brush samples and bile.[16,17] PCR is needed for definitive differentiation between these coccidia.

Cytauxzoon felis

Although multiple *Cytauxzoon* species exist,[18] the most clinically relevant is *Cytauxzoon felis*, which is a vectorborne protozoan that often causes fatal disease in cats. Cytauxzoonosis is recognized in the south-central and eastern United States.

C. felis exists in erythrocytic (piroplasm) and tissue (schizont) forms. The piroplasms are small, 1- to 1.5-μm, signet ring–shaped structures in red blood cells. Schizonts are found in giant macrophages in tissues, such as lymph node, liver, spleen, lung, and bone marrow, and rarely on peripheral blood films. They contain many developing merozoites that can appear as small, dark blue–to-purple bodies or larger ill-defined to lobulated light blue–to-purple globules (Fig. 3.21). Macrophages containing schizonts can exhibit criteria of malignancy, and it is important not to confuse these macrophages with neoplastic cells.

The morphology of the schizonts is distinctive enough to allow for confirmation of cytauxzoonosis on cytology. PCR is available for confirmation and can be used in peripheral blood when parasitemia is low.

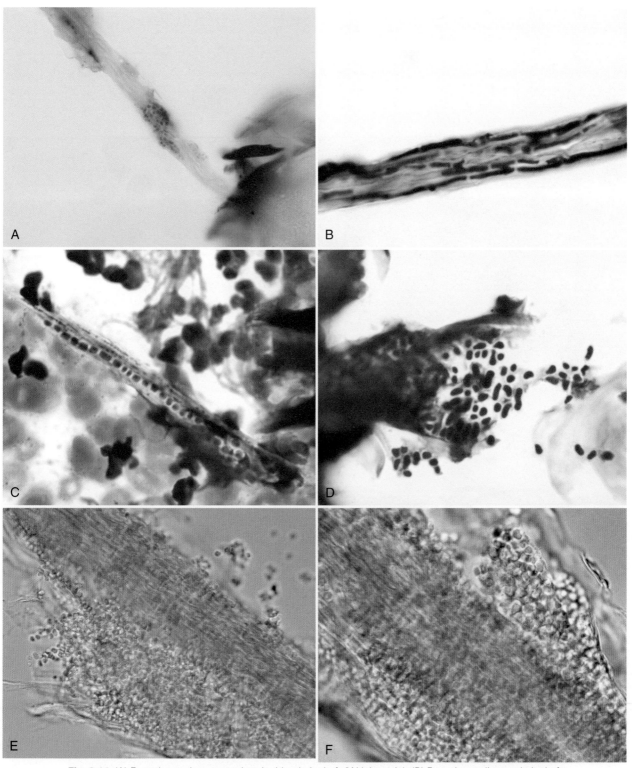

Fig. 3.14 (A) Fungal organisms associated with a hair shaft (Wright stain). (B) Fungal mycelia on a hair shaft (Wright stain). (C) High magnification of fungal mycelia. (D) Fungal spores are found adhered to the surface of epithelial cells and free in the background (Wright stain). (E and F) Fungal organisms on unstained smears (oil immersion). (A, Courtesy Amy Valenciano.)

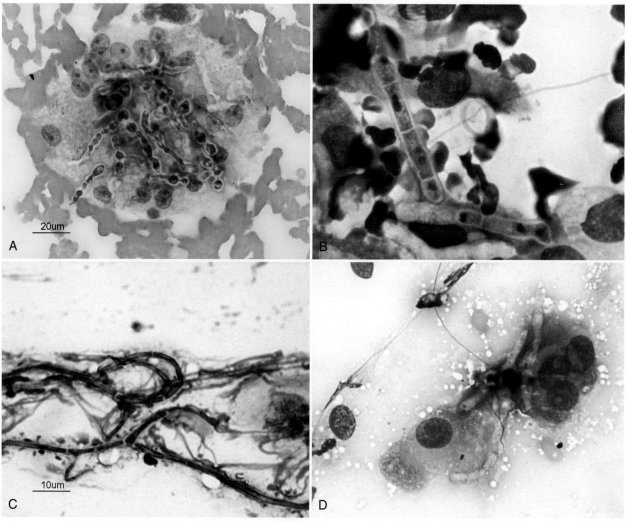

Fig. 3.15 (A) Giant multinucleated macrophage containing fungal hyphae with nonparallel walls and occasional septae (Wright stain). (B) Septate fungal hyphae in nose of a cat (Wright stain). (C) Nasal swab, branching septate fungal hyphae with parallel cell walls (Wright stain). (D) Fine-needle aspirate from a lytic bone lesion in a dog showing macrophages with nonstaining fungal hyphae (Wright stain).

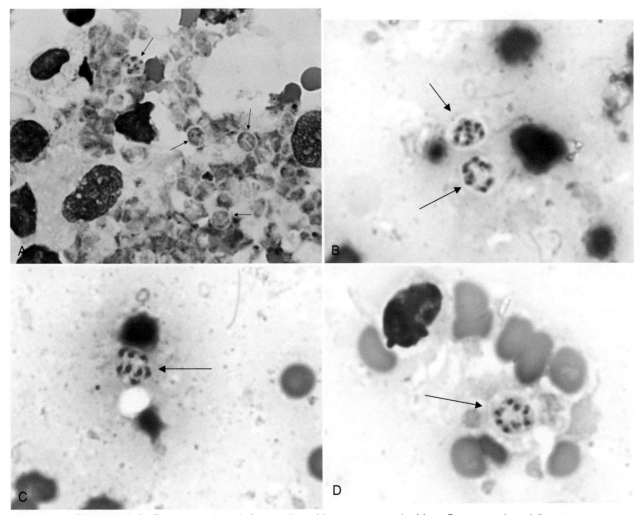

Fig. 3.16 (A–D) Transtracheal wash from a dog with pneumocystosis. Many *Pneumocystis carinii* cysts *(arrows)* containing four to eight intracystic bodies (Wright stain).

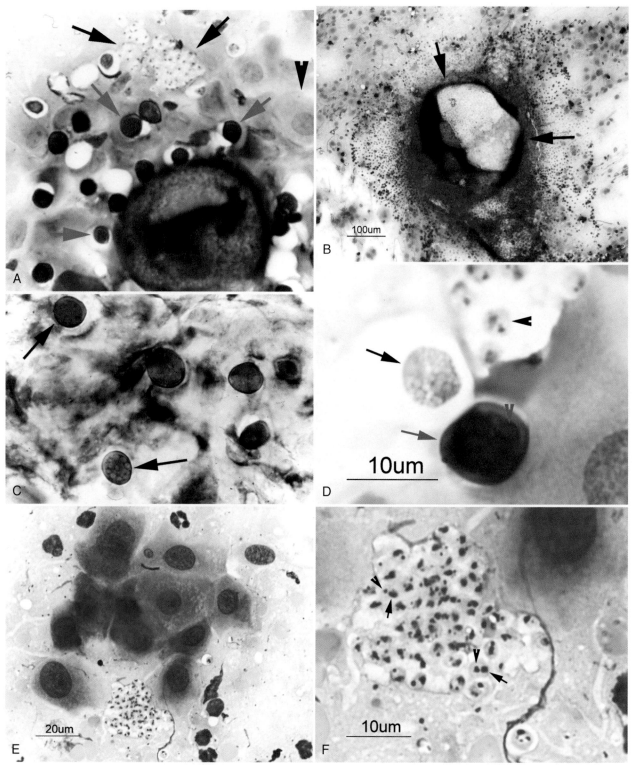

Fig. 3.17 (A) Dog with nasal rhinosporidiosis. There are numerous small pink mature endospores *(blue arrows)*, smaller immature endospores *(black arrows)*, and the large circular structure at the bottom is a relatively small sporangium. Nasal epithelial cells are present in the background *(black arrowhead)* (Wright stain). (B) Low-magnification image showing a large, ruptured sporangium *(arrows)* surrounded by many endospores (Wright stain). (C) Numerous mature endospores *(arrows)* and cellular debris (Wright stain). (D) Higher magnification of a mature endospore *(blue arrow)* with a thick cell wall and eosinophilic globular bodies *(blue arrowhead)*. Also present are immature endospores *(black arrowhead)* and an intermediate endospore *(black arrow)* (Wright stain). (E) Low-magnification image showing numerous epithelial cells with a cluster of immature endospores near the bottom of the image (Wright stain). (F) Immature endospores are spherical, lightly basophilic, with purple nuclear material *(arrows)* and one or more darker spherical structures *(arrowheads)* (Wright stain).

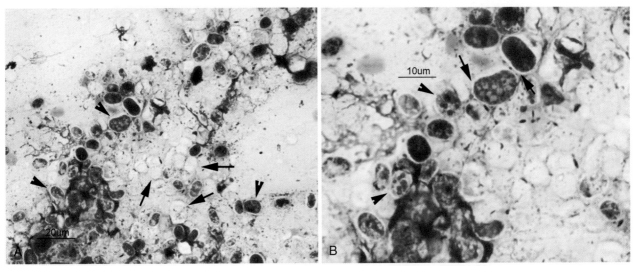

Fig. 3.18 (A) Aspirate of fluid from areas of retinal separation in a dog with protothecosis. Numerous round to oval *Prototheca* organisms *(arrowheads)* and clear, nonstaining areas representing empty casings (theca) of ruptured organisms *(arrows)* (Wright stain). (B) Higher magnification shows round to oval organisms, some of which contain endospores *(arrowheads)*. A thin, clear cell wall can be seen surrounding most organisms *(arrows)* (Wright stain).

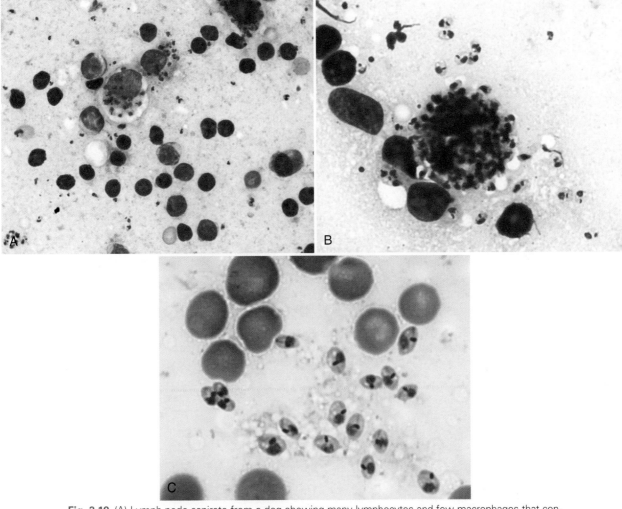

Fig. 3.19 (A) Lymph node aspirate from a dog showing many lymphocytes and few macrophages that contain *Leishmania* organisms (Wright stain). (B) Higher magnification showing *Leishmania* organisms in a macrophage and free in the background (Wright stain). (C) *Leishmania* amastigotes with purple nuclear material and rod shaped kinetoplast (Wright stain).

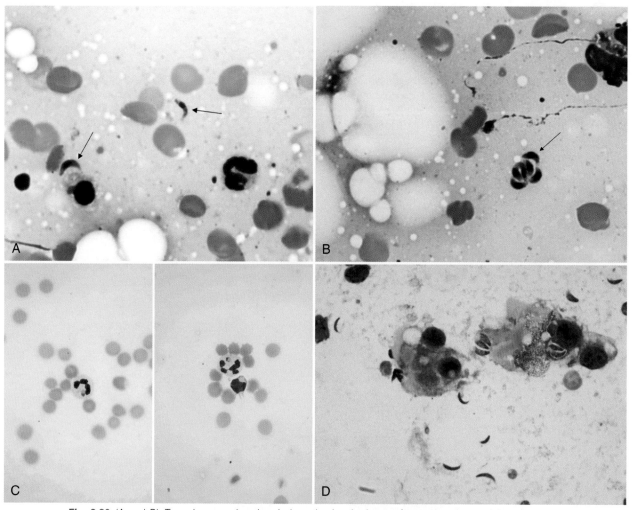

Fig. 3.20 (A and B) *Toxoplasma* tachyzoites in bronchoalveolar lavage from a cat *(arrows)* (Wright stain). (C) Composite showing ovoid Neospora tachyzoites in cerebrospinal fluid from a dog (Wright stain). (D) Ovoid and crescent shaped tachyzoites of *Hammondia heydorni* from a dog (Wright stain). (D, Courtesy Katy Jacocks.)

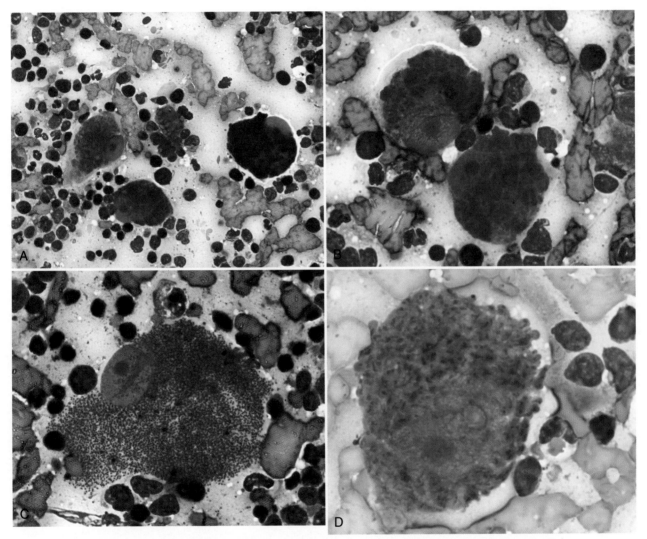

Fig. 3.21 (A–C) Lymph node aspirate from a cat with cytauxzoonosis. Large activated macrophages containing schizonts with developing merozoites of *Cytauxzoon* (Wright stain). (D) *Cytauxzoon* in cat splenic aspirate (Wright stain).

BIBLIOGRAPHY

Bottles K, Miller TR, Cohen MB, et al. Fine needle aspiration biopsy: has its time come? *Am J Med.* 1986;81:525–531.

Caruso KJ, et al. Skin scraping from a cat. *Vet Clin Pathol.* 2002;31(1):13–15.

Duprey ZH, Steurer FJ, Rooney JA, et al. Canine visceral leishmaniasis, United States and Canada, 2000–2003. *Emerg Infect Dis.* 2006;12(3):440–446.

Greene CE, ed. *Infectious Diseases of the Dog and Cat.* 4th ed. St. Louis: Elsevier; 2012.

Lester SJ, et al. Cryptococcosis: update and emergence of *Cryptococcus gattii.* *Vet Clin Pathol.* 2011;40(1):4–17.

Nelson RW, Couto G, eds. *Small Animal Internal Medicine.* 4th ed. Philadelphia: Mosby; 2009.

Raskin RE, Meyer DJ, eds. *Canine and Feline Cytology, A Color Atlas and Interpretation Guide.* 2nd ed. Philadelphia: Elsevier; 2010.

Rebar AH. Diagnostic cytology in veterinary practice, in Proceedings. 54th Annual Meet AAHA 1987; 498-504. In: Kirk RW, ed. *Current Veterinary Therapy.* vol. 7. Philadelphia: Saunders; 1980:16–27.

Sukura A, Saari S, Järvinen AK, et al. *Pneumocystis carinii* pneumonia in dogs—a diagnostic challenge. *J Vet Diagn Invest.* 1996;8:130–133.

Seybold I, Goldston RT, Wikes RD. Exfoliative cytology. *Vet Med Small Anim Clin.* 1982;77:1029–1033.

Cytology part I. Cowell RL, ed. *Vet Clin North Am Small Anim Pract.* 2002;32(6).

Cytology part II. Cowell RL, ed. *Vet Clin North Am Small Anim Pract.* 2003;32(6).

REFERENCES

1. Greene CE, ed. *Infectious Diseases of the Dog and Cat.* 4th ed. St. Louis: Elsevier; 2012.
2. Gremião ID, Menezes RC, Schubach TM, et al. Feline sporothricosis: epidemiological and clinical aspects. *Med Mycol.* 2015;53(1):15–21.
3. Schumacher LL, Love BC, Ferrell M, et al. Canine intestinal histoplasmosis containing hyphal forms. *J Vet Diagn Invest.* 2013;25(2):304–307.
4. Hanzlicek AS, Meinkoth JH, Renschler JS, et al. Antigen concentrations as an indicator of clinical remission and disease relapse in cats with histoplasmosis. *J Vet Intern Med.* 2016;30(4):1065–1073.
5. Bulla C, Thomas JS. What is your diagnosis? Subcutaneous mass fluid from febrile dog. *Vet Clin Pathol.* 2009;38(3):403–405.
6. Foy DS, Trepanier LA, Dirsch EJ, et al. Serum and urine *Blastomyces* antigen concentrations as markers of clinical remission in dogs treated for systemic blastomycosis. *J Vet Intern Med.* 2014;28(2):305–310.
7. Bemis DA, Krahwinkel DJ, Bowman LA, et al. Temperature-sensitive strain of *Cryptococcus neoformans* producing hyphal elements in a feline nasal granuloma. *J Clin Microbiol.* 2000;38(2):926–928.
8. Beaudin S, Rich LJ, Meinkoth JH, et al. Draining skin lesion from a desert poodle. *Vet Clin Pathol.* 2005;34(1):65–68.
9. Nielse C, Sutton DA, Matise I, et al. Isolation of *Cokeromyces recurvatus,* initially misidentified as *Coccidoides immitis,* from peritoneal fluid in a cat with jejunal perforation. *J Vet Diagn Invest.* 2005;17:372–378.
10. Wallin LL, Coleman GD, Froeling J, et al. Rhinosporidiosis in a domestic cat. *Med Mycol.* 2001;39:139–141.
11. Moisan PG, Baker SV. Rhinosporidiosis in a cat. *J Vet Diagn Invest.* 2001;13:352–354.
12. Brenseke BM, Saunders GK. Concurrent nasal adenocarcinoma and rhinosporidiosis in a cat. *J Vet Diagn Invest.* 2010;22(1):155–157.
13. Lane LV, Meinkoth JH, Brunker J, et al. Disseminated protothecosis diagnosed by evaluation of CSF in a dog. *Vet Clin Pathol.* 2012;41:147–152.
14. Petersen CA, Barr SC. Canine leishmaniasis in North America: emerging or newly recognized? *Vet Clin North Am Small Anim Pract.* 2009;39(6):1065–1074.
15. Nabity MB, Barnhart K, Logan KS, et al. An atypical case of *Trypanosoma cruzi* infection in a young English mastiff. *Vet Parasitol.* 2006;140:356–361.
16. Irvine KL, Walker JM, Friedrichs KR. Sarcocystid organisms found in bile from a dog with acute hepatitis: a case report and review of intestinal and hepatobiliary sarcocystidae infections in dogs and cats. *Vet Clin Pathol.* 2016;45(1):57–65.
17. Palic J, Parker VJ, Fales-Williams AJ, et al. What is your diagnosis? Duodenal brush preparation from a dog. *Vet Clin Pathol.* 2012;41(3):431–432.
18. Lloret A, Addie DD, Boucraut-Baralon C, et al. Cytauxzoonosis in cats: ABCD guidelines on prevention and management. *J Feline Med Surg.* 2015;17(7):637–641.

4

Round Cells

Kathryn Jacocks, Natalie Hoepp, and Dennis B. DeNicola

Cytologically, discrete round cell tumors are categorized separately from epithelial and mesenchymal neoplasms. Most round cell tumors are of hemolymphatic and mesenchymal origin. These neoplastic cells acquired their classification on the basis of their cytological/histological appearance of generally being individually oriented and usually lacking cellular membrane junctions or extracellular matrix adhesions. Round cell tumors customarily exfoliate extremely well for cytological evaluation.

Although few mesenchymal and epithelial neoplasms can appear discrete in fine-needle biopsy (FNB) samples, the classic tumors denoted to the round cell systemization are as follows:
Transmissible venereal tumor
Mast cell tumor
Histiocytic tumors
Lymphoma
Plasma cell tumors
Melanocytic tumors will also be briefly described in this chapter because these neoplasms share cytomorphological characteristics of traditional round cell tumors and should be considered as differentials for malignant, poorly differentiated round cell tumors.

TRANSMISSIBLE VENEREAL TUMORS

Transmissible venereal tumor (TVTs) was the first described transplantable neoplastic process. It is more commonly seen in tropical and subtropical urban areas, where free-roaming dogs are present, but are endemic in 90 countries with greater recent occurrence because of travel and movement of dogs associated with international and interstate rescues.[1] Young, sexually active dogs are most commonly affected, and although the genitalia are the typical site of neoplastic cell implantation and tumor growth, the face, eye, oral and nasal cavities, and other cutaneous locations are also reported to be associated with mechanical spread or primary tumors. TVT is generally considered a benign neoplastic process that can spontaneously regress in immunocompetent animals, with infiltration of lymphocytes (similar to histiocytoma), but it also tends to be progressive. Chemotherapy with vincristine sulfate is the treatment of choice, and surgical intervention or radiation is performed when necessary.[2,3] Metastasis is rare and may actually result from mechanical transplantation from a primary tumor, but distant metastasis involving lymph nodes, viscera, the eye, and the brain have been reported.[2,4,5]

CYTOLOGICAL APPEARANCE

TVT aspirates and impression smears are highly cellular and can have overlapping morphology with other round cell neoplasms, having the monomorphic appearance of lymphoma, more abundant cytoplasm,

and mature lymphocyte infiltrate as seen in histiocytoma or appearing plasmacytoid as a result of nuclear morphology. The consistent presence of several clear punctate cytoplasmic vacuoles, as well as the context of clinical presentation, can be a distinguishing feature in this tumor type (Fig. 4.1). TVT cells have scant to moderate amounts of basophilic cytoplasm, frequently including one to five small, 0.5- to 2-μm, round, clear, punctate vacuoles. The nuclei are round, are central to eccentric, have uniform stippled to reticulate chromatin patterns, and can include one to two prominent nucleoli (Fig. 4.2). Mitotic figures are common, and abnormal mitotic figures can be present but are not predictive of biological behavior, a feature that also overlaps with histiocytomas.

MAST CELL TUMORS

Mast cell tumors (MCTs) are common cutaneous neoplasms of dogs and cats, with both the cutaneous form and the visceral form generally considered less aggressive in the cat and associated with longer survival times. In the dog, malignant potential is determined by several factors, including histological grading, staging, growth rate (via proliferation factor assessment), and c-KIT protooncogene mutation status. In the cat, cutaneous MCT shows relatively benign behavior, except in patients with multiple or recurring tumors, and visceral involvement is often splenic (versus gastrointestinal in dogs). Positive outcomes have been achieved with splenectomy and can include regression of nonsplenic tumors.

In dogs, two histological grading schemes are in use currently, with evaluation often including combined reporting, whereas in cats, grading is not considered a reliable indicator of malignant behavior. MCTs found in subcutaneous tissue can be less aggressive, and histological grading schemes are not applied to tumors in this location. The general features of the two primary histological grading systems currently in use for canine cutaneous mast cell tumors include the three-tier grading system of Patnaik et al. and the high-low grade system of Kiupel et al.[6,7]
Three-tier system:
  Grade I: Well-differentiated cells, confined to dermis, absence of mitotic activity
  Grade II: Moderately pleomorphic cells, infiltration into deeper dermal and subcutaneous tissue, 0 to 2 mitotic cells per high-power field (hpf)
  Grade III: Pleomorphic mast cells with frequent binucleation, increased mitotic cells, extending into and replacing subcutaneous and deep tissues
High–low grading system:
  High grade: Presence of any one of the following criteria: at least seven mitotic figures per 10 hpf; at least three multinucleate cells per 10 hpf; at least three bizarre nuclei per 10 hpf; and karyomegaly.
  Low grade: Absence of high-grade criteria.

Criteria for MCT grading based on cytomorphological features have been proposed with correlation to the Kiupel grading system, as well as with use of hematoxylin and eosin (H&E) staining to better evaluate nuclear morphology.[8-11] Although these studies have demonstrated promising results and good agreement between cytological and histological grades, with karyomegaly being a consistent feature of high-grade tumors, at this time, the cytomorphological criteria and preferred staining methods are still being elucidated, and a universal system has not yet been established.

Further prognostic information can be provided by evaluation of MCTs for markers of cellular proliferation, including argyrophilic nucleolar organizing region (AgNOR), proliferating cell nuclear antigen (PCNA), Ki67, mutations of the *cKIT* protooncogene, and aberrant localization of the KIT protein.[12] Internal tandem duplications of exon 8 and 11 in *cKIT* are described, with 11 being more common, and abnormalities have been reported in up to 33% of canine tumors.[12,13]

CYTOLOGICAL APPEARANCE

The cytological diagnosis of MCT is often straightforward but can be problematic when the associated eosinophilic infiltrate or reactive fibroplasia is a greater proportion of the sample composition than the mast cell population itself or in samples where granules stain poorly. In these cases, mast cells can have a similar appearance to histiocytoma and other round cell neoplasms. In cats, cutaneous mast cell tumors have greater variation in cytological appearance and are further characterized (on histopathological examination) as mastocytic or atypical (previously histiocytic); the former is well differentiated or pleomorphic, whereas the latter includes cellular atypia, is rare, and may spontaneously regress.[14,15] Pleomorphic mastocytic and atypical forms can include eosinophilic infiltrate, a feature more commonly seen in dogs (Figs. 4.3 and 4.4).

Mast cell tumors tend to exfoliate well, leading to highly cellular samples, and in addition to discrete round cell characteristics, mast

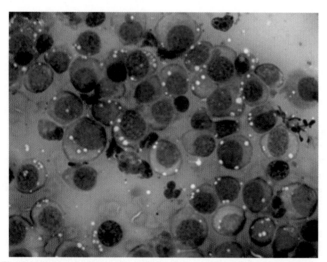

Fig. 4.1 Transmissible venereal tumor impression smear from the vulva of an intact female dog from the southern United States (×1000, oil).

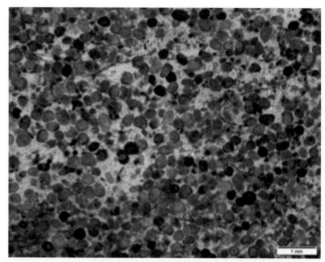

Fig. 4.3 Feline cutaneous mast cell tumor with cellular pleomorphism, variation in granulation, and mixed inflammatory (eosinophilic and neutrophilic) infiltrate (×100, oil).

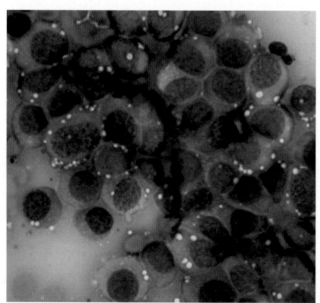

Fig. 4.2 Transmissible venereal tumor from the same patient (×1000, oil)

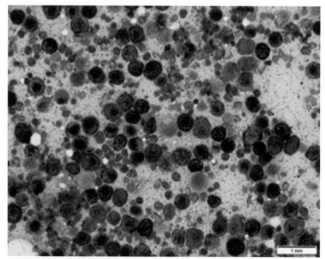

Fig. 4.4 Canine cutaneous mast cell tumor with cellular pleomorphism, variation in cytoplasmic granulation, and eosinophilic infiltrate (×500, oil).

cells have the distinction of including purple cytoplasmic granules when stained with a Romanowsky-type stain (Fig. 4.5). One of the most commonly used stains in clinical practice, Diff-Quik, may fail to adequately stain mast cell granules, making accurate distinction of MCT from other discrete round cell tumors difficult or impossible. Often, on close scrutiny of the cytoplasm, a fine dusting of purple granulation can be discerned, but confirmation by repeat sampling and staining is recommended. Lack of staining with Diff-Quik is more pronounced in mast cell populations that are poorly granulated, with well-differentiated, densely granulated mast cells having better staining quality regardless of the stain used.

Mast cells have abundant pale cytoplasm with numerous coarse, round to fine, purple granules that are often seen throughout the background of cytological preparations. The nuclei are round to slightly oval, are often obscured from view in heavily granulated mast cells, and can have a pale turquoise homogeneous tinctorial quality as a result of absorption of the stain by surrounding granules. This can be problematic for assessing chromatin patterns and nuclear morphology for cytological grading. In tumors with greater cytological atypia and less

differentiation, binucleate, trinucleate, and multinucleate cells may be present, with some mast cells exhibiting erythrophagocytosis (Fig. 4.6). Eosinophils and reactive fibroblasts are often present in the background in canine mast cell tumors and are seen to a lesser extent in cats.

Collagenolysis (resulting from chymase within mast cell granules) and reactive fibroplasia are common histological findings in MCT.[16] Fibroblasts are plump fusiform to stellate mononuclear cells, with large, oval central nuclei; uniform chromatin patterns; variably prominent nucleoli; and moderate-to-abundant amounts of deeply basophilic attenuated cytoplasm. If an area of fibroplasia is aspirated and high numbers of reactive fibroblasts and fewer well-differentiated mast cells are present, it may not be possible to distinguish MCT from a primary mesenchymal neoplasm with mast cell infiltration. In samples where eosinophils predominate, with low numbers of individualized mast cells or small groups, arthropod bite or sting with associated hypersensitivity response must also be considered. Sample acquisition from more than one area of the mass may provide a more representative sample.

LYMPHOPROLIFERATIVE DISEASE

Detailed discussion of lymphoproliferative disease is found in Chapter 11. Cytomorphological description of lymphoma (lymphosarcoma [LSA]) by cell size for prognostic purposes is often preferred and an important descriptive feature, but is no longer considered a sole predictor of biological behavior, and further characterization by immunophenotyping, biopsy with immunohistochemistry, immunocytochemistry, and/or polymerase chain reaction (PCR) for antigen receptor rearrangement (PARR) is often undertaken to make definitive prognostic comments based on lymphoma classification schemes. Lymphoma presentation is variable and includes cutaneous, multicentric, gastrointestinal (GI), hepatosplenic, renal, bladder, central nervous system (CNS), ocular, Hodgkin-like, and leukemic forms, with species dependent prevalence in cats and dogs (Figs. 4.7 through 4.10).

CYTOLOGICAL PRESENTATION

The key cytological feature of lymphoma is that the neoplastic proliferation is generally composed of a homogeneous population of lymphocytes, but some forms include a mixed population or a subpopulation of mature lymphocytes, creating a challenge for definitive cytological

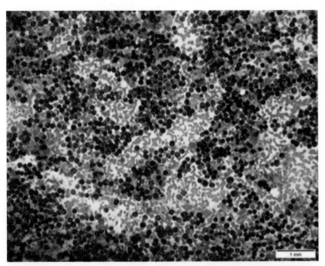

Fig. 4.5 Well-granulated canine cutaneous mast cell tumor with hemorrhage and low numbers of understained reactive fibroblasts (×100, oil).

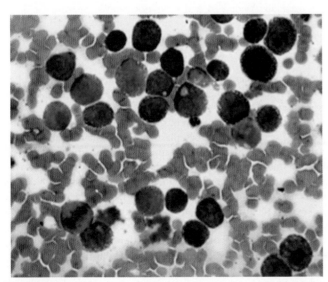

Fig. 4.6 Pleomorphic canine cutaneous mast cell tumor with erythrophagocytosis, variable granulation and mitotic figure (×500, oil).

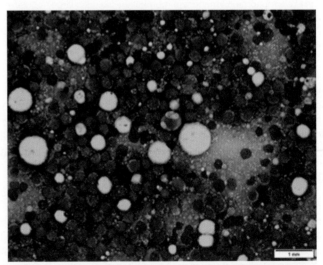

Fig. 4.7 Renal lymphoma in a feline patient. The same neoplastic population was also identified in the liver. The numerous small clear cytoplasmic vacuoles may be a feature in feline visceral and gastrointestinal lymphoma (×500, oil).

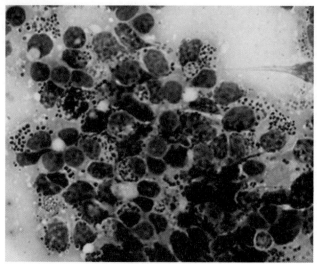

Fig. 4.8 Feline intestinal large granular lymphocyte lymphoma. On aspirates, the cells may appear similar to mast cells on initial examination but have larger, irregular, coarse magenta granules (×500, oil).

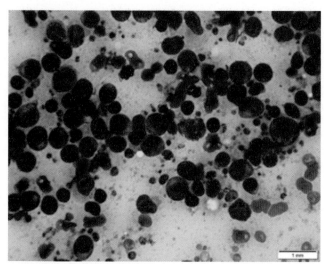

Fig. 4.10 Canine mandibular lymph node aspirate with a monomorphic population of large lymphocytes, few mature lymphocytes, and numerous cytoplasmic fragments (×500, oil).

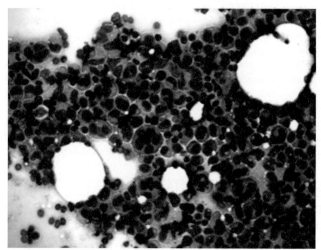

Fig. 4.9 Cervical mass from an adult male neutered cat with Hodgkin-like lymphoma. Lymphocyte morphology includes large, lobulated, and binucleate cells compatible with Reed-Sternberg-like cells and large lymphohistiocytic cells, with presence and proportions of the latter dependent on subtype (×500, oil).

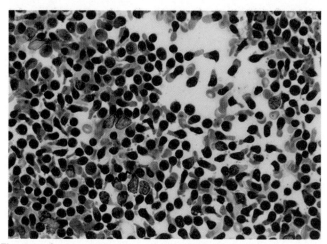

Fig. 4.11 Canine small cell lymphoma. Aspirate from a right submandibular lymph node with a history of mandibular lymphadenopathy. The slides revealed a fairly monomorphic population of small lymphocytes with expanded cytoplasm and a "mirror handle" appearance. T-cell PARR-positive lymphosarcoma (×1000, oil). (Courtesy Dr. Regan Bell, DVM, MS, DACVP.)

interpretation. Cytological specimens are often highly cellular, including those in cutaneous manifestations of disease; in skin, inflammatory or immune-mediated lymphoid infiltrate and mixed neoplastic populations can overlap significantly in cytological appearance, requiring evaluation of histopathological architecture to confirm the diagnosis and provide further distinction regarding epitheliotropic and nonepitheliotropic forms of lymphoma.

In small cell lymphoma, the malignant population is composed of mature small lymphocytes, similar to those predominating in normal lymphoid tissue, but with a monotonous appearance overall and lacking the expected spectrum of small mature, intermediate, and large lymphocytes with low numbers of plasma cells seen in normal lymph nodes or reactive hyperplasia. When microscopic features of potential reactive hyperplasia overlap with small (or intermediate) cell lymphoma as a result of expansion of one cell type, complete clinical history, including the presence or absence of additional lymph node

involvement or allergic skin disease, can aid interpretation, but often cases of suspected small cell lymphoma require additional diagnostic testing for confirmation.

On cytological examination of small cell lymphoma, the lymphocytes have scant basophilic cytoplasm and often have small cytoplasmic projections ("hand mirror" appearance) in various directions, although this feature alone is not pathognomonic and is also observed in some reactive or normal lymph nodes. The nuclei have condensed chromatin and indistinct nucleoli (Fig. 4.11). Depending on the thickness of the preparation and tinctorial quality, it can be difficult to differentiate small versus intermediate cell lymphoma because of distortion of morphology by contraction of cells in hemodilute, lipid-rich, or proteinaceous backgrounds or when disruption and flattening is present from sample preparation (Fig. 4.12). Intermediate cell lymphomas have features similar to those of small cell lymphoma, with a monomorphic population of cells of slightly larger size and

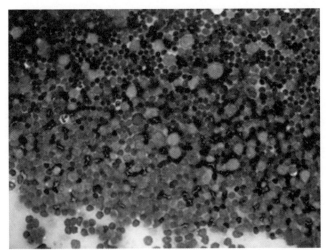

Fig. 4.12 Lymph node aspirate sample with variation in thickness that gives the appearance of intermediate lymphocytes predominating at the edges, with mature lymphocytes appearing most numerous deeper in the smear. This can be caused by contraction of cells, creating smaller size and condensed deeply stained chromatin, or flattening of small lymphocytes, making them appear larger with finer chromatin patterns, more compatible with intermediate lymphocytes (×100, oil).

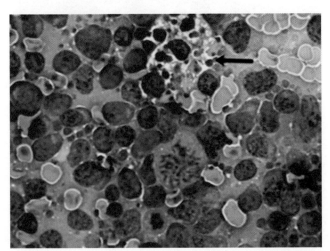

Fig. 4.13 Canine mandibular lymph node with macrophage containing phagocytosed erythrocytes and cellular debris *(arrow)*, monomorphic large lymphocytes, cytoplasmic fragments, and a mitotic figure (×1000, oil).

having ropey to stippled paler chromatin, but also lacking nucleoli. In some cases, the description will include "small-to-intermediate cell lymphoma" or "intermediate-to-large cell lymphoma" to accommodate the neoplastic population's morphological variation or sample artifact change that precludes further size delineation.

Large cell lymphomas are composed of monomorphic populations of large lymphocytes ("lymphoblasts") (see Fig. 4.10). In some variants of lymphoma, including Hodgkin-like lymphoma, the potential for cellular pleomorphism (rather than homogeneous expansion) exists; however, general criteria of malignancy for lymphoma includes lack of heterogeneity in the lymphoid population, monomorphic lymphocytic cellular infiltration of organs or nonlymphoid tissues, increased mitotic figures (although not required and also noted in normal or hyperplastic lymph nodes), and increased macrophages containing phagocytosed debris with a lack of background inflammation or other known origin for a reactive or inflammatory process (Fig. 4.13). Reactive lymphoid hyperplasia may include expansion of individual

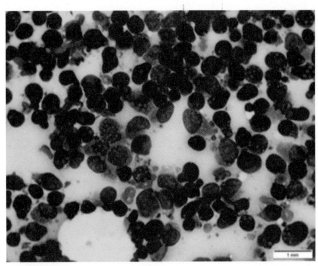

Fig. 4.14 Canine lymph node with lymphoma that includes Mott cell differentiation (×1000, oil).

cell types, particularly intermediate lymphocytes, and is not always readily discerned from lymphoproliferative disease. Similarly, plasmacytosis, an expected finding in reactive lymph nodes, can also be associated with lymphoma that includes plasma cell differentiation, but in the latter the plasmacytoid cells tend to be extremely numerous, are poorly differentiated, and may appear as atypical Mott-like cells with very few well-differentiated plasma cells (Fig. 4.14).

PLASMA CELL TUMORS

Presentation and Biological Behavior

Plasma cell neoplasms are a subset of lymphoproliferative disease. Plasma cells are fully differentiated B-cell lymphocytes that manufacture and secrete immunoglobulin. In the canine or feline patient, plasma cell tumors are categorized as multiple myeloma, cutaneous or noncutaneous extramedullary plasmacytoma, solitary plasmacytoma of bone, and extramedullary plasmacytoma (EMP) subtypes.

Multiple myeloma (MM) is the clonal proliferation of malignant plasma cells, which generally originates in bone marrow. Many patients present with hyperglobulinemia as a result of unregulated production of antibodies by myeloma cells. In dogs, two or more of the following are needed for a diagnosis of MM: osteolytic bone lesions, greater than 20% of plasma cells in bone marrow, paraproteinemia, and Bence-Jones proteinuria.

In cats, MM and advanced EMP cannot always be distinguished by the above criteria used in the dog.[17] Often, the feline patient is found to have extramedullary involvement on initial clinical presentation. EMP in cats mostly arise in the GI tract, with the colorectal mucosa overrepresented. Other reported locations include the spleen, liver, kidney, lungs, esophagus, and brain.[18] The canine patient may present with solitary plasmacytoma of visceral organs or disseminated disease (usually widespread MM).

Solitary cutaneous EMP in feline and canine patients are generally benign, and excision is curative. However, there are exceptions, which include cutaneous plasmacytosis. This is a neoplastic condition reported in dogs, in which multiple cutaneous plasma cell tumors can arise in the absence of MM.[19] There are also reported cases of progression of cutaneous plasmacytoma to multiple myeloma and plasma cell leukemia in the dog.[20]

In MM, mature, small, well-differentiated plasma cells are indicators of low-grade disease, whereas immature, blastic-appearing plasma

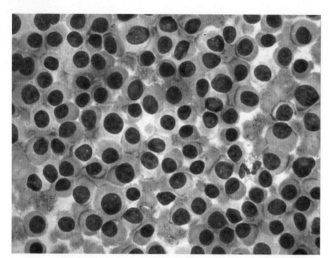

Fig. 4.15 Cutaneous skin mass from a dog—plasmacytoma. Numerous round cells noted predominantly individually with round to oval, mostly eccentric nuclei and a mild to moderate amount of moderately basophilic cytoplasm with rounded borders and a perinuclear clear zone (×1000, oil).

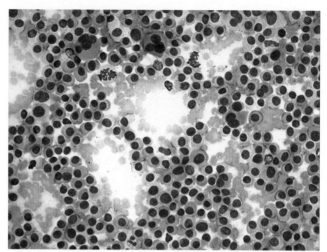

Fig. 4.16 Canine benign, cutaneous plasmacytoma. Numerous neoplastic plasma cells exhibiting mild to occasional moderate anisocytosis and anisokaryosis. Evidence of bi- and multinucleation. Few cells have pink cytoplasmic rims, which is consistent with "flaming plasma cells" (×500, oil).

cells are usually the features of high-grade malignancy. In EMP, well-differentiated forms exhibit benign behavior, whereas poorly differentiated or anaplastic-appearing plasma cells can be locally aggressive, with the potential to metastasize. Location of EMP can also be an indicator of biological behavior in dogs with cutaneous and oral cavity EMPs routinely being benign versus those arising from other locations (i.e., bone and viscera).[21]

Cytological Presentation

Plasma cells are considered round cells with round to oval eccentric nuclei, uniform to coarse chromatin, and a moderate amount of moderately to deeply basophilic cytoplasm with rounded borders. The cytoplasm is commonly deeply blue staining because of the density of cytoplasmic ribonucleic acid (RNA). Most plasma cells have a perinuclear clear zone as a result of the cytoplasmic organelle of the Golgi apparatus (Fig. 4.15). Rarely, pigmented cytoplasmic granules have been in reported in plasma cells.[22]

Plasma cells with a pink cytoplasmic rim are called "flame cells" or "flaming plasma cells." Plasma cells with retained cytoplasmic globules (Russell bodies) are referred to as *Mott cells* (see Fig. 4.14). Occasionally, pink extracellular matrix (which likely represents amyloid) is associated with the cells. Plasma cells neoplasms (EMP and MM) can present with binucleate and multinucleate cells and variable degrees of anisocytosis and anisokaryosis (Fig. 4.16).

MELANOCYTIC TUMORS

Presentation and Biological Behavior

Melanoma is a fairly common tumor of canines and relatively rare in felines. Melanoma is derived from neoplastic, pigment-generating melanocytes. Cutaneous and oral melanomas are among the most prevalent locations, with the majority of skin melanomas exhibiting benign behavior. In contrast, oral melanomas are usually malignant and are the most frequently diagnosed oral malignancy in the dog. Other reported sites for malignant melanoma include the nailbed, footpad, eye, GI system, and mucocutaneous junctions. Feline melanoma is fairly uncommon and is typically considered malignant.[23] Ocular melanoma of canines and felines is covered in Chapter 9.

Location alone is not always predictive of prognosis, but evidence of distant metastasis is associated with a poor prognosis.

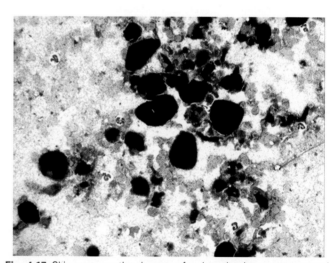

Fig. 4.17 Skin mass on the dorsum of a dog—benign cutaneous melanoma. The neoplastic melanocytes are noted individually and in loose aggregates. When visible, the cells have round to oval nuclei, stippled chromatin, and a mild to abundant amount of cytoplasm with numerous melanin granules. Note several extracellular granules from ruptured cells in the background (×500, oil).

Histopathological evaluation, especially assessment of nuclear atypia, mitotic index, degree of pigmentation, vasculolymphatic invasion, and the Ki67 index, is warranted to classify the melanocytic neoplasm as benign versus malignant. The Ki67 index is a highly objective and predictive value test, which is a measure of the growth fraction of neoplastic cells.[24]

Cytological Presentation

Unlike many of the round cell tumors that are of hemolymphatic origin, melanocytic tumors are of neural crest/neuroendocrine origin. Well-differentiated melanomas/melanocytomas can present as discrete, uniform cells that appear heavily granulated with melanosomes (melanin granules) (Fig. 4.17).

Melanoma cell morphology can range from round to polygonal to plump spindle or even stellate. Undifferentiated, non- or poorly granulated melanoma may be difficult to distinguish from other malignant

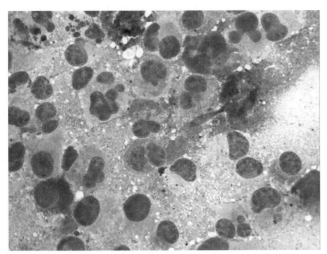

Fig. 4.18 Aspirate from a malignant oral melanoma in a dog. The neoplastic melanocytes are seen individually and in loose aggregates. The cells exhibit marked criteria of malignancy with pleomorphic nuclei, prominent and multiple nucleoli, anisocytosis and anisokaryosis, and variable granulation with variable granule sizes (×1000, oil).

round cell tumors. However, routine cytology has been found to be a reliable diagnostic method for canine oral amelanotic melanoma and metastatic amelanotic melanoma.[24]

Cell sizes can be quite variable, ranging from as small as 12 to 20 μm in greatest dimension to as large as 20 to 30 μm or greater in dimension. Nuclei are commonly paracentral in location and round to oval in shape. Nuclear chromatin patterns in the benign neoplasm are uniform and finely stippled; however, in the malignant variants, chromatin patterns are often coarsely and irregularly clumped. Nucleoli can be multiple, prominent, and irregularly shaped. Nuclear criteria of malignancy have been well documented in many of the malignant melanomas. A moderate to high number of mitotic figures may be seen with the more malignant variants of melanoma, and occasionally abnormal mitotic figures may be present (Fig. 4.18).

The cytoplasm is typically moderate to abundant in amount, giving the cells a moderate to low nuclear-to-cytoplasmic (N:C) ratio. It is granular, and stains light to moderate blue. One of the distinguishing features of this class of neoplasms is the presence of variable numbers of melanin pigment granules. In contrast to normal melanin granules, these are often rounded and variably sized and sometimes clumped to varying degrees. The granules stain black to green-black with commonly used Romanowsky stains in contrast to the purple staining granules of mast cells tumors. Histologically, a class of melanocytic tumors is identified as amelanotic melanomas because of the apparent absence of melanin pigment granules with standard histological staining procedures. Cytologically, even in the least pigmented melanomas, few melanin granules can often be identified with deliberate microscopic review of the specimen. It should be noted that simple identification of melanin granules does not mean a diagnosis of melanoma. The novice cytologist commonly misidentifies a pigmented basal cell tumor or a pigmented keratin-containing cyst as melanoma; normal melanocytes pass melanin to epithelial cells of the epidermis. Additionally, some may confuse melanin-laden macrophages (melanophages) as melanocytes.

HISTIOCYTIC TUMORS

Presentation and Biological Behavior

Histiocytic neoplastic disease is extremely complex, particularly in the dog. The wide range of clinical presentations and biological behaviors are dependent on the cell of lineage. In many cases, cytomorphological features of the neoplastic histiocytes are highly predictive of biological potential; however, tissue distribution of two of the benign histiocytic proliferative diseases cannot be predicted on the basis of cytomorphological features alone. In recent years, tremendous advances have been made in the understanding of canine histiocytic neoplastic processes, and the reader is directed to the laboratory at the School of Veterinary Medicine, University of California, Davis, California (www.histiocytosis.ucdavis.edu), for a detailed review of canine histiocytic disease. The basic presentation for histiocytic neoplasia in canine and feline patients are presented next.

Canine Cutaneous Histiocytoma

Canine cutaneous histiocytoma is typically a benign, solitary, cutaneous lesion that occurs in young dogs; however, it may be seen in dogs of any ages. Most commonly, it is seen in dogs younger than 3 years of age. Complete excision is typically curative, and spontaneous regression is usually expected. These neoplasms may be found anywhere on the body, but extremities and pinna are common locations. Metastasis of solitary a histiocytoma to dependent lymph nodes can infrequently occur, and regression is generally expected; however, in some reported cases, it failed to regress. Lymphocytic infiltration usually accompanies the resolution of the tumor. Multiple histiocytomas is a recognized syndrome in which cutaneous tumors histologically compatible with histiocytoma is observed.[25]

Reactive Histiocytosis

Cutaneous histiocytosis (CH) and systemic histiocytosis (SH) are related diseases originating from activated interstitial dendritic cells and are histiocytic–lymphocytic inflammatory disorders characterized by a degree of immune dysregulation. There is no known feline counterpart for reactive histiocytosis.[25]

Reactive histiocytosis in dogs is either noted in skin and dependent lymph nodes (CH) or involves skin and extracutaneous sites (SH). The clinical progression in both disorders can be punctuated by spontaneous remission and relapses, but it is more common with CH. Effective therapies generally involve immunosuppression and immunotherapy, and this supports the likelihood that reactive histiocytosis is a nonneoplastic, inflammatory disorder.

Histiocytic Sarcoma Complex

Histiocytic sarcoma complex (HS) occurs in both dogs and cats; however, reported feline cases are rare compared with canine cases. HS can manifest as localized lesions in skin and subcutaneous tissue, spleen, lung, lymph nodes, bone marrow, brain, and articular tissue of appendicular joints. Disseminated HS is described as HS that can occur as multiple lesions in a single organ (with overrepresentation of the spleen and skin), quickly metastasizing to encompass multiple organs.

There are two feline histiocytic disorders without canine counterparts. These include feline progressive histiocytosis (FPH) and pulmonary Langerhans cell histiocytosis (LCH). FPH is more common than pulmonary LCH and initially presents as cutaneous lesions, with either gradual progression and possible eventual multiple cutaneous lesions or potential progression to involve regional lymph nodes and, terminally, visceral organs. Pulmonary LCH is usually observed in older felines and presents as respiratory failure, which escalates to severe infiltration of the pulmonary parenchyma.

Cytological Presentation

Although significant variations exist in the clinical presentations of histiocytic proliferative disease in the dog and in the cat, cytomorphological variations are relatively few, and this makes it difficult sometimes

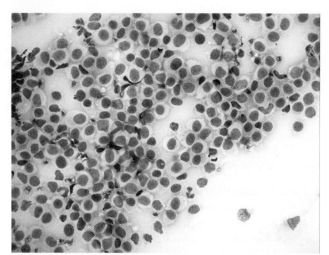

Fig. 4.19 Aspirate from a canine histiocytoma. Note numerous, relatively uniform, discrete, round, mononuclear cells with central to eccentric, round to oval, slightly indented nuclei with finely stippled and uniform chromatin patterns. The cytoplasm is moderate in amount, pale blue, and granular (×500, oil).

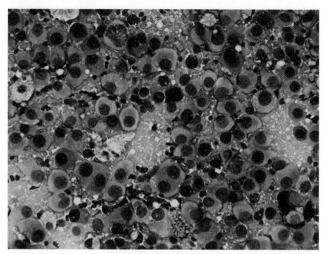

Fig. 4.20 Aspirate from an enlarged spleen in a dog with histiocytic sarcoma. The sample is highly cellular, containing a population of discrete round and mostly mononuclear cells with moderate anisocytosis, anisokaryosis, and variation in nuclear-to-cytoplasmic (N:C) ratios (×500, oil).

to make a definitive diagnosis on the basis of cytological presentation alone. All of the different variants of histiocytic proliferative disease typically present with moderate-to-high cellularity, with varying amounts of peripheral blood contamination.

Canine cutaneous histiocytoma, cutaneous histiocytosis, and systemic histiocytosis. The proliferative histiocytes in canine cutaneous histiocytoma, CH, and SH in the dog have similar morphological features. These discrete cells are relatively round and range from 12 to 30 μm in diameter. They may present with an irregular or ameboid cell shape; this is seen more in the later stages of resolution, particularly in cutaneous histiocytoma in young dogs. Nuclei are mostly round to oval in shape and central to eccentric in location, but blunt indentations of the nucleus or irregular shapes may also be seen. Nuclear chromatin patterns are finely stippled and uniform and, in many cases, resemble the nuclear chromatin patterns of normal-appearing peripheral blood monocytes. The cytoplasm is variable in amount but generally moderate to abundant. Cytoplasm stains pale blue and is granular, with rare pink granules and vacuoles (Fig. 4.19).

Low numbers of normal-appearing small lymphocytes and rarely seen macrophages and well-differentiated plasma cells may be distributed among the histiocytes. Small lymphocytes increase in numbers and become the predominant cell type as the tumor regresses.

Histiocytic sarcoma complex. Neoplastic cells within the HS of neoplasms are distinctively different from the more benign-appearing counterparts noted previously. Anisocytosis, anisokaryosis, karyomegaly, variation in N:C ratios, and overall pleomorphism are common. In addition, multinucleate giant cell formation is often seen. Nuclear chromatin patterns can be irregularly clumped and prominent; multiple, irregularly shaped nucleoli may be seen. Cytoplasm is typically moderate to abundant in amount, pale blue staining, granular, and sometimes vacuolated (Fig. 4.20). Phagocytosis of erythrocytes and leukocytes may be seen and is particularly common in a variant of HS called *hemophagocytic histiocytic sarcoma* (Fig. 4.21). A hemophagocytic syndrome, with observed anemia and possibly other peripheral cytopenias, may occur. The neoplastic histiocytes in hemophagocytic HS may appear well differentiated in bone marrow, with more atypia noted in other locations.[25]

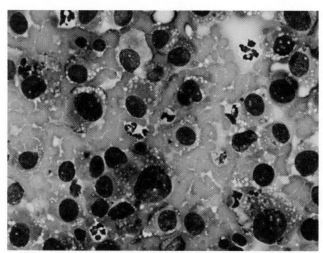

Fig. 4.21 Histiocytic sarcoma complex from a splenic aspirate in a dog. Many cells are heavily vacuolated with evidence of erythrophagia and cytophagia. Cells exhibit significant anisocytosis and anisokaryosis (×1000, oil).

REFERENCES

1. Strakova A, Murchison EP. The changing global distribution and prevalence of canine transmissible venereal tumour. *BMC Vet Res.* 2014;10:168.
2. Mukaratirwa S, Gruys E. Canine transmissible venereal tumour: cytogenetic origin, immunophenotype, and immunobiology. A review. *Vet Q.* 2003;25(3):101–111. https://doi.org/10.1080/01652176.2003.9695151.
3. Ganguly B, Das U, Das AK. Canine transmissible venereal tumour: a review. *Vet Comp Oncol.* 2016;14(1):1–12. https://doi.org/10.1111/vco.12060.
4. Ferreira AJA, Jaggy A, Varejão AP, et al. Brain and ocular metastases from a transmissible venereal tumour in a dog. *J Small Anim Pract.* 2000;41(4):165–168. https://doi.org/10.1111/j.1748–5827.2000.tb03187.x.
5. Park MS, Kim Y, Kang MS, et al. Disseminated transmissible venereal tumor in a dog. *J Vet Diagnostic Investig.* 2006;18(1):130–133. https://doi.org/10.1177/104063870601800123.
6. Patnaik AK, Ehler WJ, MacEweb EG. Canine cutaneous mast cell tumor: morphologic grading and survival times in 83 dogs. *Vet Pathol.* 1984;21(41):469–474.

7. Kiupel M, Webster JD, Bailey KL, et al. Proposal of a 2-tier histologic grading system for canine cutaneous mast cell tumors to more accurately predict biological behavior. *Vet Pathol.* 2011;48(1):147–155. https://doi.org/10.1177/0300985810386469.

8. Hergt F, von Bomhard W, Kent MS, Hirschberger J. Use of a 2-tier histologic grading system for canine cutaneous mast cell tumors on cytology specimens. *Vet Clin Pathol.* 2016;45(3):477–483. https://doi.org/10.1111/vcp.12387.

9. Scarpa F, Sabattini S, Bettini G. Cytological grading of canine cutaneous mast cell tumours. *Vet Comp Oncol.* 2016;14(3):245–251. https://doi.org/10.1111/vco.12090.

10. Ressel L, Finotello R. Cytological grading of canine cutaneous mast cell tumours: is haematoxylin and eosin staining better than May-Grünwald-Giemsa? *Vet Comp Oncol.* 2017;15(3):667–668. https://doi.org/10.1111/vco.12234.

11. Camus MS, Priest HL, Koehler JW, et al. Cytologic criteria for mast cell tumor grading in dogs with evaluation of clinical outcome. *Vet Pathol.* 2016;53(6):1117–1123. https://doi.org/10.1177/0300985816638721.

12. Webster JD, Yuzbasiyan-Gurkan V, Miller RA, Kaneene JB, Kiupel M. Cellular proliferation in canine cutaneous mast cell tumors: associations with *c-KIT* and its role in prognostication. *Vet Pathol.* 2007;44(3):298–308. https://doi.org/10.1354/vp.44-3-298.

13. Murphy S, Sparkes AH, Blunden AS, Brearley MJ, Smith KC. Effects of stage and number of tumours on prognosis of dogs with cutaneous mast cell tumours. *Vet Rec.* 2006;158(9):287–291. https://doi.org/10.1136/vr.158.9.287.

14. Sabattini S, Bettini G. Prognostic value of histologic and immunohistochemical features in feline cutaneous mast cell tumors. *Vet Pathol.* 2010;47(4):643–653. https://doi.org/10.1177/0300985810364509.

15. Wilcock BP, Yager JA, Zink MC. The morphology and behavior of feline cutaneous mastocytomas. *Vet Pathol.* 1986;23(3):320–324. https://doi.org/10.1177/030098588602300313.

16. Caughey GH. Mast cell tryptases and chymases in inflammation and host defense. *Immunol Rev.* 2007;217(1):141–154. https://doi.org/10.1111/j.1600-065X.2007.00509.x.

17. Jacocks KA, Cowell RL, Valenciano AC. Plasma cell inflammation and neoplasia. In: Norsworthy GD, ed. *The Feline Patient.* Hoboken, NJ: John Wiley and Sons, Inc.; 2018:870.

18. Mellor PJ, Haugland KC, Powell RM, et al. Histopathologic, immunohistochemical, and cytologic analysis of feline myeloma-related disorders. Further evidence for primary extramedullary development in the cat. *Vet Pathol.* 2005;45:59–173.

19. Bostrom BO, Moore AS, DeRegis CJ, et al. Canine cutaneous plasmacytosis: 21 cases (2005–2015). *JVIM.* 2017;31:1074–1080.

20. Rout ED, Shank AM, Waite AH, et al. Progression of cutaneous plasmacytoma to plasma cell leukemia in a dog. *Vet Clin Pathol.* 2017;46(1):77–84.

21. Mikiewicz M, Otrocka-Domagala I, Pazdzior-Czapula K, et al. Morphology and immunoreactivity of canine and feline extramedullary plasmacytomas. *Pol J Vet Sci.* 2016;19(2):345–352.

22. Quiroz-Rocha GF, Deravi N, Knight B, et al. What is your diagnosis? A pigmented round cell tumor. *Vet Clin Pathol.* 2017;46(3):538–539.

23. Berman PJ, Kent MS, Farese JP. Melanoma. In: Withrow SJ, DM Vail RL, eds. *Withrow and MacEwen's Small Animal Clinical Oncology.* 5th ed. St. Louis: Elsevier; 2013:321–322.

24. Smedley RC, Spangler WL, Esplin DG, et al. Prognostic markers for canine melanocytic neoplasms: a comparative review of the literature and goals for future investigation. *Vet Pathol.* 2011;48(1):54–72.

25. Moore PF. A review of histiocytic diseases of dogs and cat. *Vet Pathol.* 2014;51(1):167–184.

5

Cutaneous and Subcutaneous Lesions

David J. Fisher

Cutaneous and subcutaneous lesions are commonly sampled sites for cytological evaluation. Several reasons for this are possible, but perhaps some of the primary reasons are that these lesions are easily seen or felt by the owners of the animals and thus cause concern, and their sites are easily sampled by veterinarians. Many lesions are highly exfoliative, and skin or subcutaneous cytological samples tend to have a high diagnostic yield. In one study comparing cytological and histopathological test results of cutaneous and subcutaneous lesions in 243 specimens, diagnosis was in agreement in 90.9% of the cases.[1]

Despite the usefulness of cytological sampling, it is important to recognize that dermatological disease encompasses a broad range of inflammatory, noninflammatory, hyperplastic, and neoplastic lesions. Not all of these lesions exfoliate well, and many of the diagnoses are dependent on tissue distribution of cells, not just cytomorphological appearance. Cytology interpretation is only based on cells, organisms, and background material, but because these have no or minimal architectural arrangement, as can be evaluated in biopsy samples, the results often are less specific compared with histological interpretation (Fig. 5.1). In addition, there are instances when the cytomorphology of neoplastic cells is virtually indistinguishable from reactive or inflammatory cells (Fig. 5.2). Finally, all cytology samples have some degree of artifact, such as smudging of round cells that makes them appear spindloid, thick background material and resulting in cells shrinking and appearing more round, or artifactual aggregates of cells resembling cohesive clusters; this artifact may make it difficult to be certain about cell types in some cases.

For these reasons, histopathological analysis is often necessary for definitive diagnosis of dermatological diseases. When taking cytological samples from skin or subcutaneous lesions, it is useful to explain to the owner that the sampling process, in the best case scenario, will yield a clear-cut diagnosis, failing which it would be a preliminary step to aid in determining what needs to be done next (Table 5.1).

Although cytological evaluation is often straightforward, a better interpretation of cytological findings can often be made when all relevant clinical information is integrated. This should include signalment, history, duration, location, distribution, and other laboratory findings. If samples are to be forwarded to a clinical pathologist for review, it is important to provide this information along with the sample to allow for the best interpretation of the cytological findings. Instead of describing a lesion as a "skin" mass, it would be more helpful to describe it more completely, for example, "solitary 1 × 1 cm, round, raised, red, hairless mass confined to skin, duration 3 weeks on left pinna, in a 2-year-old Cocker spaniel dog." A clinical pathologist is likely to interpret the cytological findings for this case differently from those made in, for example, a 10-year-old dog with multiple similar-appearing lesions that had been present for several months with progressive growth.

COLLECTION TECHNIQUES

Multiple methods are used for collecting samples for cytological evaluation. These include needle aspiration, skin swabs, scrapings, and impression smears. Each method has advantages and disadvantages. For mass lesions, the most useful technique is needle aspiration

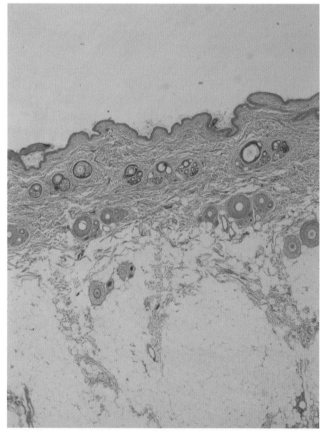

Fig. 5.1 Biopsy sample from normal skin. Skin is divided into three general areas: epidermis, dermis, and hypodermis. Adnexal structures found in skin include sebaceous glands, sweat glands, and hair follicles. The dermis contains the adnexal structures and smooth muscle, blood vessels, lymphatic vessels, collagen, and elastic fibers. This histological section shows adnexal structures in cross-section rather than longitudinally, which is related to tissue processing. The hypodermis (or subcutis) contains adipose tissue and collagen bundles. Histological diagnoses incorporate specifically what areas of the skin are being affected by inflammatory, degenerative, or neoplastic processes. This is not possible with cytological methods (hematoxylin and eosin [H&E], 2× objective).

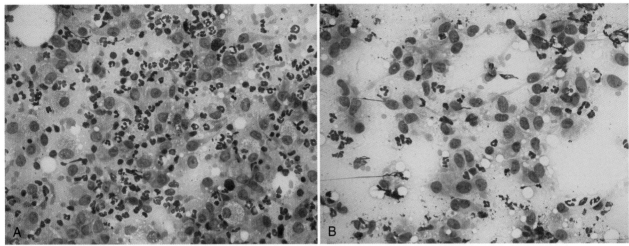

Fig. 5.2 Skin mass aspirates from two cats. (A) Skin mass near injection site present for 3 weeks. Aspirate reveals a mixture of neutrophils, small lymphocytes, larger mononuclear cells with minimally vacuolated cytoplasm, and a few mast cells. Some of the larger cells have an irregular to spindloid shape. Tissue biopsy of mass interpreted as pyogranulomatous dermatitis and panniculitis, uncertain etiology (Wright-Giemsa, 50× objective). (B) Skin mass on left thorax present for several months. Aspirate reveals a mixture of mononuclear cells, spindle cells, and neutrophils. Tissue biopsy interpreted as probable progressive histiocytosis or inflamed sarcoma (Wright-Giemsa, 50× objective).

TABLE 5.1 Cytological Findings and Follow-Up Steps

Primary Finding	Cell Types/Additional Findings	Other Findings/Conclusions	Follow-Up Steps
Low-nucleate cellularity	Acellular	Lipid droplets before staining; lipid may wash off slide during staining; possible lipoma	Continued monitoring or excision, as clinically indicated
		No lipid droplets before staining—possible cyst. Epithelial cysts usually benign. May be poorly exfoliative fibrous lesion	Diagnosis will require histopathology; however, because cystic and fibrous lesions are often benign, monitoring may be considered
	Blood	Platelets present; no erythrophagia, hemosiderin, or hematoidin	Likely blood contamination of poorly exfoliative or vascular lesion; diagnosis likely will require biopsy
		No platelets present; erythrophagia, hemosiderin, hematoidin, or all found	Likely true hemorrhage; rule out coagulopathy or trauma. May be vascular tumor, in which case diagnosis will require biopsy
Lysed cells	Only disrupted cells	Lysed cells cannot be cytologically interpreted	Evaluate smear preparation technique. Consider reaspiration. If necrosis suspected, reaspirate at the edge of lesion rather than center
Inflammatory cells	Neutrophils	Neutrophilic inflammation may occur secondary to bacterial infection as well as noninfectious causes (foreign body, keratin, immune-mediated disease)	May respond to medical therapy. If lesion is persistent and nonresponsive, surgical exploration +/– biopsy may be necessary
	Lymphocytes	Lymphocytic inflammation suggests immunological reactivity. Well-differentiated lymphoproliferative disorder should be considered	May spontaneously improve or regress. If persistent, then biopsy should be considered
	Eosinophils	Eosinophilic inflammation suggests a hypersensitivity reaction possibly caused by arthropod bite or sting. Can be seen secondary to chronic infectious agents and some tumors (particularly mast cell tumor)	May spontaneously resolve or regress. Some lesions may be corticosteroid responsive, but the possibility of fungal or protozoal infection or tumors, such as mast cell or lymphoma, should be considered
	Mixed	Mixed (pyogranulomatous, granulomatous) inflammation may be caused by chronic infectious agents but also can be secondary to foreign bodies, keratinizing cysts, immune-mediated disease	If an etiological agent cannot be identified, surgical exploration and biopsy (for both histopathology and culture) may be necessary

TABLE 5.1	Cytological Findings and Follow-Up Steps—cont'd		
Primary Finding	**Cell Types/Additional Findings**	**Other Findings/Conclusions**	**Follow-Up Steps**
Tissue cells	Minimal pleomorphism	Uniform cells, minimal pleomorphism, low mitotic rate suggest hyperplastic or benign lesion	Lack of malignant criteria does not completely exclude the possibility of malignancy, but monitoring for progression and invasiveness should be considered Mass excision should be considered, as appropriate
	Marked pleomorphism	Marked anisocytosis and anisokaryosis, open chromatin, prominent nucleoli, numerous mitotic figures, nuclear molding are features of malignancy	If large numbers of pleomorphic cells are present, malignancy should be suspected Evaluation for metastatic disease (staging) should be considered before any surgical approach
Mixed inflammatory and tissue cells	Both inflammatory cells and tissue cells are prominent	Inflammation may often cause changes in epithelial and mesenchymal cells that resemble neoplastic cells Alternatively, some tumors may cause inflammatory reactions (e.g., squamous cell carcinoma)	When prominent inflammation exists, it is difficult to ascertain the significance of tissue cells based on cytomorphology alone Surgical exploration and biopsy should be considered for further evaluation

because this allows for sampling from a variety of areas in the lesion, including cells found in deeper tissues that are not accessible by other cytological methods. Many lesions in skin and subcutaneous tissues are highly exfoliative when aspirated, and often a good cell yield is available for interpretation. Fine-needle biopsy (FNB) sampling may be done by using aspiration or nonaspiration techniques, depending on the expected degree of exfoliation and the likelihood of blood contamination. If a syringe is used to create negative pressure while the needle is embedded in the lesion of interest, then care must be taken to ensure that the pressure is released before removing the needle from the mass, because otherwise the cells may easily be lost into the syringe or surrounding normal fatty tissue may contaminate the sample. Material collected from solid masses should be carefully expelled onto a slide. A second slide or cover slip should be used to gently spread the material on the first slide into a thin layer. The sample should be allowed to air-dry before being stained with a Romanowsky-type stain. If the lesion is fluid filled, preparation of both direct and sediment smears of the fluid may be useful, but typically a complete fluid analysis (i.e., protein concentration, cell count, differential in addition to cytology) is not necessary for evaluation, and cytology alone generally will indicate whether an inflammatory, noninflammatory, or neoplastic process is present. If a solid mass is associated with a fluid-filled lesion, then the solid areas and the fluid areas of the mass should be sampled.

If the lesion is not amenable to aspiration (e.g., superficial, fistulous), then other sampling techniques such as scrapings, impression smears, or swabs should be considered. Scrapings are collected by rubbing the edge of a scalpel or spatula across the lesion and then spreading the accumulated material onto a slide. Impression smears are made by pressing the surface of a slide against the lesion with several imprints made on separate areas of the slides. If excess fluid or blood is on the surface of the lesion, then the lesion should be blotted dry before sampling. Swab samples are most commonly collected from a mucosal surface, such as the vaginal cavity. Using a sterile cotton swab, material is collected from the site of interest. After sample collection, the swab is gently rolled (not rubbed) along the surface of a slide.

Samples collected by using these latter methods may only demonstrate surface abnormalities and not underlying pathology. If a lesion is ulcerated, a swab or impression smear likely will reveal neutrophils, blood, protein, debris, and possibly some microorganisms, but these are all nonspecific findings that should be expected from an ulcerated surface. Nevertheless, with superficial or exudative lesions, these types of samples may be useful for demonstrating microorganisms, including mites, bacteria, yeast, fungal hyphae, and protozoal organisms.

GROSS APPEARANCE

Knowledge of the gross appearance of skin and subcutaneous masses is helpful in interpreting cytological findings. Descriptions of gross appearance should include location, distribution, size, shape, color, haired versus nonhaired, sessile versus pedunculated, intact epithelium versus ulceration, mobility, firmness, and duration and growth characteristics, when known. The gross appearance of the mass may aid in limiting the types of lesions that need to be considered cytologically.

GENERAL CYTOLOGICAL EVALUATION

The approach to cytological evaluation of skin and subcutaneous lesions is similar to that of other tissues. Multiple slides should be prepared for review by using standard smear preparation techniques. For the most part, cytology smears need only be stained with a Romanowsky-type stain (Wright, Wright-Giemsa, and quick stains, such as Diff-Quik). In some instances, additional stains may be required, particularly if it is thought that rare or difficult-to-see microorganisms may be present. In this circumstance, other stains, such as acid-fast stain for *Mycobacterium* or *Nocardia* and Gomori methenamine silver (GMS) or periodic acid–Schiff (PAS) stains for fungal organisms may help find these organisms. For this reason, it may be useful to leave some slides unstained in case additional staining is needed. It is possible, however, to destain slides and then restain them with a variety of different special stains and achieve adequate staining quality for interpretation.[2]

Slides should first be reviewed at low power (4–10× objective) to assess the adequacy of the smear. Degree of cellularity, adequate separation of cells, thickness of smear, and good staining quality are some of the factors that should be evaluated. The entire smear area should be reviewed on low power to review for the presence of any large structures, such as infrequent cell clusters or large fungal organisms (e.g., *Coccidioides* spherules) that could be missed with a higher-power lens. The low-power scan should also help identify areas where a higher-power review may be useful to evaluate cytomorphology.

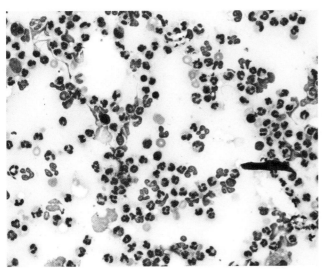

Fig. 5.3 Neutrophilic inflammation is characterized by the predominance of neutrophils (Wright stain).

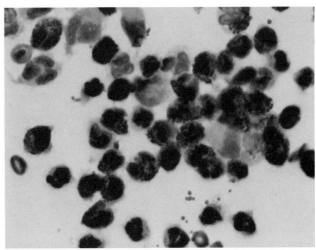

Fig. 5.4 Fine-needle aspirate from subcutaneous swelling in a dog. Mixed inflammatory cells are present, but the majority are eosinophils. Fewer macrophages and neutrophils are also noted (Wright-Giemsa, 100× objective).

Most cytological abnormalities may be seen with a good 50× oil immersion objective lens. This lens is preferable to a 40× high-dry lens, although this latter lens is an adequate alternative. The 100× oil lens is needed only to confirm small structures, such as bacteria, intercellular granules or inclusions, and small fungal spores or protozoa.

Once the adequacy of the smear has been assessed, a determination may then be made about the pathological process. On initial review, a definitive diagnosis may be made purely on the basis of the cells, any organisms present, or both. Many times, however, a clear-cut, definitive answer is not based on cytology findings alone. In these cases, a systematic approach should be taken to narrow down differentials and, just as importantly, make a decision about what the next diagnostic or therapeutic step needs to be (see Table 5.1). A consistent approach includes thorough review of all areas of the sample and then systematic classification of the type of pathological process and likely etiologies. In general, if a mass lesion is aspirated and only tissue cells are collected, then the lesion is caused by either hyperplasia or neoplasia. If only inflammatory cells are present, then the underlying cause may be determined to be infectious or noninfectious, keeping in mind that some tumors may elicit an inflammatory response. Mixtures of inflammatory and tissue cells may be difficult to interpret for this reason, in addition to the fact that inflammation may induce morphological changes in tissue cells.

INFLAMMATORY CELLS

Sampling from inflammatory lesions tends to yield large numbers of cells, often with no obvious tissue cells. Inflammatory lesions may result from infectious and noninfectious causes. Noninfectious inflammatory diseases may ultimately require histopathological analysis to further investigate underlying causes, such as immune-mediated skin disease. The types of inflammatory cells that are present, however, may aid in determining the underlying process.

Samples with primarily neutrophils are often referred to as displaying neutrophilic, suppurative, or purulent inflammation (Fig. 5.3). The neutrophils should be characterized as "well preserved" or "showing some signs of degeneration." Degenerative changes in neutrophils include nuclear swelling with paler-staining chromatin (karyolysis). Severely degenerate neutrophils may have round nuclei, and the cell type may be virtually unrecognizable. Degenerative changes are not pathognomonic for infection but should raise clinical suspicion of infection.

Neutrophilic inflammation is often caused by bacterial infection but may also be seen with fungal or yeast infection and noninfectious problems.

Samples with mostly small lymphocytes are characterized as lymphocytic inflammation, reactivity, or both. Increased numbers of mature lymphocytes suggest immunological reactivity or chronic inflammation. This pattern is often seen with vaccine reactions or arthropod bites or stings. Increased numbers of eosinophils are also noted on occasion. When lymphocytic infiltrates are persistent or progressive, a chronic lymphoproliferative disorder needs to be considered, but biopsy and analysis of these infiltrates will be required for diagnosis. Even with histopathological analysis, some well-differentiated lymphoproliferative disorders may require additional testing, including immunophenotyping and clonality assays, to aid in distinguishing between inflammatory and neoplastic populations.

Eosinophilic inflammation (Fig. 5.4) in skin has similar considerations as in other tissues. In skin, it is often related to a hypersensitivity response to the bite or sting of an arthropod (e.g., flea, bee, spider, or tick). Other parasites, including mites and nematodes, may also cause eosinophilic inflammation. It is sometimes noted as a component of inflammation secondary to infection, possibly more commonly with fungal infection, and may also be seen as a component of reaction to some vaccines. Solid masses or linear plaques with large numbers of eosinophils may be an eosinophilic granuloma, but care must be taken to rule out infectious agents or neoplasia because an eosinophilic infiltrate may also be seen as a paraneoplastic response to some tumors, most notably mast cell neoplasia and others, including lymphoma.

Granulomatous inflammation and *pyogranulomatous inflammation* are terms that should be reserved for histopathological diagnosis because these are associated with a specific type of inflammatory cell arrangement in tissues. Nevertheless, these terms are used by some cytopathologists as well. Others will use *chronic inflammation, macrophagic inflammation,* or *mixed cell inflammation.* These terms imply that macrophages are present, with some mixture of lymphocytes and possibly other cells, including sheets of epithelioid macrophages and multinucleate cells (Fig. 5.5). This type of inflammation typically is associated with chronic inflammatory disorders, and these often involve chronic infectious agents, such as higher bacteria (*Actinomyces, Nocardia,* and *Mycobacterium* spp.), fungal or protozoal organisms, or noninfectious agents, such as foreign bodies. If nothing else, this type of inflammation indicates the lesion may be unresponsive to routine antibiotic therapy alone.

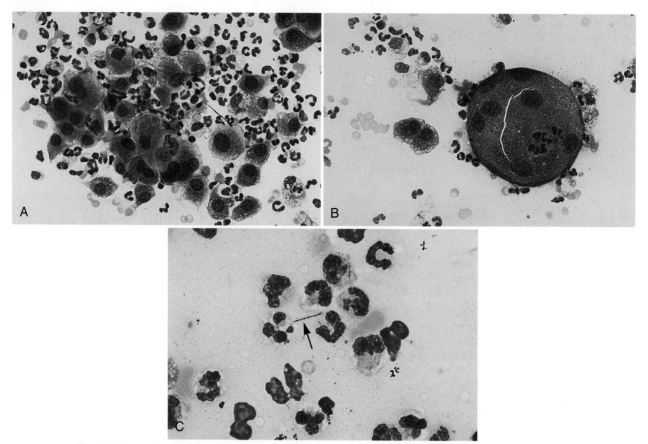

Fig. 5.5 Impression smears of a pyogranulomatous nodule in a dog. (A) Pyogranulomatous inflammation includes a mixture of neutrophils and macrophages, with the macrophages often noted in sheets (Diff-Quik, original magnification 160×). (B) Multinucleate inflammatory giant cell with scattered neutrophils and macrophages from the same lesion shown in image A (Diff-Quik, original magnification 132×). (C) Long, slender, filamentous bacterial rod *(arrow)* present among inflammatory cells (Diff-Quik, original magnification 400×).

INFECTIOUS AGENTS

Many types of infectious agents, including mites, fungi, protozoa, and bacteria, may be seen with cutaneous and subcutaneous lesions. All of these organisms may be seen either through Romanowsky staining or as a nonstaining outline. Nonstaining organisms sometimes may be highlighted with other stains.

Bacteria
Superficial or Deep Pyoderma and Bacterial Abscesses

Bacterial infection of the skin may present as surface or superficial disease or deep pyoderma. Infection may be caused by primary skin disease but may also occur secondary to bite or puncture wounds. In addition, cystic lesions and tumors may become secondarily infected, particularly if ulcerated. When stained with a Romanowsky-type stain, most bacteria will stain blue to purple, similar to chromatin. Bacterial organisms tend to be uniform in size and shape, and this is helpful in distinguishing them from particulate debris, which tends to be irregular. Further characterization of bacterial organisms may be done with Gram staining, but definitive identification requires culture. Both aerobic and anaerobic culture should be considered for subcutaneous infections.

Surface or superficial pyoderma presents with skin surface abnormalities, including pustules, papules, crusts, and erythema. Bacteria may be identified with impression smears or scrapings, but these techniques potentially could miss other underlying disease. Deeper pyoderma results from infection extending deeper into follicular tissue,

resulting in nodules and abscesses. The most common bacterial pathogen for superficial and deep pyoderma is *Staphylococcus intermedius* (Fig. 5.6, A); however, other secondary invaders may also exist, and in chronic cases, bacterial culture and sensitivity may be advisable.[3] Bacterial infection may occur as a consequence of a bite or other penetrating wound. These often result in a mixed infection with both aerobic and anaerobic organisms (see Fig. 5.6, B).

Mycobacterium spp.

Mycobacterial infection manifests in several different forms, including slow-growing tuberculous; lepromatous, cutaneous nodular; slow-growing, nontuberculous, cutaneous; and fast-growing, cutaneous and subcutaneous. All of these forms may result in cutaneous lesions. Disseminated infection may also occur, particularly with tuberculous disease. Cutaneous lesions include draining nodules, ulceration, and nodules.[3] Definitive identification of organisms requires specialized culture for both rapid growers and slow growers. In some cases, polymerase chain reaction (PCR) testing of tissue samples may be helpful.

Specific types of mycobacterial infection that is separate from tuberculous disease include canine leproid granuloma, feline leprosy syndrome, and rapid-growing mycobacterial panniculitis. Canine leproid granuloma presents as localized nodular skin disease typically involving the pinna or other head region. Aspiration reveals mixed cell inflammation with readily observable nonstaining rods found in macrophages as well as free in the background. Infection is reported most

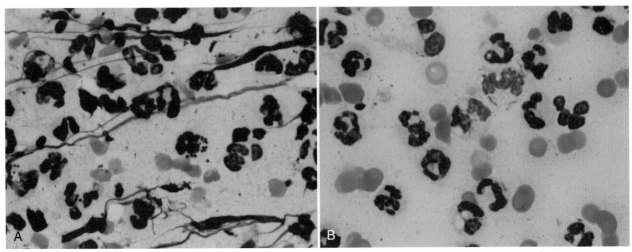

Fig. 5.6 Samples from areas with septic inflammation. (A) Most cells are degenerating neutrophils. Some contain phagocytized bacterial cocci. Streaming nuclear material is also present in addition to scattered erythrocytes (Wright-Giemsa stain, 100× objective). (B) This sample also contains many degenerating neutrophils as well as erythrocytes. Many of the neutrophils contain thin rods in the cytoplasm. Some bacteria appear to be free in the background. The organisms suggest the infection is secondary to a bite wound, foreign body, or other penetrating wound (Wright-Giemsa, 100× objective).

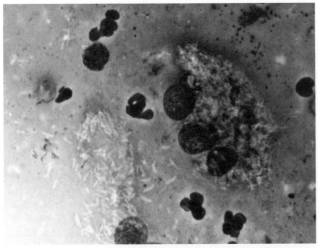

Fig. 5.7 Aspirate from a canine leproid granuloma. Large numbers of nonstaining short bacterial rods (mycobacteria) are seen within a multinucleate cell. Numerous rods are also free in the background, as well as scattered neutrophils and free nuclear material. The nonstaining rods must be distinguished from artifact or other debris and can be confirmed as bacterial organisms with an acid-fast stain (*not shown*) (Wright-Giemsa, 100× objective).

commonly in short-coated breeds. Feline leprosy syndrome presents as nodular skin disease with organisms that are difficult (or impossible) to culture. The syndrome presents variably, depending on age and sex, with different *Mycobacteria* identified by molecular methods. Finally, rapid-growing *Mycobacteria* may cause cutaneous granulomas and fistulae in dogs and cats. Lesions may occur anywhere but are most common in the inguinal or lumbar region.[3,4]

In cytological samples, *Mycobacterium* spp. may be seen, on rare occasions, as filamentous organisms but are more commonly found as short rods. Mycobacterial organisms do not stain with Romanowsky stains because of their thick lipid walls. They still may be readily identifiable on Romanowsky-stained slides as nonstaining short rods, often noted in macrophages (Fig. 5.7). These organisms will stain positive (pink to red) with an acid-fast stain.

Actinomyces spp. and *Nocardia* spp.

These organisms are often associated with chronic draining or nodular lesions. Infection is typically secondary to a bite wound or a penetrating injury by a foreign body. These filamentous bacteria are often branching and may be found in thick mats on smear preparations. *Actinomyces* and *Nocardia* spp. sometimes stain poorly with Romanowsky stains and may only be noted as a faint outline, often best visualized in the cytoplasm of epithelioid macrophages (Fig. 5.8, A). When stained, they are light blue in color with an intermittent pink beading appearance. *Nocardia* spp. also may be partially acid-fast positive, which may help distinguish them from *Actinomyces* spp. (see Fig. 5.8, B). Culture is required to definitively identify these organisms.

Yeast, Fungi, and Algae
Malassezia pachydermatitis

Overgrowth of these organisms typically occurs on the skin surface and usually is not associated with a significant exudative process. These yeast are small (3–8 micrometers [μm] diameter) and typically shaped like a "footprint" (Fig. 5.9). They are considered normal flora of skin, so just finding a few does not necessarily indicate abnormality. Greater than two organisms per 100× field has been suggested as indicative of overgrowth.[3] It is not unusual to find large numbers of organisms and large numbers of anucleate squames but minimal to no evidence for inflammation. Overgrowth of these organisms is usually thought to be secondary to other diseases, such as skin allergies, seborrhea, bacterial pyoderma, and skin conformation problems, or secondary to antibiotic use.

Dermatophytes

Dermatophyte infections may manifest in varying ways. In dogs, infection typically manifests as expanding annular areas of alopecia, scales, and crusts. Infection may be localized but may also be seen occasionally with extensive skin involvement. Infection may sometimes result in a solid, raised, nodular lesion, referred to as a *kerion*. In cats, infection usually causes one or more areas of annular to irregular alopecia with or without scales. Skin impressions or scrapings from the edge of annular lesions typically will demonstrate cellular debris and mixed inflammation, including neutrophils, macrophages, lymphocytes, and

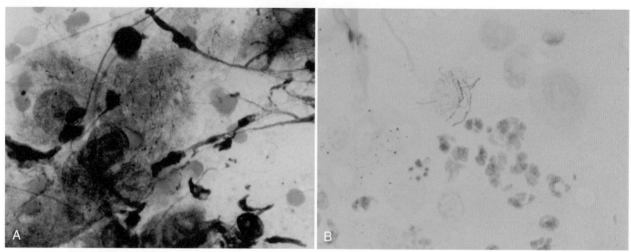

Fig. 5.8 Fine-needle aspirate from a draining nodule in a cat. (A) Large epithelioid macrophages or spindle cells mixed with degenerating cells and nuclear debris. Thin, beaded, branching bacterial rods are present and particularly evident in the cytoplasm of the central cell (Wright-Giemsa, 100× objective). (B) Slide stained with acid-fast stain. Note pink staining thin branching organisms in cell cytoplasm supporting the diagnosis of *Nocardia* spp. infection. Mycobacterial organisms more typically are short rods but, on rare occasions, may be filamentous, and definitive identification as *Nocardia* requires culture. *Actinomyces* spp. may appear morphologically similar as in image A but do not stain with acid-fast stain (100× objective).

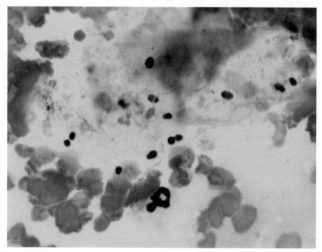

Fig. 5.9 *Malassezia* pachydermatitis from a skin lesion on a dog. Numerous small oval to "footprint"-shaped organisms are noted associated with squamous debris. Large numbers of erythrocytes are also present, as well as a single neutrophil in the lower central region (Wright-Giemsa, 100× objective).

eosinophils. Accumulations of hair follicle structures and, particularly around these areas, small fungal spores may be found, sometimes in dense aggregates (Fig. 5.10). On rare occasions, septate hyphae may be found. Similar findings may be noted with aspiration of kerion lesions. The causative agents for dermatophytosis are most commonly *Microsporum canis*, *M. gyseum*, and *Trichophyton mentagrophytes*. Fungal culture is required to definitively identify the organism.

Histoplasma capsulatum

Infection with this organism typically causes systemic disease, and animals may present with a variety of clinical signs, including fever, weight loss, anorexia, coughing, and gastrointestinal (GI) signs. Infection may also cause cutaneous lesions that are characterized by papules, nodules, ulcers, and draining tracts. Impression smears from oozing tracts or fine-needle aspirate of nodular lesions reveal mixed inflammation

with variable numbers of small (2–4 μm diameter) round yeast, with a thin nonstaining capsule and a basophilic nucleus that often is crescent shaped (Fig. 5.11). These organisms may be noted free in the background and may be phagocytized by macrophages and neutrophils.

Sporothrix schenckii

Infection by this agent may cause cutaneous, cutaneolymphatic, or disseminated lesions. In dogs, cutaneous lesions often occur on the head or trunk and typically present as nodules. These may ulcerate with purulent discharge and crusts. In cats, draining tracts are typically noted on distal limbs, head, or tail base. Samples from these sites typically reveal neutrophilic to mixed inflammation, with variable numbers of yeast organisms noted in the macrophages, in the neutrophils, and in the background. In particular, cats often will have large numbers of organisms in discharge material, and for this reason cats with this infection need to be handled with caution to prevent zoonotic spread. The yeast organisms are pleomorphic in shape, varying from round to oval to cigar shape, 2 to 10 μm in length, and 1 to 3 μm wide (Fig. 5.12). Although similar in size to *Histoplasma*, *Sporothrix* may be distinguished by its variety of shapes.

Blastomyces dermatitidis

Clinical signs associated with blastomycosis include anorexia, weight loss, cough, ocular disease, lameness, and skin lesions. Skin lesions may be found in up to 40% of cases.[3] These lesions include firm papules, nodules, plaques, ulcers, draining tracts, and abscesses. Material for cytological evaluation may be collected from draining tracts or aspirated from nodules or abscesses. These samples reveal neutrophilic to mixed inflammation with variable numbers of organisms. These are dimorphic fungi, which are typically found in the yeast phase in infected animals, although on rare occasion they may form hyphae in tissues.[5] The yeast organisms are variably sized (5.20 μm in diameter), with a thick, blue wall and a thin, nonstaining capsule (Fig. 5.13). Occasionally, broad-based budding will be seen, which is useful in distinguishing from *Cryptococcus*. Blastomyces are larger than *Histoplasma* and *Sporothrix* but typically smaller than *Coccidioides* spherules.

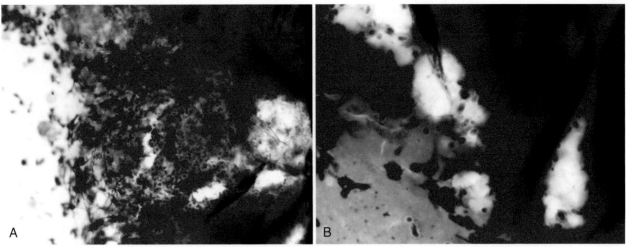

Fig. 5.10 Aspirate from a dermatophytic kerion in a dog. (A) Large numbers of small, round to slightly oval fungal spores are in the center of the figure. The spores have a small nonstaining capsule and are surrounded by a large amount of nuclear material primarily from degenerating neutrophils. Small fragments of hair are noted at the right (Wright-Giemsa, 50× objective). (B) Same lesion with 100× objective. Note the mild variation in spore shape and as the diffuse stippled internal appearance (Wright-Giemsa).

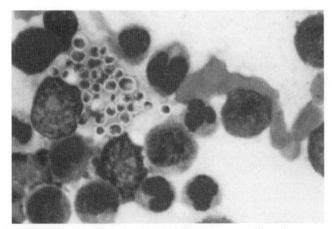

Fig. 5.11 A large macrophage containing numerous *Histoplasma capsulatum* organisms is shown (Wright stain).

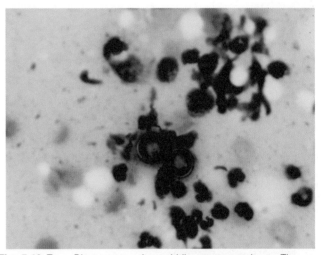

Fig. 5.13 Two *Blastomyces dermatitidis* yeast organisms. They are adjacent to one another. When budding is present *(not shown)*, it is thick and broad based. The organisms tend to be uniform in size, stain deep stippled blue, and have a thin nonstaining capsule. Scattered degenerating neutrophils, lymphocytes, macrophages, and nuclear debris are also present (Wright-Giemsa, 100× objective).

Cryptococcus spp.

Cryptococcosis is most commonly associated with nasal signs (sneezing, snuffling, nasal discharge) in cats and central nervous system (CNS) or ocular signs in dogs. Both species may also have skin lesions, which are more common in cats. The skin lesions may occur as solitary lesions or as part of disseminated disease. Lesions include papules, nodules, ulcers, abscesses, and draining tracts. Sampling from these lesions often reveals large numbers of organisms. These are yeast organisms that are round in shape (occasionally fusiform) and variably sized (2–20 μm in diameter). The organisms stain pale pink to purple and often have a granular appearance. They typically have a large nonstaining capsule, which may be up to 40 μm in diameter (Fig. 5.14). Only smaller yeast organisms with thinner capsules are sometimes found, and thus lack of a thick capsule should not be used to rule out *Cryptococcus* spp. infection. On occasion, narrow-based budding, which is a useful diagnostic feature, may be seen. Minimal

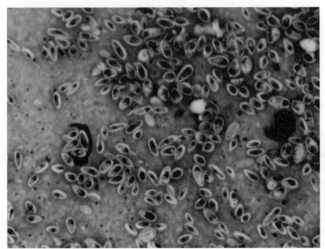

Fig. 5.12 Impression smear from a draining lesion in a cat with *Sporothrix schenckii* infection. Large numbers of small pleomorphic yeast are present. The yeast vary from round to cigar-shaped, with a thin, nonstaining capsule. A small lymphocyte is seen to the right (Wright-Giemsa, 100× objective).

associated inflammation may be present, in which case it is typically granulomatous. The etiological agent is typically *Cryptococcus neoformans;* however, *Cryptococcus gattii* has emerged as another pathogen occurring in the tropical and subtropical regions of Australia, South America, Southeast Asia, and Africa, as well as in the North American Pacific Northwest.[6] Morphological features do not distinguish these two species.

Coccidioides immitis

Infection with this organism usually causes lung disease but may disseminate systemically and cause skin involvement. Skin lesions may occur as subcutaneous nodules or draining tracts. Cytological preparations from these lesions typically contain large numbers of inflammatory cells, including neutrophils and macrophages. The organisms are often scarce, and not finding an organism does not rule out infection. When present, the organisms are usually found as spherules, which are

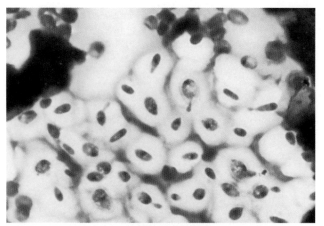

Fig. 5.14 *Cryptococcus* spp. are spherical yeast that frequently have a thick, nonstaining mucoid capsule. Organism size may vary, and the thick capsule is not always present. Narrow-based budding is a characteristic feature. This figure has numerous budding and nonbudding organisms with prominent thick capsules (Wright stain).

variable in size but may be large (10–100 μm in diameter) (Fig. 5.15). Because of the large size and low numbers of spherules in a sample, these are often easiest to find at low-power (4–10×) scans and may be missed if microscopic examination is only done at high power. The spherules have a thick, blue wall with a finely granular internal appearance (endospores). It is often necessary to focus up and down to see the internal detail because of the thickness of the spherules relative to the accompanying cells. On rare occasions, small (2–5 μm) endospores may be seen free in the background or phagocytized by cells. The smaller-sized spherules may be mistaken for *Blastomyces,* but *Coccidioides* spherules do not show budding.

Opportunistic Fungi

Many different fungal organisms may infect animals and cause either localized or disseminated skin disease and systemic disease. The terminology applied to these infections is complex and beyond the scope of what is possible to diagnose via cytology alone. Fungal skin infections typically present with chronic draining lesions or nodules. Animals with these infections frequently are immunocompromised or have a history of immunosuppressive therapy. Cytological samples from these lesions will typically reveal pyogranulomatous to granulomatous inflammation. Some cases will also have increased numbers of eosinophils. When organisms are present, usually they occur as hyphal segments (Fig. 5.16), although on occasion conidial structures may be found. Categories of opportunistic fungal infection include pheohyphomycosis (pigmented septate hyphae), hyalohyphomycosis (nonpigmented septate hyphae), mycetoma (localized nodular infections), and zygomycosis (broad, poorly septate hyphae). The structure of the hyphae (septate versus nonseptate; pigmented versus nonpigmented; hyphal width) may be helpful in suggesting a particular species of fungus, but as a rule, fungal culture is necessary to definitively identify the organism.

Pythium insidiosum

Pythium spp. are not true fungi but are water molds that infect dogs more commonly than cats. Infection results in GI signs but may also cause cutaneous lesions. Infection usually is thought to occur from

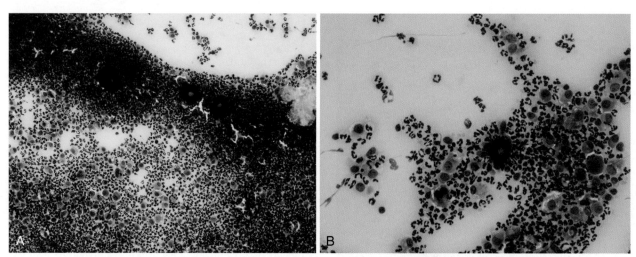

Fig. 5.15 *Coccidioides immitis* spherules, which are large, spherical structures with a thick wall and stippled blue internal appearance. (A) Low-power magnification from draining cutaneous lesion in a cat. Three large dark-blue spherules are found with marked pyogranulomatous inflammation. The spherules are thick walled and usually keep a three-dimensional shape on cytology smears. Because of this, it is usually not possible to see the spherules sharply in focus in the same plane of focus as the inflammatory cells. Focusing up and down can aid in showing the thick spherule wall and the stippled internal appearance (Wright-Giemsa, 10× objective). (B) Same lesion as image A under higher magnification (Wright-Giemsa, 20× objective).

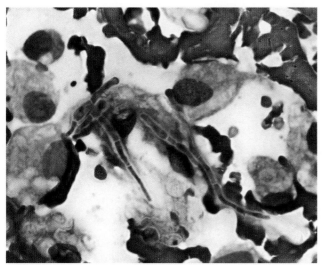

Fig. 5.16 Fungal hyphae and granulomatous inflammation are shown (Wright stain).

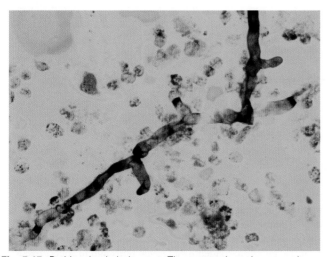

Fig. 5.17 *Pythium* hyphal element. These organisms have poorly septated, branching hyphae with relatively parallel walls ranging in diameter from 2 to 7 micrometers (μm). The hyphae stain poorly or not at all with Romanowsky stain and are easy to miss with routine cytological staining. If infection is suspected, then Gomori methenamine silver (GMS) staining should be performed. Periodic acid–Schiff (PAS) does not stain this organism (GMS, 50× objective).

standing in or drinking infected water. Cutaneous lesions often involve the extremities and typically are ulcerated nodules with draining tracts. Cytological samples from these lesions reveal mixed inflammation, usually with an eosinophilic component. When organisms are present, they are found as poorly staining, broad, poorly septate hyphae ranging from 2 to 7 μm in diameter. The hyphae do not stain well with Romanowsky stains but are easily visualized with GMS stain (Fig. 5.17). A related organism that also may cause skin infections, *Lagenidium* spp., has hyphae with broader (diameter ranging from 25–40 μm) and more irregular or bulbous hyphae than *Pythium*. Definitive identification of these organisms may require a combination of fungal culture, serology testing, and biopsy with immunohistochemical testing and other molecular diagnostics.[3]

Prototheca spp.

Prototheca spp., which are colorless algae that are ubiquitous in the southern regions of the United States, only rarely cause disease. In

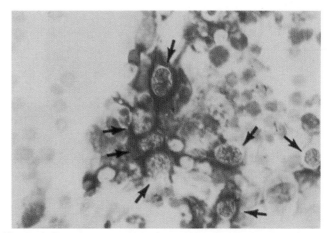

Fig. 5.18 *Prototheca* organisms *(arrows)* are round to oval and have a granular basophilic cytoplasm and a clear cell wall (Wright stain).

dogs, infection is often disseminated, but only cutaneous protothecosis has been reported in cats.[3] Cutaneous protothecosis is caused by *Prototheca wickerhamii* in both dogs and cats, whereas disseminated infections in dogs is almost always caused by *Prototheca zopfii*. Dermatological lesions include multiple papules and nodules, often over pressure points, or nodules and ulcers involving the mucocutaneous junctions (especially nostrils), scrotum, and footpads. Samples from these lesions reveal mixed cell to granulomatous inflammation, with few to numerous organisms. The organisms are found as spherules or cells (Fig. 5.18), which are round to oval and 2 to 30 μm in diameter. The organisms reproduce by endosporulation, and most commonly two to four (occasionally up to 20) endospores are visible inside the spherule. Most organisms are extracellular, but smaller organisms may be phagocytized by macrophages or neutrophils.

OTHER INFECTIOUS AGENTS

Leishmania spp.

Leishmaniasis is a disease caused by protozoal infection. It is caused by a variety of *Leishmania* species. *Leishmania* spp. infection is most commonly seen in the Mediterranean region but has also been reported elsewhere, including in the United States. Infection with this organism occurs more commonly in dogs than in cats. Skin lesions occur commonly in animals infected with *Leishmania* spp. This is typically an exfoliative dermatitis that may be generalized. Other dermatological lesions may also be seen. Other clinical findings include weight loss, muscle wasting, cachexia, intermittent fever, lameness, and lymphadenopathy, among other signs. Diagnosis may be aided by identifying the amastigotes in cytological samples. Unless nodular skin lesions are present, it may be difficult to find organisms in cytology samples from skin. Diagnosis is often made by finding organisms in draining lymph nodes or internal organs. Amastigotes are ovoid to round, 2.5 to 5 × 1.5 to 2.0 μm in size, and may be found in macrophages as well as free in the background (Fig. 5.19). They have a small nucleus, with a characteristic small, rod-shaped structure adjacent to the nucleus (kinetoplast). Although unusual, other protozoal organisms may cause cutaneous lesions also.[7] The kinetoplast aids in distinguishing this organism from other protozoal organisms or small yeasts, such as *Histoplasma* spp.

Parasites

Ectoparasites are a common cause of skin disease in both dogs and cats. Ectoparasites include fleas and mites. The diagnosis is based on a history of pruritus, direct observation of the organisms (fleas), or observation via microscopic examination of skin scraping material

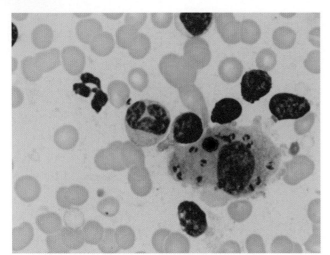

Fig. 5.19 Moderate numbers of *Leishmania* spp. organisms within a macrophage. Note the small, bar-shaped kinetoplast next to the organism nucleus. Two lymphocytes, one neutrophil, one monocyte, and several bare nuclei are also present (Wright-Giemsa, 100× objective).

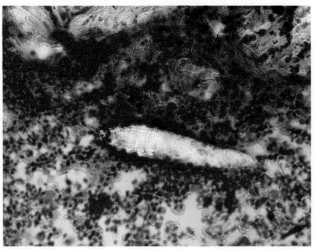

Fig. 5.20 Skin scraping from dog with chronic skin disease, including alopecia, crusts, and scaling. An adult *Demodex* spp. mite is in the center of the figure (nonstained). It is surrounded by large numbers of degenerating neutrophils and abundant cellular debris, as well as erythrocytes. The cellular elements are out of focus, as the large mite is not in the same focal plane (Wright-Giemsa, 20× objective, condenser down).

(mites). The details of mite identification are beyond the scope of a cytology textbook, and readers are referred to any veterinary parasitology text for specifics of mite identification. *Demodex* spp. are sometimes noted in superficial skin samples, including impression smears or superficial scrapings, and it is important to note that on occasion, the outline of these organisms may be seen and should not be ignored as just nonstaining debris (Fig. 5.20).

In addition to ectoparasites, other types of parasites, including different types of helminths, may also cause skin disease. Types of skin disease caused by helminths include hookworm dermatitis, *Pelodera* spp. dermatitis, *Strongyloides stercoralis*–like infection, cutaneous larval migrans, schistosomiasis, dracunculiasis,[8] and filarial infections (*Dirofilaria immitis*, *Dirofilaria repens*, *Onchocerca* spp.). Diagnosis of these conditions is often dependent on history, lesion distribution, environmental exposure, and biopsy, but on occasion, cytological methods, such as skin scraping (*Pelodera* spp. larvae) or fine-needle aspiration (Fig. 5.21) may yield a diagnosis.[9,10]

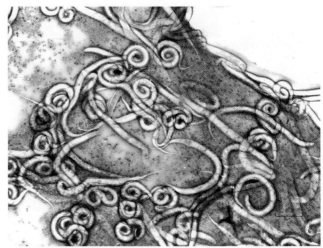

Fig. 5.21 Aspirate from subcutaneous mass in a cat. Large numbers of poorly staining curved to spiraled nematode larvae are found enmeshed in a thick background of degenerating leukocytes, predominantly neutrophils with fewer eosinophils. Findings are most consistent with *Dracunculus* spp. Cytological features that aid in identification include striated cuticle (difficult to observe in this photo) and a long, narrow, pointed tail (Wright-Giemsa). (Slide courtesy Dr. D. DeNicola, IDEXX Laboratories.)

NONINFECTIOUS INFLAMMATORY LESIONS

Inflammation in skin may occur for reasons other than infection. Inflammation may occur secondary to foreign bodies, penetrating wounds, arthropod bite or sting, trauma, allergy, immune-mediated disease, cystic lesions, and inflammation secondary to neoplastic lesions related to necrosis or a paraneoplastic effect. Noninfectious inflammatory lesions may be well-encapsulated, discrete subcutaneous lesions that are not responsive to antibiotic therapy or drainage alone. Neutrophilic, pyogranulomatous, eosinophilic, and granulomatous types of lesions are seen. Definitively diagnosing these lesions often is dependent on ruling out other underlying or systemic diseases and surgical exploration to identify a foreign body and to collect tissue for purposes of both histopathological analysis and culture.

Noninfectious inflammatory lesions may also present with nonnodular or masslike lesions. These lesions may present as macules, papules, pustules, wheals, scales, crusts, pigmentary abnormalities, plaques, excoriations or ulcerations, fissures, and draining tracts. These nonnodular lesions are the type in which cytological methods may only offer limited, if any, diagnostic information. In many instances, the distribution of the inflammatory cells in the tissue (e.g., follicular, perifollicular, vascular, epidermis–dermis interface), as well as other findings, such as edema, fibrosis, and clotting, are all important findings that help characterize disease processes, all of which are not identifiable by using cytological methods.

Injection Site and Foreign Body Reactions

Inflammatory reactions at the site of injections, most typically vaccinations, are not uncommon. Even with an unclear history of injection, these may be suspected if a nodular lesion develops in an area associated with vaccination or injection (e.g., intrascapular, hindlimb muscles). These may occur within days to several weeks after injection. Aspiration from these lesions typically is moderately cellular, with a thin proteinaceous background. Usually, a mixed inflammatory process, including lymphocytes, macrophages, and variable numbers of eosinophils and neutrophils, is present. Low numbers of moderate- to large-sized spindle cells are also usually present. Most characteristically, aspiration often will reveal abundant pink to purple, globular to amorphous material, which may be noted as being free in the background as well as in macrophages (Fig. 5.22). On occasion, the globular-to-amorphous material may be blue in color, rather than pink or purple. In cats, it may be difficult to cytologically distinguish vaccine reactions from vaccine-associated sarcomas; if a mass persists (>3 months) in the area of vaccination, then biopsy specimens should be obtained for histopathologic evaluation.

Sterile Panniculitis

Panniculitis refers to inflammation of subcutaneous fat, which results in deep cutaneous and subcutaneous nodules that may become cystic and ulcerated. The etiology is multifactorial, and this inflammation may occur in both dogs and cats. It may occur secondary to infectious agents but also from noninfectious processes and thus may be sterile.

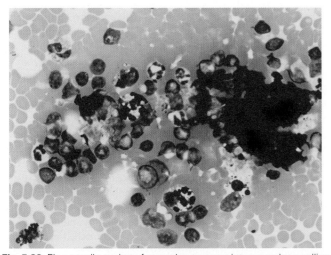

Fig. 5.22 Fine-needle aspirate from subcutaneous interscapular swelling in a dog with recent history of vaccination at the site. Mixed inflammatory cells, including small lymphocytes, macrophages, fewer neutrophils, and rare eosinophils, are present. Aggregates of globular purple material are noted extracellularly as well as irregular globular purple material in macrophages (Wright-Giemsa, 50× objective).

Noninfectious causes include trauma, foreign body, pancreatic disease, vitamin E deficiency, immune-mediated disorders, adverse drug reactions, and idiopathic disease. Aspirates from these lesions often will have large amounts of nuclear and cellular debris admixed with free lipid and a proteinaceous background. This material is sometimes noted in dense aggregates, and it may be difficult to discern intact cells. When inflammatory cells are found, they include variable numbers of neutrophils, macrophages, multinucleate inflammatory cells, and a few small lymphocytes (Fig. 5.23). A few spindle cells may also be present. Because of the large amount of cellular debris that is often present, it may be difficult to rule out whether bacteria or other organisms are present, and culture should be considered before therapy with immunosuppressive drugs.

Allergic Reactions and Arthropod Bites or Stings

Aspirates from these lesions are typically predominated by eosinophils with lower numbers of small lymphocytes as well as a few neutrophils and macrophages. A few to a moderate number of mast cells and spindle cells may also be present. In some cases, in which a moderate number of mast cells are present, it may be difficult to cytologically distinguish mast cell tumor from an arthropod bite or sting. If a moderate number of mast cells exist and the lesion is persistent, then biopsy and histopathological analysis should be considered for further evaluation.

Eosinophilic Granuloma

Eosinophilic granulomas are most common in cats but may also occur in dogs. In cats, these occur in different forms, including indolent ulcer (mucocutaneous and oral mucosal ulcerative lesion), eosinophilic plaque (plaque lesions on ventral abdomen and medial thigh), and eosinophilic granuloma (linear raised lesions on caudal thigh, face, or oral cavity). Diagnosis is typically based on the gross appearance. Samples from these lesions are predominated by eosinophils, but other mixed inflammatory cells and a few spindle cells may be present.

Reactive Histiocytosis

This is an uncommon disorder that occurs in dogs and is characterized by proliferation of dermal dendritic cells (histiocytes).[11] Two general forms occur: cutaneous and systemic. Both forms primarily result in cutaneous and subcutaneous lesions. The systemic form also has

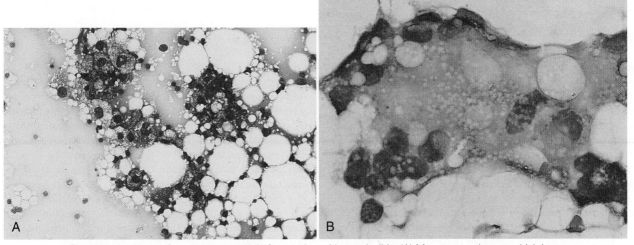

Fig. 5.23 Aspirates of a cutaneous nodule from a dog with panniculitis. (A) Many macrophages, which have foamy appearances from phagocytizing lipids, are scattered among lipid droplets (Wright stain, original magnification 100 are present). (B) Higher magnification of epithelioid macrophages or multinucleate inflammatory cells with small to large vacuoles in their cytoplasm. Cell borders are indistinct (Wright stain, original magnification 250×). (Courtesy University of Georgia, College of Veterinary Medicine.)

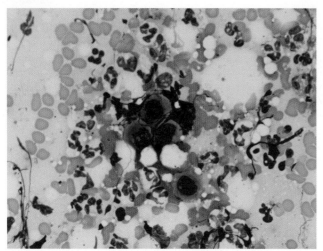

Fig. 5.24 Acantholytic cells from a dog with chronic skin disease. Four acantholytic epithelial cells are in the center of the figure. These cells are round with a large round nucleus and dark-blue cytoplasm. They are surrounded by numerous relatively well-preserved neutrophils with rare eosinophils and lymphocytes, as well as nuclear debris. The acantholytic cells should not be confused with neoplastic epithelial cells and can be found in many cases with chronic inflammatory skin disease, not just pemphigus lesions (Wright-Giemsa, 50× objective).

lesions in other tissues. The lesions are characterized by multiple, non-pruritic, haired to partially alopecic, cutaneous nodules and plaques. These are sometimes noted in linear rows. Aspirates from the nodules contain histiocytes, small lymphocytes, and neutrophils. Small lymphocytes may account for up to 50% of the cells, and neutrophils may be found in increased numbers secondary to necrosis. Because of the mixture of cells, definitive diagnosis of this disorder based on cytology alone is not possible.

Immune-Mediated Skin Lesions

Many immune-mediated skin disorders occur in dogs and cats. Examples include the pemphigus complex, lupus disorders, ischemic dermatopathy, vasculitis, and drug reactions. In general, no specific cytological findings for these disorders are made, and diagnosis is based on signalment, clinical presentation, and histopathological analysis. Acantholytic cells in pustules are a diagnostic finding in cases of pemphigus. However, these types of cells may be seen with other causes of inflammation, and these cells are not pathognomonic for pemphigus (Fig. 5.24).

NONINFLAMMATORY (TISSUE) LESIONS

The skin is a common site for neoplasia in dogs and cats. Skin tumors account for approximately 30% of all dog neoplasms and about 20% of all cat neoplasms.[9] The three most common skin tumors in dogs include lipoma, benign adenoma, and mast cell tumor, accounting for more than 50% of all skin tumors.[12] When tissue cells are the predominant finding in cytology smears, it implies that the lesion is noninflammatory in nature. That, by itself, does not mean the lesion is neoplastic because hyperplastic lesions may also form nodules or masses. Cells from hyperplastic lesions may appear similar to those from benign tumors. In addition, some benign tumors display some degree of cytological atypia. Finally, some malignant tumors may have relatively unremarkable cells, and the lack of cytological criteria of malignancy does not always rule out malignancy. Nevertheless, using cytomorphology assessing for cytological features of malignancy may aid in determining tumor type and further steps necessary for diagnostics

and therapy. Cytological features of malignancy include variable anisocytosis and anisokaryosis, open or stippled chromatin, prominent large or irregular nucleoli, nuclear molding, and mitotic figures. Prominent features of malignancy in numerous cells with no inflammatory cells suggest that the lesion is a malignant neoplasm. In many cases, biopsy and histopathological analysis will be necessary to definitively characterize a lesion as benign or malignant or to determine the cell of origin. Some features that would be looked for on biopsy samples (in histopathological analysis) that cannot be evaluated by cytological methods include invasion into the deeper subcutis, irregular borders, growth pattern, and vascular or lymphatic invasion.

When a neoplastic process is suspected on the basis of clinical presentation and the predominance of tissue cells on a cytology sample, typically the next step is to try to characterize the cells as either round cells, epithelial cells, or spindle (mesenchymal) cells. This categorization helps limit the possible differentials. However, some tumors display mixed cytomorphology. In some cases, it may be difficult to even make the limited distinction of round versus epithelial versus spindle cell neoplasia, particularly with anaplastic tumors. It may only be possible to characterize a tumor as round cell, epithelial, or spindle cell tumor and not as any specific tumor type. It is also important to note that the tumors discussed in the following sections are not a comprehensive list of all tumors that may occur in the skin or subcutaneous tissues but only those that have characteristic cytomorphology that aids in diagnosis (Table 5.2).

In general, round cell tumors have discrete, noncohesive round cells as a characteristic finding. Epithelial tumors typically have clusters of cohesive cells, although cells may also be noted individually. Cell shape varies from round to cuboidal to stellate or angular. Cytoplasmic borders are often distinct. Finally, spindle cell tumors often have cells found individually, although they are also noted in loose aggregates. The cells will typically have an irregular to wispy or spindloid shape. When found in aggregates, the cells often are enmeshed in a fibrillar background material that is usually extracellular matrix.

Round (Discrete) Cell Tumors

Round cell tumors are sometimes referred to as *discrete cell tumors* because the cells are found individually and not in cohesive clusters. They are typically highly exfoliative, and their characteristic cytological features often lead to a specific diagnosis. Round cell tumors include mast cell tumors, histiocytoma, histiocytic sarcoma, plasmacytoma, lymphoma, and transmissible venereal tumor (TVT). In some cases, epithelial or spindle cell tumors may have individual cells that may appear round.

Lymphoma

Cutaneous lymphoma is divided into two general types: epitheliotropic and nonepitheliotropic. Distinguishing these requires a biopsy sample to assess the tissue distribution of lymphocytes in relation to the epidermis, and this cannot be done with cytological samples.

Nonepitheliotropic lymphoma typically presents with nodules, which may be dermal or subcutaneous, may be alopecic, and may be red to purple in color. Usually, evidence exists for systemic involvement with this form of lymphoma. Aspirates from the nodules reveal a monomorphic population of lymphocytes, but the cells may be small to large in size and may have clumped to open chromatin. Aspirates containing a monomorphic population of cells that are large and lymphoblastic in appearance are consistent with an intermediate to high-grade lymphoma (Fig. 5.25), but those containing only small cells or a mixed cell population need biopsy and histopathological analysis to rule out the possibility of small-cell or mixed-cell lymphoma.

TABLE 5.2 Cytological Features of Cutaneous or Subcutaneous Tumors and Differential Diagnoses

Cell Shape	Characteristic Cytological Features	Cytological Interpretation	Differential Diagnoses or Other Comments
Discrete, round cells	Pale cytoplasm with no granules or vacuoles; relative uniform nuclear and cell size	Histiocytoma	Lymphoma, amelanotic melanoma, agranular mast cell tumor, plasmacytoma, transmissible venereal tumor (TVT)
	Pale cytoplasm, moderate to marked pleomorphism, variable vacuolization, multinucleate cells	Histiocytic sarcoma	Anaplastic sarcoma, fibrosarcoma, amelanotic melanoma, lymphoma
	Large cells with a high nuclear-to-cytoplasmic (N:C) ratio, open chromatin, prominent nucleoli	Lymphoma	Histiocytoma, plasmacytoma
	Blue cytoplasm with pale perinuclear zone and a few binucleate or multinucleate cells.	Plasmacytoma	Histiocytoma, osteosarcoma (rare to occur in skin)
	Fine to coarse, purple cytoplasmic granules	Mast cell tumor	Lymphoma of granular lymphocytes (rare in skin), agranular mast cell tumor may resemble histiocytic or other anaplastic tumor
	Pale cytoplasm, small numbers of punctate cytoplasmic vacuoles	TVT	Histiocytoma
Round, stellate, polygonal, columnar cells found individually and in sheets or clusters (epithelial)	Accumulations of sky blue material with angular edges and debris; anucleate squames; cholesterol crystals; +/– cell clusters and inflammation	Follicular cyst or cystic follicular tumor	Numerous epithelial tumors may have cyst formation with keratin debris accumulation
	Densely packed cells with a high N:C ratio; palisades or fronds of cells	Benign basaloid tumors (trichoblastoma, others)	Definitive diagnosis of tumor type requires histopathology
	Angular to polygonal cells; sky blue cytoplasm; N:C asynchrony	Squamous cell carcinoma	Many epithelial tumors may have areas of squamous differentiation.
	Clusters of highly vacuolated, minimally pleomorphic cells	Sebaceous adenoma	Sebaceous epithelial cells should be distinguished from highly vacuolated macrophages
	Pale granular cytoplasm, round to indistinct cell borders, cells found individually and in sheets	Sweat gland tumor	Liposarcoma, spindle cell tumor, plasmacytoma, amelanotic melanoma
	Pink granular cytoplasm with minimal pleomorphism	Perianal gland adenoma	Perianal gland adenocarcinoma
	Sheets of variably pleomorphic cells with pale cytoplasm, indistinct cytoplasmic borders	Apocrine gland tumor of anal sac origin	Neuroendocrine tumor (rare in skin)
Irregular, wispy or spindle-shaped cells found individually, in loose aggregates (spindle cell), or both	Low N:C ratio, clear cytoplasm	Lipoma	Cannot cytologically be distinguished from normal fat
	Variable N:C, pale vacuolated cytoplasm, round to irregular cells, free lipid in background	Liposarcoma	Granulomatous steatitis, sweat gland tumor, plasmacytoma, amelanotic melanoma
	Elongated cells with wispy to diaphanous cytoplasmic borders	Spindle cell tumor	Reactive fibroplasia
	Round to spindle-shaped, pleomorphic cells, giant multinucleate cells	Anaplastic sarcoma	Granulomatous inflammation, plasmacytoma
	Round to spindle-shaped cells found individually and in sheets, fine to dusty dark (black) pigment	Melanocytic tumors	Some epithelial tumors are pigmented
	Bloody sample with pleomorphic spindle cells found individually and in sheets	Hemangiosarcoma	Hematoma with secondary fibroplasia

Epitheliotropic lymphoma may present variably. These may include generalized pruritus, erythema, and scaling; depigmentation and ulceration; and solitary or multiple cutaneous plaques or nodules. Sampling from these lesions may be difficult if the lesions are not in the nodular form. The lymphocytes are often described as large or histiocytic in appearance, and associated inflammation may be present (Fig. 5.26).

Mast Cell Tumor

Mast cell tumors may be one of the easier types of tumors to diagnose by using cytological methods. Because mast cell granules typically stain well with Romanowsky-type stains, diagnosing these tumors in some ways is easier by cytology than on hematoxylin and eosin (H&E)–stained biopsy samples (Fig. 5.27). The key cytological feature is variable to large numbers of discrete, fine to coarse, purple cytoplasmic granules in a cell with a round nucleus and abundant pale cytoplasm. Sometimes, the cells are so densely granulated that it may be difficult to discern individual granules. Mast cell tumors occur in the skin of both dogs and cats but also may occur elsewhere, including the liver, spleen, and intestine. These tumors have a variable gross appearance but typically are erythematous, alopecic, edematous masses or plaques. Larger tumors may be ulcerated. Aspirates may be hemodiluted and have a variable degree of associated inflammation. Mast cells have

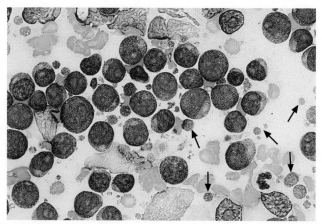

Fig. 5.25 Smear consisting primarily of large lymphoblasts from a dog with lymphoma. Scattered lymphoglandular bodies *(arrows)*, which are cytoplasmic fragments, are present in the background of the smear (Wright stain).

moderate-sized round nuclei with a moderate amount of cytoplasm. Nuclear and cytoplasmic details are often obscured by large numbers of small, round, purple granules, which are characteristic of these cells. In some cases, the cells may be poorly granulated, which is thought to be one feature of more poorly differentiated tumors (Figs. 5.28 and 5.29). It is important to note that some quick stains used in the clinic may not stain mast cell granules well. At least one study has demonstrated correlation of cytological grading with a proposed two-tier histological grading system in dogs.[13,14] Cytological features indicative of a poorly differentiated, high-grade tumor include binucleation, multinucleation, mitotic figures, anisocytosis, and anisokaryosis.

Individual mast cells may be found as part of an inflammatory reaction, so just finding a few mast cells scattered throughout a field of inflammatory cells is of questionable significance. Finding large numbers of mast cells individually but also in aggregates is more diagnostic for neoplasia. These tumors often will have a paraneoplastic infiltrate of eosinophils and may also elicit a stromal reaction with prominent spindle cells and pink fibrillar material between cells.

Histiocytoma

These tumors most commonly occur in dogs less than 2 years of age but may also be seen in older dogs.[9] Only rare anecdotal reports of this tumor in cats have been published. The tumors comprise Langerhans cells, which are intraepithelial, dendritic, antigen-presenting cells of skin. These usually occur as solitary tumors, although on rare occasions they may be multiple or involve regional lymph nodes. They are typically firm, dome or button shaped, and dermal in location. They often become ulcerated and may be secondarily infected. The majority of these tumors regress spontaneously, and increased numbers of small lymphocytes may be seen in samples from these tumors, presumably related to immunological reactivity associated with the regression. Aspirates from this tumor typically are moderately to highly cellular. Cells are found individually and have a discrete, round shape. The cells may be noted in aggregates, but they are not cohesive. The cells usually have a moderate-sized, round to slightly indented nucleus with finely reticulated to stippled chromatin and a moderate amount of pale, slightly granular cytoplasm (Fig. 5.30). It is not unusual to find low numbers of mitotic figures. The background is often proteinaceous in appearance.

Histiocytic Sarcoma (Malignant Histiocytosis)

These tumors can occur as localized masses as well as disseminated disease. The disseminated form is also referred to as *malignant*

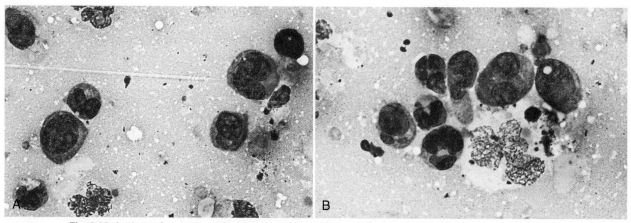

Fig. 5.26 Aspirates from a dog with epitheliotropic lymphoma. Cells from this form of lymphoma sometimes have a histiocytic appearance. (A) and (B) Blasts with irregularly shaped, monocytoid nuclei and more typical lymphoblasts (Wright stain, original magnification 250×).

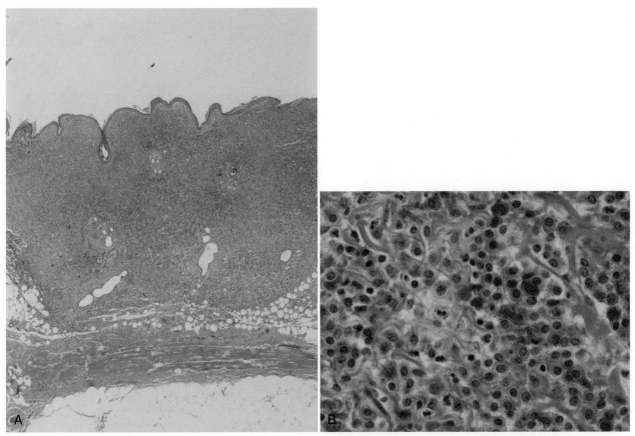

Fig. 5.27 Biopsy sample from canine mast cell tumor. (A) Low-power view (2× objective) showing intact epithelium with neoplastic round cell infiltrate just under epidermis and extending down into deeper dermis region (hematoxylin and eosin [H&E]). (B) Higher-power view (40× objective) of neoplastic round cells admixed with eosinophils. Note that purple granules are not apparent with H&E staining. Additional stains (toluidine blue or Giemsa) must be used to visualize the granules *(not shown)*. (Case material provided courtesy Dr. Shane Stiver, IDEXX Laboratories.)

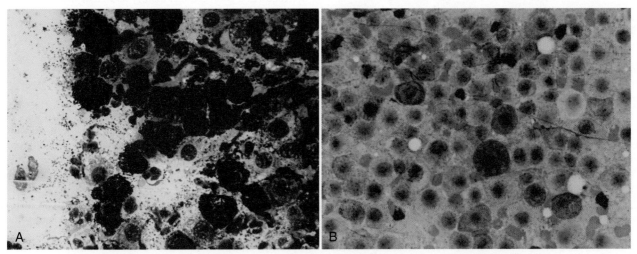

Fig. 5.28 Aspirates from canine mast cell tumors. (A) Large numbers of well-granulated mast cells are present. The numerous granules obscure the nuclear detail. Many free granules are also present in addition to neutrophils, eosinophils, and spindle cells. (Wright-Giemsa, 50× objective). (B) Numerous poorly granulated mast cells are present, suggesting a poorly differentiated mast cell tumor. Nuclear detail is more evident than in image A. The use of some quick stains may also result in poor granule staining (Wright-Giemsa, 50× objective).

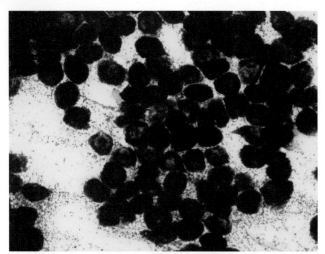

Fig. 5.29 Aspirate from feline cutaneous mast cell tumor. Large numbers of well-granulated mast cells often found in dense aggregates. Free mast cell granules are noted in the background (Wright-Giemsa, 50× objective).

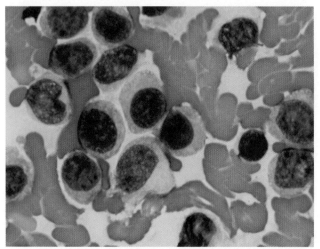

Fig. 5.30 Aspirate from a cutaneous histiocytoma. Large discrete round cells are found. They have a large round to slightly indented nucleus with a moderate amount of pale cytoplasm and stippled chromatin. Aspirates from these tumors often will have increased numbers of small lymphocytes as the tumor begins to regress or have neutrophils if the lesion is ulcerated *(not shown)* (Wright-Giemsa, 100× objective).

histiocytosis. Histiocytic sarcoma occurs more commonly in the dog than in the cat. Localized histiocytic sarcoma often originates in subcutaneous tissue but can occur as localized disease in internal organs also. The tumors are firm and often large and typically are infiltrative into surrounding tissue. Aspiration from these lesions may be moderately to highly exfoliative. Cells are often noted individually but can also be found in small, loose aggregates. The cells are large and round to spindloid in shape (Fig. 5.31). They have large round nuclei with abundant pale cytoplasm. The cytoplasm is often vacuolated, and the cells may demonstrate cytophagia. These nominally resemble macrophages but display more prominent anisocytosis and anisokaryosis. Mitotic figures are usually apparent, and multinucleate cells can sometimes be seen.

Feline Progressive Dendritic Cell Histiocytosis

This is thought to be a rare disorder in cats, as only a few cases have been reported. Cats with this disorder typically present

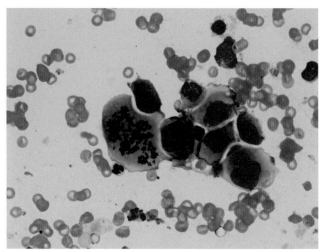

Fig. 5.31 Aspirate from dog with histiocytic sarcoma. Neoplastic cells are large (note size relative to red blood cells) with a variable nuclear-to-cytoplasmic (N:C) ratio but generally abundant blue cytoplasm. The cells may or may not be vacuolated, and erythophagia and cytophagia are sometimes found *(not shown)*. Mitotic figures *(cell on left)* are usually present and may be aberrant in appearance. The cells cannot be distinguished from other anaplastic tumor types, and definitive identification of histiocytic lineage usually requires immunophenotyping by cytological or histological methods (Wright-Giemsa, 50× objective).

with a solitary skin nodule on the head, neck, or extremities. Over time, multiple nodules develop and may be limited to one extremity or noted in more widespread locations. Nodules may wax and wane in size but do not completely regress. Clinical behavior in late disease may be similar to histiocytic sarcoma.[11] Aspirates from the lesions can contain mixed cell types, including predominantly histiocytes, some of which may be multinucleate. The cytomorphology may resemble lymphoid or plasmacytoid cells. Inflamed lesions may also contain variable numbers of neutrophils and lymphocytes. Definitive diagnosis of the disorder requires a good clinical history as well as histopathology and immunohistochemistry.

Plasmacytoma

Cutaneous plasmacytomas are common in dogs but are thought to be rare in cats. In dogs, cutaneous plasmacytomas usually are not associated with systemic multiple myeloma and often are benign. The clinical behavior in cats is less well known.

These tumors are typically found in older dogs and usually are solitary, although multiple plasmacytomas can be seen. The tumors are well circumscribed, raised, smooth, and often pink to red in color. Aspirates tend to be moderately to highly cellular and contain discrete round cells (Fig. 5.32). Aggregates of the cells may be noted, but cell-to-cell cohesion is not present. The cells have a large, round nucleus, which is typically eccentric in placement. The chromatin is coarsely reticulated to stippled, and some cells may have indistinct nucleoli. Usually, abundant blue cytoplasm is present, and many cells have a lighter staining perinuclear area (i.e., Golgi zone). Cutaneous plasmacytomas often display moderate anisocytosis and anisokaryosis. In addition, binucleate and multinucleate cells are typically found. Despite the moderate atypia these tumors may display, they usually are benign in dogs. In a small percentage of tumors, extracellular pink fibrillar material may exist, and it is often speculated to be amyloid. On rare occasions, rod-shaped to spiculated granules may be noted in the tumor cells.[15]

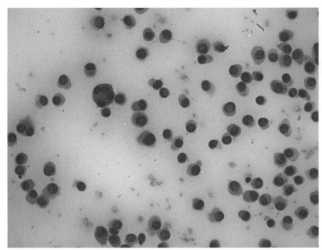

Fig. 5.32 Aspirate from cutaneous plasmacytoma in a dog. The cells from plasmacytoma often have a plasmacytoid appearance (eccentric nucleus, pale perinuclear area) but are larger and more pleomorphic than typical plasma cells. Multinucleate cells are a relatively common finding (Wright-Giemsa, 50× objective).

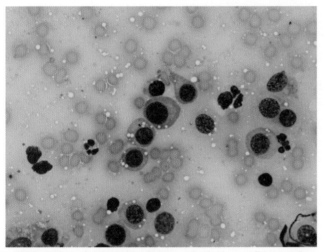

Fig. 5.33 Aspirate from a transmissible venereal tumor. Tumor cells are round and similar in appearance to histiocytes. A distinguishing feature is the presence of discrete cytoplasmic vacuoles. Several neutrophils and free nuclei are also seen in this figure (Wright-Giemsa, 50× objective).

Transmissible Venereal Tumor

TVTs occur in sexually active dogs and are most commonly found on the external genitalia, although they may also be found in skin. The cell origin is uncertain, although a histiocytic origin has been suggested. The chromosome count varies from 57 to 64 rather than the normal 78 in dogs.[16] Tumors can be single or multiple and vary from nodular to pedunculated to cauliflower-like forms. They usually are firm and friable and often ulcerated. Aspirates from these lesions usually are cellular and predominated by large discrete round cells with moderate-sized, round nuclei, stippled chromatin, small nucleoli, and a moderate amount of pale cytoplasm (Fig. 5.33). Many of the cells have a few small distinct cytoplasmic vacuoles, which is a helpful finding for distinguishing it from histiocytoma.

Epithelial Tumors

Many types of epithelial tumors can occur in skin. In general, epithelial cells tend to be cohesive, and cell clusters are often apparent

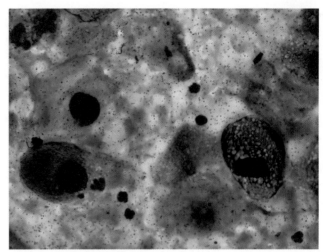

Fig. 5.34 Aspirate from a squamous papilloma. Large ovoid nucleated squamous cells are present, as well as anucleate cells, neutrophils, bare nuclei, bacteria, and precipitate debris. Despite the large nucleus, these tumors are benign and, if viral induced, may regress on their own. The cytoplasm may have a stippled purple appearance as the cell in the lower left or may appear vacuolated as the cell in the lower midright (koilocyte) (Wright-Giemsa, 50× objective).

when these tumors are aspirated. The cell shapes can vary from round to cuboidal, columnar, or stellate and can have a variable amount of cytoplasm. Epithelial cells tend to display cellular atypia in response to inflammation, and interpreting cytomorphology should be done carefully when inflammation is present. In many cases, histopathology is necessary to specifically identify the exact type of tumor.

Some epithelial tumors that have a fairly unique cytomorphological appearance include circumanal (hepatoid or perianal) gland adenoma, basal cell tumors (usually trichoblastoma), apocrine gland tumor of anal sac origin, squamous papilloma, squamous cell carcinoma, sebaceous adenoma or epithelioma, and sweat gland tumor. Keratin-producing cystic lesions are common, and aspiration from these often yields abundant keratin debris. These lesions include not only cysts but also cystic neoplasms. Cystic epithelial lesions are usually benign; however, histopathology is necessary to specifically identify them.

Papilloma

Various types of papillomas exist. They are common in dogs but rare in cats. These tumors can have a variable gross appearance, but classically, exophytic papillomas occur as single or multiple, sessile to pedunculated, or papillated masses. They often have a waxy appearance to the surface because of hyperkeratosis. These occur most commonly on the head and extremities. Aspiration from these lesions typically is moderately cellular. The cells often are found individually. In many cases, they may only resemble relatively normal squamous epithelial cells. Some epithelial cells may be large and ovoid to fusiform with a large, eccentrically placed nucleus, coarsely reticulated chromatin, and a small nucleus (Fig. 5.34). The cytoplasm may have a stippled, pink-to-purple appearance. Other cells may appear vacuolated. Mitotic figures are uncommon. The larger ovoid to fusiform cells with vacuolated or stippled cytoplasm are thought to be hypertrophied keratinocytes (also called *koilocytes*), and these are a common feature of papillomavirus infection.[17] Not all papillomas are related to papillomavirus infection.

Follicular Cysts and Cystic Follicular Tumors

Several masslike lesions, when aspirated, yield large amounts of keratin debris that is often in thick accumulations separated by a thinner

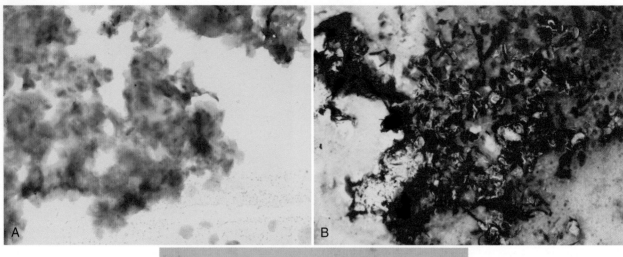

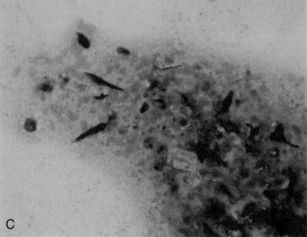

Fig. 5.35 Aspirates from follicular cysts or hair follicle tumors. Aspirates from these lesions often cannot be distinguished from each other as they are predominated by keratin and squamous material. (A) Thick accumulations of keratin and anucleate squames separated by a thin blue background material (Wright-Giemsa, 10× objective). (B) Individualized variably cornifying squames separated by a proteinaceous background and cellular debris (Wright-Giemsa, 10× objective). (C) Blood, protein, and cell debris from a cystic lesion. A cholesterol crystal is noted in the center (Wright-Giemsa, 20× objective).

proteinaceous background. The keratin material is sky blue in color and may be admixed with variable numbers of anucleate cornifying squamous epithelial cells (Fig. 5.35, A and B). In addition, cholesterol crystals are often noted as well as fragments of hair (see Fig. 5.35, C). Sometimes, sheets and clusters of relatively uniform epithelial cells may also be noted.[18] Because keratin may be irritative to surrounding tissues, if these lesions rupture, they may incite moderate to marked neutrophilic to pyogranulomatous inflammation.

Lesions that may have these types of findings include follicular cyst, dilated pore, warty dyskeratoma, trichofolliculoma, trichoepithelioma, acanthoma, and pilomatricoma. Although these all are usually benign lesions, malignant forms of pilomatricoma[19] and trichoepithelioma also exist. Distinguishing these lesions by cytology alone is generally not possible, and excision of the cyst wall or entire mass may be necessary for definitive characterization of the lesion, for resolution, and to prevent recurrent inflammation and ulceration.

Trichoblastoma (Basal Cell Tumor)

These tumors were previously referred to as *basal cell tumors* in dogs and cats. These are neoplasms that are derived from primitive hair germ and thus are thought to actually be of follicular origin.[11] Basal cell carcinoma and other epitheliomas may have a similar cytological appearance, and

definitive characterization of these tumors requires histopathology. *Basal cell tumor* continues to be a general diagnostic term to encompass these tumors for cytological diagnosis, although the majority of "basal cell tumors" are trichoblastomas. These are common in both cats and dogs. The tumors are usually solitary, firm, alopecic nodules that are dome shaped to polypoid. Larger masses may be ulcerated. The appearance in cats is similar, although the tumors also are often pigmented and may have areas of central necrosis and cyst formation. Aspirates from these lesions tend to be moderately to highly cellular. They may have a thin background separating sheets and clusters of cells, particularly if accompanied by cyst formation (Fig. 5.36, A). The clusters often form palisades, fronds, or ribbons (see Fig. 5.36, B). The cells have small- to moderate-sized, round nuclei, with a small amount of blue cytoplasm. They are often densely packed together. A small amount of fibrillar pink material may sometimes be seen along the edge of clusters, which may be basement membrane. Scattered individualized cells may be noted along with a few thin spindle cells. Mitotic figures are usually not apparent.

Squamous Cell Carcinoma

These tumors are common in both cats and dogs. They may occur anywhere in skin, but they occur most frequently in areas where sun damage can occur and thus have a higher incidence in white-furred cats

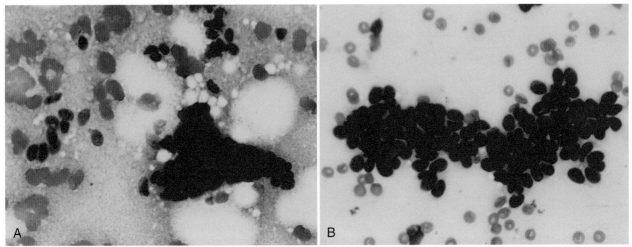

Fig. 5.36 Aspirate from trichoblastoma (basal cell tumor). (A) A dense, tightly packed cluster of cohesive cells is noted in the lower right. The cells have round to oval nuclei with a small amount of blue cytoplasm. Cells are also noted in rows *(midleft)* and sometimes found individually. Cystic lesions such as this one may have a stippled proteinaceous background (Wright-Giemsa, 50× objective). (B) Higher-power view of elongated frond of "basaloid" cells. (Wright-Giemsa, 100× objective).

and short-coated dogs. They are most common on the pinnae, nasal planum, and eyelids in cats; in dogs, tumors occur more frequently on the ventral abdomen, flank, and medial stifles. These tumors present as plaquelike, papillary, and fungiform masses, which can vary from small to large in size. They may be alopecic, erythemic, and ulcerated, and crusts are often present. Sampling from these lesions may be complicated by the lack of discrete mass lesions and ulceration. In addition, the keratin that is produced by these tumors often induces a moderate to marked inflammatory reaction, which can make interpreting the epithelial changes difficult. The tumor may be highly exfoliative if a discrete mass region is available to aspirate. If not, a scraping sample from the edge of a plaque or ulcer may be diagnostically helpful. The epithelial cells are typically found in sheets, in clusters, and individually. When found individually, the cells vary from round to large and angular (Fig. 5.37). The cells have variably sized nuclei with reticulated to open chromatin and indistinct nucleoli. Moderate to marked anisocytosis and anisokaryosis are often noted. The cytoplasm will vary from deep blue to more sky blue in coloration. In some cases, mild to moderate perinuclear vacuolization may be present. Some of the large angular cells will have large nuclei and prominent nucleoli. Large cells with abundant sky blue cytoplasm (i.e., mature cytoplasmic features) and a large nucleus with open chromatin (i.e., immature nuclear features) are present. These cells demonstrate asynchronous maturation of the nucleus and cytoplasm and are referred to as *dyskeratotic*. Sometimes, dense clusters of pleomorphic cells may be found, and often a large amount of squamous and keratin debris is noted. The lack of marked atypia does not exclude malignancy, and some of these tumors may only have well-differentiated cells. Mitotic figures are sometimes seen.

Sebaceous Adenoma and Epithelioma

These tumors are common in dogs and uncommon in cats. They occur most commonly on the limbs, trunk, and eyelids in dogs and on the head, neck, and trunk in cats. The lesions are usually solitary, well circumscribed, raised, smooth to lobular, or wartlike. Aspiration from these tumors is usually at least moderately cellular, with numerous variably sized clusters of highly vacuolated, minimally pleomorphic cells (Fig. 5.38). These vacuolated cells have a low nuclear-to-cytoplasmic (N:C) ratio, and mitotic figures are usually

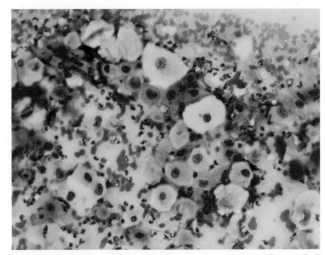

Fig. 5.37 Well-differentiated squamous cell carcinoma. The epithelial cells are noted individually in this figure but also may occur in sheets and clusters. The cells display anisocytosis and mild anisokaryosis with variably cornifying cytoplasm. Some cells with abundant cornified cytoplasm have relatively large nuclei (nuclear, cytoplasmic asynchrony) with open chromatin and nucleoli. Numerous neutrophils are present, as well as blood in the background. The presence of inflammation often makes it difficult to discern neoplastic from hyperplastic or dysplastic cells (Wright-Giemsa, 20× objective).

not evident. The cells from sebaceous adenomas are well differentiated and cannot be distinguished from hyperplastic cells. Sebaceous epithelioma has a similar cytological appearance to sebaceous adenoma, but admixed with the clusters of vacuolated cells are sheets of densely packed basophilic cells, which are smaller in size and have a higher N:C ratio.

Sweat Gland Tumor

Sweat gland tumors are uncommon in both the dog and the cat. They can occur in benign and malignant forms and have numerous histopathological classifications, including cystadenoma, glandular adenoma, ductular adenoma, and a variety of carcinoma subtypes (solitary, papillary, tubular, glandular, ductular, clear cell, and "signet

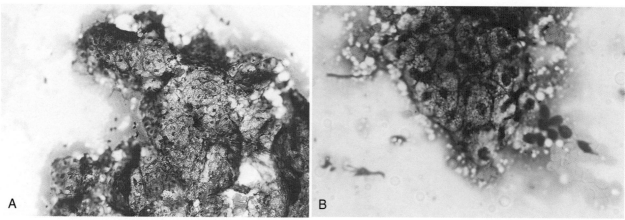

Fig. 5.38 Aspirate from a sebaceous adenoma in a dog. (A) A large cluster of cohesive sebaceous epithelial cells is present (Wright stain, original magnification 80×). (B) Higher magnification of cells in image A. The cells resemble normal sebaceous cells. Nuclei are uniform, and the nuclear-to-cytoplasmic (N:C) ratio is low. Note the vacuolation of the cytoplasm (Wright stain, original magnification 160×).

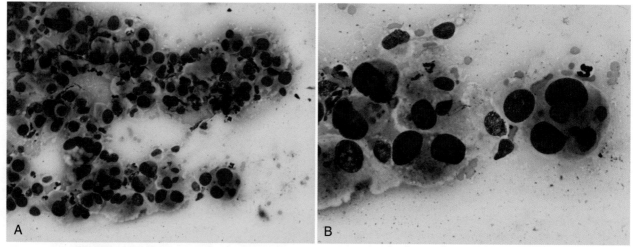

Fig. 5.39 Aspirate from a sweat gland carcinoma in the neck of a dog. (A) Cells are noted in aggregates, although it is difficult to discern whether the cells are cohesive. Many appear to be individualized and round to ovoid. Marked anisocytosis and anisokaryosis are evident, aiding in a diagnosis of malignancy in this case, although not all sweat gland tumors display this much atypia (Wright-Giemsa, 20× objective). (B) Higher-power view of image A. Note the open chromatin pattern with prominent multiple nucleoli. Low numbers of surrounding red blood cells and a single neutrophil are present and aid in emphasizing the large size of the cells. Several cells appear to be binucleate or multinucleate (Wright-Giemsa, 50× objective).

ring" types). The definitive characterization of these tumors requires histopathology, although a general diagnosis of sweat gland tumor is usually possible on the basis of cytomorphology. Grossly, these tumors are most common on the head, dorsal neck, and limbs. These tend to be solitary, well circumscribed, firm, raised tumors that often are ulcerated. On occasion, the tumors may be poorly circumscribed, infiltrative, and plaquelike.

Aspiration from these lesions tends to be moderately to highly exfoliative. Cells are noted individually and within cohesive sheets (Fig. 5.39). The cells usually have moderate-sized round nuclei, with eccentric placement and a variable amount of pale granular cytoplasm. When found individually, the cells are round to slightly angular in shape, but when found in sheets, the cytoplasmic borders may be indistinct. The cells often may be smudged and may take on a spindloid appearance, and thus aspiration from these tumors may resemble soft tissue spindle cell tumors, such as liposarcoma. Other tumors with similar cells include amelanotic melanoma and plasmacytoma.

Circumanal Gland Tumor (Perianal or Hepatoid Gland Tumor)

Circumanal gland tumors (also called *hepatoid gland* or *perianal gland tumors*) are particularly common in older intact male dogs; however, they may also occur in younger, neutered, or female dogs. They typically are found in the perianal region but also may be found on the tail, perineum, prepuce, thigh, and dorsal lumbosacral area. They may be solitary or multiple. Smaller lesions tend to be spherical to ovoid, but as they grow, these can become multinodular and ulcerated. Aspirates from these lesions tend to be highly exfoliative, characterized by sheets and clusters of large ovoid to cuboidal cells with round eccentrically placed nuclei and abundant pink granular cytoplasm (Fig. 5.40). Typically, minimal pleomorphism is present, although some admixed smaller reserve cells may also be present. These latter cells are more densely packed together with basophilic cytoplasm and have a high N:C ratio. These lesions can become secondarily inflamed or have areas of necrosis and cyst formation. This type of tumor is typically benign; however, the cytomorphology does not correlate well with clinical behavior, requiring histopathology for definitive characterization.

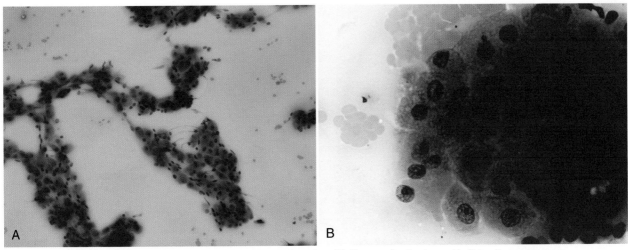

Fig. 5.40 Aspirate from a perianal gland tumor in a dog. (A) Sheets of cohesive epithelial cells are present. The cells are round to low cuboidal in shape but can have a slightly irregular or spindloid shape because of preparation technique (Wright-Giemsa, 10× objective). (B) On high-power view, the cells have pink granular cytoplasm; hence, these are also referred to as *hepatoid tumors*. Nucleoli are present, but not necessarily indicative of malignancy. The majority of hepatoid tumors are benign (e.g., adenomas), but histopathological analysis is necessary to definitively characterize malignant potential (Wright-Giemsa, 50× objective).

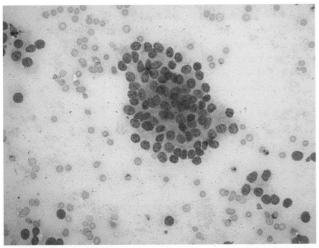

Fig. 5.41 Aspirate from apocrine adenocarcinoma of anal sac gland origin. Aspirates from these lesions can be highly cellular and often contain sheets of cells with indistinct cytoplasmic borders. The cells have round nuclei, with a moderate amount of pale blue cytoplasm. In this case, moderate anisokaryosis is present, but these tumors often have minimal anisocytosis or anisokaryosis despite being malignant (Wright-Giemsa, 50× objective).

Apocrine Gland Tumor of Anal Sac Origin

This type of tumor also is found in the perianal area but occurs in the anal sac region (ventrolateral to anus). These mostly occur in older dogs and are rare in cats. These tumors often are adenocarcinomas. They occur as an intradermal or subcutaneous mass and often invade deep into perirectal tissue along the pelvic canal. This tumor is sometimes associated with hypercalcemia of malignancy. Although usually adenocarcinomas, the cells typically do not display prominent pleomorphism. The cells are usually found in variably sized sheets, although individualized cells and free nuclei may be seen (Fig. 5.41). The cells have moderate-sized, round nuclei, with moderate to abundant pale cytoplasm. When found in sheets, the cytoplasmic borders may be indistinct, but when found individually, the cells tend to have a round shape. This morphology resembles what some cytopathologists will call a "neuroendocrine appearance." The chromatin is usually stippled, and small indistinct nucleoli may be present.

Other Epithelial Tumors

Many other epithelial tumors, for the most part, cannot be distinguished by cytomorphology alone. It is important to note that not all tumors that occur in skin or subcutaneous tissue are primary skin tumors but may, in fact, be metastatic tumors. As an example, feline lung tumors have a predisposition to metastasize to the nailbed and may be found elsewhere in skin.

Subcutaneous Glandular Tissues

Tumors and other lesions of salivary, mammary, thyroid, and parathyroid glandular tissue are discussed in Chapter 6.

Mesenchymal (Spindle Cell) Tumors

Mesenchymal tumors (sometimes referred to as *spindle cell tumors*) are characterized by cells that have irregular to wispy to indistinct cell borders, particularly when of soft tissue origin. Although these tumors are often said to be poorly exfoliative, some may be moderately to highly exfoliative. These tumors are diverse, and, for the most part, are difficult to specifically identify by cytomorphology alone. In some cases, immunocytochemical staining may be beneficial in further identifying histogenic origin.[20] In addition, although most "spindle cell tumors" are primarily mesenchymal tumors, some tumors morphologically get lumped into this category. However, they have a different histogenesis (e.g., melanocytic tumors—melanocytes that are neuroectodermal in derivation).

Of all the masses that occur in skin, probably the most care needs to be taken when evaluating spindle cells from mass lesions, as reactive spindle cells associated with fibroplasia cannot be easily distinguished from neoplastic cells. A history of progressive growth, infiltrative behavior, and irregular mass borders, along with a lack of inflammatory cells, should increase suspicion of a neoplastic process. Mesenchymal tumors have benign (e.g., fibroma) and malignant (e.g., fibrosarcoma) forms, but unless marked cytological atypia exists, making this distinction requires histopathology. Definitively characterizing a lesion as a mesenchymal neoplasm almost always requires histopathology. This is particularly true if any admixed inflammation is present.

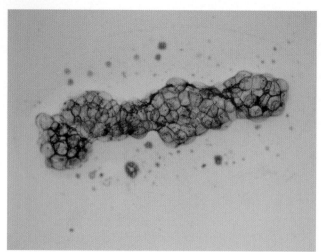

Fig. 5.42 Aspirate from a lipoma. A single large cluster of well-differentiated adipocytes is present, surrounded by small droplets of blood. Adipocytes from a lipoma cannot be distinguished from normal subcutaneous fat (Wright-Giemsa, 4× objective).

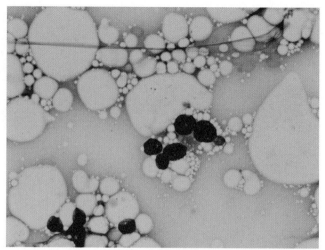

Fig. 5.43 Aspirate from liposarcoma in a dog. Aspirates from these lesions typically have a large amount of free lipid, and this sometimes results in lysis of the cells during smear preparation. The cells are often noted among the lipid material, and sometimes it may appear as if only free nuclei are present. The cytoplasm tends to be pale and can blend into the background. When cell borders are distinct, the cells may appear round to ovoid in shape rather than spindloid (Wright-Giemsa, 50× objective).

Lipoma

Lipomas are common subcutaneous tumors in dogs and less common in cats. They may be single or multiple in site and occur over the thorax, abdomen, thighs, and proximal limbs. They seldom ulcerate. Aspirates yield variable numbers of adipocytes noted individually and in variably sized clusters (Fig. 5.42). These are often admixed with a few thin spindle cells and bare nuclei. Typically, free lipid is also present. Slides with fat on them do not dry and have an oily appearance. Because most Romanowsky-type stains use alcohol as a fixative, the fat sometimes is washed off the slide during the staining process, and after staining, the slide may be essentially acellular. Adipocytes from a lipoma cannot be distinguished from normal subcutaneous fat cells, so care must always be taken when collecting samples from subcutaneous masses to avoid contamination with surrounding normal tissue.

Liposarcoma

These are rare tumors in both the dog and the cat. They are usually solitary in occurrence and are most frequently found on the ventral abdomen, thorax, and proximal limbs. These tumors tend to be poorly circumscribed, firm to fleshy, and subcutaneous. They behave similarly to other soft tissue sarcomas.

Aspiration from these tumors may be moderately to highly cellular. Typically, a variable amount of free lipid material is also present. Cells are noted individually and in sheets, and they are often found around the lipid material. The cells are round to ovoid to spindloid in shape and typically have moderate to large, round nuclei with a variable amount of pale cytoplasm. A few punctate cytoplasmic vacuoles are sometimes noted. The chromatin is stippled to lacy, and some cells may have small multiple nucleoli. Mitotic figures may be observed. The morphology of the cells can be similar to sweat gland tumor or amelanotic melanoma, and the free lipid can be a useful distinguishing finding (Fig. 5.43).

Soft Tissue Spindle Cell Tumor

These tumors encompass several types of sarcomas that are named based on their presumptive progenitor cell. A few minor cytological differences exist between these tumors, but otherwise, even with histopathology, it is not always clear what the actual origin of the neoplastic cells is. Thus, from a cytological perspective, it is probably best just to lump these tumors into the category of soft tissue spindle cell tumor, at least in the dog. These include fibrosarcoma, myxosarcoma,

hemangiopericytoma, and peripheral nerve sheath tumor. As a generalization, these tumors tend to behave similarly regardless of cell origin. In dogs, prognostic factors are related to histological grading and completeness of surgical margins. Complete surgical margins generally are associated with nonrecurrence.[21] In the cat, soft tissue sarcomas often are fibrosarcomas, which also tend to be infiltrative and recurrent with uncommon metastasis. Feline vaccine-associated sarcomas may behave more aggressively in regards to recurrence and may have a higher propensity for metastasis over time.[16]

Most of these tumors arise in subcutaneous tissue and may occur in various anatomical sites. Aspiration from spindle cell tumors vary in the degree of cellularity, but these may be moderately to highly exfoliative lesions. Cells are found both individually and within loosely arranged aggregates. The cells are usually elongated with irregular to wispy borders (Fig. 5.44). The nuclei are moderate to large in size and often centrally located with cytoplasm extending from each pole of the nucleus. The chromatin is reticulated to stippled, and small distinct nucleoli may be present. Some of these tumors (e.g., myxosarcoma) may have abundant pink-stippled to fibrillar background material, with prominent windrowing of the cells (Fig. 5.45). Others may have denser accumulations of pink fibrillar material noted between cells (e.g., fibrosarcoma). A variant of fibrosarcoma that has been reported in dogs is keloidal fibrosarcoma.[22] This may occur in a benign form also (e.g., fibroma). These have a characteristic appearance with striking accumulations of bright pink to blue, hyalinized collagen in addition to the spindle cells (Fig. 5.46).

Anaplastic Sarcoma with Giant Cells (Malignant Fibrous Histiocytoma, Giant Cell Tumor of Soft Parts)

This tumor type has a fairly distinctive cytological appearance. It has previously been called *malignant fibrous histiocytoma*, but this is considered controversial nomenclature. More recent studies have suggested this tumor is not a distinct morphological entity and likely represents a group of poorly differentiated sarcomas with morphological similarities, including fibrosarcoma, leiomyosarcoma, rhabdomyosarcoma, liposarcoma, synovial sarcoma, and histiocytic sarcoma.[11,23] These tumors appear similar to other soft tissue sarcomas and often present as large, solitary, firm, poorly circumscribed, subcutaneous and dermal masses. With aspiration, these tumors may be moderately to highly exfoliative.

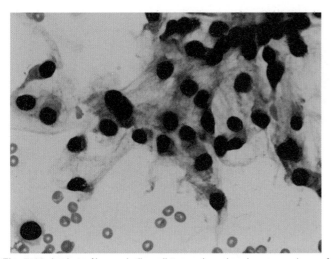

Cells are typically found individually but may be in loose aggregates. Most of the cells are large and round to slightly spindloid in shape. They usually have a large nucleus, with open chromatin and prominent nucleoli. The cytoplasm is usually abundant, pale, and granular and may be variably vacuolated. The distinctive feature is the presence of variable numbers of giant multinucleate cells (Fig. 5.47). The cells may have up to 30 nuclei and usually have abundant pale granular cytoplasm. Mitotic figures are commonly noted in the round cell population.

Melanocytic Tumors

The terminology for classifying melanocytic tumors is complex, but in general, most use the term *melanocytoma* to denote a benign tumor and *melanoma* to denote a malignant tumor. Melanocytic tumors are relatively common in both dogs and cats. When involving just skin, the majority in dogs are benign. Tumors involving the nailbed or oral cavity often have a more aggressive clinical course. In cats, benign and malignant tumors occur with about equal frequency.[9]

These tumors typically occur in older animals. They are usually solitary and mostly occur on the head, neck, trunk, and paws. The lesions are usually well circumscribed, firm to fleshy, darkly colored, and alopecic and vary from dome shaped to pedunculated or papillomatous in appearance.

Aspirates from these lesions are typically moderately to highly cellular with some degree of blood contamination. Cells are found

Fig. 5.44 Aspirate from spindle cell tumor in a dog. Large numbers of irregularly shaped spindle cells are found in loose aggregates. The cells have moderate- to large-sized nuclei with abundant pale blue cytoplasm and wispy cytoplasmic borders. Red blood cells are noted, but inflammatory cells are not apparent. After biopsy and histopathological analysis, this lesion was diagnosed as hemangiopericytoma (Wright-Giemsa stain, 50× objective).

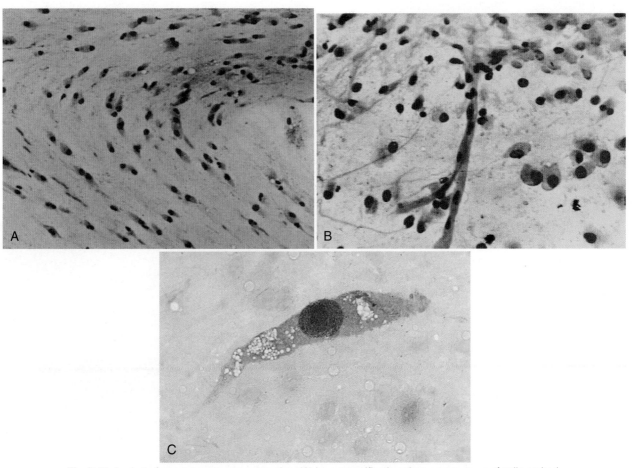

Fig. 5.45 Aspirate from a myxosarcoma in a dog. (A) Low magnification shows many rows of cells embedded in a pink substance (Wright stain, original magnification 50×). (B) Higher magnification shows many cells with a plasmacytoid appearance and a background of pink material. A few cells are spindle shaped (Wright stain, original magnification 100×). (C) Cell from a myxosarcoma, showing a large, prominent nucleolus (Wright stain, original magnification 250×).

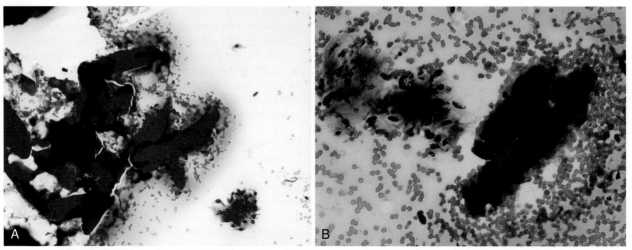

Fig. 5.46 Aspirate from keloidal fibrosarcoma. (A) Thick rectangular accumulations of pink to blue hyalinized collagen characterizes this lesion. Note small aggregates of irregular spindle cells in lower right mixed with more typical pink fibrillar matrix found with soft tissue spindle cell tumors (Wright-Giemsa, 10× objective). (B) Higher-power view of hyalinized collagen next to spindle cells (Wright-Giemsa, 20× objective). (Slide courtesy Dr. J. Johnsrude, IDEXX Laboratories.)

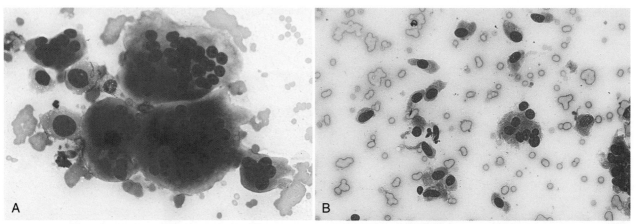

Fig. 5.47 (A) Aspirate from anaplastic sarcoma with giant cells from a cat. These tumors contain a mixture of large, multinucleate cells mixed with pleomorphic round to spindle-shaped cells (Diff-Quik, original magnification 132×). (B) Mesenchymal cells (Wright stain, original magnification 160×).

individually and in aggregates or sheets. When found individually, the cells vary from round to stellate to spindloid in shape (Fig. 5.48). They may be densely pigmented with fine to moderately coarse dark-brown to black melanin granules. The pigment may be so abundant that all other cytological details are obscured. In other cases, the cells are variably or less well pigmented, and nuclear detail may be evident. The presence of more prominent nuclear atypia, such as anisokaryosis, pleomorphism, open chromatin, and prominent nucleoli, are suggestive of a malignant process. Mitotic figures may be common in malignant tumors. Often, free pigment will also be noted in the background, as well as macrophages with phagocytized pigment. These latter cells are referred to as *melanophages*, and these may be seen in nonneoplastic lesions as well as in lymph nodes draining pigmented skin. It is also important to note that some epithelial tumors (e.g., basal cell tumors) often have large numbers of admixed melanocytes, with the epithelial cells having readily visible melanin granules, and these should not be interpreted as melanocytic tumors.

Hemangiosarcoma

This tumor is a difficult cytological diagnosis, as *hemangiosarcoma* comprises vascular tissue and may be cavernous. Aspiration often is very bloody and not very cellular, although some forms of these

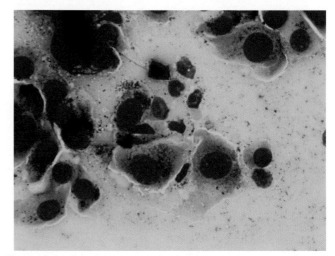

Fig. 5.48 Aspirate from melanoma. Cells are mostly noted individually in this figure but also can be found in sheets. The cell shape varies and often is irregular. The cytoplasm contains fine, dark pigment, indicating that these are melanocytes. The cellular and nuclear atypia (anisocytosis, anisokaryosis, open chromatin, and small nucleoli) suggest this is a malignant neoplasm (Wright-Giemsa, 50× objective).

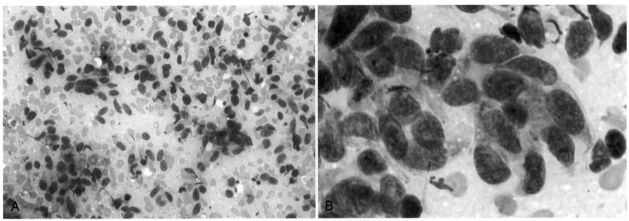

Fig. 5.49 (A) Scraping from a hemangiosarcoma. Scattered red blood cells, spindle cells, and bare nuclei are shown. (B) Higher magnification of spindle cells shown in image A (Wright stain). (Slide courtesy Dr. D. DeNicola, IDEXX Laboratories.)

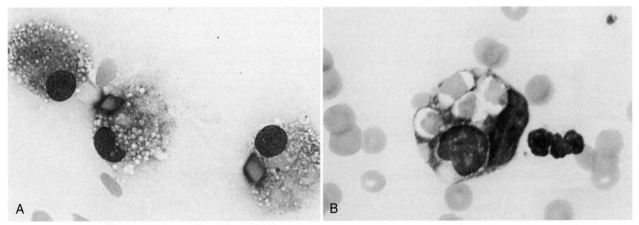

Fig. 5.50 (A) Large, vacuolated macrophages with intracytoplasmic golden hematoidin crystals. Hematoidin is a product of red blood cell breakdown and is sometimes referred to as tissue bilirubin (Wright stain). (B) A macrophage with erythrophagocytosis (Wright stain).

tumors may be densely cellular with higher cell exfoliation. The tumor cells may be found individually and in sheets. They typically have a pleomorphic appearance but usually are irregular to spindloid in shape (Fig. 5.49). As with other spindle cells, interpreting their significance based on cytomorphology alone is difficult, as reactive spindle cells found in an organizing hematoma may also appear somewhat pleomorphic. Accompanying cytological findings may include erythrophagic macrophages and extramedullary hematopoiesis.

FLUID-FILLED LESIONS

Fluid-filled lesions in skin or subcutaneous lesions may be caused by infection (abscess); trauma; cystic or necrotic or infarcted areas of glands; or neoplasia. When lesions are confined to skin, they may reflect true cysts developing from apocrine tissue. In almost all of these cases, aspiration of the fluid may aid in defining whether an inflammatory process exists or not as well as aid in finding infectious agents, if present. However, usually, tissue cells surrounding the fluid cavity do not exfoliate well into the fluid, and thus evaluation of the fluid by itself may not entirely reflect the pathological process. Examples of fluid-filled lesions with typically low to moderate numbers of nucleate cells include seroma, hematoma, hygroma, sialocele, synovial cyst, and apocrine cyst.

Seroma, Hygroma, and Synovial and Apocrine Cysts

Aspirates from these lesions are generally poorly cellular and consist of primarily macrophages or reactive mononuclear cells but no tissue cells. The fluid typically appears clear to pale yellow and may be thin or viscous. The location of the swelling aids in distinguishing these lesions: Apocrine cysts are typically superficially located in the skin; synovial cysts occur around joints; hygromas are noted over bony prominences or areas of chronic trauma; and seromas are found in areas of prior trauma, such as surgical sites.

Hematoma

The fluid from hematomas is cloudy and red to red-brown. The total protein concentration of the supernatant approaches that of peripheral blood. Smears contain primarily red blood cells (RBCs) with low numbers of leukocytes, which are primarily the same as those noted in peripheral blood. In addition, if the hematoma has been present for more than 12 to 24 hours, some macrophages should be present, including some that are more highly vacuolated and display phagocytosis of RBCs (erythrophagocytosis) as well as hemoglobin breakdown material, such as hematoidin (Fig. 5.50). Platelets are generally absent unless hemorrhage into the site has occurred within a few hours of sample collection (or if blood contamination has occurred). Some vascular

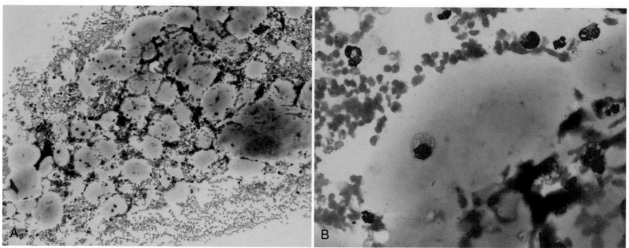

Fig. 5.51 (A) Direct smear of fluid collected from a sialocele. Large numbers of red blood cells surround different-sized thick accumulations of blue-staining mucus. The color of the mucus resembles what is seen with cornifying squames or keratin debris, and care must be taken not to interpret the material as squamous in origin. The mucous accumulations have rounded edges, unlike maturing squames. The dark structures in the mucus are cells (Wright-Giemsa, 10× objective). (B) Higher-power view of image A. Note smooth rounded margins of mucus surrounded by red blood cells and low numbers of macrophages, neutrophils, and bare nuclei. A large vacuolated macrophage is embedded mucus (Wright-Giemsa, 50× objective).

tumors (hemangioma, hemangiosarcoma) may have large cavitated areas filled with blood, and aspiration from these areas will not necessarily contain neoplastic cells; thus, the lack of overtly neoplastic cells in these samples does not exclude the possibility of neoplasia.

Sialocele

Sialoceles have characteristic findings. Aspiration from these lesions (which are found under the mandible or intermandibular space) yields a viscous fluid that is often blood tinged. Smears are bloody, with low to moderate numbers of macrophages and neutrophils. Usually, scattered thick accumulations of amorphous blue material that is consistent with mucus is present (Fig. 5.51).

MISCELLANEOUS

Calcinosis Circumscripta

These lesions are characterized by tumorlike nodules in subcutaneous tissue. They are mostly seen in young, large-breed dogs and are rare in cats. They consist of focal deposition of mineral salts forming well-circumscribed subcutaneous nodules, often over areas of chronic focal trauma. Aspirates from these lesions typically "feel" gritty. Often, a large amount of pasty material is present, but when stained, the cellularity is low. The stained surface of the slide often will have a characteristic blue chalklike appearance. On microscopic examination, usually a large amount of poorly staining irregular crystalline material with few intact cells, including macrophages and spindle cells, is seen (Fig. 5.52).

Poorly Cellular Samples

When a solid skin or subcutaneous mass is aspirated and very few cells are subsequently found on the slides, it suggests that the lesion may be poorly exfoliative. With regard to poorly cellular slides, there are other possible explanations, such as aspiration of fat, with loss of cells during the staining process. Tissues that tend to be poorly exfoliative often are densely fibrous. In many cases, these turn out to be benign lesions, such as fibromas, collagenous hamartomas, or related lesions. However, definitive identification almost always requires histopathology, and thus if the lesion is growing, feels infiltrative, becomes ulcerated, or otherwise is bothering the patient, then biopsy will be necessary for diagnosis.

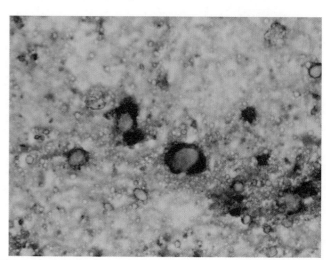

Fig. 5.52 Calcinosis circumscripta in a dog. After staining, slides from these lesions often have a dark-blue, gross appearance to the sample area, but under microscopic examination the samples are typically poorly cellular with a large amount of irregular, poorly staining calcified material (Wright-Giemsa, 50× objective).

REFERENCES

1. Ghisleni G, Roccabianca P, Ceruti R, et al. Correlation between fine-needle aspiration cytology and histopathology in the evaluation of cutaneous and subcutaneous masses from dogs and cats. *Vet Clin Pathol.* 2006;35(1):24–30.
2. Marcos R, Santos M, Santos N, et al. Use of destained cytology slides for the application of routine special stains. *Vet Clin Pathol.* 2009;38(1):94–102.
3. Greene CE. *Infectious Diseases of the Dog and Cat.* 4th ed. St Louis: Elsevier Saunders; 2012.
4. Malik R, Smits B, Rappas G, et al. Ulcerated and nonulcerated nontuberculous cutaneous mycobacterial granulomas in cats and dogs. *Vet Dermatol.* 2013;24(1):146–153.e33.
5. Bulla C, Thomas JS. What is your diagnosis? Subcutaneous mass fluid from a febrile dog. *Vet Clin Pathol.* 2009;38(3):403–405.
6. Lester SL, Malik R, Bartlett KH, et al. Cryptococcosis: update and emergence of cryptococcus gattii. *Vet Clin Pathol.* 2011;40(1):4–17.

7. Gupta A, Stroup S, Dedeaux A, et al. What is your diagnosis? Fine-needle aspirate of ulcerative skin lesions in a dog. *Vet Clin Pathol*. 2011;40(3):401–402.

8. Stowe DM, Bidwell A, Patel R. What is your diagnosis? Subcutaneous mass from a dog. *Vet Clin Pathol*. 2016;45(3):507–508.

9. Miller Jr WH, Griffin CE, Campbell K. *Muller & Kirk's Small Animal Dermatology*. 7th ed. St. Louis: Elsevier Mosby; 2013.

10. Giori L, Garbagnoli V, Venco L, et al. What is your diagnosis? Fine-needle aspirate from a subcutaneous mass in a dog. *Vet Clin Pathol*. 2010;39(2):255–256.

11. Gross TL, Ihrke PJ, Walder EJ, et al. *Skin Diseases of the Dog and Cat: Clinical and Histopathologic Diagnosis*. 2nd ed. Oxford, UK: Blackwell Science; 2005.

12. Villamil JA, Henry CJ, Bryan JN, et al. Identification of the most common cutaneous neoplasms in dogs and evaluation of breed and age distributions for selected neoplasms. *J Am Vet Med Assoc*. 2011;239(7):960–965.

13. Kiupel M, Webster JD, Bailey KL, et al. Proposal of a 2-tier histologic grading system for canine cutaneous mast cell tumors to more accurately predict biological behavior. *Vet Pathol*. 2011;48. 177–155.

14. Camus MS, Priest HL, Koehler JW, et al. Cytologic criteria for mast cell tumor grading in dogs with evaluation of clinical outcome. *Vet Pathol*. 2016;53(6):1117–1123.

15. Santos M, Canadas A, Puente-Payo P, et al. What is your diagnosis? Cutaneous ulcerated nodule in a geriatric dog. *Vet Clin Pathol*. 2017;46(3):535–537.

16. Meuten DJ. *Tumors in Domestic Animals*. 5th ed. Ames, IA: John Wiley & sons, Inc.; 2017.

17. Sprague W, Thrall MA. Recurrent skin mass from the digit of a dog. *Vet Clin Pathol*. 2001;30(4):189–192.

18. Adedeji AO, Affolter VK, Christopher MM. Cytologic features of cutaneous follicular tumors and cysts in dogs. *Vet Clin Pathol*. 2017;46(1):143–150.

19. Carroll EE, Fossey SL, Mangus LM, et al. Malignant pilomatricoma in 3 dogs. *Vet Pathol*. 2010;47(5):937–943.

20. Höinghaus R, Hewicker-Trautwein M, Mischke R. Immunocytochemical differentiation of canine mesenchymal tumors in cytologic imprint preparations. *Vet Clin Pathol*. 2008;37(1):104–111.

21. Dennis MM, McSporran KD, Bacon NJ, et al. Prognostic factors for cutaneous and subcutaneous soft tissue sarcomas in dogs. *Vet Pathol*. 2011;48(1):73–84.

22. Little LK, Goldschmidt M. Cytologic appearance of a keloidal fibrosarcoma in a dog. *Vet Clin Pathol*. 2007;36(4):364–367.

23. Fulmer AK, Mauldin GE. Canine histiocytic neoplasia: an overview. *Can Vet J*. 2007;48(10):1041–1050.

Subcutaneous Glandular Tissue: Mammary, Salivary, Thyroid, and Parathyroid

Robin W. Allison and Raquel M. Walton

Mammary, salivary, thyroid, and parathyroid glands are located in the subcutaneous fat layer. Knowledge of the normal microanatomy of these glands and of other structures in proximity is important for accurate cytological interpretation. Except for the thyroid and parathyroid glands, regional locations of these glands differ considerably. Cytologically, normal exocrine glands (mammary and salivary) may appear similar, but they differ from normal endocrine glands (thyroid and parathyroid). Lymphoid and adipose tissues may be found near any of these glands; salivary tissue may be inadvertently aspirated when attempting to aspirate submandibular lymph nodes. Thymic tissue may be near the thyroid and parathyroid tissues, especially in young animals or when any of these tissues exist in ectopic locations.

Cytological evaluation of subcutaneous glandular tissue is a valuable extension of clinical examination. Collection of samples by fine-needle aspiration (FNA) is simple and quick and avoids the trauma and anesthetic risk for surgical biopsy. Most lesions are readily palpable and, therefore, easily aspirated. Although aspiration is the usual means of obtaining specimens, cytological evaluation of mammary glands may also be performed on imprints of excised tissue, scrapings of ulcerated surface lesions, and secretions.

The primary goals of aspiration cytology are to distinguish inflammatory lesions from neoplastic lesions and to differentiate, when possible, benign neoplasms from malignant neoplasms. However, endocrine tumors (e.g., thyroid and parathyroid) frequently exhibit few cellular criteria of malignancy, appearing cytologically benign even when malignant. These tumors require histopathological evaluation of invasion and other features to determine their malignant potential.

Mammary gland lesions present special challenges because of the diversity of cell types that may be involved and the often-overlapping cell populations within hyperplastic, dysplastic, benign, and malignant lesions. Reported diagnostic accuracy for cytological differentiation of benign neoplasms from malignant mammary neoplasms in dogs varies from 33% to 93%.[1-5] Best agreement with the histological diagnosis was achieved when multiple aspirates from each lesion were evaluated collaboratively by two experienced cytologists.[1] A cytological grading system has been proposed for differentiation of benign mammary tumors from malignant mammary tumors in dogs on the basis of 10 important criteria of malignancy, but these criteria were developed for wet fixation preparations stained with a Papanicolaou stain, which is not typically used by veterinary cytopathologists.[2] In several studies, the predictive value of a positive result was higher than that of a negative result, suggesting that cytological evaluation tends to underdiagnose mammary gland malignancies.[2,3] The most recent study evaluating cytological and histological correlation showed high accuracy (93%), which may have been aided by evaluation of at least four aspirate samples per tumor and consensus diagnosis by two clinical pathologists.[1]

A high rate of false-negative results in cases of malignancies may be caused by several factors. Sampling errors occur if the needle is not directed into a representative area of the tumor. This problem is proportional to tumor size, and sampling of multiple sites in large tumors may increase the likelihood of aspirating neoplastic cells.[1] Multiple mammary tumors in an animal may be of different types, thus requiring examination of all lesions. Tumors containing an abundance of connective tissue may exfoliate poorly, leading to nondiagnostic samples. Mammary gland malignancies may be diagnosed on the basis of histopathological evidence of tissue invasion regardless of cellular atypia.[6] It is no surprise that cytological samples from such tumors may be misleading.

Conversely, some encapsulated tumors containing areas with significant cell pleomorphism may be considered benign on the basis of absence of tissue invasion. The presence of necrosis or inflammation can result in cellular atypia, and cytological samples from tumors containing necrosis or inflammation may falsely suggest a malignant process. Accuracy of evaluation will also depend on the experience of the cytologist. Samples yielding equivocal results, for example, samples of cystic fluid, tissues with nonseptic inflammatory changes, or those cytologically suggestive of benign neoplasia, should be evaluated histologically. Presence of marked criteria of malignancy makes malignant neoplasia most likely, but histopathology should still be employed to confirm the diagnosis. Samples yielding definitive nonneoplastic diagnoses may not need to be evaluated histologically.

MAMMARY GLANDS

Normal Cytological Appearance

Mammary tissue of dogs and cats consists of five pairs of modified sweat glands that extend along the ventral body wall from the cranial thorax to the inguinal region. Glands consist of secretory acini and a series of excretory ducts. Myoepithelial cells lie between glandular epithelial cells and the basement membrane. During lactation, the glands undergo marked hypertrophy to produce colostrum and then milk (Fig. 6.1). Normal mammary secretions contain large amounts of protein and lipid droplets and are of low cellularity. The predominant cell type in milk is the foam cell—a large, vacuolated epithelial cell that resembles an active macrophage (Fig. 6.2). These cells usually occur singly. Small numbers of lymphocytes and neutrophils may also be present.

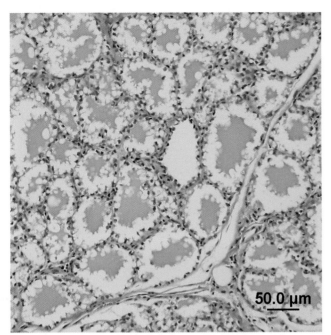

Fig. 6.1 Biopsy of mammary tissue from lactating cat. Glandular acini are hyperplastic and distended with eosinophilic secretory product (hematoxylin and eosin [H&E], 200×).

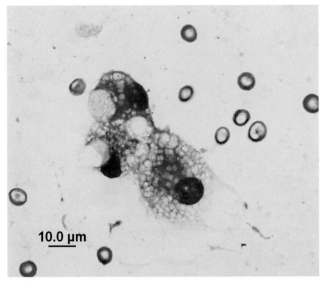

Fig. 6.2 Several vacuolated foam cells from a mammary gland aspirate contain eccentric oval nuclei and abundant vacuolated cytoplasm with a variable amount of basophilic secretory product (Wright stain, 1000×).

Aspirates of normal mammary tissue are frequently acellular or contain only blood. When mammary tissue is present, secretory cells are arranged in an acinar pattern. Individual cells have moderate amounts of basophilic cytoplasm and round, dark nuclei of uniform size. Duct epithelial cells have basal, ovoid nuclei and scanty cytoplasm and are arranged in small sheets or fragments of ductules. Myoepithelial cells appear as dark-staining, naked, oval nuclei or as spindle-shaped cells. Adipocytes and lipid droplets may be present.

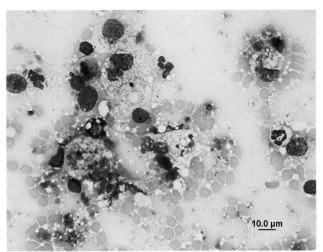

Fig. 6.3 Aspirate from an inflamed mammary gland contains macrophages, foam cells, and neutrophils with amorphous basophilic secretory material in the background (Wright stain, 1000×).

Benign Lesions
Mastitis

Mastitis, or inflammation of the mammary glands, may occur either as a diffuse form involving two or more mammae or as a focal lesion. Mastitis is usually associated with postpartum lactation or pseudopregnancy and may result from ascending or hematogenous infections.[7] Mammary secretions are usually adequate for diagnosis in cases of diffuse inflammation, whereas aspirates may be required for diagnosis of focal lesions. Smears are highly cellular and contain large amounts of debris. Inflammatory cells may include neutrophils, lymphocytes, and macrophages in variable numbers, depending on the causative agent (Fig. 6.3). Bacteria may be seen within phagocytes. Offending agents are usually coliforms, *Streptococcus* or *Staphylococcus* spp., although other bacteria and fungi may occasionally be isolated.[7]

Duct Ectasia (Cysts)

Duct ectasia results from a dysplastic process in which dilated extralobular ducts expand to form large cavitations.[6] Cyst linings may consist of single layers of flattened epithelium or may have papillary projections. Cysts may be present as single nodules or multinodular masses that grow slowly and have a bluish surface. These are common in middle-aged and older female dogs but may occasionally appear in young dogs. Aspirated fluid is usually yellow, brown, green, or blood tinged and of low cellularity unless concurrent inflammation is present. Cells are primarily vacuolated, or pigment-laden macrophages and cholesterol crystals may be evident. Duct ectasia may be secondary to occlusion of duct lumina by intraductal neoplasms; thus, cystic lesions should be evaluated histologically to exclude an underlying neoplasm.

Solid Masses

Although historically estrogen has been considered the principal ovarian hormonal risk factor for breast cancer development, recent evidence indicates that progestins also play a significant role in mammary carcinogenesis.[8] Ovariectomized dogs exposed to progestins for 6 to 12 months develop mammary gland hyperplasia and/or benign tumors, and there are reports of malignant mammary carcinomas occurring in dogs upon administration of high doses of progestins.[8] Hyperplastic/dysplastic lesions and benign epithelial neoplasms of mammary tissue include duct ectasia, lobular hyperplasia, epitheliosis, papillomatosis, adenomas, fibroadenomas, and duct papillomas, all of which contain

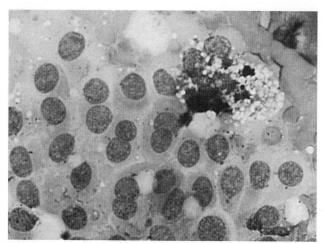

Fig. 6.4 Sheet of glandular cells exhibiting little nuclear or cytoplasmic pleomorphism and a fine granular chromatin pattern characteristic of a mammary adenoma. A large, pigment-laden macrophage is present (Wright stain, 1250×).

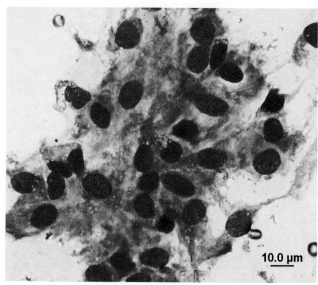

Fig. 6.6 Spindled cells and eosinophilic extracellular matrix in an aspirate of a benign mammary complex adenoma from a dog, same case as Fig. 6.5 (Wright stain, 1000×).

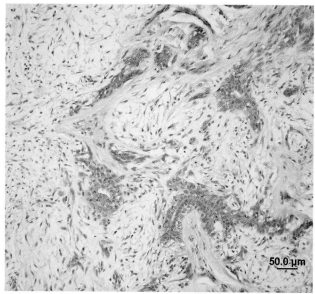

Fig. 6.5 Biopsy of a benign mammary complex adenoma from a dog contains mixed mesenchymal and epithelial components. Aspirates from this mass are shown in Figs. 6.6 to 6.8 (hematoxylin and eosin [H&E], 200×).

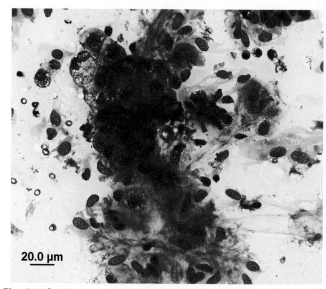

Fig. 6.7 Canine mammary complex adenoma, same aspirate as Fig. 6.6. Abundant eosinophilic matrix material and spindled mesenchymal cells near a cluster of vacuolated mammary epithelial cells. Epithelial cells exhibit moderate criteria of malignancy (Wright stain, 500×).

similar cell populations.[6] It should be noted that although there is a higher incidence of these lesions in sexually intact dogs, ovariectomized status does not preclude the presence of hyperplastic/dysplastic lesions.[9]

Smears made from aspirates of hyperplastic or benign masses contain many epithelial cells occurring singly or arranged in sheets and clusters. These cells generally exhibit little pleomorphism, having evenly dispersed chromatin and small, round nucleoli. However, dilated ducts can contain exfoliated epithelial cells that may have more criteria of malignancy than the rest of the mass.[10,11] Sampling those cells for cytological evaluation may result in a false impression of malignancy. An interpretation of carcinoma is more likely to be accurate in highly cellular samples when the majority of cells are markedly pleomorphic, rather than a few scattered aggregates. Pigment-laden macrophages may be present (Fig. 6.4). Some of these processes can also involve myoepithelial cells and connective tissue, further complicating the cytological picture. Benign tumors involving stromal and epithelial elements, such as complex adenomas (Fig. 6.5),

fibroadenomas, and benign mixed tumors, are common in dogs and sometimes seen in cats.[10] Smears of aspirates from these lesions contain spindle-shaped cells of myoepithelial or connective tissue origin, in addition to clusters of epithelial cells similar to those described previously (Fig. 6.6). These lesions can be difficult to differentiate even with histopathology because of the spectrum of cell types involved. Benign mixed tumors may produce cartilage, bone, or fat, in addition to fibrous tissue and epithelial tissue.[10,12] Aspirates from these lesions may contain all these elements, but if a single population predominates, the cytology can be misleading.[12] Additionally, individual cell pleomorphism is occasionally marked in tumors considered benign because of lack of tissue invasion (Figs. 6.7 and 6.8).[5] Spindled mesenchymal cells are not a definitive cytological characteristic of complex or mixed tumors because they may also be found in some simple tumors.[2]

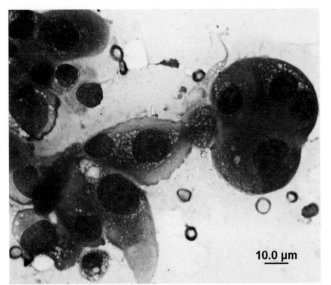

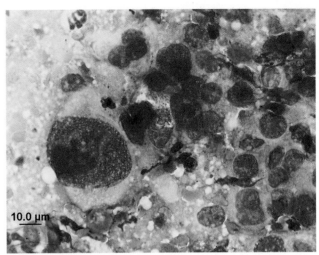

Fig. 6.9 Epithelial cells from a feline mammary carcinoma have marked variation in cell and nuclear morphology. One large nucleus contains an abnormally shaped macronucleolus (Wright stain, 1000×).

Fig. 6.8 Canine mammary complex adenoma, same aspirate as Fig. 6.6. These epithelial cells exhibit moderate to marked criteria of malignancy including anisocytosis, anisokaryosis, and multiple prominent nucleoli. Histopathology revealed this tumor to be well-encapsulated and benign despite individual cell pleomorphism (Wright stain, 1000×).

A specific form of mammary hyperplasia, termed *fibroepithelial hyperplasia* or *fibroadenomatous change*, has been recognized in cats. This condition may affect young female cats that are pregnant or actively cycling or cats of either gender that have received progesterone-containing compounds.[13,14] Typically, rapid enlargement of multiple glands occurs. Aspirates from affected mammary glands contain both uniform epithelial cells and spindled mesenchymal cells, usually associated with abundant pink extracellular matrix material.[15] The epithelial cells are of ductal origin and have a relatively high nuclear-to-cytoplasmic (N:C) ratio with dense, round nuclei and a small amount of basophilic cytoplasm. The mesenchymal cells may exhibit moderate anisocytosis and anisokaryosis.[15] Ovariohysterectomy or removal of the progesterone-containing compound is generally curative. Drug therapy with a progesterone antagonist has also been an effective treatment.[16]

Malignant Neoplasms

Mammary gland tumors are common in both dogs and cats; however, the biological behavior of the tumors varies greatly between these species. Mammary tumors comprise up to 50% of neoplasms in the canine female, and 40% to 50% of those tumors are malignant, with adenocarcinomas being the most common histological type.[10,17] Mammary tumors are the third most common neoplasm in cats and account for about 17% of all neoplasms in queens.[18] In contrast to mammary gland tumors in dogs, up to 80% of feline mammary gland tumors are malignant. As in dogs, adenocarcinomas are the most frequently diagnosed malignant neoplasm in cats.[10,18] Mammary tumors are rare in males of both species.[10,19]

A new histological classification and grading scheme was proposed for canine mammary tumors in 2011.[6] Significant histological criteria recognized for the diagnosis of malignant canine mammary tumors include tumor type; degree of pleomorphism; mitotic index; presence of random, multifocal necrosis; peritumoral or lymphatic invasion; and regional lymph node metastasis.[6] The presence of necrosis alone is not predictive of malignant potential. Necrosis can be present in benign tumors as a central lesion as a result of loss of vascular supply,

whereas it is typically random and multifocal in malignant tumors as a result of rapid cellular proliferation.[10] Multiple morphological types of carcinoma are recognized histologically on the basis of the pattern of cell arrangement and degree of cell differentiation.[6,10] Carcinomas are also graded on the basis of histological features, such as tubule formation, mitotic rate, and cellular pleomorphism. Many different types of carcinomas may contain collagenous stroma, sometimes in large amounts. Both histological type and grade, and degree of invasion, have been shown to have prognostic significance in dogs.[20,21] Similarly, in cats with mammary carcinomas, histological grade and lymph node/lymphovascular invasion are significant prognostic parameters.[22,23]

Dogs frequently have multiple tumors, which are often of different histological types.[17] A study by Sorenmo et al. provided evidence that canine mammary tumors may progress from benign to malignant over time and demonstrated a strong association between tumor size and malignancy.[24] It should be noted that lymph drainage is altered in neoplastic mammary glands in dogs.[10] Staging for mammary gland tumors should consider the potential for altered lymphatic drainage. The cranial thoracic glands, M1 and M2, normally drain to the axillary node, but neoplastic M1 and M2 can drain to the sternal node as well. In addition to the normal drainage to the axillary and superficial inguinal nodes, neoplastic M3 may drain to the medial iliac node. M4 and M5 drain to the superficial inguinal node (and M4 may drain to the iliac node); however, metastatic disease from M4 may also occur in the axillary node and from M5 in the popliteal lymph node.

Cytological criteria that best correlate with malignancy include variable nuclear size, nuclear giant forms, high N:C ratio, variable numbers of nucleoli, abnormal nucleolar shape, and the presence of macronucleoli (Figs. 6.9 and 6.10), especially when three or greater nuclear criteria are noted in a significant proportion of epithelial cells (>20%).[1,2] However, as previously discussed, mammary malignancies may be well differentiated and show little cellular pleomorphism, and moderate criteria of malignancy may be present in tumors considered benign because of lack of tissue invasion.[6] Smears of aspirates from adenocarcinomas generally contain epithelial cells occurring singly and in clusters of variable size. Adenocarcinoma cells are usually round, with round to oval, eccentrically placed nuclei and variable quantities of basophilic cytoplasm that occasionally contains vacuoles that may be

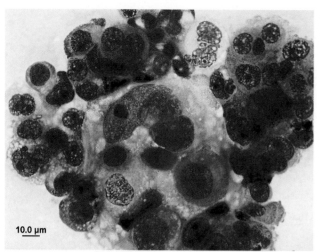

Fig. 6.10 Pleural fluid from the same cat as Fig. 6.9 contains tightly cohesive clusters of epithelial cells with marked criteria of malignancy, confirming presence of intrathoracic metastatic disease (Wright stain, 1000×).

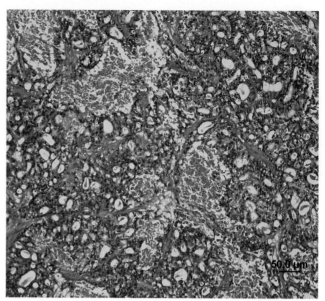

Fig. 6.12 Biopsy specimen of a ductular adenocarcinoma from a cat. Pale pink areas represent necrosis randomly distributed between neoplastic epithelial cells. Aspirates of this mass are shown in Fig. 6.13 (hematoxylin and eosin [H&E], 200×).

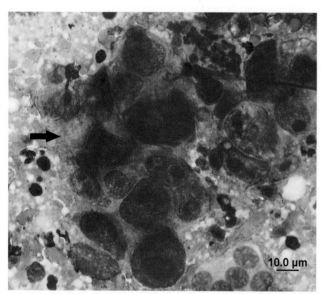

Fig. 6.11 Aspirate from a feline mammary carcinoma. Eosinophilic secretory product is visible within the cytoplasm of one cell (arrow) (Wright stain, 1000×).

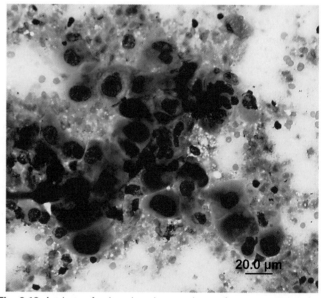

Fig. 6.13 Aspirate of a ductular adenocarcinoma from a cat, same case as Fig. 6.12. Pleomorphic cohesive malignant epithelial cells are present in an amorphous basophilic background of necrotic material (aqueous Romanowsky stain, 500×).

filled with secretory product (Fig. 6.11). Cell borders are usually distinct, and cells may be arranged in acinar or tubular patterns. Binucleate or multinucleate cells may be seen. Mesenchymal cells may be present in variable numbers. Necrosis, readily identifiable in histological sections, may also be observed in cytological samples from malignant tumors, appearing as amorphous, smudged, basophilic material (Figs. 6.12 and 6.13), but as noted previously, it is not pathognomonic for malignancy because central necrosis may occur in benign tumors as well.[10]

Anaplastic carcinomas are diffusely infiltrative tumors composed of large, pleomorphic epithelial cells with bizarre nuclear and nucleolar forms (Fig. 6.14).[6,10] These cells occur singly and in variably sized clusters and have a high N:C ratio (Fig. 6.15). Multinucleate cells and mitotic figures are common (Figs. 6.16 and 6.17). These tumors may contain abundant collagenous stroma infiltrated by inflammatory cells.[6,10] Anaplastic carcinomas are considered highly malignant, frequently metastasize, and have a poor prognosis.

Inflammatory carcinomas have distinctive clinical and histological features and are aggressive tumors associated with a poor prognosis.[25,26] These tumors may be clinically misdiagnosed as mastitis because of the marked local tissue swelling and edema with signs of systemic disease; however, inflammatory cells are not a prominent histological or cytological feature. "Inflammatory" carcinomas are so named for the gross appearance of the glands, which mimics inflammation but is actually caused by blockage of the superficial dermal lymphatics by neoplastic emboli. Inflammatory carcinomas have been reported in dogs and cats, with a variety of histological types represented.[25-28] In one report, cytology of mammary gland aspirates revealed malignant epithelial cells in 15 of 33 dogs and contributed to

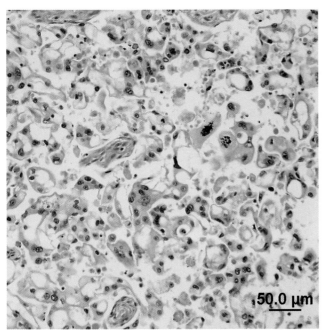

Fig. 6.14 Biopsy specimen of an anaplastic mammary carcinoma from a dog. These cells are markedly pleomorphic and variably cohesive. Aspirates from this mass are shown in Figs. 6.15 to 6.17 (hematoxylin and eosin [H&E], 200×).

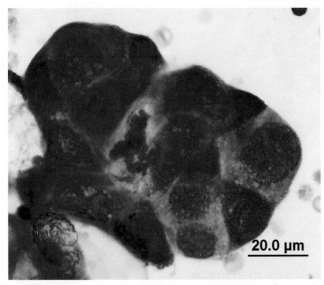

Fig. 6.15 Aspirate of an anaplastic mammary carcinoma from a dog, same case as Fig. 6.14. Cohesive cluster of malignant mammary epithelial cells with a high nuclear-to-cytoplasmic ratio and multiple prominent nucleoli. A mitotic figure is visible in the center of the cluster (Wright stain, 1000×).

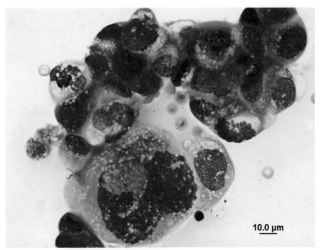

Fig. 6.16 Anaplastic mammary carcinoma, same aspirate as Fig. 6.15. Malignant epithelial cells have cytoplasmic vacuoles in this cluster, and two mitotic figures are present (Wright stain, 1000×).

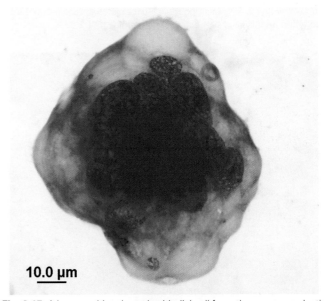

Fig. 6.17 A large multinucleated epithelial cell from the same anaplastic mammary carcinoma as Fig. 6.15. Note the nuclear fragments visible in the cytoplasm (Wright stain, 1000×).

determining the diagnosis; the other 18 cytological samples had low cellularity.[27] The hallmark of inflammatory carcinoma is the finding of dermal lymphatic involvement, and thus, it is necessarily a histological diagnosis.[6,27]

Nonglandular carcinomas may be simple, with only epithelial proliferation, or complex, with cells of epithelial and myoepithelial origin. Accordingly, cytology samples may contain predominantly epithelial cells or a mixture of cell types. In contrast to adenocarcinomas, epithelial cells from nonglandular carcinomas may not contain intracytoplasmic vacuoles (Fig. 6.18). Squamous cell carcinomas in mammary glands appear cytologically similar to those in other body regions. Tumor cells occur singly or in small sheets and may be keratinized or nonkeratinized. Nuclei are variable in size, from small and pyknotic to large with immature chromatin and prominent nucleoli. Cytoplasm is variably abundant and basophilic, appearing glassy and blue-green with keratinization (see Chapter 5 for further discussion of the features of squamous cell carcinoma). These tumors frequently adhere to the overlying dermis and may be ulcerated, leading to the presence of many inflammatory cells and bacteria in samples taken from ulcerated areas. It is important to realize that squamous metaplasia may occur in other tumor types; thus, finding squamous cells on a cytological sample is not specific for squamous cell carcinoma (Fig. 6.19).[6,10,11]

Mammary sarcomas are less common than carcinomas. They are usually large, firm tumors that have an unfavorable prognosis because of local recurrence and metastasis.[10] Osteosarcoma is the most frequent type in the dog.[6] Cells from sarcomas are often irregular or spindle shaped, occur singly or in small aggregates, and have indistinct cell borders. Pink matrix material may be

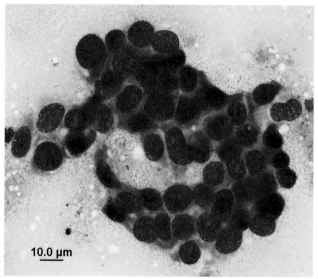

Fig. 6.18 These cohesive epithelial cells from an aspirate of a canine papillary mammary carcinoma have no cytoplasmic vacuoles and minimal cellular atypia, emphasizing the need for histopathological confirmation when neoplasia is suspected (Wright stain, 1000×).

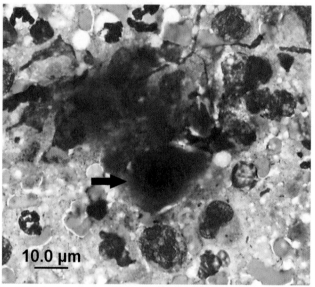

Fig. 6.19 Aspirate from a feline mammary carcinoma. A single cell contains glassy dark-blue cytoplasm and angular cytoplasm *(arrow)*, consistent with squamous differentiation (Wright stain, 1000×).

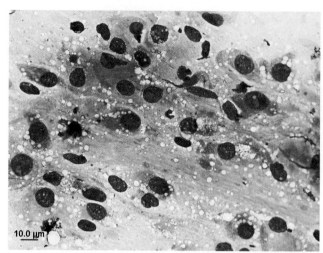

Fig. 6.20 Spindled cells and extracellular matrix in an aspirate of a malignant mixed mammary gland tumor in a dog (Wright stain, 1000×). (Glass slide courtesy Boone et al., Texas A&M University, presented at the 2000 ASVCP case review session.)

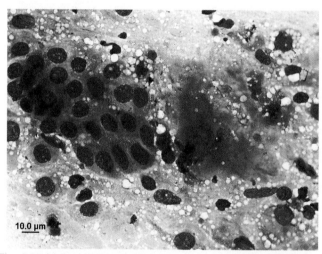

Fig. 6.21 Malignant mixed mammary gland tumor, same aspirate as Fig. 6.20. A few clusters of well-differentiated epithelial cells and an abundance of spindled cells and extracellular matrix. Despite the lack of cellular pleomorphism, neoplastic epithelial cells within lymphatics and evidence of metastases to lung and lymph node confirmed malignancy in this case (Wright stain, 1000×).

associated with cell aggregates. The degree of pleomorphism and mitotic activity is variable and indicative of tumor malignancy. In general, cytological criteria of malignancy described for carcinomas apply to sarcomas. Cytological interpretation of these cell populations may be confusing because mesenchymal cells, collagenous stroma, cartilage, and even bone formation may also be found in benign mixed tumors, mixed-type carcinomas, and carcinosarcomas (Figs. 6.20 and 6.21).[6,12] Histologically and cytologically, fibrosarcoma may be confused with other spindle cell neoplasms (spindle cell carcinoma, malignant myoepithelioma). Immunohistochemistry is required for differentiation.[6] Carcinosarcomas (malignant mixed mammary tumors) are uncommon tumors of mixed origin, containing both malignant epithelial and malignant mesenchymal populations.[6,10]

Table 6.1 presents a summary of the most common cytological findings in aspirates from mammary lesions.

SALIVARY GLANDS

Normal Cytological Appearance

The major salivary glands in dogs and cats are the parotid, mandibular, sublingual, and zygomatic glands. Minor, or buccal, salivary glands are spread over the oral mucosa. Salivary glands are composed of secretory cells arranged in acini and an extensive ductular network. A layer of myoepithelial cells lies between glandular cells and the basement membrane. Aspirated samples from normal salivary glands reveal secretory epithelial cells with small, round nuclei and abundant cytoplasm distended with clear vacuoles. Acinar cells usually occur in clusters (Fig. 6.22). When seen individually, these cells are difficult to differentiate from foamy macrophages. Ductal epithelial cells are seen less frequently and have a higher N:C ratio (Fig. 6.23). Basophilic mucin may be present in the background. Samples may also include occasional spindle-shaped myoepithelial cells, adipocytes, and lipid droplets. Hemorrhage is frequent upon aspiration of salivary glands. Erythrocytes in smears assume a characteristic linear pattern ("windrowing") caused by the mucin content of the sample.

TABLE 6.1   Common Cytological Findings in Mammary Gland Aspirates

Cell Types	Key Features	Differential Diagnoses	Comments
Foam cells Inflammatory cells: Neutrophils, lymphocytes, plasma cells, macrophages Epithelial cell clusters	Predominance of inflammatory cells Proteinaceous debris ± Bacteria Epithelial cells may be reactive	Mastitis	Mild atypia in epithelial cells expected with inflammation
Vacuolated macrophages ± Epithelial cell clusters	Low-cellularity fluid aspirated Minimal atypia in epithelial cells	Cyst	Cysts may occur along or with benign or malignant neoplasia Sample solid tissue and cystic fluid
Epithelial cell clusters Spindled mesenchymal cells Extracellular matrix	Uniform epithelial cells, high nuclear-to-cytoplasmic (N:C) ratio Mildly pleomorphic mesenchymal cells with abundant matrix	Fibroepithelial hyperplasia	Typically affects young intact female cats, or cats previously treated with progesterone drugs Affects multiple glands Rapid growth Cytological appearance similar to many benign tumors
Variable numbers of epithelial cells and mesenchymal cells ± Extracellular matrix, cartilage, or bone (osteoblasts) ± Inflammatory cells ± Necrosis (not seen with lobular hyperplasia)	Variable, depending on specific process Usually mild pleomorphism, but may be moderate to marked	Benign neoplasia (adenoma/complex adenoma, benign mixed tumors, etc.) Lobular hyperplasia	Multiple possible cell types result in confusing cytology Inflammatory nodules may occur with lobular hyperplasia Tumors exfoliating numerous atypical cells may suggest malignancy despite lack of tissue invasion Histopathological confirmation required.
Variable numbers of epithelial cells and mesenchymal cells ± Extracellular matrix, cartilage, or bone (osteoblasts) ± Inflammatory cells ± Necrosis	Variable, depending on specific process Cellular pleomorphism can be minimal or marked	Malignant neoplasia (adenocarcinoma, various carcinomas, inflammatory carcinoma, fibrosarcoma, osteosarcoma, etc.)	Canine: ≈50% are malignant Feline: ≈80% are malignant Multiple possible cell types result in confusing cytology Marked pleomorphism increases likelihood of malignancy Tumors with minimal atypia may be malignant based on tissue invasion Histopathological confirmation required

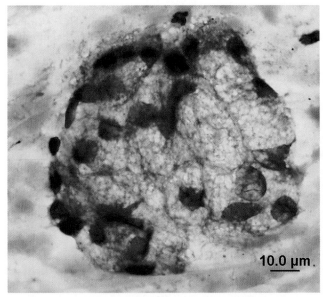

Fig. 6.22 Cohesive cluster of vacuolated secretory cells from a normal salivary gland (Wright stain, 1000×).

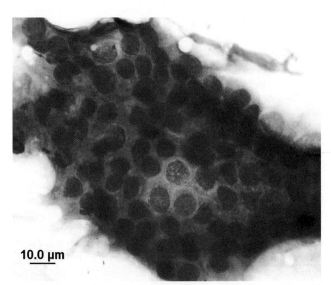

Fig. 6.23 Sheet of nonsecretory epithelial cells with a high nuclear-to-cytoplasmic ratio from a normal salivary gland most likely represent ductal epithelium (Wright stain, 1000×).

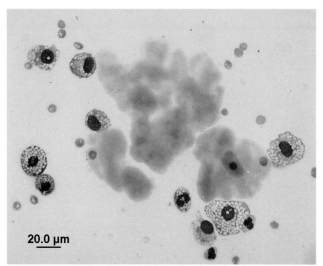

Fig. 6.24 Foamy macrophages, vacuolated epithelial cells, or both, and a few erythrocytes from a salivary sialocele. Note the extracellular clumps of amorphous basophilic material, consistent with mucin (Wright stain, 500×).

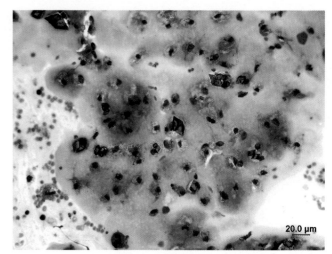

Fig. 6.25 Numerous vacuolated cells and large, golden, rhomboidal hematoidin crystals indicating previous hemorrhage in an aspirate from a sialocele. Erythrocytes and basophilic mucin are present in the background (Wright stain, 500×).

Nonneoplastic Lesions
Sialoceles

The most common salivary gland disorder in dogs is the sialocele. These are non–epithelium-lined cavities filled with salivary secretions. Leakage of salivary secretions into fascial tissues usually follows blunt trauma but may occasionally be secondary to calculi or duct obstruction by bite wounds, abscesses, and ear canal surgery. Swellings occur most commonly on the floor of the mouth (ranulae) or the cranial cervical area and less frequently in pharyngeal or retrobulbar areas. Aspirated fluid is viscous, clear, or blood tinged and contains low to moderate numbers of nucleated cells.

Cytological evaluation of sialocele aspirates usually reveals diffuse or irregular clumps of homogeneous eosinophilic to basophilic mucin. Large phagocytic cells with small, round nuclei and abundant foamy cytoplasm may be found individually or in small clusters (Fig. 6.24). Salivary gland epithelial cells may be present but are not easily distinguished from macrophages cytologically. Erythrocytes often occur in linear patterns ("windrows") because of the mucin content. Nondegenerate neutrophils are present in variable numbers, depending on the extent of the inflammatory response. Neutrophil nuclear segmentation may be difficult to appreciate because the cells often do not spread out well in the viscous fluid. Lymphocytes may increase in number with extended duration of the lesion. Macrophages containing phagocytized erythrocytes or debris may also be present. Golden, rhomboidal hematoidin crystals seen extracellularly or within the cytoplasm of macrophages result from erythrocyte degradation secondary to hemorrhage and suggest chronicity (Fig. 6.25).

Sialadenosis

Idiopathic unilateral or bilateral enlargement of the mandibular salivary glands (sialadenosis) associated with clinical signs of hypersalivation, retching/gagging or gulping, and vomiting has been reported in both dogs and cats.[29-32] Aspirates from affected glands have shown normal salivary epithelium, and histopathological evaluation has revealed normal salivary tissue with no evidence of inflammation or necrosis. These animals typically respond to oral phenobarbital therapy, suggesting a neurogenic cause.[29,30,32] Hypersalivation with salivary gland enlargement caused by acinar hyperplasia is reported as a common clinical finding associated with spirocercosis.[33]

Salivary Gland Infarction/Necrotizing Sialometaplasia

Salivary infarction has been reported in dogs and cats.[34,35] Histologically, infarction of the salivary gland appears as coagulative necrosis surrounded by a zone of congested and hemorrhagic tissue infiltrated by neutrophils and macrophages. Thrombi may be visible in vessels within the salivary glands. A hallmark feature of this disease is the marked dysplasia and squamous metaplasia of the salivary ducts adjacent to the areas of coagulative necrosis. Fine-needle aspirate in one reported case consisted of mixed salivary glandular cells, pleomorphic spindled cells, and rafts of mononuclear epithelioid cells with increased numbers of neutrophils.[36] In this case, the cytological diagnosis was sialadenitis and possible mesenchymal neoplasia, but histopathology revealed necrosis and ductal squamous metaplasia, leading to the final diagnosis. Thus accurate cytological interpretation may be limited when multiple cell types are present. The terms *sialadenosis* and *necrotizing sialometaplasia* have been used synonymously in the literature; however, it is uncertain whether these represent the same clinical entity because histological and cytological evaluation of salivary glands in cases of sialadenosis is reported to be unremarkable,[29-32] whereas salivary gland infarction/necrotizing sialometaplasia has distinctive histological features.

Sialadenitis

Inflammatory lesions of the salivary gland are uncommon.[37] Inflammation may be primary or secondary, extending into the gland from surrounding tissues. Primary inflammation is often associated with a sialocele, as described previously, or, rarely, with infarction. In both situations, mixed inflammatory cells (neutrophils, lymphocytes, and macrophages) may be present. Sialadenitis may occur with systemic viral infections (caused by canine distemper virus, rabies virus, and paramyxovirus). Viral lesions may contain significant numbers of lymphoid cells. Secondary inflammation may occur from trauma or bacterial infections in surrounding tissues. The inflammatory cell infiltrate will vary, depending on the primary process. A recent report of trichomoniasis associated with a sialocele contained an eosinophilic infiltrate.[38] In bacterial infections, degenerate neutrophils with phagocytized bacteria may be observed. Depending on the extent of the infection, salivary epithelial cells may not be evident in cytological samples.

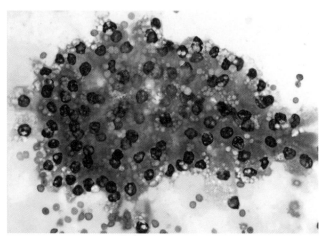

Fig. 6.26 Aspirate of a salivary cystadenoma from a cat. A cluster of poorly vacuolated epithelial cells that have a disorganized appearance despite a benign diagnosis (aqueous Romanowsky stain, 1000×).

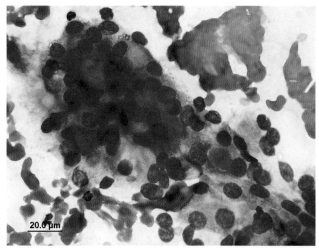

Fig. 6.27 Aspirate of a salivary adenocarcinoma from a cat. Cluster of nonvacuolated epithelial cells that have a disorganized appearance and indistinct cell borders. A small amount of eosinophilic secretory product is visible (Wright stain, 1000×).

Neoplastic Lesions

Salivary gland neoplasia is uncommon in dogs and cats. It occurs most frequently in animals age greater than 10 years, and some evidence suggests that Siamese cats may be predisposed.[39] Both the parotid and mandibular salivary glands are frequent sites for salivary neoplasia.[35,39] Benign salivary tumors occur less frequently compared with malignant tumors and include pleomorphic adenomas, oncocytomas, cystadenoma, sebaceous adenoma, canalicular adenoma, and ductal papilloma.[35] Pleomorphic adenomas contain epithelial, myoepithelial, and stromal elements and may include areas of cartilage or bone. Cells in benign tumors do not necessarily appear as well-differentiated salivary epithelial tissue on cytological evaluation, but this should not prompt an interpretation of carcinoma (Fig. 6.26).

Carcinomas occur most often (80%–90%), and a wide variety of tumor types can be recognized histologically, including acinic cell carcinomas, adenocarcinomas, squamous cell carcinomas, mucoepidermoid tumors, basal cell carcinomas, sebaceous carcinomas, and undifferentiated carcinomas.[35,39-41] Acinic cell carcinomas and adenocarcinomas in dogs and adenocarcinomas in cats represent the most common malignant neoplasms of the salivary glands.[35,39,42] Grading did not predict survival time in a small series of canine and feline salivary gland adenocarcinomas.[39]

Cytology samples from salivary carcinomas contain cohesive epithelial cells with round to oval nuclei and basophilic cytoplasm with a relatively high N:C ratio. These cells may show little differentiation toward normal vacuolated salivary epithelium (Figs. 6.27 and 6.28). Criteria of malignancy may be mild, consisting only of mild anisocytosis and anisokaryosis, or may be more pronounced with the presence of prominent nucleoli and mitotic figures in addition to marked pleomorphism.[43,44] Eosinophilic secretory product may be seen extracellularly or within the cytoplasm of the neoplastic cells in varying amounts (Figs. 6.29 to 6.31).

Squamous epithelial cells can be a component not only of salivary squamous cell carcinomas but also of mucoepidermoid carcinomas and necrotizing sialometaplasia. Salivary squamous cell carcinomas have a similar cytological appearance to squamous cell carcinomas in other locations (see Chapter 5 for further discussion of the features of squamous cell carcinoma). Mucoepidermoid carcinomas contain both squamous and mucus-producing cell types.

Malignant mixed tumors of salivary glands are rare but have been described in both dogs and cats.[35,45,46] These tumors may be the result of carcinoma arising in a previously benign pleomorphic adenoma.

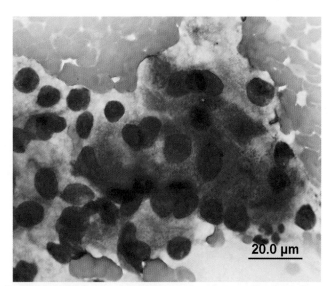

Fig. 6.28 Salivary adenocarcinoma, same aspirate as Fig. 6.27. Granular, eosinophilic, intracytoplasmic secretory material is present within epithelial cells (Wright stain, 1000×).

Rarely, true carcinosarcomas have been reported, containing both sarcoma and carcinoma elements. Cytology would be expected to reveal a mixture of epithelial and mesenchymal cell types with criteria of malignancy.

Table 6.2 presents a summary of the most common cytological findings in aspirates from salivary gland lesions.

THYROID GLANDS

Normal Cytological Appearance

The thyroid glands of dogs and cats are paired endocrine glands in the ventral cervical region. Their exact location may vary from the laryngeal region to the thoracic inlet. Ectopic thyroid tissue may also occur in the cranial mediastinum near the heart base. The normal thyroid gland is not readily palpated and is, therefore, not usually aspirated for cytological examination. Palpable abnormalities may occur unilaterally or bilaterally as diffuse swelling, multinodular swelling, or solitary nodular masses. Aspiration cytology may help differentiate

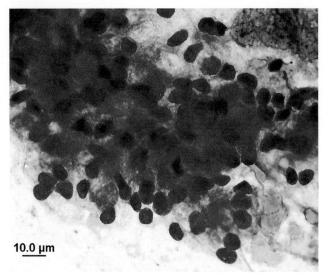

Fig. 6.29 Aspirate of a salivary adenocarcinoma from a dog contains abundant extracellular secretory material and monomorphic epithelial cells (Wright stain, 1000×).

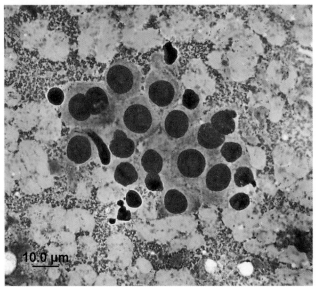

Fig. 6.30 Salivary adenocarcinoma, same aspirate as Fig. 6.29. Individual epithelial cells with round nuclei and lightly basophilic cytoplasm are present in a thick eosinophilic background of secretory material. Cellular pleomorphism is minimal (Wright stain, 1000×).

benign lesions from malignant lesions and help rule out other causes of cervical masses, including abscesses, lymphadenopathy, sialoceles, and nonthyroid neoplasms.

Thyroid tissue consists of numerous follicles lined by cuboidal to polygonal epithelial cells and filled with colloid (Fig. 6.32). Each gland is enclosed in a connective tissue capsule and has a rich vascular supply. Scrapings or imprints of normal thyroid tissue contain clusters of typical follicular epithelial cells (Fig. 6.33). Nuclei are of uniform size with finely stippled chromatin and are located centrally in a moderate amount of lightly basophilic, granular cytoplasm. Cytoplasmic borders are indistinct, and many naked nuclei from broken cells are often present. Blue-black granular pigment, thought to represent tyrosine accumulation or thyroglobulin, may be seen within the cytoplasm.[47] Large macrophages containing variable amounts of pigment believed to be digested colloid are occasionally seen. Amorphous colloid may

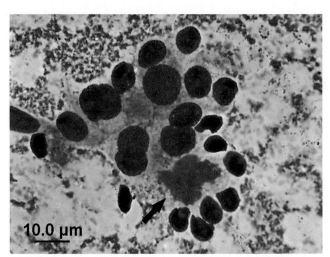

Fig. 6.31 Salivary adenocarcinoma, same aspirate as Fig. 6.29. The arrow indicates a rare acinar structure containing eosinophilic secretory material (Wright stain, 1000×).

be present extracellularly and intercellularly, usually appearing bright pink, but occasionally grayish-blue.

Benign Lesions
Inflammation
Chronic lymphocytic thyroiditis is an immune-mediated lesion that is a rare cause of thyroid gland enlargement in dogs.[48] Dogs with this syndrome usually have no signs of disease in early stages when the thyroid gland is most likely to be enlarged. When clinical signs of hypothyroidism appear, the thyroid gland has usually atrophied, is not palpable, and, therefore, is not aspirated. Affected thyroid glands contain numerous lymphocytes, plasma cells, and macrophages in addition to normal and degenerating follicular cells.

Hyperplasia and Adenoma
Functional multinodular (adenomatous) hyperplasia and functional thyroid adenoma are the most common causes of clinical hyperthyroidism in older cats.[49,50] Distinguishing between the two processes requires histopathological examination to evaluate compression of adjacent thyroid tissue and presence of a capsule, and it is likely that considerable overlap has occurred in these histological diagnoses (Fig. 6.34). In contrast to these typically functional masses in cats, thyroid adenomas in dogs are less common and generally nonfunctional.[49,51] In dogs, the majority of thyroid adenomas are incidental findings at necropsy. Cytological specimens have variable cellularity, with clusters of follicular cells and scattered naked nuclei being the predominant finding. Aspirates are often bloody because of extensive vascularity. Follicular cells are uniform in appearance, with small round nuclei placed centrally in a moderate amount of basophilic cytoplasm (Fig. 6.35). The presence of blue-black intracytoplasmic granules is variable (Fig. 6.36). Follicular cells may form acinar arrangements, sometimes surrounding central colloid (Fig. 6.37).

Uncommon causes of thyroid hyperplasia in animals include iodine deficiency, iodine excess, and errors of thyroid hormone synthesis (dyshormonogenesis).[49,52,53] Thyroid follicular cells may appear hyperplastic, and the amount of colloid present is variable.[49]

Malignant Neoplasms
The vast majority of clinically evident thyroid tumors in dogs are carcinomas (80%–90%), in contrast to only 5% in cats.[51] Thyroid carcinomas usually occur in older dogs, with no sex predilection. A breed

TABLE 6.2   Common Cytological Findings in Salivary Gland Aspirates

Cell Types	Key Features	Differential Diagnoses	Comments
Secretory epithelium Background red blood cells (RBCs)	Clusters and individual cells Low nuclear-to-cytoplasmic (N:C) ratio Abundant cytoplasmic vacuoles	Normal salivary tissue Sialadenosis	± Clusters of ductal epithelium (high N:C ratio, no vacuoles) RBCs often line up ("wind rowing")
Secretory epithelium and vacuolated macrophages Background RBCs ± Neutrophils, lymphocytes	Viscous sample Abundant amorphous basophilic mucin background	Sialocele	Sialocele may have associated inflammation Hematoidin crystals from previous hemorrhage indicate chronicity
Mostly inflammatory cells (neutrophils, lymphocytes) ± Secretory epithelium ± Bacteria	Cell types vary with cause Degenerate neutrophils suggest bacterial infection	Sialadenitis	May see bacteria phagocytized by neutrophils Epithelial cells may be lacking
Epithelial cell clusters Background RBCs ± Eosinophilic secretory material (intracellular or extracellular)	Clusters of cells with high nuclear-to-cytoplasmic ratio Cells may not be vacuolated Pleomorphism variable	Salivary carcinoma Benign cystadenoma	Carcinomas more common than benign tumors Malignant cells may have few criteria of malignancy, but often do not resemble normal salivary epithelium Histopathological confirmation warranted

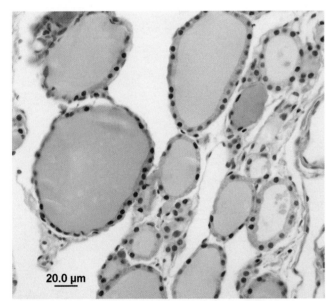

Fig. 6.32 Histological appearance of normal canine thyroid tissue. Follicles are lined by cuboidal epithelium and are filled with eosinophilic colloid (hematoxylin and eosin [H&E], 500×).

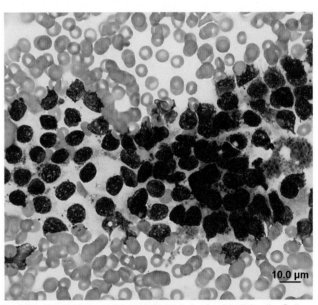

Fig. 6.33 Sheet of normal canine thyroid gland epithelial cells. Cells are slightly disrupted but have central nuclei with clumped chromatin and a small amount of basophilic cytoplasm that sometimes contains blue granular pigment (aqueous Romanowsky stain, 1000×).

predisposition has been shown for boxers, beagles, and golden retrievers.[49] Malignant tumors are poorly encapsulated and usually tightly adherent to underlying tissues because of extensive local invasion. Pulmonary metastases are frequent because of early invasion into thyroid veins.[49] Larger tumors may have a greater potential for metastasis.[54] Areas of mineralization and bone formation may be present within the tumor. Most thyroid carcinomas are nonfunctional in both dogs and cats.

A good correlation between results of aspiration cytology and histopathological examination has been found with thyroid carcinomas.[55] The problem of excessive blood contamination in many specimens may require repeated aspirations. In the absence of excessive blood contamination, smears tend to be highly cellular and may or may not contain colloid. Follicular thyroid carcinomas yield cells that occur both singly and in dense clusters, sometimes forming acinar structures (Figs. 6.38 to 6.40). Typical blue-black cytoplasmic granules

may be seen, and fine needle–shaped cytoplasmic inclusions have also been observed (Figs. 6.41 and 6.42). Anisocytosis and anisokaryosis are variable. Cytological criteria of malignancy are subtle or completely lacking in many carcinomas. Nuclei may be mildly enlarged and have indistinct nucleoli; mitotic figures are uncommon. When marked anisocytosis and anisokaryosis are present, a diagnosis of carcinoma can be made with confidence (Fig. 6.43). Otherwise, histopathological evaluation of tumor encapsulation and invasion is required to distinguish adenoma from carcinoma.

Although most carcinomas arise from follicular thyroid epithelium, medullary parafollicular C-cell tumors have also been described in dogs. Although medullary carcinomas were previously thought to be uncommon, evidence suggests that they may be recognized more frequently with increasing use of immunohistochemical stains (thyroglobulin, chromogranin A, and calcitonin).[54,56,57] Follicular tumors

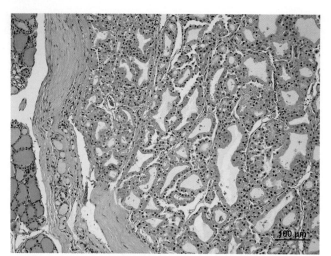

Fig. 6.34 Biopsy of a thyroid adenoma from a cat. The benign neoplasm is encapsulated and compressing normal thyroid tissue, visible on the far left (hematoxylin and eosin [H&E], 200×).

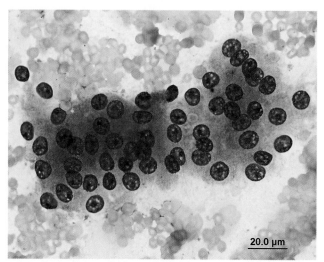

Fig. 6.35 Cluster of cells from a feline thyroid adenoma. Cells have monomorphic nuclei and abundant granular cytoplasm. Cells at the edge of the cluster have lysed (Wright stain, 1000×).

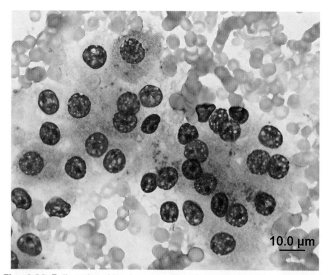

Fig. 6.36 Feline thyroid adenoma. Blue intracytoplasmic pigment is present within some of these follicular cells (Wright stain, 1000×).

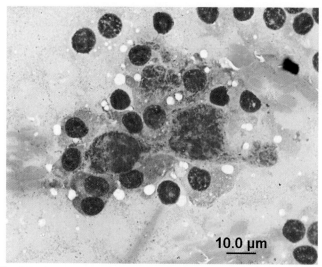

Fig. 6.37 An acinar structure surrounding eosinophilic colloid in an aspirate of a thyroid adenoma. Note the naked nuclei and lightly basophilic background from ruptured cells (Wright stain, 1000×).

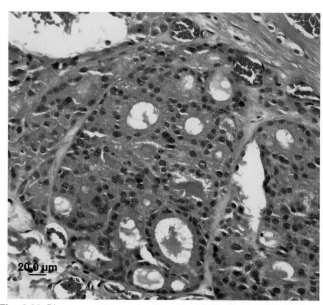

Fig. 6.38 Biopsy specimen of a functional follicular thyroid carcinoma from a dog, showing solid areas and a few follicular structures. Aspirates from this mass are shown in Figs. 6.39 to 6.41 (hematoxylin and eosin [H&E], 400×).

are expected to express thyroglobulin (Figs. 6.44 and 6.45), and medullary tumors are expected to express calcitonin (Figs. 6.46 and 6.47). Because medullary C-cell tumors tend to be well encapsulated and less likely to metastasize, differentiating them from follicular carcinomas may have prognostic implications.[56] The cytological features of medullary carcinomas are virtually identical to follicular carcinomas, with epithelial cells occurring in clusters and acinar patterns (Figs. 6.48 and 6.49).[58] Pink amorphous material consistent with colloid was observed in one case, but blue-black intracytoplasmic pigment was not.[58]

Undifferentiated carcinomas of the thyroid are rare in dogs and cats.[59] These tumors may contain spindle-shaped cells, suggestive of a sarcoma. Malignant mixed thyroid tumors are also rare, being composed of epithelial and mesenchymal elements (Figs. 6.50 and 6.51).[49,60]

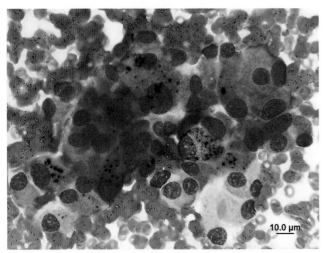

Fig. 6.39 Aspirate of a functional follicular thyroid carcinoma from a dog, same case as Fig. 6.38. Neoplastic thyroid epithelial cells are present in a cohesive cluster along with abundant erythrocytes. Some of these cells contain blue-black cytoplasmic pigment. These cells meet more criteria of malignancy than are typical for most thyroid carcinomas (Wright stain, 1000×).

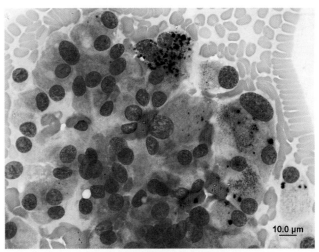

Fig. 6.41 Thyroid carcinoma, same aspirate as Fig. 6.39. Some cells contain blue-black cytoplasmic pigment, whereas others do not (Wright stain, 1000×).

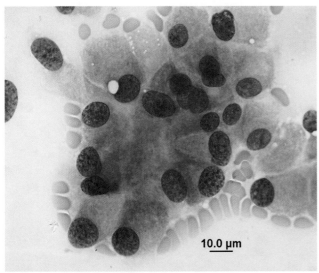

Fig. 6.40 Thyroid carcinoma, same aspirate as Fig. 6.39. An acinar structure without colloid is present (Wright stain, 1000×).

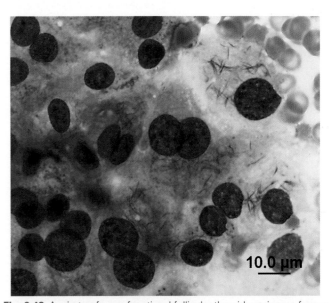

Fig. 6.42 Aspirate of a nonfunctional follicular thyroid carcinoma from a dog demonstrating needle-shaped intracytoplasmic inclusions in many cells. The significance of these inclusions is not known (Wright stain, 1000×).

Cystic Lesions

Cystic lesions have been reported in association with both thyroid adenomas and carcinomas in dogs and cats.[49,61-63] Aspirated fluid may appear serous but is more commonly brown and turbid because of previous hemorrhage and necrosis. Foamy, pigment-laden macrophages, lymphocytes, erythrocytes, and occasionally cholesterol crystals are seen along with clusters of follicular cells (Figs. 6.52 and 6.53). Thyroid hormone levels in the cystic fluid can be measured to confirm thyroid origin.[62]

THE PARATHYROID GLANDS

The parathyroid glands are located adjacent to the thyroid glands. Just as follicular and parafollicular thyroid epithelial cells cannot be distinguished on the basis of cytological evaluation, thyroid and parathyroid epithelial cells are cytologically indistinguishable. Tumors involving the parathyroid chief cells are uncommon but have been reported in both dogs and cats (Fig. 6.54).[64-66] Parathyroid tumors in dogs are not usually palpable because of their small size and location but are more often identified with ultrasonography during a search for causes of hypercalcemia in animals showing clinical signs of primary hyperparathyroidism.[67] Cats may be more likely to have a palpable parathyroid nodule.[66,68] Adenomas are diagnosed more frequently than carcinomas in both dogs and cats, and either may be functional, producing excess parathormone. Adenomas are usually encapsulated and compress adjacent normal parathyroid and thyroid tissues. Carcinomas are generally larger than adenomas and are fixed to underlying tissues because of local infiltration.[49] Because both tumors are composed of well-differentiated chief cells, differentiating adenoma from carcinoma relies on a combination of gross appearance and microscopic evidence of invasion, although cells from carcinomas may exhibit greater pleomorphism.[49]

Cells from both adenomas and carcinomas have a similar cytological appearance. Many naked nuclei are seen in a background

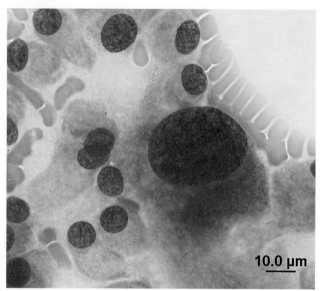

Fig. 6.43 Marked anisocytosis and anisokaryosis are present in this aspirate of a follicular thyroid carcinoma from a dog (Wright stain, 1000×).

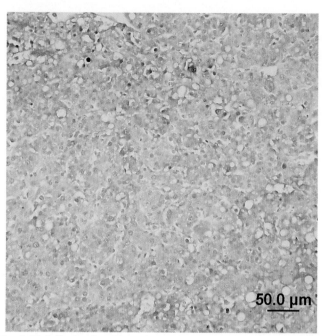

Fig. 6.45 Follicular thyroid carcinoma from a dog, same case as Fig. 6.44. Neoplastic cells have variable expression of thyroglobulin (brown stain) confirming follicular origin (immunohistochemical stain for thyroglobulin, DAB chromagen, hematoxylin counterstain, 200×).

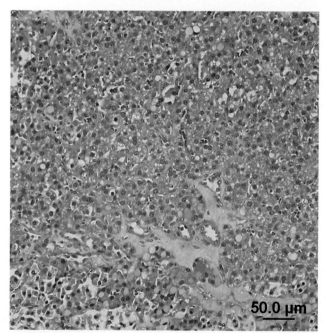

Fig. 6.44 Biopsy specimen of a follicular thyroid carcinoma from a dog. Neoplastic cells are present in solid sheets with only rare follicular structures (hematoxylin and eosin [H&E], 200×).

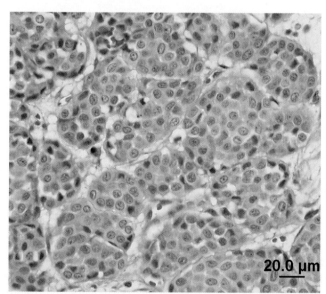

Fig. 6.46 Biopsy specimen of a medullary thyroid carcinoma from a dog. Aspirates of this mass are shown in Figs. 6.48 and 6.49 (hematoxylin and eosin [H&E], 400×).

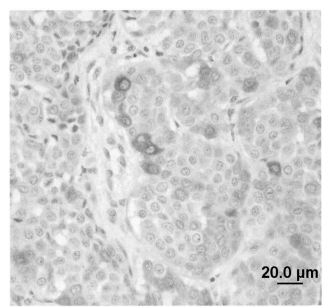

Fig. 6.47 Medullary thyroid carcinoma from a dog, same case as Fig. 6.46. Neoplastic cells have variable expression of calcitonin (brown stain) confirming C-cell origin. Immunohistochemical stain for calcitonin, DAB chromagen, hematoxylin counterstain, 400×).

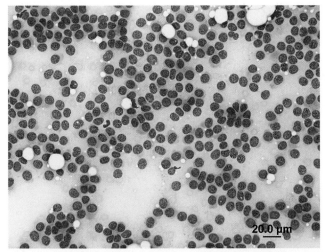

Fig. 6.48 Aspirate of a medullary thyroid carcinoma from a dog, same case as Fig. 6.46. Neoplastic cells are relatively uniform and present in loose clusters with rare acinar structures (aqueous Romanowsky stain, 400×).

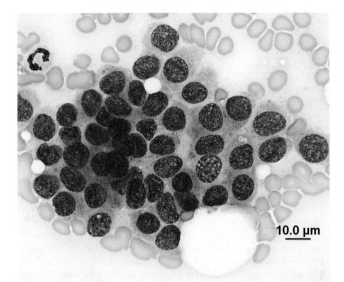

Fig. 6.49 Medullary thyroid carcinoma, same aspirate as Fig. 6.48. Faint cytoplasmic granulation is visible within this cluster of cells (aqueous Romanowsky stain, 1000×).

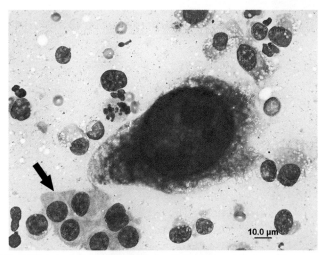

Fig. 6.50 A cluster of epithelial cells *(arrow)* and several pleomorphic mesenchymal cells in a malignant mixed thyroid tumor from a dog (Wright-Giemsa stain, 1000×). The central mesenchymal cell contains a macronucleus with two macronucleoli. (Glass slide courtesy Juopperi et al., North Carolina State University, presented at the 2002 ASVCP case review session.)

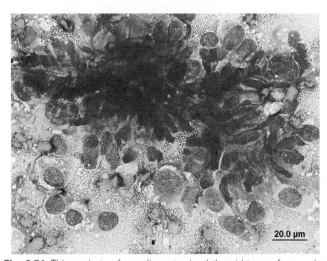

Fig. 6.51 This aspirate of a malignant mixed thyroid tumor from a dog contains only pleomorphic mesenchymal cells and abundant extracellular eosinophilic matrix, suggesting a diagnosis of sarcoma. Histopathology revealed neoplastic epithelial cells as well (Wright stain, 1000×).

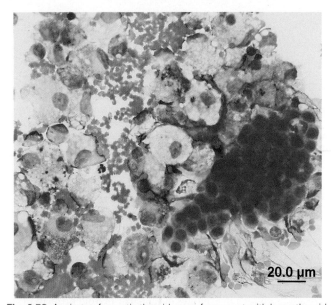

Fig. 6.52 Aspirate of a cystic thyroid mass from a cat with hyperthyroidism. A cohesive cluster of thyroid epithelial cells is present along with numerous vacuolated macrophages and erythrocytes (Wright stain, 1000×). (Glass slide courtesy Theresa Rizzi, Oklahoma State University.)

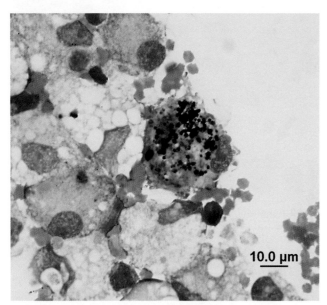

Fig. 6.53 Cystic thyroid mass, same aspirate as Fig. 6.52. Many macrophages contain blue-black phagocytized pigment, likely representing thyroglobulin (Wright stain, 1000×).

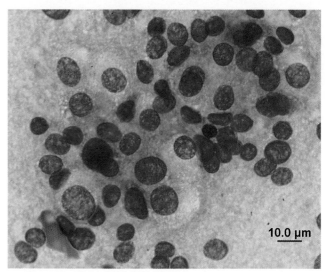

Fig. 6.55 Aspirate of a functional parathyroid carcinoma from a dog, same case as Fig. 6.54. Sheets and small clusters of cells with round nuclei, stippled chromatin, and lightly basophilic cytoplasm. Many cells are ruptured, and basophilic cytoplasm fills the background (Wright stain, 1000×).

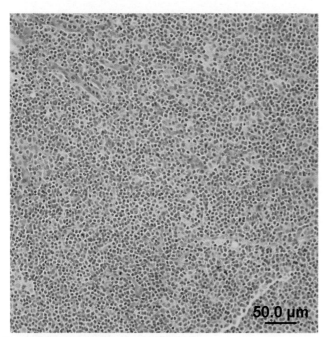

Fig. 6.54 Biopsy specimen of a functional parathyroid carcinoma from a dog. Neoplastic cells form cords and trabeculae. Aspirates from this mass are shown in Figs. 6.55 and 6.56 (hematoxylin and eosin [H&E], 200×).

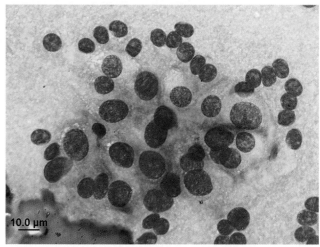

Fig. 6.56 Parathyroid carcinoma, same aspirate as Fig. 6.55. Moderate anisocytosis and anisokaryosis are seen in the intact cells (Wright stain, 1000×).

REFERENCES

1. Simon D, Schoenrock D, Nolte I, et al. Cytologic examination of fine-needle aspirates from mammary gland tumors in the dog: diagnostic accuracy with comparison to histopathology and association with postoperative outcome. *Vet Clin Path*. 2009;38:521–528.
2. Allen SW, Prasse KW, Mahaffey EA. Cytologic differentiation of benign from malignant canine mammary tumors. *Vet Pathol*. 1986;23:649–655.
3. Griffiths GL, Lumsden JH, Valli VE. Fine needle aspiration cytology and histologic correlation in canine tumors. *Vet Clin Path*. 1984;13:13–17.
4. Hellmen E, Lindgren A. The accuracy of cytology in diagnosis and DNA analysis of canine mammary tumours. *J Comp Pathol*. 1989;101:443–450.
5. Cassali GD, Gobbi H, Malm C, et al. Evaluation of accuracy of fine needle aspiration cytology for diagnosis of canine mammary tumours: comparative features with human tumours. *Cytopathology*. 2007;18:191–196.
6. Goldschmidt MH, Peña L, Rasotto R, et al. Classification and grading of canine mammary tumors. *Vet Pathol*. 2011;48:117–131.

of lightly basophilic cytoplasmic material (Fig. 6.55). Nuclei are round to oval and generally uniform in size; mild anisokaryosis may be noted in carcinomas (Fig. 6.56). When present in clusters, these cells have indistinct cytoplasmic borders and may form acinar structures. Eosinophilic needlelike structures were noted within the cytoplasm in one report of a canine parathyroid carcinoma.[69] The significance of these inclusions is not known, but they have also been seen in aspirates of follicular thyroid neoplasia (see Fig. 6.42).

7. Feldman EC, Nelson RW. Preparturient diseases. In: Feldman EC, Nelson RW, eds. *Canine and Feline Endocrinology and Reproduction.* 3rd ed. St. Louis: Saunders; 2004:831–832.

8. Rao NAS, Van Wolferen ME, Gracanin A, et al. Gene expression profiles of progestin-induced canine mammary hyperplasia and spontaneous mammary tumors. *J Physiol Pharmacol.* 2009;60(suppl 1):73–84.

9. Mouser P, Miller MA, Antuofermo E, et al. Prevalence and classification of spontaneous mammary intraepithelial lesions in dogs without clinical mammary disease. *Vet Pathol.* 2010;47:275–284.

10. Goldschmidt MH, Peña L, Zappulli V. Tumors of the mammary gland. In: Meuten DJ, ed. *Tumors in Domestic Animals.* 5th ed. Hoboken: John Wiley & Sons, Inc.; 2017:723–765.

11. Klaassen JK. Cytology of subcutaneous glandular tissues. *Vet Clin North Am Small Anim Pract.* 2002;32:1237–1266.

12. Fernandes PJ, Guyer C, Modiano JF. Mammary mass aspirate from a yorkshire terrier. *Vet Clin Path.* 1998;27:79.

13. Hayden DW, Barnes DM, Johnson KH. Morphologic changes in the mammary gland of megestrol acetate-treated and untreated cats: a retrospective study. *Vet Pathol.* 1989;26:104–113.

14. MacDougall LD. Mammary fibroadenomatous hyperplasia in a young cat attributed to treatment with megestrol acetate. *Can Vet J.* 2003;44:227–229.

15. Mesher CI. What is your diagnosis? Subcutaneous nodule from a 14-month-old cat. *Vet Clin Path.* 1997;26:4.

16. Wehrend A, Hospes R, Gruber AD. Treatment of feline mammary fibroadenomatous hyperplasia with a progesterone-antagonist. *Vet Rec.* 2001;148:346–347.

17. Sorenmo K. Canine mammary gland tumors. *Vet Clin North Am Small Anim Pract.* 2003;33:573–596.

18. Hayes AA, Mooney S. Feline mammary tumors. *Vet Clin North Am Small Anim Pract.* 1985;15:513–520.

19. Skorupski KA, Overley B, Shofer FS, et al. Clinical characteristics of mammary carcinoma in male cats. *J Vet Intern Med.* 2005;19:52–55.

20. Im KS, Kim NH, Lim HY, et al. Analysis of a new histological and molecular-based classification of canine mammary neoplasia. *Vet Pathol.* 2014;51:549–559.

21. Rasotto R, Berlato D, Goldschmidt MH, et al. Prognostic significance of canine mammary tumor histologic subtypes: an observational cohort study of 229 cases. *Vet Pathol.* 2017;54:571–578.

22. Mills SW, Musil KM, Davies JL, et al. Prognostic value of histologic grading for feline mammary carcinoma: a retrospective survival analysis. *Vet Pathol.* 2015;52:238–249.

23. Zappulli V, Rasotto R, Caliari D, et al. Prognostic evaluation of feline mammary carcinomas: a review of the literature. *Vet Pathol.* 2015;52:46–60.

24. Sorenmo KU, Kristiansen VM, Cofone MA, et al. Canine mammary gland tumours; a histological continuum from benign to malignant; clinical and histopathological evidence. *Vet Comp Oncol.* 2009;7:162–172.

25. de M Souza CH, Toledo-Piza E, Amorin R, et al. Inflammatory mammary carcinoma in 12 dogs: clinical features, cyclooxygenase-2 expression, and response to piroxicam treatment. *Can Vet J.* 2009;50:506–510.

26. Pena L, Perez-Alenza MD, Rodriguez-Bertos A, et al. Canine inflammatory mammary carcinoma: histopathology, immunohistochemistry and clinical implications of 21 cases. *Breast Cancer Res Tr.* 2003;78:141–148.

27. Perez-Alenza MD, Tabanera E, Pena L. Inflammatory mammary carcinoma in dogs: 33 cases (1995-1999). *J Am Vet Med Assoc.* 2001;219:1110–1114.

28. Perez-Alenza MD, et al. First description of feline inflammatory mammary carcinoma: clinicopathological and immunohistochemical characteristics of three cases. *Breast Cancer Res.* 2004;6:R300–R307.

29. Boydell P, Pike R, Crossley D. Presumptive sialadenosis in a cat. *J Small Anim Pract.* 2000;41:573–574.

30. Boydell P, Pike R, Crossley D, et al. Sialadenosis in dogs. *J Am Vet Med Assoc.* 2000;216:872–874.

31. Sozmen M, Brown PJ, Whitbread TJ. Idiopathic salivary gland enlargement (sialadenosis) in dogs: a microscopic study. *J Small Anim Pract.* 2000;41:243–247.

32. Stonehewer J, Mackin AJ, Tasker S, et al. Idiopathic phenobarbital-responsive hypersialosis in the dog: an unusual form of limbic epilepsy? *J Small Anim Pract.* 2000;41:416–421.

33. van der Merwe LL, Christie J, Clift SJ, et al. Salivary gland enlargement and sialorrhoea in dogs with spirocercosis: a retrospective and prospective study of 298 cases. *J S Afr Vet Assoc.* 2012;83:920–926.

34. Spangler WL, Culbertson MR. Salivary gland disease in dogs and cats: 245 cases (1985-1988). *J Am Vet Med Assoc.* 1991;198:465–469.

35. Munday JS, Lohr CV, Kiupel M. Tumors of the alimentary tract. In: Meuten DJ, ed. *Tumors in Domestic Animals.* 5th ed. Hoboken: John Wiley & Sons, Inc.; 2017:499–601.

36. Duncan RB, Feldman BF, Saunders GK, et al. Mandibular salivary gland aspirate from a dog. *Vet Clin Path.* 1999;28:97–99.

37. Brown NO. Salivary gland diseases. Diagnosis, treatment, and associated problems. *Prob Vet Med.* 1989;1:281–294.

38. Szczepaniak K, Loj.szczyk-Szczepaniak A, Tomczuk K, et al. Canine Trichomonas tenax mandibular gland infestation. *Acta Vet Scand.* 2016;58:15–18.

39. Hammer A, Getzy D, Ogilvie G, et al. Salivary gland neoplasia in the dog and cat: survival times and prognostic factors. *J Am Anim Hosp Assoc.* 2001;37:478–482.

40. Sozmen M, Brown PJ, Eveson JW. Sebaceous carcinoma of the salivary gland in a cat. *J Vet Med.* 2002;49:425–427.

41. Sozmen M, Brown PJ, Eveson JW. Salivary gland basal cell adenocarcinoma: a report of cases in a cat and two dogs. *J Vet Med.* 2003;50:399–401.

42. Carberry CA, Flanders JA, Harvey HJ, et al. Salivary gland tumors in dogs and cats: a literature and case review. *J Am Anim Hosp Assoc.* 1988;24:561–567.

43. Mazzullo G, Sfacteria A, Ianelli N, et al. Carcinoma of the submandibular salivary glands with multiple metastases in a cat. *Vet Clin Path.* 2005;34:61–64.

44. Militerno G, Bazzo R, Marcato PS. Cytological diagnosis of mandibular salivary gland adenocarcinoma in a dog. *J Vet Med.* 2005;52:514–516.

45. Perez-Martinez C, Garcia Fernandez RA, Reyes Avila LE, et al. Malignant fibrous histiocytoma (giant cell type) associated with a malignant mixed tumor in the salivary gland of a dog. *Vet Pathol.* 2000;37:350–353.

46. Smrkovski OA, LeBlanc AK, Smith SH, et al. Carcinoma ex pleomorphic adenoma with sebaceous differentiation in the mandibular salivary gland of a dog. *Vet Pathol.* 2006;43:374–377.

47. Baker R, Lumsden JH. The head and neck. In: Baker R, Lumsden JH, eds. *Color Atlas of Cytology of the Dog and Cat.* St. Louis: Mosby; 2000:119–127.

48. Graham PA, Nachreiner RF, Refsal KR, et al. Lymphocytic thyroiditis. *Vet Clin North Am Small Anim Pract.* 2001;31:1043–1062.

49. Rosol TJ, Meuten DJ. Tumors of the endocrine glands. In: Meuten DJ, ed. *Tumors in Domestic Animals.* 5th ed. Hoboken: John Wiley & Sons, Inc.; 2017:766–833.

50. Feldman EC, Nelson RW. Feline hyperthyroidism (thyrotoxicosis). In: Feldman EC, Nelson RW, eds. *Canine and Feline Endocrinology and Reproduction.* 3rd ed. St. Louis: Saunders; 2004:152–215.

51. Feldman EC, Nelson RW. Canine thyroid tumors and hyperthyroidism. In: Feldman EC, Nelson RW, eds. *Canine and Feline Endocrinology and Reproduction.* 3rd ed. St. Louis: Saunders; 2004:219–248.

52. Chastain CB, McNeel SV, Graham CL, et al. Congenital hypothyroidism in a dog due to an iodide organification defect. *Am J Vet Res.* 1983;44:1257–1265.

53. Fyfe JC, Kampschmidt K, Dang V, et al. Congenital hypothyroidism with goiter in toy fox terriers. *J Vet Intern Med.* 2003;17:50–57.

54. Leav I, Schiller AL, Rijnberk A, et al. Adenomas and carcinomas of the canine and feline thyroid. *Am J Pathol.* 1976;83:61–122.

55. Thompson EJ, Stirtzinger T, Lumsden JH, et al. Fine needle aspiration cytology in the diagnosis of canine thyroid carcinoma. *Can Vet J.* 1980;21:186–188.

56. Carver JR, Kapatkin A, Patnaik AK. A comparison of medullary thyroid carcinoma and thyroid adenocarcinoma in dogs: a retrospective study of 38 cases. *Vet Surg.* 1995;24:315–319.

57. Patnaik AK, Lieberman PH. Gross, histologic, cytochemical, and immunocytochemical study of medullary thyroid carcinoma in sixteen dogs. *Vet Pathol.* 1991;28:223–233.

58. Bertazzolo W, Giudice C, Dell'Orco M, et al. Paratracheal cervical mass in a dog. *Vet Clin Path*. 2003;32:209–212.

59. Anderson PG, Capen CC. Undifferentiated spindle cell carcinoma of the thyroid in a dog. *Vet Pathol*. 1986;23:203–204.

60. Fernandez NJ, Clark EG, Larson VS. What is your diagnosis? Ventral neck mass in a dog. *Vet Clin Path*. 2008;37:447–451.

61. Hofmeister E, Kippenes H, Mealey KL, et al. Functional cystic thyroid adenoma in a cat. *J Am Vet Med Assoc*. 2001;219:190–193.

62. Phillips DE, Radlinsky MG, Fischer JR, et al. Cystic thyroid and parathyroid lesions in cats. *J Am Anim Hosp Assoc*. 2003;39:349–354.

63. Wisner ER, Nyland TG. Ultrasonography of the thyroid and parathyroid glands. *Vet Clin North Am Small Anim Pract*. 1998;28:973–991.

64. Berger B, Feldman EC. Primary hyperparathyroidism in dogs: 21 cases (1976-1986). *J Am Vet Med Assoc*. 1987;191:350–356.

65. den Hertog E, Goossens MM, van der Linde-Sipman JS, et al. Primary hyperparathyroidism in two cats. *Vet Q*. 1997;19:81–84.

66. Kallet AJ, Richter KP, Feldman EC, et al. Primary hyperparathyroidism in cats: seven cases (1984-1989). *J Am Vet Med Assoc*. 1991;199:1767–1771.

67. Feldman EC, Hoar B, Pollard R, et al. Pretreatment clinical and laboratory findings in dogs with primary hyperparathyroidism: 210 cases (1987-2004). *J Am Vet Med Assoc*. 2005;227:756–761.

68. Feldman EC, Nelson RW. Primary hyperparathyroidism in cats. In: Feldman EC, Nelson RW, eds. *Canine and Feline Endocrinology and Reproduction*. 3rd ed. St. Louis: Saunders; 2004:711–713.

69. Ramaiah SK, Alleman AR, Hanel R, et al. A mass in the ventral neck of a hypercalcemic dog. *Vet Clin Path*. 2001;30:177–179.

7

Nasal Exudates and Masses

Maxey L. Wellman and M. Judith Radin

Cytological examination of specimens collected from the nasal cavity and nasopharynx can provide useful information in the clinical evaluation of dogs and cats presented for clinical signs of upper airway disease or facial deformity, when used in conjunction with the history and clinical findings.[1] Clinical evaluation should include a thorough examination of the nares, nasal cavity, naso- and oropharynx, hard and soft palates, and oral cavity. Visualizing the lesion increases the diagnostic potential of sample collection. Although an otoscope can be used to evaluate the rostral portion of the nasal cavity and a portion of the nasopharynx, rhinoscopy and endoscopy are essential to adequately visualize the majority of the nasal cavity.[2-4] Radiography, computed tomography (CT), magnetic resonance imaging (MRI), and other laboratory testing may be helpful.[2,5,6]

NORMAL ANATOMY

The nasal cavity extends from the nostrils to the nasopharynx, and is separated in a sagittal plane by the nasal septum.[7,8] Each nasal cavity is divided into dorsal, middle, lateral, and ventral nasal meatuses separated by dorsal and ventral turbinates and the ethmoidal labyrinth, which has a scrolled bony core covered by a richly vascular mucosa (Fig. 7.1).[8] Several frontal or paranasal sinuses extend from the nasal cavity and drain into the caudodorsal nasal cavity.[8] The maxillary sinus is a lateral diverticulum of the nasal cavity that opens at the level of the rostral roots of the fourth upper premolar tooth in dogs.[8] The nasopharynx begins at the termination of the nasal septum and extends caudal to the termination of the soft palate.[9]

The nasal vestibule is lined by keratinized squamous epithelium at the nares that transitions to nonkeratinized or slightly keratinized stratified squamous epithelium in the rostroventral and dorsal regions.[9] The caudoventral vestibule, lateral meatus, distal ends of the turbinates, and much of the nasal septum is lined by nonciliated cuboidal to low columnar transitional epithelial cells and goblet cells. Tall, pseudostratified columnar epithelial cells line the caudodorsal nasal septum and the majority of the turbinates.[9] Pseudostratified ciliated columnar epithelial cells, nonciliated columnar epithelial cells, and goblet cells line the remaining portions of the nasal cavity and the paranasal sinuses.[2,9] Nasal-associated lymphoid tissue and lymphoid follicles are present in the submucosa of the ventral, ventrolateral, and caudal areas of the nasal cavity and in the nasopharynx.[2,9]

The rostral nasal cavity contains serous, mucous, and mixed tubuloalveolar glands, and the caudal nasal cavity contains small numbers of olfactory glands.[2] Bilaterally symmetrical vomeronasal organs along the base of the rostral portion of the nasal septum comprise epithelium, glands, connective tissue, and neuronal tissue.[2,10,11] The vestibule acts as a reservoir for secretions from the lateral nasal glands and the conjunctival sac conveyed by the nasolacrimal duct.[2,12] Nasal cavity and paranasal sinus mucosae also contains neuroepithelial and neuroendocrine cells and melanocytes.[13]

SAMPLE COLLECTION AND PROCESSING

Most samples from the nasal cavity and nasopharynx are collected with the animal under general anesthesia. Rhinoscopy, endoscopy, and imaging should be performed before tissue aspiration, biopsy, brushing, or flushing techniques to minimize any effects of trauma and hemorrhage often associated with sample collection. Gauze padding of the oropharynx and tilting the animal's head downward help protect against aspiration during sampling. Care should be taken not to penetrate the cribriform plate (see Fig. 7.1).[1,2]

Obtaining a diagnostic sample depends on the type of procedure, distribution and exfoliative nature of the lesion, and the presence of inflammation or necrosis.[3] Specimens are dispersed on glass slides by using routine push or pull smear techniques, and slides are air-dried and stained with Romanowsky-type stains, which detect most infectious agents (see Chapter 1). If an infectious agent is suspected, additional samples should be collected with a sterile swab and submitted in a separate sterile tube that does not contain an anticoagulant for culture and sensitivity.[1] Cytology smears should not be exposed to formalin fumes during preparation or shipment to a reference laboratory because formalin fumes can inhibit optimal staining.

Nasal Swabs

Nasal swabs are minimally invasive and may be suitable for obtaining samples from exudates, the nares, or the rostral portion of the nasal cavity. Swabs often do not yield diagnostic specimens of deeper lesions, which may be associated with superficial ulceration, inflammation, and secondary bacterial infection that could mask the primary disease.[1,2] Direct smears are made by rolling the swab across a glass slide.

Nasal Flushing

Nontraumatic nasal flushing with sterile, nonbacteriostatic, physiological saline or lactated Ringer solution administered through a syringe or catheter is minimally invasive.[2] Nontraumatic nasal flushing may be useful for some parasite infections but often has poor diagnostic yield in others.[3] Traumatic nasal flushing may have a higher diagnostic yield. A catheter cut at an angle to create a bevel is used to dislodge tissue fragments, which are reaspirated into the syringe or collected on gauze sponges. Proper catheter length, determined by measuring the distance from the external nares to the medial canthus, is important to prevent penetration of the cribriform plate.[1] More detailed descriptions of nasal flushing methods are reviewed elsewhere.[14] Depending on cellularity, direct or concentrated smears can be made from fluid, and touch impressions can be made from tissue fragments.

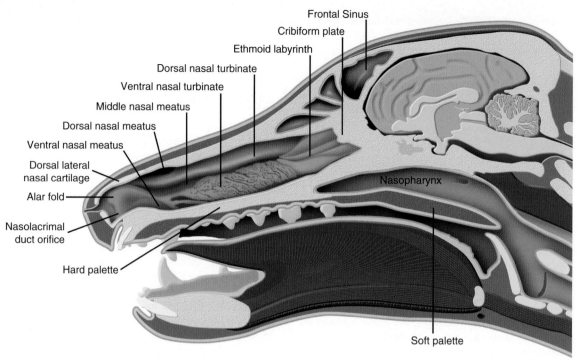

Fig. 7.1 Illustration of the nasal cavity of the dog indicating important landmarks and anatomical features (Illustration by Tim Vojt, Ohio State University.)

Nasal Brushing

Brush cytology with a small cylindrical nylon brush and endoscopic guidance can help collect cytology samples from nasal cavity lesions but may not yield samples representative of deeper lesions.[1] In one study assessing the diagnostic accuracy of nasal brushing in dogs with chronic intranasal disease that included nonneoplastic and neoplastic lesions, the sensitivity was 0.71 and specificity 0.99.[3] Diagnostic accuracy of nasal brush cytology for dogs with neoplastic disease is 70% to 88% for epithelial neoplasms and 20% to 72% for mesenchymal neoplasms.[3,15]

Fine-Needle Aspiration

Samples can be collected from masses in the rostral portion of the nasal cavity as described in Chapter 1. Diagnostic accuracy of fine-needle aspiration (FNA) has been shown to be 79% in dogs with neoplasia and evidence of facial deformity but may be higher in animals with inflammatory lesions.[15]

Biopsy and Impression Smears

Biopsy needles can be passed through the nares to sample more rostral masses, and biopsy forceps can be used to collect samples during endoscopic examination.[2,16] Small biopsy samples obtained by using endoscopic forceps and a rigid endoscope may be nondiagnostic. Larger biopsy samples can be obtained with cup biopsy forceps to grasp tissue by using CT guidance.[8] Tissue samples can be collected through small skin incisions for masses that have eroded through the dorsal or lateral wall of the nasal cavity. For masses in the frontal sinus with only marginal extension into the nasal cavity, a trephine technique can be used. A flexible endoscope that is retroflexed into the nasopharynx can be used for masses in the caudal nasal cavity.[8] In one study in dogs with intranasal malignancies, impression smears of tissue biopsies had a diagnostic accuracy of 90% for epithelial neoplasms but only 50% for mesenchymal neoplasms.[17] Biopsy remains the gold standard for diagnosing most nasal tumors.

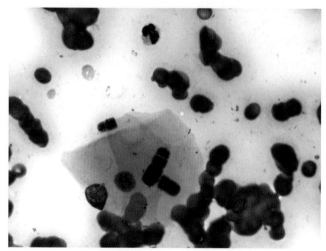

Fig. 7.2 Colonies of rod-shaped *Simonsiella* bacteria associated with the surface of a squamous epithelial cell. Additional bacterial rods are seen on the epithelial cell surface and free in the background. *Simonsiella*, a mixed bacterial population, and squamous epithelial cells indicate oropharyngeal contamination. Erythrocytes and one neutrophil *(upper center)* are likely to be present as a result of blood contamination from traumatic sampling (Wright stain).

NORMAL CYTOLOGICAL FINDINGS

Squamous epithelial cells from the rostral nasal cavity typically exfoliate as large individual cells, characterized by abundant eosinophilic to lightly basophilic cytoplasm. They can be round or appear angular, if keratinized. Nuclei are round and have condensed chromatin with inconspicuous nucleoli. Squamous epithelial cells from oropharyngeal contamination often have *Simonsiella* spp. adherent to the cytoplasmic membrane. These large, rod-shaped, gram-negative bacteria have a distinctive "stack of coins" appearance because of their alignment after division (Fig. 7.2).[2,3] Numerous species of rods and cocci that colonize the nasal cavity in healthy dogs and cats also are consistent with oropharyngeal contamination and can confound interpretation of culture results in animals with bacterial infection.[2]

Respiratory epithelial cells exfoliate individually or in clusters of columnar cells with basally located, round nuclei. Moderate amounts of basophilic cytoplasm have a ciliated brush border at the apical end (Fig. 7.3). Goblet cells are nonciliated columnar cells with a basally located round nucleus and abundant cytoplasm that contains numerous round dark purple mucin granules (see Fig. 7.3). Basal epithelial cells have a more cuboidal appearance with minimal deeply basophilic cytoplasm and round, centrally located nuclei.[2] Lymphocytes from nasal-associated lymphoid tissue typically are small lymphocytes but can include intermediate and large lymphocytes and plasma cells if there is lymphoid hyperplasia (Fig. 7.4, A).

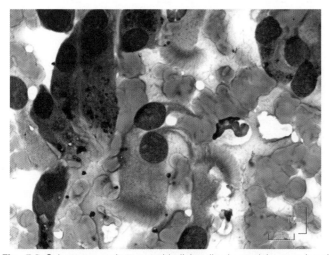

Fig. 7.3 Columnar respiratory epithelial cells *(center)* have a basal nucleus and a tuft of pink-staining cilia on the apical cell border. A cytoplasmic tail on the basal surface sometimes occurs when cells pull off the basement membrane. Several goblet cells are seen in the upper left. They have a basal nucleus and lack cilia. The cytoplasm contains variably sized, pink-to-purple mucin granules (Wright stain).

Varying amounts of mucus often are present in samples from the nasal cavity and the nasopharynx. Mucus appears as an amorphous, clear or eosinophilic to lightly basophilic, extracellular material.[2] If abundant, mucus can obscure cell morphology because it interferes with cell dispersion during slide preparation.

INFLAMMATION

Chronic inflammation from infectious or noninfectious causes is common in the nasal cavity and can be associated with epithelial hyperplasia, dysplasia, or metaplasia. Epithelial hyperplasia is characterized by numerous clusters and sheets of epithelial cells with an increased but relatively consistent nuclear-to-cytoplasmic (N:C) ratio, mild to moderate anisocytosis, and increased cytoplasmic basophilia.[2] The cytoplasmic features of epithelial metaplasia and dysplasia in the nasal cavity have not been adequately described but typically include more marked anisocytosis and anisokaryosis, increased variation in the N:C ratio, and morphological changes consistent with asynchronous maturation. These changes can be similar to those of neoplastic cells, a reminder to exercise caution in the cytological diagnosis of neoplasia, especially if there is inflammation.

Noninfectious causes of inflammation include foreign bodies, allergic rhinitis, lymphoplasmacytic rhinitis, and nasal polyps. Nasal foreign bodies most commonly are inhaled but can occur via penetration of the palate. Foreign material is rarely detected on cytology. Inflammation can be neutrophilic, macrophagic, or mixed, and secondary bacterial infection is common.[1,2]

Allergic rhinitis is characterized by a predominance of eosinophils, with variable numbers of neutrophils, goblet cells, and hyperplastic epithelial cells (Fig. 7.5). Occasional mast cells and plasma cells also can be present.[2,18] Abundant mucus can obscure visualization of eosinophil granules in thicker portions of the smear.[2] Eosinophilic inflammation also can occur with some parasitical and fungal infections and should prompt a careful search for these etiological agents. Mast cell tumors of the nasal cavity are rare and are characterized by a high proportion of mast cells (Fig. 7.6).[2,19]

Lymphoplasmacytic rhinitis is characterized by chronic unilateral or bilateral nasal discharge and can result in turbinate remodeling and bony destruction. The pathogenesis may include immune-mediated

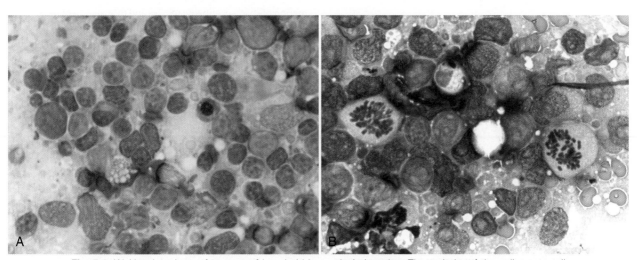

Fig. 7.4 (A) Nasal aspirate of an area of lymphoid hyperplasia in a dog. The majority of the cells are small lymphocytes along with intermediate and large lymphocytes and several plasma cells (Wright stain). (B) In comparison, lymphoma is characterized by a monomorphic population of large lymphocytes with fine chromatin, multiple prominent nucleoli, and deeply basophilic cytoplasm. Two mitotic figures are seen *(center left and right)* (Wright stain).

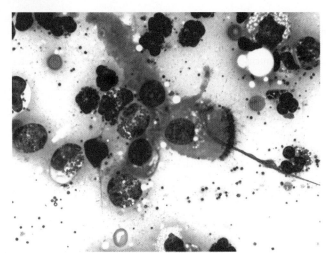

Fig. 7.5 Eosinophilic inflammation in a dog is characterized by numerous eosinophils and scattered pink extracellular granules from ruptured cells. There are three respiratory epithelial cells, one with cilia *(center)* (Wright stain).

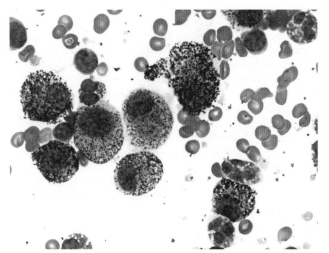

Fig. 7.6 Nasal mast cell tumor from a dog. The mast cells have fine purple cytoplasmic granules that partially obscure the nucleus. Eosinophils and lymphocytes suggest associated inflammation (Wright stain).

mechanisms, hypersensitivity reactions, disruption of normal flora, and chronic fungal infection.[2] The cause often remains unidentified. There can be increased numbers of lymphocytes and plasma cells on cytology (see Fig. 7.4, A), but histological evaluation may be necessary for a definitive diagnosis.[2,20]

Nasal polyps occur more commonly in cats than in dogs, often in cats age less than 1 year.[21,22] Polyps appear as small, smooth, well-circumscribed, pedunculated masses arising from the mucosa of the nasal cavity and are characterized by mucous membrane hyperplasia and proliferation of fibrous connective tissue. Extension into surrounding soft tissues and bone with destruction of nasal turbinates and bony lysis can occur. The cytology is characterized by mature lymphocytes, plasma cells, and epithelial cells, with variable numbers of neutrophils and macrophages. Biopsy often is necessary for a definitive diagnosis.[2]

INFECTIOUS AGENTS

Bacterial Infection

Primary bacterial rhinitis is uncommon in dogs and cats.[2] Bacterial infection secondary to other infectious agents, neoplasia, trauma,

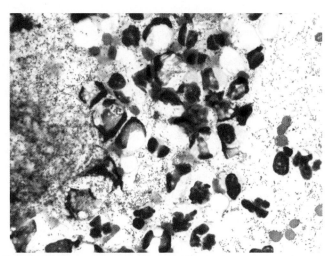

Fig. 7.7 Marked neutrophilic inflammation with intracellular and numerous extracellular bacteria in a cat (Wright stain).

foreign bodies, dental disease, or oronasal fistulation is common and is a reminder to conduct a thorough evaluation for underlying disease. Bacterial infection often is associated with marked neutrophilic inflammation and the presence of intracellular bacteria (Fig. 7.7). Although it may be possible to identify bacteria as bacilli, filamentous rods, or cocci, proper identification requires culture or more sensitive testing, such as polymerase chain reaction (PCR).

Viral Infection

The most common causes of viral rhinitis in dogs are canine distemper virus, adenovirus types 1 and 2, and parainfluenza virus. In cats, the most common causes include feline rhinotracheitis virus (feline herpesvirus), feline calicivirus, reovirus, feline leukemia virus, and feline immunodeficiency virus. The cytology often is nonspecific and can include variable numbers and types of inflammatory cells. Diagnosis is based on clinical findings, direct fluorescent antibody testing, virus isolation, or serology.[2,23]

Fungal Infection

Fungal diseases of the nasal cavity and sinuses can be primary or secondary and can cause clinical signs similar to neoplasia, including formation of space-occupying masses and destruction of nasal turbinates.[8] The nasal cavity of some clinically healthy dogs and cats can harbor *Aspergillus* spp., *Penicillium* spp., and *Cryptococcus* spp., which also can be pathogenic.[24] *Aspergillus* spp. and *Penicillium* spp. are the most common causes of mycotic rhinitis in dogs and also can be associated with disseminated respiratory infection. Infection with *Histoplasma capsulatum* and *Blastomyces dermatitidis* have been reported, but infection more commonly involves the lungs or other tissues. *Cryptococcus* spp. is the most common cause of mycotic rhinitis in cats.[2]

Infection with *Aspergillus* spp. can be associated with neutrophilic, macrophagic, or mixed inflammatory infiltrate.[2,25] Fungal hyphae can be sparse or numerous and are characterized by branching, septate structures 5 to 7 μm wide, with parallel walls and globose terminal ends (Fig. 7.8).[26] Round to oval bluish green spores are occasionally observed. Microphone-shaped conidiophores, phialides, and conidia are rarely seen.[2] Hyphae often are found in the thicker portions of the smear and sometimes appear as mats of negatively staining structures on lower magnification. In thinner areas, hyphae appear basophilic with a thin, clear outer cell wall. *Penicillium* spp. have a similar morphological appearance on cytology.[26] Definitive diagnosis is made via culture, serology, or PCR.[2]

Cryptococcus neoformans is a dimorphic fungus that exists in tissues as the yeast phase.[27] *C. neoformans* infection is more common in dogs, whereas *Cryptococcus gattii* infection is more common in cats.[28] Infection with other cryptococcal species has been described. Infection likely is from inhalation, and concurrent neurological, ocular, or cutaneous disease can occur. The yeasts typically are round, 8 to 40 μm in diameter, including the wide, nonstaining mucoid capsule (Fig. 7.9, A). However, poorly encapsulated forms occasionally occur that are only 4 to 8 μm in diameter, making the distinction from *H. capsulatum* problematic (see Fig. 7.9, B). A round, granular internal structure stains eosinophilic to purple. Narrow-based budding is characteristic but not always present. Inflammation accompanying cryptococcal infection is variable, ranging from minimal to marked pyogranulomatous inflammation, which may be related to capsule characteristics. Fungal culture and serology may be helpful for confirmation, especially for infection with poorly encapsulated forms.[2,27] A sensitive and specific latex agglutination test to detect the capsular antigen in serum has been used to monitor response to treatment.[27]

Sporothrix schenckii, a dimorphic fungus that occurs as a yeast form in tissue has been isolated from the nasal cavity of dogs and cats. Intra- and extracellular organisms are round, oval, or cigar-shaped structures, 3 to 5 μm wide and 5 to 9 μm long, and may be surrounded by a clear halo that resembles a capsule (Fig. 7.10).[27] The number of organisms is variable, but may be more numerous in cats than in dogs. Mixed inflammation with neutrophils, macrophages, lymphocytes, and eosinophils accompanies infection. Definitive diagnosis is via culture.[27]

Infection with *Alternaria* spp., one of several dematiaceous fungi causing phaeohyphomycosis, is an uncommon cause of nasal mycosis in cats. Pale staining, septate hyphae, 7 to 14 μm in diameter, with a narrow peripheral clear area and a finely stippled eosinophilic internal structure may be accompanied by neutrophils, macrophages, lymphocytes, and plasma cells.[2,29]

Other Infectious Agents

Eucoleus boehmi (formerly *Capillaria*), a nematode in the Trichuroidea family, is an uncommon cause of rhinitis in dogs and cats.[30] Infection is by ingestion of larvated eggs. Adults live and mate in the nasal cavities and sinuses and can be visualized grossly with rhinoscopy as linear, 1.5- to 4-cm-long, serpentine-shaped, white nematodes embedded in the superficial nasal mucosa.[30-32] On cytology, oval or barrel-shaped, clear to golden ova have a thick refractile wall and asymmetrical bipolar caps. *E. boehmi* ova appear similar to those of *Trichuris vulpis* and *Eucoleus aerophilis*, except for the presence of tiny pits on the surface of the wall and the slightly shorter dimension (55–60 × 30–35 μm) of *E. boehmi* eggs (Fig. 7.11).[2,32] Infection often is accompanied by neutrophils, lymphocytes, plasma cells, and variable numbers of eosinophils.[30,32,33]

Adults of *Linguatula serrata*, a wormlike arthropod, can inhabit the nasal cavity and frontal sinuses of dogs and may be associated with sneezing and nasal discharge. Prevalence is quite variable worldwide. There is zoonotic potential, so care should be taken to avoid exposure to nasal secretions and feces from infected dogs.[34]

Rhinosporidiosis is reported worldwide in dogs and cats. *Rhinosporidium seeberi* currently is classified as a member of a

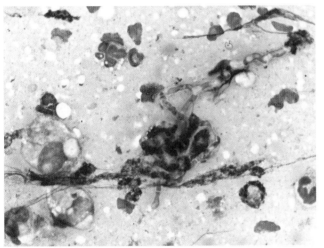

Fig. 7.8 *Aspergillus* infection in a dog is characterized by branching, septate hyphae with parallel walls and globose terminal ends. Mixed inflammation is present with neutrophils and macrophages *(lower left)* (Wright stain).

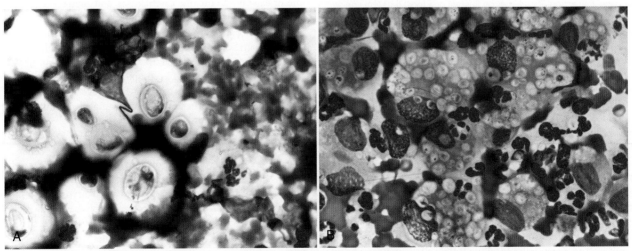

Fig. 7.9 (A) *Cryptococcus neoformans* is characterized by variably sized organisms surrounded by a wide, nonstaining capsule. Typical narrow-based budding is observed *(center left)*. (B) Poorly encapsulated *Cryptococcus* in a cat lack a nonstaining capsule, making distinction of this organism from other fungal agents challenging, requiring culture. There is marked mixed inflammation with phagocytosis of numerous organisms by macrophages (Wright stain).

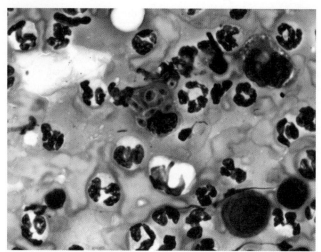

Fig. 7.10 Note the variation in shape of *Sporothrix schenckii* yeast within a macrophage from a cat *(center)*. The infection is accompanied by a mixed inflammatory response (Wright stain).

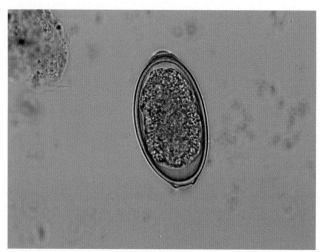

Fig. 7.11 Ova from the nematode *Eucoleus boehmi* (formerly *Capillaria*) are oval or barrel shaped, have a thick refractile wall, and asymmetrical bipolar caps. Detection of ova in nasal flushes or a fecal flotation can aid diagnosis. (Courtesy Antoinette Marsh.)

novel group of aquatic protistan parasites, and a history of water exposure is common.[35] Infection is characterized by granulomatous polypoidal masses of mucous membranes. Affected animals often present with sneezing and unilateral or bilateral nasal exudate with or without epistaxis.[35] Single or multiple polyps in the nasal cavity are covered by numerous miliary sporangia.[2] On cytology, sporangia are very large (30 to >200 µm in diameter), deeply basophilic, round structures that contain endospores. Several developmental stages of endospores have been described, the most common of which are mature endospores. Mature endospores are round to oval eosinophilic to magenta structures, 5 to 15 µm in diameter (Fig. 7.12).[2,35] The inflammatory response includes neutrophils, plasma cells, lymphocytes, macrophages, eosinophils, and mast cells. Inflammatory cells sometimes form rosettes around the spores, which is helpful in finding spores under lower magnification. Staining with periodic acid–Schiff (PAS) may enhance visualization of the spores in cytological and histological sections.[2]

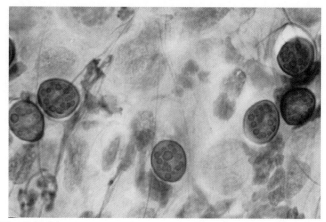

Fig. 7.12 Mature-stage endospores of *Rhinosporidium seeberi* have a thick, hyalinized cell wall, and contain small, spherical, eosinophilic, globular internal structures (Wright stain, 400×).

NEOPLASIA

Primary neoplasms of the nasal cavity and associated sinuses are uncommon in dogs and cats.[2,13,36] Benign tumors are rare, are difficult to diagnose with cytology, and include adenoma, papilloma, fibroma, chondroma, osteoma, and leiomyoma. Most tumors of the nasal cavity are malignant and locally invasive, but metastasis is uncommon.[2,8,37,38] Malignant epithelial tumors are more common than those of mesenchymal origin.[1] The most common malignant epithelial tumors are adenocarcinoma and squamous cell carcinoma.[1,2,39,40] The most common malignant mesenchymal tumors are chondrosarcoma, osteosarcoma, and fibrosarcoma.[2,13,39] Lymphoma, transmissible venereal tumor (TVT), and mast cell tumor are the most common round cell tumors. Adenosquamous carcinoma, leiomyosarcoma, histiocytic sarcoma, hemangiosarcoma, liposarcoma, melanoma, plasmacytoma, and carcinoids have been sporadically reported.[2] Of all tumors involving the nasal cavity, adenocarcinomas are the most common in dogs, and lymphoma is the most common in cats.[5,8]

Most tumors occur in the caudal two-thirds of the nasal cavity near the cribriform plate but can also involve the nasal turbinates and septum or extend into the oral cavity, orbit, and cranial vault. Tumors in the paranasal sinuses are less common. Metastasis to regional lymph nodes most commonly occurs with carcinomas, usually late during disease progression.[2] Mass lesions may be accompanied by lysis of adjacent bone, fluid in the nasal sinuses, and deviation of the nasal septum.[5] Neoplasia often is accompanied by inflammation, hemorrhage, and necrosis, which can make cytological diagnosis difficult, especially if only superficial tissues are sampled. Definitive diagnosis often requires histopathological evaluation.

Adenocarcinoma

Neoplastic cells are round to polygonal and often are present in clusters or sheets, sometimes with an acinar arrangement (Fig. 7.13). There often is marked anisocytosis and anisokaryosis, with moderate to marked variation in the N:C ratio. Deeply basophilic cytoplasm may contain variable numbers of discrete, clear vacuoles, or one large, clear vacuole, often referred to as a "signet ring" form. Nuclei are round to slightly irregular in shape and have coarse to finely stippled chromatin and single or multiple nucleoli that can vary in size and shape.[1] Single cells can appear similar to large lymphocytes, so care should be taken to look for cluster formation and intercellular junctions.[2]

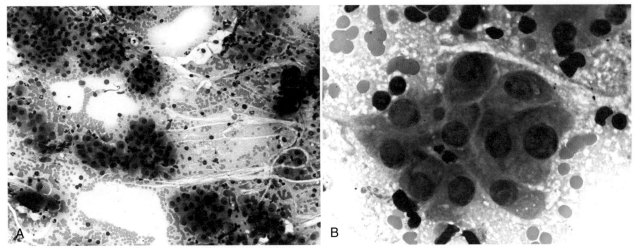

Fig. 7.13 (A) Nasal adenocarcinoma in a cat is characterized by multiple clusters of atypical epithelial cells. Note the unstained linear strands of mucus in the background (Wright stain). (B) This cluster of cells exhibits criteria of malignancy, including moderate anisokaryosis and anisocytosis, stippled chromatin, and one to several, variably sized, prominent nucleoli (Wright stain).

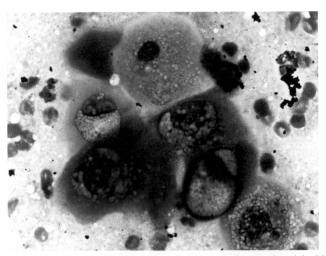

Fig. 7.14 Squamous cell carcinoma cells have round, central nuclei with irregularly condensed chromatin and single or multiple nucleoli. Cytoplasm is abundant, with perinuclear vacuolization consistent with keratohyaline granules. Several neutrophils are present, and neutrophilic inflammation may accompany this tumor as a reaction to keratin (Wright stain).

Squamous Cell Carcinoma

Squamous cell carcinoma (SCC) in the nasal cavity is locally invasive but slow to metastasize.[40] Frontal sinus SCC is extremely rare in dogs and cats and occurs more commonly as an extension of nasal SCC.[41] Cytological features of SCC include variably cohesive polyhedral cells, in which some or all cells have glassy clear to aqua cytoplasm indicative of keratinization. Perinuclear vacuolization may be present and likely represents keratohyaline granules. Nuclei are round and central and have irregularly condensed chromatin and single or multiple nucleoli. Marked anisocytosis and anisokaryosis, with moderate to marked variation in the N:C ratio, are common (Fig. 7.14).[1] Asynchronous nuclear and cytoplasmic maturation, characterized by the presence of relatively large nuclei in fully keratinized cells, and a range of immature to well-differentiated squamous epithelial cells often are observed. Keratinized debris and neutrophilic inflammation are relatively common, and there may be bacterial infection or overgrowth of commensal organisms.[27]

Chondrosarcoma

Chondrosarcomas occur most commonly in young dogs. Fine-needle aspirates typically yield moderately abundant amorphous, homogeneous, eosinophilic to magenta matrix compatible with cartilage. Cellularity may be minimal, and cells may stain poorly, especially in the presence of thick matrix. One to several chondrocytes embedded within cartilaginous lacunae is a unique feature of this neoplasm. Chondrocytes are round to oval, with round to oval nuclei, occasional binucleate cells, stippled to irregularly condensed chromatin, multiple nucleoli, and abundant variably vacuolated basophilic cytoplasm. There may be moderate to marked anisokaryosis, with moderate to marked variation in the N:C ratio.[42]

Osteosarcoma

Cytological smears are minimally to markedly cellular. Neoplastic osteoblasts occur as individual round to oval cells with round to oval eccentric nuclei, finely stippled chromatin, prominent single or multiple nucleoli, and abundant basophilic cytoplasm that occasionally contains irregularly shaped magenta granules (Fig. 7.15).[43] Moderate to marked anisocytosis and anisokaryosis are often present, as well as marked variation in the N:C ratio. Variable numbers of large, multinucleate osteoclasts are present, as is a variable amount of eosinophilic extracellular material suggestive for osteoid. Neoplastic osteoblasts stain positive for alkaline phosphatase, and some dogs with osteosarcoma can have increased serum levels of alkaline phosphatase.[44,45] Subtypes of osteosarcoma in dogs and cats, determined on the basis of histological features, have been described, but these types may not be associated with the prognosis.[46,47] Histological grading is prognostic.[46,47]

Lymphoma

Lymphoma most commonly involves only the nasal cavity (82% of cases), but sometimes it involves only the nasopharynx (10% of cases) or the nasal cavity and the nasopharynx (8% of cases).[5] Lymphoma of the nasal cavity and nasopharynx as part of multiorgan involvement can occur, as can extension into the central nervous system (CNS).[3,5] The histological pattern is almost always diffuse immunoblastic lymphoma (91%), although diffuse large cell lymphoma has been described. Biopsy is considered the gold standard for diagnosis, but cytology can be very helpful in the initial evaluation. Typically, there is

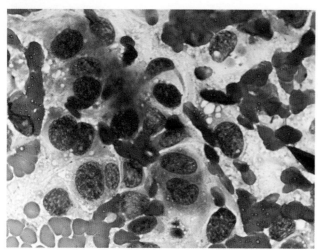

Fig. 7.15 Cells in this chondroblastic osteosarcoma from a dog are round to oval to spindle shaped with basophilic cytoplasm. There is moderate anisokaryosis, and there are occasional binucleate cells. Nuclei contain stippled chromatin and one to several prominent nucleoli. Pink extracellular matrix *(upper left)* is suggestive of osteoid formation (Wright stain).

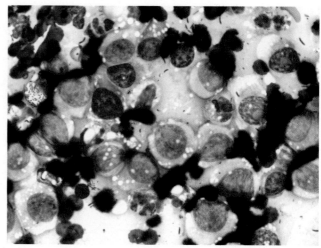

Fig. 7.17 Cells from the transmissible venereal tumor of dogs have a single round nucleus with coarse chromatin, a single prominent nucleolus, and lightly basophilic cytoplasm that contains multiple, small, clear vacuoles. Although most commonly found in the genital region, nasal implantation can occur as a result of social behaviors (Wright stain).

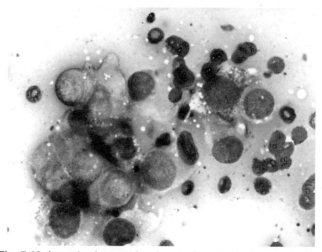

Fig. 7.16 A poorly pigmented melanoma in a dog is characterized by round cells with a single round nucleus, fine chromatin, and a large prominent nucleolus. The cytoplasm is scant to moderately abundant and lightly basophilic. Fine black melanin granules are best seen in the cytoplasm of the cell in the upper right (Wright stain).

a uniform population of intermediate to large cells with round to oval nuclei, finely stippled chromatin, single or multiple prominent central or peripheral nucleoli, and scant to moderate amounts of basophilic cytoplasm (see Fig. 7.4, B). Punctate cytoplasmic vacuoles may be observed on cytology, likely as an artifact of fixation. Most nasal cavity and nasopharyngeal lymphoma in cats are of B-cell origin (61%), although T-cell lymphoma has been reported (5%–29%).[3,5]

Melanoma

Primary intranasal melanoma is rare in dogs and may be limited to the nasal cavity or be associated with extension to the CNS.[48] Nasal discharge may appear dark brown, and the mass may be grossly dark brown or black.[48] Neoplastic cells are pleomorphic round to spindloid cells. The cytoplasm contains variable numbers of dark brown melanin pigment granules (Fig. 7.16). Nuclei are round or oval, with moderately condensed chromatin nasd single or multiple prominent nucleoli. There may be marked anisocytosis and anisokaryosis, with

variable numbers of mitotic figures. Some melanomas are amelanotic, in which case cell lineage can be confirmed via immunohistochemistry for Melan-A, an antigen present on the surface of melanocytes.[49] Clinical behavior varies from marked aggression with invasion of surrounding tissues to minimal aggression and minimal tissue invasion. Metastasis is variable, but very few cases have been described.[48]

Transmissible Venereal Tumor

Canine transmissible venereal tumor (TVT) has been reported worldwide but most commonly occurs as a contagious tumor in dogs in tropical and subtropical countries and is transmitted by viable cancer cells during social behaviors.[50] Tumors are most commonly located in and around the external genitalia but also are found in other areas, including the nasal cavity. In some cases of extragenital TVTs, it may be difficult to differentiate TVTs from other round cell tumors and poorly differentiated carcinoma. TVT cells are discrete, round cells with large round nuclei that have coarse chromatin and single, prominent nucleoli (Fig. 7.17). Moderate amounts of pale blue cytoplasm often contain numerous well-demarcated vacuoles. There may be mild to moderate anisocytosis and numerous mitotic figures.[51,52] TVT cells contain a unique long, interspersed nuclear element inserted upstream of the *myc* gene, which can be detected via PCR, which allows for a diagnosis differentiated from other round cell neoplasms.[50]

Neuroendocrine Tumors

Neuroendocrine tumors of the nasal cavity and nasopharyngeal region are rare in dogs and cats. Samples may be highly cellular, but often the cells are broken. When intact, round to polygonal cells are moderately pleomorphic with scant to moderate amounts of eosinophilic to amphophilic, faintly granular cytoplasm, with round to ovoid hyperchromatic nuclei, coarsely clumped chromatin, and single nucleoli (Fig. 7.18). The neoplastic cells rarely form small rosettelike structures and may be accompanied by minimal to marked stromal response. Differentiation from olfactory neuroblastoma may be difficult with routine staining. Neoplastic neuroendocrine cells display positive reactivity for chromogranin A and neuron-specific enolase and lack neurofilament immunoreactivity. Cytokeratin staining is variable.[13,53-55]

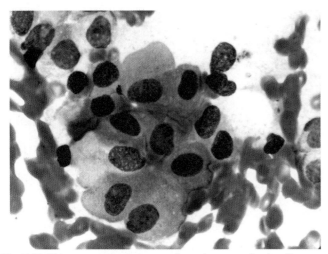

Fig. 7.18 This neuroendocrine tumor from the nose of a dog illustrates clustering of round to polygonal cells that have round to oval nuclei, coarsely granular chromatin, and a single nucleolus. Cytoplasm is amphophilic with a fine, pink granularity (Wright stain).

REFERENCES

1. Arndt TP. Nasal exudates and masses. In: Valenciano AC, Cowell RL, eds. *Diagnostic Cytology and Hematology of the Dog and Cat.* 4th ed. St. Louis: Elsevier; 2014:131–138.
2. Burkhard MJ. Respiratory tract. In: Raskin RE, Meyer D, eds. *Canine and Feline Cytology: A Color Atlas and Interpretation Guide.* 3rd ed. St. Louis: Elsevier; 2016:138–190.
3. Caniatti M, da Cunha NP, Avallone G, et al. Diagnostic accuracy of brush cytology in canine chronic intranasal disease. *Vet Clin Pathol.* 2012;41:133–140.
4. Johnson LR, Clarke HE, Bannasch MJ, et al. Correlation of rhinoscopic signs of inflammation with histologic findings in nasal biopsy specimens of cats with or without upper respiratory disease. *J Am Vet Med Assoc.* 2004;225:395–400.
5. Little L, Patel R, Goldschmidt. Nasal and nasopharyngeal lymphoma in cats: 50 cases (1989–2005). *Vet Pathol.* 2007;44:885–892.
6. Petite AF, Dennis R. Comparison of radiography and magnetic resonance imaging for evaluating the extent of nasal neoplasia in dogs. *J Small Anim Pract.* 2006;47:529–536.
7. Evans H, de Lahunta A. The head. In: Evans H, de Lahunta A, eds. *Guide to the Dissection of the Dog.* 8th ed. St. Louis: Elsevier; 2017:218–276.
8. Weeden AM, Degner DA. Surgical approaches to the nasal cavity and sinuses. *Vet Clin Small Anim.* 2016;46:719–733.
9. Harkema JR, Carey S, Wagner JG. The nose revisited: a brief review of the comparative structure, function, and toxicologic pathology of the nasal epithelium. *Toxicol pathol.* 2006;34:252–269.
10. Dennis JC, Allgier JG, Desouza LS, et al. Immunohistochemistry of the canine vomeronasal organ. *J Anat.* 2003;203:329–338.
11. Salazar I, Sanchez Quinteiro P, Cifuentes JM, et al. The vomeronasal organ of the cat. *J Anat.* 1996;188(Pt2):445–454.
12. Hirt R, Tektas OY, Carrington SD, et al. Comparative anatomy of the human and canine efferent tear duct system—impact of mucin MUC5AC on lacrimal drainage. *Curr Eye Res.* 2012;37:961–970.
13. Koehler JW, Weiss RC, Aubry OA, et al. Nasal tumor with widespread cutaneous metastases in a golden retriever. *Vet Pathol.* 2012;49:870–875.
14. Smallwood LF, Zenoble RD. Biopsy and cytological sampling of the respiratory tract. *Semin Vet Med Surg (Small Anim).* 1993;8:250–257.
15. Morrison T, Read R, Eger C. A retrospective study of nasal tumours in 37 dogs. *Austr Vet Pract.* 1989;19:130–134.
16. Elie M, Sabo M. Basics in canine and feline rhinoscopy. *Clin Tech Small Anim Pract.* 2006;21:60–63.
17. Clercx C, Wallon J, Gilbert S, et al. Imprint and brush cytology in the diagnosis of canine intranasal tumors. *J Small Anim Pract.* 1996;37:423–427.
18. Venema CM, Williams KJ, Gershwin LJ, et al. Histopathologic and morphometric evaluation of the nasal and pulmonary airways of cats with experimentally induced asthma. *Int Arch Allergy Immunol.* 2013;160:365–376.
19. Khoo A, Lane A, Wyatt K. Intranasal mast cell tumor in the dog: a case series. *Can Vet J.* 2017;58:851–854.
20. Windsor RC, Johnson LR. Canine chronic inflammatory rhinitis. *Clin Tech Small Anima Pract.* 2006;21:76–81.
21. Holt DE, Goldschmidt MH. Nasal polyps in dogs: five cases (2005–2011). *J Small Anim Pract.* 2011;52:660–663.
22. Moore AS, Ogilvie GK. Tumors of the respiratory tract. In: Moore AS, Ogilvie GK, eds. *Feline Oncology: A Comprehensive Guide to Compassionate Care.* Trenton: Veterinary Learning Systems; 2001:368–384.
23. Moise NS. Viral respiratory diseases. *Vet Clin North Am Small Anim Pract.* 1985;15:919–928.
24. Duncan C, Stephen C, Lester S, et al. Sub-clinical infection and asymptomatic carriage of cryptococcus gatti in dogs and cats during an outbreak of cryptococcosis. *Med Mycol.* 2005;43:511–516.
25. Johnson LR, Drazenovich TL, Herrara MA, et al. Results of rhinoscopy alone or in conjunction with sinoscopy in dogs with aspergillosis: 46 cases (2001–2004). *J Amer Med Assoc.* 2006;228:738–742.
26. De Lorenzi D, Bonfanti U, Masserdotti C, et al. Diagnosis of canine nasal aspergillosis by cytological examination: a comparison of four different collection techniques. *J Small Anim Pract.* 2006;47:316–319.
27. Sharkey LC, Wellman ML. Diagnostic cytology in veterinary medicine: a comparative and evidence-based approach. *Clin Lab Med.* 2011;31:1–19.
28. Trivedi SR, Sykes JE, Cannon MS, et al. Clinical features and epidemiology of cryptococcosis in cats and dogs in California: 93 cases (1988–2010). *J Am Vet Med Assoc.* 2011;239:357–369.
29. Tennent K, Patterson-Kane J, Boag AK, et al. Nasal mycosis in two cats caused by Alternaria species. *Vet Rec.* 2004;155:368–370.
30. Manzocchi S, Spiranelli E, Bertazzolo. What is your diagnosis? Nasal cavity imprint from a dog. *Vet Clin Pathol.* 2016;45:719–720.
31. Baan M, Kidder AC, Johnson SC, et al. Rhinoscopic diagnosis of *eucoleus boehmi* infection in a dog. *J Am Anim Hosp Assoc.* 2011;47:60–63.
32. Piperisova I, Neel JA, Tarigo J. What is your diagnosis? Nasal discharge from a dog. *Vet Clin Pathol.* 2009;39:121–122.
33. Veronesi F, Lepri E, Morganti G, et al. Nasal eucoleosis in a symptomatic dog from italy. *Vet Parasitol.* 2013;195:187–191.
34. Villedieu E, Sanchez RE, Jepson RE, et al. Nasal infestation by *linguatula serrata* in a dog in the UK: a case report. *J Sm Anim Pract.* 2017;58:183–186.
35. Meier WA, Meinkoth JH, Brunker J, et al. Cytologic identification of immature endospores in a dog with rhinosporidiosis. *Vet Clin Pathol.* 2006;35:348–352.
36. Mukaratirwa S, van der Linde-Sipman JS, Gruys E. Feline nasal and paranasal sinus tumours: clinicopathological study, histomorphological description and diagnostic immunohistochemistry of 123 cases. *J Feline Med Surg.* 2001;3:235–245.
37. Madewell BR, Priester WA, Gillette EL, et al. Neoplasms of the nasal passages and paranasal sinuses in domesticated animal as reported by 13 veterinary colleges. *Am J Vet Res.* 1976;37:851–856.
38. Ogilvie GK, LaRue SM. Canine and feline nasal and paranasal sinus tumors. *Vet Clin North Am Small Anim Pract.* 1992;22:1133–1144.
39. Lana SE, Turek MM. Tumors of the respiratory system: nasisal tumors. In: Withrow SJ, MacEwen EG, eds. *Small Animal Clinical Oncology.* 5th ed. Philadelphia: Saunders; 2013:435–437.
40. Turek MM, Lana SE. Canine nasosinal tumors. In: Withrow SJ, Vail DM, Page RL, eds. *Small Animal Clinical Oncology.* 5th ed. St. Louis: Elsevier; 2013:435–451.
41. Grimes JA, Pagano CJ, Boudreaux BB. Primary frontal sinus squamous cell carcinoma in a dog treated with surgical excision. *Can Vet J.* 2017;58:79–82.
42. Lin T, Hosoya K, Drost WT, et al. What is your diagnosis? Fine-needle aspirate of an aggressive bone lesion from a dog. *Vet Clin Pathol.* 2010;39:297–298.
43. Simerdova V, Vavra M, Skoric M, et al. What is your diagnosis? Multilobate nasal mass in a 5-month-old Sphynx cat. *Vet Clin Pathol.* 2017;46:369–370.

44. Barger A, Graca R, Bailey K, et al. Use of alkaline phosphatase staining to differentiate canine osteosarcoma from other vimentin-positive tumors. *Vet Pathol.* 2005;42:161–165.

45. Sternberg RA, Pondenis HC, Yang X, et al. Association between absolute tumor burden and serum bone-specific alkaline phosphatase in canine appendicular osteosarcoma. *J Vet Intern Med.* 2013;27:955–963.

46. Dimopoulou M, Kirpensteijn J, Moens H, et al. Histologic prognosticators in feline osteosarcoma: a comparison with phenotypically similar canine osteosarcoma. *Vet Sur.* 2008;37:466–471.

47. Kirpensteijn J, Kik M, Rutteman GR, et al. Prognostic significance of a new histologic grading system for canine osteosarcoma. *Vet Pathol.* 2002;39:240–246.

48. Lemetayer J, Al-Diessi A, Tryon K, et al. Primary intranasal melanoma with brain invasion in a dog. *Can Vet J.* 2017;58:391–396.

49. Smedley RC, Lamoureaux J, Sledge DG, et al. Immunohistochemical diagnosis of canine oral amelanotic melanocytic neoplasms. *Vet Pathol.* 2011;48:32–40.

50. Setthawongsin C, Techangamsuwan S, Tangkawattana S, et al. Cell-based polymerase chain reaction for canine transmissible venereal tumor (CTVT) diagnosis. *J Vet Med Sci.* 2016;78:1167–1173.

51. Levy E, Mylonakis ME, et al. What is your diagnosis? Nasal and oral masses in a dog. *Vet Clin Pathol.* 2006;35:115–118.

52. Rogers KS, Walker MA, Dillon HB. Transmissible venereal tumor: a retrospective study of 29 cases. *J Am Anim Hosp Assoc.* 1998;34:463–470.

53. Ninomiya F, Suzuki S, Tanaka H, et al. Nasal and paranasal adenocarcinomas with neuroendocrine differentiation in dogs. *Vet Pathol.* 2008;45:181–187.

54. Patnaik AK, Ludwig LL, Erlandson RA. Neuroendocrine carcinoma of the nasopharynx in a dog. *Vet Pathol.* 2002;39:496–500.

55. Sako T, Shimoyama Y, Akihara Y, et al. Neuroendocrine carcinoma in the nasal cavity of ten dogs. *J Comp Pathol.* 2005;133:155–163.

8

Oropharynx and Tonsils

Deborah C. Bernreuter

Cytology is a useful, rapid screening test for lesions in the oropharynx, including masses, ulcers, draining tracts, plaques, and enlarged tonsils. It can be performed alone or in conjunction with biopsy and/or sampling for bacterial and fungal testing. Sedation or anesthesia may be necessary for complete examination of the oropharynx and to obtain adequate, representative samples. For mass lesions and plaques, aspiration of the deeper layers of the lesion to avoid any superficial secondary inflammation is usually most rewarding. If a mass lesion is nonexfoliative, scraping the lesion might yield adequate numbers of cells; however, excisional biopsy is usually necessary for determining a definitive diagnosis and prognosis. For flat lesions, including ulcers, biopsy of the entire lesion, or at least of the edge of a lesion to evaluate early, primary abnormalities, is usually necessary to obtain an adequate number of representative cells for evaluation. However, impression smears or scrapings of ulcerative lesions can occasionally yield cells or organisms that are distinctive and can be identified as the primary cause of the lesion, rather than as secondary opportunists, and eliminate the need for biopsy. Because the oropharynx and tonsils are highly vascular, care must be taken to avoid hemodilution of the sample at the time of collection.

TECHNIQUES

For mass lesions and plaques, fine-needle aspiration (FNA) should be attempted after the surface has been cleaned with a disinfectant that is nontoxic to the digestive system of the patient. If the lesion is fibrous and nonexfoliative, scraping the lesion with a scalpel blade and transferring the cells to a slide can be rewarding if the cells are immediately thinned into a monolayer by smearing them with another slide or by using a saline-moistened sterile swab to roll (not rub) the cells along a slide. Draining tracts can also be swabbed and the cells rolled onto a slide for cytological examination. If a biopsy is performed, impression smears of the cut surface can be made after the surface has been blotted on a paper towel to remove excessive blood and tissue fluids. For flat lesions, such as ulcers, any superficial pus and fibrin should be removed before impression smears or scrapings of the surface are made. As for all cytology samples, the smears should be thin enough to dry within 30 to 60 seconds, and they should be completely dry before encasing them in a slide holder for transport to a diagnostic laboratory. Areas of the sample that are more than one cell thick cannot be adequately evaluated, and slow drying in the slide holder causes distortion and disintegration, which could ruin otherwise excellent smears.

NORMAL FINDINGS

To correctly identify abnormal criteria, recognition of normal findings is essential. The oropharynx and tonsils are covered by mature squamous epithelial cells (Fig. 8.1). These are large, flat, and round to slightly angular. They have abundant pale cytoplasm and small round nuclei that exhibit condensed chromatin. Nucleoli are not visible, and some cells are anuclear. The presence of occasional intermediate squamous cells with slightly larger, less condensed nuclei is normal (Fig. 8.2).

Normal squamous cells frequently exhibit a mixed bacterial population adhered to their surfaces (Fig. 8.3). These bacteria are also usually present in the background between cells. The normal flora

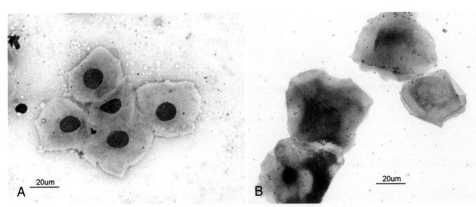

Fig. 8.1 Mature squamous cells have cornified cytoplasm that has sharp angular borders. Mature squamous cells can be nucleated or anucleate. (A) Mature nucleated squamous cells have abundant light blue-to-gray cytoplasm that has an angular appearance. (B) Mature squamous cell with a pyknotic nucleus *(lower left)* and anucleate, mature squamous cells from a scraping of oral tissue.

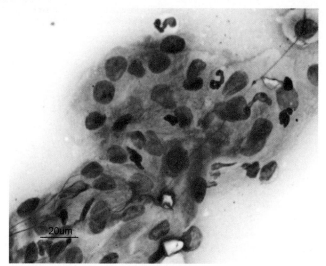

Fig. 8.2 Intermediate (less differentiated) squamous cells. These are also a normal finding from the oropharynx, particularly with samples collected by scraping. Cells are more cohesive and have large, noncondensed nuclei and a more deeply basophilic cytoplasm that does not have angular borders.

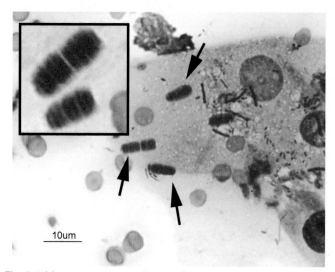

Fig. 8.4 Mature squamous cells with *Simonsiella* spp. *(arrows)*. *Simonsiella* spp. are normal inhabitants of the oropharynx and must not be mistaken for pathogens. What appears to be one very large organism is actually numerous slender bacterial rods lined up side to side. *Inset,* Higher magnification of *Simonsiella* organisms in which the individual organisms can be seen.

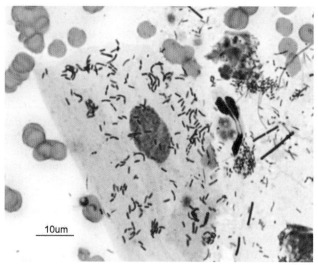

Fig. 8.3 Mature squamous cell with adherent bacteria. Extracellular bacteria are also present. Bacteria adherent to squamous cells and bacteria free in the background of the smear that are not associated with an inflammatory response are usually normal flora.

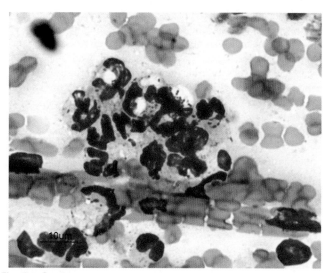

Fig. 8.5 Septic, purulent inflammation. Scraping of a lesion in the oral cavity of a cat shows many neutrophils with phagocytized bacteria. Bacteria that are associated with an inflammatory reaction and are phagocytized by neutrophils likely represent pathogens (primary or secondary).

includes aerobic and anaerobic bacterial rods and cocci. Observation of spirochetes is considered normal. Yeast organisms are never considered normal. One bacterium, *Simonsiella* spp., has a characteristic palisading appearance and is a normal inhabitant of the oropharynx (Fig. 8.4). It should never be mistaken for a pathogen. If the bacterial population is dominated by only one type of bacteria, that would be considered abnormal.

The normal appearance of smears made from the tonsils is typical of other lymphoid organs. Usually, greater than 80% of the lymphoid cells are small and appear mature. The remaining lymphoid cells are intermediate-sized lymphocytes and occasional lymphoblasts. Plasma cells, neutrophils, macrophages, eosinophils, and squamous cells from the epithelial surface can be rarely observed. Occasional granules of iron pigment can be normal.

OROPHARYNX

Nonneoplastic Lesions
Inflammation
Acute (neutrophilic) inflammation is characterized by a predominance of neutrophils. They can be degenerate or nondegenerate. Neutrophils are most frequently degenerate if bacterial endotoxins are present. Macrophages, lymphocytes, plasma cells, fibrocytes, and eosinophils can also be present in low numbers.

Infectious agents can be observed; however, their absence from a sample does not rule out the possibility of an infectious etiology. If the inflammatory lesion is caused by a primary bacterial infection or complicated by secondary bacterial infection, a homogeneous population of bacteria is often seen, and many will be phagocytized within neutrophils (Fig. 8.5).

If the inflammation is superficial, secondary overgrowth of oropharyngeal bacterial flora is common. Secondary opportunistic bacterial inflammation can also be observed in association with primary, noninflammatory lesions. The presence of a heterogeneous population of bacteria that are extracellular or adhered to epithelial cells suggests overgrowth of flora.

If the lesion is granulomatous, as from a foreign body or yeast or fungal infection, a more evenly mixed population of neutrophils, macrophages, lymphocytes, and plasma cells is observed, with variable numbers of fibrocytes and fibroblasts that are indicative of physiological fibroplasia. In some areas of the United States, histoplasmosis in cats can present with oral lesions as the predominant physical examination finding. In these cases, a diagnosis can be made on the basis of identification of organisms from proliferative oral lesions (Figs. 8.6 and 8.7).

An inflammatory infiltrate, characterized by a predominance of mature lymphocytes and plasma cells with scattered other inflammatory cells, is seen in samples from cats with chronic gingivitis or stomatitis (i.e., lymphocytic-plasmacytic gingivitis or stomatitis). The characteristic inflammatory cells are typically admixed with normal or dysplastic epithelial cells (Fig. 8.8).

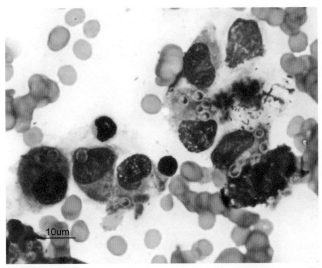

Fig. 8.6 Scraping of an oral lesion of a cat with histoplasmosis. The lesion was pyogranulomatous, yielding a mixture of neutrophils and macrophages. In this image, many macrophages are present and contain phagocytized *Histoplasma* organisms.

Reactive hyperplasia of the tonsils is characterized by a population of lymphoid cells that are predominantly small mature lymphocytes, with variably increased numbers of plasma cells (Fig. 8.9). Lymphoblast numbers remain low. Variable numbers of neutrophils and macrophages may be present, depending on the degree of concurrent inflammation. Bacterial or fungal organisms can be present. Because tonsils have no afferent lymphatic vessels, malignancies and inflammation in the oropharynx drain into the submandibular and pharyngeal lymph nodes rather than the tonsils.

Eosinophilic Granuloma Complex

Eosinophilic ulcers, granulomas, and plaques are common within the oropharynx. Cytologically, they are identified by a predominance of eosinophils (Fig. 8.10). Macrophages, fibroblasts, lymphocytes, and plasma cells can also be observed in variable numbers because they are all normal components of eosinophilic granuloma lesions. As with other oropharyngeal lesions, secondary opportunistic bacterial inflammation can be observed if the sample is superficial. Eosinophils can also be the dominant cell type in some mycotic lesions, foreign-body reactions, and, rarely, in marked inflammatory reactions to bacteria (Splendore-Hoeppli phenomenon). Rarely, numerous eosinophils are found within sites of malignant lymphoma, as a paraneoplastic syndrome caused by production of interleukin-5 by malignant lymphocytes. For this reason, these possibilities must be differentiated from eosinophilic granuloma complex on the basis of the gross appearance of the lesion, fungal culture, fungal serology, or biopsy.

Neoplastic Lesions

Tumors in this region can be classified cytologically as being of epithelial origin, of mesenchymal origin, or as discrete round cell tumors. They can be evaluated for malignant criteria and for any secondary inflammation caused by tissue necrosis from an expanding tumor or by opportunistic bacterial infection. Malignant tumors in the oropharynx can have a poor prognosis unless they are detected early and completely excised before any microscopic metastasis has occurred.

Tumors of Epithelial Origin

Epithelial tumors of the oropharynx include papillomas, epulides, squamous cell carcinomas (SCCs), adenocarcinomas, and oncocytomas. Cytologically, epithelial origin of a tumor is suggested by cells that display adhesion (i.e., cell clustering, although this may be variable, depending on the specific tumor and degree of differentiation), round

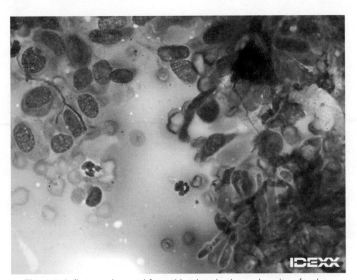

Fig. 8.7 Inflammation and fungal hyphae in the oral cavity of a dog.

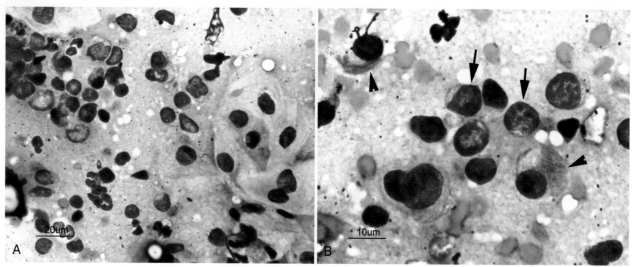

Fig. 8.8 Scrapings of a cat with lymphocytic-plasmacytic gingivitis. (A) Low-magnification image shows normal squamous cells *(right)* and a dense infiltrate of inflammatory cells. (B) Higher-magnification image of inflammatory cells shows a predominance of small lymphocytes *(arrows)* and increased numbers of mature plasma cells *(arrowheads)*.

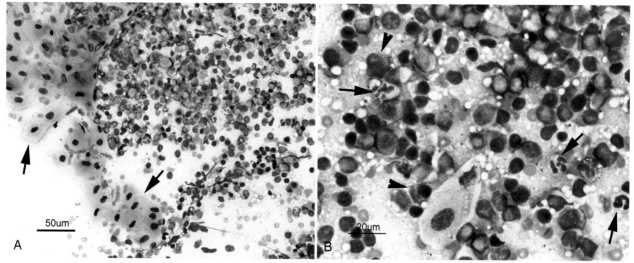

Fig. 8.9 Impression smears of a biopsy of an enlarged tonsil from a dog with a hyperplastic, inflamed tonsil. (A) Low-magnification image shows normal surrounding squamous epithelium *(arrows)* and a lymphoid population from the tonsil itself. (B) Higher-magnification image shows the lymphoid population to be a predominance of small lymphocytes. Increased numbers of neutrophils *(arrows)* and plasma cells *(arrowheads)* are present.

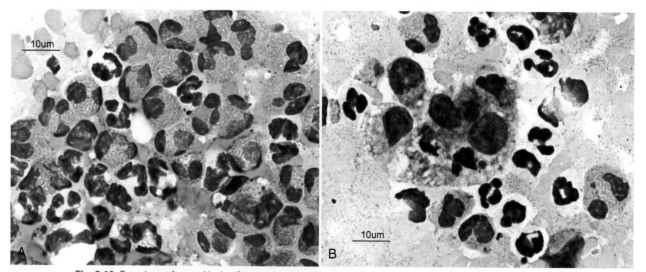

Fig. 8.10 Scrapings of an oral lesion from a cat with an eosinophilic granuloma complex lesion ("rodent ulcer"). (A) High-magnification image of the inflammatory cells shows a predominance of eosinophils and some neutrophils. The eosinophils can be easily differentiated from the neutrophils by the orange color of their cytoplasm imparted by the granules. In contrast, the cytoplasm of the neutrophils is clear. The eosinophil granules are so densely packed in the cell that individual granules are often difficult to see. (B) Another field from the same slide. Although eosinophils predominate in these lesions, variable numbers of macrophages are also present.

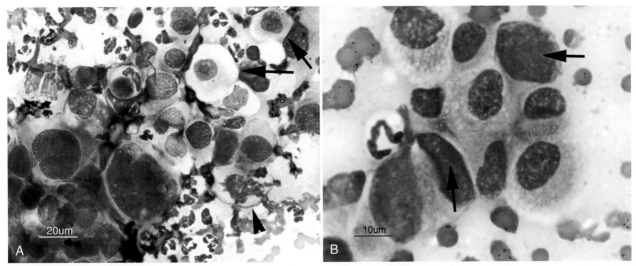

Fig. 8.11 Aspirates from a poorly differentiated squamous cell carcinoma (SCC) in the oral cavity of a cat. (A) A pleomorphic population of epithelial cells is present. Two large, karyomegalic cells are present. Only rare cells show evidence of squamous differentiation having more abundant, lightly colored cytoplasm that is beginning to show angular borders *(arrows)*. A mitotic figure is present *(arrowhead)*. (B) Poorly differentiated squamous cells with elevated nucleus:cytoplasm ratio and prominent large nucleoli *(arrows)*.

nuclei with stippled chromatin, and sparse to abundant amounts of moderately basophilic cytoplasm with generally distinct cell margins.

Canine oral papillomas are caused by a transmissible papovavirus and usually occur in animals age less than 1 year. They are usually identified by their gross appearance. When aspirated, they yield variable numbers of squamous cells that appear intermediate to mature, with keratinization of the superficial cells.

Epulides are a group of benign tumors, or tumorlike masses, that are located on the gingiva. They are common in dogs and less common in cats. They can be caused by developmental abnormalities, inflammation, hyperplasia, or neoplasia. All tumors are characterized by epithelial cells that can exhibit many criteria of malignancy or can appear rather well differentiated. They are identified and classified only by histopathological examination of the tissue architecture, not by cytology. Because epulides are frequently composed of squamous epithelium and fibrous tissue, aspirates of these tumors are composed of variable numbers of mature squamous cells and occasional small spindle cells. The fibrous portion of the epulis is nonexfoliative or minimally exfoliative, and this causes many aspirates to be nondiagnostic because they consist entirely of blood or are almost acellular. The more cellular samples are usually composed almost entirely of intermediate and mature squamous cells. Ossifying epulides can exhibit some eosinophilic, amorphous, extracellular material representing osteoid. Excisional biopsy is the diagnostic test of choice for epulides so that they can be classified correctly on the basis of the tissue architecture of an adequate number of representative cells. This can lead to complete resolution, although some can recur at the same site and some can invade alveolar bone. Biopsy will also differentiate an epulis from a well-differentiated SCC and aid in further classifying an epulis as fibromatous, ossifying, or acanthomatous (peripheral or acanthomatous ameloblastoma).

SCCs are the most common oropharyngeal malignant neoplasm. They can occur in any squamous epithelial tissue, including the squamous covering of the tonsils. The individual appearance of malignant squamous cells varies widely, depending on the degree of differentiation of the tumor and the amount of associated tissue necrosis or underlying bone involvement. Some squamous carcinoma cells (e.g., from poorly differentiated tumors) are round and exhibit sparse to moderate amounts of moderately to deeply basophilic, finely granular cytoplasm with elevated nuclear-to-cytoplasmic (N:C) ratio and prominent large nucleoli (Fig. 8.11). In addition, perinuclear, punctate

hyaline vacuoles are frequently observed in SCCs (Fig. 8.12). Mitotic figures and abnormal nuclear and cellular division can be observed. Other more well-differentiated but malignant carcinomas yield cells that have a more mature squamous appearance with fewer malignant criteria (see Fig. 8.12). These can exhibit lighter basophilia and more abundant cytoplasm; however, moderate anisocytosis, anisokaryosis, and variability of the N:C ratio remain. With well-differentiated tumors, diligent searching can reveal low numbers of cells with marked criteria of malignancy admixed among more well-differentiated cells. Because such cells can be rare to nonexistent, biopsy should be performed on any oropharyngeal squamous cell neoplasm for examination of the tissue architecture before the tumor is classified as benign. When inflammation is present, epithelial cells can exhibit some criteria that are common to epithelial hyperplasia, dysplasia, and malignancy. In that case, biopsy may be necessary to differentiate a primary malignancy with secondary inflammation from a site of primary inflammation from secondary epithelial dysplasia.

Adenocarcinomas are rarely observed in the oral cavity, although tumors of salivary epithelium are possible. Refer to Chapter 6 for characteristics of benign and malignant salivary epithelial cells.

Oncocytomas have been reported in dogs and cats. Oncocytes are epithelial cells characterized by the presence of numerous large mitochondria. They can be found in multiple anatomical sites. Their origin is uncertain but might be neuroendocrine, ductal, or glandular epithelium. Oncocytomas in dogs are reported most often in the larynx. In cats, they have been reported in the nose, nasopharynx, and mandibular salivary gland. Cytologically, oncocytes are large cells with a large round central nucleus, faint nucleolus, finely reticular chromatin, and abundant, pale, foamy cytoplasm. They are very similar in appearance to cells of granular cell tumors and rhabdomyomas. Electron microscopy may be necessary for confirmation of oncocytes on the basis of their numerous mitochondria. Oncocytomas are usually benign and excision can be curative, although some tumors can be locally invasive.

Tumors of Mesenchymal Origin

Fibrosarcomas are common mesenchymal tumors in cats and dogs, even in young dogs (Fig. 8.13). Because they are fibrous, they can be poorly exfoliative. If inadequate numbers of cells are obtained via FNA, a scraping can yield more numerous cells. However, care must be taken to spread the scraped cells into a monolayer for evaluation. Malignant

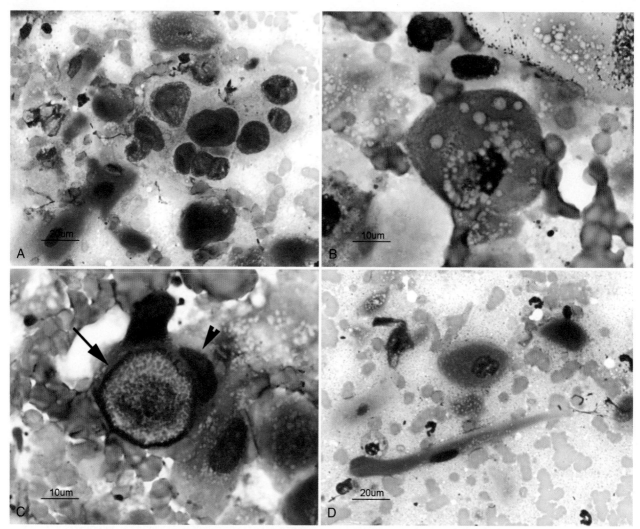

Fig. 8.12 Images from an aspirate of a well-differentiated squamous cell carcinoma (SCC). (A) Cells from a SCC exhibit significant atypia including marked anisocytosis, nuclear pleomorphism, and large prominent nucleoli. Although these cells were present, they were in low numbers and required diligent searching to find. (B) Squamous cell showing perinuclear vacuolization. Note the pink-to-purple color of the cytoplasm, which is seen in some cells undergoing keratinization. (C) Large eosinophilic cytoplasmic inclusion. This is a common finding in aspirates from a SCC. (D) An elongated epithelial cell. This morphological presentation is seen in some SCCs.

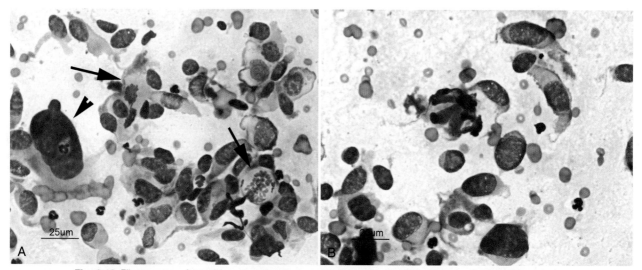

Fig. 8.13 Fibrosarcoma from the oral cavity of a cat. (A) Dense population of mesenchymal cells. A large, karyomegalic cell *(arrowhead)* and two mitotic figures *(arrows)* are present. (B) Another image from same aspirate shows cellular pleomorphism, moderate anisokaryosis, and variation of nuclear-to-cytoplasmic (N:C) ratio.

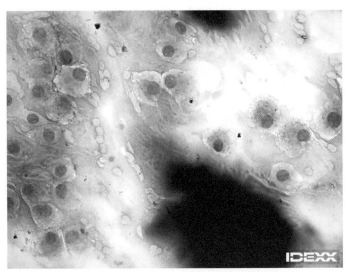

Fig. 8.14 Oral chondrosarcoma in a dog.

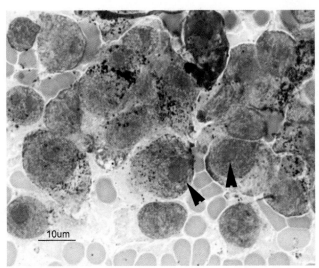

Fig. 8.15 Aspirate from a melanoma in the oral cavity of a dog. A population of melanocytes shows the marked atypia common with oral melanoma. The cells appear poorly differentiated, being large cells with a high nuclear-to-cytoplasmic (N:C) ratio, noncondensed chromatin, and large prominent nucleoli (arrowheads). Although the tumor is poorly pigmented, melanin granules are present in most cells.

fibroblasts are large spindle cells that exhibit oval nuclei, reticular chromatin, and one or more prominent, large nucleoli. Sometimes, the nucleoli can be larger than erythrocytes. Mitotic figures and abnormal nuclear and cytoplasmic division can be observed. Anisocytosis and anisokaryosis can be moderate to marked. Occasional multinucleate cells can be observed. More primitive fibrosarcoma cells can appear almost round; however, cytoplasmic tails can eventually be found upon careful examination. Fibrosarcomas that are better differentiated can yield cells with fewer malignant features. If inflammation and spindle cells are present concurrently, biopsy could be necessary to differentiate a primary, well-differentiated fibrosarcoma with secondary inflammation from primary inflammation with secondary reactive fibroplasia.

Other soft tissue sarcomas, including liposarcomas and hemangiosarcomas, can rarely occur in the oral cavity, including the tongue. Liposarcomas of the tongue that are rather well differentiated can cytologically resemble a granular cell tumor, with round nuclei, moderate anisocytosis and anisokaryosis, coarsely reticular chromatin and moderate to abundant, slightly eosinophilic, finely granular cytoplasm containing variable numbers of lipid vacuoles. Histopathology and special stains can be necessary to differentiate liposarcoma from rhabdomyoma and granular cell tumor. Most poorly differentiated soft tissue sarcomas exhibit poorly exfoliative spindle cells that exhibit oval nuclei and several features of malignancy. Histopathological examination of the tissue architecture is necessary for correct classification and prognosis. Hemangiosarcomas are typically nonexfoliative, and aspirates usually consist entirely of peripheral blood.

The bones and joints around the oropharynx can be the source of osteosarcomas and chondrosarcomas. Their appearance is identical to those described in Chapter 13 (Fig. 8.14). Oral SCCs can also metastasize to bone.

Benign fibromas can occur in the oropharynx. They are composed of poorly exfoliative, elongated small spindle cells that do not exhibit features of malignancy. Because they are very fibrous, they usually require biopsy so that an adequate number of representative cells can be evaluated.

Melanomas are traditionally discussed with tumors of mesenchymal origin, although they are of neural crest origin, and many exhibit cytological morphology that is more epithelioid than spindle shaped. Greater than 90% of oral melanomas are malignant. If detected early, they can be completely excised. However, at the time of detection, they have frequently metastasized to the submandibular lymph nodes and then to the thorax. In fact, thoracic metastatic lesions are the ultimate cause of death from malignant melanoma. For this reason, if a melanoma is identified in the oropharynx, evaluation of the submandibular lymph nodes and thoracic radiography should be included in the workup. If the submandibular lymph nodes are enlarged, cytology or biopsy can be performed to check for metastasis. Individual cellular morphology of malignant melanomas can vary from round to spindle-shaped large cells. They exhibit reticular chromatin, frequently with prominent large nucleoli (Fig. 8.15). The N:C ratio is high. The cytoplasm is usually light blue in color and finely granular, with variable numbers of punctate, round, black melanin granules. The nuclear shape varies from round to oval. Some malignant melanomas are very poorly melanotic or completely amelanotic (Fig. 8.16), which can make definitive identification almost totally dependent on histopathological examination. However, such tumors are readily identified as malignant on cytology, and the possibility of an amelanotic melanoma should be considered if cytology demonstrates malignant tumor cells that have variable characteristics, including some cells that are epithelioid, some slightly more spindle shaped, or large discrete histiocytic cells. Wide excisional biopsy would be warranted. The highly variable cytological and histological appearance of melanomas can make their identification and prognosis problematic with both methods. Ancillary diagnostic techniques, such as immunohistochemical stains and monoclonal antibodies to melanocytes, can be helpful in identifying some melanomas. Currently, no single diagnostic technique can help differentiate all benign melanocytic neoplasms from malignant ones or predict survival time.

Granular cell tumors can rarely occur in the oral cavity, including the tongue, in dogs and cats. The origin of granular cells is uncertain; however, neural tissue, especially Schwann cells, is suspected. The cytological features of granular cells include a histiocytic appearance, moderate anisocytosis, frequently eccentric small nuclei, occasional multinucleate cells, and abundant slightly eosinophilic to amphophilic granular cytoplasm. Histopathology, special stains, and, occasionally, electron microscopy can be necessary for definitive identification of granular cell tumors, differentiating them from oncocytomas and rhabdomyomas.

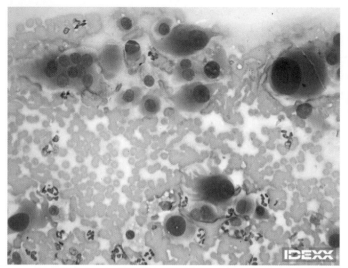

Fig. 8.16 Poorly differentiated oral amelanotic melanoma.

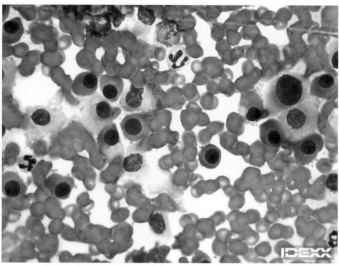

Fig. 8.17 Oral plasmacytoma in a dog.

In dogs, rhabdomyomas can rarely occur in the larynx. The cytological features are described in Chapter 13. Histopathology and staining with special stains should be performed for definitive identification. Benign and malignant tumors of skeletal muscle have also been reported in the tongue and oral cavity.

Malignant Lymphoma

Malignant lymphoma can be found in any lymphoid tissue, and it is the most common tumor of the tonsils. In high-grade lymphoma, greater than 50%, and usually greater than 90%, of the lymphoid cells are large lymphoblasts that exhibit one or more large, prominent nucleoli. The cytoplasm is sparse and deeply basophilic. In some lymphomas, punctate lipid vacuoles are observed in the cytoplasm. The remaining cells are small- and intermediate-sized lymphocytes that appear mature. Small cell and intermediate cell lymphomas comprise less than 10% of canine lymphomas but are more frequent in cats. These are characterized by a predominance of small lymphocytes or intermediate lymphocytes (approximately the size of a neutrophil), and for this reason they cannot be identified with cytology alone. By definition, low- and intermediate-grade lymphomas are identified on the basis of abnormalities in the tissue architecture. If small cell or intermediate cell lymphoma is suspected in the oropharynx, biopsy will be necessary for accurate diagnosis and for differentiation from lymphoid hyperplasia caused by nonspecific immune stimulation.

Discrete Round Cell Tumors

Histiocytomas can occur in dogs of any age, although most occur in young dogs. When evaluating histiocytic cells from the oropharynx, it should be remembered that some amelanotic melanoma cells can closely resemble histiocytes. Mastocytomas or mast cell tumors occur in the mouth; many are poorly granulated. Some are almost agranular,

although careful examination will usually lead to the identification of a few granules that are necessary to differentiate mastocytomas from other discrete round cell tumors. When an oral mastocytoma is identified, the submandibular lymph nodes should be checked for any evidence of metastasis. Consultation with an oncologist for possible treatment options would also be warranted because of difficulty in obtaining adequate margins when excising a mastocytoma from the oropharynx. Polymerase chain reaction (PCR) testing can be performed on biopsy samples and on some cytology samples to predict the success of chemotherapy. Oral plasmacytomas can occur, and most are benign. However, some are infiltrative and can recur locally or invade underlying bone if incompletely excised. Some are malignant and can metastasize to the regional lymph nodes and lungs. They sometimes exhibit marked anisocytosis with giant mononuclear cells (Fig. 8.17). Transmissible venereal tumors (TVTs) are occasionally observed in the oropharynx. All discrete round cell tumors in the mouth are cytologically identical to those in the subcutaneous tissues. Refer to the cytological description of these tumors in Chapter 4.

ALGORITHMIC INTERPRETATION OF SAMPLES

A logical approach to the evaluation of cytology samples is necessary to minimize evaluation time and especially to ensure that the evaluation is thorough and the interpretation is logical. One example of a logical algorithm is presented in Fig. 8.18. Ultimately, if cytology determines that a tumor is possible or likely, biopsy (excisional, if possible) will be warranted, in addition to evaluation of regional lymph nodes and thoracic radiography. If inflammation is present, bacterial culture, fungal culture, or both can be considered. If appropriate treatment does not lead to complete resolution, biopsy should be performed for further evaluation and possibly to remove any nidus of inflammation.

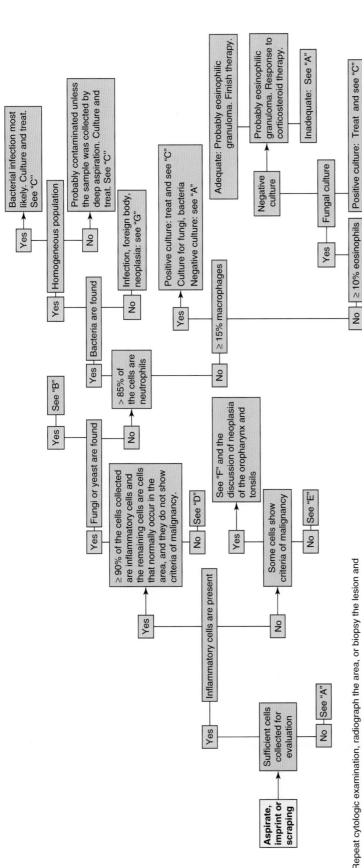

A. Repeat cytologic examination, radiograph the area, or biopsy the lesion and submit the biopsy for histopathologic evaluation.

B. Identify as:

Blastomyces dermatitidis (See Figure 3-10, page 53)
Histoplasma capsulatum (See Figure 3-9, page 52)
Cryptococcus neoformans (See Figure 3-11, page 54)
Sporothrix schenckii (See Figure 3-8, page 51)
Coccidioides immitis (See Figure 3-12, page 55)

Culture, or refer the slide if unsure of the organism or if specific identification of a hyphating fungus is needed.

C. If there is no response to therapy, the patient should be re-evaluated. Occasionally, tumors become infected and yield cytologic samples containing inflammatory cells and bacteria, but not cells from the tumor. In these cases, antibiotic therapy often eliminates the infection, and subsequent cytologic samples contain sufficient tumor cells to diagnose neoplasia.

D. When there is an admixture of inflammatory cells and noninflammatory cells, the lesion should be evaluated for causes of inflammation and for indications of neoplasia. The more the shift of the admixture is an one direction, the more likely that process is occuring (i.e., if 85% of the cells are inflammatory cells, then inflammation is very likely and neoplasia is less likely). On the other hand, if 15% of the cells are inflammatory and 85% are noninflammatory cells, neoplasia with secondary inflammation is more likely.

Also, the greater the proportion of inflammatory cells, the stronger the criteria of malignancy must be in cells suspected to be neoplastic for neoplasia to be diagnosed.

Re-evaluation by cytologic, radiographic and/or histopathologic examination after treatment of the inflammatory condition may be necessary.

E. If no inflammatory cells are present and no cells show criteria of malignancy, the lesion is probably due to hyperplasia, benign neoplasia, cyst formation (such as salivary cysts) or collection from normal tissue surrounding the lesion, but malignant neoplasia cannot be ruled out. Re-evaluation by cytologic, radiographic and/or histopathologic examination may be necessary.

F. If no inflammatory cells are present and some of the cells show criteria of malignancy, neoplasia is likely. The morphology of the cells collected should be evaluated to determine, if possible, the tumor cell type and the level of criteria of malignancy. Depending on the tumor cell type and level of criteria of malignancy present, a prediction of the malignant potential of the tumor may be possible. However, histopathologic examination may be necessary for definitive diagnosis.

G. Infection (mycotic or bacterial), neoplasia or foreign body are all possible. At this time, the cytologic preparation may be referred for interpretation, another sample may be collected, the lesion may be cultured and treated accordingly, or radiographic examination or biopsy with histopathologic examination may be performed. If the patient is treated, a cytologic sample collected 1-2 weeks after therapy is begun may reveal the true nature of the lesion.

Fig. 8.18 An algorithm for cytological evaluation of oropharyngeal lesions.

BIBLIOGRAPHY

Baker R, Lumsden JH. *Color Atlas of Cytology of the Dog and Cat*. St. Louis, MO: Mosby; 2000.

Bernreuter DC. Cytology of the skin and subcutaneous tissues. In: Ettinger SJ, Feldman EC, eds. *Textbook of Veterinary Internal Medicine*. 6th ed. St. Louis, MO: Elsevier; 2005:305–307.

Kaewamatawong T, Banlunara W, Wangnaitham S. *Canine Granular Cell Tumor of the Tongue Proceedings, The 15th Congress of FAVA FAVA-OIE Joint Symposium on Emerging Diseases*. ; 2008:P345–P346.

Piseddu E, De Lorenzi D, Freeman K, Masserdotti C. Cytologic, histologic and immunohistochemical features of lingual liposarcoma in a dog. *Vet Clin Pathol*. 2011;40:393–397.

Raskin RE, Meyer DJ. *Atlas of Canine and Feline Cytology*. St. Louis, MO: Saunders; 2001.

Smith SH, Goldschmidt MH, McManus PM. A comparative review of melanocytic neoplasms. *Vet Pathol*. 2002;39:6651–6678.

You MH, Kim YB, Woo GH, et al. Nasopharyngeal oncocytoma in a cat. *J Vet Diagn Invest*. 2011;23:391–394.

9

Eyes and Associated Structures

Karen M. Young and Leandro B. C. Teixeira

Cytological evaluation of specimens collected from diseased ocular structures may be a valuable aid in the diagnosis and management of ocular diseases. Although cytological analysis alone may provide a diagnosis, it is often used in conjunction with other tests, such as culture, immunofluorescent staining, polymerase chain reaction (PCR) assays, and surgical biopsy. Proper collection (including following appropriate precautions when sampling damaged tissue), sample processing (including concentration techniques), slide preparation, and staining are prerequisites to obtaining accurate and useful information from the microscopic evaluation, as is familiarity with the normal cytological appearance of the sampled site. If possible, several slides containing adequate sample volume should be prepared to allow for the use of special stains, if indicated. When slides are sent to a cytopathologist, it is essential to identify the source of the specimen (e.g., cornea or conjunctiva). The first slide prepared often contains the best material for evaluation and should be included even if it has been stained. In this chapter, cytological findings are reviewed by anatomical location taking into account some general considerations. Certain lesions, particularly of the eyelids and orbit, are common to other body systems, and illustrations may appear elsewhere in the text.

GENERAL CONSIDERATIONS

Stains

Romanowsky stains are standard and, in general, are excellent for observing the morphological characteristics of cells, organisms, and other structures. The major artifact is stain precipitate, which can mimic clusters of bacterial cocci. Quick stains (e.g., Diff-Quik) are often adequate but do not stain cytoplasmic features as well as do parent stains, especially methanolic stains. In some instances, for example, mast cell granules do not stain with quick stains, and the presence of these cells may go undetected if other stains are not used. Also, quick stains must be maintained well, or the stains themselves may contain certain organisms, such as *Malassezia*, from previously stained specimens or from contamination. Other stains that may be used as adjuncts include stains for fungal organisms, such as periodic acid–Schiff (PAS) and Gomori methenamine silver stain (GMS). Gram stain may be used to determine whether bacteria are gram positive or gram negative. Gram-stained slides can be tricky to read and require experience to avoid misinterpretation. Indirect fluorescent antibody (IFA) staining requires special reagents and a fluorescence microscope.

Microscopic Evaluation

Ocular specimens are often small in volume, so examination of the entire sample is easy. The observer should be familiar with the normal cytological and histological characteristics of the tissue sampled and recognize cellular patterns, other structures, and background material.[1,2] Identification of specific types of inflammatory cells permits classification of inflammation as neutrophilic (synonyms include *suppurative* and *purulent*); eosinophilic (often accompanied by mast cells); lymphocytic–plasmacytic; mixed, including pyogranulomatous; and granulomatous. If neoplasia is suspected on the basis of the presence of a mass and a homogeneous population of noninflammatory cells, the observer should be able to identify the cell type (epithelial, mesenchymal or connective tissue, and discrete round cells) and the cytological features of benign and malignant tumors. It is important to recognize that neoplasms can induce an inflammatory response. Finally, the observer should be familiar with the cytological characteristics of cysts, acute and chronic hemorrhage, and degenerative diseases.

When identifying cell types, it is essential to examine cells in an area where they can be evaluated individually. However, thick collections of material—often consisting of clustered epithelial cells, aggregates of mesenchymal cells, or necrotic material—tend to be understained, and cells with granules that stain more readily than other components (mast cell and eosinophil granules), naturally pigmented elements (melanin), bacteria, and fungal hyphae may be visualized within or on top of the thick tissue. Inclusions found in epithelial or inflammatory cells may be normal elements, artifacts of treatment, or evidence of the pathological process or etiology (Table 9.1). Normal tissue also may be present.

Once a category is identified, a more specific diagnosis may be possible. For example, search for an etiological agent is indicated if inflammation is present. At the very least, the category can guide additional testing or therapy. Special cytological features of neutrophils, epithelial cells, and extracellular material (Table 9.2) often provide additional information about the pathological process; misinterpretation of these features (e.g., mistaking free mast cell granules for bacterial cocci) could lead to erroneous conclusions.

EYELIDS

The eyelid comprises layers of skin and mucous membrane (palpebral conjunctiva) separated by muscle and specialized glands, particularly of the sebaceous type. Lesions of the eyelids for which cytological evaluation is useful include ulcerative and exudative lesions of the epidermal surface (blepharitis) and discrete masses on either the epidermal or conjunctival surface. Conjunctivitis and conjunctival cytology are described later.

Fine-needle aspiration (FNA) of ulcerated lesions and discrete masses usually provides diagnostic specimens. Frequently, specimens from eyelid lesions contain abundant blood. Scraping may be a reasonable means of sample collection for diffuse exudative epidermal lesions of the eyelid, such as parasitic blepharitis. Touch imprints of

TABLE 9.1   Inclusions in or on Cells from Ocular Tissue

Inclusions	Significance
Inclusions in or on Epithelial Cells	
Melanin granules	Normal in pigmented tissue Small granules may be confused with *Mycoplasma* organisms
Mucin or mucin granules	Normal goblet cells
Surface mixed bacteria	Contaminants
Drug inclusions	Artifact of treatment with topical ophthalmic ointments
Mycoplasma spp.	Pathogen
Chlamydophila spp.	Pathogen
Neutrophils	Intact neutrophils within squamous cells: no known significance
Inclusions in Neutrophils	
Bacteria	Pathogen
Small fungal organisms (e.g., *Histoplasma* spp.)	Pathogen
Pyknotic nuclei	Aging-related change or accelerated apoptosis
Inclusions in Macrophages	
Red blood cells (erythrophagia)	Hemorrhage
White blood cells (leukophagia): whole or degraded	Long-standing inflammation
Iron pigment (macrophages are termed *hemosiderophages*)	Chronic or previous hemorrhage
Melanin (macrophages are termed *melanophages*)	Pigmented tissue with release of melanin from ruptured or degraded epithelial cells
Certain bacteria (e.g., *Mycobacterium* spp.)	Pathogen
Some fungal organisms (e.g., *Histoplasma* spp.)	Pathogen
Protozoal organisms (e.g., *Leishmania* spp.)	Pathogen

TABLE 9.2   Special Cytological Features and Their Significance

Cytological Feature	Significance
Neutrophils	
Nondegenerate: well-lobulated condensed nuclei, intact nuclear and plasma membranes	Neutrophilic or purulent inflammation: septic or nonseptic
Degenerate: swollen hypolobulated nuclei, fragmented nuclear or cytoplasmic membrane	Septic inflammation likely
Pyknotic: shrunken, condensed, rounded, and disconnected nuclear lobes	Aging-related change or accelerated apoptosis
Intracytoplasmic bacteria	Usually pathogen(s)
Epithelial Cells	
Dysplastic change: nuclear-to-cytoplasmic (N:C) asynchrony	Secondary to inflammation; differentiate from epithelial neoplasia with secondary inflammation
Cornification or keratinization; keratin does not stain with Romanowsky stains; its presence is inferred when squamous cells are angular or folded	Abnormal for corneal epithelial cells; occurs in keratitis
Extracellular Material	
Bacteria	Possible contaminants, but may be significant, especially if found in corneal samples or if many bacteria of a single morphology are noted
Fungal organisms: yeast forms of *Blastomyces*, *Cryptococcus*, *Coccidioides*, *Histoplasma*; hyphae of *Aspergillus* and other fungi	Pathogens
Parasites: larvae rarely seen cytologically	Pathogens
Free eosinophil, mast cell, or melanin granules	Indicate presence of ruptured eosinophils, mast cells, or epithelial cells; granules may be mistaken for bacteria
Cell fragments, especially stringy nuclear chromatin	Artifact of slide preparation; may resemble fungal hyphae when surrounded by mucus
Cholesterol crystals	Epithelial degeneration
Stain precipitate	Artifact; may be mistaken for bacterial cocci
Mucus	Normal in areas where goblet cells are located; may be increased with some pathological processes

exudative skin lesions may reflect the cause of the lesion or may contain only surface debris. Therefore, both touch imprints of the exudate and samples collected after cleaning the surface of the lesion should be examined.

Blepharitis

Blepharitis may be focal or diffuse and acute or chronic; bacterial, mycotic, parasitic, allergic, or immune-mediated blepharitis may occur. The objectives in cytological examination of lesions of blepharitis are to characterize the type of exudate (neutrophilic, lymphocytic–plasmacytic, eosinophilic, or granulomatous) and search for the causative agent. Agents that may be encountered in scrapings are *Sarcoptes* spp., *Demodex* spp., dermatophytic yeast, and bacteria. *Demodex folliculorum* causes minimal exudation. Bacterial blepharitis, particularly staphylococcal blepharitis, has a neutrophilic exudate. Certain fungi, such as *Blastomyces dermatitidis*, cause either a primarily neutrophilic or a pyogranulomatous exudate, whereas others cause a granulomatous exudate composed of macrophages, including

epithelioid forms, and giant cells. Foreign bodies may elicit a pyogranulomatous or granulomatous response (Fig. 9.1).

Immune-mediated disease usually is characterized by a neutrophilic exudate, but eosinophilic types also occur. The presence of either bacteria or a primarily neutrophilic exudate does not exclude allergic and immune-mediated causes, especially if the lesion is ulcerated. In

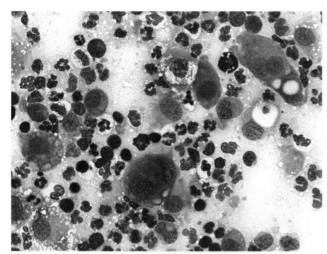

Fig. 9.1 Pyogranulomatous inflammation in the eyelid of a dog. Note neutrophils and epithelioid macrophages, including binucleate forms. Lymphocytes and low numbers of red blood cells also are present (Wright stain, original magnification 600×).

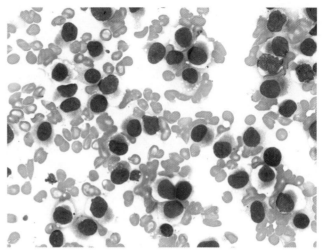

Fig. 9.2 Discrete round cell tumor with cytological characteristics of a histiocytoma on the eyelid of a dog (Wright stain, original magnification 600×).

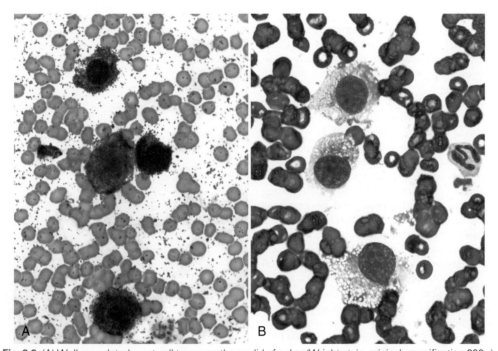

Fig. 9.3 (A) Well-granulated mast cell tumor on the eyelid of a dog (Wright stain, original magnification 600×). (B) The same specimen stained with a quick stain. Note that mast cell granules did not stain (Diff-Quik stain, original magnification 600×).

cats, eosinophilic plaques may manifest as periocular blepharitis. A fine-needle aspirate contains primarily eosinophils, some mast cells, and a mixture of other white blood cell (WBC) types.

Discrete Masses

Discrete masses on the eyelids may be neoplastic (benign or malignant) or nonneoplastic. Among neoplasms, benign sebaceous gland tumors (sebaceous/meibomian adenoma, sebaceous epithelioma) are the most common type on canine eyelids. The glands of Zeis and Moll at the eyelid margin and the meibomian glands, which lie beneath the palpebral conjunctiva and open at the lid margin, are all of the sebaceous type; tumors arising from them are similar to cutaneous sebaceous gland tumors. The cells are readily recognized by their voluminous vacuolated cytoplasm that nearly obscures small rounded

nuclei (see Chapter 5). The malignant counterpart of these tumors is rare on the eyelids. In cats, apocrine cystadenomas (hidrocystomas) develop and may form multifocal tumors around the lids; these tumors are common in Persian cats.

Other tumors frequently encountered on the eyelids and readily diagnosed by cytological examination include cutaneous melanocytoma or melanoma, cutaneous histiocytoma (Fig. 9.2), lymphoma, papilloma, squamous cell carcinoma (frequently ulcerated), and cutaneous mast cell tumor (Fig. 9.3). In cats, ocular mast cell tumors are often benign. In dogs, location of the tumor is important: cutaneous mast cell tumors on the lid are classified and behave in the same manner as do mast cell tumors elsewhere in the skin, whereas conjunctival tumors exhibit a much more benign biological behavior and have a better prognosis. Note that in mast cell tumors, mast

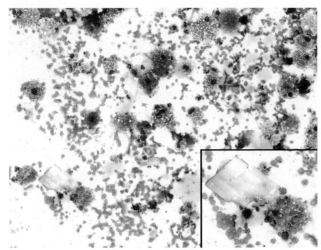

Fig. 9.4 Cytocentrifuged material from a cyst on the eyelid of a dog. Note the foamy macrophages and cholesterol crystals (Wright stain, original magnification 200×, inset 600×).

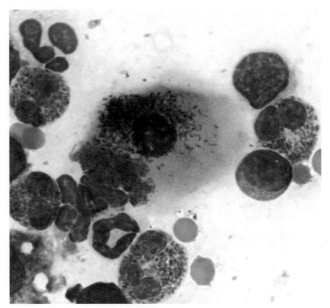

Fig. 9.5 Conjunctival scraping from a cat. An epithelial cell contains numerous melanin granules (Wright stain, original magnification 1000×). (From Young KM, Taylor J. Laboratory medicine: yesterday-today-tomorrow. Eye on the cytoplasm. *Vet Clin Pathol.* 2006;35:141. Reprinted with permission from the American Society for Veterinary Clinical Pathology.)

cell granules sometimes are not visible if aqueous quick stains are used (see Fig. 9.3, B). In cats, peripheral nerve sheath tumors are the most common periocular (lid, conjunctiva, and orbit) tumor. Other carcinomas and connective tissue tumors (fibrosarcoma, hemangiosarcoma, histiocytic sarcoma) occur less frequently and are discussed in Chapter 2.

Nonneoplastic discrete masses unique to the eyelid include the hordeolum, a localized purulent lesion of sebaceous glands, and the chalazion, a lipogranuloma of the meibomian gland. FNA of these lesions yields numerous foamy macrophages and a few giant cells and lymphocytes. The macrophages are apparently phagocytosing glandular secretory product; cytophagia is not prominent. Variable numbers of sebaceous epithelial cells also are found. Differentiating a hordeolum or chalazion from sebaceous gland adenoma via cytological examination may be difficult if the latter has ruptured internally and caused secondary inflammation. A hordeolum or chalazion may contain inspissated secretory product or mineralized debris that appears as amorphous granular material on cytological preparations.

Ocular idiopathic adnexal granulomas may simulate neoplasms, be bilateral, and be a component of systemic granulomatous disease.[3] Reactive histiocytosis of Bernese Mountain Dogs causes periocular granulomatous masses.[4,5] True cysts can occur on the eyelids and typically contain foamy macrophages and cholesterol crystals from epithelial degeneration (Fig. 9.4). In dogs, mesenchymal hamartomas may occur at the lateral canthus.

CONJUNCTIVA

The primary goals for conjunctival cytological evaluation are characterization of an exudate and identification of the cause of conjunctivitis. Certain anatomical structures affect the types of cells found on all preparations from normal eyes and diseased eyes. The conjunctiva is composed of two continuous layers of epithelium that lie in apposition. The inner epithelial layer of the eyelid, called the *palpebral conjunctiva*, is composed of pseudostratified columnar epithelium and interspersed goblet cells. Cilia may be found on the columnar cells. At the fornix, deep within the conjunctival sac, the epithelium reflects back over the globe. This bulbar conjunctiva is composed of stratified squamous epithelium. Bulbar conjunctiva is continuous with the corneal epithelium at the limbus. The squamous cells are noncornified and often contain melanin granules (Fig. 9.5). In most conjunctival

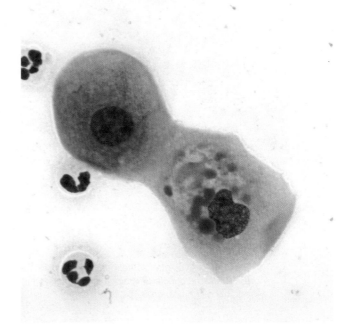

Fig. 9.6 A corneal scrape contains squamous cells with dense, homogeneous, blue cytoplasmic inclusions believed to be a consequence of treatment with ophthalmic ointment (Wright stain, original magnification 600×). (From Young KM, Taylor J. Laboratory medicine: yesterday-today-tomorrow. Eye on the cytoplasm. *Vet Clin Pathol.* 2006;35:141. Reprinted with permission from the American Society for Veterinary Clinical Pathology.)

scrapings, squamous cells are more numerous than columnar cells. In animals treated with topical ophthalmic ointments (particularly neomycin), epithelial cells may contain dense basophilic homogeneous or glassy cytoplasmic inclusions (Fig. 9.6).[6] Such inclusions must be differentiated from infectious agents. At the fornix, conjunctival lamina propria contains lymphoid tissue; various types of lymphoid cells may be found in any conjunctival scraping. Without clinical signs of

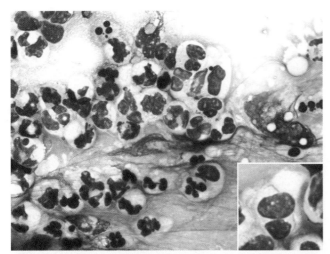

Fig. 9.7 Conjunctival scrape from a dog with neutrophilic bacterial conjunctivitis. Both well-segmented nondegenerate neutrophils and degenerate neutrophils with swollen nuclei are present (Wright stain, original magnification 600×). *Inset,* A degenerate neutrophil with two thin bacterial rods. (Wright stain, original magnification 1000×).

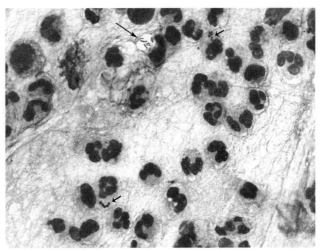

Fig. 9.8 Conjunctival scrape from a dog. Note many neutrophils and bacterial rods *(long arrow)* and cocci *(short arrows)* (Wright stain, original magnification 1000×).

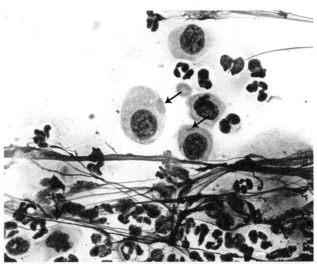

Fig. 9.9 Conjunctival scrape from a dog. Variably sized distemper viral inclusions *(arrows)* are found within epithelial cells. Note neutrophils and small bacterial rods and cocci (Wright stain, original magnification 1000×). (Photomicrograph by Judith Taylor; from Young KM, Taylor J. Laboratory medicine: yesterday-today-tomorrow. Eye on the cytoplasm. *Vet Clin Pathol.* 2006;35:141. Reprinted with permission from the American Society for Veterinary Clinical Pathology.)

conjunctivitis, little emphasis should be placed on the observation of lymphocytes or plasma cells among epithelial cells.

Cytological preparations from the conjunctiva should include freshly derived cells. If external debris within the conjunctival sac is present, imprints of the debris should be made because this material may contain the etiological agent, such as *Blastomyces* spp. More often, the debris obscures the primary lesion; therefore, after imprints are made, the debris should be removed and conjunctival scraping performed with a flat, round-tipped spatula. Preparation of bulbar conjunctival imprints using filter strips following topical anesthesia has been reported in dogs.[7]

Neutrophilic Conjunctivitis

Canine and feline conjunctivitis frequently is neutrophilic and results from bacterial or viral infections, allergic disease, or other causes. Pseudomembranous (ligneous) conjunctivitis is neutrophilic.[8] Cytological evaluation may not reveal the cause. Neutrophils may be nondegenerate or degenerate (Fig. 9.7); in cats, the latter are rarely encountered. In both dogs and cats, intact neutrophils may be found within squamous cells, and the significance of this finding is unknown. Mucus is a common component of neutrophilic exudates and may cause cells to be aligned in rows on the smear.

The exudate of canine neutrophilic conjunctivitis often contains bacteria, regardless of the primary cause. Bacteria are often large or small cocci and less frequently rods (Fig. 9.8). The dilemma is determining whether the bacteria are of primary importance or are merely opportunistic. Normal bacterial flora of the canine conjunctival sac have been described.[9] Keratoconjunctivitis sicca is a common canine disorder causing neutrophilic exudate in which bacteria frequently are encountered. The disease is diagnosed readily by the Schirmer tear test. In contrast to that of dogs, the exudate of feline neutrophilic conjunctivitis rarely contains bacteria. When observed, bacteria should be considered clinically significant in feline conjunctivitis.

Distemper is the most important viral cause of canine neutrophilic conjunctivitis. Canine distemper is diagnosed on the basis of its classic clinical signs and fluorescent antibody staining of conjunctival smears. Canine distemper inclusion bodies in epithelial cells are found rarely (Fig. 9.9), and a search for them has limited diagnostic value.

A common cause of feline neutrophilic conjunctivitis is herpesvirus infection. Diagnosis is confirmed by PCR analysis, fluorescent antibody staining of conjunctival smears, or viral isolation. Multinucleate epithelial cells may be found, but intranuclear inclusion bodies are seen rarely, if ever, cytologically.

Neutrophils also predominate in the conjunctival exudate of feline chlamydial infection. In experimental *Chlamydophila felis* infections, organisms were found on postinoculation day 6, after clinical signs first appeared.[10] Solitary, large (3–5 micrometers [μm]), basophilic particulate forms initially are found in the cytoplasm of squamous epithelial cells (Fig. 9.10). The particulate nature of the initial body is an important observation to distinguish *C. felis* from incidental foci of homogeneous cytoplasmic basophilia found in squamous epithelial cells (see Fig. 9.6); organisms also may appear as aggregates of coccoid basophilic bodies (elementary bodies), sometimes in a paranuclear location and measuring 0.5 to 1 μm in diameter (see Fig. 9.10).[11] In experimental infections, organisms rarely were found by postinoculation day 14, and in chronic conjunctivitis, intracytoplasmic

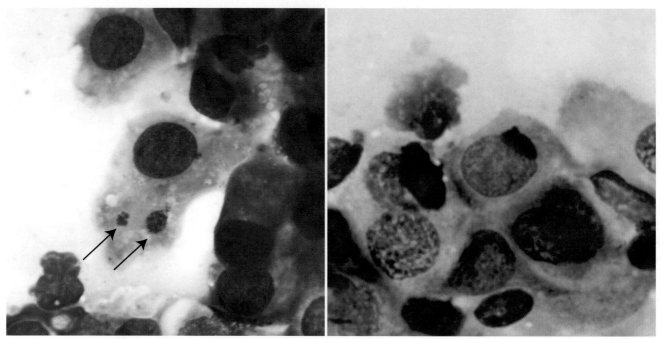

Fig. 9.10 Conjunctival scraping from a cat with chlamydial conjunctivitis. Elementary bodies of *Chlamydophila felis* are found in an epithelial cell *(arrows, left image)* and in a paranuclear location *(right image)* (Wright stain, original magnification 1000×). (*Left image* from Young KM, Taylor J. Laboratory medicine: yesterday-to-day-tomorrow. Eye on the cytoplasm. *Vet Clin Pathol.* 2006;35:141. Reprinted with permission from the American Society for Veterinary Clinical Pathology.)

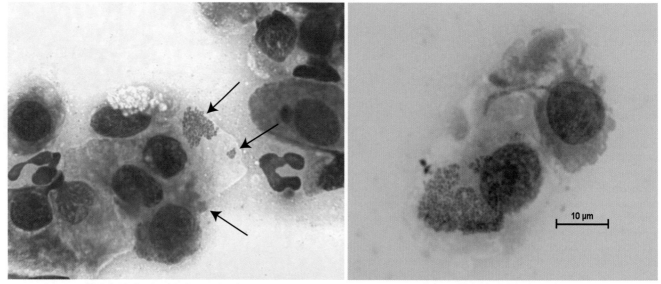

Fig. 9.11 Conjunctival scraping from a cat with mycoplasmal conjunctivitis. *Mycoplasma felis* organisms *(arrows)* are visible on the surface of and adjacent to an epithelial cell *(left image)* and overlying the nucleus *(right image)*. Note neutrophilic inflammation (Wright stain, original magnification 1000×). (*Left image* from Young KM, Taylor J. Laboratory medicine: yesterday-today-tomorrow. Eye on the cytoplasm. *Vet Clin Pathol.* 2006;35:141. Reprinted with permission from the American Society for Veterinary Clinical Pathology.)

organisms are present only infrequently.[10,12] Chlamydial conjunctivitis may be confirmed with PCR analysis or fluorescent antibody staining. Chlamydiae other than *C. felis* also may play a role in ocular disease in cats.[13]

Feline mycoplasmosis, another cause of neutrophilic conjunctivitis, may be diagnosed by finding the organisms on epithelial cells on routinely stained smears. In one study, mycoplasmosis was diagnosed in nine naturally infected cats by isolation and identification

of *Mycoplasma* spp. Of samples from 16 eyes, the organisms were found on Romanowsky-stained smears from 15 eyes, suggesting a high degree of diagnostic sensitivity for routine cytological evaluation in *Mycoplasma* infection.[14] Other studies have found cytological examination to be less reliable in the diagnosis of mycoplasmosis.[11] The basophilic organisms, 0.2 to 0.8 μm long, may be found in clusters adherent to the outer limits of the plasma membrane or over the flattened surface of squamous epithelial cells (Fig. 9.11). They also may

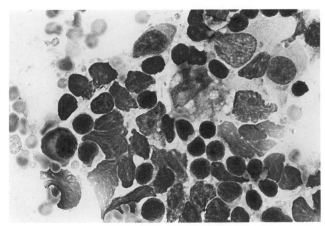

Fig. 9.12 Conjunctival scraping from a cat with lymphocytic–plasmacytic conjunctivitis. Note numerous lymphocytes, a plasma cell *(left margin)*, and a macrophage *(top right center)* (Romanowsky-type stain, original magnification 1000×).

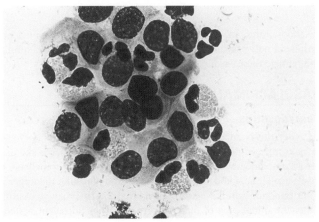

Fig. 9.13 Eosinophils and squamous cells in a conjunctival scraping from a cat with eosinophilic conjunctivitis (Romanowsky-type stain, original magnification 1000×).

be seen in clusters between cells. *Mycoplasma* organisms should not be confused with melanin granules (see Fig. 9.5).

Lymphocytic–Plasmacytic Conjunctivitis

Conjunctivitis in which lymphoid cells predominate is less common than purulent conjunctivitis. Lymphocytic–plasmacytic conjunctivitis occurs in allergic and chronic infectious conjunctivitis (Fig. 9.12). Follicular conjunctivitis yields cells typical of reactive lymphoid hyperplasia (see the section "Nictitating Membrane").

Eosinophilic and Mast Cell Conjunctivitis

Eosinophilic conjunctivitis is encountered in both dogs and cats (Fig. 9.13). It has been observed in cats as a sole entity and concomitant with eosinophilic keratitis. In conjunctival smears from both dogs and cats, mast cells also may be present. Some cases test positive for feline herpesvirus on PCR analysis. In cats, epitheliotropic mastocytic conjunctivitis may occur after spreading from the nictitating membrane. In preparations stained with aqueous quick stains, sometimes neither eosinophil granules nor mast cell granules stain well, and eosinophils may be mistaken for neutrophils. In addition, free eosinophil granules, which are rod shaped in cats, and mast cell granules from ruptured cells should not be mistaken for bacterial rods and cocci, respectively (see the section "Eosinophilic Keratitis").

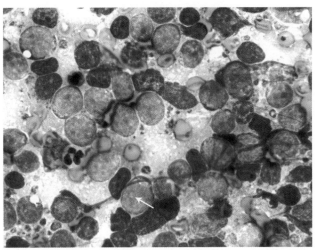

Fig. 9.14 Conjunctival lymphoma from a dog. Note the predominance of large lymphocytes with visible nucleoli *(arrow)*. Free nuclei and cytoplasmic fragments from ruptured cells are present in the background (Wright stain, original magnification 1000×).

Granulomatous Conjunctivitis

Granulomatous or pyogranulomatous inflammation may be caused by fungal organisms, some bacteria, or foreign bodies. In cats, lipogranulomatous conjunctivitis may occur.

Noninflammatory Lesions of the Conjunctiva

Neoplasms of the conjunctiva include papilloma,[15] squamous cell carcinoma, melanoma, lipoma, lymphoma (Fig. 9.14), mast cell tumors,[16] and others. In cats, peripheral nerve sheath tumors can occur in the conjunctiva. Feline conjunctival surface adenocarcinoma (mucoepidermoid carcinoma) can also affect the nictitating membrane; this tumor is a highly infiltrative and potentially metastatic neoplasm. In cases of conjunctival melanocytic tumors, location is important. In dogs, almost all conjunctival melanocytic tumors are malignant and often recur because of intraepithelial (pagetoid) spread, whereas cutaneous eyelid melanocytic tumors are more often benign. Conjunctival melanoma is much less common in cats; this tumor exhibits a malignant behavior despite benign cellular features. A unique form of mast cell neoplasia occurs in canine conjunctiva, manifests as severe diffuse swelling of the conjunctiva, and shows a benign biological behavior.[17] Cytological examination of mast cell tumors is discussed in Chapters 2 and 4. Conjunctival hemangioma and hemangiosarcoma occur most frequently within the nonpigmented epithelium of the temporal bulbar conjunctiva in dogs or the nictitating membrane in dogs and cats.[18,19]

Cystlike swellings of the conjunctiva are uncommon and include dacryops (see discussion on nasolacrimal apparatus later in this chapter), zygomatic mucocele, deposteroid granuloma, tumors, staphyloma, and inclusion cysts. The cytological findings for a mucocele are identical to salivary cysts described in Chapter 6.

NICTITATING MEMBRANE

The nictitating membrane, or "third eyelid," is composed of T-shaped cartilage covered by conjunctiva that is continuous with the bulbar and palpebral conjunctiva on its inner and outer surfaces. The gland of the third eyelid, a seromucous gland, envelops the base of the cartilage. Lymphoid tissue is located on the bulbar surface superior to the gland. Consequently, finding cells on nictitans scrapings depends on which surface is sampled. Scrapings of the bulbar

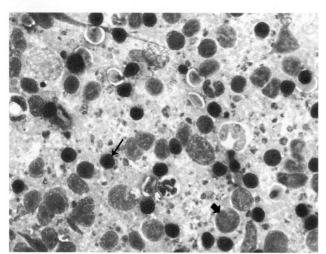

Fig. 9.15 Corneal scrape from a dog with follicular conjunctivitis. Small lymphocytes *(thin arrow)* are numerous, and large lymphocytes *(thick arrow)* also are present. Again, free nuclei and cytoplasmic fragments from ruptured cells are present in the background (Wright stain, original magnification 1000×).

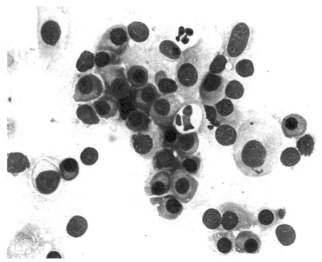

Fig. 9.16 Numerous plasma cells in a scraping of the third eyelid from a German Shepherd with plasmacytic conjunctivitis (Wright stain, original magnification 600×).

surface of the membrane in normal or diseased eyes may resemble cytological preparations from lymph nodes with all expected types of lymphoid cells.

As a conjunctival surface, the nictitating membrane may be affected by most of the diseases of the conjunctiva described previously. A few specific lesions of the membrane occur. Cytological evaluation of follicular hyperplasia reveals lymphoid hyperplasia (Fig. 9.15). A specific lesion in German Shepherds is plasmacytic conjunctivitis, in which scrapings of the third eyelid reveal many plasma cells and some lymphocytes (Fig. 9.16); this condition is sometimes referred to as *atypical pannus*. Nodular granulomatous episcleritis (nodular fasciitis) may involve the third eyelid, particularly in Collies (see the section "Sclera" and "Episclera" later in this chapter), and reactive histiocytosis occurs in the gland of the third eyelid in dogs. Feline epitheliotropic mastocytic conjunctivitis affecting the nictitating membrane has been described recently.[20]

The nictitating membrane may be the site of primary tumors, such as squamous cell carcinoma, adenoma or adenocarcinoma (mixed carcinomas and complex carcinomas) of the gland of the third eyelid,

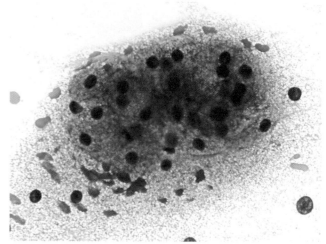

Fig. 9.17 Cells from a lacrimal gland adenoma in a dog. Note the cluster of secretory tumor cells with a uniform appearance (Wright stain, original magnification 600×).

melanoma, and, in cats, conjunctival surface adenocarcinoma and peripheral nerve sheath tumor. Cytological examination is helpful to differentiate these lesions.

NASOLACRIMAL APPARATUS

Dacryocystitis

Dacryocystitis is inflammation of the lacrimal sac. Inflammatory exudates, composed primarily of neutrophils and macrophages and usually accompanied by bacteria, may obstruct the puncta, canaliculi, or nasolacrimal sac. Exudates may be retrieved by flushing the upper or lower punctum with saline through a blunt 22- to 23-gauge cannula. Either the initial plug of material or particularly flocculent material should be examined.

Lacrimal Gland Cysts (Dacryops)

A dacryops contains serosanguineous fluid of low cellularity. On smears, red blood cells (RBCs) and small numbers of neutrophils, monocytes, and other WBCs without bacteria are found. Mucus is usually present and may cause the cells to appear in rows. A breed predisposition may be present in young Basset Hounds.

Parotid Transposition Cysts

A unique noninflammatory cystic lesion may occur in the lateral canthus as a complication of parotid duct transposition. The cyst may occur if the orifice of the transplanted duct becomes occluded. Cyst contents are similar to those of a naturally occurring salivary mucocele and include large foamy macrophages and exfoliated salivary epithelial cells. Variable numbers of neutrophils also may be found; bacteria are absent.

Lacrimal Gland Tumors

Neoplasms of the lacrimal gland are rare.[21] Lacrimal adenoma may have a benign cytological appearance (Fig. 9.17) or may be composed of pleomorphic cells. Histopathological examination provides a definitive diagnosis.

SCLERA AND EPISCLERA

The sclera is the noncorneal fibrous tunic of the eye. The scleral stroma is continuous with the corneal stroma. The fibrovascular episclera overlies the scleral stroma and is covered partly by bulbar conjunctiva.

These tissues are rich in collagen and nearly free of cells. Fibrocytes and melanocytes increase in number in the inner scleral layers, which merge with the choroid.

A nodular or dome-shaped chronic inflammatory lesion affects the episclera and sclera of dogs. It has been called *nodular fasciitis, nodular episcleritis, nodular granulomatous episclerokeratitis, fibrous histiocytoma,* and *proliferative keratoconjunctivitis,* among other terms. It primarily involves the episclera and sclera, most often near the limbus deep to the bulbar conjunctiva. FNA yields lymphocytes, plasma cells, macrophages, multinucleate inflammatory giant cells, and a few neutrophils. Other scleral masses are caused by *Onchocerca* spp., in which the granulomas contain eosinophils, reactive histiocytosis, and necrotizing scleritis, in which collagen fibers may be present.[4,22] Scleral staphylomas may be mistaken for melanocytic masses because of their dark color; if aspirated, aqueous humor may be obtained and may leak from the aspiration site. Neoplasms that involve the sclera or episclera include lymphoma, mast cell tumor, squamous cell carcinoma, limbal melanocytoma/melanoma, and infiltrating intraocular melanocytoma/melanoma.

CORNEA

The cornea is composed of thick collagenous stroma covered by noncornified stratified squamous epithelium on the outer surface and a thick basal lamina (Descemet's membrane) deep to a single layer of flattened epithelial cells (endothelium) on the inner surface. The cornea is subject to a wide variety of lesions, including congenital malformation, opacification, proliferative changes, ulcerations, and exudative keratitis. Many corneal lesions have a classic appearance, and the diagnosis is made on the basis of the history and gross examination findings.

Cytological examination is most useful to characterize exudative lesions and may aid in the differentiation of certain proliferative lesions. After application of a topical anesthetic, samples most often are acquired by scraping or may be obtained with a hypodermic needle if the lesion is very small or focal. Considerable caution must be taken in collecting samples from areas of the cornea that are very thin secondary to the disease process. Several diseases may affect the cornea and conjunctiva concurrently; some of these are described in the earlier section "Conjunctiva."

Infectious Ulcerative Keratitis

The exudate associated with ulcerative corneal lesions is typically neutrophilic and should be examined carefully for organisms. Organisms are sometimes found only extracellularly, rather than within neutrophils, as a result of bacterial defensive mechanisms. If the sample is collected appropriately, any bacterial organisms, including ones found extracellularly, are considered significant. The combination of cytological examination and culture is most effective for diagnosing and managing bacterial diseases.[23] Certain gram-negative rods, such as *Pseudomonas* spp., produce collagenase, which causes keratomalacia, often referred to as a "melting ulcer." Neutrophils may be degenerate if exposure to bacterial toxins is prominent (Fig. 9.18), and high numbers of pyknotic neutrophils may be present as an aging change in neutrophils or if apoptosis is accelerated (Fig. 9.19). Examination of all samples collected is essential because features may vary from slide to slide (Fig. 9.20). Corneal ulceration has been associated with canine herpesvirus-1 infections in dogs.[24] Corneal epithelial cells in areas of intense neutrophilic inflammation may exhibit dysplastic changes that can resemble features of malignancy.

Exudates in keratomycosis may vary in character from being nearly devoid of WBCs to having a neutrophilic or granulomatous composition. Scrapings may reveal certain organisms, such as *Aspergillus*

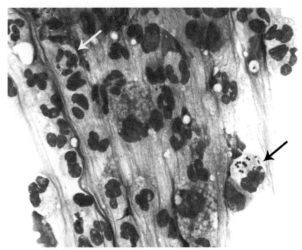

Fig. 9.18 Degenerate *(black arrow)* and nondegenerate *(white arrow)* neutrophils in a corneal scrape from a dog with infectious ulcerative keratitis. The degenerate neutrophil contains bacterial cocci (Wright stain, original magnification 1000×).

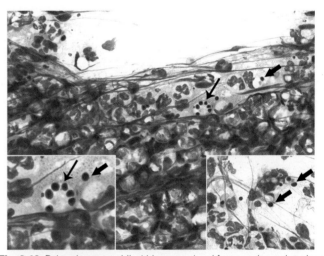

Fig. 9.19 Pyknotic neutrophils *(thin arrows)* and free condensed nuclear lobes *(thick arrows)* in a corneal scrape from a dog with infectious keratitis. Pyknosis represents an aging change or accelerated apoptosis (Wright stain, original magnification 600×, *insets* 1000×).

(Fig. 9.21) or *Candida* (Fig. 9.22), which are the most common species involved in keratomycosis. Pigmented fungi are rare, but dematiaceous fungi have been reported in infections involving multiple ocular structures in both dogs and cats.[25] In corneal scrapings with few WBCs, large clumps of corneal epithelium or necrotic cellular debris should be closely studied because hyphae may be embedded in this material (Fig. 9.23). Fragmented nuclei, often an artifact of slide preparation, may result in stringy chromatin that, when surrounded by mucus, may resemble hyphae. Hyphae have a definitive internal structure that should be recognized (see Fig. 9.23). Special stains for fungi (PAS and GMS) may be useful.

Eosinophilic Keratitis

Eosinophilic keratitis is a corneal disease of cats, and cytological examination is usually diagnostic. The raised granular vascular lesion is usually not ulcerated and has small foci of gray-to-white deposits on the surface. Scrapings reveal an impressive number of mast cells among

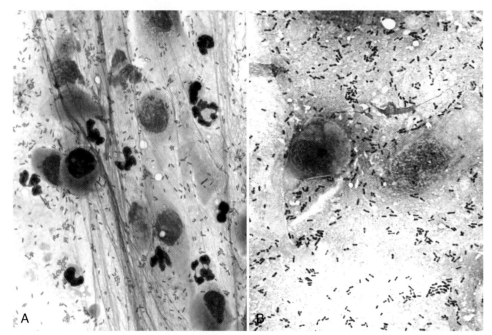

Fig. 9.20 Infectious ulcerative keratitis caused by *Pseudomonas* infection in a dog. (A) The first slide prepared contained numerous neutrophils and many extracellular bacteria of a single morphology (Diff-Quik stain, original magnification 1000×). (B) The second slide prepared had many organisms, similar to those in image (A) but only rare neutrophils (Wright stain, original magnification 1000×).

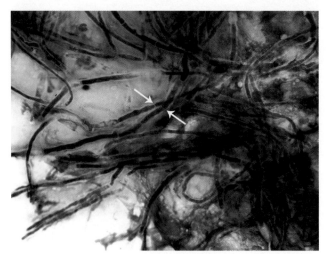

Fig. 9.21 Mycotic keratitis caused by *Aspergillus* spp. infection in a dog. Note that the fungal hyphae have internal structure and septa *(arrows)* (Wright stain, original magnification 600×).

corneal epithelial cells and eosinophils or free eosinophil granules (Fig. 9.24). When the gray-to-white surface deposits are examined, cell debris composed primarily of fragmented stringy nuclear material and numerous free eosinophil granules (and sometimes mast cell granules) are found (Fig. 9.25). Free eosinophil and mast cell granules should not be mistaken for bacteria (see Fig. 9.25, inset). In scrapings from ulcerated lesions or more deeply scraped nonulcerated lesions, eosinophils predominate, and lymphocytes and plasma cells also may be numerous. Eosinophilic keratitis (or keratoconjunctivitis) has been linked to infection with feline herpesvirus type 1.[26]

Chronic Superficial Keratitis

Chronic superficial keratitis, or pannus, is a common proliferative canine corneal lesion seen predominantly in German Shepherds.

Scrapings, although not necessary for diagnosis, reveal a mixture of WBC types, including lymphocytes, plasma cells, macrophages, and neutrophils. Lipid corneal degeneration and mineralizing corneal degeneration are two common opacifying corneal lesions of dogs. Each lesion may cause plaquelike or granular thickening of the cornea. Scraping of lipid keratopathy is nondiagnostic and not indicated because the lipid does not readily exfoliate. Scraping of mineralizing corneal degeneration may reveal crystalline unstained material (Fig. 9.26) that may stain positively with von Kossa stain, a method of demonstrating calcium.

Corneal Tumors

Tumors of the cornea are rare in dogs and cats. FNA, rather than scraping, is recommended. Corneal neoplasms include squamous cell carcinoma (Fig. 9.27), papilloma, melanoma, and various sarcomas. The cytological characteristics of these tumors are described in Chapter 2. In squamous cell carcinomas, keratin released from ruptured cells can incite neutrophilic inflammation. Distinguishing primary neutrophilic inflammation with secondary epithelial dysplasia from squamous cell carcinoma with secondary inflammation can be challenging, and histopathological evaluation may be required.

Epithelial Inclusion Cysts

A raised stromal epithelial inclusion cyst occurs in the canine cornea.[27] The cyst is thought to occur secondary to trauma. Clear acellular fluid may be aspirated from such cysts. In dogs and cats, lipogranulomatous stromal keratitis may occur.

UVEA

The uvea is the layer of the eye that lies between the corneosclera and the retina and collectively consists of the iris and ciliary body, termed the *anterior uvea*, and the choroid, termed the *posterior uvea*. The diagnosis of anterior uveitis is made clinically, and in some cases aspiration

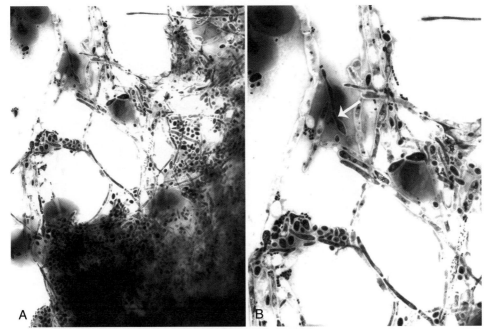

Fig. 9.22 Mycotic keratitis caused by *Candida* spp. infection in a dog. Note pseudohyphae with constrictions between segments *(arrow)* (Wright stain, original magnification 600× [A], 1000× [B]).

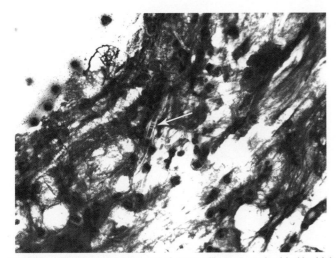

Fig. 9.23 Hyphal element *(arrow)* of *Aspergillus* spp. embedded in thick necrotic debris (Wright stain, original magnification 600×).

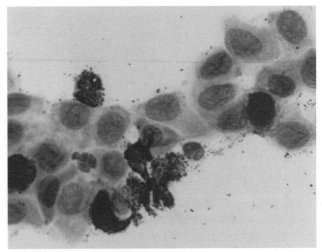

Fig. 9.24 Squamous cells, mast cells, and free eosinophil granules in a corneal scraping from a cat with eosinophilic keratitis (Romanowsky-type stain, original magnification 1000×).

of aqueous humor from the anterior chamber is performed with the goal of achieving a specific diagnosis. Posterior uveal disease is indicated by changes in the vitreous, which also can be aspirated for diagnostic purposes.

Aqueous Humor

Aspiration of aqueous humor for cytodiagnostic purposes may be indicated when the fluid is cloudy or opaque. However, clinical examination without cytological examination is sufficient to discern hyphema, hypopyon, flare, and the presence of lipid. In feline anterior uveitis, no distinguishing cytological features exist among various causes, such as toxoplasmosis and infection with feline infectious peritonitis virus. Lymphoma may be diagnosed by examination of aqueous or iris aspirates; however, most other intraocular tumors, either primary or secondary, do not exfoliate into aqueous humor (see the following section "Iris and Ciliary Body"). In most cases of infectious endophthalmitis, identification of organisms

from aspirates of vitreous is more productive compared with examination of aqueous humor (see later discussion).

Under general anesthesia, aspiration of the anterior chamber is done with a 25-gauge or smaller needle attached to a 3-milliliter (mL) syringe. Except in hyphema, the protein content of aqueous humor is very low; consequently, in vitro disintegration of cells may be rapid. Sediment smears or cytocentrifuged preparations should be made soon after aspiration. Total cell counts and protein concentration may be determined if enough volume is obtained.

Neutrophilic infiltration of aqueous humor is characteristic of most causes of anterior uveitis, including lens-induced uveitis and viral infections. A few lymphocytes and monocytes may be found. In cases of hypopyon, bacteria may or may not be found among the neutrophils. Infection with *Bartonella* spp. has been suspected as a cause of anterior uveitis in cats and of anterior uveitis and

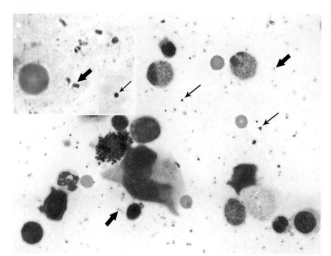

Fig. 9.25 Numerous free rod-shaped eosinophil *(thick arrows)* and round mast cell *(thin arrows)* granules are found in a corneal scrape from a cat with eosinophilic keratitis (Wright stain, original magnification 1000×).

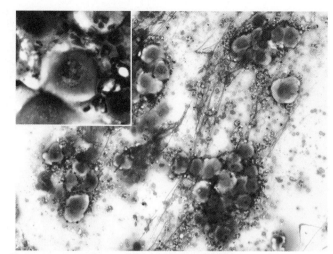

Fig. 9.27 Squamous cell carcinoma on the cornea of a dog. Note the monolayer sheets of neoplastic squamous cells and numerous neutrophils (Wright stain, original magnification 600×). *Inset,* Perinuclear vacuolation in a neoplastic squamous cell (Wright stain, original magnification 1000×).

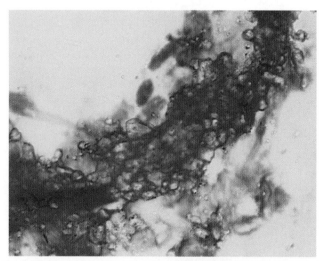

Fig. 9.26 Amorphous nonstaining crystalline material and cell debris in a corneal scraping from a dog with mineralizing corneal degeneration (Romanowsky-type stain, original magnification 1000×).

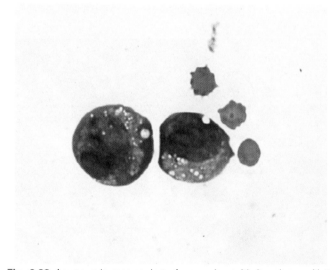

Fig. 9.28 Aqueous humor aspirate from a dog with lymphoma. Note the large lymphocytes with bizarre nucleoli and basophilic cytoplasm (Wright-Giemsa stain, original magnification 1000×).

choroiditis in a dog on the basis of positive serological titers.[28,29] *Blastomyces dermatitidis, Prototheca* spp., and *Leishmania donovani* may be found in aqueous humor. Ocular toxoplasmosis in cats with anterior uveitis is diagnosed on the basis of serological testing, and its definitive diagnosis remains challenging.[30] Phagocytosis of melanin by neutrophils is an infrequent finding of unknown significance. Hyphema is characterized by the presence of either cells typical of fresh blood or, in protracted cases, blood with macrophages containing RBCs and hemosiderin. Tumors metastatic to the anterior uvea include carcinomas, sarcomas, canine transmissible venereal tumor, and feline myeloproliferative neoplasms. Cytological examination of aqueous humor is most helpful for diagnosing lymphoma (Fig. 9.28), which may be part of systemic lymphoma.

Iris and Ciliary Body

Space-occupying masses on the anterior uvea may be an indication for cytological examination of fine-needle aspirates. Direct aspiration of the iris nodule is performed with the animal under general anesthesia, as described in the previous section on aqueous humor.

Melanoma

Melanoma is the most common primary intraocular tumor. The preparation should contain melanocytes that exhibit cytomorphological features of malignancy to be diagnostic because free melanin and some melanocytes are a component of all uveal aspirates. In cats, progressive iris hyperpigmentation may represent diffuse iris melanoma (Fig. 9.29, A–F). Melanosis (Fig. 9.30), with accumulation of melanocytes forming a freckle, may undergo a transition to iris melanoma, a diagnosis that can be challenging to make. FNA (with a 25-gauge or smaller needle) of the anterior surface of the iris lesion, without needle penetration of the iris, may yield diagnostic cells.[31] Dilution of the sample with aqueous should be avoided. In iris melanoma, the most consistent cytological findings are variability in the size and shape of nuclei and nucleoli (Fig. 9.31). Binucleate cells may be found. Both normal and tumor cells are pigmented. Normal cells have uniform nuclei and small uniform

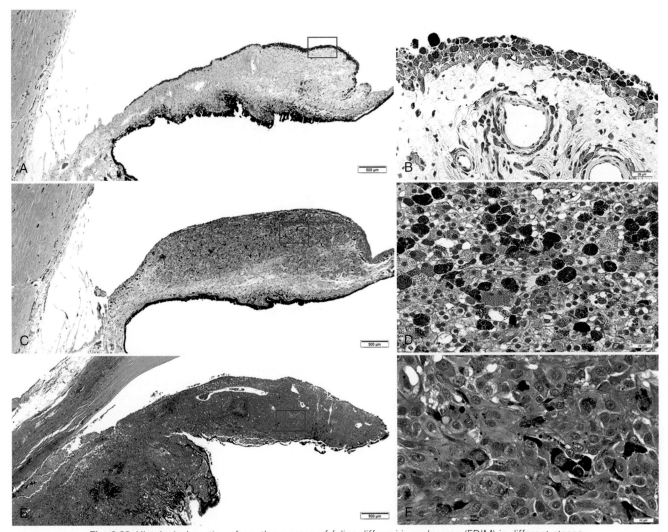

Fig. 9.29 Histological sections from three cases of feline diffuse iris melanoma (FDIM) in different stages of development. (A and B) Iris melanosis. (A) Low magnification of the affected iris profile with pigmented neoplastic cells carpeting the iris surface. (B) Higher magnification of the red box in (A). Pigmented neoplastic cells carpet but do not infiltrate the iris stroma, characterizing melanosis. (C and D) Early FDIM. (C) Low magnification of the affected iris profile. Neoplastic cells infiltrate the iris stroma but do not extend beyond the iris, characterizing the "early" stage. (D) Higher magnification of the red box in image (C). Neoplastic cells are pleomorphic with variable cytoplasmic pigmentation and vacuolation. (E and F) Extensive FDIM. (E) Low magnification of the affected iris profile. Neoplastic cells infiltrate the iris, ciliary body, and sclera, characterizing the "extensive" stage. (F) Higher magnification of the red box in image (E). Neoplastic cells are pleomorphic and poorly pigmented and often have one large central nucleolus (hematoxylin and eosin [H&E] stain, original magnification 40× [A, C, E]; 400× [B, D, F].)

nucleoli. In dogs, both melanocytomas and malignant melanomas occur, and Cairn Terriers may develop uveal melanosis.

Lymphoproliferative Diseases

Lymphoma also occurs as a diffuse or nodular iris lesion. Large lymphocytes with visible nucleoli, lymphocytes with broad pseudopodia, and mitotic figures often are present, and small lymphocytes and plasma cells also may be seen (see Chapter 11 for discussion and additional photomicrographs of lymphoma). Ocular lymphoma is usually part of multicentric disease. When it is suspected, the disease should be staged by evaluating the animal for systemic lesions that may be more easily sampled for diagnostic purposes. Extramedullary plasmacytoma in the iris of a cat with mandibular lymph node involvement but no other evidence of disease has been reported.[32]

Epithelial Tumors

Adenomas and adenocarcinomas may originate from the iris or ciliary body epithelium (Figs. 9.32 and 9.33). Among primary intraocular tumors, these are second to melanomas in frequency.

Other Common Uveal Tumors

Other common uveal tumors in dogs include anterior uveal Schwannoma of blue-eyed dogs and histiocytic sarcoma, and primitive neuroectodermal tumor (PNET) or medulloepithelioma has also been described. The anterior uvea also is a site for metastasis of systemic tumors,[33] including metastasis from oral and digital malignant melanoma and hemangiosarcoma in dogs, squamous cell carcinoma in cats, and respiratory carcinoma (lung and nasal) in both cats and dogs.

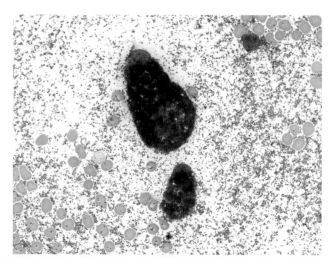

Fig. 9.30 Fine-needle aspirate of an iris freckle from a cat. Abundant melanin is found within melanocytes and extracellularly (Wright stain, original magnification 600×).

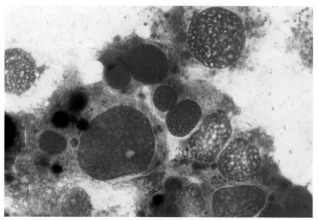

Fig. 9.31 Fine-needle aspirate of the surface of a pigmented lesion on a feline iris. Cells have marked anisocytosis and anisokaryosis and contain melanin pigment. The diagnosis is feline iris melanoma (Romanowsky-type stain, original magnification 1000×).

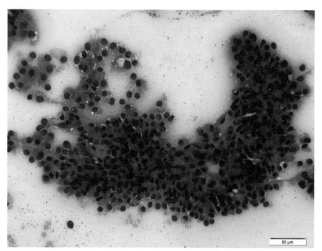

Fig. 9.32 Fine-needle aspirate of an iridociliary adenoma in a dog. Cells are a monomorphic population of low cuboidal to columnar cells situated on an eosinophilic basement membrane. The cytoplasm is lightly basophilic and sometimes contains small vacuoles. Nuclear chromatin is condensed, and nucleoli are indistinct (Wright stain, original magnification 400×).

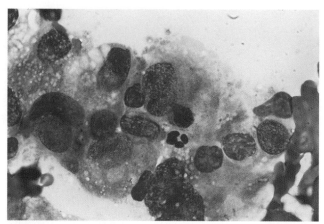

Fig. 9.33 Fine-needle aspirate of an iridociliary carcinoma in a cat. Cells exhibit anisokaryosis, irregularly shaped nuclei, nuclear molding, and distinct cytoplasmic vacuoles of variable size. (Romanowsky-type stain, original magnification 1000×).

CHOROID

Choroidal melanocytoma/melanoma occurs in dogs. Vogt-Koyanagi-Harada (VKH) syndrome in dogs is believed to be an autoimmune disorder involving T cells. Cytological characteristics have not been specifically described, but VKH is characterized histologically as lymphocyte-rich lymphoplasmacytic inflammation with the presence of free melanin and macrophages containing melanin. In some cases, the iris/choroidal tissue may be very thick, and this thickening may be mistaken for a tumor.

VITREOUS BODY

Opacity in the vitreous body is an indication for aspiration and cytological examination. However, aspiration of the vitreous body is not an innocuous procedure. If a potentially visual eye is aspirated, care must be taken not to cause hemorrhage or other sequelae that could jeopardize vision. Under general anesthesia, a 23-gauge or smaller needle is used to penetrate the eye 6 to 8 millimeters (mm) caudal to the limbus: the needle is directed into the middle of the vitreous toward the optic nerve. The lens must be avoided to prevent disruption of the lens capsule and induction of lens-induced uveitis. Aspiration of 0.5 to 1.0 mL of fluid is recommended. Sediment smears or cytocentrifuged preparations should be made immediately after aspiration. After air-drying and before staining, the glass slide can be heated on a slide warmer. Heat fixation helps vitreous body material adhere to the slide.

Vitreous body material is normally acellular, although most samples contain a few RBCs and scattered melanin granules, which, in this location in dogs, are oblong with pointed ends (Fig. 9.34). The background on stained smears is an eosinophilic, granular precipitate. Lens fibers may be found in sediment smears in cases of pars planitis ("snowbanking") (Fig. 9.35). Microfilariae may be found in samples that contain blood from microfilaremic dogs, but they are not associated with ocular disease. Melanin-laden cells may be found in samples from normal or diseased eyes. Asteroid hyalosis is a degenerative disease of the vitreous consisting of calcium and lipid complexes. It is not an indication for cytological examination.

Endophthalmitis

Bacterial endophthalmitis is purulent, and organisms are usually demonstrable in the exudate on vitreous smears. Neutrophilic exudate

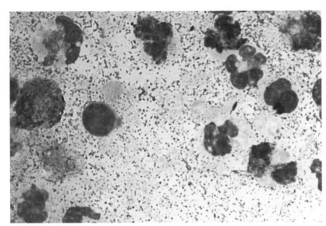

Fig. 9.34 Vitreous smear from a dog. Background granular precipitate is characteristic of all vitreous smears. Note the oblong melanin granule *(right center)* and neutrophils (Romanowsky-type stain, original magnification 1000×).

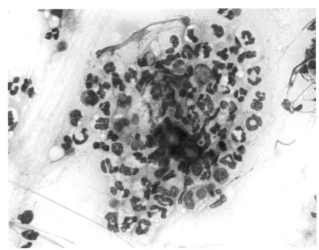

Fig. 9.36 Vitreous aspirate from a dog. Note the broad-based budding yeast of *Blastomyces dermatitidis* surrounded by neutrophils (Romanowsky-type stain, original magnification 1000×).

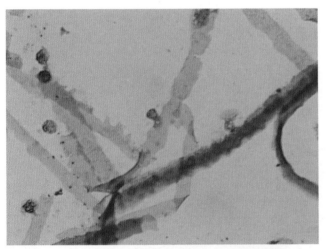

Fig. 9.35 Lens fibers in the sediment of a vitreous body aspirate from a dog. Several red blood cells provide a size reference (Romanowsky-type stain, original magnification 400×).

without organisms may be seen in lens-induced endophthalmitis and trauma. Mycotic endophthalmitis with opacification of the vitreous body is relatively common in dogs. Ocular lesions were found in 41% of dogs with blastomycosis.[34] Affected dogs had a neutrophilic exudate and *B. dermatitidis* yeast in vitreous body smears (Fig. 9.36). Sometimes the organisms are found in the absence of inflammatory cells. Other fungi that may be found in the vitreous body include *Cryptococcus neoformans* (Fig. 9.37), *Coccidioides immitis* (Fig. 9.38), and *Histoplasma capsulatum.* In cryptococcal infection, in particular, little to no inflammation may be present because of the protective mechanisms associated with the capsule, and care must be taken not to overlook the yeast forms. The use of India ink to highlight the yeast of *Cryptococcus* is sometimes suggested but is unnecessary and may even result in misinterpretation of a sample. The clear capsule around the yeast can be seen even in the presence of a pale background (see Fig. 9.37, left), and lipid droplets coated by India ink may be mistaken for organisms. Prototheosis also may affect the vitreous body. The organisms are usually systemic, although ocular manifestations because of chorioretinitis may be the initial clinical problem. A neutrophilic exudate and *Prototheca* organisms may be found on vitreous smears (see Chapter 3).

Other conditions included phacoclastic inflammation, which involves free and phagocytosed lens protein and the presence of epithelioid macrophages, and intraocular xanthogranuloma. The latter is secondary to hyperlipidemia and is usually seen in diabetic hyperlipidemic Miniature Schnauzers. The lesion appears as an intraocular mass and is composed of lipid droplets with granulomatous inflammation, including many multinucleate giant cells, cholesterol crystals, and chronic hemorrhage.

Hemorrhage

Cytological findings in vitreous smears are similar to those in hematomas or other sites of hemorrhage. In addition to RBCs, monocytes and macrophages exhibiting erythrophagia and containing hemosiderin predominate. Histologically, cholesterol crystals from RBC membranes are noted. Causes of hemorrhage can be systemic or local; for example, bleeding disorders, hypertension, rickettsial disease, retinal detachment, and intraocular tumor.

Intraocular Tumors

Posterior segment intraocular tumors can be diagnosed on cytological examination of vitreous smears. Cats may develop intraocular sarcomas after trauma.[35] This may be a sequela of metaplasia of the lens epithelium and subsequent proliferation and migration.[36] Primary intraocular chondrosarcoma and intraocular osteosarcoma[37] have been reported in cats and dogs, respectively. In dogs, histiocytic sarcoma with free-floating cells in the vitreous occurs, and both dogs and cats develop lymphoma in this location. Absence of neoplastic cells does not exclude intraocular tumor from consideration.

RETINA

Rarely, cells from the retina are obtained accidentally if retinal detachment has occurred or if the subretinal space is aspirated when cloudy material is visualized in that location. Nuclei and segments of photoreceptor cells from the outer nuclear layer and cells from the retinal pigment epithelium (RPE) might be identified in an aspirate of subretinal fluid (Fig. 9.39). Retinal hemorrhage, infection (organisms are the same as those described in the vitreous), and tumors, such as retinal/optic nerve glioma, occur; however, cytological examination of the retina is rare.

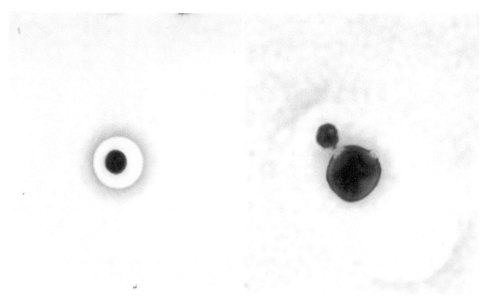

Fig. 9.37 Vitreous aspirates from a cat with cryptococcosis. *Cryptococcus* organisms have a capsule and exhibit narrow-based budding *(right)*. The clear capsule is evident even though the background material is pale *(left)*, and staining with India ink is unnecessary. Inflammatory cells may be absent (Wright strain, original magnification 1000×).

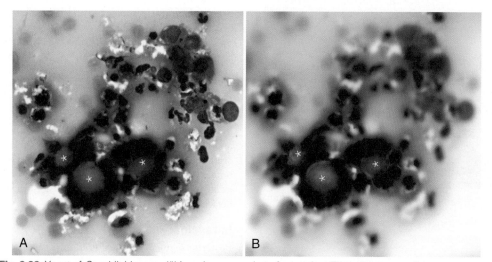

Fig. 9.38 Yeast of *Coccidioides* spp. (*) in a vitreous aspirate from a dog. These large yeast forms appear out of focus when the inflammatory cells are in focus (A); conversely, the inflammatory cells are blurred when the yeast wall is in focus (B) (Wright-Giemsa stain, original magnification 600×).

ORBIT

Exophthalmos

Exophthalmos results from a space-occupying lesion in the orbit. Causes include abscesses and orbital cellulitis from fungal infections (*Blastomyces*, *Cryptococcus*, *Coccidioides*, and, in cats, opportunistic/dematiaceous fungi), retrobulbar *Toxocara canis* infection with larval migration (reported in a dog[38]), foreign bodies, or extensions of inflammatory diseases from the sinus or oral cavity; osteomyelitis' hematomas; mucoceles; extensions of neoplastic diseases from the sinus or oral cavity; and primary tumors. Retrobulbar FNA and cytological examination are indicated. Traumatic proptosis is not an indication for retrobulbar aspiration.

Imaging with survey radiography or ultrasonography and orbital palpation can help localize the lesion. Aspirates can be obtained directly from the orbit or through the mouth, caudal to the last molar. The critical structures to avoid are the optic nerve and the globe. Principles of diagnostic cytology, described throughout the text and in detail in the beginning chapters, are applicable in differentiation of the various lesions.

Orbital Tumors

Dogs or cats with orbital tumors are presented with either exophthalmos or enophthalmos. The quantity of material obtained from retrobulbar tumors is sparse compared with an abscess or mucocele. Orbital neoplasms include feline restrictive orbital myofibroblastic sarcoma (FROMS), an aggressive tumor despite the benign appearance of the myofibroblasts (Fig. 9.40), lymphoma, plasmacytoma, squamous cell carcinoma, salivary adenocarcinoma, lacrimal adenoma/adenocarcinoma (both from the orbital lacrimal gland and the gland of the third eyelid), osteoma and osteosarcoma, chondroma and chondrosarcoma,

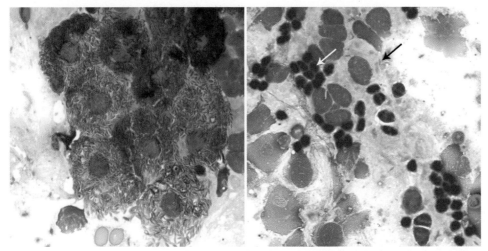

Fig. 9.39 Retinal tissue in an aspirate of subretinal fluid from a dog. Note cells from the retinal pigment epithelium (RPE) *(left)*, nuclei of photoreceptor cells *(right, white arrow)*, and free spiculate melanin granules *(right, black arrow)* from the RPE cells (Wright-Giemsa stain, original magnification 1000×).

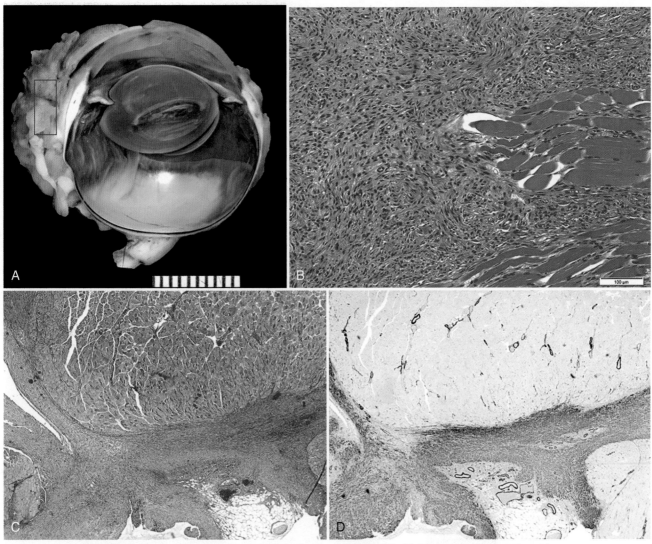

Fig. 9.40 Feline restrictive orbital myofibroblastic sarcoma (FROMS). (A) Gross image of a sectioned formalin-fixed globe. Note the poorly delineated tan neoplastic tissues infiltrating the episclera and subconjunctival tissue (scale: 1 cm). (B) Histological section of the neoplastic tissue highlighted in the red box in image A. Note streams and bundles of well-differentiated neoplastic spindle cells dissecting between normal striated muscle fibers (H&E stain, original magnification 200×). (C) Low magnification of the neoplastic tissue surrounding normal extraocular muscle *(top)* (H&E stain, original magnification 100×). (D) Immunohistochemical staining (same region as image C) highlighting α-smooth muscle actin (α-SMA)–positive neoplastic tissues *(brown)* (anti-α-SMA, 3,3′-diaminobenzidine [DAB], original magnification 200×).

multilobular tumor of bone (dogs), hemangioma (dogs), melanoma, fibrosarcoma, optic nerve meningioma in dogs (Fig. 9.41), peripheral nerve sheath tumors (Fig. 9.42), canine orbital rhabdomyosarcoma (Fig. 9.43),[39] canine orbital hibernoma (Fig. 9.44),[40] and carcinomas and sarcomas of unknown type. In dogs, a unique neoplasm in the orbit is canine lobular orbital adenoma; the origin is unclear and may be lacrimal gland, gland of the third eyelid gland, or zygomatic salivary gland (Fig. 9.45).[41] The tumor is benign but is friable and difficult to excise completely; thus it continues to grow, and the mass reappears in 1 to 2 years. The most common orbital tumor in cats is squamous cell carcinoma.[42]

Postenucleation Orbital Lesions

Conjunctival epithelial cysts are an infrequent complication of enucleation. A possible mechanism of cyst formation is implantation or incarceration of conjunctival epithelium or the gland of the third eyelid at the time of enucleation. Cytological examination reveals basal, intermediate, and mature noncornified squamous cells, large foamy macrophages, and abundant mucus (Fig. 9.46).

Frontal sinus osteomyelitis may extend into the orbit after enucleation. Osteoclasts, osteoblasts, and leukocytes are found. Mucocele and emphysema may affect the orbit after enucleation.

Acknowledgments

Thanks to Dr. Ellison Bentley, University of Wisconsin, Madison, for valuable input, and to Dr. Keith Prasse, Dean Emeritus, University of Georgia, one of the original authors of this chapter, for use of some of his original images.

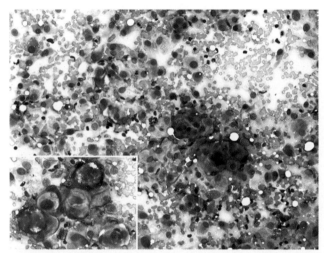

Fig. 9.41 Fine-needle aspirate of an orbital mass from a dog with an orbital meningioma. Note the large cells with abundant cytoplasm that sometimes form whorls *(inset)* (Wright stain, original magnification 200×, *inset* 600×).

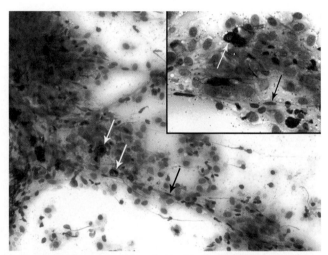

Fig. 9.42 Fine-needle aspirate of an orbital mass from a dog with an orbital peripheral nerve sheath tumor. An endothelial-lined vessel *(black arrows)* courses through the polyhedral tumor cells that aggregate around vessels. Mast cells *(white arrows)* are sometimes found in these tumors. (Wright stain, original magnification 200×, *inset* 600×).

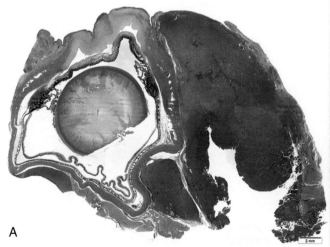

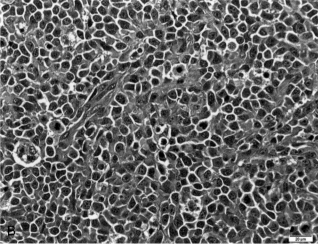

Fig. 9.43 Histological section from a canine orbital rhabdomyosarcoma. (A) Subgross image of the globe depicting the orbital neoplastic tissue surrounding and compressing the globe. (B) Higher magnification of the mass showing individualized highly pleomorphic and haphazardly arranged polygonal cells with scant cytoplasm and anisokaryosis and many mitotic figures (H&E stain, original magnification 20× [A]; 400× [B]).

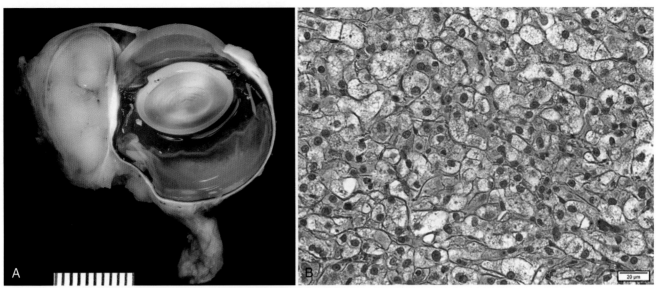

Fig. 9.44 Canine orbital hibernoma. (A) Gross image of a sectioned formalin-fixed globe. Note the well-delineated yellow neoplastic tissues expanding the episclera and subconjunctival tissue (Scale: 1 cm). (B) Histological section of the neoplastic tissue. Note a sheet of round well-differentiated neoplastic cells containing granular eosinophilic cytoplasm with few to many clear, lipidlike vacuoles (H&E stain, original magnification 400×).

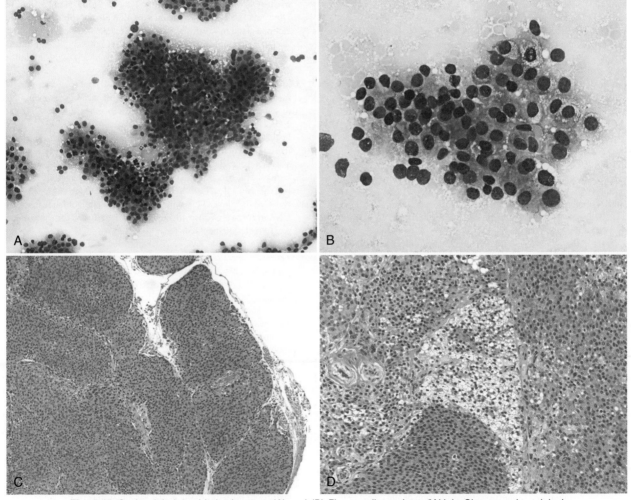

Fig. 9.45 Canine lobular orbital adenoma. (A) and (B) Fine-needle aspirate (Wright-Giemsa stain, original magnification 200× [A] and 600× [B]). Note cohesive clusters of monomorphic epithelial cells, some of which contain secretory vacuoles. (C) and (D) Histological section (H&E stain, original magnification 100× [C] and 200× [D]). Note neoplastic cells arranged in lobules; some cells are vacuolated.

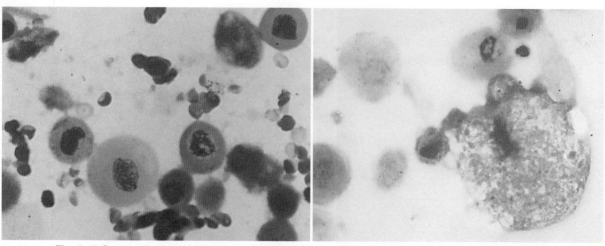

Fig. 9.46 Postenucleation orbital cyst in a dog. Note the variably sized noncornified squamous cells, red blood cells, and cellular debris *(left)* as well as the degenerating squamous cells and a large foamy macrophage *(right)* (Romanowsky-type stain, original magnification 1000×).

REFERENCES

1. Dubielzig RR, Ketring KL, McLellan GJ, et al. *Veterinary Ocular Pathology. A Comparative Review*. St. Louis, MO: Saunders; 2010.
2. Ketring KL, Glaze MB. *Atlas of Feline Ophthalmology*. ed 2. Ames, IA: Blackwell Publishing; 2012.
3. Collins BK, MacEwen EG, Dubielzig RR, et al. Idiopathic granulomatous disease with ocular adnexal and cutaneous involvement in a dog. *J Am Vet Med Assoc*. 1992;201:313–316.
4. Scherlie Jr PH, Smedes SL, Feltz T, et al. Ocular manifestation of systemic histiocytosis in a dog. *J Am Vet Med Assoc*. 1992;201:1229–1232.
5. Rosin A, Moore P, Dubielzig R. Malignant histiocytosis in Bernese mountain dogs. *J Am Vet Med Assoc*. 1986;188:1041–1045.
6. Streeten BW, Streeten EA. "Blue body" epithelial cell inclusions in conjunctivitis. *Ophthalmology*. 1985;92:575–579.
7. Bolzan AA, Brunelli AT, Castro MB, et al. Conjunctival impression cytology in dogs. *Vet Ophthalmol*. 2005;8:401–405.
8. Ramsey DT, Ketring KL, Glaze MB, et al. Ligneous conjunctivitis in four Doberman pinschers. *J Am Anim Hosp Assoc*. 1996;32:439–447.
9. Gelatt KN. Ophthalmic examination and diagnostic procedures. In: Gelatt KN, ed. *Textbook of Veterinary Ophthalmology*. Philadelphia, PA: Lea & Febiger; 1981:206–261.
10. Hoover EA, Kahn DE, Langloss JM. Experimentally induced feline chlamydial infection (feline pneumonitis). *Am J Vet Res*. 1978;39:541–547.
11. Hillström A, Tvedten H, Källberg M, et al. Evaluation of cytologic findings in feline conjunctivitis. *Vet Clin Pathol*. 2012;41:283–290.
12. Nasisse MP, Guy JS, Stevens JB. Clinical and laboratory findings in chronic conjunctivitis in cats: 91 cases (1983-1991). *J Am Vet Med Assoc*. 1993;203:834–837.
13. von Bomhard W, Polkinghorne A, Lu ZH, et al. Detection of novel chlamydiae in cats with ocular disease. *Am J Vet Res*. 2003;64:1421–1428.
14. Campbell LH, Snyder SB, Reed C, et al. Mycoplasma felis-associated conjunctivitis in cats. *J Am Vet Med Assoc*. 1973;163:991–995.
15. Beckwith-Cohen B, Teixeira LBC, Ramos-Vera JA, et al. Squamous papillomas of the conjunctiva in dogs: a condition not associated with papillomavirus infection. *Vet Pathol*. 2015;52:676–680.
16. Fife M, Blocker T, Fife T, et al. Canine conjunctival mast cell tumors. A retrospective study. *Vet Ophthalmol*. 2011;14:153–160.
17. Johnson BW, Brightman AH, Whiteley HE. Conjunctival mast cell tumor in two dogs. *J Am Anim Hosp Assoc*. 1988;24:439–442.
18. Pirie CG, Knollinger AM, Thomas CB, et al. Canine conjunctival hemangioma and hemangiosarcoma: a retrospective evaluation of 108 cases (1989-2004). *Vet Ophthalmol*. 2006;9:215–226.

19. Pirie CG, Dubielzig RR. Feline conjunctival hemangioma and hemangiosarcoma: a retrospective evaluation of 8 cases (1993-2004). *Vet Ophthalmol*. 2005;9:227–231.
20. Beckwith-Cohen B, Dubielzig RR, Maggs DJ, et al. Feline epitheliotropic mastocytic conjunctivitis in 15 cats. *Vet Pathol*. 2017;54:141–146.
21. Hirayama K, Kagawa Y, Tsuzuki K, et al. A pleomorphic adenoma of the lacrimal gland in a dog. *Vet Pathol*. 2000;37:353–356.
22. Zarfoss MK, Dubielzig RR, Eberhard ML, et al. Canine ocular onchocerciasis in the United States: two new cases and a review of the literature. *Vet Ophthalmol*. 2005;8:51–57.
23. Massa KL, Murphy CJ, Hartmann FA, et al. Usefulness of aerobic microbial culture and cytologic evaluation of corneal specimens in the diagnosis of infectious ulcerative keratitis in animals. *J Am Vet Med Assoc*. 1999;215:1671–1674.
24. Ledbetter EC, Riis RC, Kern TJ, et al. Corneal ulceration associated with naturally occurring canine herpesvirus-1 infection in two adult dogs. *J Am Vet Med Assoc*. 2005;229:376–384.
25. Bernays ME, Peiffer Jr RL. Ocular infections with dematiaceous fungi in two cats and a dog. *J Am Vet Med Assoc*. 1998;213:507–509.
26. Nasisse MP, Glover TL, Moore CP, et al. Detection of feline herpesvirus 1 DNA in corneas of cats with eosinophilic keratitis or corneal sequestration. *Am J Vet Res*. 1998;59:856–858.
27. Schmidt GM, Prasse KW. Corneal epithelial inclusion cyst in a dog. *J Am Vet Med Assoc*. 1976;168:144.
28. Lappin MR, Black JC. Bartonella spp. infection as a possible cause of uveitis in a cat. *J Am Vet Med Assoc*. 1999;214:1205–1207.
29. Michau TM, Breitschwerdt EB, Gilger BC, et al. *Bartonella vinsonii* subspecies *berkhoffi* as a possible cause of anterior uveitis and choroiditis in a dog. *Vet Ophthalmol*. 2003;6:299–304.
30. Davidson MG. Toxoplasmosis. *Vet Clin North Am Small Anim Pract*. 2000;30:1051–1062.
31. Grossniklaus HE. Fine-needle aspiration biopsy of the iris. *Arch Ophthalmol*. 1992;110:969–976.
32. Michau TM, Proulx DR, Rushton SD, et al. Intraocular extramedullary plasmacytoma in a cat. *Vet Ophthalmol*. 2003;6:177–181.
33. Miller PE, Dubielzig RR. Ocular tumors. In: Withrow SJ, Vail DM, eds. *Withrow & MacEwen's Small Animal Clinical Oncology*. ed 4. St. Louis, MO: Saunders; 2007:686–698.
34. Legendre AM, Walker M, Buyukmihci N, et al. Canine blastomycosis: a review of 47 clinical cases. *J Am Vet Med Assoc*. 1981;178:1163–1168.
35. Dubielzig RR, Everitt J, Shadduck JA, et al. Clinical and morphologic features of post-traumatic ocular sarcomas in cats. *Vet Pathol*. 1990;27:62–65.

36. Zeiss CJ, Johnson EM, Dubielzig RR. Feline intraocular tumors may arise from transformation of lens epithelium. *Vet Pathol.* 2003;40:355–362.

37. Heath S, Rankin AJ, Dubielzig RR. Primary ocular osteosarcoma in a dog. *Vet Ophthalmol.* 2003;6:85–87.

38. Laus JL, Canola JC, Mamede FV, et al. Orbital cellulitis associated with Toxocara canis in a dog. *Vet Ophthalmol.* 2003;6:333–336.

39. Scott EM, Teixeira LBC, Flanders DJ, et al. Canine orbital rhabdomyosarcoma: a report of 18 cases. *Vet Ophthalmol.* 2016;19:130–137.

40. Ravi M, Schobert CS, Kiupel M, et al. Clinical, morphologic, and immunohistochemical features of canine orbital hibernomas. *Vet Pathol.* 2014;51: 563–568.

41. Headrick JF, Bentley E, Dubielzig RR. Canine lobular orbital adenoma: a report of 15 cases with distinctive features. *Vet Ophthalmol.* 2004;7: 47–51.

42. Gilger BC, McLaughlin SA, Whitley RD, et al. Orbital neoplasms in cats: 21 cases (1974-1990). *J Am Vet Med Assoc.* 1992;201:1083–1086.

10

The External Ear Canal

Koranda A. Walsh, Heather L. DeHeer, and Reema T. Patel

ANATOMY OF THE EXTERNAL EAR

The external ear consists of cartilage and the overlying skin, which create the pinna and external acoustic meatus (between the base of the pinna to the tympanic membrane). The auricular cartilage determines the shape and appearance of the pinnae and supports the vertical ear canal. The annular cartilage, found at the base of the auricular cartilage, supports the horizontal and external ear canal. The skin covering the cartilage within the canal contains sebaceous glands, tubular ceruminous glands, and small hair follicles (Fig. 10.1).[1]

ETIOLOGY AND PATHOGENESIS OF OTITIS EXTERNA

Otitis externa, inflammation of the skin and adnexal structures of the ear canal, is commonly encountered in veterinary patients. Approximately 10% to 20% of canines and 2% to 6% of felines presented for veterinary care are thought to be affected with otitis externa.[2,3]

Causes of otitis externa are multifactorial and are commonly divided into primary, predisposing, and perpetuating factors, which are discussed briefly below.

Primary Factors

Primary factors are factors that initiate inflammation of the external ear canal and include parasites, allergic skin disease, foreign bodies, disorders of keratinization, autoimmune diseases, trauma, sebaceous adenitis, zinc-responsive dermatoses, juvenile cellulitis, and certain endocrine disorders (Box 10.1).[4-7]

Predisposing Factors

Predisposing factors facilitate the development of otitis externa by promoting an environment suitable for the survival of the perpetuating factors. Predisposing factors not only include such factors as ear conformation, hypertrichosis of the ear canal, and breed predispositions, which are congenital, environmental, or both, but also iatrogenic trauma, excessive moisture, and obstructive ear disease (Box 10.2).[3,4]

Perpetuating Factors

Rather than initiating the otitis externa, perpetuating factors sustain the established disease; once the ear canal has been altered by primary and predisposing factors, opportunistic infections and progressive changes occur to prevent resolution of disease. These factors include bacteria, yeast, otitis media, and progressive hyperplastic changes of the ear canal caused by the disease (Box 10.3).[3,4]

DIAGNOSIS OF OTITIS EXTERNA

Most cases of acute otitis externa can be readily managed by using the information gained from a thorough history, physical examination, otoscopic examination, and cytological evaluation of the ear canal secretions. More advanced or chronic cases may require culture and susceptibility testing, biopsy, diagnostic imaging, endocrine testing, and assessment of allergic skin disease.

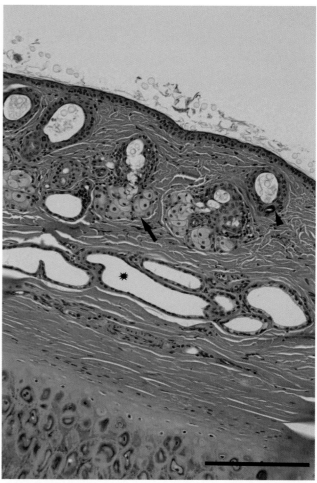

Fig. 10.1 Hematoxylin and eosin (H&E)–stained section of the normal feline vertical ear canal with hair follicle *(arrowhead)*, sebaceous glands *(arrow)*, and ceruminous glands *(asterisk)* (magnification 200×, bar ≡ 100 µm).

BOX 10.1 Primary Causes of Otitis Externa

- Parasites
  - *Otodectes cynotis (common)*
  - *Otobius megnini (found in southwestern United States)*
  - *Demodex and other mites (rare)*
- Allergic skin diseases
  - Atopy
  - Food allergy
  - Contact hypersensitivity
- Foreign bodies
  - Plant material (especially grass awns)
  - Dirt
  - Other debris
- Other skin diseases
  - Pemphigus
  - Seborrhea
  - Sebaceous adenitis
- Endocrinopathies
  - Hypothyroidism

BOX 10.2 Predisposing Causes of Otitis Externa

- Ear conformation
  - Pendulous ears
  - Long narrow ear canal
- Excessive hair in canal
- Iatrogenic trauma
- Excessive ear cleaning
- Excessive moisture
- Frequent swimming or bathing
- Obstructive ear disease
- Hyperplasia
- Benign or malignant neoplasia causing obstruction of the ear canal

BOX 10.3 Perpetuating Causes of Otitis Externa

Bacteria
- Bacterial cocci
  - *Staphylococcus (common)*
  - *Enterococcus (occasionally found)*
  - *Streptococcus (occasionally found)*
- Bacterial rods
  - *Pseudomonas (common)*
  - *Proteus (occasionally found)*
  - *Escherichia coli (occasionally found)*

Fungi
- *Malassezia (common)*
- *Candida (rarely found)*

CYTOLOGICAL EVALUATION OF EAR CANAL SECRETIONS

Cytological examination of otic secretions is a simple, inexpensive, and rapid test to assist in the diagnosis and treatment of otitis externa. Physical characteristics of secretions, if not guided by cytology, may be misleading and unreliable. The primary goal of cytology of the external

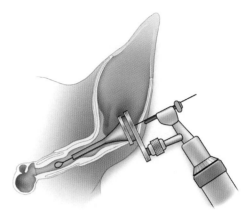

Fig. 10.2 Smears of horizontal ear canal secretions may be collected by passing a cotton-tipped swab through the cone of an otoscope after otoscopic examination.

ear is to identify overgrowth or infection that may contribute to otitis externa. Cytology should be performed at recheck examinations to monitor and adjust therapy.

Collection and Staining of Samples

Samples of ear canal secretions for cytological evaluation are collected by using separate cotton-tipped swabs for each ear canal. Samples should be collected after performing otoscopic examination, to avoid obscuring the tympanic membrane with compressed debris, and before introduction of any cleaning agents or medication. The most clinically relevant samples are obtained from the deeper horizontal canal rather than the superficial vertical canal.[3] This can be accomplished in larger patients with insertion of a cotton-tipped swab through an otoscopic cone (Fig. 10.2). However, some circumstances, such as painful ears, stenosis, and inflammation, may make acquisition in this manner difficult without sedation. Another method to obtain samples is to carefully pass a swab into the ear canal, without the aid of an otoscope, aiming for the junction of the vertical and horizontal areas of the canal. Straightening of the ear canal should be avoided to prevent damage to the tympanic membrane.[3] If the patient requires anesthesia or sedation, otoscopy and ear flushing, among other techniques, can be used to acquire samples. Samples should always be collected from both ears because animals that appear to have unilateral otitis may also have mild, less apparent disease in the contralateral ear.[8-10]

After secretion from each canal has been collected, separate slides should be prepared for parasite identification and for routine staining. The slides must be labeled to indicate which ear was sampled.

To prepare slides for routine staining, the swab is gently rolled onto a clean, dry slide in a thin layer; thick smears are difficult to evaluate. Lumps of wax should be removed and can be smeared onto a different slide, yielding additional samples, if needed, for examination. Heat fixing neither systematically increases nor decreases numbers of yeast on specimens, and although it is recommended by many to prevent loss of high lipid content, it is not necessary.[3,11,12] After the material on the slide is allowed to air-dry, it is stained with any of the usual hematological stains (e.g., Diff-Quik or Wright stain). Two sets of staining jars are recommended. One should be reserved for ear cytology, and one should be reserved for other samples (e.g., blood smears, mass aspirates), because yeast and bacteria from ear cytology may overgrow in the stain solution and contaminate other slides.

Some practitioners prefer an alternative staining procedure in which only the thiazine blue reagent counterstain of a Diff-Quik stain is used to increase rapidity and simplicity and to preserve more lipid-rich material on the slide.[12]

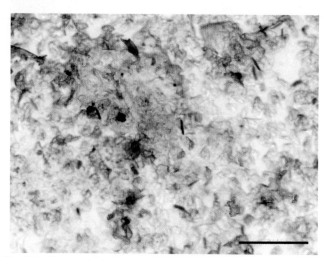

Fig. 10.3 Ear swab from a normal dog shows some staining and non-staining epithelial cells and ceruminous debris (Wright-Giemsa stain, magnification 100×, bar ≡ 200 μm).

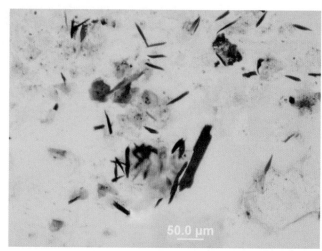

Fig. 10.4 Ear swab from a normal dog shows some staining and non-staining epithelial cells and debris. Note the absence of inflammatory cells and bacteria (Wright stain, magnification 200×).

The method was found to be sufficient for identification of bacteria, yeast, keratinocytes, and neutrophils. Eosinophils would be difficult to identify without the use of the eosin-based stain, but these are uncommon elements in ear cytology, although they may be present in cases of hypersensitivity reaction, parasitism, and, in felines, inflammatory disease.[12]

Gram staining can be used for obtaining additional information on bacterial type; however, it is more time consuming, can be difficult to interpret without practice, and may be unnecessary, given that most bacterial cocci are gram positive and most bacterial rods are gram negative.

Note that any samples collected for parasite identification should remain unstained, and the otic exudate should be mixed with a small amount of mineral oil, cover-slipped, and microscopically viewed on low power with the condenser down.

Cytological Examination
Cerumen
Cerumen, a combination of keratin, squamous epithelium, and oily secretions from underlying sebaceous and ceruminous glands, does not take up stain, given its high lipid content, and provides the background for many normal ear swab cytologies (Fig. 10.3).

Keratinocytes
Keratinocytes (keratinized squamous epithelial cell), including occasional nucleated forms, are noted in normal ears of both dogs and cats. Normal dogs were noted to have 3.9 keratinocytes per 40× high-power field (hpf) and normal cats were noted to have 8 per 40× hpf.[13] The finding of nucleated forms should not be mistaken for a pathological process (parakeratotic hyperkeratosis).

Bacteria
The ear canals of clinically normal dogs often contain small numbers of bacteria. The bacterial concentration typically is low enough that one sees only occasional or no bacteria on cytological preparations (Fig. 10.4). However, when normal conditions are altered, any of these bacteria are potentially pathogenic and may colonize the ear canal.[3,6,9,14] In animals with bacterial otitis, cytological evaluation of ear canal secretions often reveals large numbers of bacteria free in the smear (Fig. 10.5). Unfortunately, no definitive rule exists for deciding if the bacteria are clinically relevant and warrant treatment. The

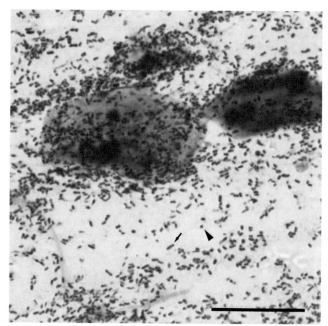

Fig. 10.5 Mixed bacterial infection characterized by large numbers of bacterial cocci *(arrowhead)* and rods *(arrow)*. Note the absence of neutrophils (Wright-Giemsa stain, magnification 1000×, bar ≡ 20 μm).

decision should be based on the severity of clinical signs and cytological findings. Semiquantitative criteria to assess the relevance of bacterial populations have been proposed on the basis of bacterial numbers per 40× hpf as follows (Table 10.1): Bacterial counts expected in normal dogs vary among studies and have been reported to be as few as zero cocci to a median of five or fewer cocci.[13-15] Abnormal numbers of organisms have been reported to be an average of 25 or greater, with 6 to 24 organisms being in the "gray zone." Bacterial counts expected in normal cats vary among studies and have been reported as a median of 0.3 cocci per 40× hpf in one study[13] and an average of four or fewer cocci in a second study.[15] Abnormal numbers of organisms have been reported to be 15 or greater, with 5 to 14 organisms being in the "gray zone." Importantly, neither study identified bacterial rods as part of the normal ear cytology of dogs or cats.

When secretions are viewed cytologically, neutrophilic inflammation may or may not be present. If neutrophils are present, bacteria

TABLE 10.1 *Malassezia* and Bacteria: Expected Quantities

	Normal	Gray Zone	Abnormal
Malassezia			
Dog	0.2* or ≤2	3–4	≥5
Cat	0.2* or ≤2	3–11	≥12
Bacteria			
Dog	0* or ≤5	6–24	≥25
Cat	0.3* or ≤4	5–14	≥15

Proposed semiquantitative criteria for assessing organisms present in otic cytology based on (*) median number per 40× high-power field (hpf) or average numbers of organisms per 40× hpf.
Data from Tater KC, Scott DW, Miller Jr WH, Erb HN. The cytology of the external ear canal in the normal dog and cat. *J Vet Med.* 2003;50:370–374; Ginel PJ, Lucena R, Rodriguez JC, Ortega J. A semiquantitative cytological evaluation of normal and pathological samples from the external ear canal of dogs and cats. *Vet Dermatol.* 2002;13:151–156; Angus JC. Otic cytology in health and disease. *Vet Clin North Am Small Anim Pract.* 2004;34:411–424.

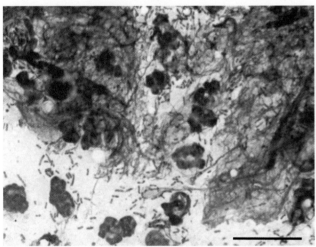

Fig. 10.6 Ear swab from a dog with a bacterial infection. Numerous bacterial rods are present phagocytized within degenerate neutrophils and free in the background (Wright-Giemsa stain, magnification 1000×, bar = 20 μm).

may be observed to be phagocytized (Fig. 10.6). True infection is still possible even in the absence of neutrophilic inflammation and/or intracellular bacteria, but the presence of neutrophilic inflammation may indicate more severe disease.

Identification of the bacterial infection involving cocci, rods, or a mixture of both, along with culture and sensitivity testing, assists with the initial selection of antibiotics and is important for antibiotic stewardship. Infections involving cocci usually represent *Staphylococcus* spp. or occasionally other species, such as *Streptococcus*.[3,9] In infections containing bacterial bacilli, *Pseudomonas* is the most common species cultured, but other species, including *Proteus* and *Escherichia coli*, are occasionally found.[3,6,9,10,14,16,17] Culture and sensitivity testing are indicated because of the high incidence of antimicrobial resistance associated with otitis externa, especially when considering *Pseudomonas* spp. Culture and sensitivity should be employed to further characterize bacterial elements that are identified cytologically but should also be considered when neutrophilic inflammation is identified in the absence of visible/identified microorganisms.[18]

Fungi

Malassezia. *Malassezia pachydermatis* is, by far, the most common yeast associated with otitis externa in dogs and cats, but it may also be found in the normal ear. *M. pachydermatis* may be found in up to 83% of dogs with otitis externa and in 15% to 49% of normal ear canals.[19,20] *Malassezia* infections may occur with or without bacterial coinfection.[3,6,8,9,10,14,16,17] In pure *Malassezia* infections, neutrophilic inflammation is not a common feature.[3,8,21]

The decision to treat *Malassezia* infection ultimately depends on the cytological findings, severity of clinical signs, and history of otitis and response to treatment. The decision may, however, be guided by semiquantitative guidelines, which were proposed on the basis of numbers of organisms per 40× hpf as follows (see Table 10.1). Amounts in normal dogs have been reported as a median of 0.2 yeasts to an average of two or fewer yeast cells, with abnormal numbers reported as five or greater, with three to four being in the "gray zone."[15] Amounts in normal cats have been reported as a median of 0.2 yeast cells, whereas another study had an average count of two or fewer yeast cells.[15] Abnormal numbers in cats have been reported as an average of 12 or greater yeast cells, with 3 to 11 being in the "gray zone."[15]

Cytologically, yeast cells identified from normal dogs and cats were broad-based, unipolar budding cells. *Malassezia* (Fig. 10.7) is a broad-based budding, basophilic-staining, oval yeast that has a characteristic "peanut" or "footprint" shape when observed during budding. *Malassezia* are small, ranging from 2 × 4 micrometers (μm) up to 6 × 7 μm.[3,8,10]

Other. Although uncommon, *Candida* and *Microsporum* have been reported in cases of otitis externa.[6,14,22,23] In addition, saprophytes, including *Penicillium* and *Aspergillus*, have been cultured from normal dogs, atopic dogs, and dogs with otitis externa. However, no cytological evidence of saprophytic fungal colonization or infection of the ear was identified in any of the samples.[24] Overall, when unidentified yeasts or hyphae are observed cytologically, culture is indicated for identification.

Mites

Ear mites are a primary cause of otitis externa and are especially common in cats. *Otodectes cynotis* reportedly accounts for at least 50% of feline cases of otitis externa and at least 5% to 10% of canine cases (Fig. 10.8).[6,8,10] In animals hypersensitized to mite antigens, clinical signs of otitis externa may develop with as few as two to three mites in the ear canal.[3,8,10,14] Typically, a dry, black, granular discharge is seen. Secondary bacterial infection, yeast infection, or both often coexist and may cause the discharge to become moist.[3,6] Larval and nymph stages of the spinous ear tick *Otobius megnini*, found in southwestern United States, may cause acute otitis externa, most commonly in dogs and infrequently in cats.[2,4] *Demodex canis*, in dogs, and *Demodex cati*, in cats, are rare causes of otitis externa, which may or may not be associated with lesions on other areas of the skin (Fig. 10.9). In these rare cases, large numbers of adult *Demodex* mites were seen in cerumen smears.[6,19,25,26] *Sarcoptes scabiei*, *Notoedres cati*, and *Eutrombicula alfreddugesi* or *Neotrobicula autumnalis* (chiggers) are other parasites that infrequently infest the ear canal and may be observed on cytology.[3,6,14]

Because small numbers of mites may not be visualized on otoscopic examination, careful cytological evaluation of unstained exudate for eggs, larvae, or adult mites should be undertaken (see Fig. 10.8). Both unstained and stained slides of ear canal secretions should always be evaluated. Mites readily wash off slides during the staining process and are seldom seen on stained slides. Hence, unstained slides are best for finding mites, and stained slides are best for recognizing increased numbers of bacteria, yeast, or both. Finding mites may be challenging,

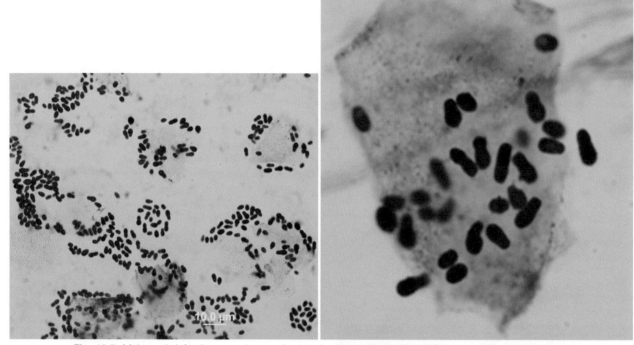

Fig. 10.7 *Malassezia* infections are characterized by large numbers of broad-based, budding yeast organisms. Image on the right displays a magnified area (Wright stain, magnification 1000×).

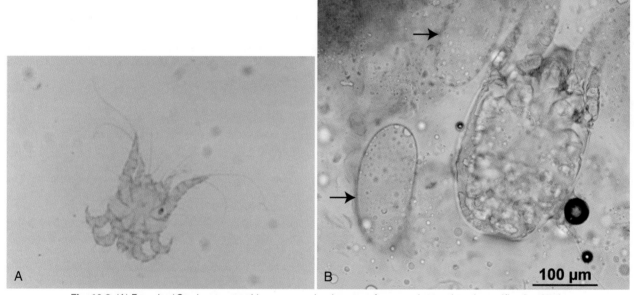

Fig. 10.8 (A) Ear mite (*Otodectes cynotis*) on an unstained smear of ear canal secretions (magnification 25×). (B) Two mite eggs *(arrows)* and an ear mite (*O. cynotis*) embedded in debris from an unstained smear of ear canal secretions (magnification 200×).

especially in hypersensitive patients with a low mite burden. Failure to find mites on cytological examination should not definitively exclude the possibility of a mite infestation.

Inflammatory Cells

Normal ears do not contain inflammatory cells, and the presence of such cells is always associated with clinical signs of otitis externa.[15] Yet, conversely, not all forms of otitis contain inflammatory cells.[15]

If identified, cells may consist of neutrophils and macrophages. These cells generally gain access to the canal because of ulceration or extension from otitis media; the presence of these cells may indicate more severe disease.[3] However, rarely, white blood cells (WBCs) may be associated with noninfectious diseases, such as pemphigus foliaceous, in which sterile pustules may rupture and exude nondegenerative neutrophils along with acantholytic cells.

Finding bacterial phagocytosis indicates infection rather than overgrowth and may warrant systemic antibiotics (see Fig. 10.6).[3]

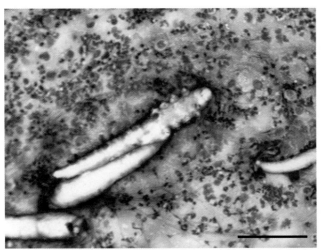

Fig. 10.9 Aspirate of lesion on canine pinna. Note several unstained *Demodex* spp. mites surrounded by numerous inflammatory cells consisting predominantly of neutrophils with rare macrophages (magnification 200×, bar ≡ 100 μm).

Data summarized from London, CA, Dubilzeig RR, Vail DM, et al. Evaluation of dogs and cats with tumors of the ear canal: 145 cases: 1978-1992. *J Am Vet Med Assoc.* 1996;208:1413–1418.

BOX 10.4 Ear Canal Tumors in Dogs and Cats

Dogs
Benign Tumors (n ≡ 33)
Benign polyps: 8
Papillomas: 6
Sebaceous gland adenomas: 5
Basal cell tumor: 5
Ceruminous gland adenoma: 4
Histiocytoma: 2
Plasmacytoma: 1
Benign melanoma: 1
Fibroma: 1

Malignant Tumors (n ≡ 48)
Ceruminous gland adenocarcinoma: 23
Carcinoma of undetermined origin: 9
Squamous cell carcinoma: 8
Round cell tumor: 3
Sarcoma: 2
Malignant melanoma: 2
Hemangiosarcoma: 1

Cats
Benign Tumors (n ≡ 8)
Benign polyp: 4
Ceruminous gland adenoma: 3
Papilloma: 1

Malignant Tumors (n ≡ 56)
Ceruminous gland adenocarcinoma: 22
Squamous cell carcinoma: 20
Carcinoma of undetermined origin: 13
Sebaceous gland adenocarcinoma: 1

Neoplasia

The ear canal can potentially develop any of the tumors that occur in skin, as well as ceruminous gland changes, including hyperplasia, adenoma, and adenocarcinoma.[8,27] In one large study of ear canal tumors in dogs and cats, the most commonly found benign neoplasms were polyps, papillomas, basal cell tumors, and ceruminous gland adenomas. The most common malignant neoplasms were ceruminous gland adenocarcinomas, squamous cell carcinomas, and carcinomas of undetermined origin (Box 10.4).[28] Unfortunately, neoplastic cells are rarely seen on cytological evaluation of external ear canal secretions. Many tumors are covered by normal epithelium, and their neoplastic cells are not available for collection by using ear swabs alone. These tumors may alter the condition of the ear canal and allow secondary infection to develop.[14]

Cytologically, inflammation may be all that is observed in an ear swab specimen. If a mass is observed upon otoscopic examination of the ear canal and if cytological examination of an ear swab specimen does not establish the cause of the mass, fine-needle aspiration (FNA) or biopsy specimens should be performed to identify the etiology of the mass (Fig. 10.10).[19] In cats, fine-needle aspirates have been shown to be useful in distinguishing inflammatory polyps from neoplasia. However, benign and malignant neoplasia may be difficult to distinguish on cytology, and histopathological confirmation is recommended.[29] (See earlier chapters for further discussion on the evaluation of cutaneous and subcutaneous masses.)

Proliferative and Necrotizing Otitis Externa of Felines

Proliferative and necrotizing feline otitis externa, an uncommon and unique proliferative dermatitis with distinct histopathological and clinical findings, affects the concave pinnae and vertical ear canal of young to middle-aged cats. The etiology is unknown but may be associated with T cell–mediated apoptosis directed against keratinocytes.[30] Patients often respond to topical tacrolimus, although in some patients, especially kittens, spontaneous regression may occur.[31]

Grossly, the lesion is characterized by large, tan-to-dark brown-black, coalescing, slightly verrucous plaques that cover the concave pinnae and external ear canal (Fig. 10.11).[30] Gentle manipulation of the plaques may result in their breaking off to reveal underlying ulcers and erosions.[31] Often, thick plugs of material within the ear canal and concurrent bacterial or yeast infection are present.[31]

Cytologically, the disease has not been well characterized. However, the ear canal exudate may often reveal bacterial and yeast infection, and treatment fails to alleviate all the clinical and gross findings (Fig. 10.12).

Histologically, the lesion is characterized by scattered and shrunken keratinocytes with hypereosinophilic and pyknotic nuclei and severe acanthosis of the outer follicular root sheath (Fig. 10.13). The lumina of the hair follicles display mild hyperkeratosis and retained corneocyte nuclei, cell debris, and neutrophils. The inflammatory infiltrates within the dermis were often mixed (neutrophilic, plasmacytic, or eosinophilic, mastocytic) but varied between cases.[31]

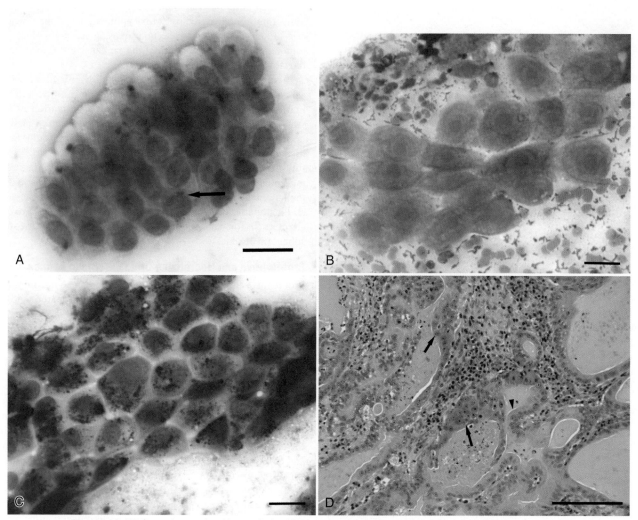

Fig. 10.10 (A) Ceruminous gland hyperplasia. Note the low columnar cells with a basally located nucleus with several cells containing globular to fine, dark-green pigment consistent with cerumen *(arrow)* (magnification 500×, bar ≡ 20 μm). (B) Ceruminous gland adenocarcinoma. Note the loss of columnar shape, very large prominent single nucleolus, anisocytosis, and anisokaryosis (magnification 500×, bar ≡ 20 μm). (C) Ceruminous gland adenocarcinoma with similar pleomorphism to image B; however, these cells also contain globular to fine, dark-green pigment consistent with cerumen (magnification 500×, bar ≡ 20 μm). (D) Ceruminous gland adenocarcinoma. Note the piling and stacking of neoplastic epithelial cells *(arrow)* displaying anisocytosis and anisokaryosis in addition to papilliferous projections into the glandular lumen *(arrowhead)* (H&E stain, magnification 200×, bar ≡ 100 μm).

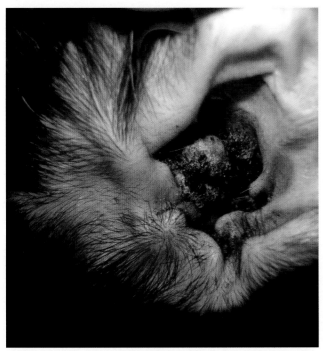

Fig. 10.11 Gross image of feline external ear canal with dark brown to black coalescing plaques. (Courtesy Dr. Andrea Lam.)

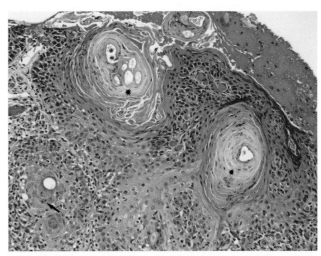

Fig. 10.13 Feline external ear canal diagnosed with proliferative and necrotizing otitis externa. Scattered and shrunken keratinocytes with hypereosinophilic cytoplasm and pyknotic nuclei (arrowhead) and follicular lumen with parakeratosis and cell debris (asterisk) are seen. The epidermis is also covered by a hemorrhagic and cellular crust (H&E stain, magnification 200×, bar ≡ 100 μm).

REFERENCES

1. Dyce KM, Sack WO, Wensing CJ. *Veterinary Anatomy*. 2nd ed. Philadelphia, PA: Saunders; 1996:339–340.
2. Saridomichelakis MN, et al. Aetiology of canine otitis externa: a retrospective study of 100 cases. *Vet Dermatol*. 2007;18:341–347.
3. Angus JC. Otic cytology in health and disease. *Vet Clin North Am Small Anim Pract*. 2004;34:411–424.
4. Kahn CM, Line S. *The Merck Veterinary Manual*. 10th ed. Whitehouse Station, NJ: Merck and Co, Inc.; 2010:482–483.
5. Noxon JO. Chapter 59 Otitis externa. In: Brichard SJ, Sherding RG, eds. *Saunders Manual of Small Animal Practice*. St Louis: MO: Elsevier Health Sciences; 2006:574–581.
6. Rosser Jr EJ. Causes of otitis externa. *Vet Clin North Am Small Anim Pract*. 2004;34:459–468.
7. Paterson S. Discovering the causes of otitis externa. *Practice*. 2016;38:7–11.
8. Scott DW, Miller WH, Griffin CE. *Muller & Kirk's Small Animal Dermatology*. 6th ed. Philadelphia, PA: Saunders; 2001:1204–1235.
9. Greene CE. *Infectious Diseases of the Dog and Cat*. St. Louis, MO: Saunders; 2006:602–606, 885–891.
10. McKeever PJ, Globus H. In: Bonagura JD, ed. *Kirk's Current Veterinary Therapy XII*. Philadelphia, PA: Saunders; 1995:647–655.
11. Griffin JS, Scott DW, Erb HN. Malassezia otitis externa in the dog: the effect of heat fixing otic exudate for cytological analysis. *J Vet Med*. 2007;54:424–427.
12. Toma S, et al. Comparison of 4 fixation and staining methods for the cytologic evaluation of ear canals with clinical evidence of ceruminous otitis externa. *Vet Clin Pathol*. 2006;35:194–198.
13. Tater KC, et al. The cytology of the external ear canal in the normal dog and cat. *J Vet Med*. 2003;50:370–374.
14. Logas DB. Diseases of the ear canal. *Vet Clin North Am Small Anim Pract*. 1994;24:905–919.
15. Ginel PJ, et al. A semiquantitative cytological evaluation of normal and pathological samples from the external ear canal of dogs and cats. *Vet Dermatol*. 2002;13:151–156.
16. Rosychuk RA. Management of otitis externa. *Vet Clin North Am Small Anim Pract*. 1994;24:921–952.
17. Graham-Mize CA, Rosser Jr EJ. Comparison of microbial isolates and susceptibility patterns from the external ear canal of dogs with otitis externa. *J Am Anim Hosp Assoc*. 2004;40:102–108.
18. Shaw S. Pathogens in otitis externa: diagnostic techniques to identify secondary causes of ear disease. *In Practice*. 2016;38:12–16.

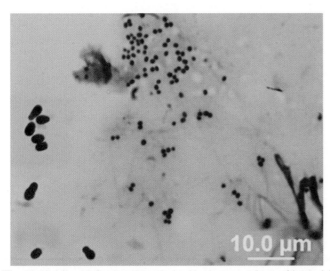

Fig. 10.12 Mixed infection characterized by large numbers of bacterial cocci. Some *Malassezia* organisms are also present (Wright stain, magnification 1000×).

19. Bond R, Saijonmaa-Koulumies LE, Lloyd DH. Population sizes and frequency of *Malassezia pachydermatis* at skin and mucosal sites on healthy dogs. *J Small Anim Pract.* 1995;36:147–150.

20. Crespo MJ, Abarca ML, Cabañes FJ. Occurrence of *Malassezia* spp. in the external ear canal of dogs and cats with and without otitis externa. *Med Mycol.* 2002;40:115–121.

21. Harvey RG, Harari J, Delauch AJ. *Diagnostic Procedure. Ear Disease of the Dog and Cat.* Ames, IA: Iowa State University Press; 2001:43–80.

22. Guedeja-Marron J, Blanco JL, Garcia ME. A case of feline otitis externa due to *Microsporum canis. Med Mycol.* 2001;39:229–232.

23. Godfrey D. *Microsporum canis* associated with otitis externa in a Persian cat. *Vet Rec.* 2000;147:50–51.

24. Campbell JJ, et al. Evaluation of fungal flora in normal and diseased canine ears. *Vet Dermatol.* 2010;21:619–625.

25. Knottenbelt MK. Chronic otitis externa due to *Demodex canis* in a Tibetan spaniel. *Vet Rec.* 1994;135:409–410.

26. van Poucke S. Ceruminous otitis externa due to *Demodex cati* in a cat. *Vet Rec.* 2001;149:651–652.

27. Fan TM, de Lorimier LP. Inflammatory polyps and aural neoplasia. *Vet Clin North Am Small Anim Pract.* 2004;34:489–509.

28. London CA, Dubilzeig RR, Vail DM, et al. Evaluation of dogs and cats with tumors of the ear canal: 145 cases: 1978-1992. *J Am Vet Med Assoc.* 1996;208:1413–1418.

29. de Lorenzi D, Bonfanti U, Masserdotti C, et al. Fine-needle biopsy of external ear canal masses in the cat: cytologic results and histologic correlations in 27 cases. *Vet Clin Pathol.* 2005;34:100–105.

30. Videmont E, Pin D. Proliferative and necrotizing otitis in a kitten: first demonstration of T-cell-mediated apoptosis. *J Small Anim Pract.* 2010;51:599–603.

31. Mauldin EA, Ness TA, Goldschmidt MH. Proliferative and necrotizing otitis externa in four cats. *Vet Dermatol.* 2007;18:370–377.

ADDITIONAL READING

Cafarchia C, Gallo S, Capelli G, Otranto D. Occurrence and population size of *Malassezia* spp. in the external ear canal of dogs and cats both healthy and with otitis. *Mycopathologia.* 2005;160:143–149.

11

The Lymph Nodes

Melissa Blauvelt and Joanne B. Messick

Extranodal lymphoid tissue is present throughout the body, but this chapter addresses the lymph node specifically.

ARCHITECTURE

When interpreting a cytological specimen of the lymph node, it is useful to keep in mind the histological structure and different cell types found in this tissue. The node is composed of a capsule, the cortex, the medulla, and the sinuses (subcapsular, cortical, and medullary).[1] The cortex, or the more peripheral area of the node, is divided into follicular and diffuse (parafollicular cortex or paracortex) regions, and the medulla, or the more central area, is divided into the medullary cords and sinuses (Fig. 11.1).

Within the parafollicular cortex are high endothelial venules through which both B and T lymphocytes from the blood enter the node. This region is also rich in interdigitating reticulum cells (IDCs), a specialized antigen-presenting cell. The initial immune response requires that the antigen presented by IDCs be recognized by T lymphocytes and early B lymphocytes in the parafollicular cortex, whereas the differentiation of B lymphocytes in response to antigen occurs in the follicular cortex.

Follicles contain predominantly B-lineage lymphocytes. The primary follicles are composed of small, dark-staining lymphocytes. In contrast, secondary follicles have a peripheral rim or mantle zone of small, dark lymphoid cells similar to those in primary follicles and a central germinal center. In the germinal center, specialized cells of the mononuclear phagocytic system (MPS), the follicular dendritic cells (FDCs), capture antigen on their surfaces to promote B-lymphocyte differentiation. Thus small resting B cells undergo mitosis and divide to become the larger, more irregular, small-cleaved, intermediate and large blast cells in the germinal center of a reactive node (follicular hyperplasia). T cells (mainly CD4+ helper cells) that play a role in stimulating B cells are also found in the follicles. Surviving B cells may eventually differentiate into plasma cells, migrating to the medullary cords or leave the node.

The parafollicular zone of the lymph node gradually transforms into medullary cords that are populated by B cells and plasma cells. Sinuses containing macrophages surround these cords. A reactive process in the lymph node may also result in hyperplasia of the parafollicular region, of sinus cells (sinus histiocytosis), or of plasma cells (plasma cell hyperplasia), alone or in combination.

Lymph nodes are strategically located at sites throughout the body and are involved in a variety of local and systemic disease processes. Antigen reaches the node via the afferent lymphatics. The lymph percolates through the sinus and sinusoidal walls into the parenchyma (Fig. 11.2), where foreign substances (antigens) are taken up and processed by specialized cells of the MPS. The sinuses (subcapsular,

cortical, and medullary) form a network of branching channels that converge at the hilus of the node to exit by the efferent lymphatics. The primary functions of the lymph nodes include filtering particles and microorganisms, exposing antigens to circulating lymphocytes, and activating B and T lymphocytes. The superficial, subcutaneous location of some lymph nodes (mandibular, superficial cervical, inguinal, and popliteal) allows for easy detection of enlargement and access for fine-needle aspiration (FNA) cytology. It is appropriate to aspirate any node that is enlarged, and in the case of lymph nodes draining areas affected by neoplasia, even in the absence of enlargement, aspiration may be justified.[2]

GENERAL CONSIDERATIONS

Lymph node aspiration cytology has become a popular procedure in human medicine in recent years because of its great convenience.[3] Similarly, this high-yield diagnostic technique is frequently used in veterinary medicine.[4-7] A few points need to be considered when obtaining nodal samples for cytological evaluation.

A normal lymph node is small and often difficult to aspirate. It is not uncommon for the cytology of a normal node to contain mostly perinodal adipose tissue and only a few or no lymphocytes. If multiple

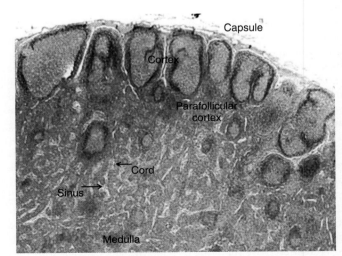

Fig. 11.1 The lymph node has two basic parts: the cortex and the medulla. The cortex has both follicular and diffuse or parafollicular regions. The parafollicular region gradually transforms into medullary cords of B lymphocytes and plasma cells, which are surround by sinuses containing macrophages attached to reticular fibers. Different populations of lymphocytes in these areas and other cells are found in nodal aspirates (hematoxylin and eosin [H&E] stain).

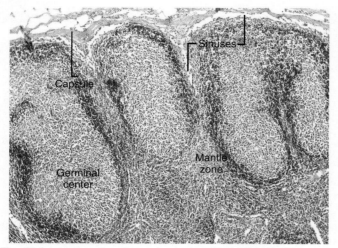

Fig. 11.2 Lymph enters the node via the afferent lymphatics, percolating through subcapsular sinuses and sinusoids, where foreign substances (antigens) are taken up and processed. The secondary follicles in this node have a peripheral rim or mantle zone and a pale-staining, central germinal center. The differentiation of B lymphocytes in response to antigen occurs in the germinal center of the follicular cortex (H&E stain).

nodes are enlarged, then sampling from several nodes is recommended. Because the submandibular nodes drain the oral cavity, they often become enlarged, reactive, and inflamed. A confusing mixture of malignant, reactive, and inflammatory cells may limit the accuracy of cytological diagnosis of lymphoma based on FNA of these nodes. Thus sampling of submandibular nodes should be avoided in cases where generalized lymph node enlargement exists. The prescapular and popliteal nodes are often a better choice. The mandibular salivary gland is quite frequently mistaken for a node and aspirated. However, the presence of large, foamy epithelial cells, either individually or in clusters, and mucus in the background allows for easy identification of salivary tissue.

Consideration also should be given to the size of the lymph node when deciding which node to aspirate—very large nodes may have areas of hemorrhage or necrosis. If the node must be sampled, the needle should be directed tangentially, avoiding the more central portions.[8] Finally, when obtaining a sample for cytological evaluation, it is important to remember that the lymph node is a heterogeneous tissue, and multiple areas within the node should be sampled to be certain that what has been obtained is representative. While keeping the needle in the node, the needle should be repeatedly advanced and withdrawn in multiple directions until a small amount of aspirate appears in the hub of the needle. This procedure may be done by using a syringe to apply gentle suction or with only the needle. If the former technique is used, the suction should be released before removing the needle from the node. Overly vigorous aspiration of the lymph node produces significant hemodilution, and cells may rupture, limiting the interpretation of the sample. A large volume of aspirate is not required; the material within the hub of the needle is sufficient for making cytological preparations. Because the lymphocytes are fragile, care must be taken to apply only minimal pressure when making slide preparations to prevent excessive rupturing of cells. The slides are air-dried (not heat-fixed) and stained for evaluation.

FINE-NEEDLE ASPIRATION

FNA is a relatively safe and painless procedure, allowing for rapid and inexpensive sampling of peripheral lymph nodes. It does not require

---

BOX 11.1 The Role of Fine-Needle Aspiration Cytology of Lymph Nodes

1. Diagnosis of infectious disease
2. Diagnosis of hyperplasia or reactive lymphadenopathy and recognition of specific conditions (i.e., lymph node hyperplasia of young cats) (If a cause for the change is not apparent, resolution does not occur, or both follow-up and subsequent biopsy are indicated.)
3. Diagnosis of metastatic neoplasia and indication of possible primary site
4. Diagnosis of lymphoma that is optimally followed by a biopsy for confirmation and accurate subtyping
5. If known malignancy, such as lymphoma or a metastatic mast cell tumor, staging and monitoring for relapse or effects of chemotherapy
6. For sampling of multiple sites as well as for obtaining samples from surgically inaccessible sites or from medically unfit patients
7. Obtaining material for clonality and research studies

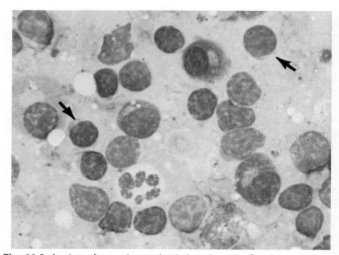

Fig. 11.3 Aspirate from a hyperplastic lymph node. Small lymphocytes *(arrows)* and plasma cells characterize the reaction. Note that the small lymphocytes are smaller than the neutrophils and their nuclei are about the size of a red blood cell. Many free nuclei, identified by pink, homogeneous chromatin and an absence of cytoplasm, are evident (Wright stain).

hospital admission or anesthesia of the animal. The role of this procedure is summarized in Box 11.1.

CYTOLOGICAL FINDINGS

Normal Lymph Node

In the absence of architectural features that can be appreciated in a histological section of a lymph node, the interpretation of cytology relies on proportions of different cell types and an understanding of what proportions are normal versus abnormal for these cell types. Small, well-differentiated lymphocytes compose greater than 75% to 85% of the total nucleated cell population (Figs. 11.3 to 11.7).[4-7] They have round nuclei that are about 1 to less than 1.5 times the size of a mature red blood cell (RBC), with an overall cell size that is smaller than that of a neutrophil. Their chromatin is densely clumped, and nucleoli are not visible. The nuclear-to-cytoplasmic (N:C) ratio is high, with a narrow rim of basophilic cytoplasm. In addition to small lymphocytes, a normal node should have low numbers (<10%–15%) of lymphocytes that are intermediate to large (often called *lymphoblasts*) in size; their nuclei are 1.5 to 3 times the size of an RBC, with

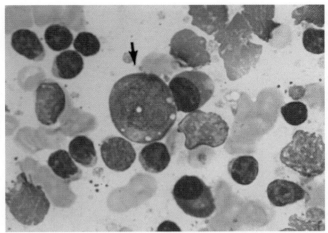

Fig. 11.4 Small lymphocytes, plasma cells, and a large transformed lymphocyte *(arrow)* characterize this aspirate from a hyperplastic lymph node. Irregular, pink nuclei from lysed cells are seen (Wright stain).

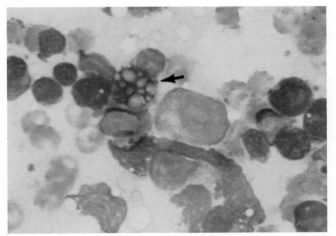

Fig. 11.5 Plasma cells, small lymphocytes, and two large lymphocytes (lymphoblasts) characterize this aspirate from a hyperplastic lymph node. The plasma cell with the vacuolated cytoplasm is a Mott cell containing Russell bodies *(arrow)*. The pink, amorphous structures are free nuclear material (Wright stain).

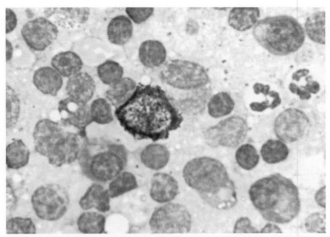

Fig. 11.6 Small lymphocytes, plasma cells, neutrophils, and a single mast cell are present in this aspirate from a hyperplastic lymph node (Wright stain).

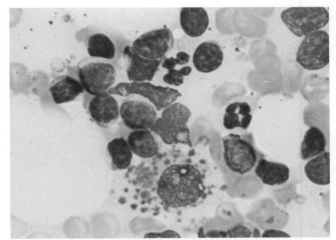

Fig. 11.7 Seen among small and medium-sized lymphocytes is a large macrophage containing phagocytized debris (Wright stain).

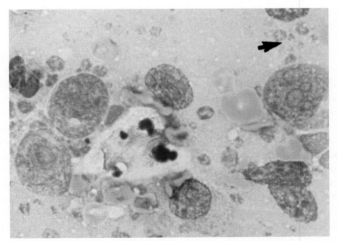

Fig. 11.8 In this aspirate from a lymphomatous lymph node are large immature lymphocytes with prominent nucleoli, dispersed chromatin, and abundant blue cytoplasm. The large cell in the center with bluish cytoplasmic globules is a tingible-body macrophage. The small blue structures *(arrow)* are lymphoglandular bodies (Wright stain).

an overall size ranging from about that of a neutrophil or larger to up to 4 times the size of an RBC (see Fig. 11.5). Their chromatin is less clumped, and nucleoli may be visible and even multiple, prominent, or both. The cytoplasm is pale blue and more abundant than in small lymphocytes.

Plasma cells have small, round, eccentric nuclei with condensed chromatin (see Figs. 11.3 to 11.6). Their abundant cytoplasm is deep blue in color and has a prominent, clear Golgi zone. Immature plasma cells (transformed B lymphocytes) are larger and have less aggregated chromatin and a higher N:C ratio (see Fig. 11.4). Their very blue cytoplasm may contain discrete vacuoles. Plasma cells in various stages of development are seen in small numbers in normal lymph nodes but typically represent less than 3% of the total nucleated cell population.

Macrophages, characterized by abundant cytoplasm often containing vacuoles and granular debris, also are found in small numbers (see Fig. 11.7). Macrophages from areas of intense lymphopoiesis and cellular turnover may contain prominent basophilic nuclear debris (tingible bodies) (Fig. 11.8). Occasionally, small numbers of neutrophils, eosinophils, and mast cells are observed in a normal node (see Fig. 11.6). Each of these cell types should represent less than 1% of the cell populations

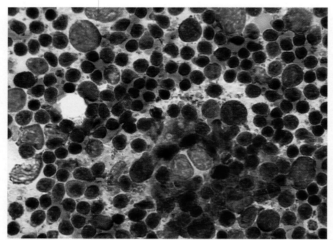

Fig. 11.9 Several reticuloendothelial cells are seen in this lymph node aspiration cytology. Their nuclei are swollen, and they are devoid of cytoplasm. Small lymphocytes are the predominant cell type in this mildly hyperplastic node.

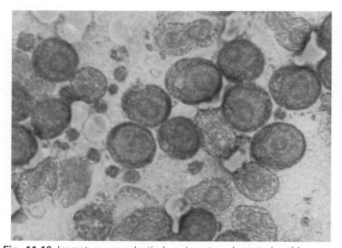

Fig. 11.10 Immature, neoplastic lymphocytes characterize this smear from a dog with malignant lymphoma. Note that the cells are much larger than the red blood cells. The pink structures lacking cytoplasm and containing prominent nucleoli are nuclei from lysed cells. Small blue lymphoglandular bodies are numerous (Wright stain).

in a normal node. It is important to consider the amount of blood contamination when making this assessment. Reticular cells and endothelial cells are common in lymph nodes, but these tissue-bound cells are rarely aspirated intact. They usually appear as large swollen nuclei, often devoid of cytoplasm (Fig. 11.9).

Because of the pressures of the aspiration technique, lymphocytes, which are very fragile, may rupture and release their nuclei. Free nuclei are swollen and uniformly pink in contrast to the blue, blocky or granular pattern of intact lymphocyte nuclei (see Figs. 11.3 to 11.5). Blue nucleoli are often exposed in the nuclear chromatin of ruptured cells. These free nuclei carry no diagnostic significance and should not be confused with large immature lymphocytes. Lymphoglandular bodies are cytoplasmic fragments and are highly characteristic of lymphoid tissue (see Figs. 11.8 and 11.10). They are round, homogeneous, basophilic structures that are similar in size to platelets.

Lymphadenopathy

One of the most common indications for performing aspiration cytology is enlargement of one or more lymph nodes. Three general

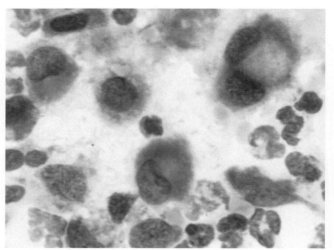

Fig. 11.11 This aspirate from an animal with blastomycosis is characterized by pyogranulomatous inflammation. Neutrophils, epithelioid macrophages, and a single multinucleate giant cell are present (Wright stain).

processes cause lymph node enlargement: (1) inflammation (lymphadenitis—suppurative, pyogranulomatous, granulomatous, and eosinophilic), (2) immune stimulation (hyperplasia or reactive lymphadenopathy), and (3) neoplasia (lymphoma or metastatic). The cytological evaluation of a sample obtained by FNA or touch imprint from the excised node usually allows for differentiation of these processes. However, these processes are not mutually exclusive and may occur simultaneously.

Lymphadenitis

Lymphadenitis or inflammation of the node may be a primary (the node itself is inflamed or necrotic) or secondary (the node is draining an area of inflammation or necrosis) finding. This process is characterized cytologically by accumulation of inflammatory cells. Neutrophils, eosinophils, and macrophages occur singly or in combination. Inflammation is probably present when the population is greater than 5% neutrophils or greater than 3% eosinophils, provided that no significant blood contamination has occurred. Macrophage numbers may increase in inflammation but also in hyperplasia and sometimes in neoplasia. Macrophages also may appear as epithelioid cells and multinucleate giant cells in granulomatous inflammation. Epithelioid macrophages are characterized by blue cytoplasm with minimal vacuolization and contain very little phagocytic debris (Fig. 11.11). Organisms may, however, be present within the cytoplasm. These cells may occur in aggregates. Inflammatory cells may represent only a small portion of the total cell population, which otherwise suggests lymphoid hyperplasia, or they may completely replace the normal cell population.

Most bacterial infections elicit a neutrophilic or purulent response (Fig. 11.12), but *Mycobacterium* spp. (Fig. 11.13) may cause a granulomatous response. An eosinophilic exudate of varying degrees is common in lymph nodes draining allergic inflammation of skin, respiratory tract, and digestive tract. Systemic fungal infections, such as histoplasmosis (Fig. 11.14), blastomycosis (Fig. 11.15), coccidioidomycosis (Fig. 11.16), and cryptococcosis (Fig. 11.17); protozoal infections, such as cytauxzoonosis (Fig. 11.18), toxoplasmosis (Fig. 11.19), and leishmaniasis (Fig. 11.20); and algal infections, such as protothecosis (Fig. 11.21) characteristically evoke a granulomatous or pyogranulomatous response (Fig. 11.22) in lymph nodes. In salmon disease (infection with *Neorickettsia helminthoeca*), lymphoid depletion and sinus macrophage hyperplasia or sinus histiocytosis occur (Fig. 11.23).

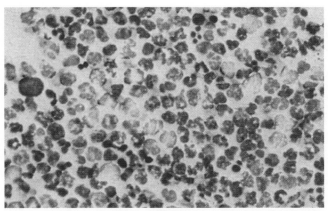

Fig. 11.12 Purulent inflammation is characterized by the predominance of neutrophils (Wright stain).

Reactive or Hyperplastic Node

No clear line of separation between a normal and a hyperplastic lymph node is evident on cytology alone. Differentiation, however, is probably a moot point because enlarged lymph nodes are reactive to some degree. Typically, a heterogeneous lymphoid cell population is usually obtained as the needle is directed through the follicular centers, paracortical area, medullary cords, and medullary sinuses. If the reactive pattern is principally follicular hyperplasia, intermediate and large lymphocytes from expanding germinal centers are found in increased numbers. These cells may constitute up to 15% to 25% or greater of the total cell population (Fig. 11.24).[4-7] However, small lymphocytes are still the predominant cell type in hyperplastic and normal lymph nodes. Plasma cell numbers may vary from none to greater than 5% to 10% of the population in some areas of the smear. They occasionally are filled with vacuoles (Russell bodies) and are referred to as Mott cells (see Fig. 11.5). Immature plasma cells or transformed

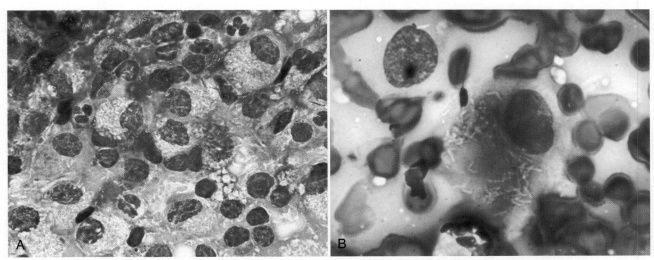

Fig. 11.13 (A) Lymph node aspirates showing a high number of macrophages containing nonstaining bacterial rods indicative of *Mycobacterium* infection. (B) Higher magnification of a single macrophage containing nonstaining bacterial rods identified as clear streaks through the cell (Wright stain). (Courtesy Dr. R. L. Cowell.)

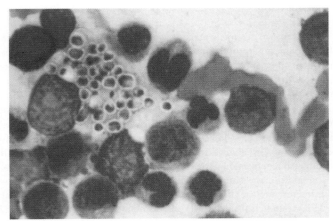

Fig. 11.14 Macrophage containing numerous *Histoplasma* organisms. *Histoplasma* organisms are small, round to oval, yeast-like organisms that have a nucleus that stains dark purple and a thin clear halo (Wright stain). (Courtesy Oklahoma State University.)

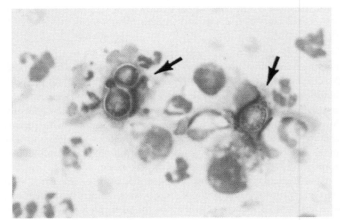

Fig. 11.15 *Blastomyces dermatitidis (arrows)* is a bluish, spherical, thick-walled, yeast-like organism. Occasionally, a single, broad-based bud may be present (Wright stain).

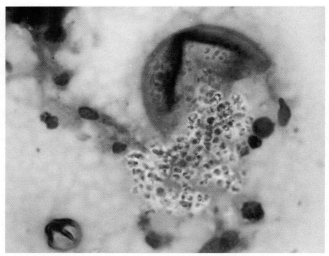

Fig. 11.16 *Coccidioides immitis* organisms are large, double-contoured, clear to blue-staining, spherical bodies that range in size from 10 micrometers (μm) to greater than 100 μm. Occasionally, endospores varying from 2 to 5 μm in diameter may be seen within some of the larger spherules (Wright stain). (Courtesy Dr. R. L. Cowell.)

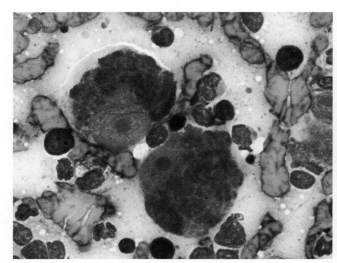

Fig. 11.18 Lymph node aspirate from a cat showing two huge mononuclear cells with abundant cytoplasm, eccentric nuclei, and prominent nucleoli. These cells contain developing cytauxzoon merozoites, which appear as either small, dark-staining bodies or larger, irregularly defined clusters (Wright stain). (Courtesy Dr. R. L. Cowell.)

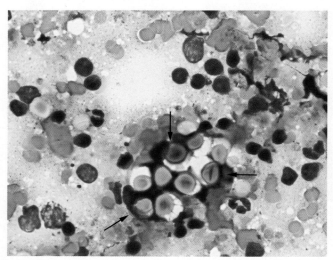

Fig. 11.17 Lymph node aspirate from a cat with cryptococcosis. Scattered red blood cells, small lymphocytes, and a group of *Cryptococcus* organisms *(arrows)* are shown. *Cryptococcus* organisms stain eosinophilic to clear and may be the smooth form (large clear capsule) or rough form (small clear capsule) as shown here (Wright stain). (Courtesy Dr. R. L. Cowell.)

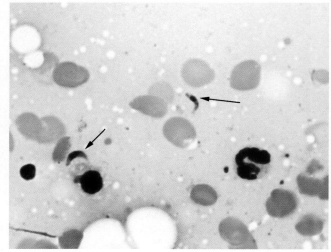

Fig. 11.19 *Toxoplasma gondii* tachyzoites *(arrows)* appear as small, crescent-shaped bodies with a light blue cytoplasm and a dark-staining pericentral nucleus (Wright stain). (Courtesy Dr. R. L. Cowell.)

lymphocytes, which are medium to large in size, also may be observed. Macrophages may on occasion represent greater than 2% of the population, particularly with hyperplasia of sinus macrophages. An aspirate from a node with parafollicular hyperplasia is also heterogeneous; however, immunoblasts are prominent in association with plasma cell hyperplasia, and tingible-body macrophages are lacking. The main cytological characteristics of the immunoblasts (parafollicular zone cells) are their medium size, fine chromatin, and large centrally located nucleolus. In reactive lymph nodes of dogs associated with mammary tumor lymphadenopathies, systemic lupus erythematosus, and leishmaniasis, these cells may be found in high numbers.[9] Any enlarged lymph node with the aforementioned cytological findings should be considered hyperplastic because a normal node should not be enlarged.

Hyperplasia occurs when antigens in high concentration reach the draining lymph node and stimulate the immune system. In some instances, these antigens also cause inflammation and attract inflammatory cells to the node (lymphadenitis). In many cases, reactions causing hyperplasia are localized, but they may be systemic and affect all nodes. Generalized lymphadenopathy with a hyperplastic cytological picture may occur in feline leukemia virus (FELV) infection, feline immunodeficiency virus (FIV) infection, bartonellosis, Rocky Mountain spotted fever, and ehrlichiosis. It may occasionally be especially difficult to distinguish reactive nodal hyperplasia from lymphoma in cats. In these cases, additional testing, such as histopathology, immunophenotyping, and polymerase chain reaction for antigen receptor rearrangement (PARR) testing, is needed for the assessment of clonality.[10-15]

Lymphoma

FNA is often sufficient for establishing a diagnosis of lymphoma in both dogs and cats. Lymphoma is caused by the predominance of

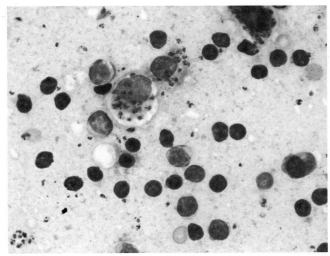

Fig. 11.20 Lymph node aspirate from a dog showing many lymphocytes and two macrophages containing numerous *Leishmania donovani* organisms. *L. donovani* organisms are small, round to oval organisms with a clear to very-light-blue cytoplasm, an oval nucleus, and a small, dark, ventral kinetoplast (Wright stain). (Courtesy Dr. R. L. Cowell.)

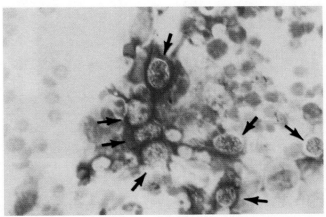

Fig. 11.21 *Prototheca* organisms *(arrows)* are round to oval and have a granular basophilic cytoplasm and a clear cell wall (Wright stain).

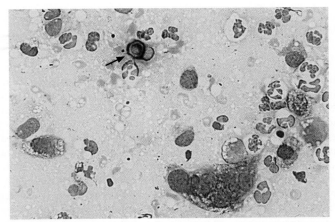

Fig. 11.22 Pyogranulomatous inflammation from a dog with blastomycosis. A *Blastomyces dermatitidis* organism *(arrow)* is in the center of the field. Neutrophils, macrophages, and an inflammatory giant cell are present (Wright stain).

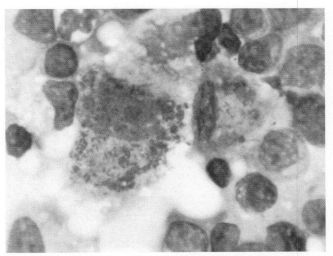

Fig. 11.23 Aspirate of a lymph node from a dog with salmon disease. Large macrophages contain the causative agent *Neorickettsia helminthoeca* (Wright stain).

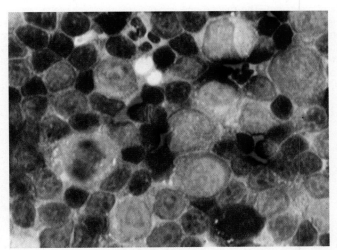

Fig. 11.24 Intermediate and large lymphocytes from expanded germinal centers are found in increased numbers in this hyperplastic node (follicular hyperplasia). However, small lymphocytes are still the predominant cell type.

monomorphic lymphoid cells that lack the polymorphism of a reactive population. Still the opportunity must not be missed at the outset of the disease process to also obtain nodal tissue for histological, immunocytochemical, and molecular evaluations. This will allow for confirmation of the diagnosis and accurate subtyping, as well as providing archival materials that may be of use to further advances in diagnosis, treatment, or both.

Lymphoma is characterized by lymphocytes that eventually replace the entire normal cell population (Figs. 11.25 and 11.26). However, not all lymphomas are the same; they are a diverse group of lymphoid neoplasms. Each of these neoplasms represents a clonal expansion of an anatomical or developmental compartment of lymphoid cells in the node, which have distinct morphological and immunophenotypic characteristics.[16-18] When immature cells compose greater than 50% of the cell population, a diagnosis of malignant lymphoma may be reliably made, but smaller numbers may be present in early stages, making a diagnosis by cytological examination alone more difficult. Usually, these neoplastic lymphocytes are larger than neutrophils and have finely granular dispersed chromatin, nucleoli, a lower N:C ratio,

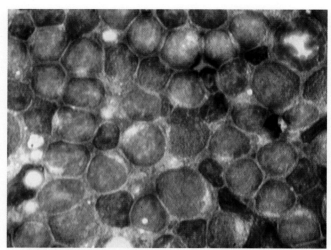

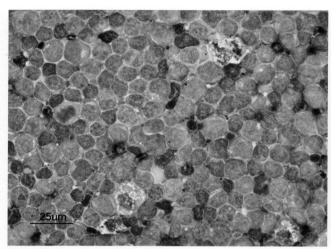

Fig. 11.25 In this aspirate from an enlarged node of a dog, a monomorphic population of immature lymphocytes that are intermediate in size is seen. Some of the nuclei in these cells are indented (clefted) and uniformly have a fine, diffuse chromatin pattern; however, nucleoli are inapparent. The mitotic rate is high. This is a high-grade, aggressive T-cell lymphoblastic lymphoma with an associated paraneoplastic hypercalcemia. The cells of B- and T-cell lymphoblastic lymphoma are not distinguishable by cytology alone but are different morphologically from other high-grade lymphomas. Immunophenotyping was done to establish the T-cell type (Wright stain).

Fig. 11.27 In this aspirate from a lymphomatous lymph node, many tingible-body macrophages were present, an indication of intense lymphopoiesis and cell turnover (Wright stain).

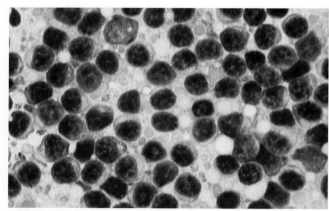

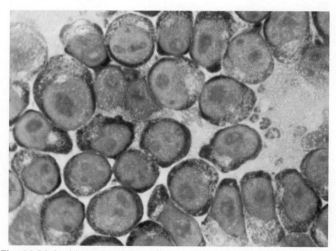

Fig. 11.26 In this nodal aspirate from a cat, a monomorphic population of immature lymphocytes that are large in size is shown. These cells have a high nuclear-to-cytoplasmic (N:C) ratio and often a single prominent nucleolus or several in a paracentral location. The cytoplasm is deeply basophilic. The histopathology showed a mitotic rate that was high with a diffuse nodal involvement. Although these high-grade lymphomas are often B-cell phenotype, the T-cell counterpart cannot be distinguished by morphology alone (Wright stain).

Fig. 11.28 A monotonous population of small, well-differentiated lymphocytes is seen in this nodal aspirate from a dog. Mitoses are not observed. Their chromatin pattern is densely clumped, nucleoli are not visible, and mitotic figures are not observed. The presence of a generalized lymphadenopathy and monomorphic lymphoid cells that lack the polymorphism of a normal node or of a reactive population is a useful characteristic that supports this diagnosis. However, the effacement of normal nodal architecture by histopathology is needed to confirm this suspicion. The cells of B- and T-cell small cell lymphoma or chronic lymphocytic leukemia cannot be distinguished by morphology alone. The cells of this low-grade lymphoma are a T-cell type (Wright stain).

and basophilic cytoplasm. The lymphocytes are considered medium and large if their nuclei are 1.5 to 2 times or more than 2 to 3 times the size of RBCs, respectively. Frequently, the percentage of the medium to large lymphocytes exceeds 80%, making the diagnosis more definitive. Mitoses may be more numerous than those in hyperplasia and tingible-body macrophages may indicate intense lymphopoiesis and cell turnover (Fig. 11.27), but neither alone is a reliable indicator of neoplasia. Lymphoglandular bodies are more numerous than those in hyperplasia.

Lymphoma is the most common hematopoietic tumor in dogs, and most of these tumors are high-grade lymphomas characterized by large immature cells but up to 20% are small cell lymphomas (Fig. 11.28). A cytological diagnosis of small cell lymphoma can sometimes be difficult to render because they comprise a predominance of small, well-differentiated lymphocytes but can often be recognized by an experienced pathologist as an excessively homogeneous or restricted population of small lymphocytes. Mitoses are extremely rare. A retrospective study describing the clinical characteristics, histopathological and immunohistochemical features of indolent lymphomas, reported that a distinct form of a small cell subtype of T-cell lymphoma, designated T-zone lymphoma, comprises up to 61.7% of indolent small cell lymphomas in dogs.[19] T-zone lymphoma is most commonly recognized in Golden Retrievers and Maltese dog breeds but can occur in many others as well as mixed breeds.[20] This form of lymphoma has a characteristic

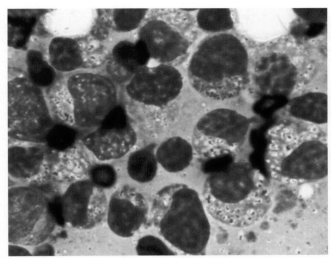

Fig. 11.29 An aspirate from an alimentary lymph node in a cat with large granular lymphoma (LGL). Most of the lymphocytes are large and contain magenta-colored intracytoplasmic granules (Wright stain). (Courtesy Dr. R. L. Cowell.)

immunophenotype pattern, which is described in the chapter on flow cytometry (see Chapter 30). T-zone lymphoma has not been described in cats. Some of the more subtle cases of small cell lymphoma may not be diagnosed until significant blood involvement occurs or with performance of additional diagnostics, such as histological examination of the node, flow cytometry, or PARR . Compared with cytology alone, histological examination offers additional features, such as determination of preservation or destruction of normal node architecture. Flow cytometry allows for investigation of large numbers of lymphocyte immunophenotypes. If there is an inappropriately expanded population of one lymphocyte population or subset (e.g., CD8-positive T cells), then lymphoma can often be confirmed. Additionally, neoplastic lymphocytes may lose or gain expression of some immunophenotype markers, indicative of lymphoma. PARR can assess for lymphocyte clonality.

Large granular lymphoma (LGL) is one form of alimentary lymphoma in dogs and cats that can be readily diagnosed on the basis of the presence of a monomorphic cell population with a distinct cytomorphology. These lymphocytes contain magenta-colored intracytoplasmic granules. However, neither the granules nor the lymphocytes are consistently large (Fig. 11.29). The unique granules are indicative of a CD8 (cytotoxic) or natural killer (NK) T-cell population.[21]

Several classification schemes have been adapted in an attempt to characterize canine and feline lymphomas.[22-25] In dogs and cats, cytomorphological classification into low (small cells and low mitotic rate) or high (large cells and high mitotic rate) grades of lymphoma has been shown to have prognostic importance.[24,25] Although low-grade lymphomas permit long survivals, they are virtually incurable and sometimes may be best left untreated in the early stages of disease. In contrast, the high-grade lymphomas initially respond well to chemotherapy, and disease remission is often achieved; yet, if left untreated, they are rapidly progressive and deadly. A predominance of high-grade lymphomas is seen in dogs and cats.[25]

The most recent iteration of the World Health Organization (WHO) system of lymphoma classification identifies these neoplasms as disease entities and not as cell types (as not all low-grade lymphomas or all high-grade lymphomas behave in the same manner). The WHO system further defines these behaviorally different lymphomas into subcategories.[18,25] A study tested accuracy and consistency in the use of these criteria for classification of canine lymphomas, including cellular

morphology, cell lineage, topography, and general biology of the neoplasm; these criteria were used to define specific disease entities, and a high degree of accuracy was achieved by veterinary pathologists.[25]

The goals of the WHO classification system are to correlate the variety of cell subtypes and architectural features of lymphoma to clinical behavior in terms of responsiveness to therapy and outlook for the patient.[18] Although there are many subcategories in human medicine, by applying this classification scheme in dogs, it was found that up to 80% of cases fell into one of only five lymphoma categories (diffuse large B-cell, marginal zone, peripheral T-cell, T-zone, and T cell–lymphoblastic)[25] (Figs. 11.30, A–E, and 11.31, A and B) (Table 11.1).

Approximately 75% of lymphoma in dogs is multicentric lymphoma.[26] It is recognized that 70% to 80% of canine lymphomas are of B-cell origin, except in the Boxer dog, in which a recent study found a predominance of T-cell lymphomas. In this study, up to 84% of lymphomas in this breed were high-grade CD4+ (helper) T-cell lymphomas.[26,27] There also appears to be a slight genetic predisposition for T-cell lymphoma in other breeds (Irish Wolfhound, Shih Tzu, Airedale, Yorkshire Terrier, Cocker Spaniel, and Siberian Husky).[28,29] T-cell lymphomas in the dog that are high-grade tumors and have a worse prognosis compared with B-cell lymphomas of the same grade.[27-30] High-grade T-cell lymphoma in dogs have been reported to have low rates of complete remission (sometimes only 40%) and shorter remission times compared with high-grade B-cell lymphoma, which has a remission rate of 90%.[27-31] Immunohistochemistry of histological preparations as well as other immunophenotyping methods, such as flow cytometry and PARR, are indicated for appropriate lymphoma classification. Surprisingly, the immunophenotype does not appear to be of prognostic significance in cats.[32]

Biomarkers, such as vascular endothelial growth factor (VEGF) and matrix metalloproteinase (MMP), have been examined as possible markers for staging, monitoring of chemotherapy effectiveness, and post-remission relapse.[33] An enzyme involved in deoxyribonucleic acid (DNA) precursor synthesis (known as *TK1*) has been studied and found to be higher in dogs with lymphoma than in healthy control dogs and dogs with nonhematopoietic neoplasia.[30,31] These levels appear to correlate with stage and prognosis.[30,31] A recent study also examined the expression of four genes in canine lymphomas, and by comparing patterns, high-grade T-cell lymphomas, low-grade T-cell lymphomas, and B-cell lymphomas could be distinguished.[31] Biomarkers for possible early detection of relapsing disease are an area of active research, and recently one biomarker in the dog has become commercially available.

If a diagnosis is equivocal, the entire lymph node should be removed, keeping the capsule intact and fixed in 10% buffered formalin. A complete cross-section is then examined to determine whether a homogeneous population of neoplastic cells has obliterated the normal nodal architecture.

A confusing mixture of malignant and reactive elements may limit the accuracy of both the histological and cytological diagnoses of lymphoma. This may be attributed to partial nodal involvement and is intrinsic to some lymphomas, such as Hodgkin disease and T-cell–rich B-cell lymphomas.[15,17] The previously mentioned ancillary techniques, including immunophenotypic assessment of smears or histological sections, immunophenotyping with flow cytometry, or PCR to determine clonality and cell lineage, are often very useful to confirm a diagnosis when cytological findings are not conclusive.[14,15,18] To exclude the possibility of a primary leukemia that has infiltrated the node, a complete blood cell count should always be performed concurrently as part of the routine workup.

A form of mixed cell lymphoma has been described in cats and has many features recognized in Hodgkin lymphoma in humans.[34]

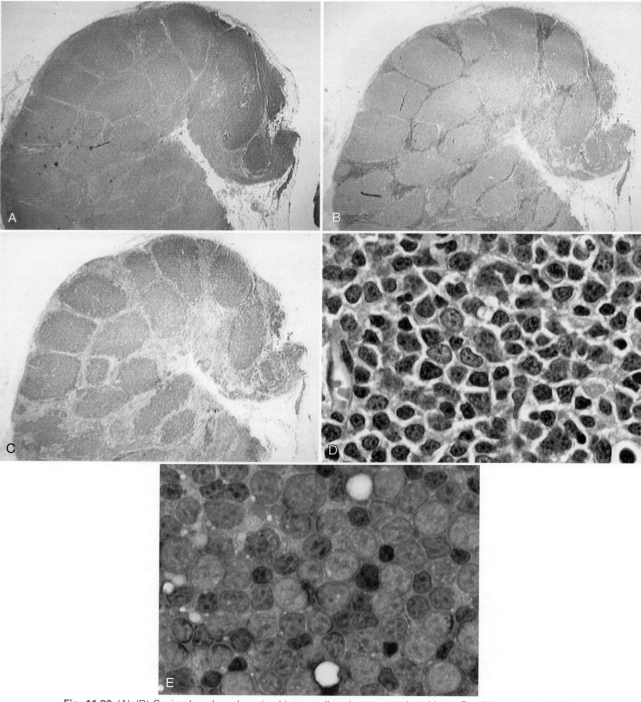

Fig. 11.30 (A)–(D) Canine lymph node, mixed intermediate (centrocytes) and large B-cell (centroblasts) follicular lymphoma. *Top left:* Histopathology mosaic photomicrograph (hematoxylin and eosin [H&E] stain). *Top right:* With CD3 staining, the interfollicular areas show residual paracortical T cells. *Bottom left:* CD79a staining distinctly marks the proliferating B cells with the interfollicular areas largely unlabeled. *Bottom right:* Cells in the follicular areas are intermediate to large in size with irregularly indented nuclei; nucleoli are multiple but often inconspicuous and sometimes impinge on the nuclear membrane. (E) Wright-Giemsa–stained fine-needle aspiration (FNA) cytology from same lymph node. Neoplastic B lymphocytes showing variability in size and multiple, inconspicuous nucleoli. A few residual small lymphocytes are also seen.

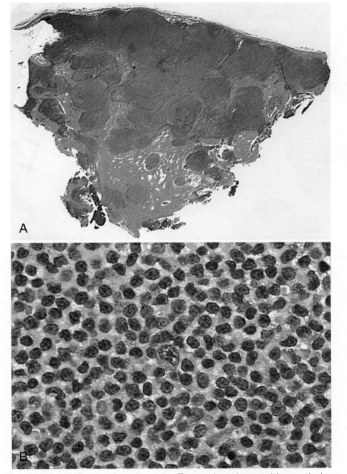

Fig. 11.31 (A) Canine lymph node, T-zone lymphoma, histopathology (hematoxylin and eosin [H&E] stain). The presence of fading germinal centers beneath the capsule and sinus ectasia helps distinguish the histological appearance of this T-zone lymphoma from small cell lymphoma, both of which are a small cell subtype. Cytologically, the lymphocytes have nuclei slightly larger than those of red blood cells and densely stained chromatin with large chromocenters and dispersed intervening areas; nucleoli are absent or small and seen in only a few cells and mitotic activity is not apparent. (B) Cytology from the same lymph node.

This form in cats is often referred to as *Hodgkin-like lymphoma*.[34] It has been classified by some as *T cell–rich B-cell lymphoma* and by others as *Hodgkin-like lymphoma*. Although this nomenclature is still considered controversial by some, the clinical presentation, behavior of the disease, and cytological and histological findings closely resemble Hodgkin lymphoma in humans.[34] This tumor is uniquely composed of a minority subpopulation of neoplastic B cells within a nonneoplastic, reactive T-cell background.

It is most often recognized as a unilateral or bilateral enlargement of a submandibular or prescapular lymph node. This disease will usually progress along contiguous lymph nodes. If caught early enough and the affected lymph node surgically removed, the disease may be cured. If allowed to progress, there will eventually be splenic, hepatic, and bone marrow involvement. This neoplasm usually occurs in cats age greater than 6 years. There is no recognized association with FELV or FIV infection.[21]

The small population of neoplastic lymphocytes in Hodgkin-like lymphoma can resemble histiocytes, but they express a B-cell immunophenotype.[34,35] Although these cells can be mononucleate, binucleate, or multinucleate, the classic appearance is that of a binucleate cell with two large nuclei and a single large nucleolus in each. This morphology has been described as resembling large "owl eyes" and are known as *Reed-Sternberg cells*. Histologically, these cells are visible, in addition to other features, which may include parafollicular sclerosis, compression of normal node architecture (as previously mentioned), and other pathological changes[35,36] (Fig. 11.32).

Plasma cells are a normal cell population of lymph nodes, but plasma cell neoplasia typically occurs in extranodal locations and is not addressed in this chapter.

Metastatic Neoplasia

In cases of nonlymphoid neoplasia, FNA of lymph nodes for evidence of metastatic neoplastic cells draining to regional lymph nodes is recommended. Tumor cells are usually obtained if metastasis has progressed to cause clinically evident enlarged nodes; however, small foci in normal-sized nodes may be missed on aspiration. Negative findings in palpably enlarged nodes should always be subordinate to clinical findings.[36] The sensitivity of detection of low numbers of metastatic cells may be increased by the use of immunocytochemical assessment of nodal preparations or by the use of molecular techniques to detect the presence of tumor antigen messenger ribonucleic acid (RNA).[37]

WHO Classification	IPT	Grade	Treatment	Average Survival With Treatment	% Patients	Significance
DLBCL	B	H	CHOP	9 months	50%	Most common
Marginal zone and Mantel cell	B	L	Surgery or prednisolone and chlorambucil	13–20 months	14%	
PTCL (NOS)	T	H	CHOP and CCNU	6 months	15%	Highest mortality
T-zone	T	L	Prednisolone and chlorambucil	20–33 months	13%	Longest survival
TLBL	T	H	CHOP and CCNU	6–8 months	4%	Highest mortality

TABLE 11.1 Classification, Approximate Percentages, and Behavior of Canine Lymphomas[22,25,31]

PTCL and TLBL survival were not statistically different.
CHOP, cyclophosphamide, doxorubicin, vincristine, and prednisone; *CCNU*, lomustine; *IPT*, immunophenotype; *NOS*, not otherwise specified; *PTCL*, peripheral T-cell lymphoma; *TLBL*, T-cell lymphoblastic leukemia.

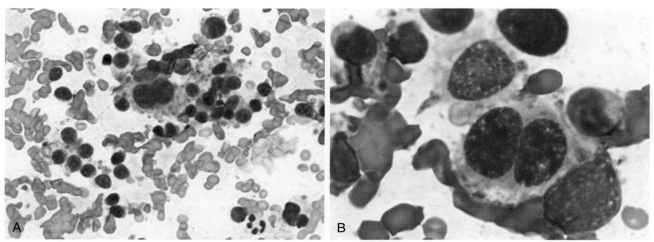

Fig. 11.32 A lymph node aspirate from a cat with Hodgkin-like lymphoma. Note the large Reed-Stenberg cell. Although this cell may sometimes appear more histiocytic than lymphocytic, it has been found to possess B lymphocyte markers. (From Steinburg J, Keating JH. Cervical mass in a cat. *Vet Clin Path J* 2008;37[3]:323-327.)

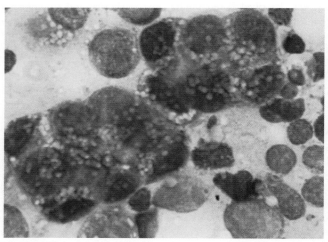

Fig. 11.33 An epithelial cell cluster from a transitional cell carcinoma that metastasized to a lymph node (Wright stain).

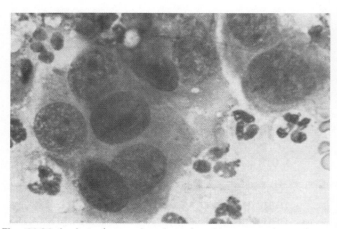

Fig. 11.34 Aspirate from a lymph node with metastatic carcinoma. Several carcinoma cells and neutrophils are present (Wright stain). (Courtesy Dr. Duncan, University of Georgia, Athens, GA.)

The presence of cells not normally found in lymph nodes or an increase in numbers of certain cell types normally present (i.e., mast cells) may suggest metastatic neoplasia (Figs. 11.33 to 11.38). Although distinguishing between a benign mast cell population and mast cell tumor metastasis is sometimes not possible, one study found that mast cell tumor metastasis is more commonly observed in patients with lymph node enlargement, mast cell clustering (three or more aggregating mast cells), or the presence of mast cells with atypical morphology[36] (see Fig. 11.36). More than 3% mast cells should also raise suspicion of mast cell tumor metastasis. Matching internal tandem duplication of the *c-kit* gene may be a more sensitive method for confirming the presence of metastasis in the node.[36-38]

Carcinomas frequently metastasize to lymph nodes. Metastatic epithelial cells (see Figs. 11.33 and 11.34) may occur singly or in groups. They are very large and bear no resemblance to cellular constituents of normal or hyperplastic nodes. Epithelial cells of any type in a lymph node aspirate indicate neoplasia, but these cells must be differentiated from epithelioid cells of granulomatous inflammation, as described previously. Salivary epithelial cells (see Fig. 11.35) from the submandibular salivary gland may be accidentally aspirated. These cells are uniform in size and have round to oval nuclei and abundant blue foamy cytoplasm and should not be confused with carcinoma cells.

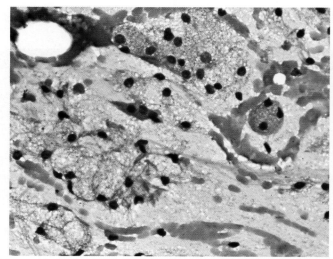

Fig. 11.35 Salivary gland aspirate. High number of red blood cells and foamy secretory cells from a normal salivary gland in a thick basophilic mucoprotein background (Wright stain). (Courtesy Dr. R. L. Cowell.)

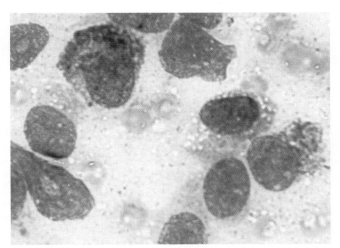

Fig. 11.36 An aspirate containing malignant melanocytes that have metastasized to the lymph node. Greenish-black cytoplasmic granules characterize these cells (Wright stain).

Transmissible venereal tumors (TVTs; Fig. 11.39) may metastasize to lymph nodes. Although sarcomas do not metastasize to lymph nodes as frequently as carcinomas do, spindle cells in significant numbers could suggest a sarcoma of some type.

Malignant melanomas also metastasize to lymph nodes. One study found that detection of metastatic melanoma in dogs to regional lymph nodes via FNA can be highly sensitive (92%) but was influenced by several factors, including use of immunostains, lymph node location, and lesion location (e.g., subcutaneous) among others.[38] The melanocyte usually is identified by its granular, brown-black cytoplasmic pigment (see Fig. 11.37). Pigment in melanocytes should not be confused with that in melanophages that have phagocytized melanin originating from pigmented structures or those from lesions in the area drained by the node. Melanophages also phagocytize pigment released by melanocytes. Differentiation may be difficult, but melanocytes usually have more attenuated and less vacuolated cytoplasm. Hemosiderin, carbon, bile, and other pigments in macrophages must not be confused with melanin.

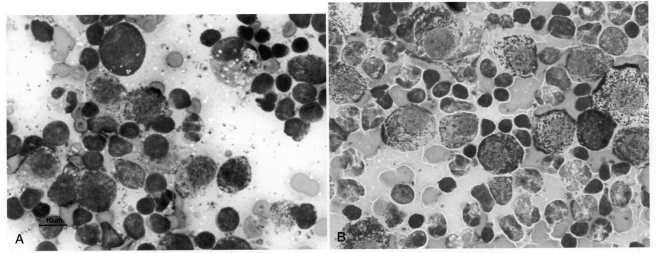

Fig. 11.37 (A) Among these small lymphocytes are a few eosinophils, a large reactive lymphoblast, and many mast cells. The presence of poorly differentiated mast cells, having fewer and less prominent granules, is supportive of metastatic disease. (Wright stain.) (B) Lymph node aspirate. Metastatic mast cell tumor with a high number of mast cells and many eosinophils along with the lymphoid cells (Wright stain). (Courtesy Dr. R. L. Cowell.)

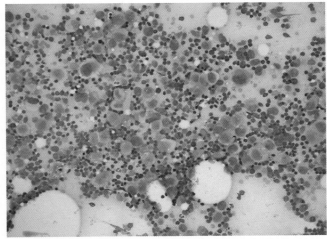

Fig. 11.38 Aspirate of a lymph node with metastatic histiocytic sarcoma (Wright stain).

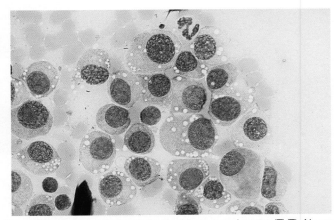

Fig. 11.39 Aspirate from a transmissible venereal tumor (TVT). Numerous TVT cells with coarse chromatin and smoky-gray vacuolated cytoplasm are seen (Wright stain).

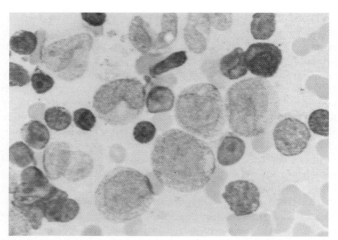

Fig. 11.40 Among small lymphocytes and a plasma cell are very immature neutrophils. This lymph node aspirate is from an animal with granulocytic leukemia (Wright stain).

Various myeloproliferative disorders may result in a leukemic hemogram and neoplastic cells in the sinuses of lymph nodes. Cytological examination of lymph node fine-needle aspirate reveals the cell population of a normal or hyperplastic node and a population of leukemic cells (Fig. 11.40). In acute leukemias, blast cells of the neoplastic myeloid cell population may be difficult to differentiate from lymphoblasts. In chronic leukemias, various maturation stages are present. Extramedullary hematopoiesis may occur in lymph nodes and contribute to cytological findings of various stages of erythroid, myeloid cells and megakaryocytes. It is a rare occurrence in chronic anemias.[39]

In conclusion, FNA cytology of the lymph node is a valuable diagnostic tool. This inexpensive, relatively painless, and rapid technique may not only help establish a primary diagnosis but also is a useful method for following up patients with known malignancies and even for guiding therapy. Fig. 11.41 presents an algorithm for evaluation of lymph node aspirates or impression smears.

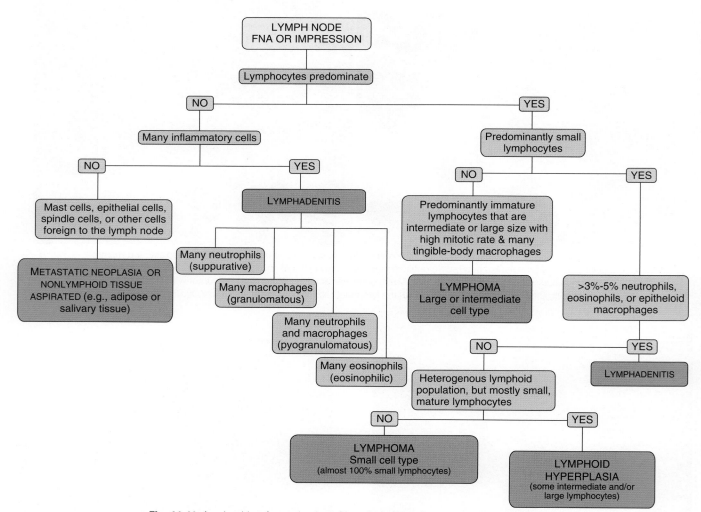

Fig. 11.41 An algorithm for evaluation of lymph node aspirates or impression smears.

REFERENCES

1. Dieter H. Blood and bone marrow. In: Eurell J, Frappier BL, eds. *Dellmann's Textbook of Veterinary Histology*. 6th ed. Ames, IA: Blackwell Publishing; 2006:143–147.
2. Soderstrom N. *Fine-Needle Aspiration Biopsy*. New York: Grune & Stratton; 1966.
3. Frable WJ. Fine-needle aspiration biopsy: a review. *Human Pathol*. 1983;14:9–28.
4. Perman V, Alsaker R, Riis R. *Cytology of the Dog and Cat*. Denver, CO: American Animal Hospital Association; 1979.
5. Rebar AH. *Handbook of Veterinary Cytology*. St. Louis, MO: Ralston Purina; 1980.
6. Thrall DE. Cytology of lymphoid tissue. *Comp Cont Educ Pract Vet*. 1987;9:104–111.
7. Raskin RE, Meyer D. *Atlas of Canine and Feline Cytology*. Philadelphia, PA: Saunders; 2001.
8. Vernau W. *Lymph Node Cytology of Dogs and Cats*. Rimini, Italy: 50th Congresso Nazionale Multisala SCIVA; 2005.
9. Fournel C, Magnol JP, Marchal T, et al. An original perifollicular zone cell in the canine reactive lymph node: a morphological, phenotypical and aetiological study. *J Comp Pathol*. 1995;113(3):217–231.
10. Werner JA, Woo JC, Vernau W, et al. Characterization of feline immunoglobulin heavy chain variable region genes for the molecular diagnosis of B-cell neoplasia. *Vet Pathol*. 2005;42(5):596–607.
11. Moore PF, Woo JC, Vernau W, et al. Characterization of feline T cell receptor gamma (TCRG) variable region genes for the molecular diagnosis of feline intestinal T cell lymphoma. *Vet Immunol Immunopathol*. 2005;106(3-4):167–178.
12. Burnett RC, Vernau W, Modiano JF, et al. Diagnosis of canine lymphoid neoplasia using clonal rearrangements of antigen receptor genes. *Vet Pathol*. 2003;40(1):32–341.
13. Lana SE, Jackson TL, Burnett RC, et al. Utility of polymerase chain reaction for analysis of antigen receptor rearrangement in staging and predicting prognosis in dogs with lymphoma. *J Vet Intern Med*. 2006;20(2):329–334.
14. Gabor LJ, Jackson TL, Burnett RC, et al. Immunophenotypic and histological characterisation of 109 cases of feline lymphosarcoma. *Aust Vet J*. 1999;77(7):436–441.
15. Fournel Fleury C, Magnol JP, Bricaire P, et al. Cytohistological and immunological classification of canine malignant lymphomas: comparison with human non-Hodgkin's lymphomas. *J Comp Pathol*. 1997;117(1):35–59.
16. Valli VE, Jacobs RM, Norris A, et al. The histologic classification of 602 cases of feline lymphoproliferative disease using the National Cancer Institute working formulation. *J Vet Diagn Invest*. 2000;12(4):295–306.
17. Valli VE, Jacobs RM, Parodi AL, et al. Tumors of lymphoid system. In: Schulman YF, ed. *Histological Classification of Hematopoietic Tumors of Domestic Animals, 2nd series*. Vol. 8. Washington, DC: Armed Forces Institute of Pathology; 2002.
18. Valli VE, San Myint M, Barthel A, et al. Classification of canine malignant lymphomas according to the World Health Organization criteria. *Vet Pathol*. 2011;48(1):198–211.
19. Wilkerson MJ, Dolce K, Koopman T, et al. Lineage differentiation of canine lymphoma/leukemias and aberrant expression of CD molecules. *Vet Immunol Immunopathol*. 2005;106(3–4):179–196.
20. Seelig D, Webb T, Avery P, Avery A. Canine T-zone lymphoma: unique immunophenotypic features, outcome and population characteristics. *JVIM*. March. 2014;28(3).
21. Valli VE, Bienzle D, Meuten DJ. Tumors of the hemolymphatic system. In: Meuten D, ed. *Tumors in Domestic Animals*. 5th ed. Ames, IA: Wiley-Blackwell; 2017:245–249.
22. Flood-Knapik KE, Durham AC, Gregor TP, et al. Clinical, histopathological and immunohistochemical characterization of canine indolent lymphoma. *Vet Comp Oncol*. 2013;11(4):272–286.
23. Ponce F, Magnol JP, Ledieu D, et al. Prognostic significance of morphological subtypes in canine malignant lymphomas during chemotherapy. *Vet J*. 2004;167(2):158–166.
24. Ponce F, et al. A morphological study of 608 cases of canine malignant lymphoma in France with a focus on comparative similarities between canine and human lymphoma morphology. *Vet Patholo*. 2010;47(3):414–433.
25. Valli VE, Kass H, San M, et al. Canine lymphomas association of classification type, disease stage, tumor subtype, mitotic rate and treatment with survival. *Vet Pathol*. 2013;50(5):738–748.
26. Modiano JF, et al. Distinct B-cell and T-cell lymphoproliferative disease prevalence among dog breeds indicates heritable risk. *Cancer Res*. 2005;65(13):5654–5661.
27. Lurie DM, Milner RJ, Suter SE, Vernau W. Immunophenotypic and cytomorphologic subclassification of T-cell lymphoma in the boxer breed. *Vet Immunol Immunopathol*. 2008;125(1-2):102–110.
28. Fournel-Fleury C, Ponce F, Felman P, et al. Canine T-cell lymphomas: a morphological, immunological, and clinical study of 46 new cases. *Vet Pathol*. 2002;39(1):92–109.
29. Franz AM. Molecular profiling reveals prognostically significant subtypes of canine lymphoma. *Vet Pathol*. 2013;50(4):693–703.
30. Moore AS. Treatment of T cell lymphoma in dogs. *Vet Record*. 2016;11(277):171–179.
31. Zandvliet M. Canine lymphoma: a review. *Vet Quarterly*. 2016;36(2):76–104.
32. Patterson-Kane JC, Kugler BP, Francis K. The possible prognostic significance of immunophenotype in feline alimentary lymphoma: a pilot study. *J Comp Pathol*. 2004;130(2–3):220–222.
33. Aresu L, Aricò A, Comazzi S, et al. VEGF and MMP-9: biomarkers for canine lymphoma. *Vet Comp Oncol*. 2012. Epub ahead of print.
34. Steinburg J, Keating JH. Cervical mass in a cat. *Vet Clinical Path J*. 2008;37:323–327.
35. Walton RM, Hendrick MJ. Feline Hodgkin's-like lymphoma: 20 cases (1992-1999). *Vet Pathol*. 2001;38:504–511.
36. Kirk EL, Billings AP, Shofer FS, Wantanabe S, Sorenmo KU. Cytological lymph node evaluation in dogs with mast cell tumors: association with grade and survival. *Vet Comp Oncol*. 2009;7(2):130–138.
37. Zavodovskaya R, Chein MB, London CA. Use of kit internal tandem duplications to establish mast cell tumor clonality in 2 dogs. *J Vet Intern Med*. 2004;18(6):915–917.
38. Doubrovsky A, Scolyer RA, Rajmohan M, et al. Diagnostic accuracy of fine needle biopsy for metastatic melanoma and its implication for patient management. *Ann Surg Oncol*. 2008;15(1):323–332.
39. Vail VE, Pinkerton ME, Young KM. Hematopoietic tumors. In: Vail DM, ed. *Withrow & MacEwan's, Small Animal Clinical Oncology*. 5th ed. St. Louis: Elsevier; 2012:641–643.

12

Synovial Fluid Analysis

Peter J. Fernandes

Synovium is essentially a living ultrafiltration membrane with fenestrated capillaries just below an intimal surface that contains wide intercellular gaps but, unlike true membranes, has no epithelial cells and no basement membrane. The fenestrated synovial capillaries, up to 50 times more permeable to water compared with continuous capillaries, allow water and small solutes into the subintima but exclude varied proportions of albumin and larger proteins, such as fibrinogen and clotting factors.

As fluid enters and leaves the joint cavity, its diffusion and composition is regulated by connective tissue of the subintima and by the cells of the intima, or synovial lining. The intima is made up mostly of secretory, fibroblast-related, synoviocytes (B cell), fewer macrophages (A cell), and very infrequent C cells, which are intermediate or stem cell–like with properties of both A and B cells. The B cells, which constitute 70% to 90% of intimal cells, secrete components for tissue interstitium and synovial fluid that include collagens, fibronectin, hyaluronan, and lubricin.[1,2] A cells are derived from bloodborne mononuclear cells and are considered resident tissue macrophages, much like hepatic Kupffer cells (Figs. 12.1 and 12.2). A cells demonstrate several macrophage linage markers, such as nonspecific esterase (NSE) activity, CD18, CD168, and CD68. B cells show immunohistochemical reactivity to heat shock protein 25 (HSP25), CD55, cadherin 11, and high activity of the enzyme Uridine diphosphate glucose dehydrogenase (UDPGD). A cells and B cells are vimentin positive and cytokeratin negative.[1]

ARTHROCENTESIS

In the verification, localization, diagnosis, and management of arthritis, synovial fluid examination is a key component of an initial medical database and includes clinical history, physical examination, radiographs, complete blood cell count, biochemical profile, and urinalysis. See Boxes 12.1 and 12.2 for indications and contraindications for arthrocentesis.

RESTRAINT

As temperament under physical immobilization and tolerance for discomfort of each individual is different, the clinician must judge which method of restraint is appropriate to allow for controlled manipulation and centesis of the joint. Complications of inadequate restraint may include damage to blood vessels, nerves, synovial membrane, and articular cartilage surfaces, along with blood contamination and retrieving a diagnostically insufficient volume of synovial fluid.

ASEPSIS

Routine aseptic technique should be followed. Normal joint spaces are sterile.

EQUIPMENT

Sterile disposable 3-milliliter (mL) syringes and 1-inch, 22-gauge or 25-gauge (for small dogs and cats), hypodermic needle are recommended. In large-breed dogs, sampling of the elbow or shoulder joints may require a 1½-inch needle and the hip joint may necessitate a 3-inch spinal needle. Microscope glass slides with frosted ends, red-top tubes, and ethylenediaminetetraacetic acid (EDTA) blood tubes should be readied and labeled with the patient's name and the joint sampled. See Box 12.3 for a complete list of materials.

APPROACHES

In most cases, arthrocentesis is performed with the patient in lateral recumbency and the joint to be sampled positioned uppermost. Palpation of the joint during manual flexion and extension helps identify the space to be entered. In all cases, the needle should be advanced gently toward and through the joint capsule to avoid damaging the articular cartilage. Once the needle is inside the joint space, the volume of fluid obtained depends on the particular joint and the disorder. Ordinarily, some synovial fluid is readily collected from the stifle joint, but it is most difficult to obtain from the carpal and tarsal joints. Obviously, when joint spaces are swollen, fluid is more easily aspirated. The plunger of the syringe should be released before the needle is removed from the joint space. This minimizes blood contamination of the sample as the needle is withdrawn.

Carpal Joint

Entry is obtained via the antebrachiocarpal joint or the middle carpal joint. In either case, the carpus is flexed to increase access to the joint's spaces. The needle is introduced from the dorsal aspect, just medial of center, then inserted perpendicular to the joint. Landmarks for the antebrachiocarpal joint are the distal radius and the proximal radial carpal bone (Fig. 12.3). The middle carpal joint is between the distal portion of the radial carpal bone and the second and third carpal bones.

Elbow Joint

Entry to the elbow may be attained with the joint in extension or flexion. Hyperextension of the elbow allows for the introduction of the needle medial to the lateral epicondyle of the humerus and lateral to the olecranon. Once in the joint space, the needle is guided cranially toward the humeral condyle (Fig. 12.4). With the elbow in a 90-degree angle of flexion, the needle can be introduced just proximal to the olecranon and medial to the lateral epicondylar crest. The needle will be inserted parallel to the olecranon and the long axis of the ulna.

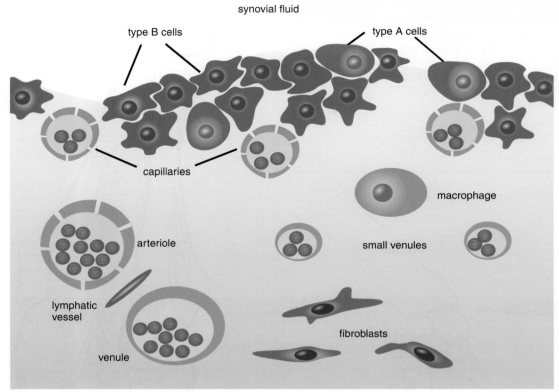

synovial fluid

type B cells   type A cells

capillaries

macrophage

arteriole   small venules

lymphatic
vessel

venule   fibroblasts

Fig. 12.1 Schematic representation of the normal synovium.

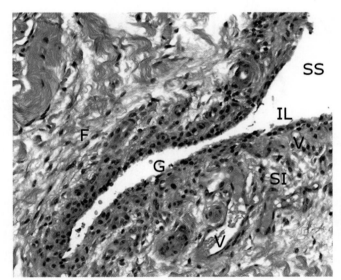

SS

IL

F   V

G

SI

V

Fig. 12.2 Histological specimen of synovial membrane showing details within the valley of a normal fold in the lining. Directly interfacing with the synovial space (*SS*) is a sparse intimal layer (*IL*), only one to two cells thick, with underlying vessels (*V*) embedded among fibrous subintima (*SI*). Note the normal acellular gap in the intimal lining (*G*) and fibrocytes (*F*) within the subintima (hematoxylin and eosin [H&E] stain, original magnification 20×). (Courtesy Dr. Dave Getzy.)

Shoulder Joint

Access is gained from the lateral aspect, with the needle introduced distal to the acromion of the scapula and caudal to the greater tubercle of the humerus. The needle is directed medially toward the

BOX 12.1 Indications for Arthrocentesis

- Fever of unknown origin
- Unexplained lameness
- Generalized pain
- Joint swelling or effusion
- Weakness
- Acute monoarthropathy
- Abnormal limb function or gait
- Shifting leg lameness or polyarthropathy

BOX 12.2 Contraindications for Arthrocentesis

Absolute: Cellulitis or dermatitis over arthrocentesis site
Relative: Bacteremia or severe coagulopathy

greater tubercle and distal to the supraglenoid tubercle of the scapula (Fig. 12.5).

Tarsal Joint

Access is gained via a cranial or caudal approach. In the cranial approach, the tarsus is slightly flexed, and the needle is introduced at the space palpated between the tibia and talus (tibiotarsal) bones, just lateral to the tendon bundle. For the caudal approach, the joint is extended and the needle can be inserted medial or lateral to the calcaneus (fibular tarsal bone) with a cranial and slightly plantar path (Fig. 12.6).

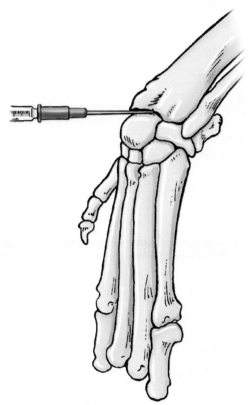

Fig. 12.3 Arthrocentesis of the carpus joint. The joint may be located by applying fingertip pressure just distal to the radius during flexion and extension. The needle is introduced between the distal radius and proximal to the radial carpal bone. (From Piermattei DL, Flo G, DeCamp C. Chapter 1: Orthopedic examination and diagnostic tools. In: *Brinker, Piermattei, and Flo's Handbook of Small Animal Orthopedics and Fracture Repair*. 4th ed. St. Louis, MO: Saunders; 2006:24.)

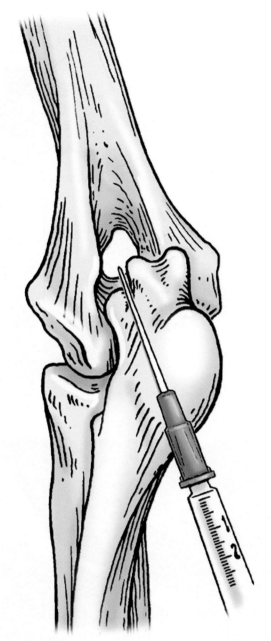

Fig. 12.4 Arthrocentesis of the elbow joint. With the elbow in hyperextension, the needle is introduced medial to the lateral epicondyle of the humerus and lateral to the olecranon. (From Piermattei DL, Flo G, DeCamp C. Chapter 1: Orthopedic examination and diagnostic tools. In: *Brinker, Piermattei, and Flo's Handbook of Small Animal Orthopedics and Fracture Repair*. 4th ed. St. Louis, MO: Saunders; 2006:23.)

Stifle Joint

The stifle is flexed, and the needle is introduced just lateral to the patellar ligament and distal to the patella. The needle is advanced in a medial and proximal direction pointing toward the medial condyle of the femur (Fig. 12.7).

Hip Joint

The femur is abducted and the leg extended caudally. The needle is introduced cranial to the greater trochanter of the femur and inserted caudal and distal or ventral toward the joint (Fig. 12.8).

SAMPLE HANDLING AND TEST PRIORITIES

Laboratory tests performed may be limited by volume of synovial fluid collected. While the sample is in the syringe, volume, color, and turbidity should be noted. Viscosity is then assessed as the sample is expelled onto a glass slide for direct smears. Direct smears are immediately made for subsequent cytological examination, nucleated cell differential count, and subjective assessment of cellularity. See Tables 12.1 and 12.2 for specific volumes needed and sequence of testing. When larger volumes of fluid are collected, a total nucleated cell count,

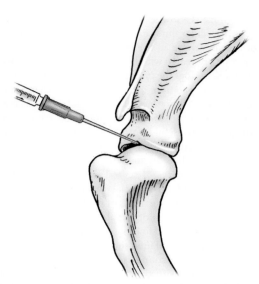

Fig. 12.5 Arthrocentesis of the shoulder joint. The needle is introduced distal to the acromion of the scapula and caudal to the greater tubercle of the humerus and then directed medially toward the greater tubercle and just distal to the supraglenoid tubercle of the scapula. (From Piermattei DL, Flo G, DeCamp C. Chapter 1: Orthopedic examination and diagnostic tools. In: *Brinker, Piermattei, and Flo's Handbook of Small Animal Orthopedics and Fracture Repair*. 4th ed. St. Louis, MO: Saunders; 2006:23.)

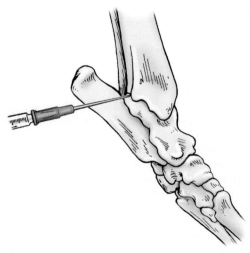

Fig. 12.6 Arthrocentesis of the tarsal joint. The joint is extended and the needle is inserted medial to the calcaneus in a cranial path. (From Piermattei DL, Flo G, DeCamp C. Chapter 1: Orthopedic examination and diagnostic tools. In: *Brinker, Piermattei, and Flo's Handbook of Small Animal Orthopedics and Fracture Repair*. 4th ed. St. Louis, MO: Saunders; 2006:22.)

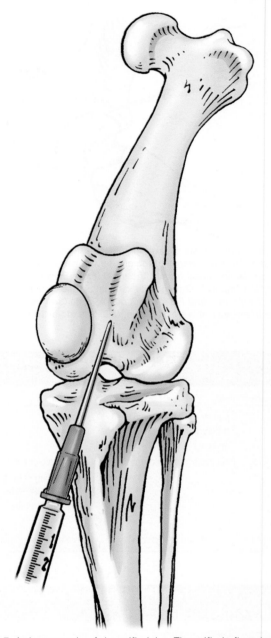

Fig. 12.7 Arthrocentesis of the stifle joint. The stifle is flexed and the needle introduced lateral to the patellar ligament and distal to the patella and advanced in a medial and proximal direction toward the medial condyle of the femur. (From Piermattei DL, Flo G, DeCamp C. Chapter 1: Orthopedic examination and diagnostic tools. In: *Brinker, Piermattei, and Flo's Handbook of Small Animal Orthopedics and Fracture Repair*. 4th ed. St. Louis, MO: Saunders; 2006:22.)

mucin clot test, and total protein estimation, in that order of priority, may be added to the aforementioned procedures.

Normal synovial fluid does not clot. However, with the possibility of incidental blood contamination, intraarticular hemorrhage, or protein exudation in various inflammatory diseases, it is best to place a portion into an EDTA anticoagulant blood tube. The smallest EDTA blood tube available should be used for storage or preservation of the synovial fluid retrieved, because gross mismatches with the use of large

EDTA tubes may lead to erroneous test results. The EDTA tube is preferred for cytological examination, whereas a heparin tube or a plain blood tube is recommended for the mucin clot test. Either anticoagulant (EDTA or heparin) is suitable for other routine tests.

When sufficient fluid is collected for cell counting, various preparations are made in accordance with the sample's cellularity. When the nucleated cell count is less than 5000 cells per microliter (cells/μL), cytological examination is enhanced by cytocentrifuge concentration. About 5 minutes at 1000 to 1500 revolutions per minute (rpm) in a cytocentrifuge is satisfactory. Fluids with nucleated cell counts greater than 5000

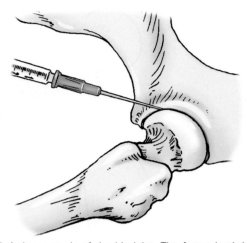

Fig. 12.8 Arthrocentesis of the hip joint. The femur is abducted with the needle introduced cranial to the greater trochanter of the femur and guided caudal and distal toward the joint. (From Piermattei DL, Flo G, DeCamp C. Chapter 1: Orthopedic examination and diagnostic tools. In: *Brinker, Piermattei, and Flo's Handbook of Small Animal Orthopedics and Fracture Repair.* 4th ed. St. Louis, MO: Saunders; 2006:21.)

TABLE 12.1	Test Priorities for Synovial Fluid ≥2 mL	
Amount	**Test**	
1 drop	Cytology and white blood cell differential with viscosity estimate	Glass slide
0.5–1.0 mL	Total nucleated cell count	Lavender top or plain
		20-mL (pediatric) Becton Dickinson BBL Septi-Chek blood culture tube
Or	Or	Or
0.5–1.0 mL	Bacterial culture and sensitivity	Sterile plain blood tube

TABLE 12.2	Test Priorities for Synovial Fluid <1 mL	
Amount	**Test**	
1 drop	Cytology and white blood cell differential with total nucleated cell estimate and viscosity	Glass slide
2 or 3 drops	Bacterial culture and sensitivity	Culturette

cells/μL are smeared directly onto glass slides. Although cytocentrifuge concentration is helpful, it is not essential to an effective evaluation, and practitioners will get accurate results from direct smears only.

Cells in sediment smears and direct smears of fluid with the normally high viscosity may not spread out well on slides, making cell identification and differential cell count difficult. If this problem is encountered, it may be overcome by mixing an equal volume of hyaluronidase at 150 international units per milliliter (IU/mL) with the synovial fluid and incubating for at least 10 minutes.[3] This helps obtain fluid that facilitates better presentation of cell morphology and more complete cytological evaluation.

A cytocentrifuge is a low-speed centrifuge that allows for concentration of poorly cellular fluids directly onto a glass slide with the least number of cells destroyed in the process. Samples with good to fair viscosity must be pretreated with hyaluronidase because otherwise the synovial fluid mucin clogs the cytocentrifuge filter paper and interferes with proper slide preparation. This technique is helpful and is used by many commercial laboratories, but it is not essential for an adequate evaluation in most cases, and the practicing veterinarian is able to obtain diagnostically useful information from a direct smear.

Slides may be stained with any Romanowsky-type stain for routine cytological evaluation. It is advisable to make synovial fluid smears soon after collection. Delays of several hours, particularly at warm temperatures, may result in artificial vacuolation of macrophages, along with pyknosis and karyorrhexis of nucleated cells.

Microbiological evaluation of samples collected aseptically can be done if cytological and clinical findings suggest that an infectious agent is present. If possible, synovial fluid should be placed into a culture system immediately after collection. Use of an EDTA tube is undesirable because EDTA interferes with growth of some bacteria; a red-top tube is not recommended because it may not be sterile.

LABORATORY ANALYSIS AND REFERENCE VALUES

Volume

An approximate or subjective estimation of fluid volume collected should be recorded. Synovial fluid volumes depend on patient size and the joint from which it is being collected (within an individual, variation exists from joint to joint). In normal animals, fluid volume can range from one drop to 1 mL in dogs and one drop to 0.25 mL in cats.[3-5] Clinical experience is an extremely valuable guide to detecting an articular effusion. This judgment is based on the degree of joint capsule distension, ease of fluid collection, and volume readily obtained. The aim of arthrocentesis for synovial fluid analysis is to collect some synovial fluid and not to drain the joint space.

Color and Turbidity

Normal synovial fluid is transparent and colorless to very light yellow or straw colored. Samples with increased cellularity exhibit variable discoloration and increased turbidity. When a fluid is blood tinged, hemarthrosis should be distinguished from iatrogenic contamination. In cases of hemarthrosis, the fluid is uniformly bloody throughout the time of collection. If the fluid was initially free of blood, but a subsequent admixture occurs during the sampling procedure, contamination should be suspected. As an alternative and when the volume is sufficiently large for centrifugation, recent hemorrhage is associated with a sediment of red blood cells (RBCs) and a clear to straw-colored supernatant. The supernatant of fluids with chronic hemorrhage has a yellow to yellow-orange discoloration because of hemoglobin breakdown products.

Viscosity

Normal synovial fluid is very viscous because of its high concentration of hyaluronic acid (HA). Viscosity may be measured using a viscometer; however, this is rarely done in small animal practice but, instead, is assessed subjectively. When slowly expressed from a needle attached to a syringe held horizontal, normal synovial fluid forms a long strand that is at least 2.5 centimeters (cm) before separating from the needle. When a drop of fluid is placed between the thumb and forefinger, a similar strand bridges the two digits as they are moved apart. Viscosity is usually recorded as normal, decreased, or markedly decreased.

Viscosity is easily assessed at the time of collection. However, if it must be evaluated after the sample is added to an anticoagulant, heparin is probably preferable to EDTA for sample preservation. EDTA tends to degrade HA and may decrease the sample's viscosity.[6]

Viscosity may also be subjectively assessed when cytologically evaluating direct or sediment smears such that smears of fluids with normally high viscosity tend to have cells aligned in a linear pattern that is sometimes referred to as "wind rowing" (Fig. 12.9). In contrast, synovial fluid samples with decreased viscosity have cells more randomly arranged on the smear (Fig. 12.10).

Mucin Quality

If sufficient sample remains after slide preparation and nucleated cell count, synovial fluid mucin quality or HA may be assessed using a mucin clot test. When the potential exists for clotting of joint fluid, heparin is recommended as an anticoagulant because EDTA interferes with the mucin clot test by degrading HA.[6]

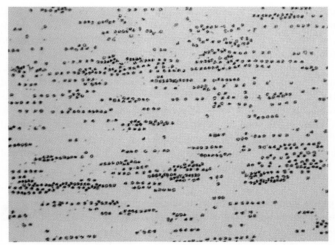

Fig. 12.9 Direct smear of synovial fluid from a dog with acute suppurative arthritis. Note the markedly increased cell count and linear arrangement of cells. The latter, referred to as *windrowing*, suggests normal viscosity (Wright stain, original magnification 160×). (From Parry BW. In Pratt PW, ed. *Laboratory Procedures for Veterinary Technicians.* 2nd ed. Goleta, CA: American Veterinary Publications; 1992.)

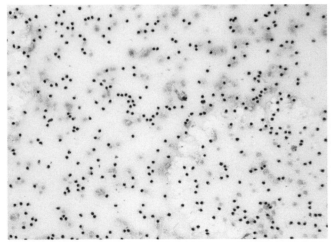

Fig. 12.10 Direct smear of synovial fluid from a dog with suppurative (neutrophilic) polyarthritis. The total nucleated cell count is increased and neutrophils are randomly distributed in the background because the normal synovial fluid viscosity is degraded secondary to inflammation (Wright-Giemsa stain, original magnification 100×).

One part synovial fluid is added to four parts 2.5% glacial acetic acid, which causes mucin to precipitate and sometimes agglutinate or clot. The test is performed in test tubes when sufficient fluid is collected or on glass slides when only a drop is available for this test. The mixture is gently agitated and the nature of the clot observed. Assessment is enhanced by reading the test against a dark background. In inflammatory arthropathies, HA is degraded by proteases from neutrophils. This results in a decreased HA or hyaluronate concentration and decreased viscosity.

The following subjective classifications are commonly used: good (normal), when a compact, ropey clot is present in a clear solution; fair (slightly decreased), with a soft clot in a slightly turbid solution; poor, with a friable clot in a cloudy solution; and very poor, with no actual clot but just some large flecks in a very turbid solution. If clot quality is initially debatable, it may be reassessed after about 1 hour at room temperature. When the solutions are gently shaken during assessment, good clots remain ropey, and poor clots fragment.

Total Cell Counts

Nucleated cell counts in normal synovial fluid vary from joint to joint within an individual animal.[3] However, surveys have not shown these differences to be either statistically significant or clinically relevant. Various canine reference intervals have been reported (Table 12.3). As a generalization from these studies, most normal joints have nucleated cell counts less than 3000 cells/µL.

A recent study of synovial fluid samples from clinically normal cats showed white blood cell (WBC) counts of 161 ± 209 cells/µL (mean ± standard deviation [SD]) and median WBC of 91 cells/µL with a range of 2 to 1134 cells/µL.[5] Samples were excluded from this study when gross evidence of blood contamination was observed, radiographic evidence of osteoarthritis, or histological evidence of synovitis was present or if postmortem physical examination revealed abnormalities. As a generalization from this study, most normal joints have nucleated cell counts less than 1000 cells/µL (Table 12.4).

A comparison of manual hemacytometer and electronic, automatic particle counting of nucleated cells in canine synovial fluid revealed that the mean electronic total nucleated cell count was statistically higher than the mean manual count.[7] Manual counting methods may demonstrate within-day and between-day analytic imprecision that is statistically higher than that of automated particle counting instruments.[8,9] In general, differences in mean cell counts and precision have not proven to be clinically relevant; therefore the efficiency and speed of automatic particle counters offer an advantage over manual methods.

EDTA is preferred as an anticoagulant and preservative for cytological examination and nucleated cell counts. In comparison of EDTA

TABLE 12.3 Reference Intervals for Synovial Fluid Total Nucleated Cell Counts in Healthy Dogs

Range (cells/microliter [µL])	Joints Sampled
33–24,953	12 joints: stifle, shoulder, carpus
0–29,004	55 joints: hip, stifle, hock, elbow, shoulder, carpus
700–440,012	20 stifles
327–145,013	14 stifles
50–272,514	58 stifles
209–20,707	19 stifles

and heparin anticoagulants as preservatives for synovial fluid, samples stored in heparin showed a fourfold and ninefold greater decrease in total nucleated cell counts over 24 hours and 48 hours at 4°C, respectively.[8] In contrast, EDTA reportedly decreases synovial fluid mucin quality; therefore, total nucleated cell counts on fluid samples collected into an EDTA tube may not be increased by hyaluronidase. Regardless of the anticoagulant or preservative used, synovial fluid should be pretreated with hyaluronidase when automated hematology analyzers are used for cell counts.[10,11]

Nucleated cell counts may also be performed by using a hemocytometer. In clear or nonturbid specimens (i.e., specimens that appear to have a low total nucleated cell count), the sample may be counted undiluted. However, if the sample is turbid and the anticipated nucleated cell count is high, the specimen should be diluted. A WBC-diluting pipette and physiological saline are suitable for this purpose. The LeukoChek test (Biomedical Polymers, Inc.) and brand Leuko-TIC test (Bioanalytic GmbH) for manual WBC counts may also be used; however, the use of an acetic acid diluent should be avoided because it causes mucin to clot and invalidates the results.

Because of lack of utility in clinical application, RBC counts are not typically reported. Samples from normal patients contain very few RBCs and are a result of incidental blood contamination at the time of collection.

Total Protein Concentration

Comparatively few studies have reported baseline values for total protein concentration, and this probably reflects the relatively low priority given to this value. Other tests are preferred because sample volume is usually insufficient to allow for protein measurement. Synovial fluid protein concentration is best measured by a quantitative biochemical assay because refractometry measures other solutes and protein. A study of normal stifle, shoulder, and carpal joints reported a total protein concentration reference interval of 1.8 to 4.8 grams per deciliter (g/dL), as measured by the refractometer.[3] Normal synovial fluid does not clot in vitro because it is essentially free of fibrinogen and other clotting factors. Joint fluid may form a thixolabile gel if left undisturbed for several hours. Because clots are not thixotropic, normal fluid can be distinguished from clotting by gently shaking the sample to restore fluidity. If a specimen forms a clot after collection, this indicates intraarticular hemorrhage or inflammation with increased vascular permeability and protein exudation into the joint space (Fig. 12.11).

CYTOLOGICAL EXAMINATION

When only a few drops of fluid are collected, cytological reports should include subjective assessments of the amount of blood present, total nucleated cell count, and sample viscosity. When cell count and mucin clot test are performed, incongruities with the subjective assessments should be reported.

Normal synovial fluid contains very few RBCs. Increased RBC numbers may result from hemorrhage associated with collection and trauma or inflammation involving the joint capsule. Generalizations regarding the cellularity of synovial fluid may be consistently made via freshly prepared direct smears. The body of the smear of normal specimens contains two 2 cells per field at 400× magnification (40× objective). Cellularity of direct smears are categorized as normal (Fig. 12.12), slightly increased, moderately increased (Fig. 12.13), or

TABLE 12.4	**Reference Intervals for Synovial Fluid in Healthy Dogs and Cats**				
	DOG[4]			**CAT[5]**	
Parameter	Range	Mean		Range	Mean
Volume (milliliter [mL])	1 drop–1.0	0.24		1 drop–0.25	—
Nucleated cell count (cells per microliter [cells/μL])	0–2900	430		2–1134	161
Neutrophils (%)	0–12	1.4		0–39	3.6
Mononuclear cells (%)	88–100	98.6		61–100	96.4

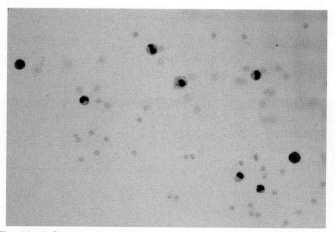

Fig. 12.11 Synovial fluid from a cat with severe blunt force trauma. A fibrin clot in the fluid suggests hemorrhage or protein exudation into the joint space. Such a fibrin bundle can entangle nucleated cells and cause unpredictably altered total nucleated cell counts and aberrant white blood cell differentials (Wright stain, original magnification 500×).

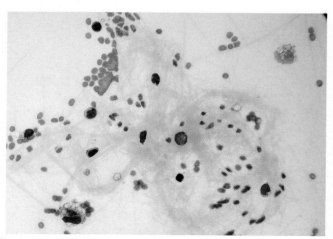

Fig. 12.12 Sediment smear of synovial fluid from a dog with degenerative arthropathy. Note the normal (low) cell count and random distribution of cells. The latter suggests decreased viscosity (May-Grünwald-Giemsa stain, original magnification 200×).

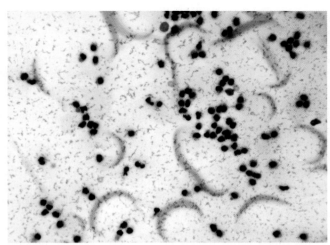

Fig. 12.13 Synovial fluid from a cat with arthritis. Fluid protein is observed as pink granular or stippled material and crescents (Wright stain, original magnification 500×).

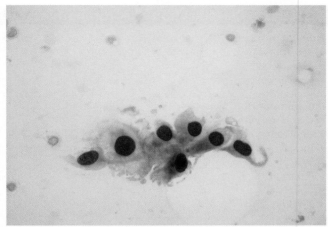

Fig. 12.14 Synovial fluid from a dog without cytological evidence of degenerative or inflammatory joint diseases. An incidental observation included a cluster of intimal cells sampled from the synovial lining with a few of the large mononuclear cells demonstrating a spindle cell–like appearance. The scanty, amorphous, pink material embedded among the cells is likely intimal matrix or stroma (Wright-Giemsa stain, original magnification 500×).

markedly increased (see Fig. 12.9). Because of unpredictable variation among processing techniques and instrumentation, such assessments are impractical with concentrated specimens (sediment and cytocentrifuge smears).

Because of the high viscosity of normal synovial fluid, cells of direct and centrifuged sediment smears tend to line up in rows (i.e., wind rowing, see Fig. 12.9). This characteristic arrangement may be used to comment on sample viscosity when volume is not sufficient for viscosity and mucin clot tests. However, in smears from synovial fluid with low cell counts, wind rowing may not be apparent, even though viscosity is normal.

Smears of normal, and sometimes abnormal, synovial fluid may have a pink granular proteinaceous background (see Figs. 12.13 and 12.28), which must not be confused with bacteria.

Nucleated cells should be classified as neutrophils, large mononuclear cells, lymphocytes, or eosinophils. On poorly made slides, it may be difficult to differentiate collapsed neutrophils from lymphocytes (see Fig. 12.13). Classification as mononuclear cells encompasses those that are phagocytically active. These cells could be derived from blood monocytes, tissues macrophages, or synovial lining cells. The origin of these cells has little practical importance with regard to clinical diagnosis and therapy. The proportion of large mononuclear cells that have phagocytized debris, cells, or microorganisms should be recorded. On smears that are freshly made or from fluid not exposed to EDTA, the degree of vacuolated large mononuclear cells should be noted and reported as mild, moderate, or marked. Sometimes, intact portions of intimal cells are directly sampled from the synovial lining, and a fraction of the large mononuclear component may have a spindle cell–like appearance. Observation of these spindloid cells may be seen in normal and diseased joints (Fig. 12.14). Overall assessment of nucleated cell morphology ought to include comments on the degree of karyolysis, pyknosis, and karyorrhexis. Delayed processing may lead to nuclear degeneration and increased numbers of markedly vacuolated large mononuclear cells.[3] Synovial fluid nucleated cell differentials are reported as percentage values and are incorporated into the interpretation of a total nucleated cell count or subjective assessment of cellularity.

Reports of normal canine synovial fluid nucleated cell differentials indicate that neutrophils make up as much as 12% of nucleated cells but frequently compose less than 5% of all nucleated cells.[3,4,12,13]

Eosinophils are absent.[3,4,12,14] Lymphocyte values may be quite variable, with studies reporting 0% to 100% (mean 44%) and 3% to 28% (mean 11%).[3,4] The balance of nucleated cells in normal joints are large mononuclear cells, ranging from 64% to 97% in one study to 60% to 92% in another study. In samples of normal joints processed immediately by direct smear, the percentage of large mononuclear cells that were markedly vacuolated was about 9%.[3] As with delayed processing, pretreatment of fluid with hyaluronidase may increase the percentage of large mononuclear cells that are markedly vacuolated to about 14% to 18%.

A study of normal feline synovial fluids reports that mononuclear cells predominate, ranging from 61% to 100% of all nucleated cells (mean 96.4%), with smaller proportions of neutrophils that vary from 0% to 39% of all nucleated cells (mean 3.6%).[5] Within the mononuclear cell component, lymphocytes or small mononuclear cells make up 0% to 45% of all mononuclear cells (mean 9.1%), and large mononuclear cells include 0% to 100% of all mononuclear cells (mean 81%). Freshly prepared smears from these cats reveal that among mononuclear cells, 0% to 100% of cells are vacuolated (mean 9.9%).

BACTERIOLOGICAL CULTURE

Conventional agar-based or broth-type bacteriological culture methods have been shown to lack sensitivity compared with blood culture methods.[15-17] Liquid blood culture media offer several advantages, including culture of larger volumes compared with culture plates, resins that decrease the inhibitory effects of antibiotics and substances intrinsic to synovial fluid, and lytic agents that release microorganisms phagocytized by inflammatory cells. Because relatively small volumes are retrieved with arthrocentesis of cats and dogs, pediatric blood culture bottles or tubes are most appropriate. Blood culture tubes or bottles should be inoculated at the time of fluid collection and incubated for 24 hours at 37°C, at which time the resulting growth is transferred to appropriate growth media.

It has been suggested that culturing a synovial membrane biopsy specimen may be superior to culture of synovial fluid, but this was not shown to be the case when stifle joints were experimentally infected with *Staphylococcus intermedius*.[17]

BOX 12.4 Classification of Arthropathies

Noninflammatory
- Degenerative
- Trauma
- Acute hemarthrosis

Inflammatory
- Chronic hemarthrosis
- Infectious
- Bacterial
- Viral
- Rickettsial
- Spirochetal
- Fungal
- Protozoal
- Mycoplasmal
- Noninfectious or immune-mediated
- Nonerosive
- Idiopathic (type I)—no identified concurrent disease
- Reactive (type II)—extraarticular infectious or inflammatory disease
- Enteropathic (type III)—primary infectious or inflammatory gastrointestinal or hepatic disease
- Malignancy-associated (type IV)—neoplasia distant from joint
- Drug-associated
- Vaccine reaction
- Polyarthritis–meningitis syndrome
- Polyarthritis–polymyositis syndrome
- Systemic lupus erythematosus
- Lymphoplasmacytic gonitis
- Juvenile-onset polyarthritis of Akitas
- Synovitis-amyloidosis of Shar-Peis
- Erosive
- Rheumatoarthritis (idiopathic erosive polyarthritis)
- Progressive feline polyarthritis

SYNOVIAL FLUID CHANGES IN DISEASED JOINTS

Because synovial fluid demonstrates a limited spectrum of response to diseases, and distinction among subcategories of long-standing disease is difficult, arthropathies are initially classified by broad categories such as inflammatory or noninflammatory and infectious or immune-mediated (Box 12.4). More definitive classification of arthritis requires supporting diagnostics that include radiography, microbial culture, serology, molecular diagnostics, and a medical database incorporating, at a minimum, history and physical examination, complete blood cell count, biochemical profile, and complete urinalysis (Fig. 12.15).

NONINFLAMMATORY ARTHROPATHIES

Degenerative Arthropathies

Degenerative arthropathies are linked to trauma, congenital or genetic bone anomalies, acquired anatomical disorders that impose abnormal stresses on articular surfaces, metabolic disturbance, nutritional disorders, or neoplasia.[18] Orthopedic diseases that may cause degenerative arthropathies include primary osteoarthritis, osteochondritis dissecans, elbow dysplasia, avascular necrosis of the femoral head, hip dysplasia, chronic patellar dislocations, and joint instabilities caused by ligament damage (e.g., rupture of the cranial cruciate ligament).

General synovial fluid changes are outlined in Table 12.5. Cytological findings may be abnormal before radiographic changes are readily apparent.[19] Cytological examination of the effusion may reveal a number of changes.[4,18,19] The total nucleated cell count is usually normal to slightly increased with a predominance of large mononuclear cells, of which greater than 10% are moderately to markedly vacuolated or phagocytic (Figs. 12.16 to 12.19). The percentage of neutrophils is typically within reference limits, although in some cases they are absent or the neutrophil percentage may be somewhat increased. The total protein concentration is frequently within the reference interval to a slightly increased level, and the fluid does not clot. Hemorrhage is marginal to absent, but in patients with capsular trauma, superimposition of transient, mild inflammation and hemorrhage may be seen. If damage to articular cartilage is severe enough, osteoclasts and chondrocytes may exfoliate into the fluid component (Fig. 12.20).

Dogs with a partial rupture of the cruciate ligament may have synovial fluid with a moderate increase in cellularity, which is predominantly caused by mononuclear cells or, in some patients, a slight increase in the percentage of neutrophils.[20,21] In contrast, cell counts in the synovial fluid of dogs with a complete rupture of the cruciate ligament were similar to those of normal dogs.[20] The volume of fluid present may vary from slightly to markedly increased.

Acute Hemarthrosis

Differential diagnoses associated with hemarthrosis include accidental iatrogenic blood contamination or concurrent hemorrhage associated with inflammatory and noninflammatory joint effusions.

In acute hemarthrosis, arthrocentesis yields bloody fluid from the time the sample first flows through the needle. With hemodilution, turbidity will increase, and fluid viscosity tends to decrease. Hemarthrosis elicits an inflammatory response, and within hours erythrophagocytosis and a mildly increased neutrophil density are evident. In a study in which canine stifle joints were injected with autologous blood (average 5.7×10^6 RBCs/μL), RBC clearance began as soon as 15 minutes and at 24 hours and 48 hours, a 71% and 96% decrease occurred in RBC concentration, respectively. In these same dogs, WBC concentrations were increased by 24 hours.[22] Lameness caused by hemarthrosis usually has an acute onset. With long-standing intraarticular hemorrhage, the joint fluid may have a xanthochromic supernatant. Recurrent hemarthrosis and resulting lameness are the most common manifestations of canine hemophilia A.[23] Intraarticular hemorrhage, for periods as short as 4 days, may cause decreases in cartilage matrix proteoglycan content and synthesis, which may interfere with cartilage metabolism and repair and eventually result in degenerative joint disease.[24]

With iatrogenic hemorrhage, synovial fluid usually is not bloody at the beginning of the procedure. But as the arthrocentesis goes on, an admixture of blood may suddenly appear, signaling puncture or rupture of a blood vessel. As soon as iatrogenic hemorrhage is recognized, collection at that joint should be ended. Blood contamination may be reduced by using minimal negative pressure for retrieval of fluid and gently releasing negative pressure of the syringe before withdrawing the needle from the joint capsule. Cytologically, only a small amount of blood is present and often without erythrophagocytosis. Platelets may be observed with recent, peracute hemorrhage or iatrogenic blood contamination (Fig. 12.21).

Hemorrhage associated with degenerative and inflammatory arthropathies is usually mild compared with true hemarthrosis.

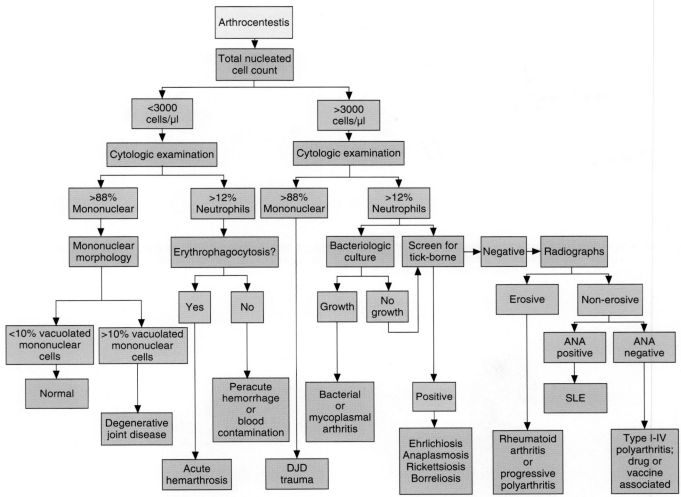

Fig. 12.15 Diagnostic plan for cytological evaluation of canine synovial fluid. *ANA*, antinuclear antibodies; *DJD*, degenerative joint disease; *SLE*, systemic lupus erythematosus.

TABLE 12.5 Characteristics of Synovial Fluid Responses to Articular Injury

Category	Color	Turbidity	Viscosity	Mucin Clot	NUCLEATED CELL DENSITY		Causes
					Total	Differential	
Acute hemarthrosis	Red	Increased proportional to amount of blood	Mild to marked decrease	Fair to poor	Increased proportional to amount of blood	Differential may be similar to peripheral blood with platelets	Coagulopathies, such as factor deficiency; severe blunt force trauma
Degenerative arthropathy	Normal	Usually normal	Normal to mildly decreased	Fair to poor	Likely increased	Mo: Normal to increased, with vacuolation and phagocytic activity PMN: Increased	Osteoarthrosis or degenerative joint diseases; trauma; neoplasia
Inflammatory arthropathy	Yellow to off-white or red-brown	Increased in relation to the amount of inflammation and hemorrhage	Mildly to markedly decreased	Fair to very poor	Increased	Mo: normal to increased PMN: Increased	Infection; immune-mediated arthropathies

Mo, Large mononuclear cells; *PMN,* neutrophils.

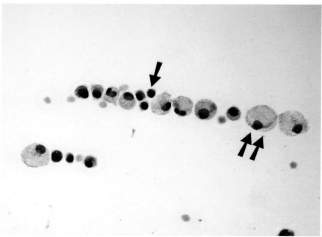

Fig. 12.16 Synovial fluid from a dog with degenerative arthropathy, showing large mononuclear cells *(double arrow)* or macrophage-type cells mingled with lymphocytes *(arrow)* (Wright stain, original magnification 500×).

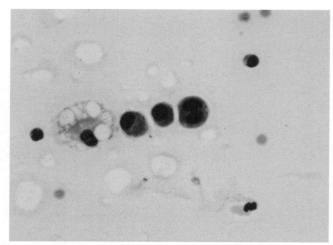

Fig. 12.19 Synovial fluid from the stifle joint of a dog with a partially ruptured cranial cruciate ligament. The array of large mononuclear cells includes a binucleate form that is suggestive of hyperplasia of the intimal cell lining (Wright-Giemsa stain, original magnification 500×).

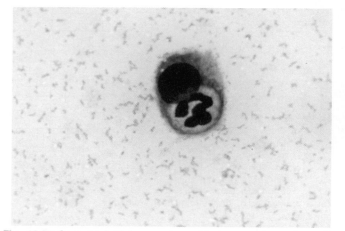

Fig. 12.17 Synovial fluid from a dog with degenerative arthropathy. Note the leukophagocytic macrophage, indicating ongoing inflammation (Wright-Giemsa stain, original magnification 1000×).

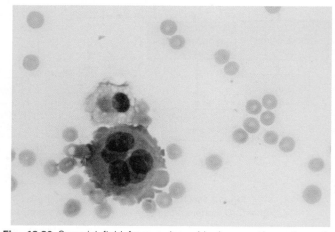

Fig. 12.20 Synovial fluid from a dog with degenerative arthropathy. Note the multinucleate, large, mononuclear cell, an osteoclast, that indicates articular cartilage erosion to subchondral bone (Wright-Giemsa stain, original magnification 500×).

Cytologically, erythrophagocytosis appears in conjunction with changes characteristic of the underlying cause (Fig. 12.22).

It is important to always send premade, direct smears, especially if the fluid sample is mailed to a laboratory because erythrophagocytosis, along with other cell changes, may occur in transit and interfere with interpretation. Submitting premade smears along with the fluid sample allows for identification of artifacts that developed in transit.

Neoplasia

Although uncommon, neoplasms may arise within joints, invade from adjacent tissues, or metastasize to joints. Neoplasms that may affect the joints include synovial cell sarcoma, histiocytic sarcoma, synovial myxoma, chondrosarcoma, osteosarcoma, fibrosarcoma, metastatic bronchial carcinoma, and lymphoma.[2,25-27] Diagnosis is made by obtaining a biopsy sample of the lesion for histopathological examination. Cytological examination of such biopsies is described in other chapters throughout this textbook. Synovial fluid changes are poorly described, but conceivably characteristics of a degenerative or inflammatory arthropathy could be present. Neoplastic cells are infrequently evident in these fluids (Fig. 12.23).

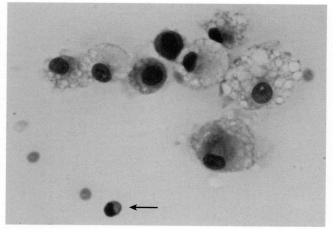

Fig. 12.18 Synovial fluid from the stifle joint of a dog with a partially ruptured cranial cruciate ligament. The majority of nucleated cells are large mononuclear, among which most show a moderate to marked density of variable-sized, colorless, clear, cytoplasmic vacuoles. A single lymphocyte is present *(arrow)* (Wright-Giemsa stain, original magnification 500×).

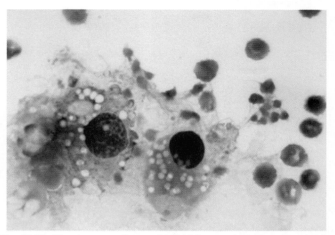

Fig. 12.21 Direct smear of synovial fluid from a dog. Note the platelet clump, indicating recent hemorrhage. The large, mononuclear cell, on the far left, is not intact and the erythrocytes along its edge are not convincing evidence of erythrophagocytosis. In this case, hemorrhage was caused by iatrogenic contamination (Wright-Giemsa stain, original magnification 1000×).

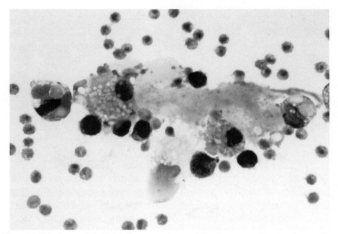

Fig. 12.22 Synovial fluid from a dog with degenerative arthropathy. Note the erythrophagocytic macrophage, on the far left, that indicates concurrent hemorrhage, and in spite of the large platelet clump this is not iatrogenic contamination (Wright-Giemsa stain, original magnification 500×).

INFLAMMATORY ARTHROPATHIES

Inflammatory arthropathies are either infectious or noninfectious and immune mediated (see Box 12.4) and associated with an exudate showing increased neutrophil numbers and variable increases in the number of large mononuclear cells, which may be vacuolated or have engulfed debris. Concurrent and often mild hemorrhagic diapedesis is common. Other findings are listed in Table 12.5.

Fundamentally, the greater the inflammatory reaction, the more discolored and turbid is the fluid, and the poorer is the viscosity. Mucin clot test results often parallel sample viscosity. The total protein concentration is increased, and the sample may readily clot. Fibrin strands often cause clumping of inflammatory cells in the smear. If not apparent on a routinely stained smear, fibrin strands may be demonstrated by staining with new methylene blue (Figs. 12.24 to 12.26).

Infectious Arthritides

Infectious arthritis is an inflammatory arthropathy, in which the causative infectious agent might be cultured or isolated from synovial membrane or joint fluid. This is not to be confused with infectious diseases that occur far from the joint and cause arthritis via a hypersensitivity disorder. Although infectious arthritides are uncommon among dogs and cats, bacteria are the most frequently isolated cause, with far fewer cases attributed to rickettsiae, spirochetes, *Mycoplasma* spp., fungi, viruses, and protozoans. Clinical presentation and history may be quite helpful because most infectious arthritides of a mature animal are monoarticular, acute in onset, and often the result of a percutaneous penetrating or surgical wound. When polyarticular infectious arthritides do occur, they are likely of hematogenous origin, as in omphalophlebitis in neonates or bacterial endocarditis in mature animals.

Bacterial Arthritides

Bacterial infectious arthritides demonstrate a markedly increased total nucleated cell count, usually greater than 50,000 cells/μL, with a predominance of neutrophils that are often greater than 75% of all nucleated cells.[28] Neutrophils are often intact and inconsistently show karyolysis or pyknosis and karyorrhexis (Fig. 12.27). Karyolytic degeneration of cells suggests a septic process; however, in many infected joints, degenerative leukocyte changes or microorganisms are not observed. When clinical observations and intuition dictate, joint fluid should be reflexively cultured. Organisms commonly cultured from dogs with an infected joint include *Staphylococcus intermedius*, *Staphylococcus aureus*, or β-hemolytic *Streptococcus* spp.[29] Among cats with bacterial arthritis, hemolytic strains of *Escherichia coli* or *Pasteurella multocida* are most common.[30] Failure to isolate organisms on culture does not necessarily exclude a bacterial cause. The absence of bacteria on cytological specimens may represent prior antibiotic therapy or an exuberant inflammatory response. Caution is warranted when attributing favorable clinical response to empiric antibiotic therapy with tetracyclines (e.g., doxycycline), because some of these drugs have immune modulatory, antiinflammatory, and chondroprotective properties.[31,32]

Rickettsial Arthritides

Granulocytic morulae have been observed in joint fluid of dogs infected with *Ehrlichia ewingii*.[33] Polymerase chain reaction (PCR) amplification of *E. ewingii* deoxyribonucleic acid (DNA) was used to differentiate it from infection with *Anaplasma phagocytophila*, formerly called *Escherichia equi*. Patients presented with fever, lameness, thrombocytopenia, and, on occasion, central nervous system signs (i.e., proprioceptive deficits, neck pain, paraparesis, or ataxia). Neutrophilic polyarthritis was diagnosed in dogs with lameness, and joint fluid contained a total nucleated cell count ranging from 16,000 to 125,000 cells/μL, of which neutrophils made up 63% to 99%. As with other rickettsial infections, polyarthritis is likely caused by immune complex–mediated disease or hemarthrosis.[34] Some reports have suggested that granulocytic morulae might be observed in 1% to 7% of neutrophils in synovial fluid and 0.1% to 26% of neutrophils in peripheral blood (Fig. 12.28).[35,36] Tentative identification of granulocytic morulae as *A. phagocytophila* may be based on geographical distribution because the tick vectors for this organism are found in western United States and Canada and upper midwestern and northeastern United States.[37]

Spirochetal Arthritides

Arthritis is the most common clinical sign in dogs with Lyme disease, which is caused by the spirochete *Borrelia burgdorferi*. Joints closest to the site of the infecting tick bite are often involved in

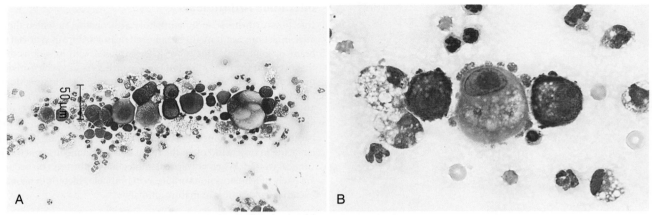

Fig. 12.23 Synovial fluid from a dog with a metastatic bronchiolar-alveolar carcinoma. (A) Low-magnification view showing a mixture of cells that includes metastatic carcinoma cells with many criteria of malignancy, including large prominent nucleoli (Wright stain, original magnification 100×). (B) Higher magnification showing metastatic carcinoma cells (Wright stain, original magnification 250×).

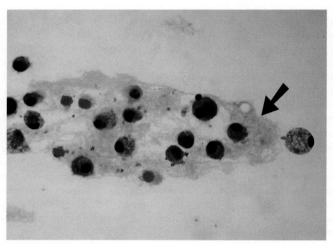

Fig. 12.24 Synovial fluid from a dog with degenerative arthropathy. Note the large clump of fibrin with enmeshed cells *(arrow)*. This is more often seen in inflammatory arthropathies (Wright stain, original magnification 500×).

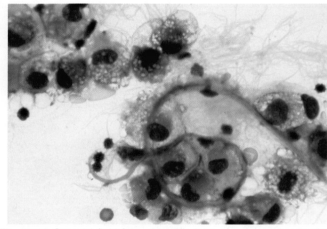

Fig. 12.26 Synovial fluid from the stifle joint of a dog with a partially ruptured cranial cruciate ligament. The large, mononuclear cells and thin band of pink-staining collagen are trapped by a clump of fibrin, which is noted in the upper right corner (Wright-Giemsa stain, original magnification 500×).

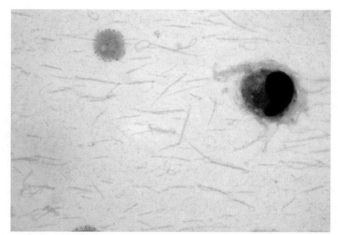

Fig. 12.25 Synovial fluid from a dog with degenerative arthropathy. The background contains numerous individualized strands of fibrin and is clumped around the right-most edge of the large mononuclear cell. This is not to be mistaken for an infectious agent (Wright stain, original magnification 1000×).

the first episodes of lameness and demonstrate the most extreme synovial fluid abnormalities. Although not observed on routine microscopy, live spirochetes are most frequently cultured from synovial membranes closest to the bite site.[38] Chronic oligoarthritis can be transient to persistent and may be caused by wider migration of spirochetes or antibody-mediated and T lymphocyte–driven responses.[39] Because acute Lyme arthritis presents with monoarthritis or oligoarthritis, synovial fluid changes may be varied from joint to joint within the same dog. Joints of limbs that demonstrate lameness may have total nucleated cell counts that range between 1400 and 76,200 cells/μL (median 12,700 cells/μL), with neutrophils composing up to 97% of all nucleated cells (median 54%). In the same dog with monoarthritis or oligoarthritis, other joints may be quite dissimilar, with total nucleated cell counts ranging between 100 and 3300 cells/μL (median 710 cells/μL) and sometimes include up to 19% neutrophils (median 0%). Dogs without lameness that are culture positive and seropositive for *B. burgdorferi* typically have total nucleated cell counts ranging between 100 and 3000 cells/μL (median 600 cells/μL) but do not contain more that 15% neutrophils (median 0%).[38]

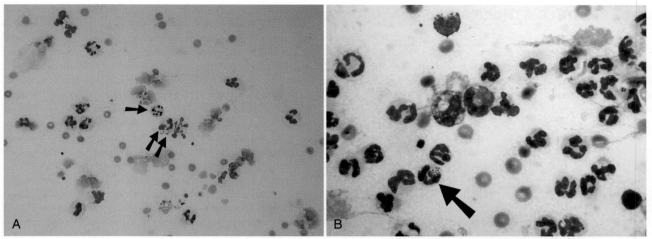

Fig. 12.27 Synovial fluid from a dog with septic suppurative (neutrophilic) arthritis. (A) Note nucleated cell with pyknotic nuclear material *(arrow)* and neutrophil with engulfed bacteria *(double arrow)*. Background contains other neutrophils with hydropic degeneration (degenerative neutrophils) along with nuclear debris and erythrocytes (Wright stain, original magnification 500×). (B) Note neutrophil with engulfed bacteria *(arrow)* (Wright stain, original magnification 1000×).

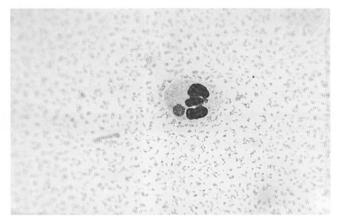

Fig. 12.28 Synovial fluid from a dog with ehrlichial polyarthritis. Note the *Ehrlichia morula* in the neutrophil and the normal granular, eosinophilic proteinaceous background (Wright stain, original magnification 1250×).

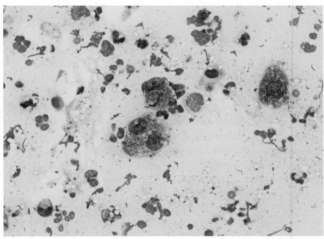

Fig. 12.29 Synovial fluid from a cat showing *Histoplasma capsulatum* engulfed by a macrophage and free in the background (Wright stain, original magnification 1000×).

Fungal Arthritides

Fungal arthritides are uncommon but have been reported as a sequela of osteomyelitis or disseminated infection by *Blastomyces dermatitidis*, *Cryptococcus neoformans*, *Aspergillus* spp., *Coccidioides immitis*, *Histoplasma capsulatum*, and *Sporothrix schenckii*.[40,41] On occasion, fungal elements might be visible in synovial fluid (Fig. 12.29).

Mycoplasmal Arithritides

Mycoplasmal arthritis has been diagnosed as a few rare cases in dogs and cats. The inflammatory reaction is neutrophilic with good cell morphology. Organisms may be observed on Romanowsky-stained smears or on mycoplasmal culture. Erosive polyarthritis of young Grayhounds has been associated with *Mycoplasma spumans*.[42] *Mycoplasma gateae* and *Mycoplasma felis* have been isolated from synovial fluid of immunocompromised cats with polyarthritis.[30,43]

Protozoal Arthritides

Polyarthritis has been documented with canine visceral leishmaniasis that is caused by geographical variants of the *Leishmania donovani* complex, *L. donovani*, or *L. infantum*. Synovial fluid sometimes shows mononuclear inflammation and *Leishmania* spp. amastigotes in synovial fluid macrophages (Fig. 12.30).[44,45]

Viral Arthritides

Feline calicivirus infection has been associated with lameness in kittens.[46] However, synovial fluid changes in experimental infections were minimal, with synovial fluid macrophage numbers subjectively increased to a moderate degree, and some leukophagocytosis exhibited.[47] Occasionally, cellularity may be markedly increased, but a predominance of macrophages with many exhibiting leukophagocytosis will still be present.[48]

IMMUNE-MEDIATED ARTHROPATHIES

Immune-mediated arthritides of dogs and cats are generally considered to be a type III hypersensitivity phenomenon.[49,50] Emerging evidence suggests concurrent cell-mediated or genetic mechanisms.[51,52] Arthritis is caused by immune complexes that are composed of circulating antigen and immunoglobulin G (IgG) or IgM antibodies. Much like renal glomeruli, synovial capillaries ultrafilter plasma, and as a result, immune complexes

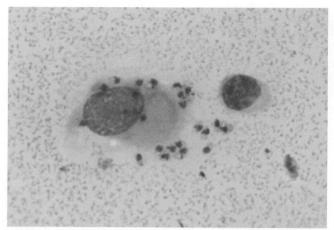

Fig. 12.30 Synovial fluid specimen showing *Leishmania* spp. amastigotes engulfed by a macrophage and free in the background (Wright stain, original magnification 1000×).

commonly are deposited at these locations. Deposited immune complexes activate inflammatory cells to secrete cytokines that increase vascular permeability, augmenting immune complex deposition and further accelerating tissue and vessel damage via complement and Fc (Fragment, crystallizable) receptor–mediated pathways. Clinicopathological features of immune-mediated arthritides are a reflection of immune complex predisposition for certain sites and are not determined by the primary source of the antigen. Because antibodies involved in immune-mediated arthropathies are not usually against fixed cells or tissue antigen, these immune complex–mediated diseases tend to have a systemic component, affecting multiple joints either concurrently or consecutively. Signals of systemic disease in patients with immune-mediated arthritis include fever, generalized stiffness, peripheral blood cytopenias, difficult-to-localize pain, neck or back pain, lymphadenopathy, or proteinuria.[53] Polyarthritis, associated with systemic immune-complex disease, is sometimes subclinical, and a patient may not demonstrate joint swelling or pain; therefore four or more joints should be sampled with sufficient volume for complete fluid analysis.[41,54] See Boxes 12.5 and 12.6 for summaries of diagnostic features.

NONEROSIVE ARTHROPATHIES

Idiopathic (Type I) Polyarthritis

Idiopathic, or immune-mediated, polyarthritis is diagnosed by exclusion of other possible causes or specific disease and breed associations. Among canine immune-mediated arthritides, idiopathic type I polyarthritis is the most common.[49] Dogs frequently present with stiffness, pyrexia, lymphadenopathy, and inappetence. Clinical signs of joint inflammation are commonly observed in all limbs, or less often just the hind legs, with carpal, hock, or stifle joints typically affected.[55] It

---

BOX 12.5 Diagnostic Features of Nonerosive, Immune-Mediated Arthritides

Idiopathic Polyarthritides for Which Other Causes of Inflammatory Arthropathy Have Been Ruled Out

- Type I—no evidence of types II, III, or IV
- Type II—Concurrent inflammatory process distant from joint (i.e., respiratory, urogenital, or integumentary systems)
- Type III—Associated with gastroenteritis of various causes or hepatopathy
- Type IV—Polyarthritis associated with malignancy remote from joint

Drug-Associated Reaction

- Arthritis develops in association with drug administration
- Previous exposure or long-term therapy
- Most commonly antibiotics, such as potentiated sulfonamides, penicillins, and cephalosporins
- Signs resolve within 7 days of discontinuation

Vaccine Reaction

- 5 to 7 days after first dose of primary immunization
- Self-limiting, lasting 1 to 3 days
- Noted with feline calicivirus and canine polyvalent modified live virus vaccines

Polyarthritis–Meningitis Syndrome

- Concurrent signs of polyarthritis and neck pain
- Cerebrospinal fluid pleocytosis
- Reported with Bernese Mountain Dog, Boxer, Corgi, German Shorthair Pointer, Newfoundland, or Weimaraner
- Negative antinuclear antibody test

Polyarthritis–Polymyositis Syndrome

- Exercise intolerance and stiffness
- Myositis diagnosed in at least two muscle biopsies

Systemic Lupus Erythematosus

- Positive antinuclear antibody (ANA) test
- Diagnosis of multisystemic immune-mediated disease (three of the following, serially or concurrently):
  - Polyarthritis
  - Mucosal or cutaneous lesions
  - Anemia, leukopenia, or thrombocytopenia
  - Glomerulonephritis or persistent proteinuria
  - Polymyositis
  - Serositis

Lymphoplasmacytic Gonitis

- Linked to subset of dogs with cranial cruciate ligament rupture

Juvenile-Onset Polyarthritis of Akitas

- Clinical signs before age 8 months, most before age 1 year
- Neutrophilic arthritis noted with:
  - Cyclic pain
  - Generalized lymphadenopathy
  - Nonregenerative anemia
  - Rarely concurrent meningitis

Synovitis–Amyloidosis of Shar-Peis

- Swollen joints with recurrent fever
- Glomerular disease from amyloidosis (proteinuria)

BOX 12.6 Diagnostic Features of Erosive, Immune-Mediated Arthritides

Canine and Feline Idiopathic Erosive Polyarthritis (Rheumatoid Arthritis)
- Seropositive for rheumatoid factor
- Joint tenderness, pain, or swelling (one or more joints)
- Additional joints affected within 3 months of first joint being affected
- Eventual symmetrical joint swelling
- Inflammatory joint fluid, often neutrophilic
- Subcutaneous nodules
- Radiographic evidence of perichondral or subchondral osteolysis, cyst formation, and erosion
- Lesions confirmed via histopathologic examination of synovial membrane or subcutaneous nodules

Progressive Feline Polyarthritis
- More common among young adult male cats
- Concurrent infection with feline leukemia and foamy viruses
- Periosteal proliferative bone lesions (common type)
- Neutrophilic inflammatory joint fluid
- Erosive bone lesions
- Variable joint fluid; normal to neutrophilic or mixed and mononuclear inflammation

would not be unusual for the likelihood of type I polyarthritis to be overestimated because of limitations of a patient's medical workup; therefore, this diagnosis and subsequent immunosuppressive therapy should be employed with caution. Reported cases indicate that synovial fluid total nucleated cell counts ranged from 3700 to 130,000 cells/µL (mean 41,900 cells/µL) and are composed of approximately 20% to 98% neutrophils.[55]

Reactive (Type II) Polyarthritis

Reactive polyarthritis is defined as an aseptic inflammatory joint disease associated with extraarticular sites of infection such as urogenital tracts, respiratory tract, and skin.[41,56] Research suggests that difficult to culture bacteria may persist within the articular cavity, evading complete removal by the immune system through antigenic modulation, intracellular localization, molecular mimicry, and T-helper-cell imbalances (Th1/Th2 imbalance).[57] Because the evasion is incomplete, intraarticular inflammation may be caused by persistent bacterial antigens, such as lipopolysaccharides and portions of free bacterial DNA.[57] Reactive polyarthritis has been linked to various tick-transmitted diseases, including bartonellosis, borreliosis, Rocky Mountain spotted fever, canine and feline ehrlichiosis, and canine and feline anaplasmosis.[33,58-63]

Enteropathic (Type III) Polyarthritis

Enteropathic arthritis is associated with inflammatory bowel diseases. The specific pathogenesis is unknown, but current hypothesis suggests an impaired barrier function of intestinal mucosa to bacterial antigens and defective local immune regulation. Clinical signs of polyarthritis are occasionally noted in dogs with colitis and only rarely observed in cats and dogs with idiopathic inflammatory bowel diseases.[64] Hepatopathic arthropathy, considered a variant of enteropathic polyarthritis, has been observed in dogs with chronic active hepatitis and cirrhosis.[49]

Malignancy-Associated (Type IV) Polyarthritis

Polyarthritis linked to extraarticular neoplasms has been reported with canine tumors, such as mammary adenocarcinoma, squamous cell carcinoma, chemoreceptor neoplasia (heart base tumor), leiomyoma, and feline myeloproliferative disease.[41]

Polyarthritis–Meningitis Syndrome

Polyarthritis–meningitis syndrome is observed in both cats and dogs, among which cases are reported in the Bernese Mountain dog, Boxer, Corgi, German Shorthaired Pointer, Newfoundland, and Weimaraner.[41] This condition has been called *polyarteritis nodosa*.[49] Polyarthritis and meningitis have shared clinical signs, such as fever, cervical rigidity, and stiff gait. Therefore patients diagnosed with nonerosive, nonseptic polyarthritis and spinal pain could benefit from cerebrospinal fluid (CSF) analysis because untreated meningitis may result in permanent neurological deficits. Reports indicated that dogs diagnosed with concurrent steroid-responsive meningitis–arteritis and polyarthritis did not have lameness or joint swelling.[65] In these patients, 25% to 100% of joints sampled demonstrated inflammation that was typically neutrophilic or, sometimes, mixed inflammation.

Polyarthritis–Polymyositis Syndrome

Polyarthritis–polymyositis syndrome is of unknown etiology. Dogs diagnosed with this syndrome have symmetrical nonerosive neutrophilic polyarthritis, inflammatory myopathy found in two or more individual muscles (>6 individual muscles sampled per patient), and systemic lupus erythematosus (SLE), rheumatoid arthritis, or bacterial endocarditis are excluded. In some patients, plasma creatine phosphokinase (CPK) and plasma aldolase concentrations are increased above the reference intervals; however, the increases are inconsistent and should not be relied on to rule out the presence of polymyositis. The syndrome is assumed to have an immune-mediated component because of the absence of a detectible infectious cause and favorable response to immunosuppressive therapy.[66]

Drug-Associated Polyarthritis

Drug-associated polyarthritis is most commonly linked to antibiotics, such as sulfonamides, and, to a lesser degree, to cephalosporins, penicillins, erythromycin, and orlincomycin.[49] Doberman Pinchers, Miniature Schnauzers, and Samoyeds are especially prone to systemic hypersensitivity reactions associated with sulfonamides and their potentiated formulations.[67] Unlike Doberman Pinchers, among which all reported cases have polyarthritis, Miniature Schnauzers and Samoyeds less frequently demonstrate an associated arthropathy. More common abnormalities include fever, thrombocytopenia, hepatopathy (i.e., necrosis and cholestasis), transient neutropenia, keratoconjunctivitis sicca, and hemolysis. Among patients with a sulfonamide hypersensitivity reaction, those with an associated thrombocytopenia or hepatopathy are less likely to recover.[67]

Vaccine-Associated Polyarthritis

Vaccine-associated polyarthritis is reported in dogs and cats. Polyarthritis and radiographic lesions or clinical signs similar to hypertrophic osteodystrophy have been reported in young Weimaraners. Clinical signs typically appear within 7 days of polyvalent modified-live virus vaccine. All Weimaraners have a low serum immunoglobulin concentration that includes IgG or IgM and infrequently IgA.[68,69] Cats vaccinated against or infected with feline calicivirus have been reported to develop polyarthritis, which is often transitory and completely resolving within 48 hours.[70]

Systemic Lupus Erythematosus

Polyarthritis is the most consistent pathological finding among dogs with SLE, with carpal and tarsal joints more severely affected than elbow and stifle joints.[49] Cats with SLE can have arthritis, although less frequently than dogs, and some cats may not demonstrate lameness. Detection of antinuclear antibodies (ANAs) is paramount to the diagnosis of SLE, but no universally accepted criteria exist for further classification. In addition to polyarthritis, dogs will demonstrate one or two systemic manifestations involving the kidneys and skin or peripheral blood cytopenias, such as anemia and thrombocytopenia. Feline SLE is most commonly diagnosed on the basis of the presence of a characteristic dermatopathy or glomerulonephritis, as well as by polyarthritis, anemia, or central nervous system dysfunction with lower frequency.[71] Patients with SLE have a dysregulated immune system and are more likely to form autoantibodies, which can result in a type II hypersensitivity reaction against RBCs, platelets, or coagulation proteins.[49] Lupus erythematosus (LE) cells are rarely seen in synovial fluid, but when present are highly suggestive for SLE (Fig. 12.31).[49] LE cells can be confused with leukophagocytic macrophages (see Fig. 12.17) or neutrophils containing particulate nucleic acid (Figs. 12.32 and 12.33), which are erroneously referred to as "ragocytes." The term *ragocyte* refers to a neutrophil with numerous, small, dark intracytoplasmic granules observed on unstained wet preparations, not on stained smears. The granules in ragocytes are phagocytized immunoglobulin and complement. To avoid confusing terminology, the contents of neutrophils observed on a stained smear should be described. The LE cell preparation test detects serum antibodies to DNA histone complexes and has been used to diagnose SLE, but because of difficulties with test interpretation and poor performance characteristics, LE preps have been replaced by ANA testing. Low ANA titers may be detected with neoplastic, inflammatory, or infectious diseases and sometimes in clinically normal animals.[72]

Lymphoplasmacytic Gonitis

Lymphoplasmacytic gonitis has been linked to a small proportion of dogs that eventually develop, or have been diagnosed with, a cranial cruciate ligament rupture.[49] Among dogs with naturally occurring cranial cruciate ligament rupture and histologically confirmed lymphoplasmacytic synovitis, only 2% have lymphocytes detected in synovial fluid.[73] Although the etiology or sequence of lesions are unclear, evidence suggests a primary immune-mediated disease.[21]

Juvenile-Onset Polyarthritis of Akitas

Clinical signs of polyarthritis syndrome in Akitas typically appear before age 8 months and include neutrophilic arthritis, cyclical pain, generalized lymphadenopathy, and nonregenerative anemia. Rarely dogs have concurrent meningitis, have positive ANA test results, or are positive for rheumatoid factors.[74] It is speculated that this may be a canine overlap syndrome, in which patients have concurrent SLE and rheumatoid arthritis.

Polyarthritis–Amyloidosis of Shar-Pei Dogs

Unlike other breeds affected by amyloidosis, Chinese Shar-Pei dogs with familial amyloidosis may have swollen joints and recurrent fever that precedes glomerular disease.[75] Lameness and arthritis may be monoarticular and sometimes pauciarticular, which typically affects tarsal joints and, less often, carpal joints.[76]

EROSIVE ARTHROPATHIES

Idiopathic Erosive Polyarthritis (Rheumatoid Arthritis)

Rheumatoid factors (RFs) are autoantibodies directed against the Fc fragment of autologous IgG. Most RFs tests detect IgM autoantibodies, as these are most common; however, IgG or IgA autoantibodies do occur in disease. The significance of RFs in the pathogenesis of rheumatoid arthritis is currently unknown. Immune complexes involving

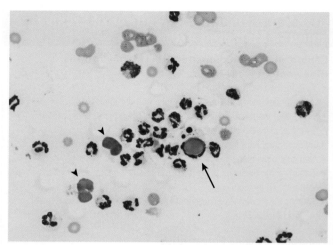

Fig. 12.31 Synovial fluid from a dog with immune-mediated polyarthritis. Most neutrophils have engulfed very small fragments of what appears to be nuclear material and one neutrophil *(arrow)* has an individual, homogeneous inclusion with a smooth border, which is a lupus erythematosus cell. The arrowheads point to free nuclear material from smudged inflammatory cells (Wright stain, original magnification 100×).

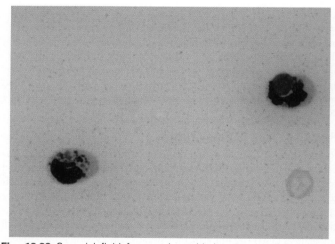

Fig. 12.32 Synovial fluid from a dog with immune-mediated polyarthritis. The neutrophil on the right is a lupus erythematosus cell, and the neutrophil on the left has engulfed very small fragments of what appears to be nuclear material (Wright-Giemsa stain, original magnification 1000×).

RFs are, in part, a cause of polyarthritis, and patients are often seropositive for RFs. See Box 12.6 for the diagnosis of rheumatoid arthritis.[77] On occasion, patients may have a low positive or transient ANA titer. Serum RFs and ANA are nonspecific autoantibodies and can be detect in patients with osteoarthritis and chronic inflammatory, neoplastic, or infectious diseases. Synovial fluid analysis reveals inflammation with a predominance of neutrophils, among which many have karyorrhetic and pyknotic nuclei.[78]

Progressive Feline Polyarthritis

The two types of progressive feline polyarthritis are (1) an erosive form, clinically similar to canine erosive arthritis; and (2) a more commonly diagnosed periosteal proliferative form. This disease most frequently affects young adult male cats. Feline foamy (syncytium-forming) virus

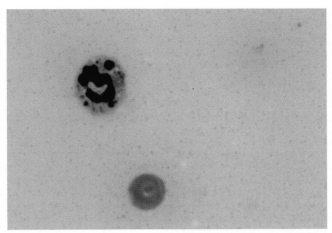

Fig. 12.33 Synovial fluid from a dog with immune-mediated polyarthritis. Note the neutrophil containing phagocytized material, probably nucleic acid. This material must be distinguished from bacteria (Wright-Giemsa stain, original magnification 1000×).

infection is consistently isolated from cats with chronic progressive polyarthritis, among which a majority are coinfected with feline leukemia virus.[79] Synovial fluid analysis reveals an inflammatory arthropathy with a predominance of neutrophils. Cats with the erosive form may have total nucleated cell counts within the reference interval or more prominent fractions of lymphocytes and large mononuclear cells.

REFERENCES

1. Smith MD. The normal synovium. *Open Rheumatol J.* 5:100–106. Published online December 30, 2011.
2. Craig LE, Thompson KG. Tumors of joints. In: Meuten DJ, ed. *Tumors in Domestic Animals.* 5th ed. Ames, IA: John Wiley & Sons Inc.; 2017:337–355.
3. Fernandez FR, Grindem CB, Lipowitz AJ. Synovial fluid analysis: preparation of smears for cytological examination of canine synovial fluid. *J Am Anim Hosp Assoc.* 1983;19:727–734.
4. Sawyer DC. Synovial fluid analysis of canine joints. *J Am Vet Med Assoc.* 1963;143:609–612.
5. Pacchiana PD, Gilley RS, Wallace LJ, et al. Absolute and relative cell counts for synovial fluid from clinically normal shoulder and stifle joints in cats. *J Am Vet Med Assoc.* 2004;225(12):1866–1870.
6. Ogston AG, Sherman TF. Degradation of the hyaluronic acid complex of synovial fluid by proteolytic enzymes and by ethylenediaminetetra-acetic acid. *Biochem J.* 1959;72(2):301–305.
7. Atilola MA, Lumsden JH, Rooke F. A comparison of manual and electronic counting for total nucleated cell counts on synovial fluid from canine stifle joints. *Can J Vet Res.* 1986;50(2):282–284.
8. Salinas M, Rosas J, Iborra J, et al. Comparison of manual and automated cell counts in EDTA preserved synovial fluids. Storage has little influence on the results. *Ann Rheum Dis.* 1997;56(10):622–626.
9. de Jonge R, Brouwer R, Smit M, et al. Automated counting of white blood cells in synovial fluid. *Rheumatology (Oxford).* 43(2):170–173.
10. Sugiuchi H, Ando Y, Manabe M, et al. Measurement of total and differential white blood cell counts in synovial fluid by means of an automated hematology analyzer. *J Lab Clin Med.* 2005;146(1):36–42.
11. Aulesa C, Mainar I, Prieto M, et al. Use of the Advia 120 hematology analyzer in the differential cytologic analysis of biological fluids (cerebrospinal, peritoneal, pleural, pericardial, synovial, and others). *Lab Hematol.* 2003;9(4):214–224.
12. Atilola MA, Lumsden JH, Hulland TJ, et al. Intra-articular tissue response to analytical grade metrizamide in dogs. *Am J Vet Res.* 1984;45(12):2651–2657.
13. Warren CF, Bennett GA, Bauer W. The significance of the cellular variations occurring in normal synovial fluid. *Am J Path.* 1935;11:953–968.
14. McCarty Jr DJ, Phelps P, Pyenson J. Crystal-induced inflammation in canine joints. I. An experimental model with quantification of the host response. *J Exp Med.* 1966;124(1):99–114.
15. MacWilliams PS, Friedrichs KR. Laboratory evaluation and interpretation of synovial fluid. *Vet Clin North Am Small Anim Pract.* 2003;33(1):153–178.
16. Shirtliff ME, Mader JT. Acute septic arthritis. *Clin Microbiol Rev.* 2002;15(4):527–544.
17. Montgomery RD, Long Jr IR, Milton JL, et al. Comparison of aerobic culturette, synovial membrane biopsy, and blood culture medium in detection of canine bacterial arthritis. *Vet Surg.* 1989;18(4):300–303.
18. Johnson KA, Watson ADJ. Skeletal diseases. In: Ettinger SJ, Feldman EC, eds. *Textbook of Veterinary Internal Medicine: Diseases of the Dog and Cat.* 6th ed. St. Louis, MO: Saunders; 2005:1965–1991.
19. Lewis DD, Goring RL, Parker RB, et al. A comparison of diagnostic methods used in the evaluation of early degenerative joint disease in the dog. *J Am Anim Hosp Assoc.* 1987;23:305–315.
20. Griffen DW, Vasseur PB. Synovial fluid analysis in dogs with cranial cruciate ligament rupture. *J Am Anim Hosp Assoc.* 1992;28:277–280.
21. Hayashi K, Manley PA, Muir P. Cranial cruciate ligament pathophysiology in dogs with cruciate disease: a review. *J Am Anim Hosp Assoc.* 2004;40(5):385–390.
22. Jansen NWD, Roosendaal G, Wenting MJG, et al. Very rapid clearance after a joint bleed in the canine knee cannot prevent adverse effects on cartilage and synovial tissue. *Osteoarthr Cartil.* 2009;14:433–440.
23. Mansell P. Hemophilia A and B. In: Giger U, ed. *Schalm's Veterinary Hematology.* 5th ed. Baltimore, MD: Lippincott Williams and Wilkins; 2000:1026–1029.
24. Hooiveld M, Roosendaal G, Vianen M, et al. Blood-induced joint damage: long term effects in vitro and in vivo. *J Rheumatol.* 2003;30(2):339–344.
25. Thompson KG, Pool RR. Tumors of bones. In: Meuten DJ, ed. *Tumors in Domestic Animals.* 4th ed. Ames, IA: Iowa State University Press; 2002:245–317.
26. Wilson DW, Dungworth DL. Tumors of the respiratory tract. In: Meuten DJ, ed. *Tumors In Domestic Animals.* 4th ed. Ames, IA: Iowa State University Press; 365–399.
27. Lahmers SM, Mealey KL, Martinez SA, et al. Synovial T-cell lymphoma of the stifle in a dog. *J Am Anim Hosp Assoc.* 2002;38(2):165–168.
28. Marchevsky AM, Read RA. Bacterial septic arthritis in 19 dogs. *Aust Vet J.* 1999;77(4):233–237.
29. Clements DN, Owen MR, Mosley JR, et al. Retrospective study of bacterial infective arthritis in 31 dogs. *J Small Anim Pract.* 2005;46(4). 171–171.
30. Liehmann L, Degasperi B, Spergser J, et al. *Mycoplasma felis* arthritis in two cats. *J Small Anim Pract.* 2006;47(8):476–479.
31. Jauernig S, Schweighauser A, Reist M, et al. The effects of doxycycline on nitric oxide and stromelysin production in dogs with cranial cruciate ligament rupture. *Vet Surg.* 2001;30(2):132–139.
32. Greene CE, Watson ADJ. Antibacterial chemotherapy. In: Greene CE, ed. *Infectious Disease of the Dog and Cat.* 3rd ed. St. Louis, MO: Saunders; 2006:274–301.
33. Goodman RA, Hawkins EC, Olby NJ, et al. Molecular identification of *Ehrlichia ewingii* infection in dogs: 15 cases (1997–2001). *J Am Vet Med Assoc.* 2003;222(8):1102–1107.
34. Greene CE, Budsberg SC. Musculoskeletal infections. In: Greene CE, ed. *Infectious Diseases of the Dog and Cat.* 3rd ed. Philadelphia, PA: Saunders; 2006:823–841.
35. Goldman EE, Breitschwerdt EB, Grindem CB, et al. Granulocytic ehrlichiosis in dogs from North Carolina and Virginia. *J Vet Intern Med.* 1998;12(2):61–70.
36. Stockham SL, Schmidt DA, Curtis KS, et al. Evaluation of granulocytic ehrlichiosis in dogs of Missouri, including serologic status to *Ehrlichia canis, Ehrlichia equi* and *Borrelia burgdorferi. Am J Vet Res.* 1992;53(1):63–68.
37. Poitout FM, Shinozaki JK, Stockwell PJ, et al. Genetic variants of *Anaplasma phagocytophilum* infecting dogs in Western Washington State. *J Clin Microbiol.* 2005;43(2):796–801.
38. Straubinger RK, Straubinger AF, Härter L, et al. *Borrelia burgdorferi* migrates into joint capsules and causes an up-regulation of interleukin-8 in synovial membranes of dogs experimentally infected with ticks. *Infect Immun.* 1997;65(4):1273–1285.

39. Straubinger RK, Straubinger AF, Summers BA, et al. *Borrelia burgdorferi* induces the production and release of proinflammatory cytokines in canine synovial explant cultures. *Infect Immun.* 1998;66(1):247–258.

40. Huss B, Collier L, Collins B, et al. Polyarthropathy and chorioretinitis with retinal detachment in a dog with systemic histoplasmosis. *J Am Anim Hosp Assoc.* 1994;30:217–224.

41. Bennett D. Immune-mediated and infective arthritis. In: Ettinger SJ, Feldman EC, eds. *Textbook of Veterinary Internal Medicine: Diseases of the Dog and Cat.* 6th ed. St. Louis, MO: Saunders; 2005:1958–1965.

42. Barton MD, Ireland L, Kirschner JL. Isolation of *Mycoplasma spumans* from polyarthritis in a greyhound. *Aust Vet J.* 1985;62(6):206–207.

43. Moise NS, Crissman JW, Fairbrother JF. *Mycoplasma gateae* arthritis and tenosynovitis in cats: case report and experimental reproduction of the disease. *Am J Vet Res.* 1983;44(1):16–21.

44. Gaskin AA, Schantz P, Jackson J, et al. Visceral leishmaniasis in a New York foxhound kennel. *J Vet Intern Med.* 2002;16(1):34–44.

45. Agut A, Corzo N, Murciano J, et al. Clinical and radiographic study of bone and joint lesions in 26 dogs with leishmaniasis. *Vet Rec.* 2003;153(21):648–652.

46. TerWee J, Lauritzen AY, Sabara M, et al. Comparison of the primary signs induced by experimental exposure to either a pneumotrophic or a limping strain of feline calicivirus. *Vet Microbiol.* 1997;56(1–2):33–45.

47. Pedersen NC, Laliberte L, Ekman S. A transient febrile limping syndrome of kittens caused by two different strains of feline calicivirus. *Feline Pract.* 1983;13:26–35.

48. Levy JK, Marsh A. Isolation of calicivirus from the joint of a kitten with arthritis. *J Am Vet Med Assoc.* 1992;201(5). 753–735.

49. Pedersen NC. A review of immunologic diseases of the dog. *Vet Immunol Immunopathol.* 1999;69(2–4):251–342.

50. Bennett D. Immune-based non-erosive inflammatory joint disease of the dog. III. Canine idiopathic polyarthritis. *J Small Anim Pract.* 1987;28:909–928.

51. Ollier WE, Kennedy LJ, Thomson W, et al. Dog MHC alleles containing the human RA shared epitope confer susceptibility to canine rheumatoid arthritis. *Immunogenetics.* 2001;53(8):669–673.

52. Hewicker-Trautwein M, Carter SD, Bennett D, et al. Immunocytochemical demonstration of lymphocyte subsets and MHC class II antigen expression in synovial membranes from dogs with rheumatoid arthritis and degenerative joint disease. *Vet Immunol Immunopathol.* 1999;67(4):341–357.

53. Goldstein RE. Swollen joints and lameness. In: Ettinger SJ, Feldman EC, eds. *Textbook of Veterinary Internal Medicine: Diseases of the Dog and Cat.* 6th ed. St. Louis, MO: Saunders; 2005:83–87.

54. Center SA. Fluid accumulation disorders. In: 4th ed. Willard MD, Tvedten H, Turnwald GH, eds. *Small Animal Clinical Diagnosis By Laboratory Methods.* St. Louis, MO: Saunders; 2004:263–266.

55. Clements DN, Gear RN, Tattersall J, et al. Type I immune-mediated polyarthritis in dogs: 39 cases (1997–2002). *J Am Vet Med Assoc.* 2004;224(8):1323–1327.

56. Rondeau MP, Walton RM, Bissett S, et al. Suppurative, nonseptic polyarthropathy in dogs. *J Vet Intern Med.* 2005;19(5):654–662.

57. Sibilia J, Limbach FX. Reactive arthritis or chronic infectious arthritis? *Ann Rheum Dis.* 2002;61(7):580–587.

58. MacDonald KA, Chomel BB, Kittleson MD, et al. A prospective study of canine infective endocarditis in northern California (1999–2001): emergence of *Bartonella* as a prevalent etiologic agent. *J Vet Intern Med.* 2004;18(1):56–64.

59. Goodman RA, Breitschwerdt EB. Clinicopathologic findings in dogs seroreactive to *Bartonella henselae* antigens. *Am J Vet Res.* 2005;66(12):2060–2064.

60. Summers BA, Straubinger AF, Jacobson RH, et al. Histopathological studies of experimental Lyme disease in the dog. *J Comp Pathol.* 2005;133(1):1–13.

61. Greene CE, Breitschwerdt EB. Rocky Mountain spotted fever, murine typhus like disease, rickettsial pox, typhus, and Q fever. In: Greene CE, ed. *Infectious Diseases of the Dog and Cat.* 3rd ed. St. Louis, MO: Saunders; 2006:232–245.

62. Breitschwerdt EB. Obligate Intracellular bacterial pathogens. In: Ettinger SJ, Feldman EC, eds. *Textbook of Veterinary Internal Medicine.* St. Louis, MO: Saunders; 2005:631–636.

63. Tarello W. Microscopic and clinical evidence for *Anaplasma (Ehrlichia) phagocytophilum* infection in Italian cats. *Vet Rec.* 2005;156(24):772–774.

64. Guilford WG. Idiopathic inflammatory bowel diseases. In: Guilford WG, Center SA, Strombeck DR, et al., eds. *Strombeck's Small Animal Gastroenterology.* 3rd ed. Philadelphia, PA: Saunders; 1996:451–486.

65. Webb AA, Taylor SM, Muir GD. Steroid-responsive meningitis-arteritis in dogs with noninfectious, nonerosive, idiopathic, immune-mediated polyarthritis. *J Vet Intern Med.* 2002;16(3):269–273.

66. Bennett D, Kelly DF. Immune-based non-erosive inflammatory joint disease of the dog. II. Polyarthritis/polymyositis syndrome. *J Small Anim Pract.* 1987;28:891–908.

67. Trepanier LA, Danhof R, Toll J. Clinical findings in 40 dogs with hypersensitivity associated with administration of potentiated sulfonamides. *J Vet Intern Med.* 2003;17(5):647–652.

68. Couto CG, Krakowka S, Johnson G, et al. In vitro immunologic features of Weimaraner dogs with neutrophil abnormalities and recurrent infections. *Vet Immunol Immunopathol.* 1989;23(1–2):103–112.

69. Foale RD, Herrtage ME, Day MJ. Retrospective study of 25 young Weimaraners with low serum immunoglobulin concentrations and inflammatory disease. *Vet Rec.* 2003;153(18):553–558.

70. Gaskell RM, Dawson S, Radford AW. Feline respiratory disease. In: Greene CE, ed. *Infectious Diseases of the Dog and Cat.* 3rd ed. St. Louis, MO: Saunders; 2006:145–154.

71. Stone M. Systemic lupus erythematosus. In: Ettinger SJ, Feldman EC, eds. *Textbook of Veterinary Internal Medicine.* 6th ed. St. Louis, MO: Saunders; 2005:1952–1957.

72. Monier JC, Ritter J, Caux C, et al. Canine systemic lupus erythematosus. II. Antinuclear antibodies. *Lupus.* 1992;1(5):287–293.

73. Erne JB, Goring RL, Kennedy FA, et al. Prevalence of lymphoplasmacytic synovitis in dogs with naturally occurring cranial cruciate ligament rupture. *J Am Vet Med Asssoc.* 2009;235:386–390.

74. Dougherty SA, Center SA, Shaw EE, et al. Juvenile-onset polyarthritis syndrome in Akitas. *J Am Vet Med Assoc.* 1991;198(5):849–856.

75. Vaden SL. Glomerular disease. In: Ettinger SJ, Feldman EC, eds. *Textbook of Veterinary Internal Medicine.* 6th ed. St. Louis, MO: Saunders; 2005:1786–1800.

76. May C, Hammill J, Bennett D. Chinese Shar Pei fever syndrome: a preliminary report. *Vet Rec.* 1992;131(25–26):586–587.

77. Allan G. Radiographic signs of joint disease. In: Thrall DE, ed. *Textbook of Veterinary Diagnostic Radiology.* 4th ed. Philadelphia, PA: Saunders; 2002:187–207.

78. Bennett D. Immune-based erosive inflammatory joint disease of the dog: canine rheumatoid arthritis. I. Clinical, radiological and laboratory investigations. *J Small Anim Pract.* 1987;28:779–797.

79. Pedersen NC, Pool RR, O'Brien T. Feline chronic progressive polyarthritis. *Am J Vet Res.* 1980;41(4):522–535.

13

The Musculoskeletal System

Susan E. Fielder

Although cytological techniques have not been used extensively in evaluating diseases of the musculoskeletal system, they may be valuable aids in the diagnosis of certain important diseases affecting this system.

BONE

Healthy bone tissue is difficult to sample and often contains few cells. However, inflammatory and neoplastic bone diseases are usually accompanied by bone lysis and increased cellularity. Both lytic and proliferative bone lesions are often easily aspirated.

Sample Collection

Collection of material from bone lesions for cytological examination may be complicated by the hardness of cortical bone. Lytic or proliferative lesions can be aspirated by techniques similar to those for any soft tissue mass. Even heavily mineralized masses can often be aspirated with a fine needle by careful palpation and exploration of the lesion surface. Examination of radiographs may reveal portions of the lesion that are less mineralized and more likely to produce useful aspirates. If the lesion cannot be sampled by fine-needle aspiration (FNA), imprints from biopsy specimens can be used for cytological evaluation.

Inflammatory Diseases

Cytological specimens from inflammatory lesions of bone are generally similar to exudates from other organs. Inflammatory lesions that are accompanied by new bone proliferation may yield cytological specimens that also contain osteoblasts and osteoclasts. Reactive osteoblasts are typically round with an eccentrically placed nucleus and dark-blue cytoplasm (Fig.13.1). They differ from neoplastic osteoblasts in that they are smaller and lack nuclear manifestations of malignancy Osteoclasts may also be found in small numbers in specimens from inflammatory lesions. These cells resemble multinucleate giant cells and arise from precursor cells of the monocyte–macrophage cell line. Osteoclasts are large and irregularly shaped with variable numbers (typically 6–10) of uniform, round nuclei arranged randomly throughout the cell and abundant, light blue cytoplasm (Fig. 13.2).

Bacterial osteomyelitis typically results in a neutrophilic or suppurative inflammatory response. Identification of intracellular bacteria confirms bacterial infection, but organisms may not be identified in all cases and culture is recommended. Some specific causes of bacterial osteomyelitis include *Actinomyces* spp. and *Nocardia* spp., often seen as branching, filamentous rods. Staphylococcal, streptococcal, and gram-negative aerobic bacterial infections are common and may be identified on cytology.[1]

Fungal osteomyelitis is typically more mixed than bacterial infections and often contains a much larger component of activated macrophages and multinucleate giant cells. Fungal organisms that may be identified include *Coccidioides immitis*, *Blastomyces dermatitidis*, *Cryptococcus neoformans*, and *Histoplasma capsulatum*. Hyphating fungal organisms, such as *Aspergillus* spp. and *Geomyces* spp., may also be seen and appear as staining or nonstaining fungal hyphae (Fig. 13.3).[1,2] Rarely, protozoal organisms, such as *Hepatozoon* spp., may be seen as gamonts within the neutrophils in inflammatory aspirates of bone.[3]

Neoplastic Diseases

Neoplasms of bone are relatively common in domestic animals, and cytological examination is useful in establishing the diagnosis in some of these diseases. As with the interpretation of histological sections of bone, evaluation of cytological specimens from bone requires knowledge of the clinical and radiographic features of a specific lesion. Cytology is probably more useful in distinguishing inflammatory bone disease from neoplasia than in identifying specific bone tumors; however, osteosarcomas and chondrosarcomas do have characteristic cytological features that aid in diagnosis.

Osteosarcoma

Osteosarcoma is the most common primary bone tumor typically affecting the appendicular skeleton. In the dog, osteosarcoma occurs more commonly in the front limbs with the distal radius and proximal humerus as the most common sites.[4] Aspirates of osteosarcomas are often cellular with cells seen individually or in aggregates. One characteristic feature that may be evident on low-power examination of the slide is the presence of islands of osteoid surrounded by tumor cells (Fig. 13.4). Osteoid appears as a somewhat fibrillar, bright-pink

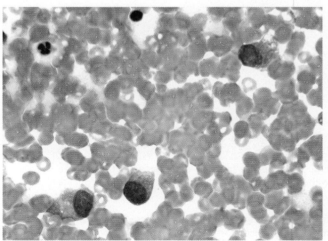

Fig. 13.1 Reactive osteoblasts with eccentrically placed nuclei and basophilic cytoplasm (Wright stain).

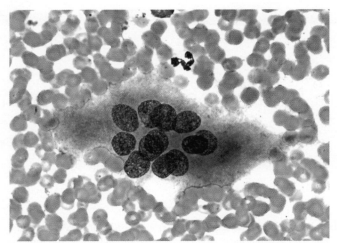

Fig. 13.2 Osteoclast with multiple, relatively uniform nuclei and abundant cytoplasm with eosinophilic stippling (Wright stain).

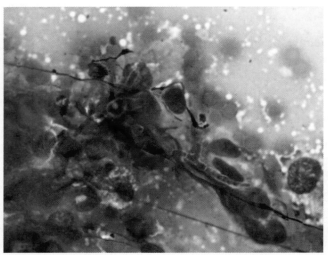

Fig. 13.3 Fungal hyphae from a lytic bone lesion in a dog. *Aspergillus* was cultured from this lesion (Wright stain).

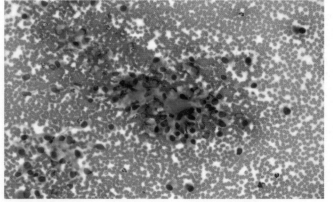

Fig. 13.4 Aspirate from an osteosarcoma. Osteoblasts interspersed with pink-staining intercellular matrix (osteoid) (Wright stain).

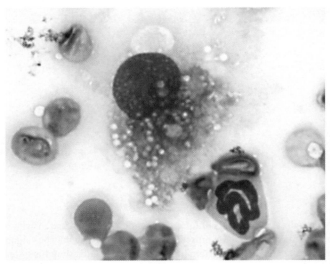

Fig. 13.5 Aspirate from an osteosarcoma. Osteoblast with vacuolated cytoplasm and fine pink cytoplasmic granules (Wright stain).

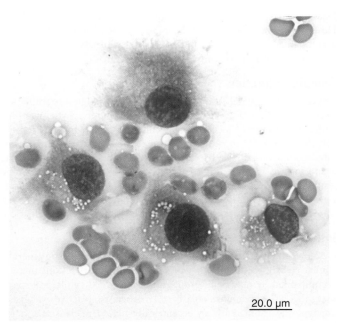

20.0 μm

Fig. 13.6 Aspirate from an osteosarcoma. Atypical osteoblasts showing anisocytosis, anisokaryosis, and multiple prominent nucleoli (Wright stain).

granules (Fig.13.5); however, these granules are not specific to osteosarcomas, and similar granules may also occur in cells from chondrosarcomas and, less commonly, fibrosarcomas. Neoplastic osteoblasts often have many of the classic cytological features of malignancy such as karyomegaly, anisokaryosis, large nucleoli, and multiple nucleoli that differ in size (Fig. 13.6). Cells from more differentiated osteosarcomas are more uniform and may be difficult to distinguish from normal or reactive osteoblasts. Small numbers of inflammatory cells, nonneoplastic osteoblasts, and osteoclasts similar to those described in the previous section on inflammation may also be found in aspirates from osteosarcomas.

Special stains are available to differentiate osteosarcoma from other mesenchymal neoplasms of the bone. Nitroblue tetrazolium chloride/5-bromo-4-chloro-3-indolyl phosphate toluidine salt (NBT/BCIP) may be used to detect alkaline phosphatase activity in osteoblasts (Fig. 13.7).[5] Because both reactive and neoplastic osteoblasts will

material on Wright-stained slides. These structures are not found in most aspirates from osteosarcomas; however, when found, their presence provides strong evidence for bone origin.

Neoplastic osteoblasts vary from round to fusiform with basophilic cytoplasm. These cells may contain scattered, pink cytoplasmic

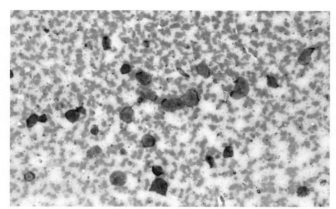

Fig. 13.7 Aspirate from an osteosarcoma. Positive alkaline phosphatase staining of a sample previously stained with Wright stain. Positive result is seen as black staining in cytoplasm (alkaline phosphatase stain).

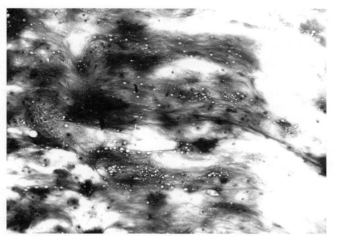

Fig. 13.8 Aspirate from a chondrosarcoma. Low-power view showing neoplastic chondrocytes surrounded by thick eosinophilic matrix compatible with chondroid (Wright stain).

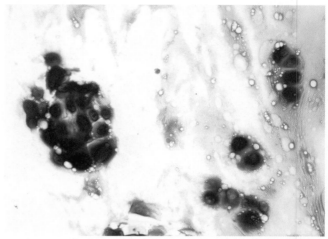

Fig. 13.9 Aspirate from a chondrosarcoma. Poorly defined neoplastic chondrocytes in thick eosinophilic matrix. These cells show anisokaryosis (Wright stain).

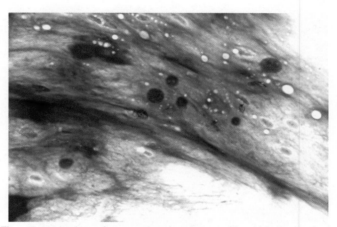

Fig. 13.10 Aspirate from a chondrosarcoma. Vacuolated neoplastic chondrocytes with a glassy appearance suggestive of cells embedded in cartilaginous lacunae (Wright stain).

stain positive, previous diagnosis of malignancy based on identification of criteria of malignancy on cytological examination is necessary. Both unstained slides and prestained slides (aqueous Romanowsky method only) may be used.[6]

Chondrosarcoma

These tumors are the second most common sarcoma of bone. The ribs, turbinates, and pelvis are the most common sites for chondrosarcomas of dogs, and the scapulae, vertebrae, and ribs are more common sites in cats.[4,7] One useful cytological feature of chondrosarcomas that may be evident on low-power examination of aspirates is the presence of chondroid (Fig. 13.8). This is seen as lakes of bright pink, smooth or slightly granular material, in which cells may be embedded (Fig. 13.9). Although the presence of this material suggests the possibility of a cartilaginous origin of a tumor, it is not a consistent finding in aspirates of chondrosarcomas. Individual chondroblasts from chondrosarcomas have cytological features that are similar to those of malignant osteoblasts (Fig. 13.10). They vary from round to fusiform, with large nuclei and blue cytoplasm. Anisokaryosis is prominent, and multinucleate tumor cells may be found. The cytoplasm often contains several small, clear vacuoles, and cells may occasionally contain fine, pink cytoplasmic granules similar to those in cells from osteosarcomas. If a tumor is causing bone lysis, osteoclasts may also be found in cytological specimens.

Other Bone Neoplasms

Fibrosarcomas and hemangiosarcomas are among the other neoplasms that arise with some frequency in bone.[7] Cytological features of these tumors are like those of the same tumors when they occur in soft tissues. Multilobular osteochondrosarcoma (also called *multilobular tumor of bone*) is a rare tumor that can appear cytologically similar to osteosarcoma; however, this tumor typically involves only the flat bones of the head and has a distinct "popcorn ball" appearance on radiographs.[8] Metastatic tumors may also present clinically as bone tumors; carcinomas exhibit this behavior most commonly. The cytological features of metastatic neoplastic cells are like those of the soft tissue tumors from which they originated. Most hematopoietic neoplasms that involve bone marrow do not present clinically as bone tumors. One major exception is the plasma cell myeloma, which may have radiographic manifestations of bone lysis. Aspirates of lytic lesions may yield sheets of neoplastic plasma cells (Fig. 13.11). These cells often appear atypical with several nuclear criteria of malignancy but may also be well differentiated and exhibit only mild pleomorphism.[9] Bone marrow aspirates from nonlytic areas may yield increased numbers of plasma cells but do not provide sufficient evidence for a definitive diagnosis of plasma cell myeloma.

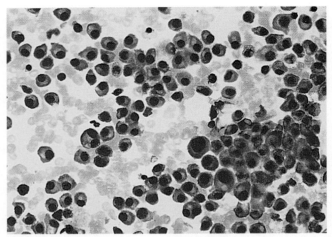

Fig. 13.11 Plasma cell myeloma. Sheets of neoplastic plasma cells with mild anisocytosis and anisokaryosis. Rare binucleate cells are present (Wright stain).

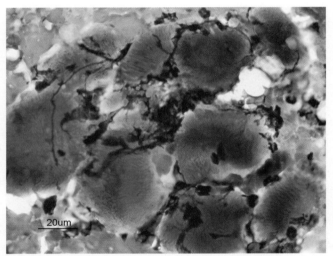

Fig. 13.12 Myocytes. Muscle fibers seen as large basophilic fragments. Cross-striations can often be seen by focusing up and down (Wright stain). (Courtesy Jim Meinkoth.)

SKELETAL MUSCLE

Striated muscle cells do not exfoliate readily, and aspirates and imprints of muscle tissue typically yield only blood. Myocytes are often rare and appear as variably sized basophilic staining fragments with cross-striations (Fig. 13.12). Relatively few clinically important inflammatory and neoplastic diseases of muscle exist compared with those of bone, and degenerative disease of muscle is not diagnosed on cytology.

Sample Collection

Cytological specimens from skeletal muscle lesions may be collected by using methods as those used for dermal and subcutaneous masses.

Myositis

When inflammatory diseases of muscle are present, they are often characterized by only a modest infiltration of inflammatory cells. Cytological samples of myositis may yield inflammatory cells and aggregates of myocytes (Fig. 13.13). Typically, histopathological evaluation is necessary to diagnose myositis.

Neoplastic Diseases

Rhabdomyomas and rhabdomyosarcomas, which are the primary skeletal muscle tumors, are rare. Canine rhabdomyomas have been primarily reported to be associated with the heart and the larynx, whereas canine rhabdomyosarcomas have been reported in numerous sites, including the myocardium, urinary bladder, urethra, vagina, perianal region, tongue, soft palate, larynx, trachea, striated muscle, and skin.[10,11] On cytology, both rhabdomyomas and rhabdomyosarcomas consist of individualized, round to polygon-shaped cells with a low nuclear-to-cytoplasmic (N:C) ratio and a large amount of eosinophilic to basophilic granular cytoplasm. Some have been described with a lighter paranuclear area. Elongated cells consistent with strap-like cells have rarely been reported on cytology. These cells sometimes have cytoplasmic cross-striations and multiple nuclei that may be linearly arranged. A second population of smaller cells with a high N:C ratio and indistinct cytoplasm is also typically seen. These cells are thought to represent undifferentiated rhabdomyoblasts and are seen in aspirates from both rhabdomyomas and rhabdomyosarcomas. Distinguishing a rhabdomyoma from a rhabdomyosarcoma on cytology is difficult, but if sufficient criteria of malignancy are present, a

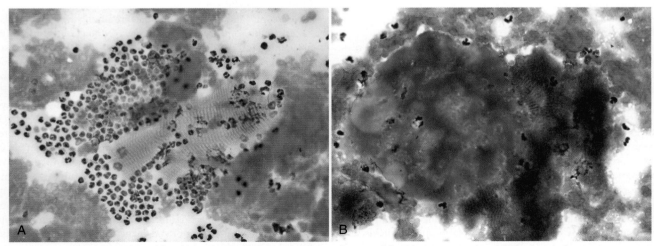

Fig. 13.13 Myositis with necrosis. (A) Large numbers of neutrophils are seen, associated with muscle fragments (Wright stain). (B) Fewer neutrophils are seen. The homogeneous appearance of some of the muscle fragments suggests necrosis (Wright stain). (Courtesy Jim Meinkoth.)

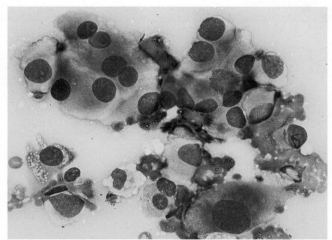

Fig. 13.14 Rhabdomyosarcoma. Neoplastic cells show criteria of malignancy, such as anisocytosis, anisokaryosis, and prominent nucleoli (Wright stain).

rhabdomyosarcoma should be suspected. Rhabdomyosarcomas often display increased pleomorphism, including spindle-shaped and ovoid cells, with marked anisocytosis and anisokaryosis and bizarre mitotic figures (Fig. 13.14).[12,13] Histopathology with special stains and immunohistochemistry are usually required for a definitive diagnosis of rhabdomyoma or rhabdomyosarcoma, although immunocytochemical methods have been used in conjunction with cytological evaluation for a diagnosis of rhabdomyosarcoma.[14]

Lipomas, fibrosarcomas, and malignant fibrous histiocytomas are among the more common tumors presenting clinically as skeletal muscle tumors. Although most of these tumors probably arise in the subcutis, they may infiltrate underlying muscle so extensively that they appear as muscle tumors on presentation.

Acknowledgment

The author wishes to acknowledge the contribution of Dr. Edward A. Mahaffey, DVM, PhD, DACVP, who authored this chapter for previous editions of the book. His contribution served as the foundation for the material appearing in this edition.

REFERENCES

1. Bubenik LJ. Infections of the skeletal system. *Vet Clin Small Anim*. 2005; 35:1093–1109.
2. Erne JB, Walker MC, Strik N, et al. Systemic infection with *Geomyces* organisms in a dog with lytic bone lesions. *J Am Vet Med Assoc*. 2007; 230:537–540.
3. Marchetti V, Lubas G, Baneth G, et al. Hepatozoonosis in a dog with skeletal involvement and meningoencephalomyelitis. *Vet Clin Pathol*. 2009; 38:121–125.
4. Thompson KG, Pool RR. In: Meuten, ed. *Tumors in Domestic Animals, Chondrosarcoma*. Ames, IA: Iowa State University Press; 2002:283–290.
5. Barger A, Graca R, Baily K, et al. Use of alkaline phosphatase staining to differentiate canine osteosarcoma from other vimentin-positive tumors. *Vet Pathol*. 2005;42:161–165.
6. Allison RW, Meinkoth JH. *Use of Alkaline Phosphatase Staining in Cytologic Specimens Previously Stained by Aqueous or Methanolic Romanowsky Methods*. Nashville, TN: ASVCP Annual Meeting Abstracts, Poster Presentation; 2011.
7. Dernell WS, Ehrhart NP, Straw RC, et al. Withrow and MacEwen's small animal clinical oncology. In: Withrow Vail, ed. *Tumors of the Skeletal System*. St. Louis, MO: Saunders; 2007:540–582.
8. Dernell WS, Straw RC, Cooper MF, et al. Multilobular osteochondrosarcoma in 39 dogs: 1979-1993. *J Am Anim Hosp Assoc*. 1998;34:11–18.
9. Patel PT, Caceres A, French AF, et al. Multiple myeloma in 16 cats: a retrospective study. *Vet Clin Pathol*. 2005;34:341–352.
10. Ueno H, Kadosawa T, Isomura H, et al. Perianal rhabdomyosarcoma in a dog. *J Small Anim Pract*. 2002;43:217–220.
11. Barnhart K, Lewis B. Laryngopharyngeal mass in a dog with upper airway obstruction. *Vet Clin Pathol*. 2000;29:47–50.
12. Fallin CW, Fox LE, Papendick RE, et al. What is your diagnosis? A 12-month-old dog with multiple soft tissue masses. *Vet Clin Pathol*. 1995;24(80):100–101.
13. Akhtar M, Ali M, Bakry M, et al. Fine-needle aspiration biopsy diagnosis of rhabdomyosarcoma: cytologic, histologic, and ultrastructural correlations. *Diagn Cytopathol*. 1992;8:465–474.
14. Avallone G, Pinto da Cunha N, Palmieri C, et al. Subcutaneous embryonal rhabdomyosarcoma in a dog: cytologic, immunocytochemical, histologic, and ultrastructural features. *Vet Clin Pathol*. 2010;39:499–504.

14

Cerebrospinal Fluid and Central Nervous System Cytology

Gwendolyn J. Levine and Jennifer R. Cook

CEREBROSPINAL FLUID

Cerebrospinal fluid (CSF) is present within the ventricular system of the brain, the central canal of the spinal cord, and the subarachnoid space (SAS) between the pia mater and the arachnoid mater. CSF is a component of, and is continuous with, the interstitial fluid of the central nervous system (CNS). It is separated from the bloodstream and from the CNS parenchyma by an intricate barrier system comprising ependymal epithelium, choroid plexus epithelium, the leptomeninges, areas of modified leptomeninges, and the arachnoid villi (the reader is referred elsewhere for a thorough discussion of these barriers and their transport mechanisms).[1,2] CSF has mechanical (protection) and metabolic (transport, excretion) functions. Sampling of the CSF is an important part of the minimum database for patients with neurological signs and may be useful in monitoring response to therapy in CNS inflammatory disease. When performed correctly, acquisition is a rapid, inexpensive, and technically simple method of sampling the local environment of the CNS extracellular space for evidence of inflammatory, neoplastic, traumatic, or degenerative disease. It is not without risk, however, and should be performed judiciously, that is, when clinical indication exists and no contraindications are present. This chapter will review the biology of CSF, methods for collection, and causes for abnormalities in parameters, such as protein concentration and nucleated cell count.

Limitations of Cerebrospinal Fluid Analysis

Analysis of CSF is an important adjunctive diagnostic tool in the workup of patients with CNS disease and must be interpreted within the context of the patient's history, clinical signs, clinicopathological data, imaging studies, and other ancillary diagnostics. Rarely is CSF solely used to provide an etiological diagnosis (exceptions include cytological visualization of infectious agents or overtly neoplastic cells), but analysis may significantly narrow the field of pathophysiological differentials, guiding further diagnostic and therapeutic options. CSF analysis is most sensitive in detecting inflammatory disease.[3] Positive findings in CSF tend to be more diagnostically helpful compared with negative findings but are often nonspecific because many different diseases may cause a common CSF pathology (e.g., neutrophilic pleocytosis).[4] Occasionally, the magnitude of change within the CSF may be as instructive as the character of the change (e.g., a marked increase in protein concentration raising diagnostic concern for feline infectious peritonitis, marked neutrophilic pleocytosis raising diagnostic concern for steroid-responsive meningitis–arteritis in a young dog in pain).[4] More frequently, however, specific disease etiologies will present with CSF changes of variable character and magnitude. CSF that falls within laboratory reference intervals should never be used to rule out a differential diagnosis because negative findings may represent early or mild disease, disease suppressed or masked by therapeutic intervention, or a disease process that does not present within the particular area of the extracellular space being sampled. CSF analysis may or may not correlate with imaging studies; a retrospective study of 92 cats receiving magnetic resonance imaging (MRI) for spinal signs showed that abnormal CSF was not a predictor for abnormal MRI.[5] In another study, approximately 25% of dogs with intracranial signs and inflammatory CSF had normal brain MRI results.[6]

Formation and Movement of Cerebrospinal Fluid

The conventionally accepted theory of CSF secretion and transport is based on the concept of active transport of ions within the ventricular ependymal cells and choroid plexi, subsequent passive flow of fluid, and circulation and drainage of CSF into dural venous sinuses. These ideas have recently come under scrutiny as potentially simplistic and inconsistent with the past 100 years of experimental evidence.[7] Analysis of past experiments, coupled with new data, supports a "global production" hypothesis—that instead of exclusive formation within the ventricles, CSF is continually created and reabsorbed diffusely by cerebral capillaries that have slight variances in hydrostatic and osmotic pressure. Canine studies have documented CSF production within the ventricular system and the SAS.[2]

Contraindications to Acquisition of Cerebrospinal Fluid

CSF should not be collected from patients with unacceptable anesthetic risk or with suspected coagulopathy, severe cervical trauma, or increased intracranial pressure secondary to edema, hemorrhage, hydrocephalus, or a large neoplasm.[8] CSF collection in the presence of elevated intracranial pressure may cause brain herniation and death secondary to compression of respiratory centers.[9] Signs of increased intracranial pressure may include stupor, coma, bradycardia, systemic hypertension, cranial nerve deficits, rigid paresis, or all of these.[10,11] Mannitol and hypertonic saline are the first-line medical therapies for elevated intracranial pressure. Head elevation, modest hyperventilation, administration of drugs to slow brain metabolism, and craniectomy with durectomy are sometimes used in cases refractory to traditional treatments. Advanced imaging before CSF collection, especially in patients presenting with intracranial neurological signs, may be useful in identifying contraindications. Imaging, in particular MRI, is exquisitely helpful in providing structural data that may be correlated to CSF results.

Collection Techniques
Collection Sites
CSF can be collected from the cerebromedullary cistern (at the atlanto-occipital space) or from the lumbar cistern in the L5-L6

interarcuate space. The cerebromedullary cistern is used more commonly because a larger volume of CSF with lower risk for blood contamination can be reliably collected.

Cerebromedullary Cistern Versus Lumbar Cistern

A study of 158 dogs with focal, noninflammatory disease showed that in cases of spinal lesions, CSF was more likely to be abnormal if collected from the lumbar cistern, that is, caudal to the lesion.[12] This observation may be explained by presupposing cranial to caudal flow of CSF, but the traditionally held theory of CSF flow has recently been contested.[7] In canines, CSF collected from the cerebromedullary cistern generally has lower microprotein concentrations compared with samples collected from the lumbar cistern.[13] Blood contamination may be more pronounced in lumbar collection, as the desired subarachnoid space is more difficult to enter and yields a smaller volume of fluid that tends to flow more slowly.[9,10] Moreover, hemodilution may contribute to increased measured protein concentration.[13]

Rare instances of CSF contamination with hematopoietic precursors have only been reported from lumbar sites.[14] A low, but potentially catastrophic, risk for puncturing the cervical spinal cord or caudal brainstem exists during cerebromedullary collection. Because the spinal cord length is variable, spinal cord puncture is a possibility during lumbar collection, but it is associated with less severe adverse effects compared with injury following cisternal puncture. In a case series of four accidental cisternal parenchymal punctures (documented by using MRI), three of the four patients suffered neurological decompensation and subsequently had to be euthanized.[15]

Equipment

The following equipment should be assembled: anesthesia and monitoring equipment, clippers, aseptic preparation materials for the skin, sterile gloves, and a spinal needle with stylet. For cerebromedullary cistern collection in dogs weighing less than 25 kg and for cats, a 22-gauge, 1.5-inch spinal needle is usually adequate, and a 22-gauge, 2.5-inch spinal needle is recommended for dogs weighing greater than 25 kg. For lumbar puncture, a 22-gauge spinal needle up to 6 inches long may be required for obese or extremely large patients. If available, fluoroscopic equipment may aid in the acquisition of cisternal or lumbar CSF. At the authors' institution, fluoroscopy is often used before cisternal CSF acquisition in toy-breed dogs to exclude the possibility of subclinical atlantoaxial subluxation.

Cerebrospinal Fluid Acquisition

The anesthetized patient is placed in lateral recumbency (it is generally easier for a right-handed clinician to have the patient in right-lateral recumbency, and vice versa), with the neck and back flush to the edge of a sturdy table. For collection from the cerebromedullary cistern, the neck is flexed such that the dorsum of the muzzle is 90 degrees to the long axis of the body (if needed, stabilizing the endotracheal tube to prevent kinking and deflating the cuff to prevent tracheal trauma), and the snout is propped up slightly, if necessary, to keep it parallel with the table and not angulated from the sagittal plane.[10] A wide area (3–5 cm) around the atlanto-occipital joint (beyond atlas wings and axis spinous process and to the external occipital protuberance) is shaved and aseptically prepared, and landmarks are palpated with a gloved, nondominant hand.[9] The needle is inserted at the intersection of two imaginary perpendicular lines that run (1) along the dorsal midline (dividing the patient sagittally) from the occipital protuberance to the cranial spinous process of the axis (C2) and (2) across the craniolateral aspects of the wings of the atlas (C1) (dividing the patient craniocaudally).

For lumbar collection, the pelvic limbs are brought forward into full flexion, and the needle is inserted cranial and parallel to the dorsal spinous process of L6 for dogs and L7 for cats, advancing the needle until the ventral aspect of the vertebral canal is encountered; the needle is then retracted slightly and CSF is collected from the ventral SAS.[10,16] The pelvic limbs may be kicked or may twitch slightly during collection because of irritation of the cauda equina or spinal cord parenchyma.

For either location, once landmarks are palpated, the needle is held stably with the dominant hand and very slowly advanced, stylet in place. The heel of the dominant hand may be supported against the table. For cisternal collection, it is important to advance the needle toward the point of the nose without angulation. The stylet is removed with the nondominant hand every 2 to 3 mm to check for fluid within the needle hub, waiting a few seconds. It is common to feel a decrease in resistance to forward needle movement once the thecal space is entered. If bone is hit or frank hemorrhage is observed from the needle, it should be withdrawn slowly and collection reattempted.[9] If clear or slightly blood-tinged fluid is observed, advancement of the needle is stopped, and open tubes are placed directly under the needle hub to collect freely falling drops. CSF is collected passively and should not be aspirated.

There are no significant objective data regarding the maximal amount of CSF that may be collected in dogs. Several authors claim that it is safe to collect 0.2 milliliters (mL) of CSF per kilogram of body weight (1 mL/5 kg); in other species much higher volumes of CSF per body weight are acquired standardly.[17] In general, 0.5 to 1 mL of CSF is adequate for routine diagnostic tests, including cell counts, protein concentration, and cytological analysis. Larger volumes are necessary for additional diagnostics (cultures, titers, polymerase chain reaction [PCR], flow cytometry, protein electrophoresis, etc.).

Two sets of tubes should be readied and ideally handled by an assistant. An ethylenediaminetetraacetic acid (EDTA)–treated (purple-top) tube is used for cell counts, flow cytometry, and PCR testing for organisms, and plain (red-top) tubes are used for protein concentration, culture, or immunologic assays.[10] Some sources indicate that plain tubes are recommended, as EDTA could increase protein concentration. If CSF analysis will occur rapidly (within 1 hour), collection into a plain tube is adequate, whereas preservation of cells may be improved with collection into EDTA if analysis will be delayed. If low volume is present, priority is given to the EDTA tube. If CSF appears red, then iatrogenic hemorrhage (puncture of a dural vessel) or actual CNS hemorrhage has occurred. In this instance, the first few drops are allowed to collect into the first set of tubes, and the second set of tubes are reserved for the latter portion of the sample, as iatrogenic hemorrhage tends to clear over time. If the hemorrhage does clear, a decision may be made about discarding the first set of tubes or keeping them for ancillary testing not affected by the hemorrhage. After collection, the needle is withdrawn without the stylet, and the CSF within the needle is allowed to drip into one of the tubes or is placed in an additional plain tube and saved for culture.

CEREBROSPINAL FLUID PROCESSING AND ANALYSIS

As with other clinicopathological and cytological samples, evaluation of a fresh specimen is preferred to minimize cellular degradation, to which CSF is particularly vulnerable because of its relatively low protein concentration. Sample degradation will affect cell differential count to a greater extent than the total nucleated cell count or the protein concentration.[18] A study of 30 canine CSF samples with pleocytosis concluded that delay of analysis up to 8 hours was unlikely to alter interpretation, especially in samples with protein concentrations above 50 milligrams per deciliter (mg/dL).[18] Preservative should be added to low protein samples unless analysis is to be completed within

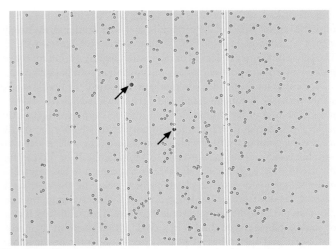

Fig. 14.1 Numerous erythrocytes and two leukocytes present on a hemacytometer. The two nuclei of the two leukocytes in the center of the field stain dark purple *(arrows)* (new methylene blue stain, original magnification 50×).

60 minutes (see next section), and a dilutional effect must then be factored into cell counts.[18] Samples to be shipped to a reference laboratory overnight should be kept at refrigeration temperature and shipped with ice packs for analysis within 48 hours.[9,16] The reference laboratory should be prenotified to ensure prompt analysis.

If analysis is likely to be delayed by more than 1 hour and the CSF sample has a protein concentration less than 50 mg/dL, one of the following may be added as a protein source to maintain cellular integrity: (1) hetastarch (add 1:1 volume), (2) fetal calf serum (3.7 g/dL protein; add 20% by volume), or (3) autologous plasma or serum (fresh or frozen; 11% by volume ≡ one drop from 25-gauge needle (approximately 0.03 mL) mixed into 0.25 mL CSF).[10,19,20] The sample should be labeled with the protein source and amount added to the sample. One study demonstrated better preservation of mononuclear cells in canine samples when fetal calf serum was used instead of hetastarch.[18] All samples should be refrigerated at 4°C to minimize cellular degradation.

Cell Counts

A hemocytometer may be employed in practice to count nucleated cells and erythrocytes. Both sides of the cover-slipped hemocytometer are loaded with unstained CSF, which is then placed in a humidified container for 10 to 15 minutes to allow cells to settle on the glass. Because the fluid is unstained, the microscope condenser is lowered to improve contrast. Erythrocytes and nucleated cells are differentiated by size, refraction, granularity, and smoothness of plasma membrane.[21] Some laboratories stain CSF samples with new methylene blue (NMB), as leukocytes will take up stain, whereas erythrocytes remain unstained, making differentiation of leukocytes (specifically small lymphocytes) and erythrocytes easier (Fig. 14.1).[22] A small volume of CSF is drawn into a capillary tube coated with NMB or a tube that has a small volume of NMB followed by an air pocket.[22] The tube containing NMB and CSF is gently rocked back and forth, allowing the cells to take up some stain without diluting the CSF with a volume of NMB.[22] The hemocytometer is then loaded, and each population is counted and totals are calculated, as follows: Neubauer chamber: (1) both areas of large nine squares are counted, and the average of the number of leukocytes and erythrocytes is found; (2) the average is multiplied by 9 to get the cells per microliter (cells/μL).[10]

The ADVIA 120 (Siemens Medical Solution, Fernwald, Germany) hematology instrument has been validated for analyzing canine CSF

samples and shows excellent correlation with manual methods used in dogs with increased total cell counts (pleocytosis), but the instrument may overestimate the cell count in samples without pleocytoses and has not been validated for the identification of eosinophils.[23] The automated differential count is also more accurate at higher cell numbers and thus should be compared with a traditional manual differential. The ADVIA 2120 hematology analyzer displayed satisfactory agreement with the standard hemocytometer method.[24] Validation experiments using 67 canine samples showed a sensitivity of 100% and specificity of 89% for accurately identifying samples with pleocytosis when manual counting was considered the gold standard (>5 cells/μL).[24] The instrument tended to be less accurate at lower (within reference interval) nucleated cell counts.[24] Erythrocytes may be a source of interference, as a red blood cell (RBC) count of 250 cells/μL was shown to elevate the nucleated cell count.[24] With regard to differential cell count, the instrument performed better in the presence of pleocytosis, whereas monocytes were overcounted at lower nucleated cell counts.[24] Automated cell counts thus should not replace a manual differential but may be used as another level of quality control. Automated instruments cannot recognize altered cell types, such as atypical neoplastic cells.

Measurement of Microprotein Concentration

Measurement of CSF specific gravity is not considered to be helpful because of low sensitivity for detecting abnormalities.[12] CSF microprotein may be semiquantitatively measured by using urine dipsticks that detect albumin. This assay has a lower detection limit of 100 mg/dL; therefore, it has low sensitivity for mild to moderate CSF protein concentration elevations (30 mg/dL to 100 mg/dL). False-positive or false-negative reactions may occur if the dipstick reads at trace or 1+, but this method is useful if other techniques are not available.[11] Reference laboratories apply a similar but more sensitive methodology to measurement of CSF microprotein as that of serum protein, using the trichloroacetic acid method, the Ponceau S red dye–binding method, or the Coomassie brilliant blue method.[22]

CSF globulin production is typically screened for with the Pandy reaction. In this test, a few drops of CSF are added to 1 mL of 10% carbolic acid solution, and the resulting turbidity is graded 0 to 4+. Any Pandy score above zero is considered elevated. Globulin concentration below 50 mg/dL will be undetectable with either test.[10,21]

Protein electrophoresis and immunoelectrophoresis may be performed on CSF and serum for maximum fractionation.[25] The utility of protein electrophoresis or immunoelectrophoresis of CSF lies in discriminating altered blood–brain barrier (BBB) permeability from increased localized production of immunoglobulin, which may be suggestive of (but not specific for) a disease entity for which an electrophoretic pattern has been established.

Cytological Slide Preparation

Cytological analysis is a critical component of CSF evaluation because the differential count (percentages) of cells may be abnormal, even if the total nucleated count is within reference interval. Cytology also enables examination for neoplastic cells, infectious agents, and evidence of prior hemorrhage. It may also serve as a quality control point, allowing for correlation between observed cellularity and the total count generated by a hemocytometer or an automated analyzer. Because of its low cellularity, CSF must be concentrated before cytological smear preparation.

Use of an in-house sedimentation chamber (Sörnäs procedure) may be very useful and preserves cell-free fluid for ancillary testing.[10] This technique will recover approximately 60% of total cells, which is sufficient for analysis.[16] A syringe barrel (with the tip and needle aseptically removed with a scalpel blade) is turned upside down and the smooth, top side is placed in warm petroleum jelly and then onto a clean slide. Once a seal has formed, fresh CSF (at least 0.5 mL) is placed in the syringe and allowed to sit for 30 minutes.[16,21] Then, the supernatant is aspirated carefully with a pipette so as not to disturb the bottom layer contacting the slide. The syringe barrel is removed, and any excess CSF is carefully absorbed with a small piece of filter paper or paper towel. The slide is completely and rapidly air-dried without heat (inadequate drying results in cellular distortion), excess petroleum jelly removed with a scalpel blade, and the slide is stained with routine Romanowsky stains (e.g., Diff-Quik).

If CSF is sent to a reference laboratory, a cytological slide will likely be prepared using cytocentrifugation (500–1000 revolutions per minute [rpm] for 5–10 minutes, either onto a slide coated with albumin or with the addition of 0.05 mL of 30% albumin for improved cell capture) for maximal concentration of nucleated cells onto one slide.[16] Cytocentrifuged cytology may show excellent cellular detail, but the preparation may enlarge cells slightly and create an artifactual foamy or vacuolated appearance.[16] Slides are air-dried and stained with conventional Romanowsky stains. Multiple cytospin preparations may be made to yield 200 intact nucleated cells for classification.

Additional Cerebrospinal Fluid Testing
Culture
As it is rare for etiologic agents to localize only within the CNS, all cases of suspected infection may be aided diagnostically by fine-needle aspiration (FNA) cytology, biopsy with histopathology, culture of nonneural lesions, or all of these.[21] Bacterial culture and sensitivity testing of CSF is recommended for most cases of neutrophilic pleocytosis, given the appropriate clinical index of suspicion for a septic lesion. Even when organisms are visualized on CSF cytology, speciation and susceptibility testing may help guide prognostic and treatment decisions. Alternatively, bacterial or fungal culture may be negative regardless of cytological observation of organisms.[10,20] It must be remembered that bacterial CNS infection is highly uncommon in dogs and cats compared with other domestic animal species.[26]

Titers and Polymerase Chain Reaction Testing for Infectious Agents
Advanced techniques for neurological disease diagnosis are expanding rapidly. Enzyme-linked immunosorbent assay (ELISA)–based assays for antibody detection and PCR-based assays for nucleic acid detection of several medically important microbes have been developed for use on CSF and may be instructive in the diagnosis of viral, rickettsial, protozoal, or fungal diseases.[20] A large canine study that included a subset of 16 dogs with neoplastic or inflammatory disease showed that CSF titer provided diagnosis in 25% of cases.[3] Antibody assays should be interpreted cautiously because the presence of antibody may indicate prior exposure or vaccination rather than active infection. Moreover, compromise to the BBB in states of inflammation may translate to the presence of antibodies within the CSF without local production. Occasionally cross-reactive antibodies may be present that do not represent presence of the disease agent under assessment. Similarly, specimens for PCR should be submitted to a laboratory with strict quality control to minimize false-negative and false-positive results. Poor collection technique may result in false-positive results, especially for bacterial species that are ubiquitous in the environment.[27] As with other aspects of CSF analysis, a negative PCR result does not definitively rule out the presence of a pathogen because of the sampling limitation of a small portion of the extracellular space.[20]

Enzymes, Neurotransmitters, and Other Molecules
CSF contains glucose, electrolytes, neurotransmitters, and enzymes, but these substances are not measured routinely, although this measurement represents a rapidly expanding area of research in the effort to give clinicians better tools for diagnosing patients and determining prognoses. CSF enzymes originate from the bloodstream, the CNS, or cells within CSF.[10] One study of 34 cats with noninflammatory CNS disease showed that measurement of CSF activities of lactate dehydrogenase (LDH), aspartate aminotransferase (AST), and creatine kinase (CK) were not diagnostically sensitive but may be useful in detection of acute injury.[28] Multiple studies have correlated elevations in CSF CK activity with poor prognosis in dogs with neurological disease or spinal cord injury.[29,30] Immunoassays for vascular endothelial growth factor (VEGF) and S-100 calcium-binding protein have shown elevations of both molecules in the CSF of experimentally induced hypothyroid dogs, suggesting endothelial and glial contribution to increased BBB permeability in this population.[31] Myelin basic protein (MBP) has been found to be elevated in lumbar CSF in dogs with degenerative myelopathy, supporting the conclusion that it is a demyelinating lesion.[32] MBP concentration is elevated in the CSF of dogs affected by intervertebral disk herniation (IVDH) and has been found to be an independent predictor of poor prognosis.[33] Beta-2-microglobulin, a major histocompatibility complex I (MHC-I)–associated molecule, has been assayed by using ELISA and found to be elevated in the CSF of dogs with IVDH and inflammatory disease and also positively correlated with normal total nucleated cell count (TNCC).[34] The amino acids tryptophan and glutamine have been found to be elevated in the CSF of dogs with portosystemic shunts because of abnormal ammonia metabolism.[35] One study found increased oxytocin in the CSF of dogs with spinal cord compression, where it is believed to have an analgesic effect.[36] Gamma-aminobutyric acid (GABA) and glutamate neurotransmitter concentrations have been measured in dogs with epilepsy.[37]

NORMAL CEREBROSPINAL FLUID PARAMETERS
Gross Examination
Normal CSF is clear and colorless, with few cellular elements and a protein concentration approximately 200 to 300 times less than that of plasma or serum. Red or yellowish coloration indicates prior lesional hemorrhage or iatrogenic hemorrhage during collection. In the latter case, a pellet of RBCs will be present after centrifugation. True xanthochromia (yellowish color of hemoglobin breakdown products) that does not clear on centrifugation, cytological evidence of erythrophagia, or both indicate prior hemorrhage into the subarachnoid space.[20] Increased bilirubin leakage into the SAS or high concentrations of CSF protein (>100–150 mg/dL) may cause xanthrochromia.[21] Increased turbidity of the sample may be caused by increased number of cells present (>400 RBCs/μL or >200 nucleated cells/μL) but is usually not affected by mild changes.[10,11]

Cell Counts
TNCC is fewer than 5 cells/μL in the dog and fewer than 8 cells/μL in the cat, and elevation above this range is termed *pleocytosis*.[10] Grading of pleocytosis is somewhat subjective: In one reference, "mild" was defined as 6 to 50 cells/μL; "moderate" as 51 to 1000 cells/μL; and "marked" as more than 1000 cells/μL.[4]

Microprotein Concentration
Depending on laboratory-specific reference intervals, normal protein concentration is usually less than 25 to 30 mg/dL for cisternal CSF and less than 45 mg/dL for lumbar CSF.[10,20] Approximately 80% to 95% of CSF protein is albumin, and 5% to 12% of CSF total protein comprises gammaglobulins.[2] Eighty percent of CSF protein is transferred from plasma, with the remainder produced within the CNS. The latter

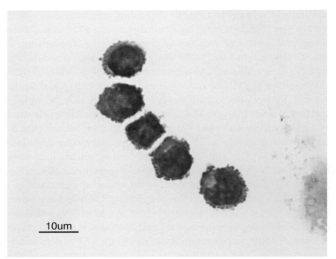

Fig. 14.2 Small lymphocytes in a cerebrospinal fluid sample (Wright-Giemsa stain).

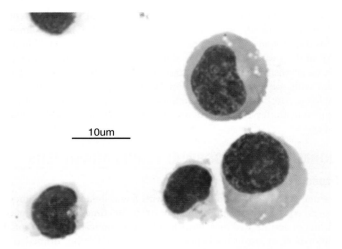

Fig. 14.3 Small lymphocytes in a cerebrospinal fluid sample. The two cells to the right have slightly increased amounts of cytoplasm (Wright-Giemsa stain).

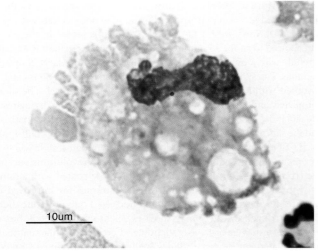

Fig. 14.4 Large mononuclear cell with cytoplasmic vacuolation in a cerebrospinal fluid sample (Wright-Giemsa stain).

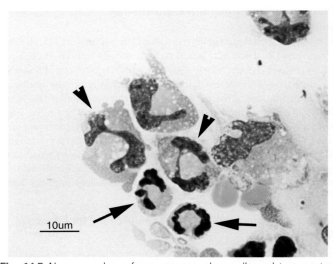

Fig. 14.5 Numerous large foamy mononuclear cells and two neutrophils (arrows) in a sample of cerebrospinal fluid. Large mononuclear cells may have nuclei that are similar in shape to band cells or neutrophils, only larger (arrowheads) (Wright-Giemsa stain).

population includes molecules also produced by other organs and proteins unique to the CSF that may potentially be used as markers of CNS tissue damage. Experimental evidence and earlier literature support a gradient of increasing protein concentration from cranial to caudal within the subarachnoid space, which has been attributed to slower flow and greater blood–CSF permeability caudally.[12]

Normal Cytology

Normal CSF is acellular or contains small numbers of small lymphocytes (Figs. 14.2 and 14.3) and large mononuclear cells (macrophages, ependymal lining cells, meningothelial lining cells, choroid plexus cells) (Figs. 14.4 and 14.5). Large mononuclear cells may be vacuolated and contain phagocytized material (Fig. 14.6). A low frequency of nondegenerate neutrophils (<25%), which are usually indicative of blood contamination during collection, may be present.[38] A study of 359 samples of canine CSF found a 7.5% incidence of meningeal, choroid plexus, ependymal, endothelial cells, or all of these.[39] No correlation existed between the presence of these cells and the presence of pleocytosis, elevated protein concentration, or the primary disease etiology.[39]

Thus it is postulated that the presence of these cells is an artifact of collection and should not be overinterpreted. The authors recommended the term "surface epithelial cells" for the combined grouping (which cannot be distinguished cytologically), although not all of these cells (meningeal, endothelial) are of epithelial origin.[39] Occasionally, anucleate superficial squamous epithelial cells may be seen; these may be caused by contamination from the skin (Fig. 14.7).

Other Parameters

Occasionally, small amounts of granular, foamy extracellular material are present and are consistent with myelin or myelin-like material, which will stain positively with Luxol fast blue stain. This material may consist of myelin fragments, which are generated from demyelination, or may consist of myelin figures (a nonspecific term for layered phospholipids exfoliated from damaged cells).[40] The two cannot be distinguished with light microscopy. The significance of this material remains unclear because it may be observed in samples from patients with no discernible cause. A study of 98 canine cerebromedullary and

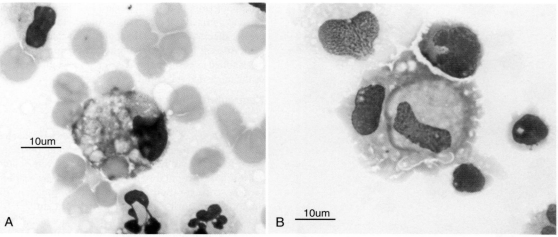

Fig. 14.6 Large mononuclear cells in cerebrospinal fluid showing evidence of (A) erythrophagia and (B) leukocytophagia (Wright-Giemsa stain).

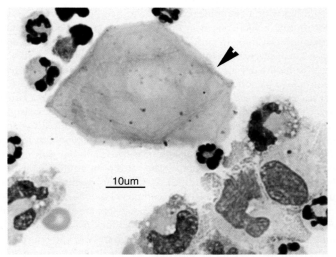

Fig. 14.7 Cerebrospinal fluid sample from a dog. A single large keratinized epithelial cell is present *(arrowhead)*. Squamous epithelial cells represent cutaneous contamination (Wright-Giemsa stain).

lumbar CSF samples showed 20% incidence of myelin-like material, with a higher percentage in samples from the lumbar cistern or from small dogs (<10 kg).[41] The presence of the material was not correlated with case outcome.[41] Similarly, in a study of 61 Cavalier King Charles Spaniels with Chiari-like malformations, myelinlike material was observed in 57% of lumbar CSF collections and 12% of cerebromedullary collections.[42] Thus myelin-like material may be a procedural artifact or may be consistent with a demyelinating (e.g., canine distemper virus, degenerative myelopathy) or potentially necrotizing disorder (e.g., IVDH, other spinal trauma, or a necrotic neoplasm).[40,41]

INTERPRETATION OF ABNORMAL CEREBROSPINAL FLUID

Blood Contamination and Hemorrhage

Normal CSF should not contain erythrocytes, but hemodilution is a common occurrence. Varying reports on the effect of blood contamination on TNCC, leukocyte differential, and protein concentration have been published.[43-46] Deciding whether increased TNCC or

protein concentration is the result of hemodilution alone or a significant change concurrent with hemodilution necessarily remains, to an extent, a subjective assessment and must be critically evaluated in light of the magnitude of CSF findings along with the other pertinent facts of the case. Correction formulas for CSF parameters in the face of hemodilution (e.g., adding 1 nucleated cell/μL per 100 or 500 RBCs/μL) are unreliable.[45,46] In a recent study of 106 canine CSF samples without pleocytosis (TNCC <5/μL) but containing at least 500 RBCs/μL, the mean percentage of neutrophils (45.2% versus 5.7%), percentage of samples with eosinophils present (36.8% versus 6.8%), and mean protein concentration (40 mg/dL versus 26 mg/dL) were found to be significantly increased in the samples with blood contamination when compared with controls.[47] Significant RBC contamination warrants repeat sampling, if possible. Marked hemorrhage or evidence of prior hemorrhage (erythrophagocytosis, xanthochromia, hemosiderin-laden macrophages) may be useful in the diagnosis of CNS trauma, which may be accompanied by neutrophilic to mixed cell pleocytosis and mild increase in protein concentration.[4]

Elevated Microprotein Concentration

Elevated protein concentration in CSF (>30 mg/dL) may occur with or without pleocytosis, and in the absence of pleocytosis is termed *albuminocytological dissociation* (ACD). High protein concentration may be the result of leakage of plasma or cellular proteins across the BBB, localized production of immunoglobulin, localized tissue damage or necrosis, decreased clearance of protein into the venous sinuses, obstruction of CSF circulation, or all of the above. As such, it is a nonspecific change that indicates CNS damage or hyperproteinemic disease and is consistent with disease of any etiology (e.g., trauma, metabolic, infectious, inflammatory, degenerative, or neoplastic). Caution should be exercised when diagnosing ACD if the sample is hemodiluted (>500 RBCs/μL).[47] As is true for pleocytosis, inflammation of the meninges and superficial regions of parenchyma will result in greater CSF protein elevations than for lesions that are more remote from the SAS.

Alterations of Leukocyte Percentages Without a Pleocytosis

Occasionally, an abnormal leukocyte differential (shifted from mononuclear predominance to neutrophil predominance) without pleocytosis occurs. This may only be detected if cytological analysis (after sedimentation or cytocentrifugation of CSF) is performed. Increased percentages of neutrophils may occur in early or mild inflammatory

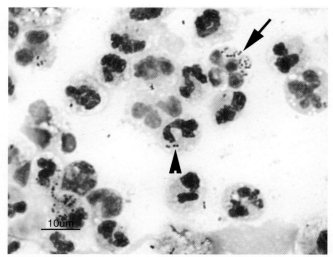

Fig. 14.8 Septic meningoencephalitis. Note the degenerate neutrophils and the presence of bacteria *(arrow)* (Wright-Giemsa stain).

disease, noninflammatory CNS disease, disease that is remote from the SAS or sampling site, or in cases of hemodilution. An increased proportion of neutrophils is present when neutrophils comprise greater than 25% of all nucleated cells, and increased percentage of eosinophils occurs when eosinophils comprise greater than 1% of the differential.[10]

Increased Neutrophil Percentage

When present (with or without increased TNCC), neutrophils should be evaluated for toxic change, degenerative change, and intracellular organisms or other inclusions (Fig. 14.8). Increased percentage of neutrophils without pleocytosis has been associated with healthy dogs, blood contamination, degenerative disk disease, neoplasia, cerebrovascular accident, fracture, CNS aspergillosis, and fibrocartilaginous embolism (FCE).[10,42,48] A study of 61 Cavalier King Charles Spaniels with Chiari-like malformation documented that those with syringomyelia were more likely to have an increased percentage of neutrophils, but it was not reported whether this subpopulation also had a concurrent pleocytosis.[42] In another study, cats with CNS neoplasia had increased percentage of neutrophils or lymphocytes without a pleocytosis.[28] Although not a classic pattern, infectious or inflammatory disease should not be ruled out if increased neutrophils are visualized without pleocytosis.

Increased Eosinophil Percentage

Increased percentage of eosinophils has been reported in parasitic and protozoal diseases, such as *Neospora caninum* infection.[38] One cat with eosinophilic meningoencephalitis (EME) of unknown etiology had an increased percentage of eosinophils and lymphocytes without pleocytosis.[49]

Increased Nucleated Cell Counts (Pleocytoses)

The specific diseases mentioned in the next section on various categories of pleocytosis are a survey of the current literature and meant to be a helpful starting point in the generation of particular differential diagnoses. Thus disease entities are listed in the section under which they are most commonly present, but it is important to note that for all disease entities, variability in the nature and the magnitude of pleocytosis may emerge in a particular patient at a particular point in time. Wherever possible, other categories of pleocytosis that have been reported for a disease have been mentioned. Generally, pleocytoses are defined by the cell type that comprises 70% or more of the nucleated

cell population. If all cell types are 50% or less, the pleocytosis is classified as a mixed cell pleocytosis. And if, for example, lymphocytes are greater than 50% but less than 70%, some pathologists will classify the pleocytosis as mixed cell, lymphocyte predominant. A pleocytosis will be classified as eosinophilic if eosinophils compose at least 10% to 20% of the nucleated cell population.[11]

Neutrophilic Pleocytosis

Infectious conditions

Bacterial meningoencephalomyelitis. Bacterial infections of the CNS are unusual and represent a small portion of neutrophilic pleocytoses. Typically, this pleocytosis is severe (could be over 1000 cells/µL), neutrophilic, and accompanied by significantly elevated protein concentration, but the cell population may change to mononuclear during the course of treatment.[10,20,50] Rare instances of brain abscessation secondary to sepsis (which may be a sequela of iatrogenic immunosuppression) may result in marked neutrophilic pleocytosis, markedly elevated protein concentration, visualization of bacterial organisms (see Fig. 14.8), and abnormal MRI findings.[51] *Staphylococcus intermedius* was cultured from the CSF of a dog presenting with a retrobulbar abscess and neurological signs.[52] The CSF showed a moderate neutrophilic pleocytosis (75 cells/µL) and borderline elevation in protein concentration (30 mg/dL).[52] Local extension of severe otitis interna resulting in meningoencephalitis and ventriculitis in a dog has been reported.[53] This patient exhibited a severe neutrophilic pleocytosis (3672 cells/µL) and protein elevation (>400 mg/dL).[53] *Pasteurella multocida* meningoencephalomyelitis in a kitten was characterized by marked neutrophilic pleocytosis (981 cells/µL) with mild protein elevation (31 mg/dL) and rare extracellular and intracellular bacterial rods.[54] Bacterial culture and susceptibility testing are recommended but may yield false-negative results if organisms are not circulating in the extracellular space or if prior antibiotic therapy had been given. Serology and CSF-PCR (using organism-specific or universal bacterial [UB] PCR) are recommended.[27,54]

Cryptococcosis in dogs. *Cryptococcus* spp. are a large genus of systemic dimorphic fungi with a predilection for CNS tissue, which is infected hematogenously or via direct penetration of the cribriform plate. Only two species at this time are medically important: (1) *Cryptococcus neoformans* (var. *neoformans* and var. *grubii*) and (2) *Cryptococcus gattii*. In a recent study of 31 dogs with cryptococcosis, 68% had CNS infection, with neurological signs being the most common reason for presentation.[55] Dogs and cats with cryptococcosis typically have pleocytoses and elevated protein concentrations, but pleocytoses may be variably neutrophilic, eosinophilic, mononuclear, or mixed. In a recent study of 15 dogs with CNS cryptococcosis, organisms were found in 11 of 15 CSF samples (Figs. 14.9 and 14.10).[56] All affected dogs had pleocytoses that were mixed to mononuclear, whereas cats tended to have neutrophilic pleocytoses.[56] Of the samples, 11 of 12 also had increased protein concentrations (mean 494 mg/dL), which were significantly higher than in cats in the same study (mean 45 mg/dL).[56] Capsular antigen latex agglutination testing on serum or CSF is highly sensitive and specific and is recommended if cryptococcosis is suspected but organisms are not visualized cytologically.[57] This test may yield negative results if disease is present but localized (i.e., within the respiratory tract), so appropriate clinical signs should guide testing. Culture of CSF may also be helpful and may distinguish *C. neoformans* from *C. gattii* with the use of selective media. The finding of inflammatory foci on MRI may be supportive of the presence of fungal disease; cryptococcosis may result in mass lesions, meningitis, or pseudocyst formation.

Cryptococcosis in cats. Cryptococcosis is the most common systemic fungal disease of cats and is believed to infect the CNS less

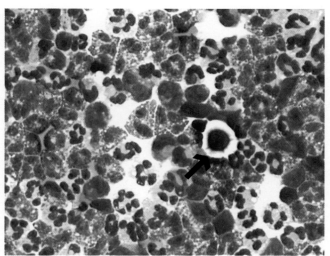

Fig. 14.9 Cryptococcosis. Note the presence of *Cryptococcus* spp. *(arrow)* and the presence of numerous eosinophils (modified Wright stain, original magnification 500×).

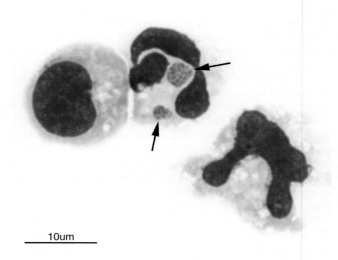

Fig. 14.11 Cerebrospinal fluid from a dog with ehrlichiosis. Two *Ehrlichia* morulae are evident in the central cell *(arrows)*.

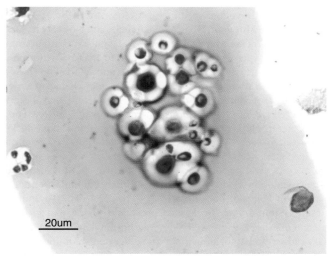

Fig. 14.10 Cryptococcosis. Numerous yeasts show a thick clear capsule. Narrow-based budding is also evident (Wright-Giemsa stain).

frequently than in the dog. A recent study found that 42% of 62 cats with cryptococcosis had CNS infection, but respiratory signs were still a more common reason for presentation.[55] Mild to marked neutrophilic or mononuclear pleocytosis may occur, with variable and occasionally normal protein concentrations.[4] A study of cats with CNS cryptococcosis showed organisms in 9 of 11 of the CSF samples, and a majority of cases (9 of 10) had neutrophilic pleocytosis and increased protein concentration (8 of 10).[56] Eosinophilic pleocytosis may also occur. Capsular antigen latex agglutination testing on serum or CSF is recommended for confirmation of *Cryptococcus* spp. infection, with rare false-negative reactions if disease is highly localized.

Histoplasmosis. *Histoplasma capsulatum* is a systemic dimorphic fungus that has been visualized in canine CSF and may be extracellular or within leukocytes.[58] A case report of an extradural *H. capsulatum* granuloma overlying spinal segments T11-L1 in a cat was associated with no cisternal CSF abnormalities.[59]

Aspergillosis. A study of dogs with systemic aspergillosis reported 4 of 8 CSF samples with neutrophilic pleocytosis (magnitude unspecified) and 1 of 8 with mononuclear reactivity.[60] Protein

concentrations were not reported.[60] A more recent study focused on dogs with CNS aspergillosis, with 4 of 6 dogs demonstrating a neutrophilic pleocytosis (range: 20–1450 cells/µL) accompanied by protein elevation (38–1682 mg/dL).[48]

Phaeohyphomycosis. Phaeohyphomycosis represents a group of darkly pigmented (typically brown, using routine stains) hyphal fungi, including neurotropic *Cladophialophora* spp. (formerly named *Cladosporidium* spp.) and *Xylohypha* spp. Acute infection may be characterized by mild to moderate neutrophilic pleocytosis and mild to moderately elevated protein concentration.[57]

Ehrlichiosis. Neutrophilic pleocytosis has been reported in cases of granulocytic *Ehrlichia* spp. in dogs (Fig. 14.11).[61] Neurological signs are uncommon in this disease, and affected dogs may display features ranging from ataxia to seizures.

Feline infectious peritonitis. Feline infectious peritonitis (FIP) has been traditionally linked to marked CSF changes, but the current literature paints a somewhat more varied picture. One study of natural FIP infection showed neutrophilic pleocytosis (as defined by >50% neutrophils) in the majority (7 of 11) of cases, with fewer cases of mononuclear (3 of 11; as defined by >80% mononuclear cells) and mixed cell (1 of 11) pleocytosis, all of variable severity.[4] Most cases (7 of 9) also had differing degrees of elevated protein concentrations.[4] Diagnosis was confirmed by histopathology or suggested by elevated feline coronavirus antibody titers and reduced albumin-to-globulin ratios in both serum and body cavity effusions.[4] A slightly older study of 16 CSF samples (natural and experimental infections) showed pleocytosis in 2 of 16 cases (neutrophilic and lymphocytic) and elevated protein concentration in 4 of 16 cases.[62] In a larger study of 67 cats with FIP or non-FIP disease, incidence of pleocytosis was highest in the neurological FIP group, but 20% of these patients did not have a pleocytosis.[63] Additionally, protein concentrations were variably elevated and not statistically different in FIP compared with non-FIP neurological disease.[63] Another study of 12 cats with CNS FIP showed 8 of 12 with unspecified pleocytosis and 3 of 12 with elevated protein concentration.[64] In cats with CNS disease, sensitivity of feline coronavirus (FeCoV) immunoglobulin G (IgG) in CSF for the diagnosis of FIP was 60%, and specificity was 93%, with a positive predictive value of 75% and a negative predictive value of 87% (FIP prevalence in this population was 25.6%).[63] Definitive diagnosis of this disease remains challenging, with virus identification (PCR or immunohistochemistry) accompanied by pyogranulomatous inflammation in tissues being the gold standard. Hypergammaglobulinemia, elevated serum α_1-acid glycoprotein (AGP), MRI abnormalities (typically involving the ventricular lining and meninges), and positive feline coronavirus IgG titer or PCR from serum, tissue, or CSF are supportive but not specifically diagnostic, and negative findings do not rule out disease.[20,63,65]

Toxoplasmosis in cats. Cats are the definitive hosts for *Toxoplasma gondii* and may be subclinically infected; thus, diagnostics should only be performed on patients with appropriate clinical signs. Cats typically present with mild neutrophilic or mononuclear pleocytosis and normal to mildly elevated protein concentration, but marked protein elevation may occur.[4] Mild lymphocytic pleocytosis is also reported.[65] Diagnosis may be confirmed by direct visualization of organisms in CSF, aspirates of other inflammatory foci, histopathology of affected tissues, or fecal examination. Serology must be interpreted cautiously because IgG may remain elevated for up to 6 years after exposure. Therefore, paired serum IgM-IgG titers, indicating acute exposure, or documentation of rising serum IgG titers are more useful, but the latter is difficult to document in the advanced state of disease.[65,66]

Spinal epidural empyema in dogs. Epidural empyema is an uncommon disease in dogs, resulting from pyogenic infection in the epidural space. One study showed 4 of 5 dogs with neutrophilic pleocytosis of variable magnitude (11–342 cells/µL).[67] No organisms were visualized on any of the samples.[67] Except for one case with a lumbar CSF protein concentration of 726 mg/dL, protein elevations were modest.[67] Three CSF samples were cultured with no growth, and two dogs for which follow-up CSF was obtained showed resolution of pleocytosis.[67] These results are not surprising, as the dura likely provides a barrier to prevent infection extending from the epidural space to the subarachnoid space.

Other infections. A case of *Sarcocystis* spp. infection has been reported in a young cat with a marked neutrophilic pleocytosis with intracellular and extracellular merozoites observed on CSF cytology.[68] Diagnosis was confirmed with decreasing paired serologic titers, and speciation to the level of *Sarcocystis dasypi* or *Sarcocystis neurona* was conducted with PCR from blood.[68] A case of systemic *Acanthamoeba* spp. infection in a young Boxer, diagnosed post mortem, had antemortem CSF with marked neutrophilic pleocytosis (4956 cells/µL), marked increase in protein concentration (259 mg/dL), and subnormal CSF IgA concentration (33 mg/dL; reference interval 35–270 mg/dL).[69] Postmortem PCR for the organism was positive on extraneural tissue but not on CSF or spinal cord.[69] The patient had been deliberately immunosuppressed on the basis of a preponderance of evidence of steroid-responsive meningitis arteritis at initial presentation and thus may have been infected either before or opportunistically after treatment.[69] Another case report of canine cerebellar *Balamuthia mandrillaris* infection (diagnosed post mortem with immunohistochemistry) displayed a marked neutrophilic pleocytosis (234 cells/µL), but other cases with lymphocytic pleocytosis have been reported.[70] Because of tissue encystment, it is suggested that extraneural tissue be used for immunohistochemistry or PCR for antemortem confirmation of amoebic infection; PCR of CSF may be diagnostic but is not widely available.[69,70] Two dogs with aberrant spinal migration of *Spirocirca lupi* nematodes had moderate to marked neutrophilic to mixed or eosinophilic pleocytoses (800 cells/µL with 91% neutrophils; 180 cells/µL with 60% neutrophils, 30% eosinophils).[71]

Noninfectious conditions

Steroid-responsive meningitis arteritis. Steroid-responsive meningitis arteritis (SRMA) is presumptively an immune-mediated

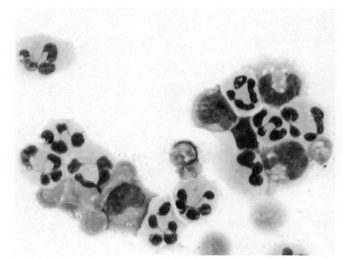

Fig. 14.12 Steroid-responsive meningitis in a Bernese Mountain Dog. Mixed inflammation with nondegenerate neutrophils and large mononuclear cells (modified Wright stain, original magnification 500×).

disease of mainly young, medium-and large- breed dogs: Beagles, Boxers, Bernese Mountain Dogs, Weimaraners, and Nova Scotia Duck Tolling Retrievers are overrepresented.[20] CSF analysis is important in diagnosis and typically features a moderate to marked neutrophilic pleocytosis (a left shift may be present) and markedly elevated protein concentration. Chronically, pleocytosis may change to a more mononuclear or mixed population (Fig. 14.12) and may become mild or even fall into reference intervals.[72] A study of 20 affected dogs showed neutrophilic pleocytosis in 12 of 20 cases and mononuclear pleocytosis in 8 of 20 cases.[72] Concurrent elevations of serum and CSF IgA titers (elevated IgG and IgM fractions may be present), serum concentration of cross-reactive protein (CRP), or serum α_2-macroglobulin is diagnostically supportive but not specific.[20,50] Increases in IgA have been linked to a T-helper 2 (Th2)–dominated immune response driven by elevated interleukin-4 (IL-4) and decreased IL-2 and interferon-gamma (IFN-γ).[73] Serum amyloid A (SAA), serum AGP, and serum haptoglobin may also be elevated.[74] Another study of 36 dogs with SRMA reported statistically significant elevations of CSF and serum CRP, but not serum α_2-macroglobulin, in dogs with SRMA compared with other neurological diseases.[75] In a study of 20 dogs, serum CRP was positively correlated with CSF TNCC.[72] Additionally, serum haptoglobin and serum and CSF IgA remained increased throughout successful treatment, indicating that these parameters are more useful for diagnosis than for monitoring therapy.[72] Serum and CSF concentrations of CRP and SAA have been documented to fall significantly during treatment, and repeat measurement of serum CRP or SAA may be used to guide therapy and predict relapse, which is less invasive and more sensitive than repeat CSF sampling.[72,74,75] Rare cases have been documented in cats with marked mononuclear or mixed pleocytosis and mild to moderate protein concentration elevations.[4]

Intervertebral disk herniation. CSF from patients with IVDH may be extremely variable; data indicate that CSF findings correlate with location of sampling, disk herniation location, chronicity of the lesion, and severity of spinal cord injury. Bearing this in mind, it is no surprise that some reports in the literature state that neutrophilic, lymphocytic, mixed, and mononuclear pleocytoses are most common in dogs with IVDH.[12,30,76] A study of 423 cases of IVDH showed 51% with pleocytosis, of which 31% were neutrophilic, 41% were lymphocytic, 20% were mixed, and 7.4% were mononuclear.[76] Of all cases, 71% had elevated protein concentrations.[76] Interestingly, a larger number of cases of lymphocytic pleocytosis were observed in the samples analyzed more than 7 days after onset of clinical signs.[76] The magnitude of pleocytosis, in general, was also shown to decrease with increasing time between clinical onset and sampling, and this observation has been corroborated by other studies.[12,76] Prior treatment with corticosteroids was observed to reduce the number of observed lymphocytes in CSF.[76] The authors also found a higher incidence of pleocytosis in thoracolumbar disease (61%) compared with cervical disease (23%), but this may have been caused by exclusive sampling of lumbar CSF closer to the lesion.[76] IVDH is rare in cats and has been reported to feature mild mixed cell pleocytosis and elevated protein concentration.[4]

Ischemic myelopathy caused by fibrocartilaginous embolism. Patients typically present with nonpainful, progressive, asymmetrical neurological signs. As only histopathology is confirmatory, it is a multimodal diagnosis of exclusion. A study of 32 dogs with presumptive FCE, based on history, clinical signs, imaging, and outcome, showed 53% with normal CSF, 25% with ACD, and 19% with mild to moderate pleocytosis (7–84 cells/µL; median 12/µL).[77] Pleocytoses were neutrophilic or mixed.[77] One study of 36 confirmed cases in dogs showed that 64% had normal CSF and the remainder displayed mild changes.[78] Another study looking at five dogs suggested that pleocytosis may be marked, up to 529 cells/µL.[3]

FCE is much less common in cats. In general, the disease process and clinical signs are similar to those in dogs, with the exception that the disease presents in cats in middle or older age, usually with cervical spinal cord signs. A case series of five cats showed CSF ranging from normal to marked neutrophilic pleocytosis with moderately elevated protein concentration and variable correlation to clinical outcome.[79] The case with the most severe CSF changes had extensive myelomalacia at necropsy.[79] It was suggested in this study that CSF is more likely to be abnormal if collected closer to the lesion and that MRI is helpful for localization and in supporting the diagnosis.[77,79]

Thiamine deficiency in cats. Thiamine deficiency is a rare nutritional disorder of patients fed noncommercial, misformulated commercial, or irradiated diets. Two case reports showed increased percentage of neutrophils or mild neutrophilic pleocytosis, presumptively from cerebrocortical necrosis.[4] Diagnosis is based on history, response to treatment, MRI features compatible with the disease (cortical and brainstem hyperintensities), or histopathology.[80]

Chiari-like malformation. A study of 61 Cavalier King Charles Spaniels with Chiari-like malformation showed that 40% of dogs with concurrent syringomyelia and cisternal CSF sampling had mild (up to 15 cells/µL) pleocytoses and increased percentages of neutrophils compared with the subpopulation without syringomyelia, but it was not specifically documented whether pleocytoses were, in fact, neutrophilic or mixed with an increased percentage of neutrophils.[42] A positive correlation was also seen to exist between TNCC and syrinx size.[42]

Neoplasia. It is important to perform CSF in neurology patients with suspected neoplasia, as definitive diagnosis may be achieved if neoplastic cells are directly observed via cytology. Inflammatory pleocytoses or elevated protein concentrations are common in patients with cancer, tend to be mild to moderate in magnitude, and may represent paraneoplastic inflammation, compromise of the BBB, lesional necrosis, or all of these.[28] Normal CSF is also a common finding in cases of neoplasia. Moreover, in the absence of overtly neoplastic cells, no defined patterns connect specific tumors with specific types of inflammatory pleocytoses. Neutrophilic pleocytosis of unspecified magnitude was found in the CSF of 2 of 11 cats with spinal lymphoma and in 3 of 7 cats with nonlymphoma spinal neoplasia (astrocytoma or osteosarcoma).[81] Additionally, the remaining four

cats with nonlymphoma spinal tumors (meningioma, peripheral nerve sheath tumor, plasma cell tumor) had either normal CSF or ACD of unspecified magnitude.[81] Metastatic tumors to the CNS should also be considered in a patient with neurological signs.

Eosinophilic Pleocytosis

Eosinophilic meningoencephalitis of dogs. EME is an idiopathic diagnosis of exclusion that is typically steroid responsive and is postulated to be triggered by an underlying hypersensitivity, allergy, or self-limiting infection. The disease may be overrepresented in Rottweilers and Golden Retrievers.[82] A study of 23 dogs with eosinophilic pleocytosis (defined by >20% eosinophils) showed 16 cases of idiopathic EME, 4 cases of infectious disease (*C. neoformans*, *N. caninum*, *Baylisascaris procyonis*), and 3 cases of IVDH.[83] The magnitude of pleocytosis or the percentage of eosinophils could not be used to distinguish infectious versus EME cases, although IVDH cases tended to have milder pleocytoses (<84 cells/µL).[83] In about half the EME cases, MRI showed abnormal findings.[83] Peripheral eosinophilia may or may not be present.

Infectious and other conditions. Eosinophilic pleocytosis is highly suggestive of protozoal (toxoplasmosis, neosporosis), fungal (cryptococcosis), parasitic (including *Cuterebra* spp., dirofilariasis), and algal (prototothecosis) infections and also rarely in cases of canine distemper and rabies viruses.[10,84] Eosinophils have also been found in cases of granulomatous meningoencephalomyelitis (GME).[85] Eosinophilic pleocytosis has been documented in bacterial encephalitis as well.[21]

Lymphocytic Pleocytosis

Infectious conditions

Toxoplasmosis in dogs. Dogs with clinical indications for *T. gondii* infection tend to have neurological or neuromuscular signs. Case reports are sporadic; documentation of mild ACD (58 mg/dL) and also a report of mild lymphocytic or eosinophilic pleocytosis (35 cells/µL) with an elevated protein concentration of 77 mg/dL exist in the literature.[86] It is important to rule out other potential causes of the neurological signs because immunocompetent dogs tend to clear subclinical infections, and therefore paired serum IgM-IgG titers or sequential serum IgG titers are preferable to a single serum IgG titer. To the author's knowledge, no data on the life span of canine IgG antibodies exist. Reports in the literature are conflicting with regard to the cross-reactivity of *T. gondii* antibodies to other agents, such as *N. caninum*.[20,86] PCR testing for *Toxoplasma* in serum, tissue, or CSF is diagnostic.[86,87]

Rabies. Pleocytoses may be lymphocytic and of varying severity. Ancillary antemortem diagnostics include viral PCR on saliva or CSF and the saliva antigen latex agglutination test. In a study of 15 dogs under quarantine for suspected natural infection (subsequently confirmed positive), 13 of 15 were saliva-PCR positive, and 4 of 15 (27%) were CSF-PCR positive.[88] All animals with positive results on CSF were also positive on saliva, and interestingly 100% correlation was seen between positive CSF-PCR and the dull clinical presentation (all aggressive clinical presentations were CSF-PCR negative).[88] Negative testing should never exclude diagnosis because viral load is highest within salivary glands and brain parenchyma.[88]

Acute canine distemper virus infection. Antemortem diagnosis of canine distemper virus (CDV) infection is difficult and is frequently made by exclusion when coupled with appropriate clinical signs. CSF and MRI findings are variable and may be normal in the acute stage of disease before inflammation has peaked.[89] In a study of 32 dogs with noninflammatory distemper, half (15 of 32) had normal

CSF.[85] A study of eight dogs with natural infection (confirmed by CNS tissue–PCR and histopathology) showed lymphocytic pleocytosis in all samples and normal protein concentrations.[90] Another case (confirmed by tissue–PCR and CSF-PCR) in a 7-month-old dog displayed marked (554 cells/μL) lymphocytic pleocytosis and a normal protein concentration.[89] Because this is a demyelinating disease, myelin-like material, which is amorphous, granular, pink, foamy, and stains positively with Luxol fast blue, may be present.[40] PCR testing of CSF, serum, urine, epithelial or tonsillar tissue is available, and immunohistochemistry on biopsy specimens of nasal mucosa, haired skin, or footpad is 88% to 96% sensitive for detection of viral antigen.[91]

Chronic canine distemper virus infection. If a pleocytosis is present, it is likely to be lymphocytic. Pleocytoses are typically mild to moderate, but severe lymphocytic pleocytoses have been reported.[89] Main differential diagnoses include other viral diseases, GME, or chronic bacterial infection. Extranigral signs related to the gastrointestinal or the respiratory system, if present, may be helpful in distinguishing this disease from GME.[89] In a study comparing four dogs with chronic CDV, six dogs with acute CDV, and controls, dogs with chronic CDV had markedly elevated CSF IgG concentration.[92] The IgG region was polyclonal, including a population of neutralizing antibodies for CDV.[92]

Coccidioidomycosis. *Coccidioides immitis* is a dimorphic fungus acquired through inhalation, and most cases in the United States are observed in the southwestern region of the country. Signs tend to involve respiratory or skeletal systems, and CNS involvement is rare. One dog had a mild to moderate lymphocytic pleocytosis.[57] Complement fixation (detecting IgG) or tube precipitation (detecting IgM), or agar-gel immunodiffusion serological testing is recommended for confirmation.

Noninfectious conditions

Necrotizing meningoencephalitis. Meningoencephalitis has been subcategorized as necrotizing meningoencephalitis (NME) and necrotizing leukoencephalitis (NLE) on the basis of histopathological appearance. Both NLE and NME are believed to have an immune-mediated basis, and recent data support that in Pugs with NME, canine leukocyte antigen gene aberrations exist.[93] Meningoencephalitis is rapidly progressive and affects a variety of generally young to middle-aged toy-breed dogs, including the Pug, Shih Tzu, Papillon, Maltese, Chihuahua, Yorkshire terrier, French bulldog, Pekingese, West Highland White terrier, Boston terrier, Japanese Spitz, and Miniature Pinscher breeds.[20,94] A study of CSF from 14 Pugs with NME showed 12 of 14 with pleocytoses of varying severity (mean 120 cells/μL).[95] Of these dogs, 66% had a lymphocytic pleocytosis, 17% had a mononuclear pleocytosis, and 17% had a mixed cell pleocytosis (Fig. 14.13)[95]; 11 of 14 dogs had elevated protein concentrations (mean 88.4 mg/dL).[95] Another study of three dogs showed one with ACD and two with moderate to marked (40–220 cells/μL) neutrophilic to lymphocytic pleocytosis.[94] MRI findings may help support a diagnosis, but only histopathological examination of lesions provides definitive proof.

Other. Four cats with ischemic encephalopathy had mild (<10 cells/μL) lymphocytic pleocytosis.[28] Another study of feline ischemic encephalopathy reported one cat with normal CSF and another with mononuclear to mixed pleocytosis (26 cells/μL).[96] A report of two cats with cerebrovascular disease (infarction or stroke) showed one with mononuclear pleocytosis and the other with ACD.[97] Cerebrovascular disease was correlated in several other cases (without CSF data) to hepatic lipidosis or FIP.[97] A prospective study of CSF from 17 Pembroke Welsh Corgis with familial degenerative myelopathy showed normal CSF in 15 samples and hemodilution in 2 samples.[98] Various

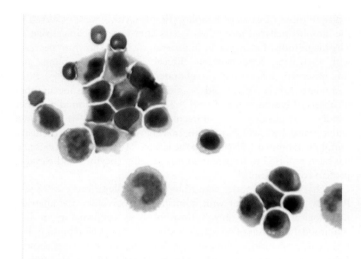

Fig. 14.13 Necrotizing meningoencephalitis in a Pug. Mixed lymphocytic and large mononuclear inflammation (modified Wright stain, original magnification 500×).

degenerative myelopathies have been described in German Shepherds, Afghan Hounds, Rottweilers, Jack Russell Terriers, and Smooth-Haired Fox Terriers and have been associated with mild CSF changes.[11]

Mononuclear Pleocytosis

Infectious conditions

Neosporosis. Dogs are the definitive host of *N. caninum*. Most clinical cases are young animals that present with CNS (especially cerebellar) signs, neuromuscular signs, or both. Two recent case reports have described protozoal tachyzoites directly visualized in the CSF intracellularly and extracellularly.[99,100] Both patients had been previously treated with glucocorticoids.[99,100] One case had a marked mixed to mononuclear pleocytosis (1450 cells/μL) with marked protein elevation (992 mg/dL), and the other case had a marked eosinophilic pleocytosis (298 cells/μL) with a markedly elevated protein concentration (392 mg/dL) protein at the time of diagnosis.[99,100] Diagnosis was confirmed in both cases by postmortem immunohistochemistry of tissue.[99,100] Another study showed six of seven naturally infected dogs demonstrating a mild to marked mononuclear pleocytosis (12–300 cells/μL) with moderately to markedly elevated protein concentrations observed in four of six dogs (60–290 mg/dL).[101] A majority of these cases displayed cerebellar neurologic signs.[101] Antemortem immunohistochemistry of CNS or muscular tissue is diagnostic but may not be practical. Increased serum liver or muscle enzymes and electromyography (EMG) may be helpful if concordant signs are present.[99] A variety of serological techniques to assay for the presence of antibody are available, and a titer greater than 1:64 is supportive of diagnosis. Antibody detection in serum or CSF, coupled with PCR of CSF or other potentially affected tissues, is currently recommended for the definitive diagnosis of CNS neosporosis.[20]

Other. A case report of a Pug with a mild mononuclear pleocytosis (8 cells/μL), mild elevation in protein concentration (89 mg/dL), evidence of hemorrhage, and direct visualization of *Angiostrongylus vasorum* helminth larvae is found in the literature.[102] Eosinophilia was not observed within the CSF or peripheral blood.[102] The organism is endemic in Europe and Canada among foxes and canids, mainly causing respiratory signs or coagulopathy; neurological signs are typically caused by hemorrhage.[102] Two dogs with paraparesis and pyogranulomatous lumbar masses (one intradural, one extradural) had lumbar CSF with

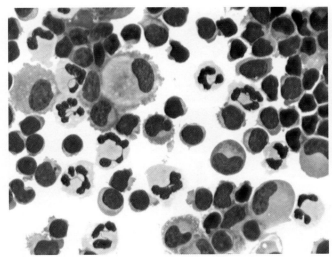

Fig. 14.14 Granulomatous meningoencephalitis. Mixed mononuclear and neutrophilic inflammation (modified Wright stain, original magnification 500×).

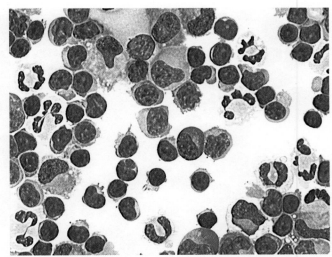

Fig. 14.15 Granulomatous meningoencephalitis. Mixed mononuclear and neutrophilic inflammation. Note the presence of a plasma cell in the center (modified Wright stain, original magnification 500×).

mild mixed cell pleocytosis (lymphocytes and nondegenrate neutrophils) or lymphocytic pleocytosis.[103] These patients were serologically PCR positive for *Bartonella vinsonii* subsp. *berkhoffi* and presented with a nodular dermatosis.[103] A dog with neurological signs and *Hepatozoon canis* infection showed marked lymphocytic pleocytosis (243 cell/μL) with mildly elevated protein concentration (37 mg/dL).[104] Organisms were not visualized in CSF but were found on cytology of peripheral blood, lymph node, bone marrow, and bony lesions. Serology and positive PCR from a bone marrow sample were diagnostic.[104]

Noninfectious conditions

Intrathecal contrast administration. Contrast media or pharmacological agents, such as epidural anesthetics, may introduce preanalytical error into CSF samples, artificially raising TNCC and protein concentrations.[105] In a study of 17 healthy dogs given either iopamidol or metrizamide for EMG, same-day CSF sampling showed that 8 of 17 developed a mild to moderate mononuclear to mixed mononuclear or neutrophilic pleocytosis (6 of 8 were from iopamidol).[106] In the same study, 3 of 17 (all metrizamide) developed mild protein elevation, but mean protein concentration for both groups stayed within the reference interval.[106] In dogs given metrizamide, 7 of 8 had an increased Pandy score after EMG, which was considered a false-positive result because of the contrast agent.[106] These data, plus histopathology from the same population, showed that the contrast agents caused low-grade leptomeningeal inflammation with no statistical difference between the two agents studied.[106] Another similar study over 30 days showed that post-EMG CSF changes reversed after approximately 5 days.[107]

Granulomatous meningoencephalitis. GME is a progressive immune-mediated disease that is overrepresented in females, Toy-breed dogs, and Terriers.[20] It is a diagnosis of exclusion and has clinical presentations and MRI findings that may be similar to various infectious and neoplastic diseases. CSF may be unaffected or may display a mononuclear to mixed pleocytosis and protein concentration elevations, both of varying severity (Figs. 14.14 and 14.15). In a study of 188 CSF samples from dogs with inflammatory neurological diseases, marked pleocytosis (>1000 cells/μL) was found in cases of SRMA, bacterial encephalitis, or GME.[85] Pleocytosis may also be lymphocytic or neutrophilic.[10] CSF protein electrophoresis may be helpful, as several cases have been shown with increased β-globulin and gammaglobulin fractions.[108]

Mixed Cell Pleocytosis

Most of the diseases described previously in this chapter may manifest as mixed cell pleocytoses, depending on the time interval between disease onset and CSF sampling, disease severity, and previous treatment administered. A mixed cell pleocytosis would be expected to occur during transition between different phases of the inflammatory response, where certain cells may predominate at specific times after injury.

Blastomycosis. Infection of the CNS by *Blastomyces dermatiditis* is typically rare and may involve chorioretinitis or focal cerebral granuloma in the cat.[109] A study of two dogs with systemic blastomycosis and neurologic signs showed mild mixed cell pleocytosis (8 cells/μL, mononuclear predominant; and 15 cells/μL, lymphocytic predominant).[110] Using CSF cytology or culture to diagnose the organism may be unrewarding. Agar-gel immunodiffusion serologic testing has high sensitivity and specificity for canine antibodies and is recommended if appropriate clinical signs (respiratory signs or lymphadenopathy) are present.[57] Agar-gel immunodiffusion testing is less sensitive (25%–33%) in the cat, as indicated by a limited number of reports.[57] Urine antigen enzyme immunoassay (EIA) has good sensitivity for dogs and has been used successfully on at least one cat.[109] EIA may also be performed on CSF. Cytology of nasal, pulmonary, or dermal lesions is more likely to yield direct visualization of organisms.

Neoplasia

Lymphoma. Lymphocytic pleocytosis of inflammatory origin may be difficult to distinguish from lymphoma exfoliating into the CSF (Fig. 14.16). The size of lymphocytes and morphological atypia may be helpful, although these may be challenging to differentiate from artifactual morphological changes secondary to cytospin preparation. Cats with neoplasia may have lymphocytic pleocytoses (suggestive of lymphoma), mild to moderate mononuclear to mixed cell pleocytoses (suggestive of nonlymphoma tumors), or normal CSF. One study examined six cases of feline CNS or multifocal lymphoma, which displayed pleocytoses of variable magnitude, absent to mildly elevated protein concentrations, and neoplastic cells visualized in 5 of 6 of the CSF samples.[4] In this study, eight cats with CNS signs that were ultimately diagnosed with nonlymphoma tumors (e.g., meningioma, carcinoma, nerve sheath tumor) had mild CSF protein elevations and either normal TNCC (1 of 8) or mild to moderate mononuclear or mixed cell

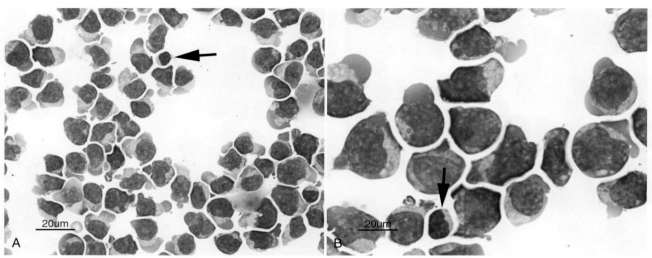

Fig. 14.16 Cerebrospinal fluid samples from a dog with central nervous system lymphoma. (A) Low magnification shows a cellular slide consisting almost entirely of large, pleomorphic lymphoid cells. A mature lymphocyte with condensed, mature chromatin is present *(arrow)*. (B) Higher magnification of the same slide. Lymphoid cells are large with pleomorphic nuclei and immature chromatin. Some cells have distinct nucleoli. A mature lymphocyte with condensed chromatin is present *(arrow)* (Wright-Giemsa stain).

pleocytosis (7 of 8).[4] Another study of 11 cats with spinal lymphoma showed neoplastic cells visualized in one case and hemodilution, ACD, or neutrophilic pleocytosis in the remainder of cases.[81] A case report of feline multiple myeloma involving lumbar vertebrae and associated soft tissues exhibited cisternal CSF with an elevated protein concentration of 290 mg/dL and mild pleocytosis (8 cells/μL) consisting of a majority of neoplastic plasma cells.[111] Diagnosis was further confirmed by abnormal urine protein electrophoresis and bone marrow aspiration.[111]

Histiocytic malignancies. Malignant histiocytosis or histiocytic sarcoma tumor cells in canine CSF have been documented in two recent case reports; CSF cytology displayed marked mononuclear pleocytoses (>500 cells/μL) and mild to moderately elevated protein concentrations (<135 mg/dL).[112,113] Tumor cells phenotypically resembled macrophages, displayed multiple criteria of malignancy, and reacted positively to CD1c on immunocytochemistry, compatible with interstitial dendritic cell origin.[112,113] Necropsy was confirmatory and found no evidence of neoplasia outside of the CNS.[112,113] A case report of a gliomatosis cerebri (GC) neoplasm in a middle-aged poodle showed CSF with a mild lymphocytic pleocytosis (20 cells/μL) and protein concentration elevation.[114] On histopathology, lymphocyte-like perivascular cuffing and meningitis were noted. Other case studies of canine GC have reported normal CSF or mild ACD.[115]

Meningioma. In a study of 56 dogs with intracranial meningioma, in which CSF analysis was performed, 29% had normal CSF, 45% had ACD, and 27% had pleocytosis (2 of 3 of these neutrophilic pleocytosis; 1 of 3 unspecified), with the overall incidence of neutrophilic pleocytosis at 18%.[116] In this study, a positive correlation existed between elevated TNCC and anatomical localization of the lesion to the caudal (versus middle or rostral) portion of the cranial fossa, and no association between pleocytosis and necrosis within the lesion was found.[116] These findings contradict prior reports of a high percentage of abnormal CSF findings in meningioma, and the authors reported that concurrent glucocorticoid therapy in some of the patients may have negatively biased the data.[11,116] A study of 26 dogs with spinal meningioma showed no cases with exfoliating tumor cells, 62% with mild pleocytosis up to 47 cells/μL (mean 11 cells/μL), and normal or variably elevated protein concentrations up to 836 mg/dL (mean 212 mg/dL).[117] Both cisternal and lumbar CSF samples were evaluated in this study and not found to

be significantly different.[117] Interestingly, tumors of the lumbar region displayed higher mean TNCC and protein concentrations compared with tumors of the cervical area (24 versus 4 cells/μL and 158 versus 98 mg/dL, respectively), which the authors postulated may be reflective of a higher number of lumbar CSF samples with proximity to the lesion.[117]

Other neoplasms. A case report of canine CSF with 240 cells/μL was characterized by atypical neoplastic round cells that were confirmed on immunocytochemistry and immunohistochemistry to be from a metastatic mammary carcinoma.[118] Inflammatory cells were of low numbers and were of a mixed population.[118] A study of CSF from 25 dogs with choroid plexus tumors showed direct observation of tumor cells in 47% of the cases of carcinoma.[119] Mild to moderate mixed-cell pleocytosis was present in all cases of papilloma and in half of the carcinomas; when pleocytosis was present, no difference in magnitude existed between benign and malignant tumors.[119] All cases had elevated protein concentrations, with median concentration for carcinoma being significantly higher (108 mg/dL) than median concentration for papilloma (34 mg/dL).[119] A cutoff protein concentration of 80 mg/dL yielded a sensitivity of 67% and a specificity of 100% for detection of choroid plexus carcinomas.[119] Another case report of canine choroid plexus carcinoma had a mononuclear pleocytosis of 165 cells/μL, mildly elevated protein concentration of 30 mg/dL, and numerous tumor cells visualized.[120]

CENTRAL NERVOUS SYSTEM CYTOLOGICAL EVALUATION

A rise in the availability of stereotactic brain biopsy has facilitated increased cytological assessments of CNS lesions. This technique offers several advantages, although significant equipment investment and time to perfect techniques is required. Stereotactic biopsy often offers application accuracy for targeting lesions that approximate 3 mm or less in all directions. In one study, diagnostic accuracy of stereotactic biopsy specimens submitted for histopathology (i.e., agreement with specimens obtained via open approaches) exceeded 90%.[121] In experienced hands, stereotactic biopsy is believed to be a relatively low-morbidity procedure.

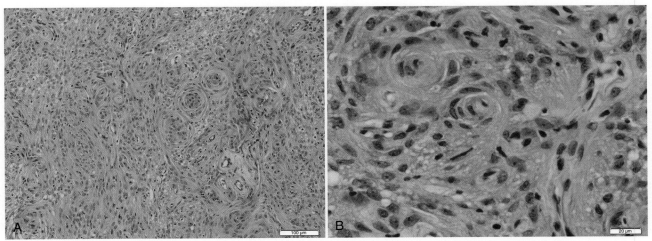

Fig. 14.17 Meningioma. (A) Low magnification shows spindle-shaped cells arranged in whorls and interweaving bundles (hematoxylin and eosin [H&E] stain, original magnification 100×). (B) High magnification of spindle-shaped cells whorling around and weaving through bright pink supporting matrix (H&E, original magnification 400×).

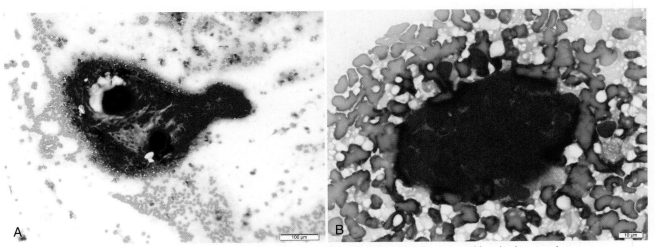

Fig. 14.18 Meningioma. (A) Low-magnification view of spindle-shaped cells arranged in whorls around centrally located mineralized material (presumed Psammoma body) (Diff-Quik, original magnification 100×). (B) Spindle cells appear to pile up on one another (Diff-Quik, original magnification 600×).

Cytological interpretation of brain biopsy specimens acquired via stereotaxy or open approaches may be challenging and does require a tumor that exfoliates well, a surgeon willing to provide multiple samples, and a cytologist with expertise in this area.[122] A study of 42 canine and feline cases of biopsy- or necropsy-confirmed CNS lesions showed squash-prep smear cytology to have 76% sensitivity in accurately determining diagnosis, with an additional 14% of cases having partial correlation between cytology and histopathology. For the remaining 10% of cases, cytological interpretation did not correlate with final diagnosis.[123] Cytological interpretation of CNS lesions may be very difficult, and biopsy with histopathological examination is recommended to confirm all diagnoses.

It is important for cytological samples to be prepared in the same manner each time to avoid introducing additional cytological variations that the pathologist has to read through. Some authors recommend wet-fixation of tissues followed by staining with hematoxylin and eosin (H&E).[122] At the authors' institution, CNS cytological samples are air-dried and stained with Diff-Quik or a modified Wright stain. The reader is referred elsewhere for a complete discussion of normal CNS cytology.[124] Clinical imaging findings, and signalment, should be considered carefully and may help the pathologist to formulate a list of potential differential diagnoses. It must be kept in mind that primary tumors may metastasize to the CNS, and these should be included in the differential diagnoses, where appropriate.

Meningioma

Meningiomas are composed of neoplastic cells arising from the meningothelial cells of the leptomeninges of the CNS.[125] These tumors are the most common primary CNS tumors of dogs and cats.[126] Histologically, these neoplasms are classified into at least nine subtypes based on appearance, and some tumors may be characterized by more than one pattern (Fig. 14.17).[125] Cytologically, smears are often characterized by spindle-shaped cells draped around vessels and arranged in large whorling structures (Fig. 14.18). Some cells may contain nuclei that display intranuclear cytoplasmic pseudoinclusions, but this is not a feature reliably seen on a majority of tumors (Fig. 14.19).[127]

Glial Tumors

As a whole, this group represents the second most common primary CNS neoplasm seen in dogs and cats.[126] Glial tumors are more

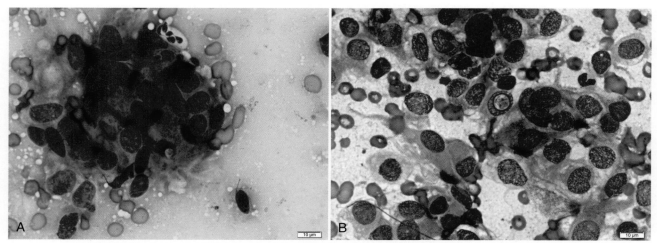

Fig. 14.19 Meningioma. (A) Cells contain plump oval to elongate nuclei, and neutrophils are occasionally observed adjacent to cell aggregates (Diff-Quik, original magnification 600×). (B) Infrequent cells *(center)* display intranuclear cytoplasmic pseudoinclusions (Diff-Quik, original magnification 600×).

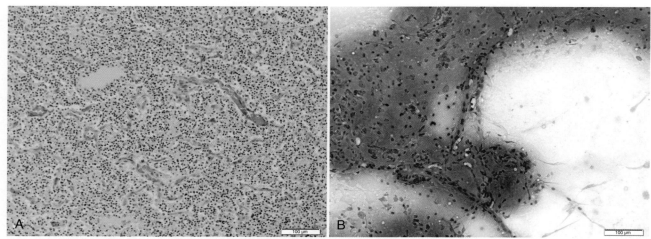

Fig. 14.20 Oligodendroglioma. (A) Tissue section showing round hyperchromatic nuclei surrounded by clear space admixed with branching capillaries and occasional lakes of basophilic mucin (H&E stain, original magnification 100×). (B) Numerous bare nuclei are seen admixed with purple fibrillar background material and branching capillary structures (Diff-Quik, original magnification 100×).

common than meningiomas in brachycephalic breeds.[126] Glial tumors arise from the supporting cells of the CNS. Astrocytomas are found most frequently in the cerebral hemispheres, although they have been reported to occur in various locations throughout the CNS.[125]

Astrocytoma

Astrocytomas arise from transformed astrocytes and are characterized cytologically by high cellularity, a high degree of nuclear pleomorphism, and fibrillar cytoplasmic processes.[125] Tumor cells will stain positively for glial fibrillary acid protein (GFAP).[125]

Oligodendroglioma

Oligodendrogliomas are derived from transformed oligodendrocytes and are found within the gray or white matter of the CNS, with the highest incidence in the cerebral hemispheres.[125] Cytological preparations are characterized by large numbers of blood vessels surrounded by neoplastic cells (Fig. 14.20).[125] Neoplastic oligodendrocytes have small amounts of eosinophilic cytoplasm surrounding uniformly round nuclei.[125]

Ependymoma

Ependymomas are derived from the ependymal lining cells found on the surface of the ventricular system of the brain and central canal of the spinal cord.[125] These tumors are rare and are found most often in the lateral ventricles.[125] Cytologically, smears are characterized by neoplastic cells palisading around branching vascular structures.[125] Cells are cuboidal to columnar in shape with high nuclear-to-cytoplasmic (N:C) ratios and eccentrically placed nuclei.[125]

Choroid Plexus Tumor

Choroid plexus tumors arise from the modified ependymal lining cells that contribute to the production of CSF. They are more common in dogs than in cats.[125] Papillomas and carcinomas have a very similar cytological appearance and may only be reliably differentiated on the basis of histopathological examination.[123] Cytological preparations contain polygonal cells arranged in rafts, columns, or papillary projections around capillary structures (Fig. 14.21).[125]

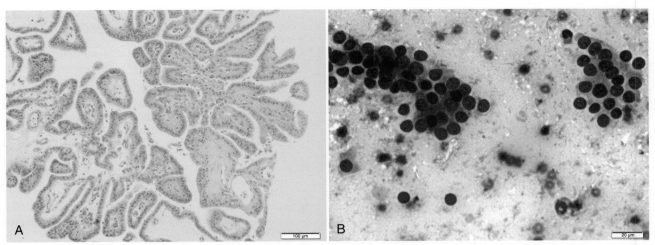

Fig. 14.21 Choroid plexus papilloma. (A) Cuboidal to columnar epithelial cells are arranged in papillary projections, which often contain small vessels (H&E stain, original magnification 100×). (B) Cuboidal epithelial cells are arranged in small sheets and papillary-like projections (Diff-Quik, original magnification 400×).

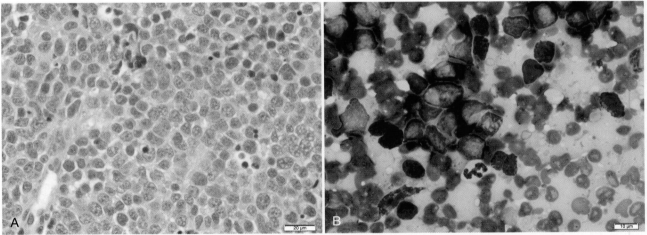

Fig. 14.22 Medulloblastoma. (A) Round cells are arranged in sheets (H&E stain, original magnification 400×). (B) Cells are large and round in shape with a high nucleus-to-cytoplasm (N:C) ratio and distinct cell borders (Diff-Quik, original magnification 600×).

Medulloblastoma

Medulloblastoma arises within the cerebellum and is a type of primitive neuroectodermal tumor derived from a germinal neuroepithelial cell.[125] Cytologically, preparations are highly cellular, composed of individual round cells that are large in size and have moderate to high N:C ratios. The appearance of these cells is reminiscent of large lymphocytes or histiocytes (Fig. 14.22).

Nephroblastoma

Nephroblastoma is a unique tumor arising in the spinal cord of young dogs (under age 4 years), usually between the T10 and L2 spinal cord segments.[125] The cytological appearance of this tumor has been described in a recent report and is characterized by three populations of cells: (1) high N:C ratio blastemal cells, (2) spindle-shaped mesenchymal cells, and (3) cuboidal epithelial cells.[128]

REFERENCES

1. de Lahunta A, Glass E, Kent M. *Veterinary Neuroanatomy and Clinical Neurology.* 4 ed. St. Louis, MO: Saunders Elsevier; 2015:600.
2. Di Terlizzi R, Platt S. The function, composition and analysis of cerebrospinal fluid in companion animals: part I–function and composition. *Vet J.* 2006;172:422–431.
3. Bohn AA, Wills TB, West CL, et al. Cerebrospinal fluid analysis and magnetic resonance imaging in the diagnosis of neurologic disease in dogs: a retrospective study. *Vet Clin Pathol.* 2006;35:315–320.
4. Singh M, Foster DJ, Child G, et al. Inflammatory cerebrospinal fluid analysis in cats: clinical diagnosis and outcome. *J Feline Med Surg.* 2005;7:77–93.
5. Gonçalves R, Platt SR, Llabrés-Díaz FJ, et al. Clinical and magnetic resonance imaging findings in 92 cats with clinical signs of spinal cord disease. *J Feline Med Surg.* 2009;11:53–59.
6. Lamb CR, Croson PJ, Cappello R, et al. Magnetic resonance imaging findings in 25 dogs with inflammatory cerebrospinal fluid. *Vet Radiol Ultrasound.* 2005;46:17–22.

7. Oreskovic D, Klarica M. The formation of cerebrospinal fluid: nearly a hundred years of interpretations and misinterpretations. *Brain Res Rev.* 2010;64:241–262.

8. Kornegay JN. Cerebrospinal fluid collection, examination, and interpretation in dogs and cats. *Compend Contin Educ Pract Vet.* 1981;3:85–90.

9. Elias A, Brown C. Cerebellomedullary cerebrospinal fluid collection in the dog. *Lab Anim.* 2008;37:457–458.

10. Di Terlizzi R, Platt SR. The function, composition and analysis of cerebrospinal fluid in companion animals: part II–analysis. *Vet J.* 2009;180:15–32.

11. Meinkoth JH, Crystal MA. Cerebrospinal fluid analysis. In: Cowell RL, Tyler RD, Meinkoth JH, eds. *Diagnostic Cytology and Hematology of the Dog and Cat.* 2nd ed. St. Louis: Mosby; 1999.

12. Thomson CE, Kornegay JN, Stevens JB. Analysis of cerebrospinal fluid from the cerebellomedullary and lumbar cisterns of dogs with focal neurologic disease: 145 cases (1985-1987). *J Am Vet Med Assoc.* 1990;196:1841–1844.

13. Bailey CS, Higgins RJ. Comparison of total white blood cell count and total protein content of lumbar and cisternal cerebrospinal fluid of healthy dogs. *Am J Vet Res.* 1985;46:1162–1165.

14. Christopher MM. Bone marrow contamination of canine cerebrospinal fluid. *Vet Clin Pathol.* 1992;21:95–98.

15. Lujan Feliu-Pascual A, Garosi L, Dennis R, et al. Iatrogenic brainstem injury during cerebellomedullary cistern puncture. *Vet Radiol Ultrasound.* 2008;49:467–471.

16. Cellio BC. Collecting, processing, and preparing cerebrospinal fluid in dogs and cats. *Compend Contin Educ Pract Vet.* 2001;23:786–792.

17. Hoerlein BF. *Canine Neurology: Diagnosis and Treatment.* Saunders; 1978.

18. Fry MM, Vernau W, Kass PH, et al. Effects of time, initial composition, and stabilizing agents on the results of canine cerebrospinal fluid analysis. *Vet Clin Pathol.* 2006;35:72–77.

19. Bienzle D, McDonnell JJ, Stanton JB. Analysis of cerebrospinal fluid from dogs and cats after 24 and 48 hours of storage. *J Am Vet Med Assoc.* 2000;216:1761–1764.

20. Nghiem PP, Schatzberg SJ. Conventional and molecular diagnostic testing for the acute neurologic patient. *J Vet Emerg Crit Care (San Antonio).* 2010;20:46–61.

21. Jamison EM, Lumsden JH. Cerebrospinal fluid analysis in the dog: methodology and interpretation. *Semin Vet Med Surg (Small Anim).* 1988;3:122–132.

22. Desnoyers M, Bedard C, Meinkoth JH, et al. Cerebrospinal fluid analysis. In: Cowell RL, Tyler RD, Meinkoth JH, eds. *Diagnostic Cytology and Hematology of the Dog and Cat.* 3rd ed. St. Louis: Mosby Elsevier; 2008:215–234.

23. Ruotsalo K, Poma R, da Costa RC, et al. Evaluation of the ADVIA 120 for analysis of canine cerebrospinal fluid. *Vet Clin Pathol.* 2008;37:242–248.

24. Becker M, Bauer N, Moritz A. Automated flow cytometric cell count and differentiation of canine cerebrospinal fluid cells using the ADVIA 2120. *Vet Clin Pathol.* 2008;37:344–352.

25. Behr S, Trumel C, Cauzinille L, et al. High resolution protein electrophoresis of 100 paired canine cerebrospinal fluid and serum. *J Vet Intern Med.* 2006;20:657–662.

26. Radaelli ST, Platt SR. Bacterial meningoencephalomyelitis in dogs: a retrospective study of 23 cases (1990-1999). *J Vet Intern Med.* 2002;16:159–163.

27. Messer JS, Wagner SO, Baumwart RD, et al. A case of canine streptococcal meningoencephalitis diagnosed using universal bacterial polymerase chain reaction assay. *J Am Anim Hosp Assoc.* 2008;44:205–209.

28. Rand JS, Parent J, Percy D, et al. Clinical, cerebrospinal fluid, and histological data from thirty-four cats with primary noninflammatory disease of the central nervous system. *Can Vet J.* 1994;35:174–181.

29. Indrieri RJ, Holliday TA, Keen CL. Critical evaluation of creatine phosphokinase in cerebrospinal fluid of dogs with neurologic disease. *Am J Vet Res.* 1980;41:1299–1303.

30. Witsberger TH, Levine JM, Fosgate GT, et al. Associations between cerebrospinal fluid biomarkers and long-term neurologic outcome in dogs with acute intervertebral disk herniation. *J Am Vet Med Assoc.* 2012;240:555–562.

31. Pancotto T, Rossmeisl JH, Panciera DL, et al. Blood-brain-barrier disruption in chronic canine hypothyroidism. *Vet Clin Pathol.* 2010;39:485–493.

32. Oji T, Kamishina H, Cheeseman JA, et al. Measurement of myelin basic protein in the cerebrospinal fluid of dogs with degenerative myelopathy. *Vet Clin Pathol.* 2007;36:281–284.

33. Levine GJ, Levine JM, Witsberger TH, et al. Cerebrospinal fluid myelin basic protein as a prognostic biomarker in dogs with thoracolumbar intervertebral disk herniation. *J Vet Intern Med.* 2010;24:890–896.

34. Munana KR, Saito M, Hoshi F. Beta-2-microglobulin levels in the cerebrospinal fluid of normal dogs and dogs with neurological disease. *Vet Clin Pathol.* 2007;36:173–178.

35. Holt DE, Washabau RJ, Djali S, et al. Cerebrospinal fluid glutamine, tryptophan, and tryptophan metabolite concentrations in dogs with portosystemic shunts. *Am J Vet Res.* 2002;63:1167–1171.

36. Brown DC, Perkowski S. Oxytocin content of the cerebrospinal fluid of dogs and its relationship to pain induced by spinal cord compression. *Vet Surg.* 1998;27:607–611.

37. Podell M, Hadjiconstantinou M. Cerebrospinal fluid gamma-aminobutyric acid and glutamate values in dogs with epilepsy. *Am J Vet Res.* 1997;58:451–456.

38. Chrisman CL. Cerebrospinal fluid analysis. *Vet Clin North Am Small Anim Pract.* 1992;22:781–810.

39. Wessmann A, Volk HA, Chandler K, et al. Significance of surface epithelial cells in canine cerebrospinal fluid and relationship to central nervous system disease. *Vet Clin Pathol.* 2010;39:358–364.

40. Bauer NB, Bassett H, O'Neill EJ, et al. Cerebrospinal fluid from a 6-year-old dog with severe neck pain. *Vet Clin Pathol.* 2006;35:123–125.

41. Zabolotzky SM, Vernau KM, Kass PH, et al. Prevalence and significance of extracellular myelin-like material in canine cerebrospinal fluid. *Vet Clin Pathol.* 2010;39:90–95.

42. Whittaker DE, English K, McGonnell IM, et al. Evaluation of cerebrospinal fluid in Cavalier King Charles Spaniel dogs diagnosed with Chiari-like malformation with or without concurrent syringomyelia. *J Vet Diagn Invest.* 2011;23:302–307.

43. Hurtt AE, Smith MO. Effects of iatrogenic blood contamination on results of cerebrospinal fluid analysis in clinically normal dogs and dogs with neurologic disease. *J Am Vet Med Assoc.* 1997;211:866–867.

44. Rand JS, Parent J, Jacobs R, et al. Reference intervals for feline cerebrospinal fluid: cell counts and cytologic features. *Am J Vet Res.* 1990;51:1044–1048.

45. Sweeney CR, Russell GE. Differences in total protein concentration, nucleated cell count, and red blood cell count among sequential samples of cerebrospinal fluid from horses. *J Am Vet Med Assoc.* 2000;217:54–57.

46. Wilson JW, Stevens JB. Effects of blood contamination on cerebrospinal fluid analysis. *J Am Vet Med Assoc.* 1977;171:256–258.

47. Doyle C, Solano-Gallego L. Cytologic interpretation of canine cerebrospinal fluid samples with low total nucleated cell concentration, with and without blood contamination. *Vet Clin Pathol.* 2009;38:392–396.

48. Taylor AR, Young BD, Levine GJ, et al. Clinical features and magnetic resonance imaging findings in 7 dogs with central nervous system aspergillosis. *J Vet Intern Med.* 2015;29:1556–1563.

49. Rand JS, Parent J, Percy D, et al. Clinical, cerebrospinal fluid, and histological data from twenty-seven cats with primary inflammatory disease of the central nervous system. *Can Vet J.* 1994;35:103–110.

50. Tipold A, Stein VM. Inflammatory diseases of the spine in small animals. *Vet Clin North Am Small Anim Pract.* 2010;40:871–879.

51. Bach JF, Mahony OM, Tidwell AS, et al. Brain abscess and bacterial endocarditis in a Kerry Blue Terrier with a history of immune-mediated thrombocytopenia. *J Vet Emerg Crit Care.* 2007;17:409–415.

52. Oliver JA, Llabres-Diaz FJ, Gould DJ, et al. Central nervous system infection with Staphylococcus intermedius secondary to retrobulbar abscessation in a dog. *Vet Ophthalmol.* 2009;12:333–337.

53. Wu CC, Chang YP. Cerebral ventriculitis associated with otogenic meningoencephalitis in a dog. *J Am Anim Hosp Assoc.* 2015;51:272–278.

54. Messer JS, Kegge SJ, Cooper ES, et al. Meningoencephalomyelitis caused by Pasteurella multocida in a cat. *J Vet Intern Med.* 2006;20:1033–1036.

55. Trivedi SR, Sykes JE, Cannon MS, et al. Clinical features and epidemiology of cryptococcosis in cats and dogs in California: 93 cases (1988-2010). *J Am Vet Med Assoc.* 2011;239:357–369.

56. Sykes JE, Sturges BK, Cannon MS, et al. Clinical signs, imaging features, neuropathology, and outcome in cats and dogs with central nervous system cryptococcosis from California. *J Vet Intern Med.* 2010;24:1427–1438.

57. Lavely J, Lipsitz D. Fungal infections of the central nervous system in the dog and cat. *Clin Tech Small Anim Pract.* 2005;20:212–219.

58. Clinkenbeard KD, Cowell RL, Tyler RD. Disseminated histoplasmosis in cats: 12 cases (1981-1986). *J Am Vet Med Assoc.* 1987;190:1445–1448.

59. Vinayak A, Kerwin SC, Pool RR. Treatment of thoracolumbar spinal cord compression associated with Histoplasma capsulatum infection in a cat. *J Am Vet Med Assoc.* 2007;230:1018–1023.

60. Schultz RM, Johnson EG, Wisner ER, et al. Clinicopathologic and diagnostic imaging characteristics of systemic aspergillosis in 30 dogs. *J Vet Intern Med.* 2008;22:851–859.

61. Meinkoth JH, Hoover JP, Cowell RL, et al. Ehrlichiosis in a dog with seizures and nonregenerative anemia. *J Am Vet Med Assoc.* 1989;195:1754–1755.

62. Foley JE, Lapointe JM, Koblik P, et al. Diagnostic features of clinical neurologic feline infectious peritonitis. *J Vet Intern Med.* 1998;12:415–423.

63. Boettcher IC, Steinberg T, Matiasek K, et al. Use of anti-coronavirus antibody testing of cerebrospinal fluid for diagnosis of feline infectious peritonitis involving the central nervous system in cats. *J Am Vet Med Assoc.* 2007;230:199–205.

64. Steinberg TA, Boettcher IC, Matiasek K, et al. Use of albumin quotient and IgG index to differentiate blood- vs brain-derived proteins in the cerebrospinal fluid of cats with feline infectious peritonitis. *Vet Clin Pathol.* 2008;37:207–216.

65. Kent M. The cat with neurological manifestations of systemic disease. Key conditions impacting on the CNS. *J Feline Med Surg.* 2009;11:395–407.

66. Lappin MR. Feline toxoplasmosis: interpretation of diagnostic test results. *Semin Vet Med Surg (Small Anim).* 1996;11:154–160.

67. Lavely JA, Vernau KM, Vernau W, et al. Spinal epidural empyema in seven dogs. *Vet Surg.* 2006;35:176–185.

68. Bisby TM, Holman PJ, Pitoc GA, et al. Sarcocystis sp. encephalomyelitis in a cat. *Vet Clin Pathol.* 2010;39:105–112.

69. Kent M, Platt SR, Rech RR, et al. Multisystemic infection with an Acanthamoeba sp. in a dog. *J Am Vet Med Assoc.* 2011;238:1476–1481.

70. Hodge PJ, Kelers K, Gasser RB, et al. Another case of canine amoebic meningoencephalitis—the challenges of reaching a rapid diagnosis. *J Parasitol Res.* 2011;108:1069–1073.

71. Dvir E, Perl S, Loeb E, et al. Spinal intramedullary aberrant Spirocerca lupi migration in 3 dogs. *J Vet Intern Med.* 2007;21:860–864.

72. Lowrie M, Penderis J, McLaughlin M, et al. Steroid responsive meningitis-arteritis: a prospective study of potential disease markers, prednisolone treatment, and long-term outcome in 20 dogs (2006-2008). *J Vet Intern Med.* 2009;23:862–870.

73. Schwartz M, Puff C, Stein VM, et al. Pathogenetic factors for excessive IgA production: Th2-dominated immune response in canine steroid-responsive meningitis-arteritis. *Vet J.* 2011;187:260–266.

74. Lowrie M, Penderis J, Eckersall PD, et al. The role of acute phase proteins in diagnosis and management of steroid-responsive meningitis arteritis in dogs. *Vet J.* 2009;182:125–130.

75. Bathen-Noethen A, Carlson R, Menzel D, et al. Concentrations of acute-phase proteins in dogs with steroid responsive meningitis-arteritis. *J Vet Intern Med.* 2008;22:1149–1156.

76. Windsor RC, Vernau KM, Sturges BK, et al. Lumbar cerebrospinal fluid in dogs with type I intervertebral disc herniation. *J Vet Intern Med.* 2008;22:954–960.

77. De Risio L, Adams V, Dennis R, et al. Magnetic resonance imaging findings and clinical associations in 52 dogs with suspected ischemic myelopathy. *J Vet Intern Med.* 2007;21:1290–1298.

78. Cauzinille L. Fibrocartilaginous embolism in dogs. *Vet Clin North Am Small Anim Pract.* 2000;30:155–167, vii.

79. Mikszewski JS, Van Winkle TJ, Troxel MT. Fibrocartilaginous embolic myelopathy in five cats. *J Am Anim Hosp Assoc.* 2006;42:226–233.

80. Marks SL, Lipsitz D, Vernau KM, et al. Reversible encephalopathy secondary to thiamine deficiency in 3 cats ingesting commercial diets. *J Vet Intern Med.* 2011;25:949–953.

81. Marioni-Henry K, Van Winkle TJ, Smith SH, et al. Tumors affecting the spinal cord of cats: 85 cases (1980-2005). *J Am Vet Med Assoc.* 2008;232:237–243.

82. Shiel RE, Mooney CT, Brennan SF, et al. Clinical and clinicopathological features of non-suppurative meningoencephalitis in young greyhounds in Ireland. *Vet Rec.* 2010;167:333–337.

83. Windsor RC, Sturges BK, Vernau KM, et al. Cerebrospinal fluid eosinophilia in dogs. *J Vet Intern Med.* 2009;23:275–281.

84. Gupta A, Gumber S, Bauer RW, et al. What is your diagnosis? Cerebrospinal fluid from a dog. Eosinophilic pleocytosis due to prototothecosis. *Vet Clin Pathol.* 2011;40:105–106.

85. Tipold A. Diagnosis of inflammatory and infectious diseases of the central nervous system in dogs: a retrospective study. *J Vet Intern Med.* 1995;9:304–314.

86. Tarlow JM, Rudloff E, Lichtenberger M, et al. Emergency presentations of 4 dogs with suspected neurologic toxoplasmosis. *J Vet Emerg Crit Care.* 2005;15:119–127.

87. Schatzberg SJ, Haley NJ, Barr SC, et al. Use of a multiplex polymerase chain reaction assay in the antemortem diagnosis of toxoplasmosis and neosporosis in the central nervous system of cats and dogs. *Am J Vet Res.* 2003;64:1507–1513.

88. Saengseesom W, Mitmoonpitak C, Kasempimolporn S, et al. Real-time PCR analysis of dog cerebrospinal fluid and saliva samples for ante-mortem diagnosis of rabies. *Southeast Asian J Trop Med Public Health.* 2007;38:53–57.

89. Amude AM, Alfieri AA, Balarin MR, et al. Cerebrospinal fluid from a 7-month-old dog with seizure-like episodes. *Vet Clin Pathol.* 2006;35:119–122.

90. Amude AM, Alfieri AA, Alfieri AF. Clinicopathological findings in dogs with distemper encephalomyelitis presented without characteristic signs of the disease. *Res Vet Sci.* 2007;82:416–422.

91. Haines DM, Martin KM, Chelack BJ, et al. Immunohistochemical detection of canine distemper virus in haired skin, nasal mucosa, and footpad epithelium: a method for antemortem diagnosis of infection. *J Vet Diagn Invest.* 1999;11:396–399.

92. Johnson GC, Fenner WR, Krakowka S. Production of immunoglobulin G and increased antiviral antibody in cerebrospinal fluid of dogs with delayed-onset canine distemper viral encephalitis. *J Neuroimmunol.* 1988;17:237–251.

93. Greer KA, Wong AK, Liu H, et al. Necrotizing meningoencephalitis of Pug dogs associates with dog leukocyte antigen class II and resembles acute variant forms of multiple sclerosis. *Tissue Antigens.* 2010;76:110–118.

94. Higgins RJ, Dickinson PJ, Kube SA, et al. Necrotizing meningoencephalitis in five Chihuahua dogs. *Vet Pathol.* 2008;45:336–346.

95. Levine JM, Fosgate GT, Porter B, et al. Epidemiology of necrotizing meningoencephalitis in Pug dogs. *J Vet Intern Med.* 2008;22:961–968.

96. Williams KJ, Summers BA, de Lahunta A. Cerebrospinal cuterebriasis in cats and its association with feline ischemic encephalopathy. *Vet Pathol.* 1998;35:330–343.

97. Altay UM, Skerritt GC, Hilbe M, et al. Feline cerebrovascular disease: clinical and histopathologic findings in 16 cats. *J Am Anim Hosp Assoc.* 2011;47:89–97.

98. Coates JR, March PA, Oglesbee M, et al. Clinical characterization of a familial degenerative myelopathy in Pembroke Welsh Corgi dogs. *J Vet Intern Med.* 2007;21:1323–1331.

99. Gaitero L, Anor S, Montoliu P, et al. Detection of Neospora caninum tachyzoites in canine cerebrospinal fluid. *J Vet Intern Med.* 2006;20:410–414.

100. Galgut BI, Janardhan KS, Grondin TM, et al. Detection of Neospora caninum tachyzoites in cerebrospinal fluid of a dog following prednisone and cyclosporine therapy. *Vet Clin Pathol.* 2010;39:386–390.

101. Garosi L, Dawson A, Couturier J, et al. Necrotizing cerebellitis and cerebellar atrophy caused by Neospora caninum infection: magnetic resonance imaging and clinicopathologic findings in seven dogs. *J Vet Intern Med*. 2010;24:571–578.

102. Negrin A, Cherubini GB, Steeves E. Angiostrongylus vasorum causing meningitis and detection of parasite larvae in the cerebrospinal fluid of a pug dog. *J Small Anim Pract*. 2008;49:468–471.

103. Cross JR, Rossmeisl JH, Maggi RG, et al. Bartonella-associated meningoradiculoneuritis and dermatitis or panniculitis in 3 dogs. *J Vet Intern Med*. 2008;22:674–678.

104. Marchetti V, Lubas G, Baneth G, et al. Hepatozoonosis in a dog with skeletal involvement and meningoencephalomyelitis. *Vet Clin Pathol*. 2009;38:121–125.

105. Widmer WR, Blevins WE, Cantwell HD, et al. Cerebrospinal fluid response following metrizamide myelography in normal dogs: effects of routine myelography and postmyelographic removal of contrast medium. *Vet Clin Pathol*. 1990;19:66–76.

106. Widmer WR, DeNicola DB, Blevins WE, et al. Cerebrospinal fluid changes after iopamidol and metrizamide myelography in clinically normal dogs. *Am J Vet Res*. 1992;53:396–401.

107. Johnson GC, Fuciu DM, Fenner WR, et al. Transient leakage across the blood-cerebrospinal fluid barrier after intrathecal metrizamide administration to dogs. *Am J Vet Res*. 1985;46:1303–1308.

108. Sorjonen DC, Golden DL, Levesque DC, et al. Cerebrospinal fluid protein electrophoresis: a clinical evaluation of a previously reported diagnostic technique. *Prog Vet Neurol*. 1991;2:261–267.

109. Smith JR, Legendre AM, Thomas WB, et al. Cerebral blastomyces dermatitidis infection in a cat. *J Am Vet Med Assoc*. 2007;231:1210–1214.

110. Lipitz L, Rylander H, Forrest LJ, et al. Clinical and magnetic resonance imaging features of central nervous system blastomycosis in 4 dogs. *J Vet Intern Med*. 2010;24:1509–1514.

111. Appel SL, Moens NM, Abrams-Ogg AC, et al. Multiple myeloma with central nervous system involvement in a cat. *J Am Vet Med Assoc*. 2008;233:743–747.

112. Tzipory L, Vernau KM, Sturges BK, et al. Antemortem diagnosis of localized central nervous system histiocytic sarcoma in 2 dogs. *J Vet Intern Med*. 2009;23:369–374.

113. Zimmerman K, Almy F, Carter L, et al. Cerebrospinal fluid from a 10-year-old dog with a single seizure episode. *Vet Clin Pathol*. 2006;35:127–131.

114. Galan A, Guil-Luna S, Millan Y, et al. Oligodendroglial gliomatosis cerebri in a poodle. *Vet Comp Oncol*. 2010;8:254–262.

115. Porter B, de Lahunta A, Summers B. Gliomatosis cerebri in six dogs. *Vet Pathol*. 2003;40:97–102.

116. Dickinson PJ, Sturges BK, Kass PH, et al. Characteristics of cisternal cerebrospinal fluid associated with intracranial meningiomas in dogs: 56 cases (1985-2004). *J Am Vet Med Assoc*. 2006;228:564–567.

117. Petersen SA, Sturges BK, Dickinson PJ, et al. Canine intraspinal meningiomas: imaging features, histopathologic classification, and long-term outcome in 34 dogs. *J Vet Intern Med*. 2008;22:946–953.

118. Behling-Kelly E, Petersen S, Muthuswamy A, et al. Neoplastic pleocytosis in a dog with metastatic mammary carcinoma and meningeal carcinomatosis. *Vet Clin Pathol*. 2010;39:247–252.

119. Westworth DR, Dickinson PJ, Vernau W, et al. Choroid plexus tumors in 56 dogs (1985-2007). *J Vet Intern Med*. 2008;22:1157–1165.

120. Pastorello A, Constantino-Casas F, Archer J. Choroid plexus carcinoma cells in the cerebrospinal fluid of a Staffordshire Bull Terrier. *Vet Clin Pathol*. 2010;39:505–510.

121. Koblik PD, LeCouteur RA, Higgins RJ, et al. CT-guided brain biopsy using a modified Pelorus Mark III stereotactic system: experience with 50 dogs. *Vet Radiol Ultrasound*. 1999;40:434–440.

122. Vernau KM, Higgins RJ, Bollen AW, et al. Primary canine and feline nervous system tumors: intraoperative diagnosis using the smear technique. *Vet Pathol*. 2001;38:47–57.

123. De Lorenzi D, Mandara MT, Tranquillo M, et al. Squash-prep cytology in the diagnosis of canine and feline nervous system lesions: a study of 42 cases. *Vet Clin Pathol*. 2006;35:208–214.

124. Raskin RE, Meyer D. *Canine and Feline Cytology—E-Book: A Color Atlas and Interpretation Guide*. Elsevier Health Sciences; 2009.

125. Meuten DJ. *Tumors in Domestic Animals*. 5th ed. Ames, IA: John Wiley & Sons Inc.; 2017.

126. Summers BA, Cummings JF, deLahunta A. *Veterinary Neuropathology*. St. Louis: Mosby; 1995.

127. Harms NJ, Dickinson RM, Nibblett BM, et al. What is your diagnosis? Intracranial mass in a dog. *Vet Clin Pathol*. 2009;38:537–540.

128. De Lorenzi D, Baroni M, Mandara MT. A true "triphasic" pattern: thoracolumbar spinal tumor in a young dog. *Vet Clin Pathol*. 2007;36:200–203.

15

Abdominal, Thoracic, and Pericardial Effusions

Amy C. Valenciano and Theresa E. Rizzi

The three primary body cavities are (1) thoracic (pleural), (2) abdominal (peritoneal), and (3) pericardial. In health, these potential cavities contain a small amount of serous fluid that acts as a lubricant allowing the free motion of internal organs against one another and body cavity walls. The body cavities are lined by mesothelial cells, which are specialized cells that play an active role in the homeostasis of these potential spaces. The abnormal accumulation of fluid within a body cavity is called *effusion*. Effusion is not a disease in itself; rather, it results from alterations in fluid production, lymphatic drainage, or a combination of both. Some of the major factors that affect production and resorption of fluid include changes in capillary hydrostatic pressure, plasma osmotic pressure, and capillary permeability.

Fluid analysis, including cytological evaluation and classification, is a quick, inexpensive, and relatively safe way to obtain useful information in the diagnosis, prognosis, and treatment of diseases that cause thoracic, abdominal, and pericardial fluid accumulations. Common causes of body cavity effusions include trauma, neoplasia, cardiovascular compromise, metabolic disorders, altered Starling forces, ruptured urinary or gall bladder, ruptured vessels or lymphatics, and bleeding diathesis, as well as infectious and inflammatory diseases.

General mechanisms of thoracic, abdominal, and pericardial effusions will be categorized in the section titled "General Classification of Effusions" and explored in detail in the section titled "Specific Disorders Causing Effusions."

THORACIC AND ABDOMINAL EFFUSIONS

Dogs and cats with thoracic effusions often exhibit dyspnea as the most common clinical sign.[1,2] Other clinical signs include a crouched, sternal recumbent position with extension of the head and neck; open-mouth breathing; tachypnea; and forceful abdominal respiration. Cyanosis may be present. With milder effusions, lethargy and lack of stamina may be the only clinical signs. Animals, especially cats, with mild to moderately severe effusions often adapt by decreasing their activity, thus concealing their illness until it is severe. With chronic pleural effusion, dogs and cats may present with coughing as the only clinical sign.[1] Physical findings depend on the amount of fluid present but include muffled heart and lung sounds.

Patients with abdominal effusions may present for lethargy, weakness, and abdominal distension—the latter may be mistaken by pet owners as weight gain, gas, or ingesta. Physical findings include a fluid wave during ballottement in high-volume effusions or pain if peritonitis is present.

PERICARDIAL EFFUSIONS

Pericardial effusion in cats is often secondary to congestive heart failure or feline infectious peritonitis but may be caused by primary cardiac neoplasia, such as lymphoma.[3] The most common causes of pericardial effusion in the dog include cardiac neoplasia and idiopathic pericardial effusion.[4,5] Hemangiosarcoma is the most common cardiac neoplasm reported, but other reported neoplasms include lymphoma, chemodectoma, and thyroid carcinoma.[4] Other less common causes include cardiac disease, inflammatory or infectious diseases, trauma, coagulopathy, and congenital defects.[9]

Clinical signs include weakness, lethargy, exercise intolerance, collapse, and coughing. Physical findings vary with the amount of fluid present but include muffled heart sounds, weak pulses, and pallor.

COLLECTION TECHNIQUES

For all fluids collected, a portion of the fluid (2–3 milliliters [mL]) should be placed in an ethylenediaminetetraacetic acid (EDTA) lavender-top Vacutainer (Becton Dickinson Vacutainer Systems, Franklin Lakes, NJ) tube for cell counts, protein analysis, and cytological evaluation. EDTA prevents clots from forming in the fluid in the event of iatrogenic blood contamination. A second portion (2–3 mL) should be placed in a sterile red-top Vacutainer tube without anticoagulant to assess for clot formation and to have on hand if aerobic or anaerobic bacterial cultures are required or biochemical analyses are desired (bilirubin, cholesterol, triglyceride, creatinine, etc.).

Thoracocentesis

Pleural effusions are typically abundant and bilateral but may be mild, unilateral, compartmentalized, or both. Radiography and ultrasonography help determine the extent and location of the effusion and guide thoracocentesis. If the fluid is not compartmentalized, thoracocentesis is performed approximately two-thirds down the chest, near the costochondral junction at the sixth, seventh, or eighth intercostal spaces.

The patient is restrained in the sternal recumbent or standing position. The site of needle insertion is shaved and aseptically prepared. Tranquilization and local anesthesia are generally not necessary for collecting a small sample for analysis but may be needed if a large amount of fluid must be drained from the chest. Large dogs may require a 1½-inch, 18- to 20-gauge needle or over-the-needle catheter, but a ⅞-inch, 19- or 21-gauge butterfly needle is preferred for cats and small dogs. The catheter unit allows the needle to be withdrawn after the catheter is introduced into the thoracic cavity, thus decreasing the chances of injury to intrathoracic organs.

The needle should be inserted next to the cranial surface of the rib to minimize the risk for lacerating the vessels on the rib's caudal border. If the needle or catheter is below the fluid line, air will not be aspirated into the thoracic cavity. If only a single syringe of fluid is to be collected, the syringe may be attached to the catheter, the fluid aspirated, and the catheter withdrawn with the syringe attached. If a larger

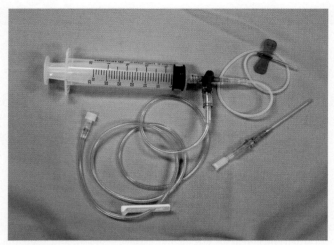

Fig. 15.1 Basic equipment for thoracocentesis, abdominocentesis, or pericardiocentesis: syringe, three-way stopcock, extension tubing, butterfly catheter, and over-the-needle catheter.

volume of fluid is to be removed or the syringe is to be repeatedly filled, extension tubing and a three-way stopcock should be attached (Fig. 15.1).

Abdominocentesis

The ventral midline of the abdomen, 1 to 2 cm caudal to the umbilicus, is the usual site of needle insertion. This site avoids the falciform fat, which may block the needle barrel. The urinary bladder is emptied to help avoid accidental cystocentesis. The site of needle insertion is shaved and aseptically prepared. Neither local nor general anesthesia is usually needed. With the animal in lateral recumbency, a ventral midline puncture is made using a 1- to 1½-inch, 20- to 22-gauge needle, or a 16- to 20-gauge, 1½- to 2-inch plain or fenestrated over-the-needle catheter without the syringe attached. Free-flowing fluid should be collected into appropriate collection tubes. The needle may be rotated if fluid is not visible in the needle hub or a syringe may be attached and gentle negative pressure applied.[6] If a scar from a previous surgical incision is present, the needle should be inserted at least 1.5 cm away from the site to avoid abdominal viscera that may have adhered to the abdominal wall in the area of the scar. To enhance fluid collection, abdominal compression may be applied when an over-the-needle catheter is used after the stylet has been removed, leaving only the catheter in the abdominal cavity. Although the catheter may kink, sufficient fluid can usually be collected for analysis.

If the technique described above fails to yield fluid, four-quadrant paracentesis or diagnostic peritoneal lavage (DPL) may be performed. In four-quadrant paracentesis, the umbilicus serves as a central point, and centesis, as previously described, is performed in the right and left cranial and caudal quadrants.[7] If DPL is performed, the animal is placed in dorsal recumbency, the area is clipped and aseptically prepared, and a small 2-cm incision caudal to the umbilicus is made. A peritoneal lavage catheter without the trocar is inserted into the abdominal cavity and directed caudally into the pelvis. A syringe is attached and gentle suction applied. If no fluid is obtained, 20 mL/kg of warm sterile saline may be infused into the abdominal cavity. The patient is then rolled from side to side and the fluid collected via gravity drainage.[6,7]

Pericardiocentesis

Pericardiocentesis may be performed with the animal in the standing position or in sternal or left lateral recumbency. Adequate restraint is needed to avoid cardiac puncture, coronary artery laceration, or pulmonary laceration. Sedation is used as necessary. Electrocardiography (ECG) monitoring is recommended but not essential. Cardiac contact with the catheter or needle usually causes an arrhythmia. A large area of the right hemithorax from the third rib to the eighth rib is shaved and aseptically prepared. Local anesthesia, including infiltration of the pleura with lidocaine, may be used to minimize discomfort associated with pleural penetration. Puncture is generally made between the fourth and fifth intercostal spaces at the costochondral junction. The needle is attached to a three-way stopcock, extension tubing, and syringe, and gentle negative pressure is applied.[5,8]

SLIDE PREPARATION AND STAINING

Preparation of the sample for cytological evaluation depends on the character and quantity of the fluid, the type of stain used, and whether the cytological evaluation will be performed in the hospital or sent to a diagnostic laboratory.

Clear, colorless fluids are usually transudates (low protein content and low cellularity). Preparation of sedimented or cytocentrifuged concentrated slides from low cellularity fluids aid in cytological evaluation. Clear-amber and mildly opaque fluids are often effusions of low to moderate cellularity. Moderately to markedly opaque fluids, however, are usually exudates of moderate to very high cellularity. Slide preparation and staining techniques are detailed in Chapter 1.

Sediment smears should be made on all nonturbid fluid specimens. This is done by centrifuging the fluid for 5 minutes at 165 to 360 gravity (G). This may be achieved in a centrifuge with a radial arm length of 14.6 cm by centrifuging the fluid at 1000 to 1500 revolutions per minute (rpm). After centrifugation, most of the supernatant is poured off, leaving only about 0.5 mL of fluid with the pellet in the bottom of the tube. The supernatant may be used for total protein and chemical analysis (EDTA samples should be avoided because EDTA interferes with chemical analyses). The pellet is then resuspended in the remaining 0.5 mL of fluid by gentle agitation, a drop of the suspension is placed on a glass slide, and a routine pull smear or squash prep is made (see Chapter 1). The smear is air-dried and then stained with an appropriate hematological stain.

Opaque fluids may need only a direct smear because of high cellularity. Direct smears may be made by making either pull smears or squash preps on well-mixed, uncentrifuged fluid.

LABORATORY DATA

Cell Counts and Counting Techniques

Accurate nucleated cell counts may be determined at commercial laboratories on many modern automated cell counters or by manual methods with use of a hemacytometer; however, cell clumping, cell fragmentation, and noncellular debris may cause counting errors with automated and manual techniques.[10] Determination of nucleated cell counts should be performed on EDTA-preserved fluid to prevent clot formation or clumping of the sample. Serum separator tubes may introduce artifact to the count and therefore should not be used. A nucleated cell differential may be made on cytology preparations and often aids in classification of the effusion type.

Automated red blood cell (RBC) counts may help determine the amount of blood in the effusion. If grossly bloody fluid is obtained, a packed cell volume (PCV) may be performed. The RBC count, together with cytological assessment (identification of platelets, erythrophagocytosis, and intracellular and extracellular heme pigments, e.g., hemosiderin and hematoidin), may aid in determination of the origin of the blood as far as iatrogenic blood contamination, per-acute hemorrhage, chronic hemorrhage, and increased capillary permeability with diapedesis of RBC into the cavity.

TABLE 15.1	Ancillary Tests: Biochemical Analysis of Effusion Fluid	
Biochemical Test	**Indications**	**Interpretation**
Bilirubin	Bile peritonitis	Twofold or greater concentration in effusion fluid than serum supports bile peritonitis. (Mucocele rupture may not have concentration differences.)
Creatinine	Uroperitoneum	Twofold or greater concentration in effusion fluid versus serum supports uroperitoneum
Triglyceride	Chylous effusion	Triglyceride level greater than 100 milligrams per deciliter (mg/dL) in fluid supports chylous effusion.
Cholesterol	Nonchylous effusion	Higher concentration of cholesterol in effusion fluid versus serum supports nonchylous effusion (not common in veterinary species).

Total Protein Measurement and Techniques

Fluid total protein concentration is used with the nucleated cell count to classify effusions and to estimate the severity of inflammation, if present. The total protein content may be determined biochemically or estimated by using refractometry. For ease and accuracy, the method of choice for determining total protein concentrations in effusions is refractometry. If the fluid is opaque, it is best to determine the refractive index of the supernatant after centrifugation, as the refraction of light by suspended nonprotein particles (i.e., lipoproteins, urea, cholesterol, and glucose) may result in an erroneous total protein reading.[10,11] It must be kept in mind that chylous or lipemic fluids may not separate sufficiently to allow total protein to be estimated by using refractometry or chemical methods.

Biochemical Analysis

In conjunction with fluid analysis, measurement of abdominal effusion supernatant bilirubin and creatinine and comparison with serum values may be performed to diagnose bile peritonitis and uroperitoneum, respectively. Additionally, when a white, opaque effusion is obtained, measurement and comparison of effusion supernatant and serum triglyceride and cholesterol values may be used to distinguish between chylous and pseudochylous effusions (Table 15.1). Specific biochemical analyses performed on effusions will be highlighted in the section titled "Specific Disorders Causing Effusions."

Microbiological Cultures

Effusion fluid may be submitted for either bacterial or fungal cultures. It is best to contact the laboratory for specific information regarding submission protocol, types of transport containers, and media, as many laboratories will provide special transport tubes and, in the case of anaerobic bacterial culture, special anaerobic tubes or media. In general, if the cytological evaluation of an effusion suggests bacterial infection caused by the presence of large numbers of neutrophils or if definitive bacteria are identified, the fluid should be cultured for both aerobic and anaerobic bacteria. Fluid samples for aerobic and anaerobic cultures should be collected by using aseptic technique to avoid contamination. Fluid should be placed into a sterile tube (i.e., sterile red-top tube) without EDTA, which may be bacteriostatic or bactericidal. Note that some transport systems support both aerobic and anaerobic bacteria. Submission of fluid for fungal culture should be performed as in the case of fluid submitted for aerobic bacterial culture. Chapter 1 contains a detailed discussion of methods for collection and transportation of samples for microbiological culture.

CELLS AND STRUCTURES SEEN IN EFFUSIONS

Neutrophils

Neutrophils are present to some degree in most effusions and tend to predominate in effusions associated with inflammation. Cytologically, two general classes of neutrophils exist: degenerate and nondegenerate.

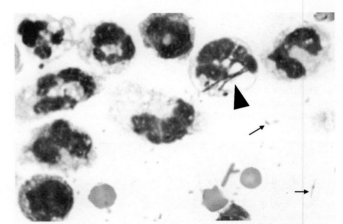

Fig. 15.2 Numerous degenerate neutrophils with swollen nuclear chromatin. Phagocytized bacterial rods *(arrowhead)* and extracellular bacteria are in the background *(arrows)*.

Degenerate neutrophils are neutrophils that have undergone hydropic degeneration. This is a morphological change that occurs in tissue and effusions secondary to bacterial toxins that alter cell membrane permeability. The toxins allow water to diffuse into the cell and through the nuclear pores, causing the nucleus to swell, fill more of the cytoplasm, and stain homogeneously eosinophilic. This swollen, loose, homogeneous, eosinophilic nuclear chromatin pattern characterizes the degenerate neutrophil (Fig. 15.2). Although all cell types are exposed to the same toxin, degenerative change is evaluated only in neutrophils.

Nondegenerate neutrophils, such as peripheral blood neutrophils, are those with tightly clumped, basophilic nuclear chromatin (Fig. 15.3). Some neutrophils in effusions may be hypersegmented. Hypersegmentation is an age-related change; the nuclear chromatin condenses and eventually breaks into round, tightly clumped spheres (pyknosis) (Fig. 15.4). These aged neutrophils are often seen phagocytized by macrophages (cytophagia) (Fig. 15.5). The presence of nondegenerate neutrophils suggests that the fluid is not septic; however, bacteria that are not strong toxin producers, for example, *Actinomyces* spp., may be associated with nondegenerate neutrophils. Also, some infectious agents, such as *Ehrlichia* and *Toxoplasma* spp. and various fungi, may be associated with nondegenerate neutrophils.

Effusions may also contain toxic neutrophils. Toxic changes (i.e., Döhle bodies, toxic granulation, diffuse cytoplasmic basophilia, foamy cytoplasm) develop in bone marrow in response to accelerated granulopoiesis caused by inflammation. Toxic neutrophils in peripheral blood migrate into the body cavity and are observed in effusions of the cavity. Although foamy cytoplasm is considered a toxic change, cytoplasmic vacuolation may be seen in neutrophils of peritoneal or thoracic fluid smears because of age-related change or EDTA-induced artifact.

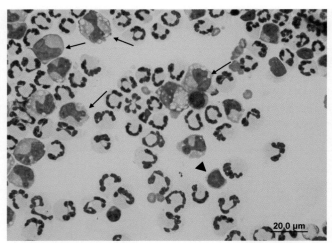

Fig. 15.3 Feline abdominal fluid. Numerous nondegenerate neutrophils. The chromatin is clumped and segmented. Also present are macrophages *(arrows)* and a small lymphocyte *(arrowhead)*.

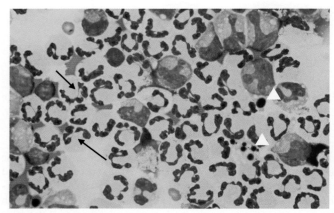

Fig. 15.4 Feline abdominal fluid. Numerous nondegenerate neutrophils are present; some are hypersegmented with only thin chromatin strands connecting the segments *(small arrows)*. Pyknotic nuclei *(arrowheads)* are also present.

Mesothelial Cells

Mesothelial cells line pleural, peritoneal, and pericardial cavities, as well as visceral surfaces, and are present in variable numbers in most effusions. Mesothelium easily becomes activated and reactive or hyperplastic in the face of inflammation or fluid accumulation of any type. In effusions, mesothelial cells are large, round, with moderate amounts of pale to dark basophilic cytoplasm and singular, round, central nuclei. Multinucleation can occur when cells are reactive (Fig. 15.6). The nuclear chromatin has a fine reticular pattern, and nucleoli may be present. Reactive mesothelial cells may have a pronounced, pink, cytoplasmic coronal fringe (Fig. 15.7). Mesothelial cells may be present in low or moderate numbers, as individual cells, in small clusters, and sometimes in large, three-dimensional aggregates (Fig. 15.8). Reactive mesothelial cells may have several morphological characteristics of malignancy and may be easily confused with neoplastic cells.

Macrophages

Macrophages found in effusions generally have a single oval to bean-shaped nucleus and resemble tissue macrophages. The nuclear chromatin is lacy and cytoplasm is frequently vacuolated and may contain phagocytized debris or degenerate cells (Figs. 15.9 and 15.10).

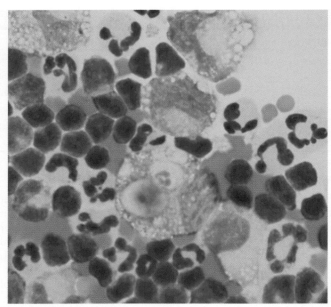

Fig. 15.5 Abdominal fluid from a cat. A large macrophage is present in the center, with a phagocytized remnant of cellular material. Numerous small lymphocytes, neutrophils, and macrophages are also present.

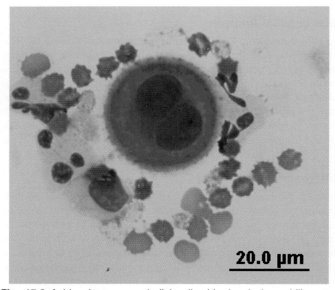

Fig. 15.6 A binucleate mesothelial cell with deeply basophilic cytoplasm and an encircling eosinophilic fringe border.

Lymphocytes

Lymphocytes are commonly seen in effusions and are often the predominant cells in lymphocytic and chylous effusions (Fig. 15.11) and neoplastic effusions secondary to lymphoid malignancy (Fig. 15.12). Small to intermediate or medium-sized lymphocytes present in body cavity fluids will appear similar to peripheral lymphocytes, with a scant rim of blue cytoplasm, round nucleus with evenly clumped to coarse chromatin, and no apparent nucleoli. Normal fluids will have low numbers of lymphocytes. Reactive lymphocytes may be seen in inflammatory effusions and are usually larger than small lymphocytes, with deeply basophilic cytoplasm imparting a plasmacytoid appearance (Fig. 15.13).

Eosinophils

Eosinophils are readily recognized by their rod-shaped (in cats) or variably sized, round (in dogs), pink granules (Fig. 15.14). When

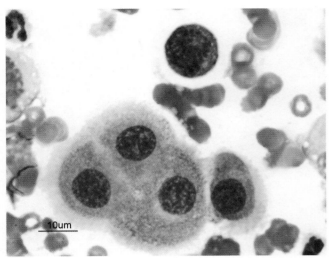

Fig. 15.7 A small cluster of mesothelial cells with prominent eosinophilic corona.

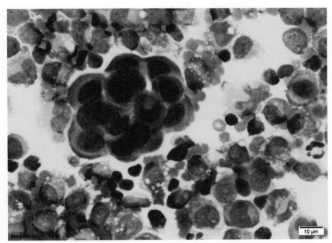

Fig. 15.8 Pericardial fluid from a dog. In a concentrated cytocentrifuge specimen, a three-dimensional aggregate of mildly pleomorphic mesothelial cells is present and surrounded by small lymphocytes, monocytes, macrophages, few red blood cells and rare nondegenerate neutrophils. Pleomorphic mesothelial cells are often present in pericardial fluid.

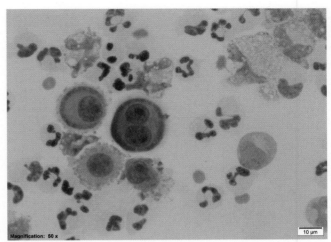

Fig. 15.9 Several macrophages with varying morphology. In the upper right and left, the macrophages are vacuolated. Macrophages in the lower right area are monocyte-like. In addition, there are few mesothelial cells, including one that is binucleate and a few nondegenerate neutrophils.

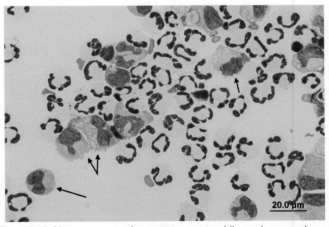

Fig. 15.10 Numerous nondegenerate neutrophils and macrophages with variable nuclear morphology *(arrows).*

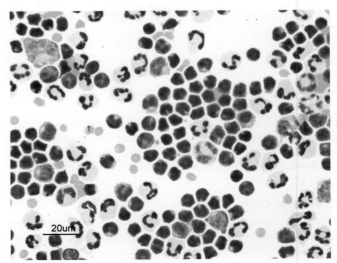

Fig. 15.11 Chylous pleural effusion from a cat. Small lymphocytes are the predominant cells. The small lymphocytes are typically smaller than neutrophils. They have round or indented nuclei and a small amount of cytoplasm.

eosinophils are present in moderate to high numbers in effusions, differentials could include: Parasitical disease (heartworm infection), allergic or hypersensitivity disease, a paraneoplastic response to lymphoma or mast cell neoplasia, a foreign body, infectious etiologies or idiopathic hypereosinophilic syndrome.[12]

Mast Cells

Mast cells (Figs. 15.15 and 15.16) are readily identified by their numerous, round, red-purple cytoplasmic granules. Mast cells may be found in low numbers in effusions in dogs and cats with many different inflammatory disorders. Mast cell tumors within body cavities may be associated with effusions and may exfoliate large numbers of mast cells into the effusion. Visceral forms of mast cell neoplasia are rare in the dog.[12,13] Visceral forms of mast cell tumors in cats most often involve the spleen[14] or the gastrointestinal (GI) tract.[15]

Erythrocytes

Erythrocytes may be seen cytologically within effusions secondary to overt hemorrhage or contamination with peripheral blood. It is

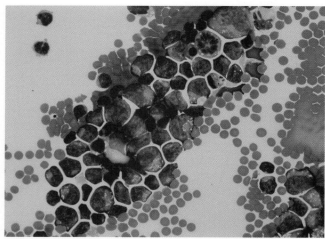

Fig. 15.12 Feline thoracic fluid with many lymphoblasts, which are large, with a scant rim of basophilic cytoplasm, eccentric round nuclei with smooth chromatin and visible nucleoli. The high cell yield and large numbers of lymphoblasts are compatible with a neoplastic effusion secondary to high-grade lymphosarcoma.

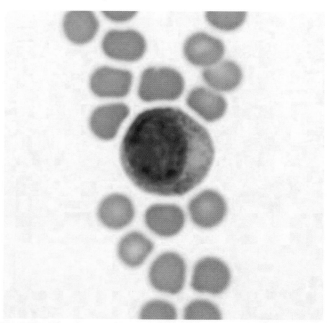

Fig. 15.13 Reactive lymphocyte. This cell is slightly larger than a small lymphocyte with deeply basophilic cytoplasm and a perinuclear clearing (plasmacytoid features).

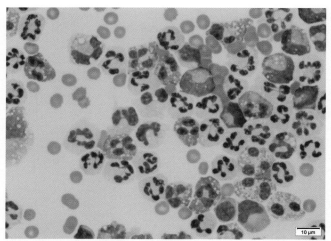

Fig. 15.14 Canine pleural effusion with numerous eosinophils, neutrophils, several monocytes, and red blood cells.

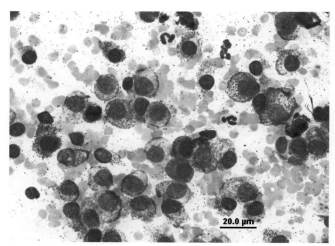

Fig. 15.15 Many heavily granulated mast cells in an effusion secondary to mast cell neoplasia.

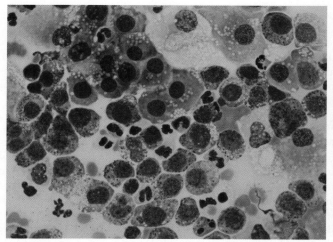

Fig. 15.16 Canine abdominal effusion secondary to mast cell neoplasia. Note the large numbers of heavily granulated mast cells, with fewer admixed vacuolated macrophages, eosinophils and few mature lymphocytes.

important to differentiate iatrogenic causes from true intracavity hemorrhage, on the basis of clinical signs, laboratory data, and the presence or absence of erythrophagia, hemosiderin or hematoidin pigments, and platelets in the effusion, as described in the discussion of hemorrhagic effusions later in this chapter.

Neoplastic Cells

Neoplastic cells may be observed in low to high numbers in effusions secondary to many different types of neoplasia. Various carcinomas and adenocarcinomas (epithelial cell tumors), lymphoma and mast cell tumors (discrete cell tumors), hemangiosarcoma (vascular endothelial–derived neoplasia), and mesothelioma may exfoliate neoplastic cells into the pleural, peritoneal, or pericardial cavity. Identification of the neoplastic cells depends on the viewer's ability to recognize the cell type and signs of malignancy. (See the discussion of neoplasia later in this chapter and the general criteria of malignancy in Chapter 1.)

Miscellaneous Findings
Glove Powder

Cornstarch (glove powder) may be seen on slides made from effusion fluid (Fig. 15.17). Typically, it is a clear-staining, large, round to hexagonal structure with a central fissure and may be slightly refractile. Glove powder is a contaminant and should not be confused with an organism or cell.

Microfilariae

Microfilariae may occasionally be seen within hemorrhagic effusions. These are generally *Dirofilaria* or *Acanthocheilonema* (formerly *Dipetalonema*) larvae that have entered the cavity with the peripheral blood (see Fig. 15.42 later in the chapter).

Basket Cells (Broken Cells)

Basket cells are free cell nuclei from ruptured nucleated cells. When cells rupture, the nuclear chromatin spreads out and stains eosinophilic. Nucleated cells may rupture because of the stresses induced in slide preparation; however, certain effusions (i.e., chylous effusions and septic exudates) cause increased cell fragility and may result in increased numbers of ruptured cells. Neoplastic effusions may contain fragile neoplastic cells, and increased cellular rupture may be seen (especially true for neoplastic immature lymphocytes).

GENERAL CLASSIFICATION OF EFFUSIONS

Traditionally, abdominal, thoracic, and pericardial fluid accumulations have been classified as transudates, modified transudates, or exudates, on the basis of the total nucleated cell count (TNCC) and total protein (TP) concentration (Fig. 15.18). If overlap occurs in these

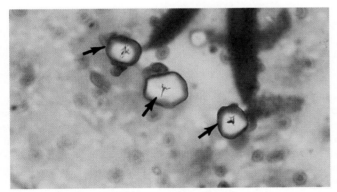

Fig. 15.17 Glove powder artifact *(arrows).*

classifications (i.e., a fluid may have TNCC in the transudate range and TP in the modified transudate range), TP is the more important criterion in separating transudates from modified transudates, and cellularity is more important in separating modified transudates from exudates. Modified transudates often are the least specific categorization from a diagnostic standpoint. Various other classification schemes have been proposed, such as those based on etiology, septic versus nonseptic exudate, vascular or lymphatic disruption, internal organ rupture, or by the presence of particular cells exfoliated into the effusion.[16] Additionally, some schemes classify transudative effusions as protein-poor or protein-rich, addressing the general pathological mechanism of the effusions.[10]

Classifying the effusion helps direct the clinician to the general mechanism of fluid accumulation and may provide a preliminary list of differential diagnoses. However, whatever schema is used, the effusion should always be interpreted in light of clinical signs, history, physical examination findings, laboratory data, imaging information, and importantly, results of cytological examination of the fluid. The results of the effusion fluid examination may be diagnostic for specific conditions, such as neoplasia or infection, or may simply indicate a process. The following sections will initially characterize effusions mechanistically as transudates, modified transudates, and exudates, followed by specific etiologies.

Transudates

Protein-poor transudative effusions are generally clear and colorless, with TP concentrations less than 2.0 g/dL, and often contain less than 1500 cells/µL. Cells found in transudative effusions consist primarily of mononuclear cells (macrophages and small lymphocytes), mesothelial cells, and low numbers of neutrophils. The general mechanism is fluid shifts caused by changes in oncotic and/or hydraulic pressure or impaired lymphatic drainage. Conditions associated with these mechanisms include severe hypoproteinemia (primarily hypoalbuminemia) (<1.0 g/dL) secondary to protein-losing nephropathy, hepatic insufficiency, protein-losing enteropathy, malnutrition, malabsorption, portal hypertension, and early myocardial insufficiency (more common in cats). Early bladder rupture may result in a fluid classified as a transudate; however, the nature of the effusion will change rapidly because uroperitoneum often induces a rapid chemical peritonitis. Intravenous fluid administration after marked blood loss may result in an acute and marked hypoproteinemia, which, in turn, may cause a transudative process triggered by an acute disruption in oncotic pressures and insufficient lymphatic drainage.[10]

Modified transudates (also known as *protein-rich transudates*) occur because of increased hydraulic pressure caused by venous congestion in the lungs or liver.[10] TP concentration is greater than 2 g/dL, and the effusion often contains less than 5000 cells/µL. Effusion fluid color and turbidity may vary. Cells found in this effusion are reactive mesothelial cells, neutrophils, macrophages, and few small lymphocytes. Common conditions associated with modified transudates are congestive heart failure and portal hypertension.

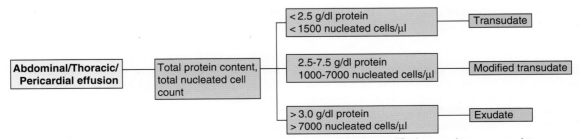

Fig. 15.18 Traditional algorithm to classify effusions as transudates, modified transudates, or exudates, based on total protein content and nucleated cell count.

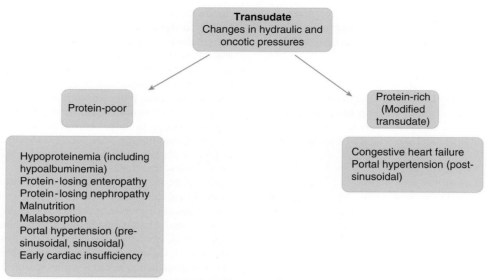

Fig. 15.19 Classification and causes of transudative effusions.

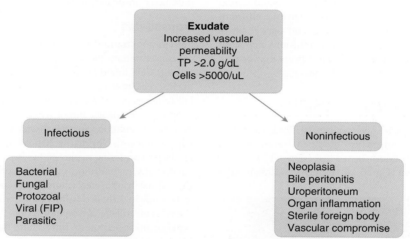

Fig. 15.20 Classification and causes of exudative effusions.

Dogs develop abdominal effusion secondary to right-sided heart failure, and cats often develop pleural effusion. Effusions caused by congestive heart failure are multifactorial and result from changes in vascular pressure, poor cardiac output, and retention of excess water. With portal hypertension, there is increased intrahepatic pressure and decreased lymphatic drainage, causing congestion and subsequent leakage of high-protein hepatic lymph into the abdominal cavity. No cytological finding in these effusions is pathognomonic for these conditions. Physical examination findings and imaging studies often help confirm functional abnormalities.

Fig. 15.19 is a flow chart of the more common causes of transudative effusions.

Exudates

Exudates typically have TP concentrations greater than 2 g/dL and contain greater than 5000 cells/µL. Exudates may vary in color but are often turbid to cloudy. A flow chart of the more common causes of exudative effusions is outlined in Fig. 15.20. Exudates are inflammatory in nature and occur because of vascular permeability caused by the release of inflammatory mediators from the inflamed tissue. Neutrophils are typically the predominant cell type in most exudates, but macrophages and, to some extent, lymphocytes are

also increased. Exudates may be infectious (septic) or not (nonseptic). Septic exudates are most often caused by bacteria but may be caused by fungi, protozoa, or parasites. Nonseptic exudates may be associated with a wide range of pathological conditions that elicit an inflammatory response, such as tumor necrosis; chemical irritants, such as urine and bile; or the presence of a sterile foreign body.

In the case of a predominantly neutrophilic exudate, a thorough investigation for an infectious agent is warranted. Degenerate neutrophils may be present in cases of sepsis; however, the presence of nondegenerate neutrophils does not preclude the possibility of an infectious etiology, and neither does the absence of cytologically visible organisms. Previous or concurrent antibiotic use may reduce bacterial numbers. Whenever a significant neutrophilic inflammatory component is present, regardless of the cytological presence or absence of bacteria, bacterial culture should be considered.

Occasionally, because of abundant exfoliation of neoplastic cells or secondary to a chronic chylous effusion, an effusion that has not yet been cytologically examined may fit into the exudative category solely on the basis of high cellularity. Once examined, these effusions are named according to etiology.

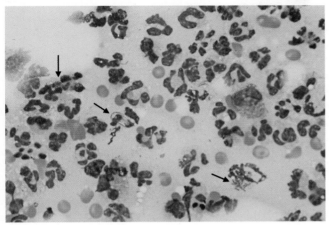

Fig. 15.21 Septic exudate showing degenerate neutrophils and phagocytized bacteria *(arrow)*.

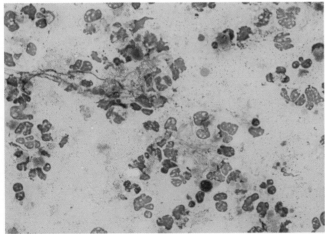

Fig. 15.22 Feline pyothorax. Large numbers of markedly degenerate neutrophils and abundant phagocytized and extracellular mixed bacteria consisting of cocci and long strands of bacilli.

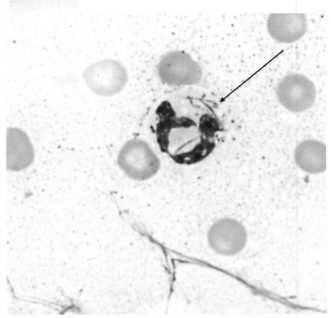

Fig. 15.23 Phagocytized filamentous bacterial rods *(arrow)*.

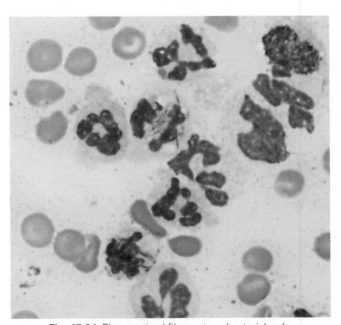

Fig. 15.24 Phagocytized filamentous bacterial rods.

SPECIFIC DISORDERS CAUSING EFFUSIONS

Septic Exudates

Inflammation is associated with the production of inflammatory mediators released from tissue causing increased neutrophil and monocyte or macrophage migration and the influx of protein-rich fluid as a result of increased vascular permeability. A septic effusion may result from hematogenous or lymphatic spread from systemic sepsis, from extension of pleuropneumonia or GI compromise or perforation, or by introduction of organisms via penetration of the body cavity (i.e., trauma, foreign body, surgery, and prior centesis).

Degenerate neutrophils may predominate in bacterial infections; organisms may be intracellular or extracellular (Figs. 15.21 and 15.22). The presence of long, slender, filamentous rods in a fluid with "tomato soup–like" characteristics is highly suggestive of *Actinomyces* spp., *Nocardia* spp., *Fusobacterium* spp., or any combination of the three (Figs. 15.23 and 15.24). Spirochetes are occasionally seen in association with bacterial peritonitis and pleuritis secondary to bite wounds. Although bacterial infections are the most common causes of septic exudates, mycotic infections associated with *Histoplasma* spp. (Fig. 15.25), *Blastomyces* spp. (Fig. 15.26), *Coccidioides* spp. (Figs. 15.27 and 15.28), *Candida* spp. (Figs. 15.29 to 15.31), and other fungal infections (Fig. 15.32) may occur. Fungal culture can be used to further define the fungal infection when hyphae are found. Additionally, effusions

secondary to protozoal infections (*Neospora* spp., *Toxoplasma* spp., *Leishmania* spp.) (Fig. 15.33) have been reported.[17,18]

Tissue Inflammation

Inflammation of an intracavity organ (liver, pancreas, lungs), or a walled-off abscess may cause an exudative effusion. Inflammatory mediators released from affected tissue results in increased vascular permeability, increased neutrophil and monocyte or macrophage migration, and the influx of protein-rich fluid. In effusions caused by tissue inflammation, nondegenerate neutrophils generally predominate, but macrophages, mesothelial cells, and some lymphocytes are also present. Macrophages, however, may become the predominant cell type in some chronic inflammatory processes. Cytological examination of these effusions readily identifies the inflammatory process but may not be able to determine a specific etiology.

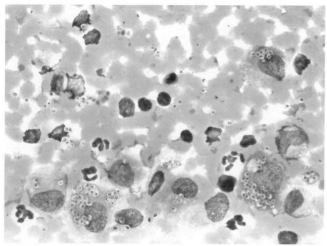

Fig. 15.25 Numerous *Histoplasma capsulatum* organisms are both phagocytized by macrophages and present extracellularly.

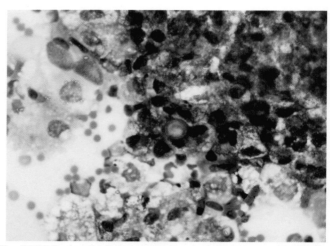

Fig. 15.28 Pericardial fluid from a dog. In the center, a singular *Coccidioides* spp. yeast is present in the extracellular space. There are surrounding macrophages that contain intracellular hemosiderin and hematoidin. Extracellular rhomboid, golden hematoidin crystals are also evident.

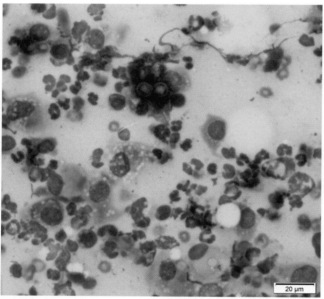

Fig. 15.26 Pleural fluid from a dog. Several *Blastomyces* spp. organisms are surrounded by inflammatory cells (macrophages and degenerate neutrophils). The organisms exhibit broad-based budding.

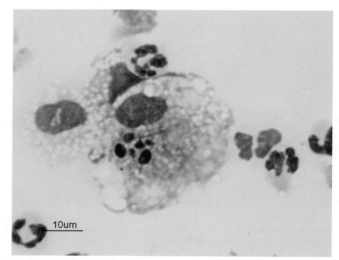

Fig. 15.29 Abdominal fluid from a dog. A large foamy macrophage with intracellular *Candida* spp. yeast. (Courtesy Dr. James Meinkoth, Oklahoma State University.)

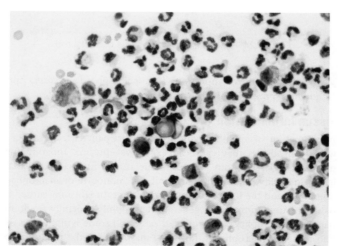

Fig. 15.27 Pleural fluid from a dog. In the center, a singular, large, round, pale blue, round yeast with a cell wall is present extracellularly, consistent with *Coccidioides* spp. The yeast is surrounded by macrophages nondegenerate neutrophils and fewer macrophages.

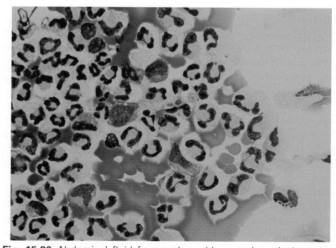

Fig. 15.30 Abdominal fluid from a dog with gastrointestinal compromise. *Candida* spp. yeast with narrow budding, phagocytized by a neutrophil in the center. *Lower right,* a degenerate neutrophil with phagocytized bacteria.

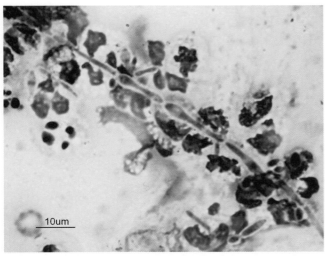

Fig. 15.31 Abdominal fluid from a dog. *Candida* spp. pseudohyphae surrounded by degenerate inflammatory cells. (Courtesy Dr. James Meinkoth, Oklahoma State University.)

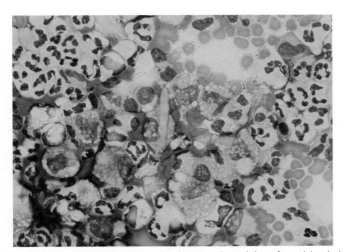

Fig. 15.32 In the center, note the large, pale-staining, fungal hyphal structure surrounded by foamy macrophages, neutrophils, and eosinophils.

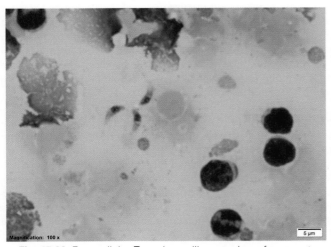

Fig. 15.33 Extracellular *Toxoplasma*-like organisms from a cat.

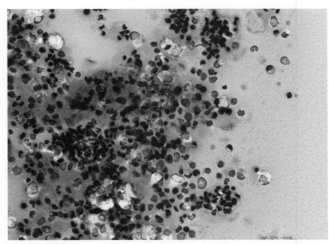

Fig. 15.34 Abdominal fluid from a cat with effusive feline infectious peritonitis. Note the nondegenerate neutrophils, macrophages, and rare small lymphocytes within a granular, stippled, proteinaceous background.

Feline Infectious Peritonitis

Effusive FIP is the classic infectious exudate in the cat, caused by a virus. The virus is not detectable with microscopic examination of the fluid. Clinical FIP may occur in cats of all ages, but the proportion of cats with FIP between ages 6 months and 2 years is significantly higher compared with the control cats in similar age groups.[19] In effusive FIP, fluid may accumulate in the abdomen, thorax, or pericardium or in all cavities. Evaluation of fluid may lend significant support to a diagnosis of FIP. The effusion is odorless, straw colored to golden, may contain flecks or fibrin strands, and foams upon agitation because of the high protein content, which is often greater than 4 g/dL. Cell counts may be variable but are typically 2000 to 6000 cells/µL, and typically hemodilution is minimal. Cytologically, the typical FIP effusion has a prominent stippled proteinaceous basophilic background (Fig. 15.34) and consists primarily (60%–80%) of nondegenerate to mildly degenerate neutrophils and lesser numbers of macrophages, small lymphocytes, and occasionally plasma cells. Effusions consisting primarily of neutrophils but with large numbers of macrophages are referred to as *pyogranulomatous* and are also common in effusions associated with FIP. Although these findings are not diagnostic of FIP, when correlated with clinical findings, a presumptive diagnosis of FIP may be made. Other diagnostic tests are often used collaboratively to diagnose FIP. These include determining the albumin-to-globulin (A:G) ratio in serum and fluid. A serum A:G ratio less than 0.8 g/dL and effusion A:G ratio less than 0.9 g/dL are often present with FIP. Anti–feline corona virus (FCoV) antibodies in serum should be interpreted with caution because many healthy cats are FCoV antibody positive.[19,20] Low to medium titers (1:25, 1:100, 1:400) of FCoV antibodies are of no diagnostic value in determining FIP infection; however, antibody titers of 1:1600 increased the probability of FIP.[20] A negative test result does not rule out the possibility of FIP infection. In one study, the anti-FCoV antibody test was negative in 10% of the cats, which did, in fact, have FIP.[20] Tests that show promise include reverse transcriptase–polymerase chain reaction (RT-PCR) performed on effusion fluids and an RT-PCR for the detection of FCoV messenger ribonucleic acid (mRNA) in peripheral blood mononuclear cells. Thus far, histological examination of affected tissue samples remains the gold standard for diagnosing FIP.

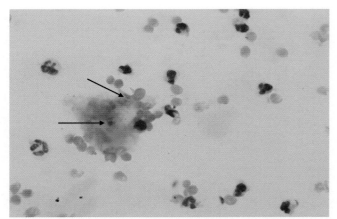

Fig. 15.35 Abdominal fluid from a dog. Extracellular bile pigment *(arrows)* and nondegenerate neutrophils.

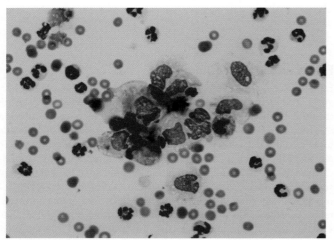

Fig. 15.36 Abdominal fluid from a dog. Dark, yellow-green, amorphous extracellular and phagocytized bile pigment, with several mildly degenerate neutrophils and macrophages.

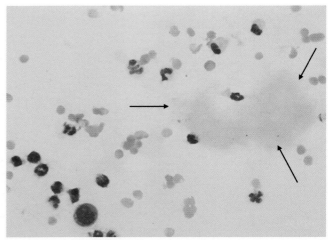

Fig. 15.37 Abdominal fluid from a dog. Extracellular homogeneous basophilic material, or "white bile" *(arrows)*.

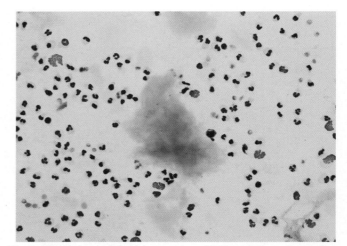

Fig. 15.38 Abdominal fluid from a dog. "White bile" seen as a large accumulations of extracellular, homogeneous, pale basophilic, mucinous-type material, with many mildly degenerate neutrophils.

Bile Peritonitis

Release of bile into the abdominal cavity secondary to gallbladder or bile duct rupture produces peritonitis. Rupture of the biliary system may occur secondary to bile duct obstruction, trauma, mucocele formation, biliary tract inflammation, and percutaneous biopsy of the liver. Bile in the peritoneal cavity causes a chemical peritonitis that is typically exudative. The effusion fluid color may be green tinged to yellow-orange. Amorphous to slightly spiculated, blue-green to yellow-green bile pigment may be present within macrophages and/or in the background fluid (Figs. 15.35 and 15.36). These pigments may resemble hemosiderin seen in hemorrhagic effusions, and caution should be exercised during interpretation. If definitive differentiation is necessary, cytochemical staining may be used to highlight the iron in hemosiderin. Bilirubin concentration can be measured in the abdominal fluid and compared with the serum concentration: If the abdominal fluid bilirubin level is at least twofold greater than concurrent serum bilirubin levels, bile peritonitis is likely.

A mucocele (mucinous cystic hyperplasia) of biliary and gallbladder epithelial cells may occur secondary to inflammation and cholelithiasis. Mucoceles may result from dysfunction of mucus-secreting cells within the gallbladder mucosa, leading to accumulation of bile and potential rupture.[21] Rupture of a biliary mucocele may cause atypical

bile peritonitis, and the effusion fluid may be yellow or red in color. The cellularity is exudative and composed of predominantly nondegenerate to mildly degenerate neutrophils and low to moderate numbers of macrophages and reactive mesothelial cells. Varying amounts of mostly extracellular amorphous, homogeneous, mucinous, basophilic material is seen in small clumps and lakes. This material has been termed "white bile," although this mucinous material does not contain bile constituents (Figs. 15.37 and 15.38). In these cases, abdominal fluid bilirubin concentrations are typically, but not always, higher than serum bilirubin concentrations.[22]

Uroperitoneum

Uroperitoneum may result from leakage of urine from the kidney, ureter, urinary bladder, or urethra. Urine released into the peritoneal cavity acts as a chemical irritant and causes inflammation that may lead to an exudative process. Uroperitoneum effusions will have varying numbers of inflammatory cells depending on the duration and dilutional effect of urine; however, nucleated cell counts are typically less than 6000 cells/μL and the total protein content is generally less than 3 g/dL as a result of the dilutional effect of urine volume. Neutrophils may be degenerate and ragged even in a nonseptic fluid because of the

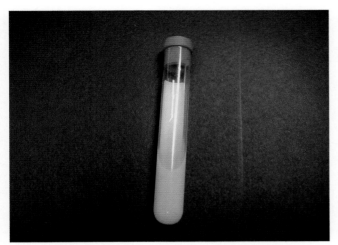

Fig. 15.39 White, opaque chylous pleural effusion from a cat.

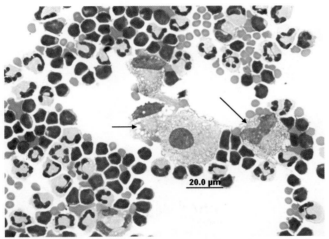

Fig. 15.40 Chylous effusion. Numerous small lymphocytes and several macrophages containing small, distinct clear cytoplasmic vacuoles (*arrows*).

chemically irritating property of urine. Bacteria and urinary crystals may be found in the abdominal fluid if they were present in the bladder at the time of rupture. Comparing serum creatinine concentrations to the concentration of abdominal fluid creatinine will confirm uroperitoneum. Creatinine of the abdominal fluid will generally be higher than the creatinine level of serum because it equilibrates more slowly compared with blood urea nitrogen (BUN). Hyperkalemia and hyponatremia are often present.[23]

Chylous Effusions

Chylous effusions contain chylomicron-rich lymph fluid (chyle) that circulates in the lymphatic system. Chylomicrons are triglyceride-rich lipoproteins absorbed from the intestines after the ingestion of food containing lipids. Chylous effusions in dogs and cats occur most frequently as bilateral pleural effusions; chylous abdominal effusions occur less frequently.[24]

The classic description of a chylous effusion is a "milky" fluid that does not clear after centrifugation and cytologically consists primarily of small lymphocytes (Fig. 15.39). Macrophages may have small, punctate clear cytoplasmic vacuoles, and plasma cells may also present (Fig. 15.40). Chylous effusions are odorless and may vary in color from classic "milky white" to an opaque-yellow or pink, depending on diet

(i.e., thin or anorectic patients may not have the characteristic opaque white fluid because of lack of dietary lipids) and the number of RBCs in the fluid. Although small lymphocytes are typically thought of as the predominant cell type, chylous effusions may occur with predominantly neutrophils, lipid-containing macrophages, or both.[24] Increased neutrophils may occur secondary to inflammation induced by repeated thoracocentesis or merely the presence of chyle in the pleural cavity. Chyle is an irritant, and chronic chylous effusions may cause an inflammatory reaction that may eventually lead to pleural fibrosis.[24] Bacterial infection in chylous effusions is uncommon because of the bacteriostatic effect of the fatty acids in chyle.[2,24,25] However, bacteria may be introduced as a result of repeated thoracocentesis.

An effusion composed of mostly small lymphocytes but not exhibiting the typical physical characteristics (opaque) of a chylous effusion can be confirmed by measuring and comparing effusion and serum triglyceride concentrations.[24,25] The chylous effusion triglyceride concentration is higher than the serum concentration.[24,25] Chyle normally drains from the thoracic duct into the venous system. Chylous effusions form when there is an obstruction (physical or functional) of lymphatic flow resulting in increased pressure within lymphatics and dilation of the thoracic duct (lymphangiectasia). Rupture of the thoracic duct (i.e., after surgery or blunt trauma) is a rare cause of chylous effusion in veterinary medicine and is usually self-limiting.[2,24] Physical obstructions of the thoracic duct may result from neoplasms (thymoma, lymphoma, lymphangiosarcoma), granulomas, or inflammatory reactions in the mediastinum that compress the thoracic duct or the vessels into which it drains, or secondary to obstruction of intralymphatic flow with neoplastic cells. Functional obstructions may occur with cardiovascular disease from increased central venous pressure (right-sided heart failure) or increased lymphatic flow from increased hepatic lymph production that exceeds drainage capability.[24,25] Cardiovascular disease (i.e., cardiomyopathy, heartworm disease, pericardial effusions) resulting in poor venous flow may also lead to chylous effusion as a functional effect.

Many other miscellaneous causes of chylous effusion, including coughing and vomiting, diaphragmatic herniation, congenital defects, trauma, and thrombosis of the thoracic duct, have been reported, and often no underlying etiology can be determined despite extensive testing (idiopathic chylous effusion).[2,24,25]

Although most opaque effusions are true chylous effusions, they may rarely be pseudochylous. True pseudochylous effusions are a debated entity; however, they are opaque effusions that do not contain chyle. Instead, the white color is classically thought to be the result of cellular debris, lecithin globulin complex, cholesterol from cell membranes, or all of these. Pseudochylous effusions described in humans are most commonly the result of long-standing pleural effusions caused by tuberculosis, rheumatoid pleuritis, and malignant effusions, with resultant cell breakdown within the fluid. Despite much discussion about differentiating these two types of fluids, pseudochylous effusions are not well described in veterinary medicine and are rare in dogs and cats.[2,24] Cytologically, the presence of cellular breakdown material, such as cholesterol crystals, and the lack of a significant lymphocytic cellular component may suggest a pseudochylous effusion (Fig. 15.41). Additionally, pseudochylous effusions have high cholesterol and low triglyceride content compared with serum.

Hemorrhagic Effusions

Hemorrhagic effusions may be seen with various primary disorders, such as hemostatic defects (congenital or acquired coagulopathies); trauma; neoplasia; and heartworm infection (Fig. 15.42). Hemorrhagic effusions secondary to neoplasia may not contain neoplastic cells, or neoplastic cells may be present in low, moderate, or high numbers.

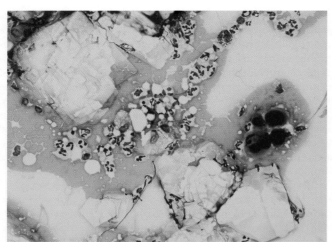

Fig. 15.41 Abdominal effusion from a dog. Large numbers of extracellular, clear, flat, notched cholesterol crystals, with red blood cells, few reactive mesothelial cells *(right center)*, and admixed nondegenerate neutrophils and macrophages.

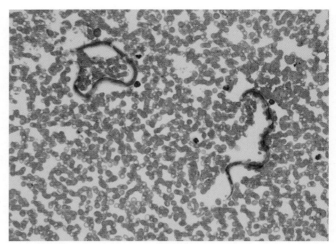

Fig. 15.42 Hemodilute background with two large, basophilic microfilaria and few scattered blood leukocytes and few small platelet clumps. (Courtesy Jennifer Neel, North Carolina State University.)

The presence or absence of neoplastic cells in a hemorrhagic effusion is often dependent on the type of neoplasm. For example, mesenchymal neoplasms such as hemangiosarcoma (splenic, hepatic, cardiac) often lack neoplastic cells or contain low numbers of neoplastic cells within the hemorrhagic effusion. In comparison, if mesothelioma is associated with a hemorrhagic effusion, moderate to high numbers of atypical mesothelial cells may be evident. However, it should be kept in mind that reactive mesothelial cells may have significant atypia and that differentiating a reactive population from a malignant population is often difficult, even for experienced cytopathologists. Determining the etiology of a hemorrhagic effusion, just as in the case of other effusion categories, requires not only cytological assessment of the fluid but also correlation with clinical signs, history, laboratory data, imaging studies, and often fine-needle aspiration (FNA) of abnormalities found in the respective body cavity. Distinguishing hemorrhagic effusions from iatrogenic blood contamination or inadvertent aspiration of an organ (i.e., liver, spleen) is of diagnostic importance. Differentiating blood contamination from per-acute or acute hemorrhage may be difficult; however, assessment of clinical signs, physical examination findings, and laboratory data are helpful. Hemorrhage of greater than 24 hours' duration may be differentiated from blood contamination by identifying erythrophagocytosis in the sample (Fig. 15.43) and by noting the presence or absence of platelets and the RBC breakdown products, hemosiderin, and hematoidin (Fig. 15.44). When blood enters a body cavity, the platelets quickly aggregate, degranulate, and disappear. Also, RBCs are phagocytized and digested by macrophages. Therefore the presence of platelets and lack of erythrophagocytosis or heme breakdown products suggests either per-acute hemorrhage or iatrogenic blood contamination. Concurrent identification of platelets and erythrophagocytosis, with or without heme breakdown products, suggests either chronic hemorrhage or previous hemorrhage with iatrogenic contamination. The absence of platelets, with evidence of erythrophagocytosis, heme breakdown products, or a combination of both, supports chronic or previous hemorrhage.

In cases of inadvertent organ aspiration, inadvertent major vessel puncture, or frank intracavity hemorrhage, the fluid obtained will be grossly bloody. With a major vessel or splenic aspirate, the PCV of the fluid is generally equal to (vessel puncture) or greater than (splenic aspirate) the peripheral blood PCV. With severe intracavity hemorrhage, clinical signs of hemorrhagic shock are expected.

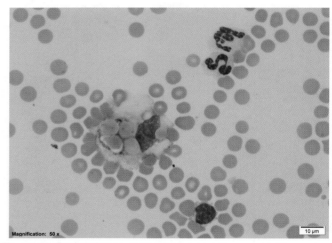

Magnification: 50 x   10 µm

Fig. 15.43 Erythrophagocytosis. Note macrophage containing several intact phagocytized red blood cells.

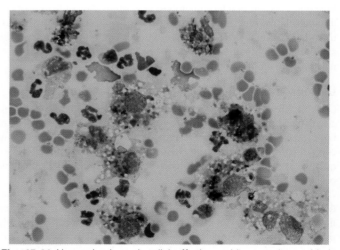

Fig. 15.44 Hemorrhagic pericardial effusion, with many hemosiderin and hematoidin-laden macrophages.

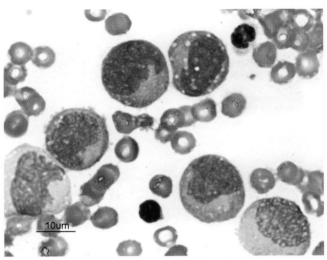

Fig. 15.45 Pericardial fluid from a dog with lymphoma. Large immature lymphocytes predominate. (Courtesy James Meinkoth, Oklahoma State University.)

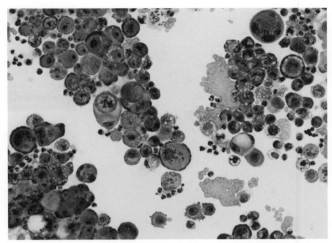

Fig. 15.46 Effusion fluid consistent with mesothelioma. Aggregates and individualized markedly pleomorphic, neoplastic mesothelial cells. Note the many features of malignancy, such as cell gigantism, multinucleation, macrokaryosis, macronucleoli, and multiple nucleoli.

Neoplastic Effusions

Effusions may occur secondary to many forms of neoplasia (lymphoma, mast cell neoplasia, sarcoma, mesothelioma, carcinoma or adenocarcinoma, etc.) and may often be diagnosed with cytological examination of the fluid. In one study, the sensitivity of cytological examination of effusions to detect malignant neoplasms was 64% in dogs and 61% in cats.[26] Poorly exfoliating tumors may have effusions in the modified transudate to exudative range if there is concurrent inflammation. Many tumors do not exfoliate neoplastic cells, and the absence of neoplastic cells within effusions does not rule out neoplasia. Similar to tissue aspirates, neoplastic cells in an effusion must be distinguished from dysplastic cells secondary to inflammation or reactive mesothelial cells. Thus the presence of concurrent inflammation in the fluid may confound the diagnosis of neoplasia, especially if neoplastic cells are not present in high numbers, do not exhibit significant cytological criteria of malignancy, or both. Distinguishing neoplastic epithelial cells (exfoliative carcinoma or adenocarcinoma) from mesothelioma, and mesothelioma from hyperplastic and reactive mesothelial cells, which are frequently found in both neoplastic and nonneoplastic fluids, is a particular challenge. This dilemma is discussed further in the section on mesothelioma below. Neoplastic effusions are inherently difficult samples to interpret for many of the reasons outlined above, and therefore in-house samples interpreted as neoplastic, or suspected of being neoplastic, should be confirmed by a veterinary clinical pathologist.

Lymphoma

A neoplastic effusion secondary to high-grade lymphoma may occur with lymphoma of the intracavitary lymph nodes, spleen, liver GI tract, kidneys, thymus, and mediastinum. Cytologically, low to high numbers of a monomorphic population of exfoliating large immature lymphocytes may be present (Fig. 15.45; and see Fig. 15.12). Immature lymphocytes are large cells, with a scant to moderate amount of basophilic cytoplasm, round to variably shape nuclei, finely stippled nuclear chromatin, and prominent nucleoli.

Mast Cell Neoplasia

Mast cell tumors within body cavities (nodal, hepatic, splenic, and GI) may cause effusions and frequently exfoliate large numbers of mast cells into the effusion (see Figs. 15.15 and 15.16). Mast cells are readily identified by large numbers of metachromatic (purple) cytoplasmic granules. In effusions, mast cells tend to have "packeted" granules, and because of the high affinity of granules for stain and stain exhaustion, the nucleus may stain poorly or not at all. Diff-Quik stain does not undergo the same metachromatic reaction as Wright-Giemsa or modified Wright stain and often does not stain mast cell granules well. Eosinophils are occasionally (but not reliably) present, as are few scattered nondegenerate neutrophils, mesothelial cells, and macrophages. It should be noted that pleomorphic (anisocytosis, anisokaryosis, prominent nucleoli, multinucleation) and poorly granular mast cell tumors may be found in an effusion.

Sarcoma

Sarcomas involving intracavity organs often do not exfoliate neoplastic mesenchymal cells into effusions and are rarely diagnosed on fluid analysis alone. Often, effusions secondary to mesenchymal tumors are hemorrhagic secondary to rupture of the tumor (i.e., splenic and hepatic hemangiosarcoma) and of low nucleated cellularity. In this case, making concentrated specimens or buffy coat preparations may aid in concentrating low numbers of neoplastic cells. In the rare event that neoplastic cells are identified, the cells have a characteristic spindle appearance and malignant features (see Chapter 2).

Mesothelioma

Mesotheliomas are uncommon tumors in domestic species and can be well differentiated or pleomorphic. Subtypes are based on histological evaluation of growth patterns (epithelioid, biphasic, sarcomatoid, and undifferentiated). Mesothelioma is often difficult to diagnose cytologically because of the moderate to marked pleomorphism exhibited by reactive mesothelial cells. Thus, when an effusion contains significant numbers of mesothelial cells where marked cytological criteria of malignancy is not evident, it is often impossible to differentiate mesothelial reactivity or hyperplasia from mesothelioma. When an effusion contains large numbers of mesothelial cells, and the cells exhibit marked criteria of malignancy—extreme macrocytosis, marked anisokaryosis, large variably shaped nucleoli, large numbers of mitotic figures, and aberrant mitoses—although diagnostic on cytology for a malignant exfoliative neoplasm, it may be nearly impossible to differentiate between mesothelioma, carcinoma, or adenocarcinoma (Figs. 15.46 and 15.47).[26] Identification of a primary carcinoma/adenocarcinoma is helpful. If a primary tumor is not identified, histopathology of the

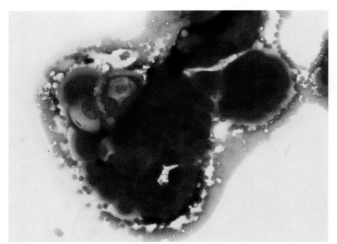

Fig. 15.47 Canine thoracic effusion secondary to mesothelioma. Histopathology was consistent with epithelioid subtype.

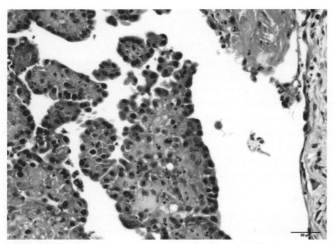

Fig. 15.48 Histological section of mesothelioma. Papillary projections of multilayer neoplastic mesothelium with significant cellular pleomorphism and frequent mitoses. (Courtesy Luke Borst, North Carolina State University.)

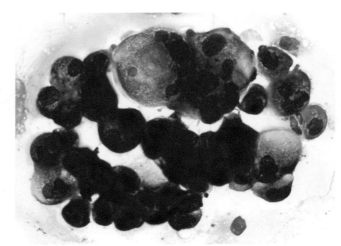

Fig. 15.49 Pleural fluid from a dog with a neoplastic effusion secondary to epithelial neoplasia. Note the clusters of pleomorphic cells, with abundant basophilic cytoplasm, significant variation in the nuclear-to-cytoplasmic (N:C) ratios, occasional multinucleation, and marked anisocytosis.

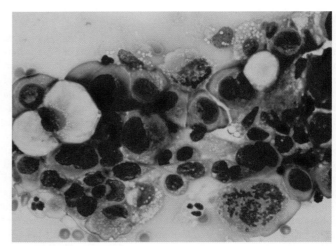

Fig. 15.50 Few neoplastic cells contain large clear vacuoles that push the nucleus to the periphery. Additionally, note the two mitotic figures. The bottom right mitotic figure is aberrant.

affected mesothelium may be necessary. Often, a combination of history, imaging findings, cytology, and histopathology is needed to diagnose mesothelioma or to distinguish mesothelioma from epithelial neoplasia. Histological differentiation of reactive or hyperplastic mesothelial cells from neoplastic mesothelial cells may also be challenging, particularly if the biopsy sample is small and not representative of the lesion. Histologically, no single defined criterion to diagnose mesothelioma exists; however, assessment for neoplastic invasion into the submesothelial tissues and immunohistochemistry may be helpful.[27] Fig. 15.48 demonstrates the histopathology of mesothelioma.

Carcinoma or Adenocarcinoma

Carcinomas and adenocarcinomas may often be diagnosed by cytological evaluation of effusions on the basis of significant numbers of exfoliating cells and numerous criteria of malignancy. Neoplastic effusions may be inflammatory or noninflammatory. Neoplastic epithelial cells often form aggregates, clusters, and sheets. Occasional glandular (acinar) arrangements may be found. Significant anisocytosis, anisokaryosis and anisonucleoliosis may exist, with cell gigantism and abundant basophilic cytoplasm (Fig. 15.49). Cytoplasm may also contain large clear vacuoles, which push the nucleus to the periphery

of the cell, or numerous fine, foamy cytoplasmic vacuoles (Figs. 15.50 and 15.51), and may also contain intracytoplasmic eosinophilic secretory material. Documenting strong nuclear criteria of malignancy is important, including anisokaryosis; nuclear gigantism; coarse nuclear chromatin; large, bizarre, or angular nucleoli; multiple nucleoli; nuclear molding; high nucleus-to-cytoplasm ratios; multinucleation (see Fig. 15.49); numerous mitotic figures; and aberrant mitoses (see Fig. 15.50). When an effusion is diagnostic for epithelial neoplasia, imaging studies of the respective body cavity may identify masses or organomegaly, prompting FNA or tissue biopsy for further characterization.

Thymoma

Thymoma is a neoplasm of thymic epithelium and is a top consideration in the differential diagnosis for a cranial mediastinal mass. Thymomas may be benign or malignant, and both invasive and noninvasive forms exist. Additionally, thymomas may be heterogeneous, cystic, or inflamed. A detailed description of the cytological appearance of aspirates from thymomas is provided in Chapter 17. When thymomas are associated with a thoracic effusion, the effusion may be inconclusive or suggestive of thymoma. An effusion associated with

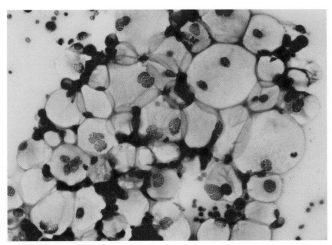

Fig. 15.51 Feline abdominal effusion secondary to epithelial neoplasia. Note the numerous, clear, small cytoplasmic vacuoles.

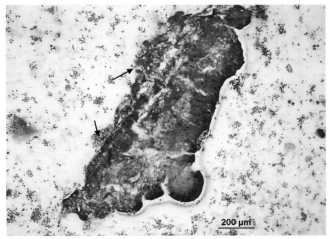

Fig. 15.52 Metacestode remnant. Note the size of the red blood cells and inflammatory cells in the background compared with this structure. The clear, nonstaining structures are calcareous corpuscles *(arrows)*.

thymoma may contain large numbers of small lymphocytes, which are often a significant and predominant nonneoplastic cell population in thymomas. The presence of a prominent population of small lymphocytes, together with low to moderate numbers of well-differentiated mast cells (also a prominent cell population in thymomas), helps lend support to a diagnosis of thymoma if a cranial mediastinal mass is evident. It is uncommon for the neoplastic epithelial component to exfoliate, and if epithelial cells are present, it may be difficult to differentiate them from reactive mesothelial cells. The neoplastic epithelial cells have somewhat ill-defined borders, are found in aggregates and sheets, and contain small to moderate amounts of pale blue cytoplasm, round central nuclei, and indistinct nucleoli. The cells often are minimally pleomorphic. Direct aspiration, tissue biopsy and histopathology, or flow cytometry of either the mass or effusion fluid may be used to differentiate thymoma from thymic small cell lymphoma. Lymphocyte coexpression of CD4 and CD8, which is characteristic of thymocytes, is suggestive of thymoma.[28]

Parasitic Effusions

Abdominal effusion caused by aberrant larval migration of the tapeworm *Mesocestoides* spp. is uncommon. Cases of canine infection are reported in northwestern United States, particularly in California, with fewer cases in Washington.[29] Clinical signs may include anorexia, vomiting, weight loss, depression, and abdominal distension. In reported cases of parasitical effusions, the gross appearance of the fluid contains small opaque flecks, which are the metacestodes.[29] Analysis

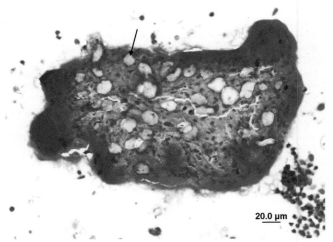

Fig. 15.53 Metacestode remnant. The clear, nonstaining structures are calcareous corpuscles *(arrow)*.

of the aspirated fluid is in the exudative range. Cytological features include numerous inflammatory cells, partial to intact metacestodes, and numerous round to angular, clear to pink refractile calcareous corpuscles (Fig. 15.52 and Fig. 15.53).

REFERENCES

1. Nelson OL. Pleural effusion. In: Ettinger SJ, Feldman EC, eds. *Textbook of Veterinary Internal Medicine*. Philadelphia, PA: Saunders; 2005:204–207.

2. Fossum TW. Surgery of the lower respiratory system: pleural cavity and diaphragm. In: Fossum TW, ed. *Small Animal Surgery*. St. Louis, MO: Mosby; 2005:788–820.

3. Zoia A, Hughes D, Connolly DJ. Pericardial effusion and cardiac tamponade in a cat with extranodal lymphoma. *J Small Anim Pract*. 2004;45:467–471.

4. Tobias AH. Pericardial disorders. In: Ettinger SJ, Feldman EC, eds. *Textbook of Veterinary Internal Medicine*. Philadelphia, PA: Saunders; 2005:1107–1111.

5. Gidlewski J, Petrie JP. Therapeutic pericardiocentesis in the dog and cat. *Clin Tech Small Anim Pract*. 2005;20:151–155.

6. Fossum TW. Surgery of the abdominal cavity. In: Fossum TW, ed. *Small Animal Surgery*. St. Louis, MO: Mosby; 2002:271–272.

7. Walters JM. Abdominal paracentesis and diagnostic peritoneal lavage. *Clin Tech Small Anim Pract*. 2003;18(1):32–38.

8. D'Urso L. Thoracic and pericardial taps and drains. In: Ettinger SJ, Feldman EC, eds. *Textbook of Veterinary Internal Medicine*. Philadelphia, PA: Saunders; 2005:380–831.

9. Johnson M, et al. A retrospective study of clinical findings, treatment and outcome in 143 dogs with pericardial effusion. *J Small Anim Pract*. 2004;45:546–552.

10. Stockham SL, Scott MA. Cavitary Effusions. In: *Fundamentals of Veterinary Clinical Pathology*. 2nd ed. Ames, IA: Blackwell Publishing; 2008:851, 849, 841, 842.

11. George JW. The usefulness and limitations of hand-held refractometers in veterinary laboratory medicine: an historical and technical review. *Vet Clin Path*. 2001;30(4):201–210.

12. Cowgill E, Neel J. Pleural fluid from a dog with marked eosinophilia. *Vet Clin Pathol*. 2003;32(4):147–149.

13. Takahashi T, et al. Visceral mast cell tumors in dogs: 10 cases (1982-1997). *J Am Vet Assoc*. 2000;216(2):222–226.

14. Spangler WL, Culbertson MR. Prevalence and type of splenic diseases in cats: 455 cases (1985–1991). *J Am Vet Med Assoc*. 1992;201:773–776.

15. Rissetto K, Villamil JA, Selting KA, Tyler J, Henry CJ. Recent trends in feline intestinal neoplasia: an epidemiologic study of 1129 cases in the veterinary medical database from 1964 to 2004. *J Am Anim Hosp Assoc*. 2011;47:28–36.

16. O'Brien PJ, Lumsden JH. The cytologic examination of body cavity fluids. *Semin Vet Med Surg (Small Animal)*. 1988;3(2):140–156.

17. Arndt Holmberg T, Vernau W, Melli AC, Conrad PA. *Neospora caninum* associated with septic peritonitis in an adult dog. *Vet Clin Pathol*. 2006;35(2):235–238.

18. Dell'Orco M, Bertazzolo W, Paccioretti F. What is your diagnosis? Peritoneal effusion from a dog. *Vet Clin Pathol*. 2009;38(3):367–369.

19. Rohrbach BW, et al. Epidemiology of feline infectious peritonitis among cats examined at veterinary medical teaching hospitals. *J Am Vet Assoc*. 2001;218(7):1111–1115.

20. Hartmann K, et al. Comparison of different tests to diagnose feline infectious peritonitis. *J Vet Intern Med*. 2003;17:781–790.

21. Pike FS, et al. Gallbladder mucocele in dogs: 30 cases (2000-2002). *J Am Vet Assoc*. 2004;224(10):1615–1622.

22. Owens SD, et al. Three cases of canine bile peritonitis with mucinous material in abdominal fluid as the prominent cytologic finding. *Vet Clin Pathol*. 2003;32(3):114–120.

23. Aumann M, Worth LT, Drobatz KJ. Uroperitoneum in cats: 26 cases (1986-1995). *J Am Anim Hosp Assoc*. 1998;34(4):315–324.

24. Meadows RL, MacWilliams PS. Chylous effusions revisited. *Vet Clin Pathol*. 1994;23:54–62.

25. Mertens MM, Fossum TW. Pleural and extrapleural diseases. In: Fossum TW, ed. *Small Animal Surgery*. St. Louis, MO: Mosby; 2002:1281–1282.

26. Hirschberger J, et al. Sensitivity and specificity of cytologic evaluation in the diagnosis of neoplasia in body fluids from dogs and cats. *Vet Clin Path*. 1999;28(4):142–146.

27. Reggeti F, Brisson B, Ruotsalo K, et al. Invasive epithelial mesothelioma in a dog. *Vet Pathol*. 2005;42:77–81.

28. Lana S, Plaza S, et al. Diagnosis of mediastinal masses in dogs by flow cytometry. *JVIM*. 2006;20:1161–1165.

29. Caruso KJ, et al. Cytologic diagnosis of peritoneal cestodiasis in dogs caused by Mesocestoides sp. *Vet Clin Pathol*. 2003;32(2):50–60.

16

Transtracheal and Bronchoalveolar Washes

Roberta Di Terlizzi, Kate English, Rick L. Cowell, Ronald D. Tyler, and James H. Meinkoth

Respiratory flushes or washes sample the contents of the airways, the trachea, bronchi, and alveolar spaces. These samples frequently provide clinically useful information of the pulmonary disease process and may also provide definitive diagnosis in some patients. Pulmonary disease is often defined by the area that it affects (e.g., bronchitis) or by the changes that may occur as a result of the disease process (e.g., bronchiectasis); however, the underlying pathology may be variable with these disease presentations, and cytology and culture of a lower respiratory tract sample may be helpful in determining the etiology. In pathologies that solely involve abnormal structure or function of the airways or in diseases that do not have direct airway involvement, which may include some primary or metastatic neoplasms, the information obtained from a flush or wash sample may be limited.[1,2] Cytology of flush or wash samples may, however, be highly sensitive in cases of inflammatory airway disease.[3]

Tracheal wash or bronchoalveolar lavage (TW or BAL) samples are quick, easy, and inexpensive ways to obtain diagnostic samples from the respiratory tree. Although complications are rare, subcutaneous emphysema, pneumomediastinum, hemorrhage, resultant hypoxia, needle tract infection, transient hemoptysis, bronchoconstriction, and other complications have been reported.[4-7]

It is frequently helpful to perform radiography in conjunction with the wash procedure, although radiographic changes may not always be apparent in the early stages of respiratory disease.[8,9] Radiography before a flush or wash procedure may be invaluable if the disease is focal because this will indicate which lung lobe is most likely to provide a diagnostic yield and allow for selective sampling, particularly if bronchoscope-guided lavage is used. If the disease is diffuse, sampling of any area of the lung may be representative, although sampling from multiple sites is more likely to provide a diagnostic yield.[10]

The cell types noted in the sample may vary, depending on the site of sampling (Tables 16.1 and 16.2).

TECHNIQUE OF TRACHEAL WASH AND BRONCHOALVEOLAR LAVAGE

Approach to the lower respiratory tract may be transtracheal or endotracheal. If the endotracheal approach is used, sampling may be performed by bronchoscopic or nonbronchoscopic (blind) methods.

The advantage of the bronchoscope is that observation of the mucosa lining the airways and quantification of mucus or secretions present may provide additional information during patient assessment. More directed sampling of the individual lobes may also be performed. Nonbronchoscopic sampling, however, does not require expensive equipment and so may be more widely available in first opinion practice.

Many reviews of the sampling techniques exist.[11-14] However, a brief summary is provided here.

Transtracheal Sampling

The transtracheal or percutaneous method is optimal for patients who are at a high risk for general anesthesia–related complications because it can be performed with local anesthesia only or with additional sedation, if required. This technique may also be less prone to oropharyngeal contamination and therefore may be preferred if obtaining a sample for culture. Small amounts of fluid are instilled, and a cough reflex is essential for fluid recovery.

- The skin over the cranioventral larynx is clipped, and the site is prepared as for aseptic surgery. Surgical gloves should be worn.
- A small amount of 1% to 2% lidocaine is injected into subcutaneous tissue. Very light sedation may be helpful in cats and small dogs[4]; intravenous ketamine has been recommended for sedation of cats.[5]
- The animal is restrained in the sitting position or in sternal recumbency, with the neck extended. Overextension of the neck, however, may result in increased oropharyngeal contamination.
- A small, triangular depression is digitally palpated just cranial to the ridge of the cricoid cartilage. This is the location of the cricothyroid ligament and of needle insertion (Fig. 16.1). Alternatively, the catheter may be inserted between two tracheal rings 1 to 3 cm below the larynx (e.g., C2 to C3, or C3 to C4).[15]
- Using a large commercial intravenous catheter set, "through the needle," or intravascular catheter and a 3.5-French (Fr) polyethylene urinary catheter, with the needle directed slightly caudal, the

TABLE 16.1 Lining Cells of the Lower Respiratory Tract That May Be Noted on Tracheal Wash or Bronchoalveolar Lavage Sampling

Airway	Lining cell
Large airway, trachea, and bronchi	Ciliated columnar epithelium, goblet cell
Bronchiole	Columnar to cuboidal epithelium, ciliated to nonciliated
Alveolus	Type I pneumocyte (not commonly observed on bronchoalveolar lavage cytology)

From Bacha WJ, Jr., Bacha LM. Respiratory system. In Anderson RC, ed. *Nematode Parasites of Vertebrates: Their Development and Transmission.* 2nd ed. Wallingford, UK: CABI Publishing; 2000.

TABLE 16.2   Average of Mean Percentage Cell Differential of Nonepithelial Populations From a Number of Studies of Bronchoalveolar Lavage Samples From Healthy Dogs and Cats

	Macrophage	Neutrophil	Eosinophil	Lymphocyte	Mast Cell
Dogs	71%	5%	5%	17%	2%
Cats	70%	6%	18%	4%	1%

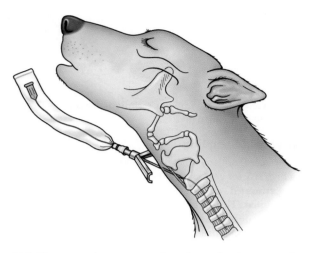

Fig. 16.1 Diagrammatic representation of needle placement through the cricothyroid ligament of the larynx.

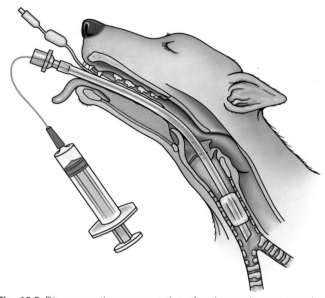

Fig. 16.2 Diagrammatic representation of catheter placement and tracheal wash or bronchoalveolar lavage collection through an endotracheal tube.

skin, subcutaneous tissue, and cricothyroid ligament of the larynx, or ligament between the tracheal rings, are penetrated.[5] Smaller catheters are recommended for cats and very small dogs.

- Once in the tracheal lumen, the needle is positioned parallel to the trachea, and the catheter is advanced through the needle and down the lumen of the trachea to a level just above the carina. Insertion of the needle and passage of the catheter induces coughing in most animals.[4,5]
- The catheter should pass through easily; if it does not, it may have become embedded in the dorsal tracheal wall or failed to enter the trachea and may be embedded in the peritracheal tissue.[16] In either case, the needle and the entire catheter should be withdrawn and the procedure repeated. Also, the catheter may bend, causing it to advance toward the oropharynx, and this results in the washing of the oropharynx, not the bronchial tree.
- Once the catheter is properly placed, the needle is withdrawn, leaving the catheter in place. With some severe pulmonary diseases, a sample may be obtained by simply aspirating after positioning the catheter. However, the infusion of saline into the bronchial tree is usually necessary before aspiration to obtain an adequate sample. A 12-mL (milliliter) or larger syringe containing 1 to 2 mL of non-bacteriostatic, sterile, buffered saline for every 5 kilogram (kg) of body weight is attached to the catheter. The saline is injected into the bronchial lumen until either the animal starts to cough or all the fluid is injected.
- The animal will typically start coughing before all the saline is injected, at which time aspiration must start. If coughing does not occur, coupage may be helpful. Only a small portion of the injected fluid will be retrieved. The injected fluid remaining in the tracheobronchial tree will be rapidly absorbed and is no cause for concern.[4]
- The operator aspirates for only a few seconds and then stops. Aspiration for a prolonged time results in more fluid being collected, but the chances of a contaminated wash are greatly increased,

because the animal will cough fluid into the oropharyngeal area and reaspirate the fluid, which now contains cellular and bacterial contaminants.

Maintaining gentle pressure on the puncture site for a few minutes generally inhibits the formation of subcutaneous emphysema.[15] Applying mild pressure to the puncture site with a gauze wrap for 12 to 24 hours also helps eliminate the formation of subcutaneous emphysema.

Endotracheal Tube Technique

Alternatively, samples are collected through an endotracheal tube (Fig. 16.2). This procedure requires general anesthesia. This technique may be used to obtain either a TW or a BAL. For a tracheal sample, the sample catheter extends beyond the end of the endotracheal tube but does not extend past the carina. The location of the carina is externally assessed as approximately the level of the fourth intercostal space.[10] For blind BAL, a sample tube of appropriate size for the patient (e.g., a 16-Fr polyvinyl chloride stomach tube in a medium- to large-sized dog, and a 5-Fr polypropylene urinary catheter in a cat) was shown to consistently maintain a snug fit between the external landmarks of the seventh and eleventh ribs, so the sample tubing should be a minimum length to reach the level of the eleventh rib.[17,18] Sterile tubing should be used. Pretreatment with bronchodilators is recommended by some authors before BAL.[7]

- Once the patient has reached a suitable plane of anesthesia, an endotracheal tube should be carefully placed with as minimal contact with the oropharynx and larynx as can be achieved.

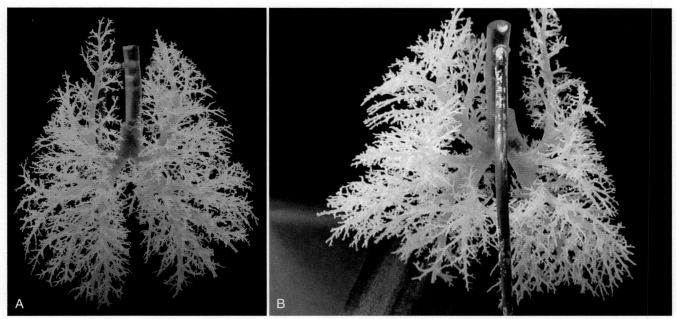

Fig. 16.3 (A) A cast of the canine bronchial tree. (B) Close-up of the area of the bifurcation of the trachea to show the bronchial branching in more detail. (A, Courtesy A. Crook, RVC, UK.)

- Preoxygenation is recommended. Fitting of a T- or Y-piece to the endotracheal tube will allow delivery of oxygen and anesthetic gas throughout the procedure. If the leakage of gas is a concern to the veterinary staff, anesthesia may be maintained by using injectable anesthetic agents administered via an intravenous (IV) catheter.
- The patient is placed in sternal or lateral recumbency; if the lateral position is used, it is preferable to place the most affected side down.[14] In some cases, use of a foam wedge to elevate the cranial part of the thorax above that of the caudal part has been recommended.[19]
- A bronchoscope, tube, or catheter through which the sample will be obtained is introduced through the endotracheal tube, ensuring this does not contact the oropharynx.

The canine bronchial tree branches in an irregular manner and has been reviewed in detail.[20] Briefly, when the patient is orientated in sternal recumbency, from the bronchial tree, the entrance to the right principal bronchus appears as almost a direct continuation of the trachea, with the left principal bronchus seen at a more acute angle. The first lobar bronchus on the right is the right cranial lung lobe, in the lateral wall of the bronchus opposite the carina. The next lobar bronchus is the right middle lung lobe, in the ventral floor, usually between the 6 and 8 o'clock positions. The right accessory lobe is located in the ventromedial to medial aspect of the right principal bronchus, just beyond the origin of the middle lobe bronchus, extending in a ventromedial direction. Beyond this bronchus is the lobar bronchus for the right caudal lung lobe. On the left the left cranial lung lobe is accessed ventrolateral to the lateral aspect of the left cranial bronchus. Beyond this, the left principal bronchus becomes the left caudal lung lobe bronchus. Fig. 16.3 shows a cast of a canine bronchial tree to provide an idea of the branching that may be seen in vivo.

The feline bronchial tree has also been reviewed.[21] The right principal bronchus is similarly a near continuation of the trachea, as in the dog, with the left principal bronchus at a slightly more acute angle. Entering the right principal bronchus, the right cranial bronchus is first encountered, arising lateral to the right principal bronchus and directly opposite the carina. Advancing caudally, the next lobar bronchus is the

right middle lung lobe located ventrally. The right accessory lobe bronchus and the first segment of the right caudal lobar bronchus arise at approximately the same level, with the right accessory lobe bronchus being located ventromedially and the right caudal bronchus dorsally. The second segment of the right caudal lobe bronchus is more dorsal and located ventrally, with the third segment more caudal and dorsal. Entering the left principal bronchus, the left cranial lobar bronchus is lateral and slightly ventral. The continuation of the left principal bronchus enters the left caudal lobe bronchus, with the segmental bronchi branching alternately dorsally and ventrally as in the right caudal lobe. It may not be possible to enter all the bronchi or even visualize the more caudal bronchi in all cats examined.

- If the patient is in lateral recumbency, the orientation and access to the lung for sampling may be altered.[22]
- When the desired level has been reached for a TW or a BAL (see previous), then fluid may be introduced. To optimize recovery of fluid from a BAL, the bronchoscope or tube should be wedged into the bronchi. This may be determined visually on a bronchoscope. If performing blind BAL, then the tube should be advanced gently until it stops; it should then be withdrawn a few centimeters, rotated gently, and readvanced until resistance is felt at a consistent level.[17]
- Once a snug fit has been achieved, a syringe with an appropriate volume of fluid and an additional 5-mL of air to ensure complete delivery of the fluid is attached to the top of the sample tube. Volumes used may vary; however, a suitable volume in cats is reported to be aliquots of 5-mL/kg.[23] This volume may be used in dogs, but volumes of 2-mL/kg have been reported to be adequate.[24,25] Repeat aliquots may be administered until sufficient fluid is retrieved; however, no more than three aliquots are generally used.
- Fluid recovery may be affected by the tightness of the fit of the bronchoscope or sample tubing in the airway. In the double catheter technique, the catheter to collect the sample is placed a few centimeters above the level of the catheter delivering the fluid aliquot; the authors describing this technique have reported good fluid recovery without the need for a snug fit.[26]

BOX 16.1 Samples for Submission to the Pathology Laboratory

- Smears prepared from the flush or wash sample within 30 minutes of obtaining the sample
- Ethylenediaminetetraacetic acid (EDTA) sample for further cytology preparations
- Plain sterile sample for culture
- Optional specific media preparations (e.g., for *Mycoplasma* culture); contact laboratory before sampling

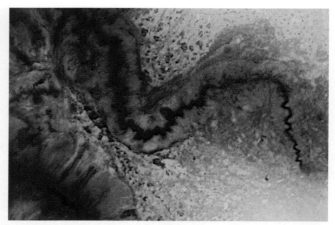

Fig. 16.4 Tracheal wash or bronchoalveolar lavage from a dog with chronic bronchial disease. Large Curschmann spiral and scattered alveolar macrophages are present in an eosinophilic mucous background (Wright stain, original magnification 50×).

Other measures that may increase fluid retrieval include tilting the head of the patient downward and rotating the patient with the lavage lung area uppermost to encourage fluid drainage.[27] This may be complicated in larger patients, and the risk for gastric dilation–volvulus in large, deep-chested dogs may also be a concern with rotation of these patients. Coupage may also be helpful.

Retrieved fluid should appear foamy if the sampling has been adequate and is reported to reflect the presence of surfactant.[14]

Other techniques of bronchoscopic sampling that have been reported are bronchial brushings and biopsy.[15] One study suggested that in some instances, bronchial brushing may be a more sensitive test to assess for inflammation, although in one patient, BAL was the more sensitive test.[28] However, the criteria to determine what constitutes inflammation with these types of samples alone is not clearly defined.

Bronchoscopy may also be used for treatment, as in the removal of tracheobronchial foreign bodies.[29] Therapeutic BAL has been described in a dog affected by pulmonary alveolar proteinosis.[30]

SAMPLE SUBMISSION

Several studies in healthy patients have shown that no significant differences exist between different lobes of the lung lavaged either in overall cell numbers or differential counts.[19,31] Therefore, increases of cells will be interpreted similarly, no matter which area of the lung the samples are derived from. The first aliquot is reported to have fewer epithelial cells and higher numbers of polymorphonuclear cells, and some authors recommend discarding the first aliquot, although it is unlikely to significantly affect clinical interpretation if the first aliquot is combined with subsequent aliquots.[23]

It is recommended that fresh smears be prepared at the time of sample collection, within 30 minutes because cell morphology is not well preserved in TW/BAL samples.[31] A direct smear of turbid fluid (or if mucous flecks are noted grossly), a smear of mucus material, and additional cytocentrifuged preparations are likely to provide the most information from the sample.

Recommendations for samples submitted to the laboratory are noted in Box 16.1. Guidelines for preparing smears from fluids are presented in Chapter 1.

If the TW/BAL is deemed unacceptable because of oropharyngeal contamination (or for any other reason) and the procedure is to be repeated, it should be repeated either immediately or after 48 hours. Even though a sterile saline solution is used for the wash, it induces a neutrophilic response that peaks about 24 hours after washing. If TW/BAL is performed the next day (i.e., 24 hours after the first wash), an inflammatory response will be present, and it may be difficult to tell whether it is secondary to the prior wash or because of an inflammatory lung disease.[32-34] However, no significant difference may exist in samples collected 48 hours apart.[24,32,34] If a contaminated wash is obtained, it is ideal to wait at least 48 hours to collect a TW/BAL again because it allows the lungs time to clear the oropharyngeal contaminants. Sometimes, however, such a delay is not practical. Although some contaminants from the previous wash may persist in the sample, if the TW/BAL is repeated immediately, the amount of oropharyngeal contamination should be minimal, and this may be preferable to waiting 48 hours.

CELL COUNTS

Cell counts are difficult to perform on TW/BAL fluids because of the mucous content, and the dilution factor may be variable.[35] The method of obtaining cell counts is also varied in many studies of TW/BAL in dogs and cats, so values may not be directly comparable, and diagnostic significance is often difficult to determine.[36] One study of cases of idiopathic pulmonary fibrosis found increased total cell counts in diseased individuals compared with controls, although differential cell counts were generally not altered.[37] Some authors recommend cell counts to determine whether an adequate sample has been obtained and to assess whether resampling is necessary. However, this may not be easily applicable in the practice setting. Qualitative estimates (normal or increased) of cellularity may be done on stained sediment smears and may be useful.

CYTOLOGICAL EVALUATION

Mucus

A small amount of mucus may be present in TW/BAL specimens from clinically normal dogs and cats. Mucus appears as amorphous sheets ranging from blue to pink or as homogeneous strands that are frequently twisted or whorled (Fig. 16.4; see also Figs, 16.7, 16.12, 16.13, 16.17, and 16.18, later in the chapter).[4,27] A granular appearance of the mucus is frequently associated with increased cellularity.[4] Inflammation, irritation, or upper airway damage, which may be a result of chronic airway disease, may result in increased numbers of goblet cells, and an increased amount of mucus is generally present, possibly with altered mucus properties.[4,32,38] In inflammatory conditions, mucus usually stains eosinophilic because of the incorporation of inflammatory proteins and material from lysed cells.[4]

Curschmann spirals (see Fig. 16.4) are mucous casts of small bronchioles that appear as spiral, twisted masses of mucus that may have perpendicular radiations, giving them a test tube–brush-like appearance.[39] They may be seen in TW/BAL specimens from patients with any disorder that results in chronic, excessive production of mucus and are an indication of bronchiolar obstruction.

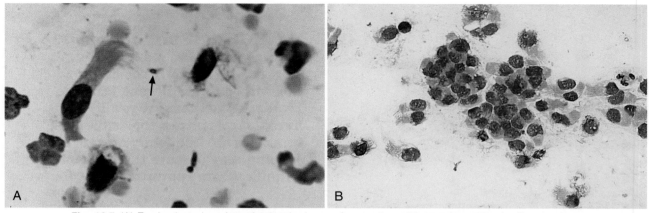

Fig. 16.5 (A) Tracheal wash or bronchoalveolar lavage from a dog with toxoplasmosis. A ciliated columnar cell, red blood cells, scattered neutrophils, and an extracellular *Toxoplasma gondii* organism *(arrow)* are shown (Wright stain, original magnification 250×). (B) Ciliated columnar cells are present both individually and in a cluster. The morphology of the cells in the cluster cannot be discerned. Cilia are evident on the cells that are well spread out. Many of the cells are traumatized as evidenced by their irregular nuclear outlines (Wright stain, original magnification 160×).

Cell Types

Many different types of cells (e.g., ciliated and nonciliated columnar cells, ciliated and nonciliated cuboidal cells, alveolar macrophages, neutrophils, eosinophils, lymphocytes, mast cells, erythrocytes, and dysplastic and neoplastic cells) may be seen in TW/BAL specimens (see Tables 16.1 and 16.2). Ciliated and nonciliated columnar and cuboidal cells and alveolar macrophages are the cell types seen in washings from normal dogs and cats. They are also seen in many disease states unless the washed area is filled with exudative secretions or the disease process has obliterated normal lung parenchyma. In one study in cats, storage of the BAL specimen for 24 hours or longer has been shown to result in decreased neutrophil percentages and increased eosinophil percentages. In a few individual cases, this change was sufficient to alter the cytological interpretation.[40] One study in dogs reported that neutrophil and eosinophil percentages were both decreased on the smears prepared at 24 hours after sampling compared with those prepared 3 hours after sampling.[41] Cytocentrifugation has been reported to affect the cell populations, particularly reducing the number of small lymphocytes present.[42] However, in one canine study, neutrophils were found to be more represented on cytospin preparations compared with direct smears of pelleted cells.[43] One canine study suggested that age may influence differential cell counts, but the group size was small and the findings were at variance with a previous study, suggesting that further work may be needed to determine whether age should be considered when assessing BAL cytology.[44,45] When determining differential cell counts, it is difficult to be consistent when assessing the epithelial population, and many do not consider this essential to assess the sample. When assessing macrophages, neutrophils, and eosinophils, counting 200 cells from a cytospin preparation, if available, has been shown to provide repeatable results.[46]

Columnar and Cuboidal Cells

Ciliated columnar cells (Figs. 16.5 and 16.6) have an elongated or cone shape, with cilia on their flattened apical ends. The nucleus, which is generally round to oval with a finely granular chromatin pattern, is present in the basal end of the cells, which often terminate in a thin tail.[39] The ciliated cuboidal cells look similar to the ciliated columnar cells except that the cuboidal cells are as wide as they are tall. Nonciliated columnar and cuboidal cells look identical to their ciliated counterparts except for the absence of cilia.

These cell types are normal findings in TW/BAL. If these cell types are predominant in a sample, the washing procedure probably sampled mainly bronchi and bronchioles (as opposed to alveolar spaces).

Cuboidal and columnar epithelial cells may be present individually or in clusters (see Fig. 16.5, B). Depending on the orientation of the cell on the slide (especially with cells in clusters), the cuboidal or columnar nature of the cells and cilia may be difficult to visualize. This is of little clinical significance, but these cells must not be interpreted as abnormal cell types.[39] Also, the majority of the columnar cells may be poorly preserved in many washes (see Fig. 16.5, B) as a result of the low protein fluid in which they are collected. Cells traumatized during slide preparation may show irregular nuclear outlines or be overtly ruptured (e.g., smudge cells).

Goblet Cells

Goblet cells (see Fig. 16.6) are mucus-producing bronchial cells that are generally elongated (i.e., columnar) with a basally placed nucleus and round granules of mucin, which frequently distend the cytoplasm.[39] Occasionally, the cytoplasm is so distended that the cell appears round. The granules stain from red to blue to clear with Romanowsky (e.g., Giemsa-Wright) stains. Free granules from ruptured goblet cells may be seen in the smear (see Fig. 16.6, B). The shape of the cells and the large size of the granules are helpful in differentiating these cells from mast cells (see Fig. 16.6, C). Goblet cells are not frequently seen; however, any chronic pulmonary irritant may result in increased numbers of goblet cells.

Macrophages

Alveolar macrophages (Fig. 16.7) (see also Figs. 16.9, 16.13, and 16.18) are readily found and are often the predominant cell type in TW/BAL samples from clinically normal animals. They are present in samples that have adequately washed the alveolar spaces and therefore are a useful indicator of sample adequacy. The nucleus is round to bean shaped and eccentrically positioned. A binucleate alveolar macrophage is rarely seen in clinically normal animals. Alveolar macrophages have abundant blue-gray granular cytoplasm. When they become activated, their cytoplasm becomes more abundant and vacuolated (i.e., foamy) and may contain phagocytized material (see Fig. 16.7, B).[31]

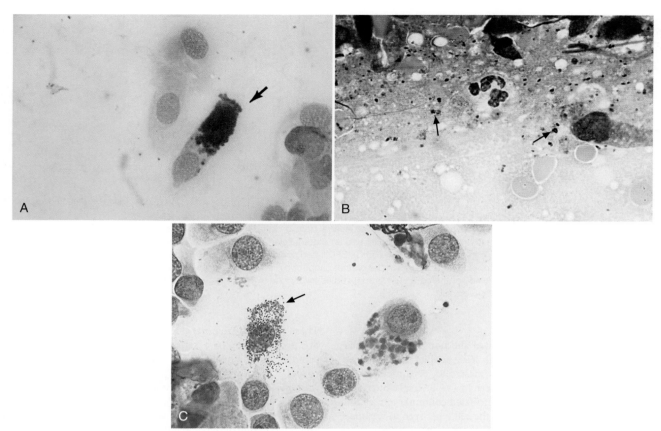

Fig. 16.6 (A) Tracheal wash or bronchoalveolar lavage from a dog. A goblet cell *(arrow)* and several ciliated columnar cells are present (Wright stain, original magnification 250×). (B) Granules from ruptured goblet cells are shown extracellularly (arrows) and must not be confused with bacterial cocci (Wright stain, original magnification 330×). (C) Goblet cells can be differentiated from mast cells *(arrow)*, which have smaller granules.

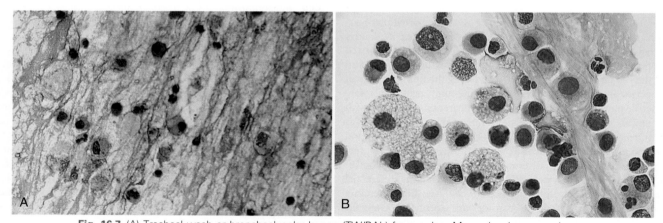

Fig. 16.7 (A) Tracheal wash or bronchoalveolar lavage (TW/BAL) from a dog. Many alveolar macrophages and some neutrophils are present in an eosinophilic mucous background (Wright stain, original magnification 132×). (B) TW/BAL from a dog. Numerous stimulated and unstimulated alveolar macrophages and scattered granulocytes and lymphocytes are present in strands of mucus (Wright stain, original magnification 250×).

Eosinophils

Eosinophils (Figs. 16.8 to 16.10) are polymorphonuclear granulocytes that contain intracytoplasmic granules, many of which have an affinity for the acid dye, eosin (i.e., eosinophilic), which stains them red with Romanowsky stains.[47] Increased numbers of eosinophils indicate a hypersensitivity reaction that is either allergic or parasitical[4]; see the discussion on hypersensitivity later in this chapter.

Careful examination is required to distinguish eosinophils from neutrophils in some wash specimens. In thick areas where the cells are not well spread out, individual granules may be hard to see. If normal neutrophils are present, the contrast in cytoplasmic color is usually evident; however, caution must be exercised because the cytoplasm of neutrophils, especially in exudative samples, sometimes stains a diffuse, uneven, eosinophilic color. When differentiating between these two cells, it is best to search for well-spread-out cells with definitive cytoplasmic granules instead of diffuse eosinophilic coloration. Individual granules are most readily observed in partially ruptured cells that are spreading out and are also free in the background of the smear (see Fig. 16.9, B). In cats, eosinophils may be difficult to recognize because they tend to be tightly packed with slender, rod-shaped granules that are not as pronounced in color as those in dogs (see Fig. 16.9, A). Eosinophils tend to be slightly larger than neutrophils, and their nuclei are less segmented (often bilobed or trilobed), which may aid in their identification (see Figs. 16.9, A, and 16.10, B).

Neutrophils

In TW/BAL samples, neutrophils look like peripheral blood neutrophils (Figs. 16.11 and 16.12), although degenerative changes may be present. Increased numbers of neutrophils indicate inflammation; see the discussion on inflammation later in this chapter.

Globule Leukocytes

Another distinct population of cells containing eosinophilic cytoplasmic granules, but with round to oval, eccentric nuclei, have been seen in bronchial wash specimens (see Fig. 16.10, B).[31] Although in one study, these cells have been identified as atypical-appearing eosinophils because of identification of specific microgranules, they may also represent the rare globule leukocyte.[48] Globule leukocytes are cells whose origin remains uncertain but have been reported in the respiratory tract of dogs and cats.[49]

Lymphocytes or Plasma Cells

Lymphocytes (Fig. 16.13) may represent a small percentage of the cells in TW/BAL samples from normal dogs and cats. Increased numbers of lymphocytes generally denote nonspecific inflammation and are of limited diagnostic value. Lymphocytes may, on occasion, appear reactive with more abundant cytoplasm staining a deeper basophilic color. Plasmacytoid differentiation, where a perinuclear clearing may develop, or mature plasma cells may also be rarely seen. Mildly increased numbers of lymphocytes reportedly occur with airway hyperreactivity, viral diseases of the tracheobronchial tree, and chronic infections.[4,50] Marked increases in lymphocyte numbers, especially lymphoblasts, may suggest pulmonary lymphoma.

Mast Cells

Mast cells (see Fig. 16.6, C), which are occasionally observed in TW/ BAL samples from dogs and cats with many different inflammatory lung disorders, are usually present in low numbers and are of little diagnostic significance. They are readily identified by their small red-purple, intracytoplasmic granules, which are frequently present in high numbers and may obscure the nucleus. Free, scattered granules from ruptured mast cells may be present on the slide and must not be confused with bacteria. A mild increase in mast cell numbers has been reported to occur with airway hyperreactivity.[50]

Superficial Squamous Cells

Superficial squamous cells are large epithelial cells with abundant, angular cytoplasm and small, round nuclei. Their presence in a TW/ BAL sample indicates oropharyngeal contamination (see Fig. 16.11), either from endotracheal sampling, or accidental catheter misdirection

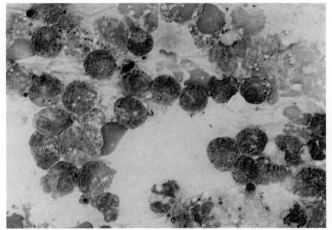

Fig. 16.8 Tracheal wash or bronchoalveolar lavage from a dog. Mucus, scattered neutrophils, and a large number of eosinophils are shown. Some extracellular bacterial rods, probably from oropharyngeal contamination, are also present (Wright stain, original magnification 330×).

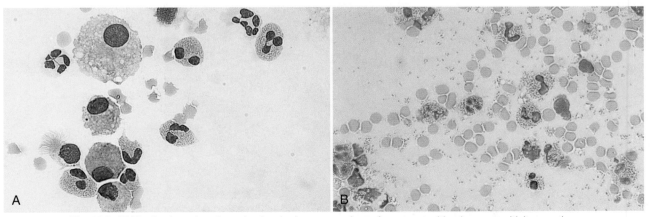

Fig. 16.9 (A) Tracheal wash or bronchoalveolar lavage specimen from a cat with a hypersensitivity reaction. Several eosinophils with bilobed and trilobed nuclei, scattered alveolar macrophages, two neutrophils with multilobulated nuclei, and a ciliated columnar epithelial cell are shown. The granules of the eosinophils are tightly packed, slender rods that may be easily overlooked. Note that the eosinophils are somewhat larger than the neutrophils and have less segmented nuclei (Wright stain, original magnification 250×). (B) Feline eosinophils. Granules are seen more easily in cells that are well spread out or partially ruptured. Many free eosinophil granules are seen in the background (Wright stain, original magnification 250×).

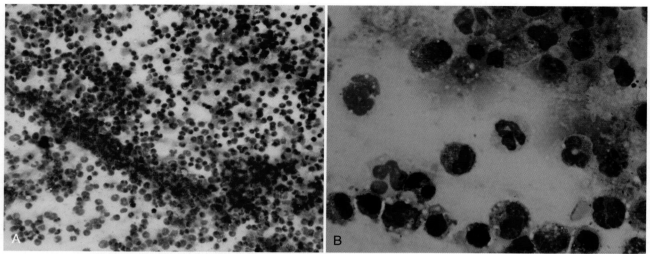

Fig. 16.10 Bronchoalveolar lavage from a dog with a hypersensitivity reaction. (A) Note the abundant brightly staining eosinophils, in conjunction with less prominently staining cells (Wright stain, original magnification 200×). (B) Higher magnification of slide shown in image A. Note the central neutrophil with pale eosinophilic staining cytoplasm and multilobulated nucleus. The eosinophils possess brightly staining eosinophilic granules, to the left an unlobulated nucleus, presumptive globule leukocyte, and to the right a trilobed nucleus, typical of eosinophils (Wright stain, original magnification, 1000×).

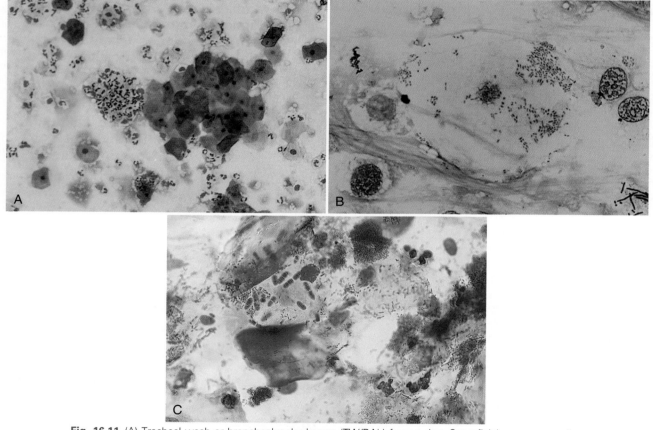

Fig. 16.11 (A) Tracheal wash or bronchoalveolar lavage (TW/BAL) from a dog. Superficial squamous cells, which denote oropharyngeal contamination, and neutrophils are shown (Wright stain, original magnification 50×). (B) Oropharyngeal contamination in a TW/BAL from a dog. Mucus, alveolar macrophages, and a large superficial squamous cell (with bacteria adhering to its surface) are present. Bacteria are also scattered throughout the slide (Wright stain, original magnification 250×) (C) TW/BAL from a cat. High numbers of bacteria, including some *Simonsiella* spp. organisms, are adhering to the surface of the squamous epithelial cells. *Simonsiella* spp. organisms are normal inhabitants of the oropharynx and indicate that the wash from this area is contaminated (Wright stain, original magnification 250×).

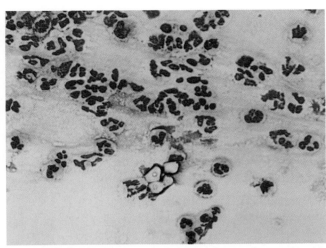

Fig. 16.12 Tracheal wash or bronchoalveolar lavage from a dog. High numbers of neutrophils, an alveolar macrophage, and a cluster of four granules of cornstarch (glove powder) are present in an eosinophilic mucous background (Wright stain, original magnification 165×).

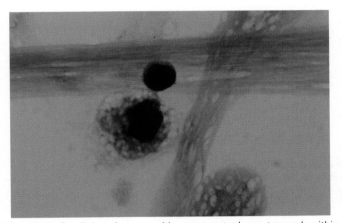

Fig. 16.13 Small lymphocyte with scant cytoplasm trapped within mucin, and macrophage with vacuolated cytoplasm noted below (Wright stain, original magnification, 1000×).

in transtracheal wash sampling. A rare differential for their presence may be a bronchoesophageal fistula, congenital or acquired.[51] See the discussion on oropharyngeal contamination later in this chapter.

Erythrocytes

Erythrocytes may be present within macrophages or free on the slide. Erythrophagocytosis (see Fig. 16.19, later in the chapter) indicates intrapulmonary hemorrhage or diapedesis. See the discussion on hemorrhage later in this chapter.

Atypical Cell Types

Atypical cells may be seen with pulmonary metaplasia, dysplasia, or neoplasia (primary or metastatic). Mild dysplasia of the respiratory epithelium may be seen whenever inflammation is present. Anticancer therapy (i.e., irradiation and chemotherapy) may result in such severe atypia of the cells of the tracheobronchial epithelium, the terminal bronchial epithelium, and the alveolar epithelium that differentiation from neoplasia is not reliable.[39] When atypical cells are observed cytologically, they should be evaluated for malignant criteria (see Chapter 2). TW/BAL samples collected after cancer therapy should be interpreted with caution.

Metaplasia

Metaplasia is an adaptive response of epithelial cells to chronic irritation.[39] Replacement of normal pulmonary epithelial cells of the trachea, bronchi, and bronchioles with stratified squamous epithelium (i.e., squamous metaplasia) is an example of pulmonary metaplasia.[39] These metaplastic cells mimic maturing squamous epithelium and must not be confused with neoplasia.

Dysplasia

Dysplasia is, by definition, a nonneoplastic change; however, severely dysplastic changes are sometimes referred to as *carcinoma in situ*. Dysplastic changes include variation in cell size and shape, darker-staining cells, and increased nucleus-to-cytoplasm (N:C) ratio and numbers of immature cells. These changes can be difficult to differentiate from neoplasia and may progress to neoplasia.[52]

Neoplastic Cells

Neoplastic cells are not often seen on cytological evaluation of TW/BAL samples. Unless the neoplasm has invaded the tracheobronchial tree and the invaded bronchiole is not blocked by a mucous plug, they are not accessible for collection by TW/BAL. Neoplastic cells, when observed, are generally from lymphoma or a carcinoma. High numbers of lymphoblasts may be seen in animals with lymphoma involving the respiratory system (see Fig. 16.31, later in the chapter). Carcinoma cells are large epithelial cells that may be present in clusters or as single cells (see Fig. 16.30, later in the chapter). Their cytoplasm is generally basophilic and vacuolated, and they show marked variation in cellular and nuclear size, often with grossly enlarged nuclei. They have a high N:C ratio, coarse nuclear chromatin, and prominent nucleoli that are frequently large and angular. Care must be taken not to confuse inflammation-induced cell dysplasia with neoplasia.

Miscellaneous Findings
Corn Starch

Corn starch (glove powder) is occasionally seen cytologically on slides from TW/BAL. It is typically a large, round to hexagonal structure that stains clear or blue and has a central fissure (see Fig. 16.12). Corn starch is an incidental finding and should not be confused with an organism or cell.

Plant Pollen

Plant pollen or plant cells may occasionally be present in TW/BAL samples and should not be confused with infectious organisms or cells.

Barium Sulfate

Aspirated barium sulfate has been reported to occur as greenish granular refractile material, most commonly noted in macrophages.[53]

CYTOLOGICAL INTERPRETATION

Fig. 16.14 presents an algorithm to aid in the evaluation of TW/BAL samples. Integrating historical, physical, and radiographic findings with the results of other diagnostic tests may allow for further diagnostic refinement. TW/BAL specimens are interpreted according to the type, quantity, and proportion of cells recovered. Cell proportions often differ between transtracheal aspirates and BAL samples.

Cellular patterns can generally be categorized as follows:
- *Insufficient sample*—no cells or an inadequate number of cells for evaluation
- *Oropharyngeal contamination*—superficial squamous cells, *Simonsiella* spp. of bacteria, or both (see the discussion on oropharyngeal contamination later in this chapter)

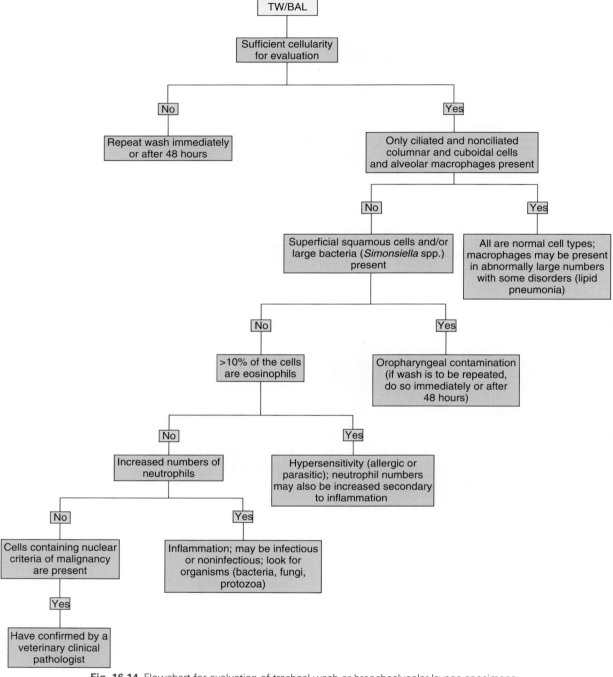

Fig. 16.14 Flowchart for evaluation of tracheal wash or bronchoalveolar lavage specimens.

- *Eosinophilic infiltrate*—increased numbers of eosinophils (see the discussion on hypersensitivity later in this chapter)
- *Neutrophilic infiltrate*—increased numbers of neutrophils (see the discussion on inflammation later in this chapter)
- *Macrophage (histiocytic or granulomatous) infiltrate*—very cellular sample of primarily macrophages (see the discussion on inflammation later in this chapter)
- *Presence of atypical cells*—evaluation for criteria of malignancy (see the discussion on neoplasia later in this chapter)

These categories, aside from insufficient samples, are not mutually exclusive. Classification of TW/BAL samples into one or more of these categories may allow the process or processes to be identified.

Insufficient Sample

The absence of cells on a smear or concentrated preparation may indicate that this sample is not truly representative of the cytology of the respiratory tract. Additionally, when assessing a BAL sample in which only columnar respiratory epithelial cells are noted, the absence of macrophages would indicate that only the airways and not the alveolar space had effectively been sampled.

Oropharyngeal Contamination

Oropharyngeal contamination is much more likely to occur when a TW/BAL sample is collected by passing a catheter through an endotracheal tube than when a transtracheal sample is taken and the oropharyngeal area is bypassed. Regardless of the procedure used, careful attention must be paid to technique to avoid oropharyngeal contamination.

Superficial squamous cells and certain large bacteria (e.g., *Simonsiella* spp.) are the hallmark of oropharyngeal contamination (see Fig. 16.11).[54] Superficial squamous cells are large epithelial cells with abundant, angular cytoplasm and small, round nuclei. Many bacteria may adhere to the surface of squamous epithelial cells (see Fig. 16.11, B and C). *Simonsiella* spp. organisms (see Fig. 16.11, C) are bacteria that divide lengthwise, thus lining up in parallel rows that give the impression of a single large bacterium. These are nonpathogenic organisms that may adhere to superficial squamous cell surfaces or be free in smears. When superficial squamous cells or *Simonsiella* spp. organisms are present, indicating oropharyngeal contamination, whatever cellular constituents and bacterial organisms were present in the oropharyngeal area may also be present in the contaminated wash. Therefore a variety of bacterial rods and cocci may be present in a contaminated wash (see Fig. 16.11, B). Bacteria are generally present without neutrophils when the wash primarily consists of oropharyngeal contaminants. Neutrophils may occur in a TW/BAL sample secondary to oropharyngeal contamination if the animal has a purulent or ulcerative oropharyngeal lesion. Therefore oropharyngeal contamination may significantly alter the cytological evaluation and culture results.

Hypersensitivity

Increased numbers of eosinophils in a TW/BAL specimen indicate a hypersensitivity response. Normal animals of most species, including dogs, generally have very low numbers of eosinophils (<5%) in bronchial wash specimens, but clinically normal cats may have significantly higher numbers of eosinophils compared with other species.[23,55,56] In some studies, eosinophils comprised an average 20% to 25% of the cells present in bronchial wash specimens from asymptomatic cats with no evidence of pulmonary disease or parasitism. In a few of these animals, eosinophils were the predominant cell type present. Whether these findings are truly normal or merely represent a subclinical hypersensitivity response is not known, but these animals were asymptomatic throughout the observation periods; thus, the clinical significance of a cytological diagnosis of hypersensitivity reaction, when based on relatively low numbers of eosinophils (10%–25% of cells present), may depend on the clinical and radiographic findings of the case.

Clinically normal dogs typically have wash specimens of less than 5% eosinophils.[31,45,57] Many of the studies describing normal BAL cytology were done on dogs reared in closed environments. One study showed that random source dogs had significantly higher percentages of eosinophils (24%) compared with dogs reared in an isolated environment with routine prophylactic anthelmintic treatment (<5%).[58] It was suggested that previously heavy parasitical burdens may have been responsible for the high numbers of eosinophils in these animals; however, other studies have also found increased eosinophil percentages in apparently healthy dogs.[59,60] These authors' experience suggests that such a significant percentage of eosinophils is unusual in most clinically normal dogs. Specimens composed of greater than 10% eosinophils are indicative of a significant hypersensitivity component of the disease process.

Increased numbers of neutrophils, macrophages, or both may be seen along with increased numbers of eosinophils if tissue irritation is sufficient to induce an inflammatory response. Cells are not always evenly distributed throughout wash specimens, especially if thick mucus strands are present. Eosinophils, trapped in strands of mucus, often predominate in certain areas of the slides, whereas other areas may be predominantly neutrophilic. A careful examination of the entire slide is necessary for an accurate evaluation.

Allergic bronchitis or pneumonitis, feline asthma, lungworm and heartworm infestations, and eosinophilic bronchopneumopathy (previously pulmonary infiltrates with eosinophils [PIEs]) are some of the disorders that frequently cause the hypersensitivity responses seen in TW/BAL specimens.[61,62] Specimens should be scanned on low power (10× objective) for parasitical larvae or ova (Fig. 16.15). If present, parasitical larvae (e.g., *Filaroides* spp., *Aelurostrongylus abstrusus*, *Angiostrongylus vasorum*, and *Crenosoma vulpis*) and ova (e.g., *Eucoleus aerophilus* and *Paragonimus* spp.) are large and readily identified, but sometimes only an eosinophilic exudate is present. Multiple fecal examinations (including Baermann and zinc sulfate flotation techniques) may be helpful in identifying infestations. Even when not found in wash specimens, larvae may sometimes be identified in brushings or biopsies of parasitical nodules visible in the bronchi of affected animals.

Free eosinophil granules, which stain eosinophilic and should not be confused with bacteria, may be seen secondary to cell rupture in the smear. These granules may coalesce into a large crystal known as a Charcot-Leyden crystal (Fig. 16.16), which may occur in any condition that causes large numbers of eosinophils to accumulate.

Inflammation

Neutrophils are present only in very low numbers (generally <5%) in TW/BAL specimens from normal dogs and cats.[4,31] Cytologically, neutrophils in bronchial mucus look like peripheral blood neutrophils, but they may show degenerative changes because of bacterial toxins or be smudged (ruptured) secondary to trauma from collection and preparation. An influx of neutrophils occurs early in an inflammatory response, making neutrophils from TW/BAL a sensitive indicator of inflammation.[32] Even very mild insults, such as sterile saline TW/BAL, result in marked influxes of neutrophils. As a result, neutrophil numbers are increased in nearly all conditions (infectious and noninfectious) that cause inflammation. Infectious disorders include bacterial (Fig. 16.17), mycotic (see Fig. 16.25, later in the chapter), viral, or protozoal (see Fig. 16.28 and discussion later in the chapter) diseases. Noninfectious disorders include tissue irritation or necrosis secondary to inhalation of a toxic substance (e.g., smoke), as well as neoplasia that has outgrown its blood supply and developed a necrotic center. Whenever neutrophil numbers are increased, one should look closely (and, especially, intracellularly) for bacteria and other microorganisms (see Fig. 16.17). Organisms may be found cytologically in most bacterial infections, but noninfectious inflammation is typified by the absence of microorganisms. Increased neutrophils on BAL are one of the criteria for the diagnosis of acute respiratory distress syndrome (ARDS), although it is often not practical to obtain this type of sample from presenting patients.[63]

Increased numbers of macrophages are seen with many subacute and chronic lung disorders (e.g., congestive heart failure, granulomatous and lipid pneumonia). Alveolar macrophage numbers frequently increase with chronic persistent inflammation.[32] Binucleate and multinucleate giant cell macrophages (Fig. 16.18) may be seen in conditions that produce chronic lung disease.[39] Large, lipid-containing vacuoles may be present within macrophages in lipid pneumonia.[39] Dark or black granules (anthracotic pigment) may be present within macrophages in clinically normal animals living in large cities or other areas with polluted air. Phagocytized erythrocytes (i.e., erythrophagia) and erythrocyte-breakdown products (e.g., hematoidin or hemosiderin) may be seen within macrophage cytoplasm in conditions that cause pulmonary hemorrhage or red cell diapedesis (Fig. 16.19). Macrophages are also important to defend against microorganisms, and phagocytized microorganisms (e.g., mycotic, protozoal, or bacterial) may be seen.

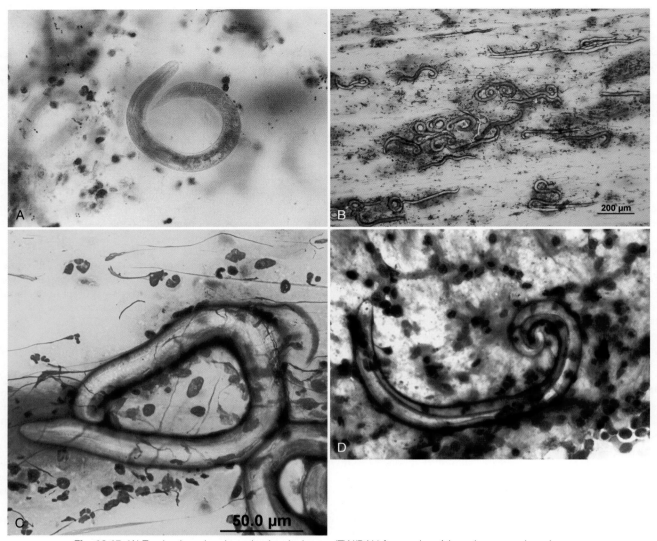

Fig. 16.15 (A) Tracheal wash or bronchoalveolar lavage (TW/BAL) from a dog. A large lungworm larva is present (Wright stain, original magnification, 100×). (B) TW/BAL from a cat. Low-power magnification showing large numbers of lungworm larvae (*Aelurostrongylus* spp.) (Wright stain). (C) Higher magnification from the same case shown in image B. Lungworm larvae (*Aelurostrongylus* spp.) and scattered inflammatory cells are shown (Wright stain). (D) TW/BAL from a dog. Although the tail of the lungworm larva (*Angiostrongylus vasorum*) may be observed on BAL cytology, it is not always possible to see enough detail to speciate. Wet preparations are preferred for identification (Wright-Giemsa stain, original magnification 400×). (B and C, Courtesy Dr. T. Rizzi. D, Slide courtesy A. Leuschner, TDDS, UK.)

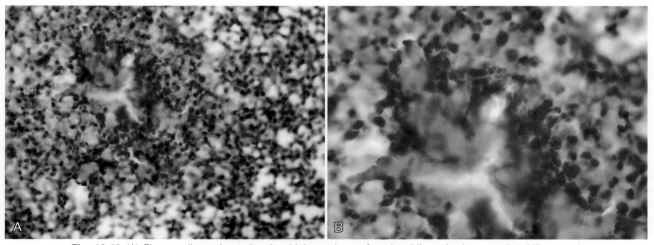

Fig. 16.16 (A) Fine-needle aspirate showing high numbers of eosinophils and a large eosinophilic crystal thought to be a Charcot-Leyden crystal. (B) Higher magnification of same slide (Wright stain). (Courtesy Dr. Peter Fernandes.)

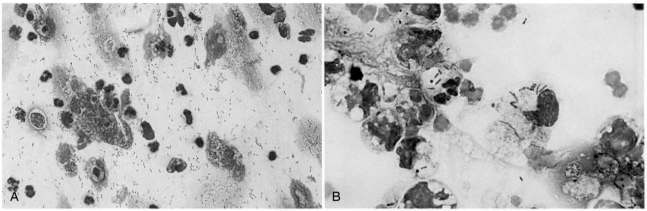

Fig. 16.17 (A) Tracheal wash or bronchoalveolar lavage (TW/BAL) from a dog with bacterial tracheobronchitis. Many neutrophils and some mucus strands are shown. High numbers of bacterial rods are present, mostly extracellularly (Wright stain, original magnification 250×). (B) TW/BAL from a dog with bacterial pneumonia. A mixed population of bacteria is present; some bacteria are phagocytized within neutrophils (Wright stain, original magnification 400×).

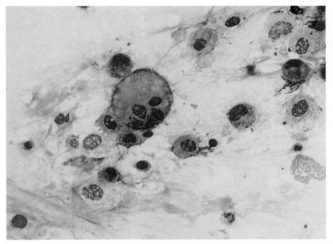

Fig. 16.18 Tracheal wash or bronchoalveolar lavage from a dog with chronic lung disease. Many alveolar macrophages, two neutrophils, and one multinucleate giant cell macrophage are present in an eosinophilic mucous background (Wright stain, original magnification 132×).

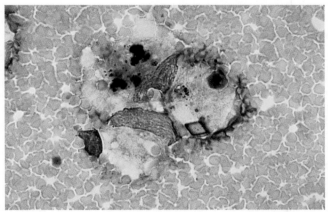

Fig. 16.19 Tracheal wash or bronchoalveolar lavage from a dog. Many red blood cells (RBCs) and three macrophages that contain phagocytized RBCs and RBC breakdown products (dark-staining hemosiderin and golden hematoidin crystals) are present. This finding indicates intrapulmonary hemorrhage or diapedesis of erythrocytes (Wright stain, original magnification 330×).

Hemorrhage

Erythrocytes may be seen in TW/BAL washes from dogs and cats with disorders that cause vascular damage or erythrocyte diapedesis in the lung (see Fig. 16.19). Iatrogenic hemorrhage (i.e., hemorrhage caused by the sampling procedure) may also result in erythrocytes noted on the smear. To demonstrate that the hemorrhage is a result of pulmonary pathology (intrapulmonary hemorrhage), erythrophagocytosis, hemosiderophages, or heme-pigment should be identified on the smears. Hemosiderophages have been referred to as "heart failure cells"; however, in one recent study in cats, in which the presence of hemosiderophages was specifically assessed with Prussian blue staining to identify the presence of iron, hemosiderosis was not a consistent feature in the tracheal wash specimens from cats with cardiac disease. Hemosiderosis was noted in cats with feline asthma, neoplasia (primary and metastatic), pneumonia (bacterial, parasites) secondary to inhaled irritants, bleeding diathesis, trauma, spontaneous pneumothorax, collapsed trachea, neurological disease, and uncomplicated rhinitis.[64] Other causes of intrapulmonary hemorrhage that may be considered include other infectious agents (e.g., fungi), pulmonary embolism, and lung lobe torsion.

INFECTIOUS AGENTS

Bacteria

The culture of bacteria from a lower respiratory tract specimen should be assessed in conjunction with the clinical presentation because the tracheobronchial tree may not be regarded as sterile even in healthy individuals.[65] A number of studies have reported gram-negative rods as the most common type of bacterial infectious agent.[66,67] Greater than 60% of dogs with lower respiratory tract disease are reported to have only a single agent isolated.[66] Quantitative assessment of culture results and the cytological examination of a BAL sample may provide increased diagnostic specificity.[66] A wide variety of bacteria have been reported as causative agents of bacterial (septic) pneumonia; these are too many to be covered adequately here; organisms discussed later are highlighted with regard to specific culture requirements or concerns over identification. See Chapter 3 for more illustrations of infectious agents.

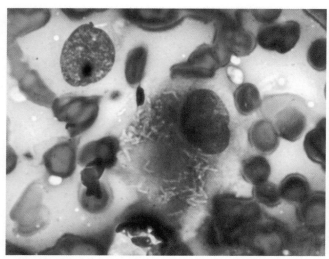

Fig. 16.20 Fine-needle aspirate showing many red blood cells and a large macrophage. The macrophage contains many small, nonstaining, bacterial rods indicative of *Mycobacterium* spp. (Wright stain). (Courtesy Dr. R. L. Cowell, IDEXX Laboratories.)

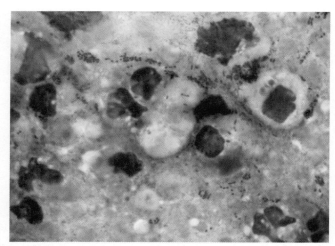

Fig. 16.21 Tracheal wash or bronchoalveolar lavage from a dog with *Mycoplasma* pneumonia. High numbers of the small coccobacilli are noted extracellularly, with degenerate neutrophils and other poorly preserved cells also present (Wright-Giemsa stain, original magnification 1000×).

Mycobacteria

Mycobacteria do not readily take up Romanowsky stains, and on the majority of preparations they appear as negative-staining rods generally located within macrophages but sometimes noted in neutrophils (Fig. 16.20). These bacteria may be particularly hard to identify on flush or wash samples, and staining with a specific stain (e.g., Ziehl-Neelsen [acid-fast stain]) is recommended to assess for these bacteria. The bacteria stain red with a beaded appearance with Ziehl-Neelsen stain. Calcospherite-like bodies, which are concentrically laminated crystalline structures, have been reported in a single case of canine tuberculosis.[68] Mycobacterial culture duration may be prolonged, generally for at least 3 weeks, particularly if phenotyping is attempted. If submitting unfixed material, it should be clearly labeled because the organism has zoonotic potential. It is necessary to specifically request culture for these bacteria on submission, and it is recommended that the laboratory be contacted before submission because not all laboratories have appropriate containment facilities to culture the organism.

Mycoplasma

Mycoplasma organisms are small bacteria that may have a variable appearance, as cocci or coccobacilli (Fig. 16.21).[69] These organisms have been associated with respiratory tract disease in both dogs and cats.[70-72] Specific conditions are required for culture of these organisms, and culture for these organisms should be requested by the submitting clinician if a clinical suspicion exists. Also, many laboratories supply culture medium for submission of specimens. The laboratory should be contacted before obtaining the sample for advice on submission and to allow time for media to be supplied, if appropriate.

Bordetella

Bordetella bronchiseptica (Fig. 16.22) is a cause of respiratory infections in a wide range of mammals. It is of interest as a common etiological agent in kennel cough syndrome in dogs and may also be a cause of respiratory disease in cats.[73,74] In young kittens, and rarely in older cats, it may cause a severe pneumonia, which may be fatal.[75] In community-acquired pneumonia in puppies, it may present as a more severe disease compared with other etiological agents.[76] Recent reports have suggested that this organism may be considered a zoonosis, even if it occurs rarely.[77]

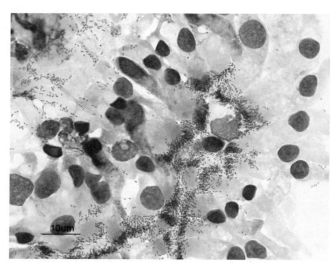

Fig. 16.22 Tracheal wash from a dog with *Bordetella*. High numbers of the rods, or coccobacilli are noted often associated with the cilia of the columnar respiratory epithelial cells (Wright stain). (Courtesy Dr. R. L. Cowell, IDEXX Laboratories.)

Fungi

TW/BAL sampling may provide definitive diagnoses of mycotic infections. The systemic mycotic infections blastomycosis, histoplasmosis, and coccidiomycosis frequently involve the lungs, and *Aspergillus* and *Cryptococcus* may also be observed. One study has suggested that lavage of multiple lung lobes is most likely to obtain a diagnosis of mycotic infection, and that BAL may be more sensitive than TW.[10]

Aspergillus

Aspergillus is uncommonly noted in the lung. It appears as branching septate hyphae. In other species, calcium oxalate crystals have also been noted in the BAL sample in *Aspergillus* infections.[78] This organism is a frequent environmental contaminant, and if cultured from a lower respiratory specimen, careful patient assessment is required to determine whether this is a likely etiological agent.

Blastomyces

Blastomyces is a fungal organism, which appears as blue, round, medium-sized (5–20 micrometers [μm] in diameter), thick-walled yeast. Occasional broad-based budding may be observed (Fig. 16.23). In one review of cases, 85% of the affected dogs had lung involvement.[79] Transtracheal aspiration allowed identification of organisms in patients with pulmonary involvement, and this resulted in diagnosis in more than 65% of cases sampled in two separate studies.[80,81] Although aspiration of other lesions may provide a diagnosis, BAL may also be helpful.[10]

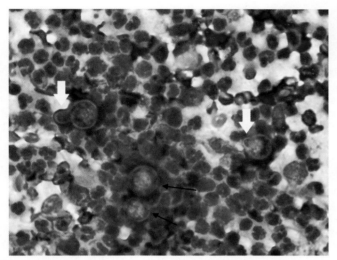

Fig. 16.23 Four *Blastomyces dermatitidis* organisms (*arrows*) surrounded by high numbers of neutrophils, scattered macrophages, and some red blood cells. *Blastomyces* organisms are spherical, thick-walled, yeast-like organisms that stain basophilic. The organisms are 5 to 20 micrometers in diameter and occasionally, a single, broad-based bud may be present *(broad arrows)* (Wright stain). (Courtesy Dr. R. L. Cowell, IDEXX Laboratories.)

Coccidioides

Coccidioides immitis and *Coccidioides posadasii* may infect dogs and cats residing in, or with a history of visiting, an endemic area in the past 3 years. In vivo, two morphological forms are noted: (1) the thick-walled, blue-staining, spherical sporangia, which are 10 to greater than 100 μm in diameter; and (2) the smaller endospores, which may be observed in some of the larger sporangia. The endospores are 2 to 5 μm in diameter and may also be noted individually, released from ruptured sporangia (Fig. 16.24). These highly infectious organisms may take 1 to 2 weeks to culture, and submission of the sample should be discussed with the laboratory because alternative diagnostic methods are always preferable for identifying this organism.[82]

Cryptococcus

Cryptococcus organisms are yeast organisms that are extremely variable in size but are generally 4 to 15 μm in diameter without their capsule and 8 to 40 μm with their capsule (smooth form of *Cryptococcus*). The yeast stains pink to blue-purple and may be slightly granular. The capsule is usually clear (nonstaining) and homogeneous (Fig. 16.25). Also, nonencapsulated forms of *Cryptococcus* may be observed (rough form of *Cryptococcus*). These appear similar but have a thin clear capsule. Occasional organisms showing narrow-based budding may be found. A case report in a cat demonstrated organisms 3 to 15 μm diameter, with a thick nonstaining wall in the BAL sample, although the organisms from the lymph node of the patient were reported as 8 to 12 μm in size with a 1- to 6-μm nonstaining capsule.[9] Pulmonary involvement is not the most frequent presentation of this disease.[83]

Histoplasma

Histoplasma organisms may be more likely to be noted in BAL samples in the acute presentation of the disease, compared with a more chronic presentation. These organisms are most commonly noted intracellularly, but extracellular organisms may be observed on smears because of cell rupturing.

Histoplasma organisms are small (approximately 2–4 μm diameter), with a thin, clear halo surrounding a darker staining, round-to-oval, yeast-like organism (Fig. 16.26).[84] Coughing may not be reported in many patients with pulmonary lesions of histoplasmosis.[85]

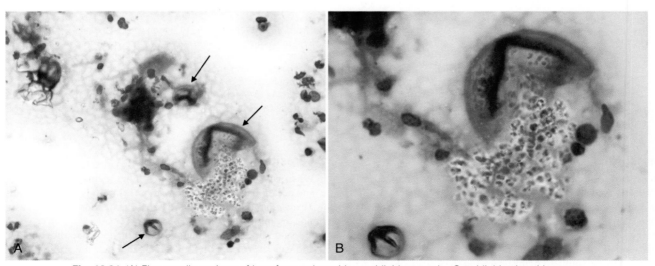

Fig. 16.24 (A) Fine-needle aspirate of lung from a dog with coccidioidomycosis. *Coccidioides immitis* organisms *(arrows)* are large, double-contoured, clear to blue-staining, spherical bodies that range in size from 10 micrometers (μm) to greater than 100 μm. Occasionally, endospores varying from 2 to 5 μm in diameter may be seen within some of the larger spherules. (B) Higher magnification of larger spherule containing endospores (Wright stain). (Courtesy Dr. R. L. Cowell, IDEXX Laboratories.)

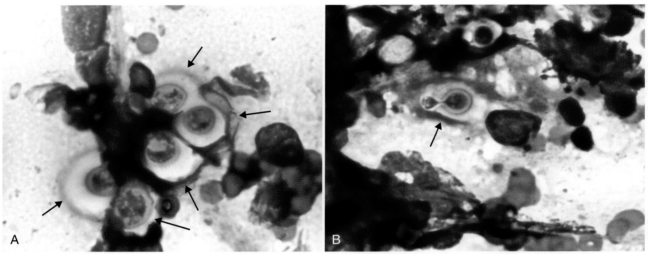

Fig. 16.25 (A) *Cryptococcus neoformans* is a spherical, yeast-like organism that frequently has a thick, clear-staining, mucoid capsule. Five *Cryptococcus* organisms *(arrows)* with nonstaining capsules are shown. (B) *Cryptococcus* organism with a single narrow-based bud *(arrow)*. (Wright stain). (Courtesy Dr. R. L. Cowell, IDEXX Laboratories.)

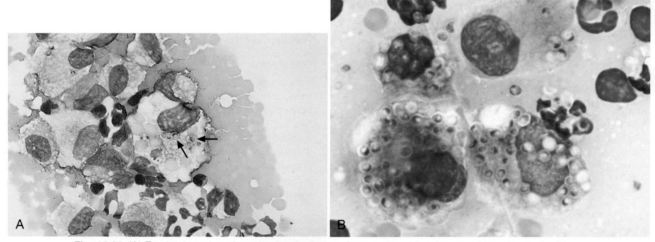

Fig. 16.26 (A) Tracheal wash or bronchoalveolar lavage from a cat with pulmonary histoplasmosis. Many macrophages, some of which show the yeast phase of *Histoplasma capsulatum (arrows)*; scattered neutrophils and lymphocytes; and red blood cells are seen. A macrophage also displays erythrophagocytosis (Wright stain, original magnification 250×). (B) Fine-needle aspirate of lung showing large macrophages containing numerous *H. capsulatum* organisms. *Histoplasma* organisms are small (1–4 micrometers [μm] in diameter), round to oval, yeast-like organisms that have a dark blue to purple staining nucleus. The organism is often surrounded by a thin, clear halo (Wright stain). (Courtesy Dr. R. L. Cowell, IDEXX Laboratories.)

Pneumocystis

Pneumocystis is an opportunistic fungal pulmonary pathogen, which may be observed in either cyst form (5–10 μm diameter with up to eight intracystic bodies) (Fig. 16.27) or troph form (1–2 μm).[86] Cytologically, it may appear morphologically similar to a protozoal organism, and this led to misclassification in the past. Particular breeds have been overrepresented in the literature—the Miniature Dachshund in the southern hemisphere and the Cavalier King Charles Spaniel in the northern hemisphere.[87,88] However, this is likely related to the underlying immunodeficiencies that are reported in these breeds because any breed may be affected by this organism. It is not possible to culture this organism on media.

Parasites

When considering parasites of the lungs, nematodes (see Fig. 16.15) and occasionally trematodes are most commonly considered, although *Toxoplasma* (Fig. 16.28), a protozoal agent, is also classified as a parasitic organism.

An outline of the nematode and trematode parasites noted in dogs and cats is provided in Table 16.3, although the sizing of the larvae differs among authors. If specific identification is required, it is recommended that expert opinion be sought.

Although eosinophilic inflammation may be expected with these organisms, many patients will present with only neutrophilic inflammation.[89,90]

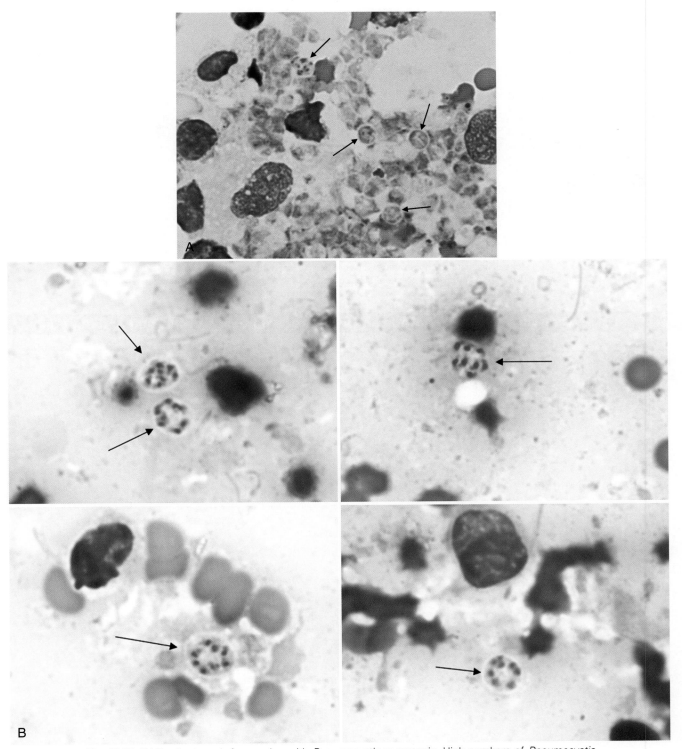

Fig. 16.27 (A) Tracheal wash from a dog with *Pneumocystis* pneumonia. High numbers of *Pneumocystis* cysts *(arrows)* are present. *Pneumocystis* cysts are 5 to 10 micrometers (μm) in diameter and usually contain four to eight intracystic bodies that are 1 to 2 μm in diameter. (B) Composite showing high-magnification pictures of *Pneumocystis* cysts (Wright stain). (Courtesy Dr. R. L. Cowell, IDEXX Laboratories.)

Oslerus osleri (*Filaroides osleri*) and *Filaroides hirthi* ova and larvae noted in respiratory washings are very similar in appearance (see Fig. 16.15). Differentiation may be undertaken by identification of nodules formed by *O. osleri*, particularly at or in the area surrounding the bifurcation of the trachea, whereas *F. hirthi* organisms are more likely to form subpleural nodules.[89,91] The airway nodules may be noted on bronchoscopy, and either may be noted on radiography. In some instances, the nodules may be difficult to distinguish radiographically from neoplastic foci. *Filaroides milksi* is almost identical to *F. hirthi*, and whether these are two separate species is still being debated.[92]

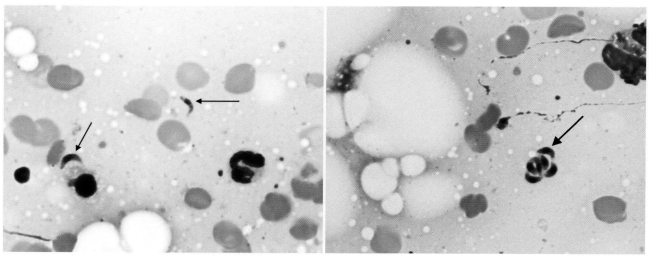

Fig. 16.28 Tracheal wash or bronchoalveolar lavage from a cat with toxoplasmosis. *Toxoplasma gondii* tachyzoites *(arrows)* appear as small crescent-shaped bodies with a light blue cytoplasm and a dark-staining pericentral nucleus. (Courtesy Dr. R. L. Cowell, IDEXX Laboratories.)

TABLE 16.3   Overview of the Nematode and Trematode Parasites of the Dog and Cat Lung

	Host	Location in Lung	Stage in Lung Commonly Observed by Flush or Wash Sample
Nematode Parasite			
Aelurostrongylus abstrusus	Cat	Terminal and respiratory bronchioles, alveolar ducts	Ova and larvae
			Ova 70–80 micrometers (μm) by 50–75 μm, with thin shell, embryonated
			L1, 360–400 μm, short thick larvae with sinus wave shaped kink and dorsal spine on tail, granular contents
			L3, 460–530 μm
Angiostrongylus vasorum	Dog	Pulmonary arteries, right heart	L1
			310–400 μm length, sharply pointed tail with distinct notch on dorsal surface "dorsal notch" cephalic button on anterior end; not regularly identified in more recent studies
Eucoleus aerophilus (*Capillaria aerophila*)	Dog and cat	Trachea, bronchi, bronchioles	Ova
			Bipolar thick-walled, pigmented golden brown
			58–79 μm length, 29–40 μm width
Crenosoma vulpis	Dog	Trachea, bronchi, and bronchioles	L1 243–281 μm length
			L3, 458–549 μm length
			Slightly curved tail, no kink
			Adult worms, observed grossly, stout, white, ≈0.5–1 cm length
Filaroides hirthi	Dog	bronchioles alveoli, lung parenchyma	Embryonated ova and larvae
			Larvae 240–290 μm length ≈10–14 μm width, slightly kinked tail
			Adults 2.3–13 mm length ≈30–100 μm width, both stages have prominent basophilic granules internally
Oslerus osleri	Dog	Trachea and bronchial nodules, particularly nodules at bifurcation of trachea	Ova and larvae practically identical to Filaroides hirthiL1 223–267 μm Adults 6.5–13.5 mm length
Trematode Parasite			
Paragonimus spp.	Dog and cat	Primarily right caudal lung lobe	Ova 75–118 μm length, 42–67 μm width
			Ovoid with single flattened operculum, golden brown

From Anderson RC, ed. *Nematode Parasites of Vertebrates: Their Development and Transmission.* 2nd ed. Wallingford, UK: CABI Publishing; 2000.

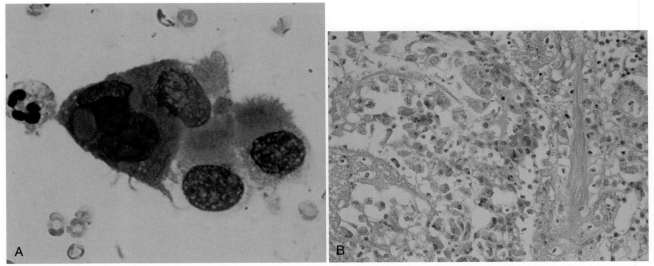

Fig. 16.29 (A) Fine-needle aspirate from the lung of a cat with cowpox viral pneumonia with presumptive viral intracytoplasmic type A inclusions (May Grunwald Giemsa stain, original magnification 1000×). (B) Histology section of the lung obtained post mortem from the same case showing high numbers of the cytoplasmic eosinophilic inclusions (hematoxylin and eosin [H&E] stain, original magnification 400×). (Courtesy Prof. E. Milne, Edinburgh, UK, ESVCP case 2010.)

Angiostrongylus vasorum is reported in many areas worldwide, including Europe, South America, North America (Newfoundland), and Africa, with the geographical range likely to continue to expand.[93] Associated clinical signs may include hypercalcemia and bleeding diatheses from prolongation of prothrombin time, activated partial thromboplastin time, or both, resolving on successful treatment of the worm burden.

Toxoplasma gondii infection in cats may frequently involve the lung. Identification of tachyzoites both extracellularly and within macrophages, which may be numerous, have been reported in the BAL samples of cats with both experimentally induced and spontaneous clinical disease.[94-96] *T. gondii* tachyzoites appear as small crescent-shaped bodies, with a light-blue cytoplasm and a dark-staining pericentral nucleus (see Fig. 16.28).

Viral Diseases

Many viral respiratory diseases may cause lung damage and allow for secondary bacterial infection. Cytologically, increased numbers of neutrophils indicate inflammation. Lymphocytes may be increased, but the numbers are often low and nonspecific. If a secondary bacterial infection has occurred, bacterial organisms may be seen intracellularly and extracellularly on the slides. Viral agents are not usually identified on cytological preparations of lavage fluids from the lungs of dogs and cats. Many papers describe immunohistochemical detection of various viral agents, but this is generally performed on postmortem lung samples. Viral pneumonia may be caused by viruses that are not commonly considered to affect the respiratory system[97] (Fig. 16.29).

Neoplasia

Neoplasia may exist as single, solitary nodules or a diffuse infiltration. Solitary lesions are rare in metastatic lung tumors but common in primary lung tumors. Most solid tissue pulmonary neoplasms (i.e., not lymphoid) are metastatic nodules from malignant tumors at sites other than the lungs. Because metastatic lung tumors are generally interstitial, neoplastic cells are not collected with TW/BAL unless the tumor has invaded the bronchial tree and the affected portion of the bronchial tree is not clogged by secretions or is so peripherally located that its cells cannot be collected with TW/BAL. Primary lung tumors that involve the bronchial tree are more likely to exfoliate cells that are collected by routine washings (Fig. 16.30).

Carcinomas comprise 80% or more of all primary lung tumors in dogs and cats.[98,99] Lung carcinomas tend to appear in the following three areas[99]:

- Hilus of the lungs
- Multifocal and often peripheral sites (most commonly)
- In an entire lobe or lobes

Carcinomas are epithelial cell tumors; when cytological evidence of acini formation or secretory product production is seen, they are classified as adenocarcinomas. Lymphoma is a common neoplasm in both dogs and cats. It is typically multicentric and may involve the pulmonary parenchyma in dogs. Large numbers of lymphoblasts may be diagnostic of lymphoma. Scattered large lymphoid cells, when they are part of a generalized inflammatory reaction, are not sufficient for a diagnosis. TW/BAL specimens may be useful in diagnosing pulmonary involvement of lymphoma (Fig. 16.31). In one study, 31 of 47 dogs with multicentric lymphoma (66%) had pulmonary involvement, as determined by examination of BAL fluid collected with a bronchoscope.[100] In the same group of dogs, examination of TW fluid (collected by passing a urinary catheter through a sterile endotracheal tube) was much less sensitive, documenting pulmonary involvement in only four of the 46 dogs tested.

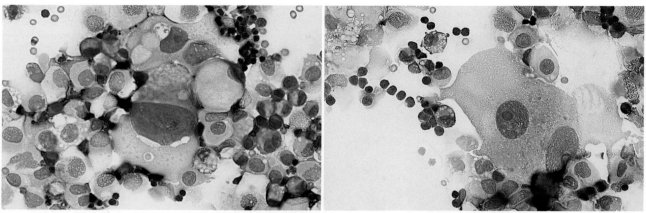

Fig. 16.30 Tracheal wash or bronchoalveolar lavage from a cat with a bronchoalveolar adenocarcinoma. A few large epithelial cells showing macronuclei and large prominent nucleoli are among the inflammatory cells (Wright stain, original magnification 160×).

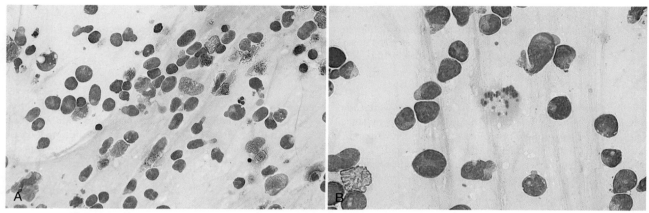

Fig. 16.31 Tracheal wash or bronchoalveolar lavage from a dog with multicentric lymphoma. (A) Highly cellular slide containing many lymphoid cells in strands of mucus (Wright stain, original magnification 160×). (B) Higher magnification of the slide in image A. The lymphoid cells are a population of pleomorphic lymphoblasts. A cluster of goblet cell granules is also present in the center of the field (Wright stain, original magnification 250×).

REFERENCES

1. Norris CR, Griffey SM, Samii VF, et al. Comparison of results of thoracic radiography, cytologic evaluation of bronchoalveolar lavage fluid, and histologic evaluation of lung specimens in dogs with respiratory tract disease: 16 cases (1996-2000). *J Am Vet Med Assoc.* 2001;218:1456–1461.
2. Norris CR, Griffey SM, Samii VF, et al. Thoracic radiography, bronchoalveolar lavage cytopathology, and pulmonary parenchymal histopathology: a comparison of diagnostic results in 11 cats. *J Am Anim Hosp Assoc.* 2002;38:337–345.
3. Cocayne CG, Reinero CR, DeClue AE. Subclinical airway inflammation despite high-dose oral corticosteroid therapy in cats with lower airway disease. *J Feline Med Surg.* 2011;13:558–563.
4. Creighton S, Wilkins R. Transtracheal aspiration biopsy: technique and cytologic evaluation. *J Am Anim Hosp Assoc.* 1974;10:219–226.
5. Turnwald GH. *Scientific Presentations of the 53rd Annual Meeting of the American Animal Hospital Association.* New Orleans, Louisiana; 1986:52–55.
6. Cooper ES, Schober KE, Drost WT. Severe bronchoconstriction after bronchoalveolar lavage in a dog with eosinophilic airway disease. *J Am Vet Med Assoc.* 2005;227:1257–1262.
7. Johnson LR, Drazenovich TL. Flexible bronchoscopy and bronchoalveolar lavage in 68 cats (2001-2006). *J Vet Intern Med.* 2007;21:219–225.
8. Saunders HM, Keith D. Thoracic imaging. In: King LG, ed. *Textbook of Respiratory Disease in Dogs and Cats.* St. Louis, MO: Elsevier; 2004.
9. Hamilton TA, Hawkins EC, DeNicola DB. Bronchoalveolar lavage and tracheal wash to determine lung involvement in a cat with cryptococcosis. *J Am Vet Med Assoc.* 1991;198:655–656.
10. Hawkins EC, DeNicola DB. Cytologic analysis of tracheal wash specimens and bronchoalveolar lavage fluid in the diagnosis of mycotic infections in dogs. *J Am Vet Med Assoc.* 1990;197:79–83.
11. McCullough S, Brinson J. Collection and interpretation of respiratory cytology. *Clin Tech Small Anim Pract.* 1999;14:220–226.
12. Hawkins EC. Bronchoalveolar lavage. In: King LG, ed. *Textbook of Respiratory Disease in Dogs and Cats.* St. Louis, MO: Elsevier; 2004:118–128.
13. Creevy KE. Airway evaluation and flexible endoscopic procedures in dogs and cats: laryngoscopy, transtracheal wash, tracheobronchoscopy, and bronchoalveolar lavage. *Vet Clin North Am Small Anim Pract.* 2009;39:869–880.
14. Hawkins EC, DeNicola DB, Kuehn NF. Bronchoalveolar lavage in the evaluation of pulmonary disease in the dog and cat. State of the art. *J Vet Intern Med.* 1990;4:267–274.
15. Boon D. In: *Scientific Presentations of the 52nd Annual Meeting of the American Animal Hospital Association.* San Diego, CA 2009:388–394.

16. O'Brien. Transtracheal aspiration in dogs and cats. *Mod Vet Prac.* 1983;64:412–413.

17. Hawkins EC, Berry CR. Use of a modified stomach tube for bronchoalveolar lavage in dogs. *J Am Vet Med Assoc.* 1999;215(1620):1635–1639.

18. Hawkins EC, DeNicola DB. Collection of bronchoalveolar lavage fluid in cats, using an endotracheal tube. *Am J Vet Res.* 1989;50:855–859.

19. Vail DM, Mahler PA, Soergel BS. Differential cell analysis and phenotypic subtyping of lymphocytes in bronchoalveolar lavage fluid from clinically normal dogs. *Am J Vet Res.* 1995;56:282–285.

20. Amis TC, McKiernan BC. Systematic identification of endobronchial anatomy during bronchoscopy in the dog. *Am J Vet Res.* 1986;47:2649–2657.

21. Caccamo R, Twedt D, Buracco P, et al. Endoscopic bronchial anatomy in the cat. *J Feline Med Surg.* 2007;9:140–149.

22. Padrid P. Bronchoalveolar lavage in the evaluation of pulmonary disease in the dog and cat. *J Vet Intern Med.* 1991;5:52–55.

23. Hawkins EC, Kennedy-Stoskopf S, Levy J, et al. Cytologic characterization of bronchoalveolar lavage fluid collected through an endotracheal tube in cats. *Am J Vet Res.* 1994;55:795–802.

24. Pinsker K, Norris AJ, Kamholz SL, et al. Cell content in repetitive canine bronchoalveolar lavage. *Acta Cytologica.* 1980;24:558–563.

25. Melamies MA, Jarvinen AK, Seppala KM, et al. Comparison of results for weight-adjusted and fixed-amount bronchoalveolar lavage techniques in healthy Beagles. *Am J Vet Res.* 2011;72:694–698.

26. McCauley M, et al. Unguided bronchoalveolar lavage techniques and residual effects in dogs. *Aust Vet J.* 1998;76:161–165.

27. Moise B. Bronchial washings in the cat: procedure and cytologic evaluation. *Comp Cont Ed.* 1983;5:621–627.

28. Hawkins EC, Rogala AR, Large EE, et al. Cellular composition of bronchial brushings obtained from healthy dogs and dogs with chronic cough and cytologic composition of bronchoalveolar lavage fluid obtained from dogs with chronic cough. *Am J Vet Res.* 2006;67:160–167.

29. Tenwolde AC, Johnson LR, Hun GB, et al. The role of bronchoscopy in foreign body removal in dogs and cats: 37 cases (2000-2008). *J Vet Intern Med.* 2010;l24:1063–1068.

30. Silverstein D, Greene C, Gregory C, et al. Pulmonary alveolar proteinosis in a dog. *J Vet Intern Med.* 2000;14:546–551.

31. Rebar A, DeNicola D, Muggenburg B. Bronchopulmonary lavage cytology in the dog: normal findings. *Vet Pathol.* 1980;17:294–304.

32. Henderson RF. Use of bronchoalveolar lavage to detect lung damage. *Env Health Perspect.* 1984;56:115–129.

33. Carre P, Laviolette M, Belanger J, et al. Technical variations of bronchoalveolar lavage (BAL): influence of atelectasis and the lung region lavaged. *Lung.* 1985;163:117–125.

34. Damiano V, Cohen A, Tsang A, et al. A morphologic study of the influx of neutrophils into dog lung alveoli after lavage with sterile saline. *Am J Pathol.* 1980;100:349–364.

35. Mills PC, Litster AL. Using urea dilution to standardize components of pleural and bronchoalveolar lavage fluids in the dog. *N Z Vet J.* 2005;53:423–428.

36. Johnson LR, Vernau W. Bronchoscopic findings in 48 cats with spontaneous lower respiratory tract disease (2002-2009). *J Vet Intern Med.* 2011;25:236–243.

37. Heikkila HP, Lappalainen AK, Day MJ, et al. Clinical, bronchoscopic, histopathologic, diagnostic imaging, and arterial oxygenation findings in West Highland White Terriers with idiopathic pulmonary fibrosis. *J Vet Intern Med.* 2011;25:433–439.

38. Thornton DJ, Sheehan JK. From mucins to mucus: towards a more coherent understanding of this essential barrier. *Proc Am Thorac Soc.* 2004;1:54–61.

39. Johnston W. Cytologic diagnosis of lung cancer: principles and problems. *Path Res Pract.* 1986;181:1–36.

40. Nafe LA, DeClue AE, Reinero CR. Storage alters feline bronchoalveolar lavage fluid cytological analysis. *J Feline Med Surg.* 2011;13:94–100.

41. Vallim de Mello MF, Ferreira AM, Nascimento A. Cytologic analysis of bronchoalveolar lavage fluid collected through an endotracheal tube in dogs. *Acta Scientiae Veterinariae.* 2002;30:119–125.

42. Thompson A, Teschler H, Wang Y, et al. Preparation of bronchoalveolar lavage fluid with microscope slide smears. *Eur Respir J.* 1996;9:603–608.

43. Dehard S, Bernaerts F, Peeters D, et al. Comparison of bronchoalveolar lavage cytospins and smears in dogs and cats. *J Am Anim Hosp Assoc.* 2008;44:285–294.

44. Mercier E, Bologin M, Hoffman AC, et al. Influence of age on bronchoscopic findings in healthy beagle dogs. *Vet J.* 2011;187:225–228.

45. Mayer P, Laber G, Walzl H. Bronchoalveolar lavage in dogs; analysis of proteins and respiratory cells. *Zentralblatt fur Veterinarmedizin Reihe A.* 1990;37:392–399.

46. De Lorenzi D, Masserdotti C, Bertoncello D, et al. Differential cell counts in canine cytocentrifuged bronchoalveolar lavage fluid: a study on reliable enumeration of each cell type. *Vet Clin Pathol.* 2009;38:532–536.

47. Young KM. Eosinophils. In: Feldman BF, Zinkl JG, Jain NC, eds. *Schalm's Veterinary Haematology.* 5th ed. Baltimore, MD: Lippincott Williams and Wilkins; 2000:297–307.

48. Baldwin F, Becker A. Bronchoalveolar eosinophilic cells in a canine model of asthma: two distinctive populations. *Vet Pathol.* 1993;30:97–103.

49. Spoor MS, Royal AB, Berent LM. The elusive globule leukocyte. *Vet Clin Pathol.* 2011;40:136.

50. Hirshman C, Austin D, Klein W, et al. Increased metachromatic cells and lymphocytes in bronchoalveolar lavage fluid of dogs with airway hyperreactivity. *Am Rev Respir Dis.* 1986;133:482–487.

51. Della Ripa M, et al. Canine bronchoesophageal fistulas. *Compendium (Yardley, PA).* 2010;32:E1–E10.

52. Slauson D, Cooper B. In: Slauson D, Cooper B, eds. *Mechanisms of Disease: A Textbook of Comparative General Pathology.* St. Louis, MO: Mosby; 2002.

53. Nunez-Ochoa L, Desnoyers M, Lecuyer M. What is your diagnosis: iatrogenic aspiration of barium sulphate preparation. *Vet Clin Pathol.* 1993;22:122–123.

54. Nyby M, Gregory DA, Kuhn DA, et al. Incidence of *Simonsiella* in the oral cavity of dogs. *J Clin Microbiol.* 1977;6:87–88.

55. Lecuyer M, Dube PG, DiFruscia R, et al. Bronchoalveolar lavage in normal cats. *Can Vet J.* 1995;36:771–773.

56. Padrid PA, Feldman BF, Funk K, et al. Cytologic, microbiologic, and biochemical analysis of bronchoalveolar lavage fluid obtained from 24 healthy cats. *Am J Vet Res.* 1991;52:1300–1307.

57. Brown N, Noone K, Kurzman I. Alveolar lavage in dogs. *Am J Vet Res.* 1983;44:335–337.

58. Baudendistel L, Vogler G, Frank P, et al. Bronchoalveolar eosinophilia in random-source versus purpose-bred dogs. *Lab Anim Sci.* 1992;42:491–496.

59. Clercx C, Peeters D, German AJ, et al. An immunologic investigation of canine eosinophilic bronchopneumopathy. *J Vet Intern Med.* 2002;16:229–237.

60. Boothe HW, Jones SA, Wilkie WS, et al. Evaluation of the concentration of marbofloxacin in alveolar macrophages and pulmonary epithelial lining fluid after administration in dogs. *Am J Vet Res.* 2005;66:1770–1774.

61. Nafe LA, DeClue AE, Lee-Fowler TM, et al. Evaluation of biomarkers in bronchoalveolar lavage fluid for discrimination between asthma and chronic bronchitis in cats. *Am J Vet Res.* 2010;71:583–591.

62. Clercx C, Peeters D. Canine eosinophilic bronchopneumopathy. *Vet Clin North Am Small Anim Pract.* 2007;37:917–935.

63. Kelmer E, Love LC, DeClue AE, et al. Successful treatment of acute respiratory distress syndrome in dogs. *Can Vet J.* 2012;53:167–173.

64. DeHeer HL, McManus P. Frequency and severity of tracheal wash hemosiderosis and association with underlying disease in 96 cats: 2002-2003. *Vet Clin Pathol.* 2005;34:17–22.

65. McKiernan BC, Smith AR, Kissil M. Bacterial isolates from the lower trachea of clinically healthy dogs. *J Am Anim Hosp Assoc.* 1984;20:139–142.

66. Peeters DE, McKiernan BC, Weisiger RM, et al. Quantitative bacterial cultures and cytological examination of bronchoalveolar lavage specimens in dogs. *J Vet Intern Med.* 2000;14:534–541.

67. Epstein SE, Mellema MS, Hopper K. Airway microbial culture and susceptibility patterns in dogs and cats with respiratory disease of varying severity. *J Vet Emerg Crit Care.* 2010;20:587–594.

68. Bauer N, O'Niell E, Sheahan B, et al. Calcospherite-like bodies and caseous necrosis in tracheal mucus from a dog with tuberculosis. *Vet Clin Pathol.* 2004;33:168–172.

69. Carter GR, Wise DJ. *Mycoplasmas in Essentials of Veterinary Bacteriology and Mycology*. Blackwell: Iowa State Press; 2004.

70. Randolph J, Moise NS, Scarlett JM, et al. Prevalence of mycoplasmal and ureaplasmal recovery from tracheobronchial lavages and prevalence of mycoplasmal recovery from pharyngeal swab specimens in dogs with or without pulmonary disease. *Am J Vet Res*. 1993;54:387–391.

71. Williams M, Olver C, Thrall MA. Transtracheal wash from a puppy with respiratory disease. *Vet Clin Pathol*. 2006;35:471–473.

72. Foster SF, Martin P, Braddock JA, et al. A retrospective analysis of feline bronchoalveolar lavage cytology and microbiology (1995-2000). *J Feline Med Surg*. 2004;6:189–198.

73. Mochizuki M, Yachi A, Ohshima T, et al. Etiologic study of upper respiratory infections of household dogs. *J Vet Med Sci / Jap Soc Vet Sci*. 2008;70:563–569.

74. Cohn LA. Feline respiratory disease complex. *Vet Clin North Am Small Anim Prac*. 2011;41:1273–1289.

75. Egberink H, Addie D, Belak S, et al. *Bordetella bronchiseptica* infection in cats: ABCD guidelines on prevention and management. *J Feline Med Surg*. 2009;11:610–614.

76. Radhakrishnan A, Drobatz KJ, Culp WT, King LG. Community-acquired infectious pneumonia in puppies: 65 cases (1993-2002). *J Am Vet Med Assoc*. 2007;230:1493–1497.

77. Register KB, Sukumar N, Palavecino EL, et al. *Bordetella bronchiseptica* in a paediatric cystic fibrosis patient: possible transmission from a household cat. *Zoonoses Public Health*. 2012;59:246–250.

78. Muntz F. Oxalate-producing pulmonary aspergillosis in an alpaca. *Vet Pathol*. 1999;36:631–632.

79. Legrende A, Walker MNB. Canine blastomycosis: a review of 47 clinical cases. *J Am Vet Med Assoc*. 1981;178:1163–1168.

80. Crews LJ, Feeney DA, Jessen CR, et al. Utility of diagnostic tests for and medical treatment of pulmonary blastomycosis in dogs:125 cases (1989-2006). *J Am Vet Med Assoc*. 2008;232:222–227.

81. McMillan CJ, Taylor SM. Transtracheal aspiration in the diagnosis of pulmonary blastomycosis (17 cases: 2000-2005). *Can Vet J*. 2008;49:53–55.

82. Graupman-Kuzma A, Valentine B, Subitz LF, et al. Coccidioidomycosis in dogs and cats: a review. *J Am Anim Hosp Assoc*. 2008;44:226–235.

83. Lester SJ, Malik R, Bartlett KH, et al. Cryptococcosis: update and emergence of *Cryptococcus gattii*. *Vet Clin Pathol*. 2011;40:4–17.

84. Ford R. Canine histoplasmosis. *Comp Cont Ed*. 1980;11:637–642.

85. Bromel C, Sykes JE. Histoplasmosis in dogs and cats. *Clin Tech Small Anim Pract*. 2005;20:227–232.

86. McCully R, Lloyd J, Kuys D, et al. Canine *Pneumocystis* pneumonia. *J South Afr Vet Assoc*. 1979;50:207–213.

87. Lobetti R. Common variable immunodeficiency in miniature dachshunds affected with *Pneumocystis carinii* pneumonia. *J Vet Diagn Invest*. 2000;12:39–45.

88. Watson PJ, Wotton P, Eastwood J, et al. Immunoglobulin deficiency in Cavalier King Charles Spaniels with *Pneumocystis* pneumonia. *J Vet Intern Med*. 2006;20:523–527.

89. Outerbridge CA, Taylor S. *Oslerus osleri* tracheobronchitis: treatment with ivermectin in 4 dogs. *Can Vet J*. 1998;39:238–240.

90. Chapman P, Boag AK, Guitian J, et al. *Angiostrongylus vasorum* infection in 23 dogs (1999-2002). *J Small Anim Pract*. 2004;45:435–440.

91. Carrasco L, Hervas J, Gomez-Villamandos JC, et al. Massive *Filaroides hirthi* infestation associated with canine distemper in a puppy. *Vet Rec*. 1997;140:72–73.

92. Conboy G. Helminth parasites of the canine and feline respiratory tract. *Vet Clin Small Anim*. 2009;39:1109–1126.

93. Koch J, Willesen JL. Canine pulmonary angiostrongylus: an update. *Vet J*. 2009;179:348–359.

94. Hawkins EC, Davidson MG, Meuten DJ, et al. Cytologic identification of *Toxoplasma gondii* in bronchoalveolar lavage fluid of experimentally infected cats. *J Am Vet Med Assoc*. 1997;210:648–650.

95. Barrs VR, Martin P, Beatty JA. Antemortem diagnosis and treatment of toxoplasmosis in two cats on cyclosporin therapy. *Aust Vet J*. 2006;84:30–35.

96. Brownlee L, Sellon RK. Diagnosis of naturally occurring toxoplasmosis by bronchoalveolar lavage in a cat. *J Am Anim Hosp Assoc*. 2001;37:251–255.

97. Schoniger S, Chan DL, Hollinshead M, et al. Cowpox virus pneumonia in a domestic cat in Great Britain, he. *Vet Rec*. 2007;160:522–523.

98. Hahn F, Muggenburg B, Griffith W. Primary lung neoplasia in a Beagle colony. *Vet Pathol*. 1996;33:633–638.

99. Moulton J, von Tscharner C, Schnieder R. Classification of lung carcinomas in the dog and cat. *Vet Pathol*. 1981;18:513–528.

100. Hawkins EC, Morris WB, DeNicola DB, et al. Cytologic analysis of bronchoalveolar lavage fluid from 47 dogs with multicentric malignant lymphoma. *J Am Vet Med Assoc*. 1993;203:1418–1425.

The Lung and Intrathoracic Structures

Carolyn N. Grimes, Michael M. Fry, Casey J. LeBlanc, and Silke Hecht

Fine-needle aspiration (FNA) of the lungs or intrathoracic structures may be diagnostically useful in patients with many types of pulmonary or other intrathoracic lesions. Complications may occur, but intrathoracic FNA is generally a safe procedure that results in the cytological diagnosis of neoplasia, inflammatory conditions, or specific infectious agents. Aspirated material may also be submitted for culture or evaluation via molecular techniques (e.g., polymerase chain reaction [PCR]).

This chapter discusses intrathoracic FNA techniques, including various imaging methods used to guide sampling, and cytological diagnosis of a variety of conditions (normal, inflammatory, infectious, neoplastic, other) affecting the lungs, mediastinal structures, pleura or pleural space, and intrathoracic chest wall. Pleural effusion, washes of the respiratory tract, and thoracic lymph node cytology are covered in other chapters.

SAMPLE COLLECTION

Equipment and Technique

Intrathoracic FNA is performed by using 20- to 25-gauge (most commonly 22-gauge) needles of variable length, depending on the size and depth of a lesion. Superficial lesions may usually be sampled using a 1.5-inch needle. A 2.5- to 3.5-inch (spinal) needle may be needed to reach lesions in deeper locations. A 5- to 12-mL (milliliter) syringe is attached to the needle either directly or by means of an extension tube. Additional equipment needs include glass slides with or without culture media.[1]

The procedure is performed after a lesion has been identified, most often by means of thoracic radiography. Although diffuse intrathoracic lesions, such as infiltrative pulmonary disease, may be amenable to blind sampling, image guidance is invaluable in obtaining targeted samples from focal or multifocal lesions associated with mediastinal structures and the pleura or pleural space, thoracic wall, diaphragm and lung.[2-4] Imaging modalities most commonly used to obtain intrathoracic tissue samples in veterinary patients include fluoroscopy, ultrasonography, and computed tomography (CT).[5-12] Although magnetic resonance imaging (MRI) is increasingly used in veterinary medicine, MRI-guided tissue sampling is, at this point, not commonly performed because of the need for expensive specialized nonferromagnetic biopsy equipment. Depending on the individual patient and the method used for tissue sampling, the procedure may be performed with the animal under sedation or may require general anesthesia. Intubation and breath-hold techniques are recommended when sampling small or deeply located lesions to minimize adverse effects from sliding of aerated lung against the needle during respiration. The thoracic wall at the sampling site is clipped and thoroughly cleaned of hair and debris (e.g., by scrubbing the skin with a soap-based disinfectant and alcohol). Samples can be obtained using aspiration or nonaspiration ("pincushion") technique.[13,14] After the procedure, the needle is withdrawn, the sample is gently expelled onto a glass slide, and smears are prepared in a routine fashion.[1]

Once the specimen is within the bore of the needle, it is important to deliver the specimen efficiently to a clean glass slide. The next task is to convert the focally distributed specimen into a monolayer of intact cells that is easily evaluated by light microscopy. To create the monolayer, a second glass slide should be gently laid atop the specimen in a parallel or perpendicular fashion. Then, with no applied downward force besides the weight of the second slide, the two slides are gently pulled apart. Last, the smears are allowed to air-dry; no fixation is necessary. Air-drying should be complete within a short period, usually just a few seconds. If a slide takes longer than a minute or so to dry, then the preparation is likely too thick.

Special Considerations for Image-Guided Fine-Needle Aspiration

Positioning of the patient is variable and dictated by the location of the lesion and the imaging modality used to guide tissue sampling.

1. Ultrasonography is an excellent, inexpensive, and noninvasive modality to obtain guided fine-needle aspirates, which allows monitoring of needle placement in real time.[6,7,9,11] The major disadvantage of this method is that ultrasound is unable to penetrate aerated lung tissue or free air in the pleural space. Ultrasound-guided sampling is therefore limited to superficial lesions in contact with the thoracic wall (Fig. 17.1). Especially for small and deep-seated lesions, use of a needle guide is strongly recommended. Needle guides consist of probe attachments and needle channels, which dictate the course of the needle in a predetermined direction, thus minimizing risk for injury to surrounding structures and assuring needle placement in the area of interest (Fig. 17.2). The use of contrast agents is advocated by some because it allows differentiation of necrotic from viable areas within a lesion, which may increase the diagnostic yield of ultrasound-guided sampling.[15]

2. Fluoroscopy allows for intermittent radiographic monitoring of needle placement as it is advanced toward a lesion.[8] This technique initially showed promising results, but the potential radiation exposure to the clinician and the necessity to rotate the patient or x-ray tube to achieve an orthogonal view to verify needle placement are disadvantages in comparison with CT.

3. CT is a cross-sectional imaging technique, which allows for visualization of deep intrathoracic lesions and controlled placement, even of long needles.[10,12] After a diagnostic scan of the thorax, a table (scan) position that is deemed most suitable for needle

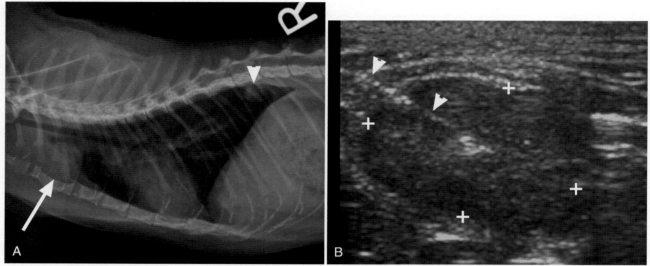

Fig. 17.1 (A) Lateral thoracic radiograph, cat, cranial mediastinal mass *(arrow)*. Note also a pulmonary nodule in the caudal lung fields *(arrowhead)*. (B) Ultrasonographic image of same case, obtained during ultrasound-guided sampling of the mass. The needle is recognized as a strongly hyperechoic line entering the oval mass from the left top corner of the image *(arrowheads)*. The cytology results were suggestive of a malignant fibrous histiocytoma.

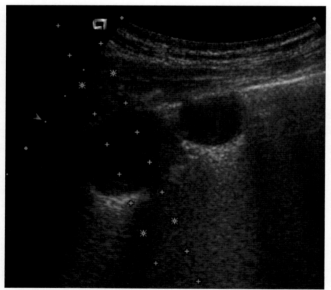

Fig. 17.2 Ultrasonographic image demonstrating use of a needle guide before ultrasound-guided aspiration of a pulmonary nodule. The guide is attached to the probe and dictates course of the needle in a predetermined direction indicated by the dotted lines. Use of this technique minimizes risk for injury to surrounding structures and assures appropriate needle placement.

placement (usually at the largest extent of the lesion and avoiding vascular structures) is identified. After identification of the target, a laser light in the CT gantry is switched on to indicate the site of needle placement in the long axis of the patient. Additionally, marking the skin with ink, radiopaque markers (barium strips), or both before inserting the needle may be helpful to ensure appropriate needle placement. After the insertion site for the needle is identified, repeat CT images are obtained at the same table position to monitor advancement of the needle until the lesion is reached

(Fig. 17.3, A). Bronchoscopic transparenchymal nodule access (BTPNA) is a new technique in which specific navigation software is used to guide tissue sampling by combining CT data sets with live fluoroscopic images to achieve a straight-line path from a central airway through parenchymal tissue.[16,17] This approach has been successfully tested in canine models and may be available for clinical use in veterinary patients in the future.

Complications

FNA of intrathoracic structures is generally considered a safe procedure. Potential complications include pneumothorax (see Fig. 17.3, B) and hemorrhage, which are usually mild and self-limiting.[1,8,12,18] More severe cases of pneumothorax may require placement of a thoracic drain, and animals should be monitored closely for dyspnea or other clinical signs after the procedure. One case of death from severe pneumothorax occurring after fluoroscopy-guided aspiration of a thoracic lesion has been reported.[8] BTPNA has proven to be a very safe technique in preliminary studies in research dogs, with minimal blood loss and no evidence of pneumothorax after the procedure.[16,17] Needle-tract implantation during FNA of thoracic lesions is extremely rare but has been reported in a dog with a pulmonary carcinoma.[19]

Diagnostic Yield

General diagnostic limitations of cytopathology in any tissue (e.g., lack of tissue architecture, varying cellularity of samples, limited ability to speciate certain organisms) apply to FNA cytology of the lung. Although a rate of nondiagnostic samples as high as 35% has been reported, FNA of thoracic lesions is considered a useful technique with a sensitivity ranging from 77% to 91% and a specificity as high as 100%.[8,11,12,20,21] FNA cytopathology of the lung correlates reasonably well (82%–83%) with histopathology.[3,21]

CYTOLOGY OF THE LUNG

FNA of lung tissue is most often performed when pulmonary lesions are detected by using various imaging modalities (previously discussed). Specific indications include (1) presence of a focal pulmonary

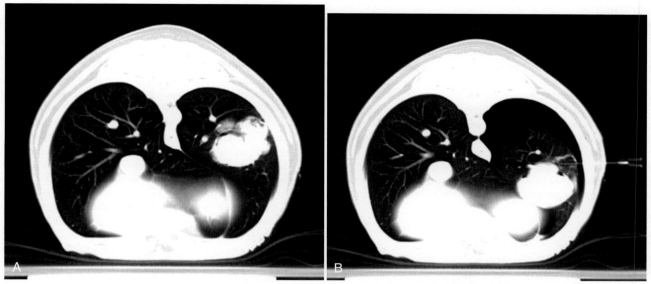

Fig. 17.3 (A) Transverse computed tomography image of a large left caudal lung lobe mass in a dog. A needle was advanced into the mass at this predetermined location and aspirates were obtained. (B) Repeat image at the same level during a second attempt of fine needle aspiration reveals a moderate left-sided pneumothorax as indicated by a hypoattenuating *(black)* area surrounding the left lung. Note also change in position of the pulmonary mass secondary to atelectasis, which resulted in placement of the needle dorsal to the current position of the mass. Cytological diagnosis of the mass was carcinoma. The pneumothorax did not result in clinical signs and resolved without treatment.

lesion; (2) presence of diffuse pulmonary parenchymal disease; (3) suspicion of pulmonary neoplasia (primary or metastatic); (4) need to obtain material for microbial culture; and (5) avoidance of more invasive procedures (e.g., biopsy, thoracotomy).[2,22] For diffuse lesions, aspiration of the caudal right lung lobe is recommended.[23] Ultrasound guidance (previously discussed) may help minimize complications and maximize diagnostic yield, particularly when a focal lesion is present. Contraindications for FNA of lung tissue include bleeding disorders, bullous emphysema, fractious or otherwise uncontrollable patients (sedation may be needed to achieve adequate restraint), severe uncontrolled coughing, and pulmonary hypertension.[24]

Normal Lung

Samples from healthy pulmonary tissue are typically contaminated with a variable amount of blood and may contain small amounts of mucus, which appears as foci of extracellular, pink to lightly basophilic, amorphous or ribbonlike material (Fig. 17.4). Nucleated cells are typically present in very low numbers and are predominantly well-differentiated, respiratory epithelial cells. Epithelial cells are arranged individually or in small clusters and may have cilia on their apical surface. They are cuboidal to columnar with lightly basophilic, finely granular cytoplasm and a single, round, eccentric (basal) nucleus with condensed or coarsely stippled chromatin (Fig. 17.5). In addition to respiratory epithelium, low numbers of scattered alveolar macrophages are also commonly observed. Occasionally, very low numbers of goblet cells may be present. Goblet cells are columnar (or occasionally round) and frequently contain many pale, dark-pink or blue, discrete, cytoplasmic mucin granules (Fig. 17.6). The nucleus of the goblet cell (when not obscured by its cytoplasmic granules) is small, round to oval, and eccentrically located. Occasional mucin granules may be present extracellularly and should not be confused with microorganisms or mast cell granules. The number of leukocytes present should not significantly exceed that which is expected with blood contamination.

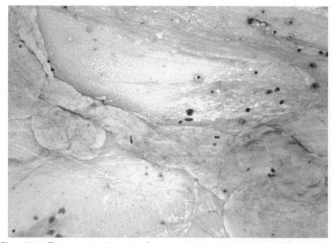

Fig. 17.4 Transtracheal wash, from a dog. Low numbers of poorly preserved, mixed nucleated cells within a pink, granular background matrix are scattered around a moderate amount of amorphous to ribbonlike, ice-blue material consistent with mucus (Wright stain, original magnification 200×).

Common contaminants of pulmonary samples include those observed for many other tissues—for example, ultrasound gel, cornstarch (glove powder), and skin contaminants (squamous cells, keratin bars, low numbers of bacteria not associated with inflammatory cells). However, samples collected via transthoracic lung FNA may also contain elements from the pleura (mesothelial cells), pleural space (substances from effusion, if present), or both (Fig. 17.7). Additionally, well-differentiated hepatocytes (Fig. 17.8), skeletal muscle (Fig. 17.9), or both are sometimes observed. These findings are most consistent with inadvertent aspiration of the liver, diaphragm, or intercostal muscle and should not be confused with a pathological process.

Inflammation
Neutrophilic Inflammation

As in other tissues, increased proportions of neutrophils are associated with acute and chronic inflammation. Common causes of neutrophilic inflammation include bacterial infection, neoplasia, necrosis, and the presence of foreign material or other (nonbacterial) infectious agents. The cause of inflammation may or may not be evident cytologically, but care should be taken to look for intracellular bacterial organisms, neoplastic cells, necrotic debris, foreign material, and other infectious agents. Cytologically, necrotic debris appears as amorphous, bluish-gray material that may be present scattered throughout the smear or in dense aggregates (Fig. 17.10). Foreign material may be of varying morphology; its presence may be suspected on the basis of the observation of unidentified, nonorganismal material that may be surrounded by

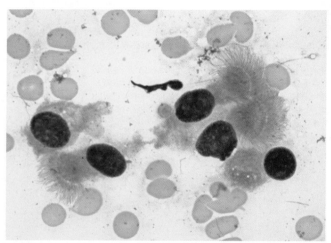

Fig. 17.5 Lung fine-needle aspirate, from a dog. Uniform, well-differentiated, columnar epithelial cells with an oval, eccentric (basal) nucleus, and apical cilia are the predominant cell type in samples from healthy pulmonary tissue (Wright stain, original magnification 1000×).

dense aggregates of inflammatory cells. Cytological findings associated with specific infectious and neoplastic lesions are discussed later in the chapter.

Macrophagic, Granulomatous, and Mixed Inflammation

Increased proportions of macrophages may be observed in both acute and chronic inflammatory lesions. They may represent the sole inflammatory cell type or may be present among varying proportions of neutrophils, eosinophils, and lymphocytes. Whether present as the sole inflammatory cell or as part of a mixed population, differentials for macrophagic inflammation include necrosis, atelectasis, lung lobe torsion, hemorrhage, neoplasia, inhalation pneumonia, lipid pneumonia, and the presence of foreign material or infectious agents.

The term *granulomatous inflammation* is often used to describe lesions that contain multinucleate giant cells and epithelioid macrophages. In some cases, lower numbers of other inflammatory cells, for example, neutrophils (i.e., pyogranulomatous inflammation), lymphocytes, and eosinophils may also be seen. Granulomatous or pyogranulomatous inflammation is most commonly associated with certain infectious agents, including fungi, protozoa, algae (pythiosis), some bacteria (e.g., mycobacteria, filamentous bacteria, such as *Actinomyces* spp.), or the presence of foreign material.

Lipid pneumonia (LP) is an uncommon disorder that has been observed in both dogs and cats.[25,26] It may be caused by inhalation of oily materials (exogenous LP) or may develop secondary to other disease processes (endogenous LP), in particular airway obstruction (e.g., secondary to a neoplasm).[25] Cytologically, LP is characterized by accumulations of highly vacuolated macrophages and, on occasion, fewer numbers of lymphocytes and neutrophils. Characteristics of granulomatous inflammation (e.g., multinucleate giant cells, epithelioid macrophages) may also be seen.

Eosinophilic Inflammation

When eosinophils are a prominent feature of the sample (>10% of all nucleated cells in the absence of peripheral eosinophilia), etiologies of eosinophilic inflammation should be considered (Fig. 17.11). Causes

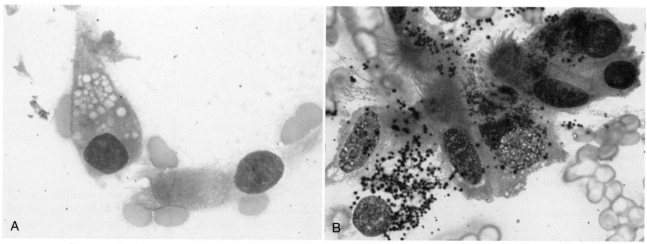

Fig. 17.6 Goblet cells are a normal resident population in pulmonary tissue and are typically present in fewer numbers than ciliated columnar epitheliocytes. Goblet cells are columnar to round and contain many pale (A), dark-purple (B), blue, or magenta mucin-containing cytoplasmic granules. (A) Nasal mass, fine-needle aspirate, from a dog. A single goblet cell with pale, cytoplasmic granules is next to a ciliated, columnar epithelial cell (Wright stain, original magnification 1000×). (B) Lung mass, fine-needle aspirate, from a cat. Ciliated columnar epithelial cells are loosely aggregated with two intact goblet cells which contain many small, dark purple cytoplasmic granules. A third goblet cell is disrupted and several mucinous granules are scattered extracellularly (Wright stain, original magnification 1000×).

of eosinophilic inflammation include allergic or hypersensitivity disorders, parasite infestation, and some fungal, bacterial, protozoal, and neoplastic diseases. It is not unusual to find low numbers of scattered mast cells in lesions with eosinophilic inflammation.

Eosinophilic bronchopneumopathy, pulmonary infiltration with eosinophils (PIE), eosinophilic pneumonia (EP), and pulmonary eosinophilia (PE) have been used to describe various disorders characterized by eosinophilic infiltration of pulmonary parenchyma with unknown etiology. Inconsistent use of this terminology has led to confusion. Clercx and Peeters used the term *eosinophilic bronchopneumopathy* (EBP) to describe eosinophilic infiltration that affects both the airway and pulmonary interstitium and suggested the term *simple eosinophilic pneumonia* (SEP) for cases (although not described in veterinary species) in which only the parenchyma is affected.[27] EBP encompasses those lesions traditionally described as PIE or PE in the veterinary literature. EBP is associated with a bronchointerstitial radiographic pattern. A complete blood count (CBC) in these patients may or may not reveal peripheral eosinophilia.[28] EBP is believed to be a hypersensitivity disorder; however, its cause has not been definitively determined.[27] It is most often suspected when eosinophilic inflammation is observed on cytological analysis of bronchoalveolar fluid (BAL) (see Chapter 16); however, identification of increased proportions of eosinophils (and exclusion of other causes of eosinophilic inflammation) on FNA samples of pulmonary parenchyma should prompt inclusion of EBP in the differential diagnosis.

Eosinophilic granulomatous pneumonia (EGP, or pulmonary eosinophilic granulomatosis) is a parenchymal disorder described in dogs; it is characterized by multiple pulmonary masses (granulomas) composed of eosinophils, macrophages, multinucleate giant cells, lymphocytes, and plasma cells.[29,30] Although EGP is considered an idiopathic disorder, an association with dirofilariasis has been suggested.[29] Additionally, other diseases that could cause eosinophilic inflammation with associated granulomatous inflammation (e.g., pythiosis,[31] immune-mediated hypersensitivity) could have a similar cytological presentation and should be considered in the differential diagnosis.

Lymphocytic Inflammation

Inflammation characterized by a predominance of well-differentiated small lymphocytes is not common. If cytology reveals a predominance of lymphocytes, neoplastic lymphoid proliferations and differentials for lymphocytic inflammation in general (e.g., viral infection, local antigenic stimulation) should be considered. However, the possibility of inadvertent aspiration of an intrathoracic lymph node or the thymus should also be considered.

Infectious Diseases
Bacterial Infection

Cytological specimens that aid in the diagnosis of bacterial pneumonia are most commonly obtained via a transtracheal wash (TW) or BAL (see Chapter 16). However, FNA of infected pulmonary tissue (diffuse disease or large focal lesions) may also be diagnostically valuable.[32] A wide spectrum of bacterial organisms can cause pulmonary infections in the dog and cat.[33] Extracellular bacteria may be true pathogens or contaminants. Observing bacteria within neutrophils, macrophages, or both suggests that they are true pathogens. Common pulmonary bacterial pathogens of the dog and cat may be rod shaped or coccoid. Bacterial morphology is not sufficient to identify its genus and species; culture, molecular diagnostics, or both are necessary to definitively identify the organism. However, few bacteria do exhibit morphology or staining characteristics that allow a presumptive etiological diagnosis. For example, beaded, filamentous bacteria are consistent with an infection of *Actinomyces* spp., *Nocardia* spp., or (rarely) *Fusobacterium* spp. origin (Fig. 17.12). *Mycobacterium* spp. is suspected when slender, nonstaining, rod-shaped elements are seen within macrophages or extracellularly (Fig. 17.13). *Mycobacterium* spp. organisms do not stain with routine Romanowsky-type stains but will stain reddish-pink with acid-fast stains.[34]

Viral Infection

Viral infection is a rare cytological diagnosis. Common viruses, such as canine distemper virus and canine adenovirus, have been associated with intracellular inclusion bodies seen histologically, but these inclusions are very rarely seen on cytological specimens.[35]

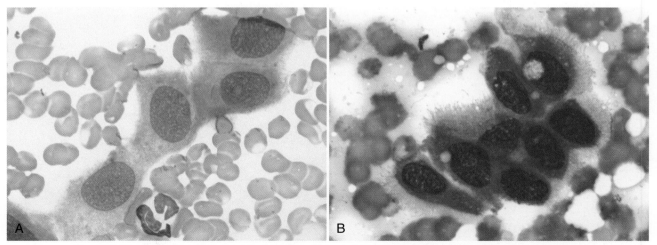

Fig. 17.7 Visceral and parietal mesothelial cells may be incidentally aspirated when performing fine-needle aspiration (FNA) of an intrathoracic lesion. (A) Lung, fine-needle aspirate, from a dog. Small sheets of normal mesothelium consist of uniform, polygonal cells with light blue, finely granular cytoplasm and a central, round to oval nucleus (Wright stain, original magnification 1000×). (B) Lung, fine-needle aspirate, from a dog. Reactive mesotheliocytes often appear round to polygonal with dark blue cytoplasm that may have a peripheral, pink halo or "fringe" (Wright stain, original magnification 1000×).

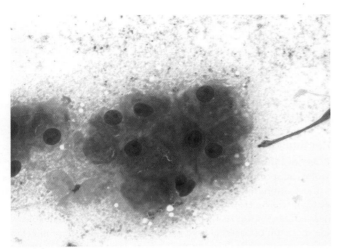

Fig. 17.8 Lung fine-needle aspirate, from a dog. The presence of hepatocytes is suggestive of inadvertent, transdiaphragmatic aspiration of the liver and should not be confused with a pathological process (Wright stain, original magnification 500×).

Observation of secondary inflammation, bacterial infections, or both is more commonly found in cytological specimens from virally infected animals.

Fungal Infection

Pulmonary parenchyma may be infected by many different mycotic organisms. When infections result in the formation of morphologically distinct yeast, the genus of the fungus may typically be definitively determined via cytology (Table 17.1; Figs, 17.14 to 17.18).[36-40] An exception to this is *Blastomyces helicus* (formerly *Emmonsia helica*) (Fig. 17.19), which can appear morphologically very similar to *Histoplasma capsulatum* when small but can greatly enlarge in vivo and may be confused with *Coccidioides immitis*.[41,42,42a] In contrast, when intralesional hyphae are observed, the causative organism cannot be definitively determined by routine cytological evaluation because visually distinct characteristics are not commonly observed. A relatively common hyphae-forming fungal organism that has been diagnosed via FNA of the pulmonary parenchyma is *Aspergillus* spp. (Fig. 17.20).[43]

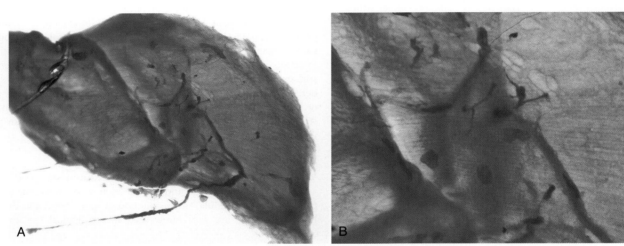

Fig. 17.9 Lung fine-needle aspirate, skeletal muscle, from a dog. Low-magnification (A) (200×) and high-magnification (B) (500×) images (Wright stain). Aggregates of well-differentiated striated skeletal myocytes often appear bright blue with compressed nuclei and visible striations. Most commonly, this is an incidental finding consistent with aspiration of intercostal muscle or the diaphragm.

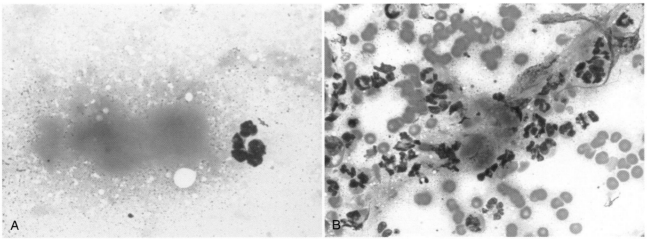

Fig. 17.10 Lung fine-needle aspirate, from a dog. Necrotic debris often appears as amorphous, bluish-gray material. In (A), a single small focus of necrotic debris is next to a neutrophil (Wright stain, original magnification 1000×). In (B), the necrotic debris is associated with neutrophilic inflammation and blood contamination (Wright stain, original magnification 1000×).

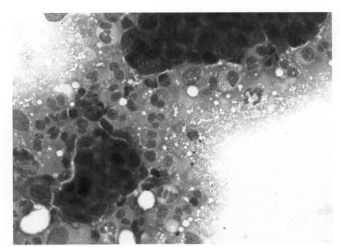

Fig. 17.11 Lung fine-needle aspirate, from a dog. Moderate numbers of eosinophils surround clusters of neoplastic epithelial cells in a dog with a carcinoma (Wright stain, original magnification 500×).

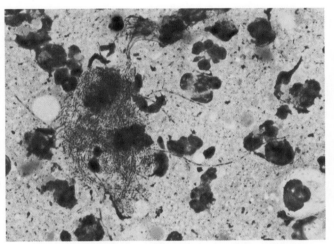

Fig. 17.12 Thoracic fluid from a dog with actinomycosis. Several degenerate neutrophils surround a mat of bacteria. These beaded filamentous bacteria are consistent with *Actinomyces, Nocardia*, or *Fusobacterium* spp. (Wright stain, original magnification 1000×).

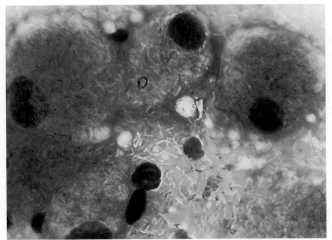

Fig. 17.13 Skin, impression smear, cat, mycobacteriosis. Epithelioid macrophages contain many negatively stained rod-shaped bacteria consistent with *Mycobacterium* spp. These bacteria are commonly more visible when extracellular in a proteinaceous background (Wright stain, original magnification 1000×).

Protozoal Infection

Tachyzoites of *Toxoplasma gondii* or *Neospora caninum* may be seen on inspection of pulmonary cytological specimens from infected dogs and cats.[44] The crescent or banana-shaped tachyzoites of these two organisms are not distinguishable from each other as their size (1 × 3–7 micrometers [μm]) and morphology are very similar (Fig. 17.21). Tachyzoites may be found extracellularly (individually or in clusters) or within phagocytes (usually macrophages). *Cytauxzoon felis* infection in cats results in a tissue phase characterized by large, distended macrophages that contain a cytoplasm-consuming schizont packed with many morphologically indistinct merozoites. The nuclei of the infected macrophages typically contain very large and prominent nucleoli. These cells may be found in tissues throughout the body but are most commonly identified on histopathological samples from the spleen, liver, and lungs.[45,46] Protozoa of the genus *Acanthamoeba* may also infect the pulmonary parenchyma of cats and dogs[47]; trophozoites, cysts, or both may (rarely) be seen cytologically (Fig. 17.22).

Helminthic Infection

Lungworms are uncommonly diagnosed by cytological evaluation of BAL or TW fluid. Very rarely, evaluation of pulmonary parenchymal aspirates results in the identification of helminthic infections. Ova are more commonly found (Fig. 17.23), but aspiration of lungworm larvae has been reported.[48]

Neoplasia

Hypertrophy (increased cell size), hyperplasia (increased number of cells), metaplasia (replacement of one cell type by another), and dysplasia (abnormal pattern of tissue growth with asynchronous nuclear and cytoplasmic maturation) are reversible, preneoplastic changes.[49] Distinguishing these changes from well-differentiated neoplasia with certainty is best accomplished histologically.

Canine and feline primary tumors of the lung are most commonly epithelial in origin.[50-52] Histological classification of primary pulmonary epithelial tumors may be a complex process.[52] With the exception of squamous cell carcinoma, cytological differentiation of various primary epithelial tumors is usually not possible (see Fig. 17.11; Figs. 17.24 and 17.25). Observing acinar structures may suggest a glandular cell origin (adenoma, adenocarcinoma), but this arrangement of cells is often not apparent. Furthermore, differentiating a primary from a metastatic epithelial tumor in the lung is typically not achievable. Aspiration of primary malignant and metastatic epithelial lung tumors often yields highly cellular smears that consist of clusters of round to polygonal, basophilic cells with malignant criteria. However, primary malignant epithelial tumors may also appear quite uniform, exhibiting minimal anisokaryosis and nuclear atypia (see Fig. 17.24). Last, any tumor may be associated with necrosis, inflammation (most often neutrophilic or pyogranulomatous), or both. Necrotic material appears cytologically as bluish-gray, amorphous, extracellular debris and, in the lung, is most commonly observed in association with primary epithelial tumors (see Fig. 17.10; Fig. 17.26).

Primary mesenchymal tumors of the lung are not common. Histiocytic sarcoma may manifest as a primary lung tumor or as a metastatic lesion in the disseminated variant of this malignancy.[53] Cytologically, histiocytic sarcomas may consist of individual round cells or spindle to pleomorphic cells. Typically, these cells have an abundant amount of lightly to moderately basophilic cytoplasm that is often, but not always, vacuolated (Fig. 17.27). The nuclear-to-cytoplasmic (N:C) ratio is variable. A common and often distinguishing feature of these tumors is the presence of large, multinucleate cells. Although other tumors may contain multinucleate cells, when these cells are in the

TABLE 17.1   Common Yeast-Forming Fungal Pathogens of the Lungs

Name	Typical size (µm)	Predominant location	Characteristics[a]
Blastomyces dermatitidis	5–15 diameter	Extracellular	Round, basophilic when viable at time of aspiration, coarsely stippled, thin poorly stained cell wall, broad-based budding commonly noted (see Fig. 17.14)
Cryptococcus spp.	5–20 diameter (including capsule)	Extracellular	Round, commonly deeply basophilic, thick nonstaining capsule, occasional narrow-based budding (see Fig. 17.15)
Coccidioides immitis	10–80 diameter	Extracellular	Round, basophilic, thick double-walled spherules that may or may not contain many visible endospores (see Fig. 17.16)
Blastomyces helicus (formerly *Emmonsia helica*)	2–4 diameter; can become enlarged to 40–500	Intracellular and extracellular	Round to oval, round to irregularly shaped eccentric nucleus, pale cytoplasm, thin poorly stained cell wall (see Fig. 17.19)
Histoplasma capsulatum	2 wide, 4 long	Intracellular	Round to oval, round to crescent-shaped eccentric nucleus, pale cytoplasm, thin poorly stained cell wall (see Fig. 17.17)
Sporothrix schenckii	1–3 wide, 3–9 long	Intracellular	Similar to *Histoplasma*, but more pleomorphic, with occasional elongate or cigar-shaped yeast
Pneumocystis carinii	3–5 diameter (cyst)	Intracellular and extracellular	Small, round, poorly stained cysts containing many small, pleomorphic, basophilic trophozoites, often in a circular arrangement (see Fig. 17.18)

[a]When stained with a Romanowsky-type stain.

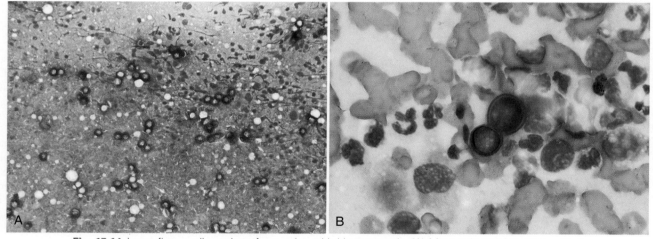

Fig. 17.14 Lung, fine-needle aspirate from a dog with blastomycosis. (A) Many pale-staining, thick-walled yeast can be seen at low-power magnification (Wright stain, original magnification 200×). (B) Basophilic, broad-based budding *Blastomyces dermatitidis* yeast with thick walls are surrounded by poorly preserved neutrophils and macrophages (Wright stain, original magnification 1000×).

presence of the cells described above, histiocytic sarcoma should be one of the top differential diagnoses.

Lymphomatoid granulomatosis is a term that has been used to describe a spectrum of pulmonary diseases, usually lymphomas, in which the neoplastic cells have an atypical morphology with histiocytic features. The term *lymphomatoid granulomatosis* is controversial because it has been applied to lesions with varying cytological and molecular features. In dogs, the term has been applied to tumors consisting of large, pleomorphic, mononuclear cells admixed with few to many eosinophils and lower numbers of plasma cells and small lymphocytes.[54,55]

Lung carcinoids are primary pulmonary tumors that arise from neuroendocrine cells in the airway epithelium. These tumors are also rare but have been presumptively diagnosed via FNA and cytological evaluation.[56]

Because the pulmonary capillaries are the first filter met by many tumor emboli, secondary tumors in the lung are relatively common.[57]

Common practices in monitoring veterinary patients with cancer allow for pulmonary metastases to be readily identified and frequently aspirated. Essentially, any tumor may metastasize to the lungs, but tumors more likely to do so include oral and nail bed melanoma, thyroid carcinoma (Fig. 17.28), osteosarcoma, mammary carcinoma, and high-grade soft tissue sarcoma (personal communication, Dr. Amy K. LeBlanc).[33]

Other

Hemorrhage

Hemorrhage is indicated by the presence of erythrophagia (consistent with acute hemorrhage, Fig. 17.29, A), the presence of pigmented hemoglobin breakdown products (associated with chronic hemorrhage), or both. Hemoglobin breakdown products include hemosiderin (globular to irregular, bright-blue to black, pigmented material within macrophages; see Fig. 17.29, B) and hematoidin (small, rhomboid, bright-orange crystals present extracellularly or within macrophages; see Fig. 17.29, B). Hemorrhage may be secondary to another

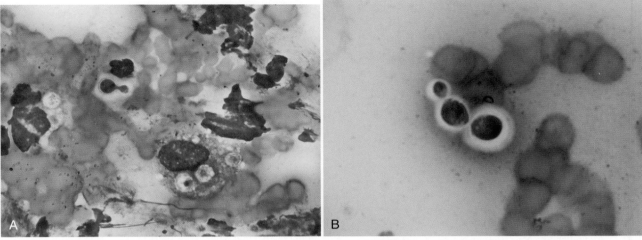

Fig. 17.15 Nose, impression smear from a cat with cryptococcosis. (A) Narrow-based budding *Cryptococcus* spp. yeast with a thick, nonstaining capsule are found extracellularly and surrounded by poorly preserved neutrophils, a macrophage, and cellular debris. Also present within the macrophage are three, poorly stained acapsular yeast. (B) Three extracellular *Cryptococcus* spp. yeast of variable size exhibit a thick, nonstaining capsule (Wright stain, original magnification 1000×).

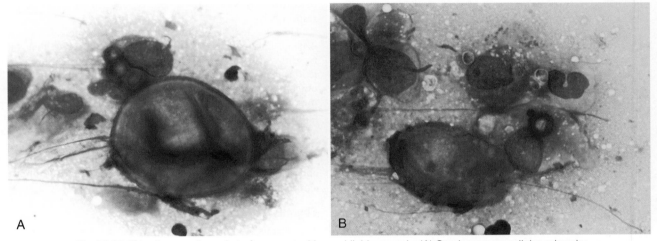

Fig. 17.16 Skin, fine-needle aspirate from a cat with coccidioidomycosis. (A) One large extracellular spherule (measuring 35 μm in diameter) with a thick, well-demarcated wall is adjacent to a macrophage containing three smaller spherules. (B) One large extracellular, partially folded spherule is adjacent to a macrophage containing one small spherule. Few small extracellular endospores (3–5 μm) are also present (Wright stain, original magnification 1000×). (Glass slide courtesy Sharon Dial).

process (e.g., neoplasia, inflammation) or may be the primary pulmonary lesion (e.g., in patients with coagulopathy).

Benign Epithelial Cells

As cytology from normal lung tissue is typically of low cellularity, a sample with increased numbers of goblet cells or respiratory epitheliocytes that lack striking features of malignancy is suggestive of atelectasis or hyperplasia (a benign proliferation of epithelial cells secondary to chronic irritation or some other stimulus, discussed previously). However, a well-differentiated carcinoma should be considered in the differential diagnosis if historical or clinical findings are suggestive.

Benign Mesenchymal Cells

When cytology reveals a predominance of fusiform (mesenchymal) cells that lack striking criteria of malignancy and that are sometimes associated with small amounts of amorphous, pink, extracellular

matrix material, a benign mesenchymal proliferation should be considered. Fibroplasia and fibrosis are nonspecific, secondary changes wherein mesenchymal cells proliferate (most commonly) in response to chronic irritation. In such cases, evidence of the primary disease process (inflammation, neoplasia, necrosis, etc.) may not be seen. Fibrosis may also represent a specific clinical entity, for example, canine pulmonary fibrosis (CPF) in West Highland White Terriers.[58] CPF is, however, rarely diagnosed cytologically because of the tendency of these lesions to be poorly exfoliative. Benign mesenchymal neoplasms of the pulmonary parenchyma are rare.

CYTOLOGY OF THE MEDIASTINUM

The mediastinum is the structure of tissues and organs between the pleural spaces. It contains the heart, which separates the cranial and caudal portions of the mediastinum; lymphoid tissue, including thymus

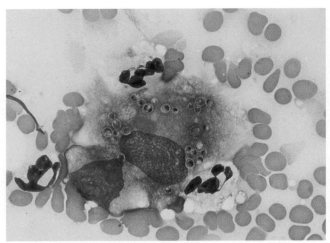

Fig. 17.17 Lung, fine-needle aspirate from a cat with histoplasmosis. A macrophage contains many small, round to oval yeast with an eccentric, often crescent-shaped nucleus consistent with *Histoplasma capsulatum* (Wright stain, original magnification 1000×).

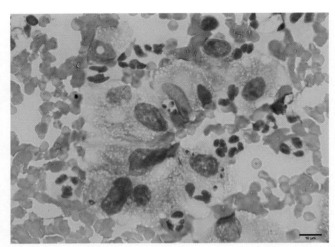

Fig. 17.19 Lung, fine-needle aspirate from a cat with *Blastomyces helicus* pneumonitis. Few macrophages containing low numbers of small, round to oval yeast with eccentric round to irregularly shape nuclei, similar to *Histoplasma capsulatum* (Wright-Giemsa stain, original magnification 1000×). (Courtesy Dr. Caitlyn Martinez, case from 2016 ASVCP case review session.)

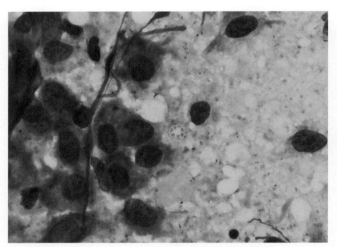

Fig. 17.18 Lung, impression smear from a dog with *Pneumocystis* infection. One extracellular, round cyst consisting of seven basophilic bodies arranged in a circular fashion is shown in the center of the photograph. Many small pleomorphic, poorly defined trophozoites are also found adjacent to many necrotic epithelial cells (Wright stain, original magnification 1000×). (Glass slide from 2005 ASVCP case review session, submitted by Drs. Tara Holmberg and Sonjia Shelly.)

and lymph nodes; portions of trachea, bronchi, esophagus, and major blood vessels, lymphatic vessels, and nerves; fat; and loose connective tissue.[59,60]

FNA sampling of mediastinal lesions is feasible, but the deep intrathoracic location, presence of vital structures, and cardiorespiratory movement carry associated risks. Sampling should be performed under imaging guidance to minimize the likelihood of major complications. See the techniques section earlier in this chapter for more information on imaging-guided sample acquisition.

Indications for cytology of mediastinal lesions include the presence of a mass, organomegaly, and abnormal accumulation of fluid. Contraindications for FNA of mediastinal lesions are similar to those previously described for pulmonary lesions. Cytology of many mediastinal lesions is covered below; lymph node and pericardial effusion cytology are covered in Chapters 11 and 15, respectively.

The expected cellularity of FNA samples of mediastinal lesions depends on the nature of the lesion. Lymphoid and epithelial lesions typically yield samples of higher cellularity than connective tissue lesions. Potential contaminants in mediastinal samples include cells or other material from tissues pierced by the needle (e.g., skin, blood, fat, mesothelium, effusion fluid, mucus, microbes) and introduced contaminants (e.g., glove powder, ultrasound gel).

A retrospective study of 58 cases (all but one of them neoplastic, mostly lymphoma and thymoma) found good agreement between cytological and histological diagnoses of mediastinal masses in dogs and cats. There was complete agreement in 46 cases and complete disagreement in 2 cases.[61]

Thymus

The thymus is located principally in the cranial mediastinum. (The shape and exact location of the thymus vary among domestic animals.[60] Cats may have cervical and thoracic thymic lobes; the cervical lobe is usually small but may extend along the lateral surfaces of the cervical trachea. Dogs do not have a cervical lobe.) The normal size of the organ varies with age: It is largest in relation to body mass at birth, and involutes after sexual maturity. After involution, thymic tissue is replaced by loose connective tissue and fat, but microscopic remnants of the original tissue remain.[60]

In addition to being a primary lymphoid organ essential for normal development of T lymphocytes, the thymus has an epithelial component. Hassall corpuscles, foci of epithelial cells in the thymic medulla, are a characteristic histological feature of the organ.[60] Interactions between the thymic epithelial cells and lymphocytes are critical to normal thymic function and may also play a role in some diseases (see "Thymoma," below). Thymic lymphocytes (sometimes called *thymocytes*) have a characteristic CD4+ CD8+ phenotype, which distinguishes them from lymphocytes in other organs.[62] Fig. 17.30 shows the normal thymic microanatomy.

Thymic lesions reported in dogs and cats include thymoma, lymphoma, cysts, and other disorders that occur more rarely (Box 17.1).[62-81]

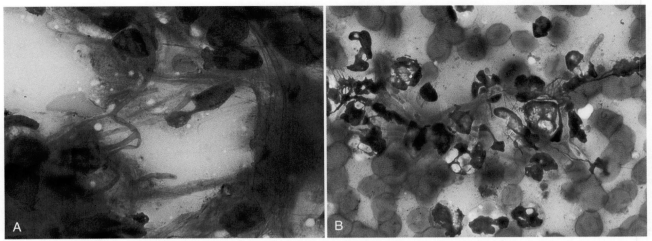

Fig. 17.20 Nose, fine-needle aspirate, dog, aspergillosis. Lightly stained, branching fungal hyphae are seen admixed with respiratory epithelial cells (A) and poorly preserved neutrophils (B) (Wright stain, original magnification 1000×).

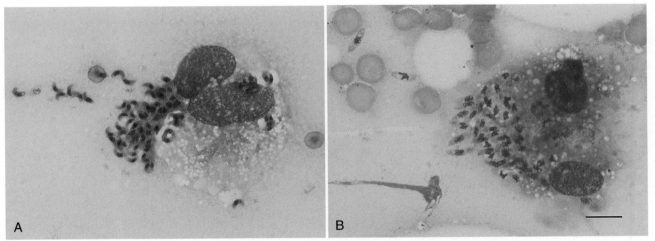

Fig. 17.21 (A) Lung, impression smear from a cat with toxoplasmosis. (B) Lung, fine-needle aspirate from a dog with neosporosis (Wright stain, original magnification 1000×). Both photomicrographs consist of vacuolated macrophages containing intracellular, banana- to cigar-shaped tachyzoites with centrally located oval nuclei. Extracellular tachyzoites are also seen in both cases. (A, Glass slide from 2005 ASVCP case review session, submitted by Dr. Deborah Davis.)

Thymoma

Thymoma is a major differential diagnosis for a cranial mediastinal mass; rare reports of ectopic thymomas in dogs and cats have been published.[82,83] Thymomas are thymic epithelial neoplasms that may be benign or malignant (malignant thymoma is also referred to as *thymic carcinoma*) and often have a nonneoplastic lymphoid component.[63] In vitro experiments have shown that neoplastic thymic epithelial cells induce differentiation of CD4− CD8− T-lymphocyte precursors to those with the CD4+ CD8+ phenotype typical of cortical thymocytes.[84] In fact, in dogs and cats with thymomas, lymphocytes usually comprise the majority population of nucleated cells in FNA cytology samples, whereas epithelial cells are often absent or present in relatively low numbers. Presumably, lymphocytes predominate in these cases because the neoplastic thymic epithelial cells produce cytokines that promote lymphoid hyperplasia and because lymphocytes exfoliate readily. Classifying thymomas as benign or malignant or according to the predominant cell type is most reliably accomplished histologically.[85,86] The system proposed by the World Health Organization

(WHO) has gained wide acceptance for histological classification of thymomas and thymic carcinomas in people.[84,87]

Most lymphocytes in thymomas are well-differentiated, small, CD4+ CD8+ lymphocytes. Relatively low numbers of larger lymphocytes may also be present. Flow cytometric immunophenotyping has been used to discriminate thymomas from aspirates of other lymphocyte-rich mediastinal lesions in dogs.[62] Another common feature of thymomas is the presence of low numbers of well-differentiated mast cells. Thymic epithelial cells may be variably shaped—from round or oval to polygonal to fusiform—and present individually and in more cohesive arrangements, or both. These cells typically have round to oval nuclei, inconspicuous nucleoli, and moderate amounts of lightly basophilic cytoplasm. They usually lack striking morphological features of malignancy. Foci of pink extracellular material, perhaps originating from the capsule of the tumor or from intralesional septae, may also be present in aspirates of thymomas.[88] Fig. 17.31 shows classic cytological findings of a canine thymoma; Fig. 17.31, C shows an example of a sample containing high numbers of thymic epithelial cells.

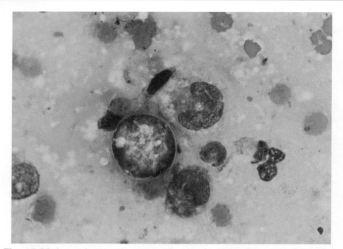

Fig. 17.22 Lung, impression smear from a dog with *Acanthamoeba* infection. A 28-μm–diameter cyst is seen adjacent to few macrophages and a small amount of cellular debris. Note the thin, nonstaining wall and the coarsely granular internal structure of the cyst (modified Wright stain). (Glass slide from 2010 ASVCP case review session, submitted by Dr. Katie Boes.)

Thymomas are often associated with the autoimmune disorder myasthenia gravis in humans and in dogs and cats.[63,64,84,] The exact mechanism responsible for this association is not clear but may involve development of altered T-lymphocyte repertoires.[84] Hypercalcemia and other paraneoplastic disorders have also been reported in dogs and cats with thymomas.[63-65]

Thymic Lymphoma

The interpretive principles that apply to cytological diagnosis of lymphoma in lymph nodes and other organs also apply to diagnosis of lymphoma in the thymus, mediastinal lymph nodes, and other intrathoracic locations. Cytological diagnosis of lymphoma is covered in detail in Chapter 11.

Other major differentials for mediastinal samples consisting mostly of lymphocytes include thymoma, as discussed above, and lymphoid hyperplasia (also covered in Chapter 11).

Thymic Cysts

The thymus originates during embryogenesis from pharyngeal (branchial) pouches, and remnants of these structures may be associated

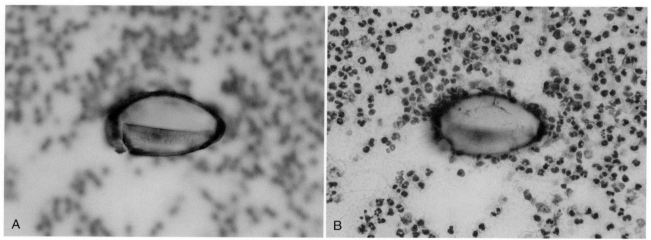

Fig. 17.23 Lung, fine-needle aspirate from a cat with paragonimiasis. (A) Focused on ovum. (B) Focused on background cellularity. A large (45 × 75 μm) single-operculated ovum is surrounded by many neutrophils, eosinophils, and few macrophages (Wright-Giemsa stain, original magnification 400×).

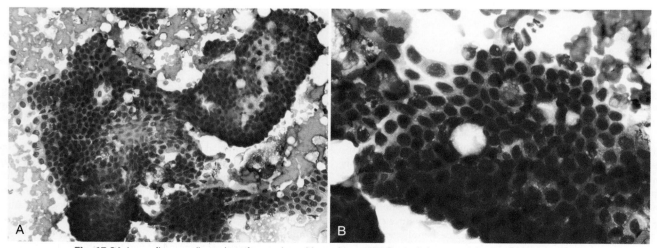

Fig. 17.24 Lung, fine-needle aspirate from a dog with carcinoma. (A) Several clusters to sheets of very basophilic epithelial cells with high nuclear to cytoplasmic ratio. Anisokaryosis is minimal (Wright stain, original magnification 200×). (B) Although a benign lesion or a metastatic lesion cannot be ruled out, the cellularity and uniformity of this tumor is most consistent with primary pulmonary epithelial neoplasia (original magnification 500×).

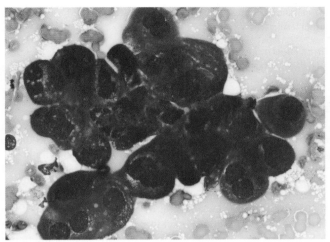

Fig. 17.25 Lung, fine-needle aspirate from a dog with carcinoma. Epithelial cells exhibiting many malignant criteria (Wright stain, original magnification 1000×).

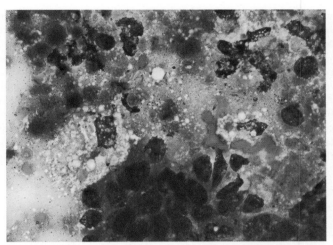

Fig. 17.26 Lung, fine-needle aspirate from a dog with carcinoma. A cluster of malignant epithelial cells is associated with few highly vacuolated macrophages and a large amount of amorphous cellular debris consistent with necrosis (Wright stain, original magnification 500×).

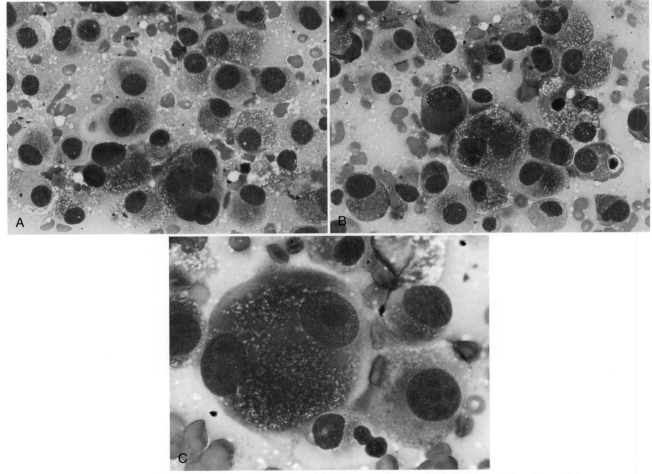

Fig. 17.27 Lung, fine-needle aspirate from a dog with histiocytic sarcoma. (A) & (B) Many histiocytes exhibiting malignant criteria are seen. Occasional large multinucleated cells are also present. Phagocytic activity (B) is rarely noted (Wright stain, original magnification 500×). (C) Higher-power magnification of a large binucleate histiocyte with coarse chromatin and multiple prominent nucleoli (original magnification 1000×).

with cysts, neoplasms, or both. Thymic branchial cysts have been reported in dogs and cats, including some cases in which the cysts were associated with thymic neoplasia.[63,66-71] Histologically, they are lined with ciliated columnar epithelial cells, and some of these cells may be present in aspirates obtained for cytological evaluation, but aspirates of these cystic lesions are likely to consist mostly of low-cellularity fluid. A report on branchial cysts in people that included results of FNA biopsy in 36 patients described varying proportions of inflammatory cells, mature squamous epithelial cells, cholesterol crystals, and cellular debris.[89] Mediastinal cysts of nonthymic origin (e.g., parathyroid, thyroglossal, pleural) may also occur and are likely to have similarly

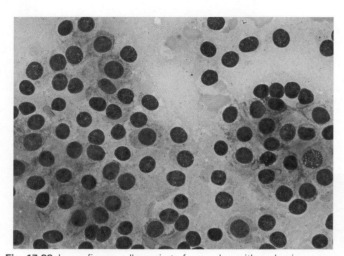

Fig. 17.28 Lung, fine-needle aspirate from a dog with endocrine or neuroendocrine carcinoma. Loosely cohesive clusters of uniform cells with indistinct cytoplasmic borders are consistent with a tumor of endocrine or neuroendocrine origin. The extracellular pink material is consistent with colloid, suggesting a metastatic thyroid carcinoma (Wright stain, original magnification 500×).

low-cellularity fluid.[90,91] Fig. 17.32 shows an aspirate of a cystic mediastinal lesion in a cat.

Other Thymic Lesions

Other thymic lesions reported in dogs, cats, or both are listed in Box 17.1.

Mediastinal Lymph Nodes

Clinically relevant thoracic lymph nodes are present in the mediastinum and include the sternal, cranial mediastinal, and tracheobronchial lymph nodes. The presence or absence and number of intrathoracic lymph nodes varies considerably between individuals.[92] Lymph node cytology is covered in Chapter 11.

Other Mediastinal Lesions

Cardiac and Chemoreceptor Tumors

FNA sampling of cardiac lesions for cytological evaluation is uncommon. The lesions sampled most often are heart base tumors, particularly chemodectoma (a form of paraganglioma arising from aortic or carotid body chemoreceptor organs) and hemangiosarcoma.

Chemodectoma cytological findings have been reported in dogs and cats.[93,94] Like other neuroendocrine tumors, chemodectomas are composed of cells that frequently lyse during sample collection, leaving many free nuclei among a background of free cytoplasm. Intact cells are often present both individually and in sheets or clusters. The cells are typically round to polygonal and have round to oval nuclei that are often eccentrically placed, and small to moderate amounts of lightly basophilic cytoplasm that often contains very fine pink granules (Fig. 17.33, A); a report of a chemodectoma in a cat describes some cells with numerous round cytoplasmic vacuoles. Anisocytosis and anisokaryosis are usually mild to moderate. The nuclei typically have stippled chromatin and often have one to several discernible nucleoli. Special stains (e.g., Churukian-Schenk stain; see Fig. 17.33, B) may be used to confirm the argyrophilia of the cytoplasmic granules.

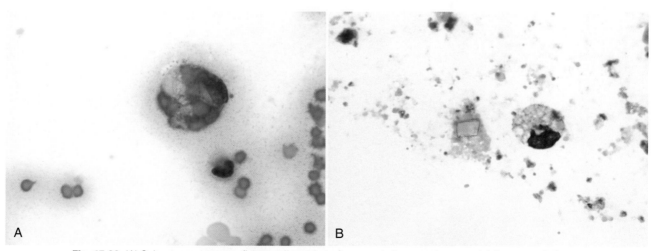

A   B

Fig. 17.29 (A) Subcutaneous mass, fine-needle aspirate from a cat. A macrophage containing several phagocytized erythrocytes indicates acute hemorrhage (Wright stain, original magnification 1000×). (B) Subcutaneous mass, fine-needle aspirate from a dog. Bright blue, irregular, pigmented material (hemosiderin) is present extracellularly and within macrophages, and a single, hematoidin crystal is present extracellularly, indicating chronic hemorrhage (Wright stain, original magnification 1000×).

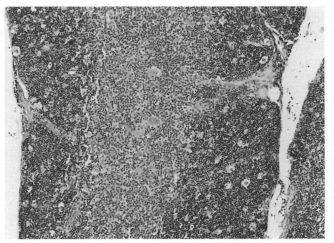

Fig. 17.30 Normal thymus in a juvenile dog. The cortex is darker because it contains a higher concentration of T lymphocytes (thymocytes) compared with the medulla. Hassall's corpuscles, evident here as round, pink foci in the center of the image, are a characteristic feature of the medulla but are usually not detectable in thymic aspirates. The large cells with abundant pale cytoplasm that are scattered throughout the cortical areas are cytophagic ("tingible body") macrophages (hematoxylin and eosin [H&E]). (Courtesy Dr. Linden Craig.)

BOX 17.1 Thymic Lesions Reported in Dogs and Cats

- Neoplastic lesions
- Thymoma/thymic carcinoma[62-65,72]
- Thymic lymphoma[62,63]
- Thymolipoma/thymofibrolipoma[73,74]
- Thymic carcinoid (in a Bengal tiger)[75]
- Squamous cell carcinoma[76,77]
- Lymphangiosarcoma[78]
- Nonneoplastic
- Amyloidosis[72]
- B-lymphoid follicles[79]
- Cysts[63,66-70]
- Hematoma/Hemorrhage[63,71,80,81]
- Hyperplasia[63,71]
- Hypoplasia[63]

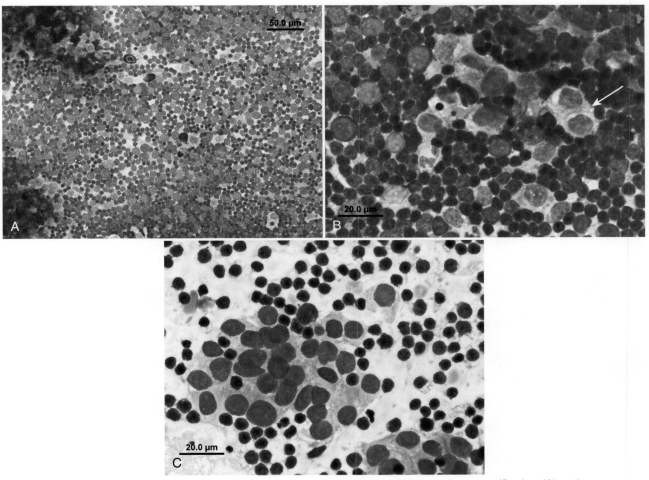

Fig. 17.31 Cranial mediastinal mass, fine-needle aspirate, dog, thymoma. Low-magnification (A) and high-magnification (B) images. The sample consists mostly of a mixed population of lymphocytes, including many small lymphocytes. Also present are thymic epithelial cells *(white arrow)*, which in image A are present mainly as poorly defined clusters *(in the upper and lower left corners)*, and a few well-differentiated mast cells *(present near the center of image A)*. An aspirate from a different canine thymoma (C) shows a higher concentration of thymic epithelial cells (Wright stain). (C, Slide courtesy Dr. David F. Edwards.)

The right atrium is a site of predilection for hemangiosarcoma in dogs, but it is more common to sample hemangiosarcoma lesions for cytological evaluation from abdominal organs (especially spleen or liver) than from the heart. The morphology of hemangiosarcoma cells does not tend to vary greatly, depending on the anatomical location of the tumor; regardless of location, cytological samples of hemangiosarcoma are usually bloody and otherwise of relatively low cellularity. Hemangiosarcoma cytology is covered in more detail in Chapters 20 and 21.

Pericardial Lesions

Mesothelioma, which may arise from or progress to involve the pericardial surface, is covered under "Pleural Lesions" below.

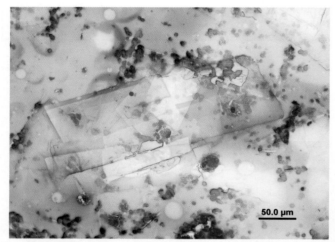

Fig. 17.32 Cystic mediastinal lesion, fine-needle aspirate from a cat. Some large cholesterol crystals and a few hemosiderin-laden macrophages are present, similar to what is often seen in aspirates of cystic fluid from other anatomical locations. It was not determined whether this lesion was associated with a tumor (Wright stain).

Other Neoplasms

A partial list of other neoplasms that may arise in the mediastinum (in addition to thymoma, lymphoma, chemodectoma, and hemangiosarcoma), but which are more often diagnosed in other anatomical locations, includes the following:

- Mesothelioma—usually diagnosed cytologically in effusion fluid (see Chapter 15)
- Neoplasms of ectopic thyroid or parathyroid tissue[95] (see Chapter 6)
- *Spirocerca lupi*–associated esophageal sarcoma (see below)
- Lipoma or liposarcoma[96,97]
- Histiocytic sarcoma[98,99]
- Chondrosarcoma[100,101]
- Leiomyoma or leiomyosarcoma[102,103]

Figs. 17.34, 17.35, and 17.36 are examples of mediastinal sarcomas. Of course, many different tumor types have the potential to metastasize to mediastinal lymph nodes or other mediastinal locations.

Hemorrhage

Mediastinal hematomas have been reported in dogs with possible elastin dysplasia, and mediastinal hemorrhage was reported in a dog with rodenticide intoxication.[71,104] Cytological features of hemorrhage are discussed in the earlier section on cytology of the lung.

Esophageal Lesions

Esophageal granulomas are among the classic lesions associated with canine spirocercosis, a disease with worldwide distribution in tropical and subtropical regions.[105,106] Cytological preparations from these lesions are likely to show evidence of pyogranulomatous inflammation and may contain *S. lupi* ova (Fig. 17.37).[107] Affected dogs are strongly predisposed to developing esophageal sarcomas (especially osteosarcoma or fibrosarcoma).[108]

A case of a dog with a large, encapsulated, inflamed, cystlike (fluid-filled but not epithelial-lined), caudal mediastinal mass suspected to have originated from an esophageal perforation has been reported.[109]

Esophageal lesions are covered in more detail in Chapter 18.

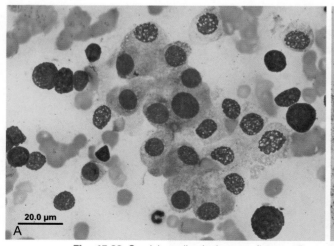
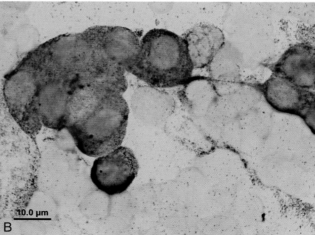

Fig. 17.33 Cranial mediastinal mass, fine-needle aspirate from a dog with chemodectoma. (A) The neoplastic cells have a typical neuroendocrine morphology—round to polygonal in shape, present individually and in clusters, with lightly basophilic cytoplasm containing fine pink granules; the free nuclei are also a characteristic feature of neuroendocrine tumor aspirates (Wright stain). (B) Another slide from the same aspirate, showing the argyrophilia of the cytoplasmic granules (also present in the background from lysed cells) (Churukian-Schenk stain).

Infectious Diseases

Although uncommon, certain infectious diseases may manifest as mediastinal lesions. A partial list includes cryptococcosis, blastomycosis, paecilomycosis, basidiomycosis, aspergillosis, bartonellosis, and oomycosis.[110-116]

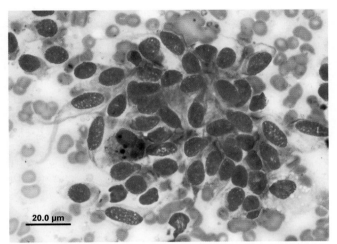

Fig. 17.34 Mediastinal mass, fine-needle aspirate from a dog, histologically diagnosed with anaplastic sarcoma. The fusiform cell morphology and loosely aggregated arrangement of the cells are characteristic of mesenchymal tumors. A cell to the left of center contains two intracytoplasmic (likely phagocytized) erythrocytes and some dark globular material that may be hemosiderin; it is not clear whether this cell is an activated macrophage or part of the neoplastic population (Wright stain). Immunohistochemical staining of the tumor for CD18 and von Willebrand factor (to identify histiocytic and endothelial cell origin, respectively) was negative.

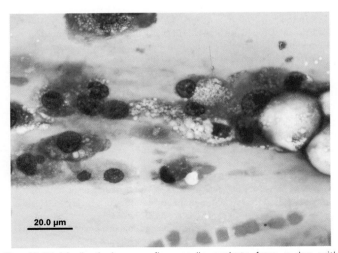

Fig. 17.35 Mediastinal mass, fine-needle aspirate from a dog with myxoid liposarcoma. These tumors produce a mucinous extracellular matrix that may cause the cells to form linear patterns ("wind rows"), as shown affecting the erythrocytes at the bottom of this image. The vacuoles in liposarcoma cells will stain positive with cytochemical stains for lipid, such as Oil red O *(not shown here)* (Wright stain).

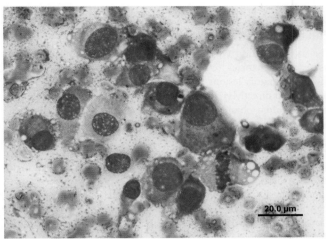

Fig. 17.36 Cranial mediastinal mass, fine-needle aspirate from a dog with sarcoma. This mass apparently originated from the manubrium. Findings were diagnostic for sarcoma based on the striking features of malignancy. Histopathological confirmation of the cell type was unavailable in this case, but osteosarcoma was considered most likely based on the cytomorphology and extracellular matrix consistent with osteoid (see Chapter 13) and on the anatomical location (Wright stain).

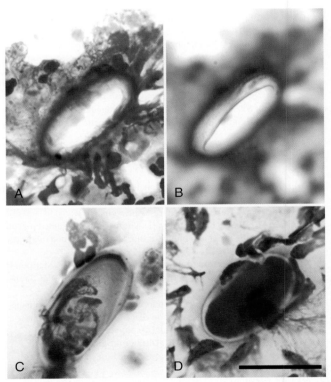

Fig. 17.37 Esophageal nodule, fine-needle aspirate from a dog with spirocercosis. *Spirocerca lupi* egg (A). Same egg, in a different plane of focus (B); note the longitudinal fold on egg surface. Note the filamentous (C) or homogeneous (D) material filling the eggs (May-Grünwald-Giemsa stain, bar = 20 mm). (From De Lorenzi D, Furlanello T. What is your diagnosis? Esophageal nodules in a dog. *Vet Clin Pathol.* 2010;39(3):391–392. Used with permission.)

CYTOLOGY OF OTHER INTRATHORACIC LESIONS

Pleural Lesions

The most common types of pleural lesions are reactive mesothelial lesions, malignancies (especially mesothelioma or carcinomatosis), and inflammatory lesions. Cytological specimens of these lesions may be obtained directly via aspiration or biopsy (impression smears) but are more often obtained indirectly via sampling of pleural effusion fluid (see Chapter 15).

Chest Wall Lesions

Nonpleural intrathoracic lesions include neoplasms and inflammatory lesions associated with the chest wall. More reports have been made of primary chest wall tumors in dogs than in cats. A partial list of cases reported in dogs includes osteosarcoma (see Fig. 17.36), chondrosarcoma, hemangiosarcoma, and fibrosarcoma.[117-121]

Diaphragmatic Hernias

Diaphragmatic hernias may cause displacement of abdominal contents into the mediastinum or the pleural cavity. Therefore cytological features consistent with that of abdominal organs should prompt consideration of diaphragmatic hernia as a differential diagnosis. A report of ectopic hepatic parenchyma in the thorax of a cat has also been published.[122]

REFERENCES

1. Cole SG. Fine needle aspirates. In: King SG, ed. *Respiratory Disease in Dogs and Cats*. St. Louis, MO: Saunders; 2004.
2. Roudebush P, Green RA, Digilio KM. Percutaneous fine-needle aspiration biopsy of the lung in disseminated pulmonary disease. *J Am Anim Hosp Assoc*. 1981;17:109.
3. Teske E, Stokhof AA, Vandeningh TSGAM, et al. Transthoracic needle aspiration biopsy of the lung in dogs with pulmonic diseases. *J Am Anim Hosp Assoc*. 1991;27:289.
4. Smallwood LJ, Zenoble RD. Biopsy and cytological sampling of the respiratory tract. *Semin Vet Med Surg (Small Anim)*. 1993;8:250.
5. Finn-Bodner ST, Hathcock JT. Image-guided percutaneous needle biopsy: ultrasound, computed tomography, and magnetic resonance imaging. *Semin Vet Med Surg (Small Anim)*. 1993;8:258.
6. Hecht S, Pennick D. Thorax. In: Pennick D, d'Anjou MA, eds. *Atlas of Small Animal Ultrasonography*. 2nd ed. Ames, IA: Wiley Blackwell; 2015.
7. Kirberger RM, Stander N. Interventional procedures. In: Barr F, Gaschen L, eds. *Bsava Manual of Canine and Feline Ultrasonography*. Gloucester, UK: British Small Animal Veterinary Association; 2011.
8. Mcmillan MC, Kleine LJ, Carpenter JL. Fluoroscopically-guided percutaneous fine-needle aspiration biopsy of thoracic lesions in dogs and cats. *Vet Radiol*. 1988;29:194.
9. Nyland TG, et al. Ultrasound-guided biopsy. In: Nyland TF, Mattoon JS, eds. *Small Animal Diagnostic Ultrasound*. Philadelphia, PA: W.B. Saunders; 1995.
10. Tidwell AS, Johnson KL. Computed tomography-guided percutaneous biopsy in the dog and cat: description of technique and preliminary evaluation in 14 patients. *Vet Radiol Ultrasound*. 1994;35:445.
11. Wood EF, O'Brien RT, Young KM. Ultrasound-guided fine-needle aspiration of focal parenchymal lesions of the lung in dogs and cats. *J Vet Intern Med*. 1998;12:338.
12. Zekas LJ, Crawford JT, O'Brien RT. Computed tomography-guided fine-needle aspirate and tissue-core biopsy of intrathoracic lesions in thirty dogs and cats. *Vet Radiol Ultrasound*. 2005;46:200.
13. Menard M, Papageorges M. Ultrasound corner: technique for ultrasound-guided fine needle biopsies. *Vet Radiol Ultrasound*. 1995;36:137–138.
14. Papageorges M, et al. Ultrasound-guided fine-needle aspiration: an inexpensive modification of the technique. *Vet Radiol*. 1988;29:269.
15. Linta N, Baron Toaldo M, Bettini G, et al. The feasibility of contrast enhanced ultrasonography (CEUS) in the diagnosis of non-cardiac thoracic disorders of dogs and cats. *BMC Vet Res*. 2017;13:141.
16. Silvestri GA, Herth FJ, Keast T, et al. Feasibility and safety of bronchoscopic transparenchymal nodule access in canines: a new real-time image-guided approach to lung lesions. *Chest*. 2014;145:833.
17. Sterman DH, Keast T, Rai L, et al. High yield of bronchoscopic transparenchymal nodule access real-time image-guided sampling in a novel model of small pulmonary nodules in canines. *Chest*. 2015;147:700.
18. Bigge LA, Brown DJ, Penninck DG. Correlation between coagulation profile findings and bleeding complications after ultrasound-guided biopsies: 434 cases (1993–1996). *J Am Anim Hosp Assoc*. 2001;37:228.
19. Vignoli M, Rossi F, Chierici C, et al. Needle tract implantation after fine needle aspiration biopsy (FNAB) of transitional cell carcinoma of the urinary bladder and adenocarcinoma of the lung. *Schweiz Arch Tierheilkd*. 2007;149:314.
20. Bonfanti U, Bussadori C, Zatelli A, et al. Percutaneous fine-needle biopsy of deep thoracic and abdominal masses in dogs and cats. *J Small Anim Pract*. 2004;45:191.
21. DeBerry JD, Norris CR, Samii VF, et al. Correlation between fine-needle aspiration cytopathology and histopathology of the lung in dogs and cats. *J Am Anim Hosp Assoc*. 2002;38:327.
22. Cowell RL, et al. The lung and intrathoracic structures. In: Cowell RT, Tyler RD, Meinkoth JH, DeNicola D, eds. *Diagnostic Cytology and Hematology of The Dog and Cat*. 3rd ed. St. Louis, MO: Mosby; 2008.
23. Burkhard MJ, Millward LM. Respiratory tract. In: Raskin RE, Meyer DJ, eds. *Canine and Feline Cytology: A Color Atlas and Interpretation Guide*. 2nd ed. St. Louis, MO: Saunders Elsevier; 2010.
24. Roudebush P, Green RA, Digilio KM. Percutaneous fine-needle aspiration biopsy of the lung in disseminated pulmonary disease. *J Am Anim Hosp Assoc*. 1981;17:109.
25. Jones DJ, et al. Endogenous lipid pneumonia in cats: 24 cases (1985–1998). *J Am Vet Med Assoc*. 2000;216:1437.
26. Raya AI, Fernandez-de Marco M, Nunez A, et al. Endogenous lipid pneumonia in a dog. *J Comp Pathol*. 2006;135:153.
27. Clercx C, Peeters D. Canine eosinophilic bronchopneumopathy. *Vet Clin North Am Small Anim Pract*. 2007;37:917.
28. Clercx C, Peeters D, Snaps F, et al. Eosinophilic bronchopneumopathy in dogs. *J Vet Intern Med*. 2000;14:282.
29. Calvert CA, et al. Pulmonary and disseminated eosinophilic granulomatosis in dogs. *J Am Anim Hosp Assoc*. 1988;24:311.
30. Von Rotz A, et al. Eosinophilic granulomatous pneumonia in a dog. *Vet Rec*. 1986;23:631.
31. Kepler D, Cole R, Lee-Fowler T, et al. Pulmonary pythiosis in a canine patient. *Vet Radiol Ultrasound*. 2017. https://doi.org/10.1111/vru.12516. [Epub ahead of print].
32. Sauve V, Drobatz KJ, Shokek AB, et al. Clinical course, diagnostic findings and necropsy diagnosis in dyspneic cats with primary pulmonary parenchymal disease: 15 cats (1996–2002). *J Vet Emerg Crit Care*. 2005;15:38.
33. Cohn L. Pulmonary parenchymal disease. In: Ettinger SJ, Feldman EC, eds. *Textbook of Veterinary Internal Medicine*. 7th ed. St. Louis, MO: Saunders; 2010.
34. Rufenacht S, Bogli-Stuber K, Bodmer T, et al. *Mycobacterium mycroti* infection in the cat: a case report, literature review and recent clinical experience. *J Feline Med Surg*. 2011;13:195.
35. Rodriguez-Tovar LE, Ramirez-Romero R, Valdez-Nava Y, et al. Combined distemper-adenoviral pneumonia in a dog. *Can Vet J*. 2007;48:632.
36. Crews LJ, Feeney DA, Jessen CR, et al. Utility of diagnostic tests for and medical treatment of pulmonary blastomycosis in dogs: 125 cases (1989–2006). *J Am Vet Med Assoc*. 2008;232:222.
37. Barron PM, Rose A. Cryptococcal pneumonia in a boxer without obvious extrapulmonary dissemination. *Aust Vet Pract*. 2008;38:108.
38. Graupmann-Kuzma A, Valentine BA, Shubitz LF, et al. Coccidioidomycosis in dogs and cats: a review. *J Am Anim Hosp Assoc*. 2008;44:226.
39. Kobayashi R, Tanaka F, Asai A, et al. First case report of histoplasmosis in a cat in Japan. *J Vet Med Sci*. 2009;71:1669.
40. Watson PJ, Wotton P, Eastwood J, et al. Immunoglobulin deficiency in Cavalier King Charles Spaniels with pneumocystis pneumonia. *J Vet Int Med*. 2006;20:523.

41. Schwartz IS, Kenyon C, Feng P, et al. 50 years of Emmonsia disease in humans: the dramatic emergence of a cluster of novel fungal pathogens. *PLoS Pathog.* 2015;11:11.
42. Emmon CW, Jellison WL. *Emmonsia crescens* sp. n. and adiaspiromycosis (haplomycosis) in mammals. *Ann N Y Sci.* 1960;89:91.
42a. Schwartz IS, Wiederhold NP, Hanson KE, et al. *Blastomyces helicus*, a new dimorphic fungus causing fatal pulmonary and systemic disease in humans and animals in Western Canada and the United States. *Clin Infect Dis.* 2019;68:188.
43. Harkin KR. Aspergillosis: an overview in dogs and cats. *Vet Med.* 2003;98:602.
44. Dubey JP, Carpenter JL. Histologically confirmed clinical toxoplasmosis in cats: 100 cases (1952–1990). *J Am Vet Med Assoc.* 1993;203:1556.
45. Snider TA, Confer AW, Payton ME. Pulmonary histopathology of Cytauxzoon felis infections in the cat. *Vet Pathol.* 2010;47:698.
46. Meinkoth JH, Kocan AA. Feline cytauxzoonosis. *Vet Clin North Am Small Anim Pract.* 2005;35:89.
47. Greene CE, Howerth EW, Kent M. Nonenteric amebiasis: acanthamebiasis, hartmannelliasis, and balamuthiasis. In: Greene CE, ed. *Infectious Diseases of The Dog and Cat.* 3rd ed. St. Louis, MO: Saunders; 2006.
48. Palic J, Busch K, Unterer S. What is your diagnosis? Fine-needle aspirate of a lung nodule and bronchoalveolar lavage from a dog. *Vet Clin Pathol.* 2017;46:533.
49. Kuseeit D. Neoplasia tumor and biology. In: Zachary JF, McGavin MD, eds. *Pathologic Basis of Veterinary Disease.* 5th ed. St. Louis, MO: Mosby; 2012.
50. Ogilvie GK, Haschek WM, Withrow SJ, et al. Classification of primary lung tumors in dogs: 210 cases (1975–1985). *J Am Vet Med Assoc.* 1989;195:106.
51. Reichle JK, Wisner ER. Non-cardiac thoracic ultrasound in 75 feline and canine patients. *Vet Radiol Ultrasound.* 2000;41:154.
52. Wilson DW, Dungworth DL. Tumors of the respiratory tract. In: Meuten DJ, ed. *Tumors in Domestic Animals.* 4th ed. Ames, IA: Iowa State Press, Blackwell Publishing; 2002.
53. Affolter VK, Moore PF. Localized and disseminated histiocytic sarcoma of dendritic cell origin in dogs. *Vet Pathol.* 2002;39:74.
54. Bain PJ, et al. An 18-month-old spayed female boxer dog: lymphomatoid granulomatosis. *Vet Clin Pathol.* 1997;26(55).
55. Berry CR, Moore PF, Thomas WP, et al. Pulmonary lymphomatoid granulomatosis in 7 dogs (1976–1987). *J Vet Intern Med.* 1990;4:157.
56. Choi US, Alleman AR, Choi JH, et al. Cytologic and immunohistochemical characterization of a lung carcinoid in a dog. *Vet Clin Pathol.* 2008;37:249.
57. Lopez A. Respiratory system, mediastinum, and pleurae. In: Zachary JF, McGavin MD, eds. *Pathologic Basis of Veterinary Disease.* 5th ed. St. Louis, MO: Mosby; 2012.
58. Norris AJ, Naydan DK, Wilson DW. Interstitial lung disease in West Highland White Terriers. *Vet Pathol.* 2005;42:35.
59. *Dorland's Illustrated Medical Dictionary.* 27th ed. Philadelphia: W.B. Saunders; 1988.
60. Zachary JF, McGavin MD. Diseases of white blood cells, lymph nodes, and thymus. In: Zachary JG, McGavin MD, eds. *Pathologic Basis of Veterinary Disease.* 5th ed. St. Louis, MO: Elsevier; 2012.
61. Pintore L, Bertazzolo W, Bonfanti U, et al. Cytological and histological correlation in diagnosing feline and canine mediastinal masses. *J Small Anim Pract.* 2014;55:28.
62. Lana S, Plaza S, Hampe K, et al. Diagnosis of mediastinal masses in dogs by flow cytometry. *J Vet Intern Med.* 2006;20:1161.
63. Day MJ. Review of thymic pathology in 30 cats and 36 dogs. *J Small Anim Pract.* 1997;38:393.
64. Atwater SW, Powers BE, Park RD, et al. Thymoma in dogs: 23 cases (1980–1991). *J Am Vet Med Assoc.* 1994;205:1007.
65. Zitz JC, Birchard SJ, Couto GC, et al. Results of excision of thymoma in cats and dogs: 20 cases (1984–2005). *J Am Vet Med Assoc.* 2008;232:1186.
66. Newman AJ. Cysts of branchial arch origin in the thymus of the Beagle. *J Small Anim Pract.* 1971;12:681.
67. Liu S, Patnaik AK, Burk RL. Thymic branchial cysts in the dog and cat. *J Am Vet Med Assoc.* 1983;182:1095.
68. Parnell PG, Andreasen CB. What is your diagnosis? Cranial mediastinal mass from a dog. *Vet Clin Pathol.* 1992;21:9.
69. Levien AS, Summers BA, Szladovits B, et al. Transformation of a thymic branchial cyst to a carcinoma with pulmonary metastasis in a dog. *J Small Anim Pract.* 2010;51:604.
70. Uchida K, Awamura Y, Nakamura T, et al. Thymoma and multiple thymic cysts in a dog with acquired myasthenia gravis. *J Vet Med Sci.* 2002;64:637.
71. Rickman BH, Gurfield N. Thymic cystic degeneration, pseudoepitheliomatous hyperplasia, and hemorrhage in a dog with brodifacoum toxicosis. *Vet Pathol.* 2009;46:449.
72. Aronsohn MG, et al. Clinical and pathologic features of thymoma in 15 dogs. *J Am Vet Med Assoc.* 1984;184:1355.
73. Vilafranca M, Font A. Thymolipoma in a cat. *J Feline Med Surg.* 2005;7:125.
74. Morini M, Bettini G, Diana A, et al. Thymofibrolipoma in two dogs. *J Comp Pathol.* 2009;141:74.
75. Powe J, Castleman W, Fiorello C. A thymic carcinoid in a Bengal tiger (*Panthera tigris*). *J Zoo Wildl Med.* 2005;36:531.
76. Anilkumar TV, Voigt RP, Quigley PJ, et al. Squamous cell carcinoma of the feline thymus with widespread apoptosis. *Res Vet Sci.* 1994;56:208.
77. Carpenter JL, Valentine BA. Squamous cell carcinoma arising in two feline thymomas. *Vet Pathol.* 1992;29:541.
78. Hinrichs U, Puhl S, Rutteman GR, et al. Lymphangiosarcomas in cats: a retrospective study of 12 cases. *Vet Pathol.* 1999;36:164.
79. Ploemen JP, Ravesloot WT, van Esch E. The incidence of thymic B lymphoid follicles in healthy beagle dogs. *Toxicol Pathol.* 2003;31:214.
80. Liggett AD, Thompson LJ, Frazier KS, et al. Thymic hematoma in juvenile dogs associated with anticoagulant rodenticide toxicosis. *J Vet Diagn Invest.* 2002;14:416.
81. Van der Linde-Sipman JS, van Dijk JE. Hematomas in the thymus in dogs. *Vet Pathol.* 1987;24:59.
82. Faisca P, Henriques J, Dias TM, et al. Ectopic cervical thymic carcinoma in a dog. *J Small Anim Pract.* 2011;52:266.
83. Lara-Garcia A, Wellman M, Burkhard MJ, et al. Cervical thymoma originating in ectopic thymic tissue in a cat. *Vet Clin Pathol.* 2008;37:397.
84. Okumura M, Fujii Y, Shiono H, et al. Immunological function of thymoma and pathogenesis of paraneoplastic myasthenia gravis. *Gen Thorac Cardiovasc Surg.* 2008;56:143.
85. Dell'Orco M, Bertazzolo W, Caniatti M, et al. Cytological features of 11 cases of canine and feline thymoma and correlation with a human histologic classification. *Veterinaria (Cremona).* 2008;22:23.
86. Rae CA, Jacobs RM, Couto CG. A comparison between the cytological and histological characteristics in thirteen canine and feline thymomas. *Can Vet J.* 1989;30:497.
87. Ströbel P, et al. Thymoma and thymic carcinoma: an update of the WHO Classification 2004. *Surg Today.* 2005;35:805.
88. Andreasen CB, Mahaffey EA, Latimer KS. What is your diagnosis? Mediastinal mass aspirate from a 10-year-old dog. *Vet Clin Pathol.* 1991;20:15.
89. Kadhim AL, et al. Pearls and pitfalls in the management of branchial cyst. *J Laryngol Otol.* 2004;118:946.
90. Zekas LJ, Adams WM. Cranial mediastinal cysts in nine cats. *Vet Radiol Ultrasound.* 2002;43:413.
91. Swainson SW, et al. Radiographic diagnosis: mediastinal parathyroid cyst in a cat. *Vet Radiol Ultrasound.* 2000;41:41.
92. Miller M, Evans H, eds. *Miller's Anatomy of the Dog.* 3rd ed. Philadelphia, PA: Saunders; 1993.
93. Zimmerman KL, et al. Mediastinal mass in a dog with syncope and abdominal distension. *Vet Clin Pathol.* 2000;29:19.
94. Caruso KJ, Cowell RL, Upton ML, et al. Intrathoracic mass in a cat. *Vet Clin Pathol.* 2002;31:193.
95. Patnaik AK, MacEwen EG, Erlandson RA, et al. Mediastinal parathyroid adenocarcinoma in a dog. *Vet Pathol.* 1978;15:55.
96. Messick JB, Radin MJ. Cytologic, histologic, and ultrastructural characteristics of a canine myxoid liposarcoma. *Vet Pathol.* 1989;26:520.
97. Woolfson JM, Dulisch ML, Tams TR. Intrathoracic lipoma in a dog. *J Am Vet Med Assoc.* 1984;185:1007.

98. Kohn B, Arnold P, Kaser-Hotz B, et al. Malignant histiocytosis of the dog: 26 cases (1989–1992). *Kleintierpraxis*. 1993;38:409.

99. Walton RM, Brown DE, Burkhard MJ, et al. Malignant histiocytosis in a domestic cat: cytomorphologic and immunohistochemical features. *Vet Clin Pathol*. 1997;26:56.

100. Cohen JA, Bulmer BJ, Patton KM, Sisson DD. Aortic dissection associated with an obstructive aortic chondrosarcoma in a dog. *J Vet Cardiol*. 2010;12:203.

101. Mellanby RJ, Holloway A, Woodger N, et al. Primary chondrosarcoma in the pulmonary artery of a dog. *Vet Radiol Ultrasound*. 2003;44:315.

102. Fews D, Scase TJ, Battersby IA. Leiomyosarcoma of the pericardium, with epicardial metastases and peripheral eosinophilia in a dog. *J Comp Pathol*. 2008;138:224.

103. Rollois M, Ruel Y, Besso JG. Passive liver congestion associated with caudal vena caval compression due to oesophageal leiomyoma. *J Small Anim Pract*. 2003;44:460.

104. Boulineau TM, Andrews-Jones L, Van Alstine W. Spontaneous aortic dissecting hematoma in two dogs. *J Vet Diagn Invest*. 2005;17:492.

105. Van der Merwe LL, Kirberger RM, Clift S, et al. Spirocerca lupi infection in the dog: a review. *Vet J*. 2008;176:294.

106. Mylonakis ME, Rallis T, Koutinas AF, et al. Clinical signs and clinico-pathologic abnormalities in dogs with clinical spirocercosis: 39 cases (1996–2004). *J Am Vet Med Assoc*. 2006;228:1063.

107. De Lorenzi D, Furlanello T. What is your diagnosis? Esophageal nodules in a dog. *Vet Clin Pathol*. 2010;39:391.

108. Ranen E, Lavy E, Aizenberg I, et al. Spirocercosis-associated esophageal sarcomas in dogs: a retrospective study of 17 cases (1997–2003). *Vet Parasitol*. 2004;119:209.

109. Aulakh KS, et al. What is your diagnosis? A large soft tissue mass measuring approximately 15 X 12 X 13 cm is present in the caudodorsal aspect of the thorax, just right of midline, extending from the tracheal bifurcation to the diaphragm. *J Am Vet Med Assoc*. 2011;238:699.

110. Magstadt D, Fales-Williams A, Palerma J, et al. Severe disseminated necrotizing and granulomatous lymphadenitis and encephalitis in a dog due to *Sporotrichum pruinosum* (Teleomorph: *Phanerochaete chrysosporium*). *Vet Pathol*. 2018;55:298.

111. Meadows RL, et al. Chylothorax associated with cryptococcal mediastinal granuloma in a cat. *Vet Clin Pathol*. 1993;22:109.

112. Schmiedt C, Kellum H, Legendre AM, et al. Cardiovascular involvement in 8 dogs with *Blastomyces dermatitidis* infection. *J Vet Intern Med*. 2006;20:1351.

113. Nakagawa Y, Mochizuki R, Iwasaki K, et al. A canine case of profound granulomatosis due to *Paecillomyces* fungus. *J Vet Med Sci*. 1996;58:157.

114. Wood GL, Hirsh DC, Selcer RR, et al. Disseminated aspergillosis in a dog. *J Am Vet Med Assoc*. 1978;172:704.

115. Saunders GK, Monroe WE. Systemic granulomatous disease and sialometaplasia in a dog with *Bartonella* infection. *Vet Pathol*. 2006;43:391.

116. Grooters AM, Hodgin EC, Bauer RW, et al. Clinicopathologic findings associated with *Lagenidium* sp. infection in 6 dogs: initial description of an emerging oomycosis. *J Vet Intern Med*. 2003;17:637.

117. Liptak JM, Kamstock DA, Dernell WS, et al. Oncologic outcome after curative-intent treatment in 39 dogs with primary chest wall tumors (1992–2005). *Vet Surg*. 2008;37:488.

118. Halfacree ZJ, Baines SJ, Lipscomb VJ, et al. Use of a latissimus dorsi myocutaneous flap for one-stage reconstruction of the thoracic wall after en bloc resection of primary rib chondrosarcoma in five dogs. *Vet Surg*. 2007;36:587.

119. Baines SJ, Lewis S, White RA. Primary thoracic wall tumours of mesenchymal origin in dogs: a retrospective study of 46 cases. *Vet Rec*. 2002;150:335.

120. Matthiesen DT, Clark GN, Orsher RJ, et al. En bloc resection of primary rib tumors in 40 dogs. *Vet Surg*. 1992;21:201.

121. Feeney DA, Johnston GR, Grindem CB, et al. Malignant neoplasia of canine ribs: clinical, radiographic, and pathologic findings. *J Am Vet Med Assoc*. 1982;180:927.

122. Dhaliwal RS, Lacey JK. Ectopic hepatic parenchyma attached to the diaphragm: simulating a pulmonary mass in a cat. *J Am Anim Hosp Assoc*. 2009;45:39.

18

The Gastrointestinal Tract

Jamie L. Haddad, Devorah A. Marks Stowe, and Jennifer A. Neel

The gastrointestinal (GI) tract is an endoderm-derived structure, consisting of the esophagus, stomach, small intestine, and large intestine. Although the primary purpose of the GI tract is the digestion and absorption of food, it also has important secondary roles, including immune functions, elimination of waste products, and endocrine effects. As such, diseases of the GI tract are a major cause of morbidity and mortality in companion animals and include a wide variety of conditions, such as infectious diseases, neoplasia and other mass lesions, motility disorders, congenital disorders, and effects of medications. This chapter will focus on diseases and conditions of the GI tract that can be diagnosed via cytological examination of various sample types. The discussion will include sampling techniques, normal findings, and common or important diagnostic dilemmas and introduce important aspects of histopathology of the GI tract. Because infectious organisms are an important cause of GI disease and will be discussed throughout the chapter, a detailed description of the most common organisms, their location within the GI tract, and additional useful diagnostic testing may be found in Table 18.1.[1-3]

SAMPLING TECHNIQUES FOR THE GASTROINTESTINAL TRACT

When evaluating a patient for GI conditions, it is important to rule out diseases of other organs, such as the liver, pancreas, kidneys, and adrenal glands, which may cause secondary GI disease or overlapping clinical signs. Once sampling of the GI tract is determined to be appropriate, several methods are used for obtaining cytological and histological samples, including ultrasound-guided aspirates or tissue biopsies; those from endoscopy, laparoscopy, or direct sampling during abdominal exploratory surgery; rectal scrapings; and examination of fecal material.

Ultrasound-Guided Sampling

Ultrasonography is commonly used to evaluate the intestinal tract in dogs and cats and is often used to obtain aspirates and, less commonly, tissue biopsy samples. Ultrasonographic evaluation is very helpful in aiding the diagnosis of GI diseases, particularly infiltrative GI neoplasia. It is important to note, however, that ultrasonography is not entirely specific and that overlap exists between the ultrasonographic appearance of neoplastic and nonneoplastic diseases.[4] Cytology from aspiration of the wall of the GI tract usually has a low yield unless a significant lesion, mass effect, or increased wall thickness is present. Ultrasound-guided aspiration has the advantage of being less invasive and less expensive than obtaining endoscopic or full-thickness biopsies; however, depending on the type of lesion, it may not be of as high of a diagnostic yield.

Endoscopy

Endoscopy is a well-established procedure for examining the GI tract and serves as an important alternative to exploratory surgery for direct examination of tissues and anatomy. It is minimally invasive and allows for visualization and sample collection of the luminal surface of the esophagus, stomach, proximal and distal small intestine (duodenum and ileum, respectively), and distal large intestine.[5] Access to the remainder of the intestinal tract (and, in particular, the jejunum) is limited or impossible during an endoscopic procedure. Endoscopic mucosal brushing and endoscopic biopsies are the main sample types that are collected during this procedure and predominantly evaluate the mucosal surface. Squash preparations for cytological evaluation may be performed by using endoscopic samples and may provide diagnostic information.[6,7] In general, although endoscopic samples are useful for detecting surface or mucosal inflammation and mucosal neoplasia, lesions that are deep to the mucosal surface may not be identified with this modality.

Laparoscopy and Abdominal Exploration

Laparoscopy is an operative procedure that is performed through a keyhole opening with a rigid endoscope. It allows for visual inspection of the organs and, in specialized settings, may allow for laparoscopy-assisted full-thickness biopsies of the GI tract. Abdominal exploration is a more invasive surgical procedure that is often used to obtain full-thickness biopsy samples of the GI tract. Although this procedure is more invasive, full-thickness biopsies may provide the best opportunity for obtaining a definitive diagnosis, particularly in cases where the lesion is more prominently within the deeper layers of the stomach or the intestinal wall. In addition, the generally larger biopsy size obtained via these techniques may provide an easier opportunity to make touch imprints of the tissue for cytology, before placing the sample in formalin. Cytological evaluation of touch imprints may provide a preliminary or definitive diagnosis before histopathology results are available. In some cases, such as with mast cell tumor or granulated lymphoma, cytological evaluation may provide cellular details that are not as readily apparent with histopathology of a biopsy sample. Although care must be taken to preserve the integrity of the biopsy sample, it is important to gently wipe or blot blood and serum off the tissue before making the touch imprints to achieve proper adhesion of the cells to the slide. It is also possible to make touch imprints or squash preparations of ultrasound-guided or endoscopically obtained tissue biopsies, but the smaller size and greater fragility of these types of samples make this more difficult and may increase the risk for damage to the tissue.

Text continued on p. 294

TABLE 18.1   Infectious Agents of the Gastrointestinal Tract

Category	Organism	Cytological Description	Common Location for Diagnosis	Additional Diagnostic Tests (if applicable)
Bacteria: spirochetes	*Helicobacter* spp.	Gram-negative, motile; "S" shape to corkscrew appearance	Stomach	Culture and isolation; rapid urease test, using a biopsy sample and special media; urea breath test (humans and research animals)
	Campylobacter spp.	Gram-negative; distinct gull-wing appearance	Feces	Culture; polymerase chain reaction (PCR)
Bacteria: spore-forming bacilli	*Clostridium perfringens*[a]	Gram-positive large rod with a central to terminal spore that gives the organism a "safety pin" appearance	Feces	Fecal enterotoxin immuno-detection with enzyme-linked immunosorbent assay (ELISA) or reverse passive latex agglutination, PCR

TABLE 18.1   Infectious Agents of the Gastrointestinal Tract—cont'd

Category	Organism	Cytological Description	Common Location for Diagnosis	Additional Diagnostic Tests (if applicable)
Fungi	*Candida* spp. 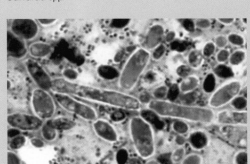	Yeast (3–6 micrometers [μm] basophilic round to oval or elongated, clear cell wall, basophilic interior), pseudo-hyphae (chains of elongated yeast that remain attached end to end), true hyphae (well-septated 3–5 μm wide structures with parallel walls, occasional branching)	Stomach, intestine	Fungal culture, PCR (limited availability)
	Cryptococcus neoformans 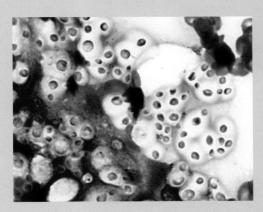	Extracellular 5–25 μm yeast with a refractile cell wall, wide nonstaining to poorly staining capsule, narrow-based budding and often a folded appearance	Intestine	Mayer mucicarmine staining to highlight the capsule; fungal culture; cryptococcal polysaccharide capsular antigen detection using latex agglutination; PCR
	Histoplasma capsulatum 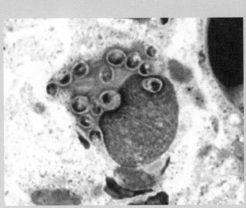	Intracellular 2–4 μm round yeast organisms with a clear cell wall and a "half empty, half full" interior appearance; multiple organisms within macrophages	Large intestine, feces	Fungal culture; antigen detection assay; PCR

Continued

TABLE 18.1   Infectious Agents of the Gastrointestinal Tract—cont'd

Category	Organism	Cytological Description	Common Location for Diagnosis	Additional Diagnostic Tests (if applicable)
	Cyniclomyces guttulatus 	Individual or short branching or forking chains of cylindrical yeast, 5–7 × 15–20 μm in size, with a clear cell wall and an interior that stains uniformly purple, mottled or vacuolated, or has a broad, transverse, poorly staining central region	Feces	
Protozoa	*Cryptosporidium parvum*[b] 	Small, 2- to 4-μm oocysts or trophozoites on the surface of enterocytes, often with a stippled appearance with Romanowsky stains; typically only oocysts are seen in feces	Feces	Acid-fast staining (organisms stain red-pink), direct fluorescence antibody detection, PCR, concentration techniques, such as Sheather sucrose flotation, zinc sulfate flotation, saturated sodium chlorine methods
	Giardia spp.[a] 	Pear-shaped, flagellated (four pairs: one anterior, two posterior, one caudal) trophozoites, 15–10 μm in length, "smiling face" appearance formed by two anterior nuclei, a longitudinal axoneme running between them and a transverse median body situated in the posterior portion of the cell	Feces	Multiple fecal examinations may be required (shed intermittently), ELISA (IDEXX SNAP *Giardia* antigen detection test), PCR, zinc sulfate centrifugation float, direct fluorescent antibody test

TABLE 18.1	**Infectious Agents of the Gastrointestinal Tract—cont'd**			
Category	Organism	Cytological Description	Common Location for Diagnosis	Additional Diagnostic Tests (if applicable)
	Entamoeba histolytica	Large (12–50 μm) round to oval trophozoites with a small round, eccentrically placed nucleus with evenly distributed peripheral chromatin, a central compact karyosome and baso-philic cytoplasm, with possible phagocytosis of red blood cells (RBCs)	Large intestine, feces	Trichrome or iron-hematoxylin stained fecal smears, methylene blue, specific culture media is available
	Pentatrichomonas hominis	Spindle- to pear-shaped, highly motile, flagellated organism with five anteriorly directed flagella and a single posteriorly directed flagellum, and an undulating membrane	Feces	PCR
	Tritrichomonas fetus	Oval to pear-shaped, 5–20 × 3–14 μm, highly motile, flagellated organism with three anteriorly directed flagella, a single posteriorly directed flagellum, an undulating mem-brane, oval anterior nucleus, and an axostyle protruding from the posterior end	Large intestine, feces	Culture using the InPouch TF test (Biomed Diagnos-tics, White City, OR), PCR

Continued

TABLE 18.1   Infectious Agents of the Gastrointestinal Tract—cont'd

Category	Organism	Cytological Description	Common Location for Diagnosis	Additional Diagnostic Tests (if applicable)
Algae	*Prototheca* spp.	Oval algal organisms with granular basophilic to magenta internal structure surrounded by a clear capsule ("jelly bean" appearance) with internal endosporulation	Large intestine, feces	Culture
Oomycete	*Pythium insidiosum*	Wide, nonstaining to poorly staining, occasionally branching, hyphal-like structures with parallel cell walls and infrequent septation	Stomach, small intestine, and ileocolic junction	Culture, serology, PCR

[a]Image courtesy Rick Cowell.
[b]Slide courtesy Jody Gookin.
From Broussard JD. Optimal fecal assessment. *Clin Tech Small Anim Pract.* 2003;18:218; Greene CE. *Infectious Diseases of the Dog and Cat.* 4th ed. St. Louis, MO: Saunders; 2012; Marks SL, Rankin SC, Byrne BA, et al. Enteropathogenic bacteria in dogs and cats: diagnosis, epidemiology, treatment, and control. *J Vet Int Med.* 2011;25:1195.

Fecal Examination

Fecal testing is a common diagnostic procedure in the clinical evaluation of GI disease. Timing of sample collection and preparation is very important. Feces are altered after stool is passed, and significant degeneration of cells and some organisms, such as *Giardia* spp. or *Tritrichomonas fetus*, can occur rapidly, making identification increasingly difficult with time (Fig. 18.1).[1] If processing of the fecal sample is delayed, some nematode eggs will release larvae, and bacterial overgrowth may occur. Processing of a fresh sample immediately is best.

Several collection techniques are used for either the luminal contents or the surface mucosa of the rectum. Defecated feces and feces obtained during a digital rectal examination or with a fecal loop represent the rectal lumen, whereas rectal lavage or rectal scrape samples are representative of the mucosal surface. If defecated feces are used, it is critical that they be fresh and not heavily contaminated with debris. Additional fecal diagnostics include fecal flotation, fecal sedimentation, and the Baermann technique. Consultation of a veterinary parasitology text is recommended for additional information about these techniques.

When sampling feces or the rectal mucosa, lubricant gel should be used sparingly or avoided entirely because the lubricant material could complicate evaluation of the cytological specimen. Cytologically, lubricant has the appearance of thick extracellular magenta aggregates of material that may obscure the cells and organisms within the sample (Fig. 18.2).

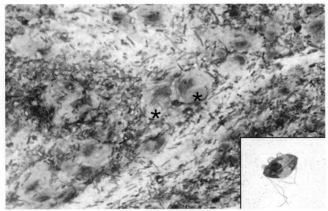

Fig. 18.1 Feline fecal smear; degenerating *Tritrichomonas fetus* organisms. Many degenerating organisms are present *(two are indicated by asterisks [*])* on a background of fecal material. The degenerating trophozoites are large round structures with round, dark, basophilic nuclei and an abundant amount of light basophilic cytoplasm. These could easily be mistaken for debris, degenerating tissue cells, or histiocytes. *Tritrichomonas* degenerates quickly on exiting the body; thus it is imperative that smears or wet mount preparations be made with fresh feces. The inset image is of a cytology preparation made from cultured *T. fetus* trophozoites. Typical morphological features may be seen, including three anterior flagella, an undulating membrane, a longitudinal axostyle, an anterior nucleus, and a single posterior flagellum (modified Wright-Giemsa stain, original magnification 50× objective. *Inset:* Wright-Giemsa stain, original magnification 100× objective). (*Tritrichomonas* culture courtesy Katie Tolbert.)

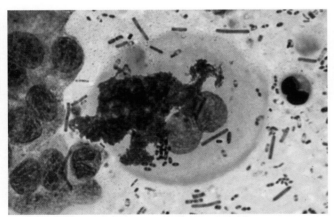

Fig. 18.2 Fecal sample from a dog; abundant lubricant gel. Few columnar epithelial cells are present at the left of the image with two squamous epithelial cells in the center. The morphological characteristics of the squamous epithelial cells are partially obscured by bright pink–magenta granular to globular lubricant material (Wright-Leishman stain).

Direct Smears of Fecal Material

Direct smears from a luminal sample are made by spreading a small amount of feces thinly and evenly across the slide. The sample should not be heat-fixed; it is unnecessary and could cause significant damage to cells and organisms.[1] After air-drying, the slide may be stained with a standard Romanowsky-type stain (e.g., Wright stain, Giemsa stain, rapid stains) and evaluated like any cytological sample. If using a rapid stain (e.g., Diff-Quik), it is recommended that a separate "dirty" staining station be set up for fecal and ear cytology so as to not contaminate the station where "clean" cytology and hematology samples are stained.

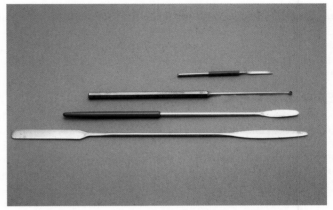

Fig. 18.3 Various instruments used to perform rectal mucosal scrapings include *(top to bottom)* a conjunctival scraper, an ear curette, and two blunt chemistry spatulas.

Rectal Lavage

To perform rectal lavage, the end of a lubricated red rubber catheter is inserted into the rectum and approximately 6 to 12 milliliters (mL) of saline is infused and aspirated multiple times until the sample has a mudlike appearance.[1] Rectal lavage yields a small sample but allows the sample to be directly examined as an unstained wet mount preparation rather than as a stained dry fecal smear.

Rectal Scraping

To obtain a sample via rectal scraping, the rectum is cleaned of feces; use of lubricant gel is minimized or avoided; and a rigid instrument, such as a conjunctival scraper or chemistry spatula, is used to obtain the specimen (Box 18.1 and Fig. 18.3). The sample should be obtained cranially enough to reach the rectum, avoiding sampling of the anal mucosa. Pressure should be applied firmly enough to sample the mucosa, rather than just the surface material, while care is taken to not perforate the rectal wall. Slides are prepared, dried, and stained in a manner similar to the process for a fecal smear.

ESOPHAGUS

Normal Esophagus

The esophagus consists of the mucosal epithelium, the submucosa, and the muscular wall. The esophageal mucosa is lined by nonkeratinizing stratified squamous epithelium. Submucosal mucous glands are present throughout the esophagus in the dog and are located only at the pharyngeal–esophageal junction in the cat.[8]

Cells from multiple layers of the squamous epithelium may be identified in cytological specimens (Fig. 18.4). Progressing from the superficial layer to the deep layer, superficial squamous cells are angular with a pyknotic to absent nucleus, intermediate cells are somewhat angular with a larger nucleus, and deep intermediate and parabasal cells have a smaller volume of more deeply basophilic cytoplasm with rounded borders.[9] Cytology of normal esophageal brushings and washings consists of predominantly intermediate squamous cells with occasional superficial squamous cells. Cells from the deeper layers, including deep intermediate cells, parabasal cells, and rarely submucosal glandular epithelial cells, may also be seen cytologically, depending on the aggressiveness of the sampling technique, but this finding is typically an indicator of disease.[10] Oropharyngeal contamination may be seen in normal or abnormal esophageal samples and may consist of a mixed bacterial population, including *Simonsiella* spp. and, rarely, respiratory epithelial cells. *Simonsiella* organisms are gram-negative, large (6–8 micrometers [μm] long and 2–3 μm wide), rod-shaped bacteria with a distinctive cytological appearance because of their barcode-like or stacked-disk arrangement.

Esophageal Inflammation

Esophagitis occurs with injury to the esophageal mucosa as a result of a variety of underlying causes, including foreign bodies, infectious etiologies, and mucosal irritants (Box 18.2). Although esophagitis often has an erosive or ulcerative component, lack of a discernible superficial lesion at endoscopy does not rule out underlying esophagitis.

In addition to ingestion of substances damaging to the esophageal mucosa, an important cause of esophagitis with mucosal injury is reflux esophagitis. This condition, which is most common in the distal esophagus, results from the effect of gastric acid, pepsin, and possibly bile salts and pancreatic enzymes on the esophageal mucosa.[11] Reflux of these substances into the esophagus may occur with relaxation of the lower esophageal sphincter under anesthesia, a hiatal hernia, or chronic vomiting.[12] In addition to esophageal inflammation, a possible sequela of gastroesophageal reflux is metaplasia of the distal esophageal stratified squamous epithelium to a more acid-friendly simple columnar epithelium with interspersed goblet cells (Fig. 18.5). This lesion has been reported in dogs and cats; grossly or endoscopically, the appearance may range from a region of hyperemia to a polypoid mass, which could be mistaken for neoplasia (Table 18.2).[13] In humans, this condition is known as *Barrett esophagus*, and the lesion may progress and transform into a distal esophageal adenocarcinoma.

Cytological findings with esophagitis are typically nonspecific, with the presence of neutrophils amid the squamous epithelial cells. Eosinophils in esophageal cytology may occur with neoplastic, parasitical, or fungal disease; with reflux esophagitis; as a part of eosinophilic gastroenteritis; or with eosinophilic esophagitis (Fig. 18.6). Eosinophilic esophagitis has been reported in dogs, may be associated with allergic skin disease, and is a diagnosis of exclusion after eliminating the aforementioned causes of eosinophils within an esophageal sample.[14]

Pyogranulomatous esophagitis may occur with pythiosis in dogs (see "Gastric Inflammation"). *Spirocerca lupi* infection causes a mass-like granulomatous lesion in the distal esophagus of dogs because of the presence of adult nematodes in the esophageal submucosa.

BOX 18.2 Causes of Esophagitis

- Foreign body
- Irritant (caustic agent, medication lodged)
- Thermal injury (radiation, hot ingesta)
- Gastroesophageal reflux
- Eosinophilic esophagitis
- Infectious etiology
- Neoplasia

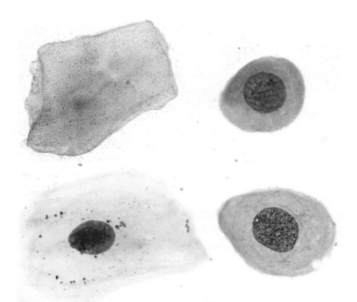

Fig. 18.4 Esophageal brushings from normal dogs; various stages of esophageal squamous cells. *Beginning at the top right and moving clockwise:* A parabasal cell, a deep intermediate cell, an intermediate cell, and a superficial cell. Intermediate cells are most numerous in normal esophageal samples and, compared with superficial cells, are characterized by a less angular shape, a similar amount abundant cytoplasm that is nonkeratinized and a round, medium-sized nucleus (Wright-Giemsa stain, original magnification 50× objective). (Slides courtesy Sally Bissett.)

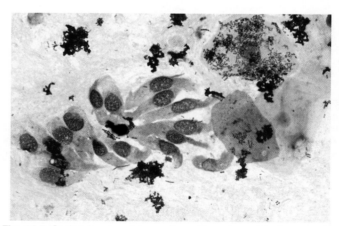

Fig. 18.5 Canine brush cytology of a midesophogeal lesion; esophageal metaplasia. The presence of uniform columnar epithelial cells *(left side of image)* indicates metaplasia has occurred. Note *(right side of the image)* the three superficial squamous epithelial cells with adhered bacteria and free bacteria in the background, indicating oropharyngeal contamination, and the small scattered clumps of magenta extracellular material consistent with lubricant gel. This pet was suffering from chronic vomiting (Wright-Giemsa stain, original magnification 50× objective).

Typically, a single mass is present in the caudal thoracic portion of the esophagus, occasionally with surface ulceration or protrusion of adult worms into the esophageal lumen. An association exists between spirocercosis and the subsequent development of esophageal fibrosarcoma or osteosarcoma.

Esophageal Neoplasia

Primary esophageal neoplasia, which is rare in dogs and cats, includes squamous cell carcinoma and smooth muscle tumors, with rare reports of adenocarcinoma, neuroendocrine carcinoma, primary extraskeletal osteosarcoma, or plasma cell neoplasia.[15,16] Fibrosarcoma and osteosarcoma are associated with *S. lupi* infection (see "Esophageal Inflammation"). Rarely, esophageal involvement of canine oral papillomavirus infection may occur.[15]

Squamous cell carcinoma arising from the esophageal mucosal epithelium typically appears as an ulcerated nondiscrete mass and may be confused with ulcerative esophagitis.[15] Cytologically, this tumor resembles squamous cell carcinoma elsewhere in the body and often will have superimposed inflammation or evidence of superficial infection. Esophageal adenocarcinoma is rare but may arise from the submucosal esophageal glands or from regions of glandular metaplasia, as with reflux esophagitis. Leiomyomas and leiomyosarcomas, which are smooth muscle tumors, may occur in the esophagus, particularly in dogs, and are most commonly found confined to the muscular wall in the distal esophagus.[16,17]

STOMACH

Normal Stomach

The stomach in dogs and cats is glandular and, from proximal to distal, contains cardiac, fundic, and pyloric regions. The layers of the stomach wall consist of the mucosa, muscularis mucosae, submucosa, and smooth muscle wall (tunica muscularis). The largest portion of the stomach is the fundus, which consists of a surface columnar foveolar epithelium with subjacent glandular cells, including parietal cells and chief cells, which secrete hydrochloric acid and pepsinogen, respectively (Fig. 18.7). The pyloric region consists of a similar surface foveolar epithelium with predominantly mucous glands in the deeper mucosa (see Fig. 18.7).

Normal gastric cytology usually consists of small to rarely large sheets of surface epithelium that have a characteristic honeycomb appearance (Fig. 18.8). These columnar cells have round to oval basally oriented nuclei with an abundant amount of finely vacuolated cytoplasm.[9] Parietal and chief cells may be seen in gastric cytology samples collected from brushing techniques that access the deeper mucosal tissue (see Fig. 18.7). Parietal cells have abundant granular eosinophilic to vacuolated cytoplasm, whereas chief cells have many well-staining basophilic cytoplasmic granules.[9,10] Particularly in the pyloric region, mucus-secreting cells may be identified in cytological samples (see Fig. 18.7).

Helicobacter spp. are spiral bacteria that are commonly identified in samples of the gastric surface of dogs and cats, often in close association with surface mucus (Fig. 18.9). The possible clinical significance of finding *Helicobacter* organisms in the stomach is discussed below (see "Gastric Inflammation"). Gastric samples may be easily contaminated by food material, or material from the oral cavity and esophagus, which is indicated by the presence of *Simonsiella* organisms and squamous epithelial cells. Ciliated columnar respiratory epithelium may be noted if the patient swallowed sputum, whereas red blood cells (RBCs) may be identified with traumatic sample collection and blood contamination.

Gastric Inflammation

Gastritis is a nonspecific finding that may occur with a variety of causes (Table 18.3).[18] Most cases in dogs and cats are likely a component of inflammatory bowel disease (IBD), which may have predominantly lymphoplasmacytic, eosinophilic, or, rarely, granulomatous inflammation, although the presence of inflammation is not specific for IBD. Normal endoscopic appearance of the gastric mucosa does not rule out underlying inflammation.

TABLE 18.2 Benign Nonneoplastic Lesions That May Be Confused With Neoplasia	
Organ	**Lesion**
Esophagus	Barrett esophagus (metaplasia resulting from reflux esophagitis)
	Parasitic granuloma (*Spirocerca lupi*)
Stomach	Gastric polyps
	Chronic hypertrophic gastropathy
	Chronic hypertrophic pyloric gastropathy
	Pyloric stenosis
	Granulomatous gastritis (pythiosis)
	Feline gastrointestinal eosinophilic sclerosing fibroplasia
	Idiopathic eosinophilic gastrointestinal masses
	Scirrous eosinophilic gastritis
Intestine	Granulomatous enteritis or colitis (histoplasmosis, pythiosis, feline infectious peritonitis, prototheecosis)
	Intestinal polyps
	Histiocytic ulcerative colitis of Boxers
	Feline gastrointestinal eosinophilic sclerosing fibroplasia
	Idiopathic eosinophilic gastrointestinal masses
	Anomalous cystic duct remnants

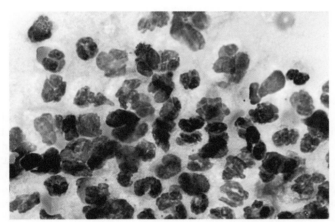

Fig. 18.6 Esophageal brushing from a dog; eosinophilic esophagitis. The sample has a mix of eosinophils and neutrophils on a background of mucus. Eosinophilic inflammation of the esophagus is not specific for the entity of eosinophilic esophagitis and other causes, such as neoplasia, parasitic or fungal disease, reflux esophagitis, and eosinophilic gastroenteritis, must be ruled out. In this case no improvement was seen after treatment with a proton pump inhibitor, but significant improvement occurred after corticosteroid administration (Wright Giemsa stain, original magnification 100× objective).

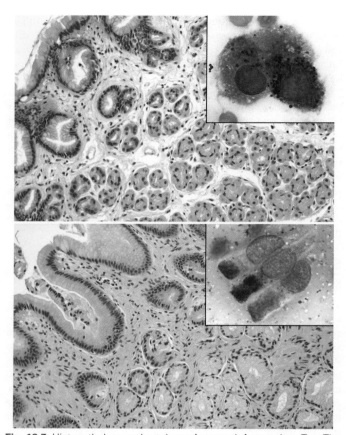

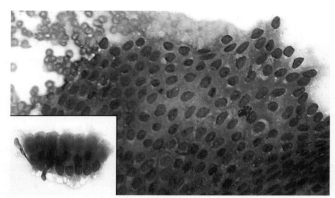

Fig. 18.8 Cytology of normal gastric epithelium. A large cluster of normal epithelium is present. Cells are uniform and have a honeycombed appearance within the cluster. The inset image is of a smaller cluster in which the columnar appearance of the cells can be appreciated. Cells are uniform with basilar oriented small round nuclei and abundant cytoplasm (modified Wright-Giemsa stain, original magnification 50× objective. *Inset:* Wright-Giemsa stain, original magnification 100× objective).

Fig. 18.7 Histopathology and cytology of stomach from a dog. *Top:* The mucosa of the fundus is covered by a simple columnar epithelium with vacuolated cytoplasm (foveolar epithelium) that invaginates to form gastric pits. Deeper within the mucosa, glandular structures are present, with an inner rim of cuboidal basophilic to vacuolated chief cells (pepsinogen-secreting cells) and an outer rim of round eosinophilic parietal cells (hydrochloric acid-secreting cells) (hematoxylin and eosin [H&E] stain, original magnification 20× objective). The inset of a cytological specimen has a chief cell with basophilic to purple cytoplasmic granules *(right)* and likely a parietal cell with pink cytoplasmic granules *(left)* (modified Wright stain, original magnification 100× objective). *Bottom:* The mucosa of the pylorus is covered by a similar epithelium to the fundus, but the deeper mucosa contains predominantly mucus-secreting glands lined by pale, highly vacuolated epithelial cells (H&E stain, original magnification 20× objective). The inset of a cytological specimen has few mucus-secreting columnar epithelial cells, which contain apical pink-magenta cytoplasmic mucus-containing granules (Wright-Giemsa stain, original magnification 100× objective).

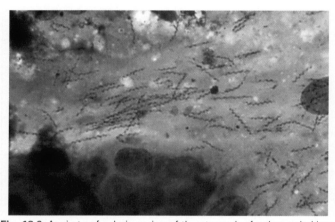

Fig. 18.9 Aspirate of pyloric region of the stomach of a dog; spiral bacteria consistent with *Helicobacter* spp. The S-shaped spiral bacteria are embedded in thick streaming clumps of mucus; note the gastric epithelial cells at the bottom of the image. The significance of this finding is unknown because *Helicobacter* spp. is commonly found in the stomachs of dogs and cats and may or may not be associated with inflammation (Wright-Giemsa stain, original magnification 50× objective).

Neutrophilic Inflammation

Neutrophilic inflammation in gastric samples may occur with a variety of lesions but is seen most often with gastric ulcers; for a more complete list of common causes, see Table 18.3. Ulcers in the stomach or proximal small intestine may occur as the result of mechanical or chemical irritation, drug administration, or hormone secretion (e.g., gastrin hypersecretion or histamine release). Ulceration caused by nonsteroidal antiinflammatory drugs (NSAIDs) is secondary to compromise of mucosal protective mechanisms, whereas with excess exogenous or endogenous corticosteroids, ulceration may be caused by reduced mucosal perfusion.[11] Uremic gastropathy is not typically an inflammatory lesion histologically but may cause gastric congestion, hemorrhage, and edema, possibly with ulceration, necrosis, and mineralization of the mucosa.[11]

Lymphoplasmacytic Inflammation

Lymphoplasmacytic gastritis is the most common histopathological finding in abnormal gastric biopsy samples from dogs and cats and has a variety of causes and disease associations, including IBD and hyperplastic, hypertrophic, or atrophic conditions, among others (Fig. 18.10).[19] For a more complete list of potential causes, see Table 18.3. Because of the potential for increased mucosal-associated lymphoid tissue (MALT) with underlying gastric disease, increased numbers of mixed lymphocytes may be identified in cytological samples with MALT hyperplasia, even in the absence of true lymphocytic gastritis.

Several hyperplastic or hypertrophic gastric conditions occur in dogs and cats (see Table 18.3). In addition to a potential lymphoplasmacytic inflammatory component, these conditions often have a component of mucosal epithelial proliferation, with or without thickening or muscular hypertrophy of the stomach wall; therefore, increased mucosal epithelium may be noted cytologically in these conditions. Because of their gross or endoscopic appearance as a diffuse or regional masslike thickening of portions of the stomach, these hyperplastic and

TABLE 18.3 Causes of Gastric Inflammation

Type of Inflammation	Disease Process	Potential Causes
Neutrophilic	Mechanical ulceration	Gastric foreign body, hairball
	Chemical gastritis	Ingestion of irritating plants or chemicals
	Gastric or gastrointestinal (GI) ulcers	Hypersecretion of acid (liver disease, gastrin-secreting tumor)
		Histamine release (mast cell tumor, medications, and hormones)
		Drug therapy (nonsteroidal antiinflammatory drugs [NSAIDs], corticosteroids)
		Sepsis, burns, hypoadrenocorticism, surgery
Lymphoplasmacytic	Inflammatory bowel disease	
	Hyperplastic or hypertrophic conditions	Benign gastric polyps
		Pyloric stenosis
		Chronic hypertrophic gastropathy of Drentsche Patrijshond and Basenji dogs
		Chronic hypertrophic pyloric gastropathy
	Atrophic conditions	Chronic atrophic gastritis of Norwegian Lundehund dogs
	Healing gastric ulcers	
	Helicobacter infection	
	Parasite infestation	*Physaloptera* and *Gnathostoma* in dogs and cats
		Ollulanus and *Cylicospirura* in cats
	Secondary to other conditions	Neoplasia
Eosinophilic	Inflammatory bowel disease	
	Allergy or hypersensitivity disorders	
	Neoplasia	Mast cell tumor, T-cell lymphoma
	Infectious agents	Pythiosis, parasitism, *Toxocara canis* larval migration
	Miscellaneous	Feline hypereosinophilic syndrome
		Feline gastrointestinal eosinophilic sclerosing fibroplasia
		Canine idiopathic eosinophilic gastrointestinal masses
		Scirrhous eosinophilic gastritis
Granulomatous	Infectious etiologies	Mycobacteriosis, histoplasmosis, pythiosis
	Inflammatory bowel disease	Rare

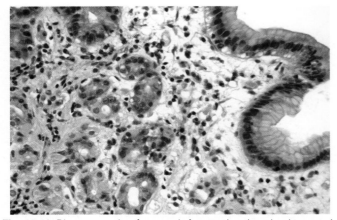

Fig. 18.10 Biopsy sample of stomach from a dog; lymphoplasmacytic gastritis as a component of inflammatory bowel disease. Within the lamina propria of the superficial gastric mucosa, increased numbers of lymphocytes and plasma cells are seen, with mild edema and increased connective tissue (hematoxylin and eosin [H&E] stain, original magnification 40× objective).

hypertrophic lesions may be confused with gastric adenocarcinoma (see Table 18.2).[15] For this reason, it is important to consider these benign conditions when increased mucosal epithelium is seen in cytology specimens.

Helicobacter spp. are highly prevalent spiral bacteria found in the stomach of dogs and cats; however, it is controversial whether a causal association exists between the presence of *Helicobacter* and the presence of gastritis in these species (see Fig. 18.9 and Table 18.1). In cats, an association seems to exist between *Helicobacter* and lymphoid follicle formation or epithelial proliferation in the stomach, and possible associations have been made between *Helicobacter* infection and gastric MALT lymphoma.[20,21] *Helicobacter* may be present in higher numbers and easier to identify in cytological specimens than in histological samples because of their presence in the surface mucus, which is readily sampled for cytological evaluation.

Eosinophilic Inflammation

Eosinophilic inflammation in stomach samples may occur as a component of IBD or with other diseases typically associated with eosinophils (see Table 18.3). Other conditions with predominance of eosinophils include feline GI eosinophilic sclerosing fibroplasia, idiopathic eosinophilic GI masses, and scirrhous eosinophilic gastritis. An important feature of these diseases is their tendency to form a thickened or masslike region in the stomach, giving the impression of neoplasia (see Table 18.2). Feline *gastrointestinal eosinophilic sclerosing fibroplasia* is a masslike lesion, occurring most commonly at the pyloric sphincter but also at the ileocecocolic junction, and it may also involve the mesenteric lymph nodes. Cytologically, this lesion has increased eosinophils, alone or in combination with large spindle cells amid pink, extracellular matrix, occasionally with neutrophils and intracellular and extracellular, rod-shaped or coccoid bacteria with fewer lymphocytes, plasma cells, and mast cells (Fig. 18.11).[22] The term *idiopathic eosinophilic gastrointestinal masses* (IEGMs) refers to a rare condition in dogs, with a predisposition in Rottweiler dogs, in which one or multiple mass lesions consisting of eosinophilic inflammation are present in the GI tract, with intervening eosinophil-free regions.[23] *Scirrhous eosinophilic gastritis* in dogs is a thickening of the gastric wall with granulation tissue and eosinophils.[15]

Granulomatous Inflammation

Granulomatous inflammation in stomach samples may occur with infectious etiologies, or, rarely, with IBD (see Table 18.3). Because granulomatous inflammation can cause a thickening of the gastric wall, these lesions may be mistaken for neoplasia grossly or endoscopically (see Table 18.2). *Pythiosis*, caused by the aquatic oomycete *Pythium insidiosum*, typically causes a transmural, masslike, obstructive or nonobstructive thickening most commonly in the stomach, small intestine, or ileocolic junction. Mesenteric lymph nodes are also commonly involved, and hypercalcemia may occur.[24] Cytologically, pyogranulomatous inflammation is seen along with eosinophils and nonstaining to poorly staining hyphal structures with fairly parallel 4 to 8 μm wide walls with infrequent septation (Fig. 18.12). Cytology alone cannot definitively distinguish among *Pythium*, *Lagenidium* (another aquatic oomycete), and zygomycete organisms (fungi); therefore, additional diagnostics such as culture or polymerase chain reaction (PCR) may be required (see Table 18.1). *Candida* spp. are typically opportunistic invaders of the mucosal epithelium in immunocompromised patients. This organism has yeast, pseudohyphal, and true hyphal forms, and finding all three forms together is supportive of *Candida* spp. (Fig. 18.13; see Table 18.1).

Although not known to cause significant inflammation, *Sarcina ventriculi*, a large gram-positive coccoid bacterium, has been associated with abomasal bloat in small ruminants and calves and may be associated with acute gastric dilatation in dogs.[25] This organism has a characteristic appearance with formation of packets and bundles of very large cocci and is not a component of the normal gastric bacterial flora in dogs (Fig. 18.14).

Gastric Neoplasia

Gastric tumors are uncommon in dogs and cats and include epithelial, mesenchymal, and round cell tumors (Table 18.4). In dogs, gastric carcinoma is most common, whereas in cats, lymphoma is most common.[26]

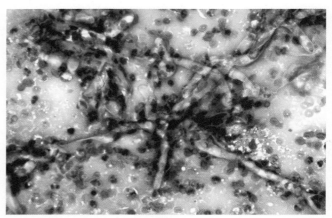

Fig. 18.12 Cytology from a dog; pythiosis. A mat of wide, poorly staining hyphal structures with parallel walls and infrequent septation is present on a background of neutrophilic inflammation and blood. Cytological appearance alone cannot be used to definitively distinguish between *Pythium* and *Lagenidium* (oomycetes), and zygomycete organisms (true fungi). In this case culture of the lesion and immunohistochemistry performed on biopsy samples using anti–*Pythium insidiosum* specific antibodies confirmed infection with *P. insidiosum* (modified Wright stain, original magnification 40× objective). (Case from American Society of Veterinary Clinical Pathology, Mystery Slide Conference, 1998 Case 10, submitted by Casey LeBlanc.)

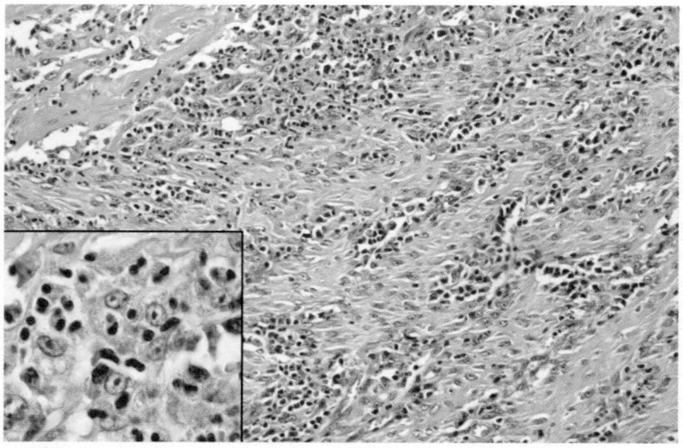

Fig. 18.11 Biopsy of pyloric region of the stomach from a cat; feline gastrointestinal eosinophilic sclerosing fibroplasia. The majority of the masslike lesion is composed of thick bands of dense collagenous or fibrous stroma, with plump proliferating fibroblasts and intervening aggregates of numerous eosinophils. The inset is a closer view of the inflammatory cells and fibroblasts with predominantly eosinophils and fewer macrophages, lymphocytes, plasma cells, and mast cells. (hematoxylin and eosin [H&E] stain, original magnification 20× objective. *Inset:* H&E stain, original magnification 100× objective). (Case from Joint Pathology Center Veterinary Pathology Services [formerly AFIP], Wednesday Slide Conference 2011–2012, Conference 15, Case 1.)

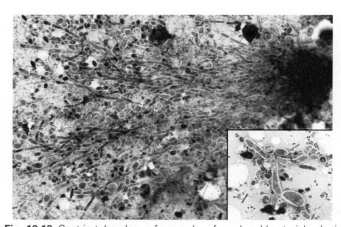

Fig. 18.13 Gastric tube plaque from a dog; fungal and bacterial colonization and overgrowth. A large fungal plaque consisting of round yeast and long, slender, septate hyphae is present. The inset image consists of round to elongated chaining yeast (pseudohyphae) on a background of cocci and rod-shaped bacteria. Finding yeast, hyphae, and pseudohyphae together is consistent with *Candida* spp. In this case the lack of inflammation and location of the plaque within the lumen of the gastric tube were consistent with colonization and overgrowth rather than a true infection (Wright-Giemsa stain, original magnification 10× objective. *Inset:* Wright-Giemsa stain, original magnification 50× objective).

On endoscopic examination, gastric neoplasia may appear as a mass, a polypoid lesion, an area of ulceration, or a regional or diffuse infiltrative process. The infiltrative endoscopic appearance or the presence of a stenotic lesion in the pylorus with gastric neoplasia may be difficult to differentiate from hyperplastic/hypertrophic or eosinophilic gastric lesions (see Table 18.2). Neoplasia in the stomach may also be secondary to extension of neoplasia from an adjacent organ, metastasis from a distant site, or gastric involvement in carcinomatosis. GI tumors, whether in the stomach or intestines, can have significant ulceration or necrosis and may lead to perforation with subsequent peritonitis.

Epithelial Neoplasia

Epithelial proliferations include both benign and malignant lesions, with malignant tumors occurring more commonly.[15] Gastric polyps (a nonneoplastic benign lesion) and adenomas typically are solitary lesions, most commonly arising from the pylorus. It may be difficult to distinguish one from the other, even histologically.[15] Gastric adenocarcinomas are most common in the pylorus and may present as a plaque-like ulcerated thickening, diffuse nonulcerating thickening, or a raised polypoid mass. Gastric carcinomas often have annular thickening and stenosis of the pyloric lumen caused by a scirrhous or fibrous response with contraction of the tissue. The neoplastic cells are typical of an adenocarcinoma and, cytologically, may have cytoplasmic vacuolation (Fig. 18.15). In some cases, gastric carcinomas may be mucinous with abundant production of extracellular mucin or have a "signet ring" morphology, with intracellular mucin accumulation that displaces

the nucleus to the periphery of the cell[16] (Fig. 18.16). Gastric adenocarcinomas most commonly metastasize to the regional lymph nodes but may also seed the abdomen with subsequent carcinomatosis. Less often they metastasize to the lungs or other distant sites.[15]

Neuroendocrine carcinoma (carcinoid) of the stomach is rare and has a typical neuroendocrine cytological appearance (Fig. 18.17). In the rare chronic atrophic gastritis of Norwegian Lundehund dogs, the mild chronic inflammation with fundic gland atrophy may be associated with subsequent development of gastric neuroendocrine carcinoma (carcinoid).[27]

Mesenchymal Neoplasia

Mesenchymal neoplasia in the stomach primarily includes smooth muscle tumors and gastrointestinal stromal tumors (GISTs). These tumors are most common in dogs and rare in cats and have been associated with paraneoplastic hypoglycemia caused by tumor production of insulin-like growth factor II (IGF-II), or paraneoplastic erythrocytosis caused by tumor production of erythropoietin.[11] In dogs, smooth muscle tumors are more common in the stomach compared with GISTs, which are more common in the intestine.[15] Leiomyomas and leiomyosarcomas arise from the smooth muscle wall of the stomach. Leiomyomas are more common and may be multiple, whereas leiomyosarcomas are typically single, larger symptomatic tumors. Compared with leiomyosarcomas, leiomyomas have more well-defined borders and bland morphological features, though leiomyosarcomas are often well-differentiated, and even histological distinction may be difficult.[15] Typically more pleomorphic than leiomyomas, leiomyosarcomas are characterized by plump spindle cells with elongated, blunted, cigar-shaped nuclei (Fig. 18.18). GISTs may have a similar morphology but often have a more haphazard arrangement with a looser, pale pink stroma histologically (Fig. 18.19). Although leiomyosarcomas and GISTs may have slightly different features, significant morphological overlap exists and definitive differentiation usually requires immunohistochemistry (Table 18.5).[28,29] Immunohistochemistry may identify some sarcomas that are neither GISTs nor leiomyosarcomas and may reflect another type of sarcoma of neuroidal origin.[29] Metastasis of these malignant mesenchymal tumors is slow and typically occurs only late in the disease, with lymph node and liver as potential sites of spread.

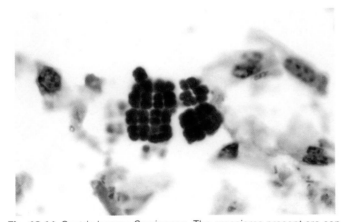

Fig. 18.14 Gastric lumen; *Sarcina* spp. The organisms present are consistent with *Sarcina* spp. and are very large cocci arranged in characteristic packets and bundles. These organisms have been associated with abomasal bloat in calves and lambs and with gastric dilatation in dogs (hematoxylin and eosin [H&E] stain, original magnification 100× objective). (Slide courtesy Kara Corps.)

TABLE 18.4 Types of Gastric or Intestinal Neoplasia	
Category of Neoplasm	**Most Common Neoplasms**
Epithelial	Adenoma, adenocarcinoma, neuroendocrine carcinoma (carcinoid)
Mesenchymal	Leiomyoma, leiomyosarcoma, gastrointestinal stromal tumors
Round cell	Lymphoma, mast cell tumor, plasma cell tumor

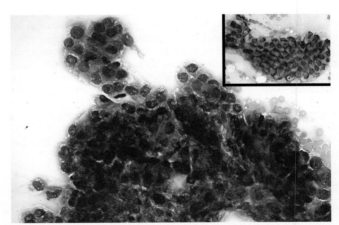

Fig. 18.15 Aspirate from a gastric mass in a dog; gastric carcinoma. The large cohesive aggregate of polygonal epithelial cells is typical of a carcinoma. Note the occasional cytoplasmic vacuoles, which can be seen with gastrointestinal carcinomas. Compare the decreased differentiation and increased pleomorphism within this population to the inset, which is a group of normal foveolar epithelial cells found in the same sample from this dog (Wright-Giemsa stain, original magnification 50× objective). (Courtesy Andrea Siegel.)

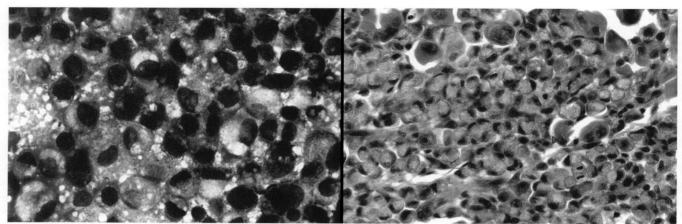

Fig. 18.16 Imprint cytology *(left)* and biopsy sample *(right)* from a gastric thickening in a dog; "signet ring" carcinoma. *Left:* Abundant background bright magenta material is seen, likely reflecting mucin production in this carcinoma. The sample is a tissue imprint, and therefore, there is slight dissociation of the cell connections with some cell rupture, but the round cell morphology with clear to magenta cytoplasmic material peripheralizing the nucleus is typical of a "signet ring" carcinoma phenotype (Wright-Giemsa stain, original magnification 100× objective). *Right:* The "signet ring" morphology is readily apparent in this histopathology sample with solid sheets of rounded epithelial cells with cytoplasmic pale gray mucin material peripheralizing the nucleus. There is moderate pleomorphism in this population with occasional mitotic figures (hematoxylin and eosin [H&E] stain, original magnification 40× objective). (Courtesy Taryn Donovan.)

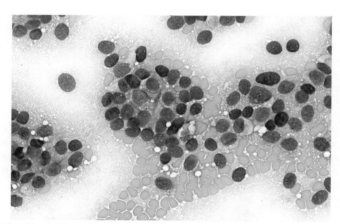

Fig. 18.17 Touch imprints of the serosal surface at the ileocecal junction from a dog; gastrinoma. The cell population has a neuroendocrine appearance characterized by relatively uniform cell size, loosely cohesive clusters with many bare nuclei, pale, delicate, and mildly vacuolated cytoplasm, and round nuclei with finely stippled chromatin. These features are seen in many different neuroendocrine tumors; a diagnosis of gastrinoma in this case was supported by positive immunohistochemical staining for gastrin on the surgical biopsy specimen (modified Wright-Giemsa stain, original magnification 50× objective). (Case from American Society of Veterinary Clinical Pathology, Mystery Slide Conference, 2011 Case 10, submitted by Sarah Colledge.)

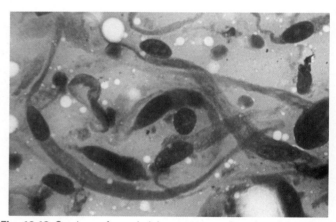

Fig. 18.18 Cytology of gastric leiomyosarcoma in a dog. Spindle cells are elongated with extensive thin cytoplasmic projections and oval to flattened nuclei. The cytological appearance is diagnostic for a spindle cell neoplasm; a definitive diagnosis of leiomyosarcoma was made with histopathology and immunohistochemistry in this case (Wright stain, original magnification 100× objective).

Round Cell Neoplasia

Round cell neoplasia in the stomach includes lymphoma, mast cell tumor, and, rarely, plasma cell tumor. Gastric lymphoma may present as a diffuse infiltrative process or as one to multiple transmural plaques or nodules. Lymphoma may be primary in the stomach or stomach can be involved with more widespread GI or multicentric lymphoma (Figs. 18.20 and 18.21). In cats, gastric lymphoma is usually of B-lymphocyte origin.[30] Mast cell tumors are less common in the stomach than in other parts of the GI tract, and arise from mucosal mast cells. This is distinct from cutaneous mast cell tumors, which arise from connective

tissue mast cells (see "Intestinal Neoplasia" for further discussion). A rare variant of mast cell tumor in cats, known as *feline sclerosing mast cell tumor*, may occur in the stomach but is more often reported in the intestine (see "Intestinal Neoplasia").

SMALL AND LARGE INTESTINES

Normal Intestine

The intestinal tract consists of mucosa with underlying muscularis mucosae, submucosa, and smooth muscle wall (tunica muscularis). The small intestine comprises the duodenum, jejunum, and ileum, and the large intestine is composed of the cecum, colon, and rectum. Unremarkable small and large intestinal mucosae consist of a surface simple columnar epithelium with underlying crypts and variable numbers of goblet cells, whereas unremarkable anal mucosa consists of

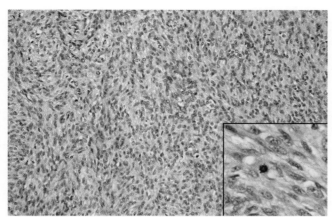

Fig. 18.19 Biopsy of gastrointestinal stromal tumor (GIST) in a dog. The neoplastic cells are arranged in haphazard interwoven fascicles among a loose, pale eosinophilic stroma. Cells are spindle shaped, with eosinophilic fibrillar cytoplasm and an oval nucleus with clumped chromatin and one to three prominent nucleoli. Pleomorphism is mild in this population, with occasional mitotic figures *(inset)*. Immunohistochemistry was positive for c-kit, which is diagnostic for a GIST. (hematoxylin and eosin [H&E] stain, original magnification 20× objective. *Inset:* H&E stain, original magnification 100× objective).

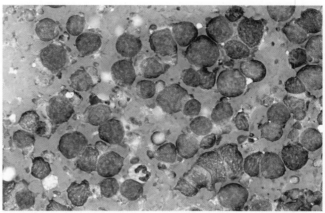

Fig. 18.20 Aspirate of stomach from a dog; lymphoma. Classic appearance of lymphoma. Cells are primarily large and have open, dispersed chromatin, variably prominent nucleoli, and a thin rim of basophilic cytoplasm. Scattered lymphoglandular bodies are also present in the background (Wright-Giemsa stain, original magnification 50× objective).

TABLE 18.5 Differentiating Leiomyosarcomas and Gastrointestinal Stromal Tumors (GISTs)

	Leiomyosarcoma	GISTs
Origin	Smooth muscle cells	Interstitial cells of Cajal (pacemaker cells of the GI tract)
Immunohisto-chemistry	C-kit negative, smooth muscle actin positive, +/– desmin positive	C-kit positive, +/– smooth muscle actin positive, desmin negative
Most common locations	Stomach (pylorus), small intestine	Large intestine
Expected behavior	Locally invasive (particularly with poorly differentiated (vimentin-negative) tumors); low potential for metastasis	Locally invasive; higher potential for metastasis (e.g., to liver, lymph node)

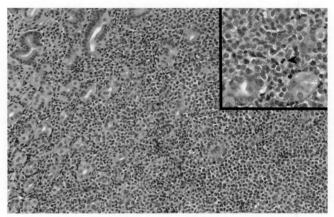

Fig. 18.21 Biopsy sample of stomach from a cat; lymphoma. The gastric mucosa from the fundus region is largely effaced by sheets of larger-sized lymphocytes that have prominent nucleoli and mitotic activity *(inset; arrowhead indicates mitotic figure)*. Few background remaining glandular structures can be seen with brightly eosinophilic parietal cells and basophilic chief cells. Gastric lymphoma in cats is most commonly a large B-cell phenotype (hematoxylin and eosin [H&E] stain, original magnification 40×).

squamous epithelial cells. Goblet cells in the surface and crypt epithelium are typically present in increasing numbers distally within the GI tract. The small intestine has villi projecting from the mucosal surface, whereas the large intestine lacks villi (Fig. 18.22).[8] Lymphoid nodules, called *Peyer's patches*, are present in the submucosa throughout the intestinal tract, especially in the ileum, as part of the MALT (Fig. 18.23).

The cytological appearance of the small intestinal epithelial cells consists of honeycomb-like sheets of absorptive enterocytes admixed with lesser numbers of goblet cells (mucus-secreting cells). The absorptive enterocytes appear as tall columnar cells with basally located nuclei and a distinct striated microvillous border, or terminal bar, at the apical surface. Goblet cells often appear as large pale or vacuolated cells (Fig. 18.24).[9]

The epithelium of the large intestine is similar to that of the small intestine with a honeycomb pattern of tall columnar glandular epithelial cells but with higher numbers of goblet cells compared with the small intestine. If sampled, cytology of the Peyer's patches will consist of a mixed lymphoid population, including small, intermediate, and large lymphocytes along with rare plasma cells. Given how large Peyer's patches may be, even in healthy animals, particularly in young animals, this is an important consideration with intestinal aspirates yielding a lymphoid-predominant cell population (see Fig. 18.23). At any level of the intestinal tract, fine-needle aspirates of the intestines may contain rare spindle-shaped cells that may represent submucosal fibrocytes or smooth muscle cells from the muscularis layers.[9] Magenta-staining gel or lubricant products may be seen as a contaminant in intestinal samples, depending on the method of sample collection (e.g., ultrasound-guided, rectal scraping) (see Fig. 18.1).

Intestinal Inflammation

Enteritis, typhlitis, colitis, and enterotyphlocolitis may be idiopathic, immune mediated, or caused by infectious etiologies or neoplasia.

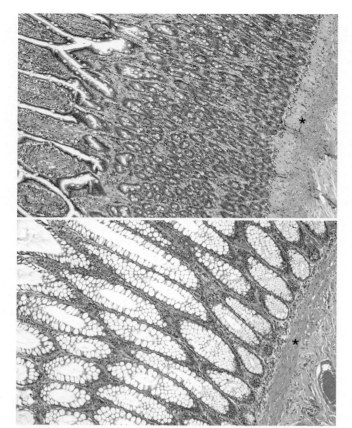

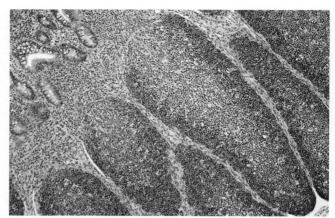

Fig. 18.23 Histopathology of ileum with Peyer's patches in a young animal. The Peyer's patches within the submucosa are very large and have prominent germinal centers, which are lighter-staining than the peripheral rim of smaller lymphocytes. It is feasible that on aspiration of the intestinal wall in this region, a robust lymphoid population could be identified cytologically. If the majority of the cells aspirated are from the germinal center, the presence of large lymphocytes could be confused with a diagnosis of lymphoid neoplasia (hematoxylin and eosin [H&E] stain, original magnification 10× objective). (Slide courtesy Jody Gookin.)

Fig. 18.22 Histopathology of small intestine *(top)* and large intestine *(bottom)* from a dog. The small intestinal mucosa *(top image)* has surface villi lined by absorptive enterocytes with few mucin-containing pale-gray goblet cells and has numerous tightly packed crypts in the deeper mucosa. The large intestinal mucosa *(bottom image)* lacks villi and has numerous tightly packed crypts containing more numerous goblet cells than in the small intestine. Both the small and large intestines have a muscularis mucosae composed of smooth muscle (*), which separates the mucosa from the submucosa (hematoxylin and eosin [H&E] stain, original magnification 20× objective).

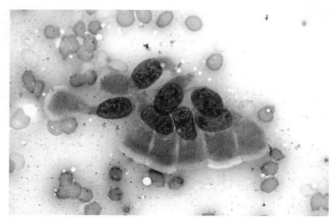

Fig. 18.24 Intestinal aspirate from a cat. Uniform enterocytes characterized by a columnar shape, round basilar oriented nuclei, basophilic cytoplasm and a microvillus brush border *(terminal bar)* are present (Wright-Giemsa stain, original magnification 100× objective). (Slide courtesy Jaime Tarigo.)

Types of inflammation may include lymphoplasmacytic, neutrophilic, eosinophilic, or granulomatous inflammation, and the nature of the inflammation depends on the underlying etiology; for more specific details on causes for each type of inflammation, see Table 18.6.

Lymphoplasmacytic Inflammation

IBD is a common cause of enterocolitis in dogs and cats. The inflammation is most commonly lymphoplasmacytic, but eosinophilic and rare macrophage-predominant or granulomatous forms also occur (Fig. 18.25). IBD is thought to be caused by dysregulation of mucosal immunity in predisposed animals with loss of tolerance to certain antigens; therefore, an immune-mediated component to the pathogenesis is likely.[31] The World Small Animal Veterinary Association (WSAVA) has published guidelines for the standardization of GI inflammation on histological examination of biopsy specimens to help pathologists better categorize the severity and type of inflammatory disease.[32] Cytological evidence of inflammation is a typical finding with IBD but is not specific for this disease process. Lymphoplasmacytic inflammation often predominates with protein-losing enteropathies (PLEs).

A rare cause of lymphocytic inflammation deep within the muscular wall of the intestinal tract is an entity known as *chronic intestinal pseudo-obstruction* (CIPO), which is an immune-mediated lymphocytic intestinal leiomyositis (inflammation of the smooth muscle wall).[33] This lesion does not affect the mucosa but leads to a decrease in motility with marked dilation of the intestinal loops mimicking an obstructive lesion. Cytological sampling of this lesion would be unlikely because there is often thinning of the intestinal wall in this condition, making aspiration very difficult.

Neutrophilic Inflammation

Although neutrophil transmigration into the GI lumen is the main route of neutrophil elimination from the body, finding numerous neutrophils in cytological specimens from the intestine is abnormal. Similarly, on histological examination, the presence of neutrophils in the intestinal mucosa is never considered a normal finding. Because neutrophilic inflammation in the intestine has various causes, finding a component of neutrophilic inflammation is a relatively nonspecific finding (see Table 18.6). If neutrophilic inflammation is identified as a component of IBD, it is likely secondary to epithelial damage (erosions or ulcers) or a

TABLE 18.6 Causes of Intestinal Inflammation

Type of Inflammation	Disease Process	Specific Causes
Lymphoplasmacytic	Inflammatory bowel disease (IBD)	Including protein-losing enteropathies (PLEs)
	Chronic intestinal pseudo-obstruction (CIPO)	
	Nonspecific inflammation	
Neutrophilic	Infectious agents	Bacterial (*Escherichia coli, Salmonella* spp., *Clostridium* spp.)
		Parasitic (typhlocolitis in dogs with *Trichuris vulpis* infection)
	Secondary	Erosions or ulcers of any cause (including foreign body)
	IBD	May be caused by secondary infection or epithelial injury component
	Necrotizing colitis	Glucocorticoid administration, hyperadrenocorticism, spinal trauma, uremia
Eosinophilic	IBD	
	Allergic disease	Food allergies, gluten sensitivity
	Neoplasia	Mast cell tumor, T-cell lymphoma
	Infectious	Pythiosis, parasitism, *Toxocara canis* migration
	Miscellaneous	Feline hypereosinophilic syndrome, feline gastrointestinal eosinophilic sclerosing fibroplasia, canine idiopathic eosinophilic gastrointestinal masses
Granulomatous	Infectious	Histoplasmosis, cryptococcosis, protothecosis, schistosomiasis (*Heterobilharzia*), amoebiasis, feline infectious peritonitis (FIP), salmon poisoning disease in dogs, histiocytic ulcerative colitis of Boxers, pythiosis, mycobacteriosis, leishmaniasis, or mycotic infection
	Noninfectious	Intestinal lymphangiectasia with transmural lipogranulomatous lymphangitis

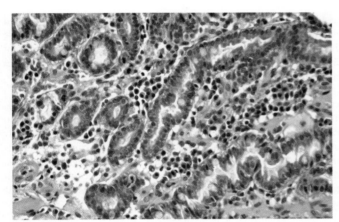

Fig. 18.25 Biopsy of small intestine from a dog; inflammatory bowel disease characterized by lymphoplasmacytic enteritis. The intestinal crypts are mildly separated by an increased amount of connective tissue and moderate numbers of lymphocytes and plasma cells, with a predominance of plasma cells, and mild edema (hematoxylin and eosin [H&E] stain, original magnification 40× objective).

secondary bacterial component, whereas a primary neutrophilic inflammatory lesion without underlying IBD is more likely caused by mucosal irritation/injury or by bacterial infection or other etiological agents.

Eosinophilic Inflammation

Eosinophilic enterocolitis may occur as a component of IBD or may be associated with other causes, particularly with underlying allergy/hypersensitivity or endoparasitism (see Table 18.6). In hypereosinophilic syndrome in cats, the associated eosinophilic enteritis, if present, predominantly involves the small intestine and is accompanied by marked smooth muscle hypertrophy of the intestinal wall, which greatly expands the wall thickness. The eosinophilic infiltrate may also involve the mesenteric lymph nodes in these cases.[11] Canine idiopathic eosinophilic GI masses and feline GI eosinophilic sclerosing

fibroplasia do occur in the intestine but are discussed elsewhere (see "Gastric Inflammation"; see Fig. 18.11).

Granulomatous Inflammation

Granulomatous enteritis and/or colitis is typically associated with a variety of infectious and some noninfectious diseases (see Table 18.6). Many granulomatous intestinal diseases cause segmental thickening of the intestinal wall and may cause a masslike lesion, which may be radiographically or ultrasonographically confused with neoplasia (see Table 18.2).

Histoplasma capsulatum, a fungal organism, causes segmental transmural granulomatous inflammation in the stomach, small intestine, or large intestine (see Table 18.1). Infection with *Prototheca zopfii* or *Prototheca wickerhamii* causes hemorrhagic and ulcerative colitis with a mild lymphohistiocytic inflammatory response relative to the marked numbers of algal organisms present (see Table 18.1). Canine schistosomiasis, caused by the trematode *Heterobilharzia americana*, results in granulomatous enteritis in response to the transmigration of eggs across the intestinal wall. The adult trematodes live in the mesenteric vessels and release their eggs into the mucosal venules, and the eggs migrate to the intestinal lumen to be excreted in feces. An association may exist between this infection and hypercalcemia (see Table 18.1).[34] *Entamoeba histolytica*, an amoeba, causes ulcerative and granulomatous colitis with numerous trophozoites and cyst forms (see Table 18.1). Although rare in the intestinal tract, infection with the fungal agent *Cryptococcus neoformans* may be associated with granulomatous enterocolitis (Fig. 18.26; see Table 18.1).

Feline infectious peritonitis (FIP) can cause multifocal granulomatous lesions on the serosal surface of the intestines (Fig. 18.27) but also may present as regional granulomatous colitis with involvement of the colic lymph node. This presentation of FIP may be isolated to the colon and associated lymph node and may not be accompanied by more widespread FIP lesions. In these cases, ultrasonographic appearance could be mistaken for neoplasia (see Table 18.2). In some cases, FIP can be more prominently lymphoplasmacytic or neutrophilic, without as prominent a granulomatous component. Salmon poisoning disease

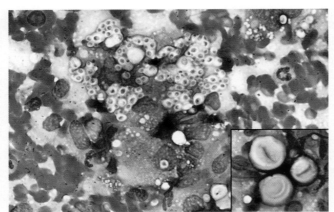

Fig. 18.26 Intestinal aspirate from a dog; *Cryptococcus neoformans* infection. A cluster of epithelioid macrophages and few neutrophils are present, along with many small extracellular yeast organisms characterized by a pale interior and a variably wide nonstaining capsule. Because of the small size of the organisms and somewhat petite capsule, they could be confused with other fungal agents, such as *Histoplasma capsulatum* or the yeast form of *Candida*. The inset is of organisms from a different region of the sample characterized by larger size and a distinctive fold in the cell wall giving the cell the appearance of a partially deflated kick-ball or a folded contact lens (Wright-Giemsa stain, original magnification 50× objective. *Inset:* Wright-Giemsa stain, original magnification 50× objective).

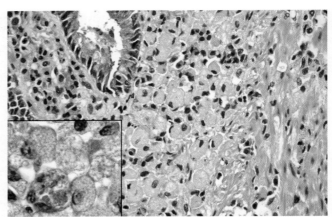

Fig. 18.28 Biopsy of colon from a Boxer; histiocytic ulcerative colitis. A dense infiltrate of foamy macrophages separates and elevates the colonic crypts. The macrophages contain granular eosinophilic to basophilic cytoplasmic material, which is suggested to be phagocytized membranous or cellular debris and stains positive with periodic acid–Schiff (PAS; *not pictured*). This condition is thought to be associated with, and is likely caused by, bacterial infection with *Escherichia coli* (hematoxylin and eosin [H&E] stain, original magnification 40× objective. *Inset:* H&E stain, original magnification 100×). (Case from Joint Pathology Center Veterinary Pathology Services [formerly AFIP], Wednesday Slide Conference 2010–2011, Conference 7, Case 1.)

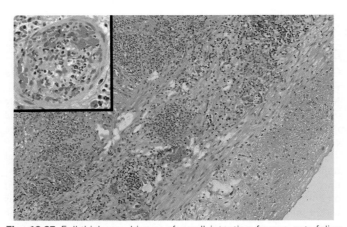

Fig. 18.27 Full-thickness biopsy of small intestine from a cat; feline infectious peritonitis (FIP). Pockets of suppurative to pyogranulomatous inflammation are present multifocally throughout the intestinal wall. Note that vasculitis is also present *(inset)* and is a characteristic feature of FIP. FIP should be considered as a differential for inflammatory lesions in the GI tract in cats, particularly if signalment and clinical history are supportive (hematoxylin and eosin [H&E] stain, original magnification 40× objective).

is caused by the rickettsial organism *Neorickettsia helminthoeca* transmitted to dogs by the trematode *Nanophyetus salmincola*. It is associated with granulomatous enteritis resulting from the presence of the fluke and intralesional intrahistiocytic rickettsial organisms, although the more damaging lesion occurs in lymphoid tissues.

Histiocytic ulcerative colitis (or granulomatous colitis) of Boxer dogs, although not exclusive to that breed, is characterized by transmural thickening of the colon with mucosal and submucosal dense infiltrates of macrophages containing numerous periodic acid–Schiff (PAS)–positive granules in the cytoplasm (Fig. 18.28). The inflammatory lesion may also affect the mesenteric lymph nodes. Originally thought to be

an idiopathic or immune-mediated disease, it has since been associated with, and is likely caused by, infection with an adherent and invasive *Escherichia coli* organism.[35] Infection may be confirmed with fluorescent in situ hybridization (FISH). The PAS-positive material in macrophages may consist of broken-down cell membranes and bacterial organisms.

Pythiosis (discussed in more detail earlier in "Gastric Inflammation") causes segmental transmural granulomatous inflammation (see Fig. 18.12). Mycobacterial infection and leishmaniasis are uncommon causes of intestinal granulomatous inflammation and more commonly cause disease elsewhere in the body. An occasional cause of granulomatous colitis is a fungal infection such as with *Aspergillus*, *Candida*, or zygomycete organisms. Often, these represent a secondary infection from immunocompromise or other primary GI disease, as may occur with panleukopenia virus infection in cats.[11]

Other Inflammatory or Noninflammatory Conditions

Other infectious agents associated with inflammation in the intestine in cats include *Clostridium piliforme*, *Anaerobiospirillum*, and *Tritrichomonas fetus*. In *C. piliforme* colitis in cats, surface colonic epithelial cells contain multiple, fine, linear, rod-shaped bacteria in the cytoplasm. In *Anaerobiospirillum* infections numerous spiral bacteria are associated with ileocolitis. *T. fetus* infection is associated with many luminal organisms within colonic crypts and associated inflammation and is of the highest prevalence in cattery-housed cats (see Table 18.1).[11,36]

Several infectious agents in dogs and cats are associated with diarrhea, although they do not always cause marked inflammatory lesions. They include whipworms in the large intestine (*Trichuris vulpis* in dogs) and small intestinal protozoal infections, such as giardiasis, cryptosporidiosis, and coccidiosis caused by *Cystoisospora* spp. in dogs and cats (see Table 18.1). Infection with other nematodes in the small intestine may be associated with disease or ill-thrift, particularly in younger animals, including roundworms (*Toxocara canis* in dogs, *Toxocara cati* in cats, *Toxascaris leonina* in dogs and cats) and hookworms (*Ancylostoma caninum* in dogs, *Ancylostoma tubaeformae* in cats). *Toxoplasma gondii* is a protozoal organism with cats serving as the definitive host, so various stages of developing organisms may be found in the small intestine of clinically normal cats.

Intestinal Neoplasia

Intestinal tumors in dogs and cats include epithelial, mesenchymal, and round cell tumors (see Table 18.4). In dogs, intestinal neoplasia is more often malignant than benign, and intestinal adenocarcinoma is the most common tumor. In cats, lymphoma is most common, and adenocarcinoma is second most common.[15] In cats that do have epithelial neoplasia, malignant tumors are far more common than are benign neoplasms.[15,16] Besides primary neoplasia arising from the intestine, the intestine may be involved in secondary neoplasia caused by extension from an adjacent tissue, including the pancreas, urinary bladder, biliary system, or stomach. Intestine may also be involved secondarily with carcinomatosis, which predominantly affects serosal tissue, or with metastatic disease as a part of widespread metastasis from a distant site. As mentioned previously, GI tumors can have significant ulceration or necrosis and may lead to perforation with subsequent peritonitis.

Epithelial Neoplasia

Epithelial proliferations in the intestine include hyperplastic or adenomatous polyps, adenomas, adenocarcinomas, and rare neuroendocrine carcinomas (carcinoids). Controversy exists in the literature with regard to the criteria for diagnosing a nonneoplastic polyp versus a benign epithelial neoplasm versus an in situ adenocarcinoma. Polypoid lesions in the intestine occur most commonly in the rectum and are often multiple. Most of these lesions are *rectal papillary adenomas*, although if increased atypia is noted, these may be interpreted as in situ carcinomas. This distinction may not be of prognostic significance, particularly compared with invasive adenocarcinomas.[15] Rectal adenomas or in situ carcinomas protrude into the rectal lumen and are composed of proliferative columnar epithelial cells. The cellular morphology may be somewhat pleomorphic; therefore, the tissue architecture on histopathology is required to differentiate an

infiltrative adenocarcinoma from a papillary adenoma or in situ carcinoma (Figs. 18.29 and 18.30).[15,16] Infiltrative adenocarcinoma is confirmed if there is evidence of tissue invasion deeper into the rectal wall or into lymphatic vessels. Given the degree of pleomorphism that may be identified in papillary adenomas or in situ carcinomas, cytological distinction between this lesion and infiltrative adenocarcinoma is not likely to be accurate, and histopathology should be recommended for more definitive diagnosis, if possible. Even biopsy samples may be too superficial to definitively rule out infiltrative growth and therefore, biopsy with histopathology may still not yield definitive diagnosis, particularly with endoscopic samples.

Anomalous outpouchings from the intestine can be mistaken for neoplastic mass lesions clinically and are rarely seen in the proximal duodenum in cats (author experience [JH]). These lesions, which likely represent vitelline duct remnants or a similar anomalous structure, are typically cystic and have a proliferative to attenuated epithelial lining that could cytologically or histologically be mistaken for a neoplastic epithelial population.

Adenocarcinomas in the GI tract are more common in the intestine in cats (Fig. 18.31) and in the stomach in dogs (as discussed previously; see Figs. 18.15 and 18.16).[15] Grossly, intestinal adenocarcinomas may be intramural or intraluminal and may be plaquelike, ulcerated, or masslike. The intramural tumors are often annular or circumferential leading to stenosis because of the scirrhous response to the tumor. Because of the extensive mural involvement in some cases, sampling of the mucosal or surface component alone may miss the lesion, whether an endoscopic cytology or biopsy technique is used. Subtypes of adenocarcinoma are similar to those described for gastric carcinomas and may have acinar, tubular, or papillary structures, a mucinous variant

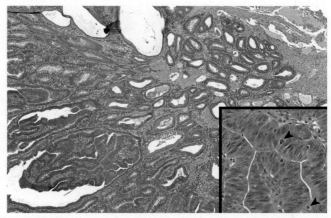

Fig. 18.30 Biopsy sample of rectum from a dog; rectal papillary adenoma/*in situ* carcinoma. A polypoid mass arising from the rectal mucosa projects into the rectal lumen. The neoplastic cells are arranged in papilliferous projections and form tubules supported by a fibrovascular stroma *(basophilic area to left of image)*. Cells are columnar with a basally located nucleus and eosinophilic cytoplasm. As identified in the inset, frequent piling of cells on one another occurs, with occasional mitotic figures *(arrowheads)*. A diagnosis of an infiltrative adenocarcinoma requires evidence of invasion of the neoplastic cells into the underlying submucosal tissue, which is not evident in this case despite the atypical morphological features of the individual cells *(note well-defined smooth muscle border of muscularis mucosae at top right of image)*. For this reason, diagnosis of malignancy based on cytological or individual cell features is not advised; histopathology with evaluation for submucosal invasion is required for more definitive diagnosis (hematoxylin and eosin [H&E] stain, original magnification 5× objective. *Inset:* H&E stain, original magnification 40× objective).

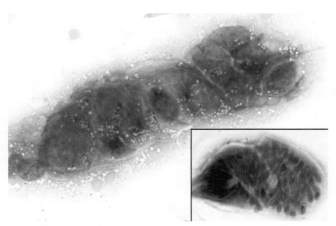

Fig. 18.29 Aspirate from a polypoid rectal mass in a dog. The sample contains regions of moderately pleomorphic epithelial cells, characterized by anisocytosis, anisokaryosis, a jumbled and crowded appearance to the cell clusters, large nuclei, visible nucleoli and fine cytoplasmic vacuolization. Although these findings may suggest a malignant process, much of the sample consists of uniform epithelial cells *(inset)*. Caution should be exercised when evaluating apparent cytological criteria of malignancy in polypoid rectal masses as papillary adenomas or in situ carcinomas may have regions of moderate pleomorphism (Wright-Giemsa stain, original magnification 50× objective. *Inset:* Wright-Giemsa stain, original magnification 50× objective).

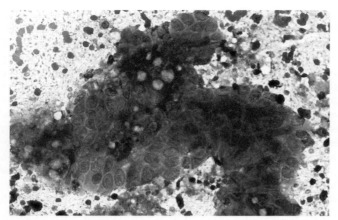

Fig. 18.31 Jejunal aspirate from a cat; adenocarcinoma. A large cluster of carcinoma cells is present on a background of necrosis and cellular debris. Cells have features typical of a carcinoma with moderate pleomorphism. Note the clear vacuoles present in the cluster suggesting there may be mucin formation by the tumor cells (Wright-Giemsa stain, original magnification 50× objective). (Slide courtesy Jamie Tarigo.)

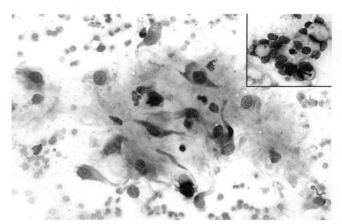

Fig. 18.33 Abdominal mass aspirate from a dog; intestinal adenocarcinoma with a scirrhous response. Many immature mesenchymal cells are admixed with bright-pink, fibrillar, extracellular matrix material. Although the cells do not have strong nuclear criteria of malignancy, the presence of primarily immature mesenchymal cells could lead to an erroneous diagnosis of sarcoma; thus, it is important to keep nonneoplastic causes of mesenchymal cell proliferation in mind, especially when cells lack overt features of malignancy. The inset image is of one of the rare clusters of adenocarcinoma cells that were present in this sample. In this particular case, the cells have a prominent signet ring appearance (Wright-Giemsa stain, original magnification 40× objective. *Inset:* Wright-Giemsa stain, original magnification 40× objective).

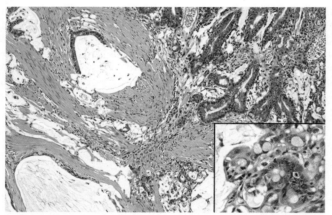

Fig. 18.32 Biopsy sample of small intestine from a dog; mucinous intestinal adenocarcinoma. The neoplastic epithelial cells form tubular and acinar structures within the mucosa and extend into the submucosal and muscularis layers of the intestinal wall. Large lakes of mucinous material accumulate within portions of the neoplasm, as depicted on the left side of the image. Individual neoplastic cells occasionally have a signet ring morphology with an intracytoplasmic accumulation of mucin material that peripheralizes the nucleus *(inset)*. (hematoxylin and eosin [H&E] stain, original magnification 10× objective. *Inset:* H&E stain, original magnification 40× objective). (Case from Joint Pathology Center Veterinary Pathology Services [formerly AFIP], Wednesday Slide Conference 2009–2010, Conference 21, Case 2.)

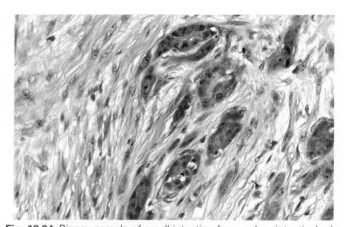

Fig. 18.34 Biopsy sample of small intestine from a dog; intestinal adenocarcinoma and desmoplasia. Few infiltrative groups of neoplastic epithelial cells form acinar/tubular structures. Surrounding the carcinoma cells, there is loose collagenous tissue with plump fibroblasts, consistent with a scirrhous host response to the neoplasm, also known as *desmoplasia* (hematoxylin and eosin [H&E] stain, original magnification 40× objective).

with abundant production of extracellular mucin, or, rarely, "signet ring" morphology with intracellular mucin accumulation that displaces the nucleus to the periphery of the cell (Fig. 18.32). Cases with extensive desmoplasia may have a component of mesenchymal cells identified cytologically, which should not be mistaken for mesenchymal neoplasia (Figs. 18.33 and 18.34). Occasionally, in cats, intestinal adenocarcinomas have osseous or chondroid metaplasia within the stromal component of the tumor.[15] Metastasis occurs typically to the mesenteric lymph nodes or by seeding of the abdomen with carcinomatosis, and there is potential for distant metastasis, such as to the liver or the lungs.

Neuroendocrine carcinomas (carcinoids) arise from enteroendocrine cells throughout the intestinal mucosa and have a typical neuroendocrine appearance cytologically (see Fig. 18.17). These tumors are rare and are typically malignant and aggressive in their behavior, with metastasis to the liver, the most common site of spread.[16]

Mesenchymal Neoplasia

Mesenchymal neoplasia in the intestinal tract includes leiomyoma, leiomyosarcoma, and GIST, with rare reports of other tumors (Fig. 18.35). These tumors are much more common in dogs than in cats.[15] Leiomyomas are typically small nodules in the outer layer of the

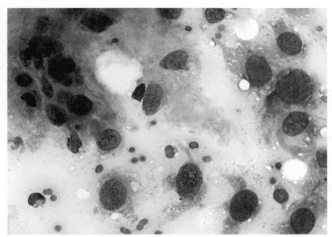

Fig. 18.35 Small intestinal tissue imprint from a dog; sarcoma. A pleomorphic population of plump sarcoma cells are admixed with pink, extracellular matrix material. Although the cells have clear mesenchymal features and criteria of malignancy, they do not have specific cytological features that may allow tumor identification beyond sarcoma. In this case, histochemical or immunohistochemical staining revealed a vimentin-positive, c-kit-negative, desmin-positive (intracytoplasmic globules present in 10% of cells), smooth muscle actin–positive (10% of neoplastic cells) neoplasm suggestive of smooth muscle origin (Wright-Giemsa stain, original magnification 50× objective). (Case from American Society of Veterinary Clinical Pathology, Mystery Slide Conference, 2009 Case 23, submitted by Rebeccah Urbiztondo.)

intestinal wall and may be multiple, whereas leiomyosarcomas are typically a larger solitary mass and may be more invasive. Differentiation of leiomyosarcomas and GISTs has been previously discussed (see Table 18.5; see Figs. 18.18 and 18.19). These mesenchymal tumors, in particular GISTs, do have the potential to metastasize to the regional lymph nodes, mesentery, or liver but still may carry a better prognosis compared with other malignant neoplasms of the intestinal tract, such as carcinomas or round cell tumors.[11] GISTs are more likely to metastasize than leiomyosarcomas and poorly differentiated leiomyosarcomas are more likely to be locally invasive than well-differentiated leiomyosarcomas.[15,29] There are rare reports of extraskeletal osteosarcoma arising within the intestine, including at the site of a retained surgical sponge.[15]

Round Cell Neoplasia

Lymphoma is the most common round cell tumor of the intestinal tract and has varying morphologies (Fig. 18.36). As with lymphoma in other locations, the size and morphological features will vary with different lymphoma subtypes, and this may have an important effect on prognosis and appropriate therapy. GI lymphoma may occur as a component of multicentric disease or, more commonly, as primary GI lymphoma. Primary GI lymphoma can be focal, multifocal, or diffuse in the GI tract, and often spreads to the mesenteric lymph nodes and to the liver. The correlation of cytology with histopathologic findings in diagnosing GI neoplasia is reported to range from 72% to 89%, but cytology is considered reasonably accurate for a diagnosis of GI lymphoma, particularly with large cell phenotypes[37] (see Fig. 18.20). In cases that are not clearly a monomorphic neoplastic lymphoid population on cytology, subsequent biopsy or other advanced diagnostic testing may be considered.

Even histologically, differentiation between intestinal inflammation and lymphoma can be a diagnostic challenge. This is particularly true of superficial endoscopic samples from early or emerging small cell lymphoma, which often develops on a background of intestinal inflammation. In these cases, histopathology is often followed by additional diagnostic testing, and, in particular, polymerase chain reaction for antigen receptor rearrangement (PARR). This test is used to detect clonality within a lymphoid population and can be performed either on cytological preparations from fine-needle aspirates, or paraffin-embedded formalin-fixed tissues from a biopsy sample. It should be noted that PARR does not provide the immunophenotype of a lymphoma (T- versus B-cell origin) in the way that immunohistochemistry does and should therefore be interpreted as a confirmatory test for lymphoma, but not an accurate method of further subtyping.[15]

In cats, GI lymphoma occurs more commonly in the small intestine, followed by the stomach, and less often the large intestine. T-cell lymphoma is most common overall.[15,38] In the small intestine, T-cell lymphoma is more common, whereas in the stomach and large intestine, B-cell lymphoma is more common.[30] An association with feline leukemia virus (FeLV) infection is typically not seen in feline gastrointestinal lymphoma. Although the literature varies as to terminology, and not all cases fit specifically into these subtypes, cats have three more common presentations of GI T-cell lymphoma: (1) mucosal T-cell lymphoma, also referred to as *enteropathy-associated T-cell lymphoma type 2* (EATL 2), (2) transmural T-cell lymphoma, also referred to as *enteropathy-associated T-cell lymphoma type 1* (EATL 1), and (3) granulated lymphoma (also referred to as large granular lymphoma [LGL]). Additional information comparing these types is provided in Table 18.7. Cytologically, these types of lymphoma have different morphological characteristics (see Fig. 18.36). Histologically, EATL 1 is a large-cell lymphoma that often effaces the mucosa and transmural tissues. In contrast, EATL 2 is a small- to intermediate-cell lymphoma, which starts within the mucosa but can subsequently infiltrate transmurally, and is often characterized by prominent epitheliotropism (Fig. 18.37). EATL 2 is the most common subtype in cats.[15] It may be difficult to definitively differentiate between IBD and small cell lymphoma histologically; features that are helpful in the identification of lymphoma include intraepithelial nest or plaque formation, a monomorphic population, altered mucosal architecture, infiltration of the submucosa, intravascular infiltration, or increased mitotic activity.[38,39] If histological distinction between lymphoma and IBD is not possible, PARR is recommended to assess for a clonal population (see previous discussion). The combination of histopathology, immunohistochemistry, and PARR increases the likelihood of successful differentiation of these entities compared with any of these diagnostic tests alone.[39] Although not always clinically possible, full-thickness biopsy samples may be preferred over endoscopic samples to allow for evaluation of mural invasion by the lymphocytes, which can be central to the histological diagnosis of lymphoma over IBD in some cases. In many cases, however, a diagnosis of lymphoma can be made with endoscopic samples alone (see Fig. 18.37).

With regard to granulated lymphoma (often referred to as LGL, although not always actually of large cell phenotype), this is a subtype of T-cell lymphoma in cats with intracytoplasmic eosinophilic to magenta granules that may be more easily seen with cytology compared with histopathology (see Fig. 18.36, A and B). With histopathology, the granules may be visible with histochemical or immunohistochemical stains (phosphotungstic acid–hematoxylin [PTAH], granzyme B, or perforin) and the neoplastic cells are often epitheliotropic.[15,38,40] These cases may have concurrent involvement of the mesenteric lymph nodes, liver, peritoneal effusion, and peripheral blood.[40]

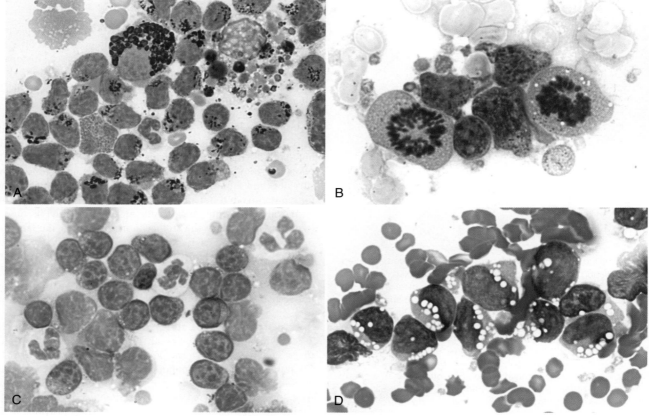

Fig. 18.36 Morphological comparison of four different intestinal lymphoma aspirates. (A) Granular lymphoma from a cat. Cells are intermediate to large in size; nuclei contain smudged chromatin but do not have obvious nucleoli; and the cytoplasm contains large, chunky magenta granules. Note the single tumor cell in the top middle of the image with many extremely large granules. To the right of this cell is a slightly disrupted macrophage with phagocytized granules and debris, and below the granulated tumor cell are a neutrophil and an eosinophil (Wright-Giemsa stain, original magnification 100× objective). (B) Granular lymphoma from a cat. Cells are intermediate to large in size, with coarse chromatin and some visible nucleolar rings, and contain few very fine magenta granules. Note the two mitotic figures and the presence of granules in the lymphoglandular body in the lower right region of the slide (Wright-Giemsa stain, original magnification 100× objective). (C) Small cell lymphoma in a cat. Cells are smaller than the neutrophils with coarse, clumped chromatin and a thin rim of basophilic cytoplasm. Because of the well-differentiated appearance of these cells, a definitive diagnosis of lymphoma could be challenging on the basis of the cytology alone (Wright-Giemsa stain, original magnification 100× objective). (D) Lymphoma in a cat. Cells in this case have typical nuclear characteristics of lymphoma but the cytoplasm contains scattered, prominent, medium-sized vacuoles (Wright-Giemsa stain, original magnification 100× objective). (A, Slide courtesy Jaime Tarigo. B, Slide courtesy Taryn Sibley. D, Slide courtesy Jaime Tarigo.)

TABLE 18.7	**Types of Gastrointestinal Lymphoma in Cats**			
Subtype of Lymphoma	**Cell of Origin/ Immunophenotype**	**Cytological Description**	**Gross/Ultrasonographic Appearance**	**Additional Findings**
Gastric lymphoma	Most commonly B-cell	Large cells, often with prominent nucleoli	Diffuse thickening or mass lesion	
Mucosal T-cell lymphoma (enteropathy-associated T-cell lymphoma type 2 [EATL type 2])	Epitheliotrophic T-cell	Cells are small to intermediate in size, often appear well differentiated	Diffuse thickening (jejunum most common)	Ultrasonography findings similar to inflammatory bowel disease (IBD)
Transmural T-cell lymphoma (EATL type 1)	T-cell (often epitheliotropic)	Large, immature cells with visible nucleoli	One to multiple masses or transmural thickening	
Granulated lymphoma (large granular lymphoma)	Intestinal intraepithelial lymphocyte origin (likely cytotoxic T-cell or natural killer cell); may be subcategory within transmural T-cell lymphoma	Variably sized (intermediate to large), variable nuclear features, magenta granules vary from fine to large and chunky	Segmental thickening of the intestinal wall or one to multiple mass lesions	Granules may not be visible with routine histopathology

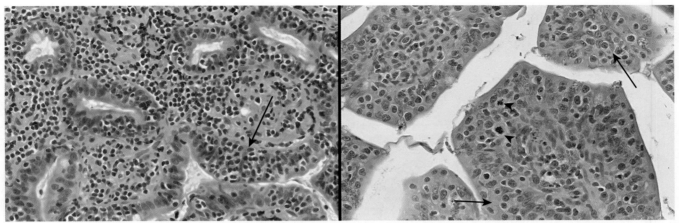

Fig. 18.37 Endoscopic biopsies of small intestine from two cats with intestinal lymphoma. *Left:* Classic histological appearance of epitheliotropic small cell lymphoma in a cat, also referred to as *mucosal T-cell lymphoma* or *enteropathy-associated T-cell lymphoma type 2* (EATL type 2). The neoplastic lymphocytes are small and are in nests and plaques *(arrow)* within the mucosal and crypt epithelium. More subtle cases may require additional diagnostic testing for confirmation, such as polymerase chain reaction for antigen receptor rearrangement (PARR) (hematoxylin and eosin [H&E] stain, original magnification 40× objective). *Right:* A more subtle intraepithelial population of intermediate to large-sized lymphoid cells can be seen. These cells have a round shape and pale gray to pale eosinophilic cytoplasm with a rounded nucleus *(arrows)*, which distinguishes them from the surrounding enterocyte population. Mitotic figures are noted *(arrowheads)*, and this is likely a more aggressive form of T-cell lymphoma, such as EATL type 1 or a granulated lymphoma. Granules are often not seen histologically even with granulated lymphomas (large granular lymphoma; LGL), and cytology can be useful to aid in this characterization, as well as potential immunohistochemistry (hematoxylin and eosin [H&E] stain, original magnification 40× objective).

In dogs, GI lymphoma affects the small intestine more than it affects the stomach and less often involves the large intestine.[15] Cytological findings are not distinct from lymphoma at other sites (see Figs. 18.20 and 18.36). In dogs, GI lymphoma is most commonly of T-cell origin and, in contrast to cats, EATL type 1 with transmural infiltration by a larger lymphocyte population is more common than EATL type 2. Because EATL 1 is a more obvious cytological and histological diagnosis given the larger size and immaturity of the lymphoid population, the distinction from IBD is a less common diagnostic dilemma in dogs. In borderline cases, if needed, a diagnostic algorithm comprising histopathology, immunohistochemistry, and PARR is still recommended.[15,41,42] In addition, with EATL type 2 in dogs, unlike that in cats, increased epitheliotropism of small lymphocytes is less specific for lymphoma and is often also seen in IBD cases, including with PLEs.[41] In dogs, some T-cell lymphomas have an intense infiltrate of eosinophils among the neoplastic lymphocytes,[43] which can also be seen in other subtypes of T-cell lymphoma in dogs and cats in the GI tract or elsewhere in the body.

Plasma cell tumors are rare in the intestine and occur more in dogs than in cats, with the rectum being the most common site (Figs. 18.38 and 18.39). They are most often considered benign lesions; however, rare reports of metastasis to the lymph nodes or distant sites of involvement have been published.[15] Mast cell tumors are more common in cats than in dogs and typically occur as distinct intestinal masses that are more often extraluminal in the outer layers of the intestinal wall but may have a varied gross appearance.[16] Because these are often not associated with the mucosa, more superficial sampling via endoscopic cytology or biopsy may not yield the neoplastic population (Figs. 18.40 and 18.41). Similar to gastric mast cell tumors, intestinal mast cell tumors arise from the mucosal mast cells and, therefore, may be less well granulated and lack the associated GI ulceration that often accompanies cutaneous mast cell tumors. Because they may be less

well granulated, tumors arising from these mucosal mast cells may be difficult to differentiate from lymphoma on histopathology, even with histochemical stains, such as Giemsa or toluidine blue (see Fig. 18.41). These cases may benefit from immunohistochemistry, such as c-kit (mast cell marker) and CD79a, CD20, and CD3 (lymphocyte markers), although feline mast cell tumors may not stain with c-kit.[15,43,44] In these cases, cytology may also be helpful in identifying subtle granularity. The presence of eosinophils is variable in GI mast cell tumors and is not specific for this tumor because eosinophils are also seen in some lymphomas. A variant of mast cell tumor in cats, known as *feline sclerosing mast cell tumor*, is a mass lesion composed of somewhat poorly granulated mast cells among a marked amount of sclerotic collagen with associated plump spindle cells and many eosinophils. Although these neoplastic mast cells have a low mitotic count, a high propensity to metastasize to the lymph nodes and liver has been reported.[45] A differential diagnosis for this entity is *feline eosinophilic sclerosing fibroplasia*, a nonneoplastic lesion, which poses a diagnostic challenge on histopathology, and the distinction between these entities remains somewhat controversial (see Fig. 18.11).

FECAL ANALYSIS

Normal Fecal Cytology

Normal fecal cytology consists of a polymorphic population of microbial flora that consists predominantly of rod-shaped bacteria with rare coccoid bacteria and occasional yeast structures with a background of mucus and debris.[1] Clusters of columnar epithelium may occasionally be noted on rectal scraping samples (Fig. 18.42). Squamous epithelium may be noted as the result of contamination from the anus. *Cyniclomyces guttulatus* is a fungal agent that is part of the normal GI flora in rodents and lagomorphs (see Table 18.1). Occasionally, low

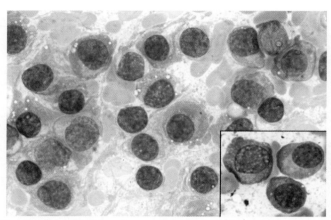

Fig. 18.38 Rectal aspirate from a dog; plasma cell tumor. This tumor is moderately well differentiated with many variably intact cells. Cells are large and round with typical plasmacytoid features, including round eccentric nuclei, moderately coarse chromatin, deeply basophilic cytoplasm, and a variably apparent perinuclear clear zone (Golgi apparatus). Cytoplasm from disrupted cells gives the background a basophilic swirling appearance. The inset is of a thicker region of the slide in which cells are better preserved (Wright-Giemsa stain, original magnification 100× objective. *Inset:* Wright-Giemsa stain, original magnification 100× objective).

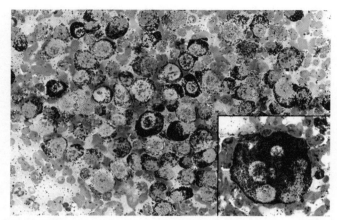

Fig. 18.40 Intestinal aspirate from a dog; mast cell tumor. Although mast cell tumors that arise from the gastrointestinal tract may be less well granulated than their cutaneous and subcutaneous counterparts, they may also be well granulated as can be seen in this image. In this case the cells are also highly pleomorphic with moderate to marked anisocytosis and anisokaryosis. The inset is of one of the rare giant multinucleate cells found in this specimen (Wright-Giemsa stain, original magnification 50× objective. *Inset:* Wright-Giemsa stain, original magnification 50× objective).

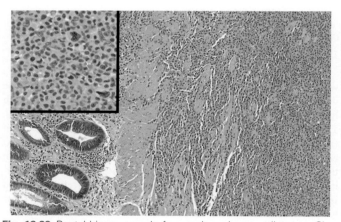

Fig. 18.39 Rectal biopsy sample from a dog; plasma cell tumor. Classic appearance of a plasma cell tumor with histopathology. Note the sheets and rows of neoplastic round cells predominantly within the submucosa. Even benign plasma cell tumors are fairly pleomorphic histologically *(see inset)*. Neoplastic plasma cells have characteristic eccentrically located nuclei, coarse chromatin, karyomegaly or multinucleation, or bizarre and convoluted nuclei (hematoxylin and eosin [H&E] stain, original magnification 10× objective; *Inset:* H&E stain, original magnification 40× objective).

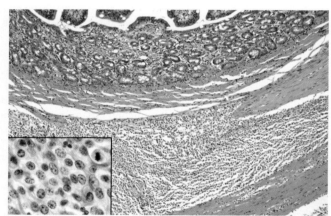

Fig. 18.41 Full-thickness biopsy sample of small intestine from a cat; intestinal mast cell tumor. Within the wall of the small intestine, separating smooth muscle bundles of the tunica muscularis and extending into the submucosa, sheets of neoplastic mast cells are pale-staining and lack very obvious granularity. This morphology is typical for tumors arising from mucosal mast cells, compared with cutaneous mast cell tumors, which are often more obviously granulated. The relative lack of granularity may make diagnosis of mast cell tumor over other round cell tumors, such as lymphoma, difficult in some cases, even with histochemical or immunohistochemical stains. In the inset, a mitotic figure is identified *(right aspect of image)* with few eosinophils *(left aspect of image)*. (hematoxylin and eosin [H&E] stain, original magnification 10× objective. *Inset:* H&E stain, original magnification 100× objective).

numbers of *Cyniclomyces* organisms may be identified in canine feces and, rarely, feline feces; the significance of this organism is not fully understood (see below discussion in "Abnormal Fecal Cytology"). Cytologically, *Cyniclomyces* are large organisms present individually or as short, forked, or branching chains (Fig. 18.43). Individual segments are approximately 5 to 7 × 15 to 20 μm, oval to cylindrical structures surrounded by a prominent clear cell wall, with an interior that stains uniformly purple, is mottled or vacuolated, or has a broad, transverse, poorly staining central region.[46]

Abnormal Fecal Cytology

Eosinophilic, neutrophilic, and lymphoplasmacytic inflammation may be noted and correspond to concurrent disease in the intestines,

such as IBD or infection (see "Intestinal Inflammation"). Because the normal flora identified in feces is a very mixed population of predominantly rod-shaped bacteria, alterations to this, including increased proportion of a specific bacterial subtype or a monomorphic bacterial proliferation, may indicate bacterial overgrowth. It is difficult to determine whether overgrowth suggested cytologically is truly causing the clinical signs in a patient because overgrowth may occur with a variety of disease processes or as a result of antibiotic therapy (Box 18.3).[47] In addition to bacterial overgrowth, overgrowth

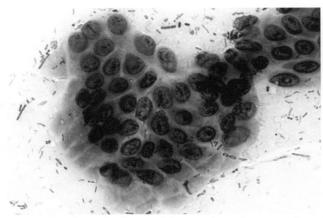

Fig. 18.42 Rectal scraping from a dog; normal rectal mucosa. A medium-sized cluster of normal columnar epithelial cells is present. Cells are uniform in appearance, with round basally oriented nuclei and moderate amounts of deeply basophilic cytoplasm. The columnar appearance is best appreciated on the left side of the cluster; in the center, the cells appear more cuboidal (Wright-Giemsa stain, original magnification 100× objective).

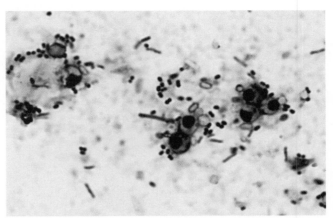

Fig. 18.44 Fecal smear from a dog; yeast overgrowth. Multiple round yeast organisms with a basophilic round eccentric nucleus and light-blue cytoplasm are present on a background of mixed bacteria and fecal debris. Polymerase chain reaction sequencing and culture indicated the organism was likely *Pichia* spp., and findings were interpreted as overgrowth of this nonpathogenic yeast (Wright-Giemsa stain, original magnification 100× objective). (Case from American Society of Veterinary Clinical Pathology, Mystery Slide Conference, 2008 Case 14, submitted by Shir Gilor.)

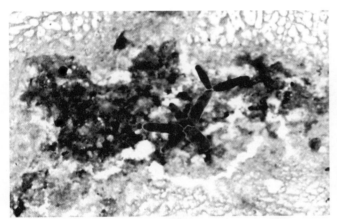

Fig. 18.43 Aspirate of a peripancreatic mass in a dog; necrotic material and *Cyniclomyces guttulatus* organisms. The underlying lesion in this animal was a full-thickness ulcer, which led to intestinal rupture and leakage of intestinal contents. Amorphous clumps of muted mauve material consistent with necrotic debris and large bacillus-shaped yeast organisms with branching or forked morphology and a banded, basophilic staining interior consistent with *C. guttulatus* were present. Organisms were considered incidental to the leakage of gastrointestinal contents and were not identified in tissue biopsy specimens (Wright-Giemsa stain, original magnification 50× objective).

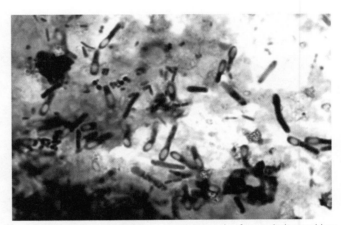

Fig. 18.45 Fecal smear from a cat; overgrowth of sporulating rod bacteria. The bacteria are large and contain a single eccentric clear spore giving them a "tennis racket" appearance. Although the presence of sporulating cells in a diarrheal patient warrants concern about *Clostridium perfringens*–associated diarrhea, studies have shown that identification of fecal endospores does not correlate with the detection of the enterotoxin. In addition, sporulation may be found in animals with or without diarrhea, and other organisms, such as *Bacillus* spp., may also sporulate (modified Wright-Giemsa stain, original magnification 100× objective).

BOX 18.3 Causes of Microbial Overgrowth in the Gastrointestinal Tract

- Idiopathic (primary)
- Antibiotic administration
- Exocrine pancreatic insufficiency
- Inflammatory bowel disease
- Intestinal stagnation or abnormal motility
- Intestinal obstruction
- Neoplasia
- Lymphangiectasia
- Impaired mucosal defense mechanisms
- Decreased gastric acid secretion
- Gastric or enteric surgical procedures

---

of yeast organisms may be identified in fecal samples (Fig. 18.44). Occasionally, animals with diarrhea are found to have large numbers of *C. guttulatus* organisms on fecal examination or smears (see Fig. 18.43). It remains unclear whether the overgrowth of this organism may cause or contribute to diarrhea or if the organism is simply flourishing in an altered environment. In some reported cases with diarrhea and high numbers of *Cyniclomyces* organisms, clinical signs did resolve with nystatin therapy.[48-50]

Bacterial agents that have been associated with diarrhea include large sporulating rod-shaped bacteria, such as *Clostridium* spp. and spirochetes, such as *Campylobacter* spp. (Figs. 18.45 and 18.46).

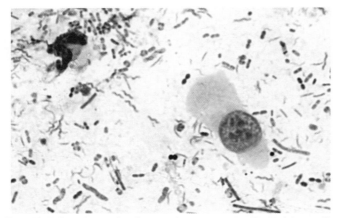

Fig. 18.46 Rectal scraping from a dog; numerous *Campylobacter*-like organisms (CLOs). A single enterocyte surrounded by a mixed population of bacteria is present. Many of the bacteria have the distinctive "gull wing" appearance characteristic of CLOs. Because pathogenic *Campylobacter* spp., nonpathogenic *Campylobacter* spp., and other organisms, such as *Arcobacter*, may all share similar morphology, additional diagnostics, including culture and polymerase chain reaction, should be used to diagnose campylobacteriosis (Wright-Giemsa stain, original magnification 100× objective).

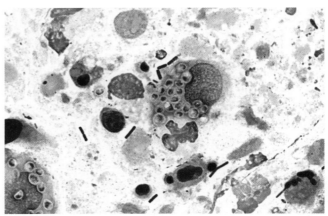

Fig. 18.47 Rectal scraping from a cat; histoplasmosis. Two macrophages containing *Histoplasma capsulatum* yeast are present. *Histoplasma* yeast are small and round with a thin clear cell wall and an interior that stains part basophilic and part clear, giving it a characteristic "half full, half empty" appearance. A monomorphic population of large rod bacteria is present, suggesting that there may be an abnormal overgrowth of bacteria as well (modified Wright-Giemsa stain, original magnification 100× objective).

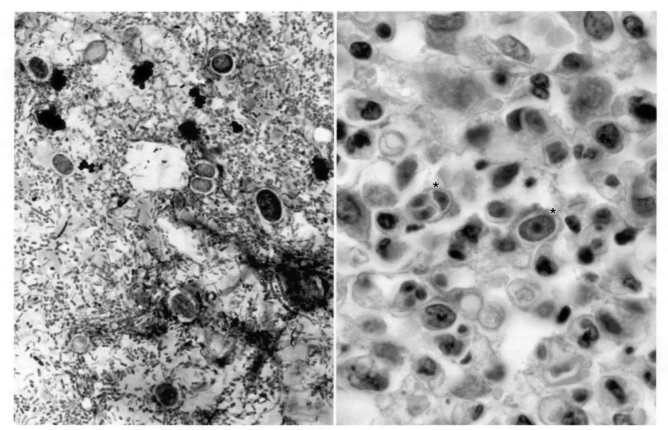

Fig. 18.48 Fecal sample *(left)* and large intestinal biopsy sample *(right)* from a dog; *Prototheca* infection. *Left:* Scattered oval shaped organisms with a thin clear cell wall and deeply basophilic granular interiors are present ("jelly bean" appearance) on a background of mixed bacteria consistent with fecal flora (Wright-Giemsa stain, original magnification 50× objective). *Right:* The inflammatory cells expanding the colonic wall consist mainly of epithelioid macrophages with fewer neutrophils and lymphocytes. Among the inflammatory cells, numerous empty cell walls of the *Prototheca* organisms are present. Several intact sporangia *(right [*])* are oval with a prominent magenta-purple nucleus and nucleolus and a clear halo of a cell wall, with occasional endosporulation *(left [*])* (hematoxylin and eosin [H&E] stain, original magnification 100× objective). (Case from Joint Pathology Center Veterinary Pathology Services [formerly AFIP], Wednesday Slide Conference 2002-03, Conference 16, Case 2.)

Although the presence of more than 3 to 5 sporulating cells per 100× field on cytological examination has previously been used to suggest *Clostridium perfringens*–associated diarrhea, several studies have shown that fecal endospore counts do not correlate with the presence of diarrhea or detection of the enterotoxin in fecal specimens and that sporulation may be found in animals with and without diarrhea.[3] In general, it may be difficult to differentiate nonpathogenic bacteria from pathogenic bacteria on fecal cytology; therefore, additional diagnostics such as culture, PCR, or toxin identification (for clostridial agents), are required for definitive identification (see Table 18.1).

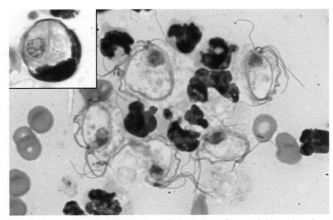

Fig. 18.49 Intestinal mass aspirate from a dog; *Pentatrichomonas hominis* infection and a carcinoma *(not pictured)*. A group of trophozoites admixed with degenerate neutrophils is present. The trophozoites are oval-shaped cells with five anterior flagella; a sixth recurrent flagellum associated with an undulating membrane that runs the length of the cell; a single anterior nucleus; and a well-developed vertical axostyle. The inset image is of an organism that has been phagocytized by a neutrophil (modified Wright-Giemsa stain, original magnification 100× objective). (Slide courtesy Valarie Pallatto.)

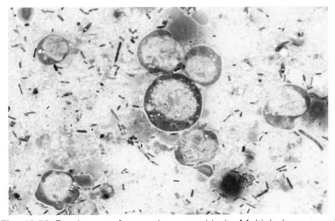

Fig. 18.50 Fecal smear from a dog; amoebiasis. Multiple large round parasitical organisms are present on a background of mixed primarily rod-shaped bacteria and are characterized by a central clear to pale staining area surrounded by a thin basophilic rim containing one to several round pink structures. The morphology is suggestive of the cyst form of *Iodamoeba bütschlii*, a typically harmless organism that may cause amoebiasis in immune-compromised individuals; however, other organisms such as *Blastocystis* can have overlapping morphology (Wright-Giemsa stain, original magnification 100× objective). (Case from American Society of Veterinary Clinical Pathology, Mystery Slide Conference, 2004 Case 20, submitted by Craig Thompson.)

Other than the normal bacterial flora, infectious agents, including *H. capsulatum*, *Prototheca* spp., *Pentatrichomonas hominis*, and *T. fetus*, may occasionally be identified in fecal samples (see Fig. 18.1; Figs. 18.47 to 18.50). Detailed descriptions, additional diagnostic testing, and images of the most common organisms in feces and throughout the GI tract are presented in Table 18.1.

REFERENCES

1. Broussard JD. Optimal fecal assessment. *Clin Tech Small Anim Pract.* 2003;18:218.
2. Greene CE. *Infectious Diseases of the Dog and Cat.* 4th ed. St. Louis, M: Saunders; 2012.
3. Marks SL, Rankin SC, Byrne BA, et al. Enteropathogenic bacteria in dogs and cats: diagnosis, epidemiology, treatment, and control. *J Vet Int Med.* 2011;25:1195.
4. Gaschen L. Ultrasonography of small intestinal inflammatory and neoplastic diseases in dogs and cats. *Vet Clin North Am Small Anim Pract.* 2011;41:329.
5. Tams TR. *Handbook of Small Animal Gastroenterology.* 2nd ed. St. Louis, MO: Saunders; 2003.
6. Ruiz G, Verrot L, Laloy E, et al. Diagnostic contribution of cytological specimens obtained from biopsies during gastrointestinal endoscopy in dogs and cats. *J Small Anim Pract.* 2016;58:17.
7. Maeda S, Tsuboi M, Sakai K, et al. Endoscopic cytology for the diagnosis of chronic enteritis and intestinal lymphoma in dogs. *Vet Pathol.* 2017;54(4):595.
8. Bacha WJ, Bacha LM. *Color Atlas of Veterinary Histology.* 2nd ed. Philadelphia, PA: Lippincott Williams & Wilkins; 2000.
9. Atkinson BF. *Atlas of Diagnostic Cytopathology.* 2nd ed. Philadelphia, PA: Saunders; 2004.
10. Drake M. *Gastro-Esophageal Cytology.* Basel, Switzerland: Karger; 1985.
11. Uzal FA, Plattner BL, Hostetter JM. Alimentary system. In: Maxie MG, eds. *Jubb, Kennedy and Palmer's Pathology of Domestic Animals.* 6th ed. St. Louis, MO: Saunders Elsevier; 2015.
12. Sellon RK, Willard MD. Esophagitis and esophageal strictures. *Vet Clin North Am Small Anim Pract.* 2003;33:945.
13. Gibson CJ, Parry NMA, Jakowski RM, et al. Adenomatous polyp with intestinal metaplasia of the esophagus (Barrett esophagus) in a dog. *Vet Pathol.* 2010;41:116.
14. Mazzei MJ, Bissett SA, Murphy KM, et al. Eosinophilic esophagitis in a dog. *J Am Vet Med Assoc.* 2009;235:61.
15. Munday JS, Lohr CV, Kiupel M. Tumors of the alimentary tract. In: Meuten DJ, ed. *Tumors in Domestic Animals.* 5th ed. Hoboken, NJ: John Wiley & Sons, Inc.; 2016.
16. Head KW, Cullen JM, Dubielzig RR, et al. *Histologic Classification of the Tumors of the Alimentary System of Domestic Animals.* series 2 Washington, D.C: Armed Forces Institute of Pathology; 2003.
17. Farese JP, Bacon NJ, Ehrhart NP, et al. Oesophageal leiomyosarcoma in dogs: surgical management and clinical outcome of four cases. *Vet Comp Oncol.* 2008;6:31.
18. Webb C, Twedt DC. Canine gastritis. *Vet Clin N Am Small Anim Pract.* 2003;33:969.
19. Lidbury JA, Suchodolski JS, Steiner JM. Gastric histopathologic abnormalities in dogs: 67 cases (2002-2007). *J Am Vet Med Assoc.* 2009;234:1147.
20. Takemura LS, et al. *Helicobacter* spp. in cats: association between infecting species and epithelial proliferation within the gastric lamina propria. *J Comp Pathol.* 2009;141:127.
21. Bridgeford EC, Marini RP, Feng Y, et al. Gastric *Helicobacter* species as a cause of feline gastric lymphoma: a viable hypothesis. *Vet Immunol Immunop.* 2008;123:106.
22. Craig LE, Hardam EE, Hertzke EM, et al. Feline gastrointestinal eosinophilic sclerosing fibroplasia. *Vet Pathol.* 2009;46:63.
23. Lyles SE, et al. Idiopathic eosinophilic masses of the gastrointestinal tract in dogs. *J Vet Int Med.* 2009;23:818.
24. LeBlanc CJ, Echandi RL, Moore RR, et al. Hypercalcemia associated with gastric pythiosis in a dog. *Vet Clin Pathol.* 2008;37:115.

25. Vatn S, et al. Possible involvement of *Sarcina ventriculi* in canine and equine acute gastric dilatation. *Acta Vet Scand*. 2000;41:333.

26. Gualtieria M, Monzeglio MG, Scanziani E. Gastric neoplasms. *Vet Clin North Am Small Anim Pract*. 1999;29:415.

27. Qvigstad G, et al. Gastric neuroendocrine carcinoma associated with atrophic gastritis in the Norwegian Lundehund. *J Comp Pathol*. 2008;139:194.

28. Russell KN, Mehler SJ, Skorupski KA, et al. Clinical and immunohistochemical differentiation of gastrointestinal stromal tumors from leiomyosarcomas in dogs: 42 cases (1990-2003). *J Am Vet Med Assoc*. 2007;230:1329.

29. Hayes S, Yuzbasiyan-Gurkan V, Gregory-Bruson E, Kiupel M. Classification of canine nonangiogenic, nonlymphogenic, gastrointestinal sarcomas based on microscopic, immunohistochemical and molecular characteristics. *Vet Pathol*. 2013;50:779.

30. Pohlman LM, et al. Immunophenotypic and histologic classification of 50 cases of feline gastrointestinal lymphoma. *Vet Pathol*. 2009;46:259.

31. Cerquetella M, Spaterna A, Laus F. Inflammatory bowel disease in the dog: differences and similarities with humans. *World J Gastroenterol*. 2010;16:1050.

32. Day MJ, Bilzer T, Mansell J, et al. Histopathological standards for the diagnosis of gastrointestinal inflammation in endoscopic biopsy samples from the dog and cat: a report from the World Small Animal Veterinary Association Gastrointestinal Standardization Group. *J Comp Pathol*. 2008;138:S1.

33. Johnson CS, Fales-Williams AJ, Reimer SB, et al. Fibrosing gastrointestinal leiomyositis as a cause of chronic intestinal pseudo-obstruction in an 8-month-old dog. *Vet Pathol*. 2007;44:106.

34. Fabrick C, Bugbee A, Fosgate G. Clinical features and outcome of *Heterobilharzia Americana* infection in dogs. *J Vet Int Med*. 2010;24:140.

35. Craven M, Mansfield CS, Simpson KW. Granulomatous colitis of boxer dogs. *Vet Clin North Am Small Anim Pract*. 2011;41:433.

36. Yaeger MJ, Gookin JL. Histologic features associated with *Tritrichomonas foetus*-induced colitis in domestic cats. *Vet Pathol*. 2005;42:797.

37. Frank JD, et al. Clinical outcomes of 30 cases (1997-2004) of canine gastrointestinal lymphoma. *J Am Anim Hosp Assoc*. 2007;43:313.

38. Moore PF, Rodriguez-Bertos A, Kass PH. Feline gastrointestinal lymphoma: mucosal architecture, immunophenotyped and molecular clonality. *Vet Pathol*. 2012;49:658.

39. Kiupel M, Smedley RC, Pfent C, et al. Diagnostic algorithm to differentiate lymphoma from inflammation in feline small intestinal biopsy samples. *Vet Pathol*. 2011;48:212.

40. Krick EL, Little L, Patel R, et al. Description of clinical and pathological findings, treatment and outcome of feline large granular lymphocyte lymphoma (1996-2004). *Vet Comp Oncol*. 2008;6:102.

41. Carrasco V, Rodriguez-Bertos A, Rodriguez-Franco F, et al. Distinguishing intestinal lymphoma from inflammatory bowel disease in canine duodenal endoscopic biopsy sample. *Vet Pathol*. 2015;52:668.

42. Fukushima K, Ohno K, Koshino-Goto Y, et al. Sensitivity for the detection of a clonally rearranged antigen receptor gene in endoscopically obtained biopsy specimens from canine alimentary lymphoma. *J Vet Med Sci*. 2009;71:1673.

43. Ozaki K, et al. T-cell lymphoma with eosinophilic infiltration involving the intestinal tract in 11 dogs. *Vet Pathol*. 2006;43:339.

44. Ozaki K, et al. Mast cell tumors of the gastrointestinal tract in 39 Dogs. *Vet Pathol*. 2002;39:557.

45. Halsey CHC, Powers BE, Kamstock DA. Feline intestinal sclerosing mast cell tumour: 50 cases (1997-2008). *Vet Comp Oncol*. 2010;8:72.

46. Neel JA, Tarigo J, Grindem CB. Gall bladder aspirate from a dog. *Vet Clin Pathol*. 2006;35:467.

47. Tarpley HL, Bounous DI. Digestive system. In: Latimer KS, ed. *Duncan and Prasse's Veterinary Laboratory Medicine Clinical Pathology*. 5th ed. Ames, IA: Wiley-Blackwell; 2011.

48. Houwers DJ, Blankenstein B. *Cyniclomyces guttulatus* (brillendoosjegist) en diarree bij honden [*Cyniclomyces guttulatus* {eyeglass box yeast} and diarrhea in dogs]. *Tijdschr Diergeneesk*. 2001;126:502.

49. Mandigers PJ, Duijvestijn MB, Ankringa N, et al. The clinical significance of cyniclomyces guttulatus in dogs with chronic diarrhea, a survey and a prospective treatment study. Wiley-Blackwell. *Vet Microbiol*. 2014;172:241.

50. Winston JA, Piperisova I, Neel J, Gookin JL. Cyniclomyces guttulatus infection in dogs: 19 cases (2006-2013). *J Am Anim Hosp Assoc*. 2016;52:42.

19

The Pancreas

Regan R. W. Bell, Jean-Sébastien Latouche, and Dori L. Borjesson

Cytology of the pancreas is increasingly used to help clinicians diagnose pancreatic disorders. This increase in pancreatic aspiration in human medicine may have resulted from increased clinician comfort with pancreatic manipulation, as well as the utility of pancreatic aspiration with its minimal complications. Previous perceptions that pancreatic manipulation may cause pancreatitis have largely been unsubstantiated. A recent study showed that fine-needle aspiration (FNA) of normal canine pancreas does not result in increased serum concentrations of trypsin-like immunoreactivity (TLI) or canine-specific pancreatic lipase (cPL).[1] This is compared with intraoperative biopsy, which was associated with increased serum TLI and sporadic, mild, peracute necrosis, inflammation, hemorrhage, and fibrin deposition,[1] as well as postoperative complications in approximately 23% of dogs and cats in one study, of which five cases were suggestive of postoperative pancreatitis.[2]

Currently, no single test conclusively differentiates inflammatory, cystic, neoplastic, and infectious diseases involving the pancreas. Patients with pancreatic disorders, except for pancreatic insufficiency, often have similar histories and clinical signs. Clinicopathological testing can frequently identify the presence of pancreatic disease in the dog.[3,4] However, in the cat, serum chemistry tests are often less useful.[5-9] In both dogs and cats, abdominal ultrasonography (AUS) is a useful diagnostic tool to visualize and assess an abnormal pancreas, guide aspirates and biopsies, and monitor response to treatment.[7,10-12] As with biochemical tests, however, AUS has variable sensitivity and specificity because ultrasonography (US) appearances of various pancreatic disorders overlap.[7,10-12] Once the pancreas is visualized, ultrasound-guided FNA is a safe and effective adjunct to imaging in the diagnosis of pancreatic disorders. The pancreas exfoliates well, and the cytology of the pancreas in small animals has proven useful in diagnosis of both neoplastic and nonneoplastic lesions, including abscesses, cysts, and pancreatitis.

NORMAL PANCREAS STRUCTURE

Anatomy and Histology

The pancreas consists of a right (duodenal) limb and a left (transverse or splenic) limb joined at the head. The number and position of the pancreatic duct(s) opening into the duodenum and the location of the duct(s) to the common bile duct varies among species and individuals within a species.[13] The pancreas consists of endocrine and exocrine components. Numerous tubuloacinar secretory units form the exocrine component of the organ (Fig. 19.1). These secretory units drain into long, narrow intercalated ducts lined by elongated, cuboidal cells. Intercalated ducts communicate directly with interlobular ducts.[14] Functionally, the tubuloacinar secretory units (exocrine pancreas) secrete digestive enzymes in an inactive proenzyme form. Pancreatic enzymes are activated by trypsin secreted by the duodenum.

The endocrine islets of Langerhans are clusters of epithelial cells scattered among the secretory units (Fig. 19.2). Normal pancreatic islets contain four cell types, each secreting different pancreatic polypeptides: (1) α-cells secrete glucagon, (2) β-cells secrete insulin, (3) D-cells secrete somatostatin, and (4) F-cells secrete pancreatic polypeptide. β-cells are the most numerous (constituting 60%–70% of the islet cells) and usually centrally located in the islet. α-cells constitute about 20% of the islet cells and are generally located peripherally.[13]

SAMPLING TECHNIQUE

Methods

In veterinary medicine, percutaneous, ultrasound-guided FNA of the pancreas is the most common method of tissue sampling.[15] In dogs, dynamic computed tomography (CT) has recently been used to assess normal and neoplastic lesions of the pancreas.[16] Endoscopic ultrasonography (EUS) has proven to be feasible and safe in medium-sized dogs, although more studies are needed to determine its diagnostic utility.[17] In cats (especially obese cats), EUS may be superior to AUS for imaging the pancreas.[18]

Methods for FNA of the pancreas are outlined in Box 19.1. The described methods are closely based on methods originally proposed by Bjorneby and Kari.[15] In brief, the pancreas and the

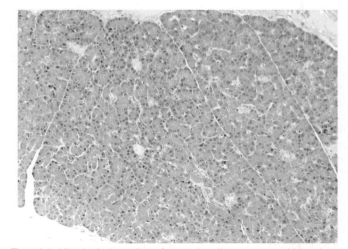

Fig. 19.1 Histological section of normal canine pancreas. Normal pancreas consists of numerous lobules separated by septa of connective tissue. Lobules are primarily composed of tubuloacinar secretory units that form the exocrine component of the organ. Acinar cells have small, dark, uniform nuclei with abundant bright-pink cytoplasm. Islets and scattered intercalated ducts are also present, which drain the epithelial cells (hematoxylin and eosin [H&E] stain, original magnification 100×).

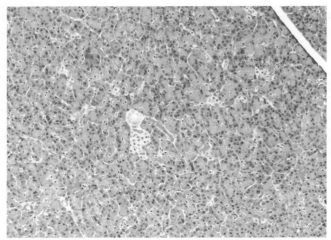

Fig. 19.2 Histological section of normal canine pancreas. A pancreatic lobule composed of exocrine tubuloacinar secretory units with a single duct and a single aggregate of pale pancreatic endocrine cells (islet of Langerhans cells) near the center of the section. Acinar cells have a distinct polarity with centrally located eosinophilia (zymogen granules) and basilar basophilia (nucleus and cytoplasm). Scattered small vessels and small intercalated ducts are also present (hematoxylin and eosin [H&E] stain, original magnification 100×).

BOX 19.1 Outline of Fine-Needle Biopsy Technique

- Use ultrasonography to visualize the area to be aspirated.
- Set out and label 6 to 10 clean glass slides.
- Draw 1 milliliter (mL) of air into a 3-mL syringe.
- Attach a ½- to 3-inch 22-gauge needle to the syringe.
- Guide the needle attached to the syringe into the pancreas.
- *Avoid* redirecting the needle; negative pressure is *not* needed.
- Quickly expel the sample onto a slide.
- Prepare multiple smears by using a variety of gentle techniques.
- Include squash preparations and blood-smear techniques.
- Sample multiple sites within the lesion.
- Rapidly air-dry the smears.
- Submit air-dried, labeled slides to a veterinary clinical pathologist.

---

surrounding abdominal structures should be thoroughly evaluated with US. If a mass is present, multiple areas within the mass and surrounding tissue should be aspirated. In dogs, inflammation (purulent or lymphocytic) has been shown to occur in discrete areas throughout the pancreas (right and left limb).[15] Therefore no specific site is preferred to sample the pancreas (and confirm pancreatitis) in the absence of a visible lesion. The following steps are then performed:

- Label clean glass slides, preferably those with frosted edges, with patient identification and site of aspiration.
- Draw 1 milliliter (mL) of air into a 3-mL syringe. Attach a 1½- to 3-inch 22-gauge needle to the syringe. This needle-and-syringe combination may permit more accurate needle placement and angle control.[19]
- Using ultrasound-guided biopsy or a freehand technique, place the needle in the desired region for aspiration, and move the needle back and forth within the pancreas.
- Be sure to visualize the needle with US guidance at all times, and maintain the needle in the same tract. For sample procurement, no additional negative pressure is required. Do not attempt to redirect

the needle because the tip of the needle may lacerate the tissue and cause excessive hemorrhage and leakage of pancreatic enzymes.[19]

- To minimize cell disruption, sample expulsion and smear preparation should be as gentle as possible.
- Expel the sample onto the middle of the slide where cells are most readily stained and visualized.
- Sample three to four different sites within the lesion/pancreas, if possible.
- To ensure the best-quality sample (and thus enhance the likelihood of a cytological diagnosis), make multiple smears by using a variety of smear techniques that result in both thin and thick preparations.
- Slide preparation techniques include the squash-smear (slide-over-slide) or the blood-smear technique. The smears should be air-dried and submitted to a veterinary clinical pathologist.[19]

In the authors' experience, this technique can be improved by using an extension set for intravenous lines that can be used multiple times and a 12-mL syringe prefilled with 5 mL of air. The extension set is draped over the shoulders with the syringe easily accessible with the nondominant hand. This makes the needle easier to hold (like a pen), produces more precise sampling, reduces the risk for laceration, and permits an expeditious transfer of the sample onto the slides.[20]

Troubleshooting

In general, pancreatic tissue exfoliates well for FNA. In case of quality concerns, a cytopathologist should be consulted about sample attainment and preparation. Ruptured cells may result from negative pressure in the syringe while aspirating or too much pressure on slides during preparation.[19] Rapid drying of slides reduces artifact on the slides. Hemodilution is common and usually will not confound diagnosis. However, if hemodilution is obscuring the diagnosis (especially distinguishing between blood contamination and inflammation), the number of times the needle is moved within the pancreas should be decreased. However, the trade-off may be poor cytological yield, which may occur if the needle biopsy technique is not aggressive enough. If clots tend to form, the needle and syringe should be flushed with an anticoagulant (i.e., ethylenediaminetetraacetic acid [EDTA]) before aspiration. Nondiagnostic samples because of poor cellularity may occur when lesions are fibrous or if the lesion was missed during aspiration. Reaspiration may be attempted if the pancreas appears active and enlarged. However, if fibrosis is likely, intraoperative biopsy will likely be required for a diagnosis. Cytological findings should always be interpreted in light of imaging, physical examination, and biochemical findings. For example, if poorly cellular, proteinaceous fluid is obtained and the lesion on imaging is compatible with a cyst, then further diagnostics may not be warranted (Fig. 19.3). However, if poorly cellular, proteinaceous fluid is obtained and the lesion is primarily solid or infiltrative with cystic or necrotic areas, reaspiration may be indicated because the primary lesion may not be represented. Without history and US findings, interpretation and recommendations can be more difficult.

Diagnostic Yield and Complications

Diagnostic yield is typically good, and significant adverse effects secondary to percutaneous FNA of the pancreas in dogs or cats are uncommon. In one recent study of 92 dogs, diagnostic yield was 73.5% (calculated as the percentage of cases in which a cytological diagnosis could be achieved), with good correlation when histopathology was available for comparison (10 of 11 cases). Seven adverse events were seen, all in dogs with significant comorbidities or undergoing other invasive procedures.[21] In cats, ultrasound-guided FNA did not increase the complication or mortality rates in those undergoing pancreatic aspiration compared with those that did not, and most complications were noted when a second organ, typically the liver, was aspirated.[22]

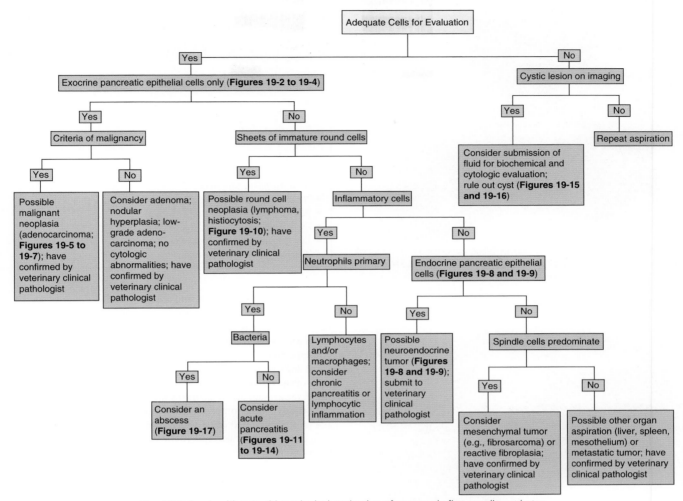

Fig. 19.3 An algorithm to aid cytological evaluation of pancreatic fine-needle aspirates.

CYTOLOGICAL EVALUATION

Normal

A decision tree to help guide initial cytological evaluation of the pancreas is depicted in Fig. 19.3. Exocrine epithelial cells are the most common cell type found on cytology of the pancreas. The background of the slide may contain blood from iatrogenic contamination, or it may be light pink, indicating the presence of a small amount of protein. Normal exocrine epithelial cells are found in small clusters to large sheets, sometimes with tubular and acinar structures (Fig. 19.4). Unlike intestinal epithelial cells, cell-to-cell junctions are not prominent, giving cells a more indistinct, fluffy appearance (Fig. 19.5). The cells are polyhedral, with abundant cytoplasm and a low nucleus-to-cytoplasm (N:C) ratio (see Figs. 19.4 and Fig. 19.5; Fig. 19.6). Nuclei are basilar, uniform, and round to oval. Chromatin is stippled, sometimes with a distinct single, small, occasionally prominent nucleolus (see Figs. 19.5 and 19.6). On high magnification, abundant pink cytoplasmic granules consistent with membrane-bound zymogen granules are noted. In preparations with abundant cell rupture, these granules may fill the background of the slide, giving a mottled blue-and-pink appearance (see Fig. 19.6). In FNA of normal pancreas, no other cell populations will be present in high numbers. Occasionally, hematopoietic precursors indicative of extramedullary hematopoiesis, small ductal cells, or uniform pancreatic endocrine cells will be seen. Interpret leukocyte numbers in light of peripheral blood cell counts to avoid interpreting peripheral neutrophilia or lymphocytosis as pancreatic inflammation.

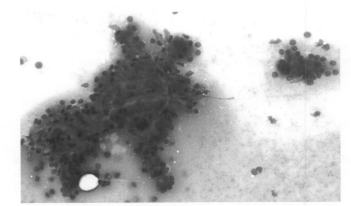

Fig. 19.4 Fine-needle aspirate of normal canine pancreas. Exocrine epithelial cells predominate and often exfoliate in small sheets and large clusters with acinar and tubular formations. Cells are polyhedral, cytoplasm is abundant, nucleus-to-cytoplasm (N:C) ratios are low, and nuclei are uniform (Wright-Giemsa stain, original magnification 200×).

Pancreatic Lesions

A summary of the World Health Organization (WHO) scheme for the histological classification of pancreatic lesions of domestic animals is presented in Box 19.2.[23,24]

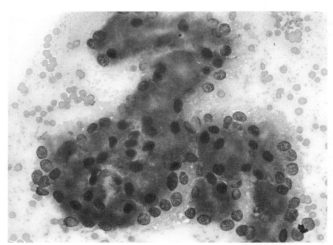

Fig. 19.5 Fine-needle aspirate of normal feline pancreas. The nuclei of exocrine epithelial cells often show a basilar distribution. Clear cell-to-cell junctions are not apparent. Nuclei are round to oval, chromatin is stippled, and single, small, uniform nucleoli can be present (Wright-Giemsa stain, original magnification 500×).

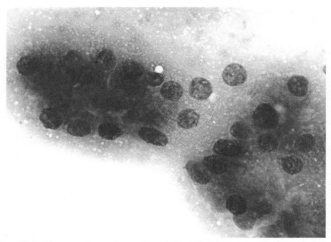

Fig. 19.6 Fine-needle aspirate of normal canine pancreas. Exocrine epithelial cells are characterized by apical, abundant, small, pink cytoplasmic granules, most consistent with membrane-bound zymogen granules. These granules give densely packed pancreatic exocrine epithelial cells a pink hue at lower magnification (Wright-Giemsa stain, original magnification 1000×).

Neoplasia

Adenoma

Benign exocrine epithelial tumors (i.e., exocrine adenomas, ductal [tubular] adenomas, or acinar adenomas) are rare in small animals and are far less common than their malignant counterparts. They tend to be small, solitary lesions found incidentally on imaging or at necropsy. Histologically, they are partially or totally encapsulated, unlike the more common lesion of nodular hyperplasia.[13,23,25] Cytologically, adenomas cannot be distinguished from normal or hyperplastic pancreatic tissue (see Fig. 19.3). If abundant, uniform, pancreatic exocrine epithelial cells are noted along with imaging findings suggestive of a solitary, solid lesion, differential diagnoses should include an adenoma, well-differentiated carcinoma, or a hyperplastic nodule (see Fig. 19.3).

Adenocarcinoma

Malignant tumors of the exocrine pancreas (i.e., adenocarcinomas, ductal [tubular] adenocarcinomas, or exocrine carcinomas) are

uncommon in dogs and cats and are rare in other domestic animals.[25] They are subtyped by the predominant arrangement of cells within the neoplasm. It is currently uncertain whether either the subtype of the neoplasm or the differentiation of cells has prognostic significance in domestic animals.[25]

In dogs, pancreatic adenocarcinomas are rare in animals less than 4 years of age with no reported sex or breed predisposition.[19] In one small study, the average age at diagnosis was 9 and 10 years for dogs and cats, respectively.[19] In another study, 85% of dogs and cats with pancreatic adenocarcinoma had distant metastases at the time of diagnosis, and 88% of the patients had metastatic disease at the time of necropsy.[19] Common metastatic sites include abdominal or thoracic lymph nodes, mesentery, adjacent gastrointestinal (GI) organs (including the liver, duodenum, and jejunum), lungs, and, less frequently, spleen, kidney, and diaphragm.[19] Local, destructive infiltration may destroy the common bile duct.

Presenting clinical signs are nonspecific, but weight loss, vomiting, abdominal pain, and anorexia are common in dogs. Jaundice and cholestasis may result from obstruction of the bile duct by tumor, secondary liver disease, or both. Clinicopathological tests often show peripheral neutrophilia and may show increased pancreatic enzyme activity, but evidence of extrahepatic biliary obstruction, including elevations in alkaline phosphatase (ALP) and alanine aminotransferase (ALT) activities, is more frequently seen.[19] Described paraneoplastic syndromes include alopecia, exocrine pancreatic insufficiency, and cutaneous and visceral necrotizing panniculitis and steatitis.[26-28]

In dogs, pancreatic adenocarcinomas are generally solitary, firm and pale. Because they are infiltrative, neoplasms can be diffusely present within the pancreas and difficult to differentiate from pancreatic parenchyma. In cats, pancreatic adenocarcinomas are most commonly solitary masses but can also be multifocal or diffusely infiltrate the pancreas.[25] In one study of 19 cats, the only imaging finding unique to malignant pancreatic tumors was the presence of a single pancreatic nodule or mass exceeding 2 cm in at least one dimension.[11] Histopathologically, pancreatic adenocarcinomas are highly variable. Some are well-differentiated, tubular adenocarcinomas that form acinar structures, whereas others may form more solid sheets of poorly differentiated cells that no longer resemble pancreatic acini (Fig. 19.7).[25]

Although pancreatic adenocarcinoma is far less common in dogs and cats than in humans, most pancreatic neoplasms are malignant as in humans. In human medicine, implementation of objective cytological criteria has resulted in a relatively high diagnostic sensitivity and

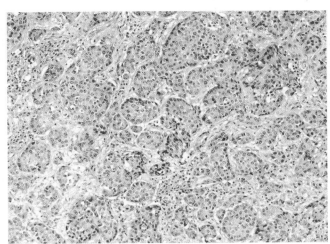

Fig. 19.7 Histopathological section of pancreatic carcinoma in a dog. The section is hypercellular and consists of variably disorganized acinar epithelial cells found in islands and primitive tubules. Neoplastic islands are separated by desmoplastic stroma (mesenchyme). A general loss of uniform acinar architecture occurs. Anisocytosis and anisokaryosis are noted, along with increased nucleus-to-cytoplasm (N:C) ratio and large, pale nucleoli (hematoxylin and eosin [H&E] stain, original magnification 100×).

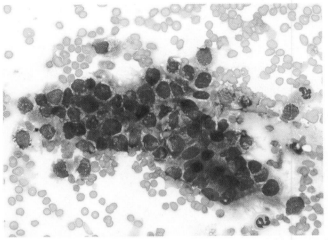

Fig. 19.8 Fine-needle aspirate of pancreatic adenocarcinoma in a cat. These cells show a markedly increased nucleus-to-cytoplasm (N:C) ratio and anisokaryosis. Additional criteria of malignancy include polygonal nuclei, nuclear overlap, irregular nuclear membranes, cytoplasmic vacuolization, and rare nucleoli (Wright-Giemsa stain, original magnification 500×).

BOX 19.3 Cytological Criteria of Malignancy

- Nuclear crowding and overlap (oval, polygonal, angular nuclei)
- Anisokaryosis (with nuclei >2.5 times red blood cell diameter)
- Nuclear membrane contour irregularities
- Irregular chromatin distribution (alcohol-fixed specimens mostly)
- Prominent nucleoli (large and irregular/macronucleoli)
- Single cells or loss of cellular cohesion
- Mitotic figures, especially aberrant mitoses
- Increased nucleus-to-cytoplasm ratio

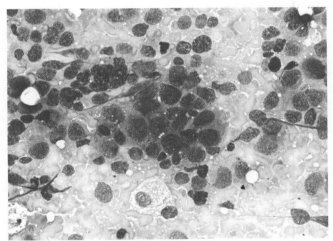

Fig. 19.9 Fine-needle aspirate of pancreatic adenocarcinoma in a dog. Cells from this sample exfoliated in loosely cohesive sheets with many single cells present. Additional criteria of malignancy included marked anisokaryosis, increased nucleus-to-cytoplasm (N:C) ratios, nuclear crowding and molding, polygonal nuclei, punctate cytoplasmic vacuoles, and occasional nucleoli (Wright-Giemsa stain, original magnification 500×).

specificity for the diagnosis of pancreatic adenocarcinoma, ranging from 80% to 98% and 93% to 100%, respectively.[29] Similar standard criteria have not been developed in veterinary medicine, although this may be a goal in small animals. Until that time, the criteria stated in human-based studies are compatible with the important criteria of malignancy noted by the authors.

Criteria of malignancy defining pancreatic adenocarcinoma are listed in Box 19.3.[30-32] The strongest indicators of malignancy that define human pancreatic adenocarcinomas include anisokaryosis, loss of cellular cohesion (single cells are common), irregular nuclear contours, nuclear crowding, prominent nucleoli, and aberrant mitoses (see Box 19.3).[29-32]

Aspirates of pancreatic carcinoma in small animals tend to be highly cellular (see Fig. 19.3; Figs. 19.8 and 19.9), and cells often show an increased N:C ratio and marked anisokaryosis (see Figs. 19.8; 19.9; Fig. 19.10). Irregular nuclear contours, nuclear molding, and polygonal and angular nuclei may be noted (see Figs. 19.8 to 19.10). Cytoplasmic vacuolization is frequently noted in carcinoma (see Figs. 19.8 to 19.10) but may also reflect epithelial reactivity secondary to pancreatitis. Chromatin varies from stippled to coarsely clumped, with occasionally prominent, irregular, and multiple nucleoli (see Figs. 19.9 and 19.10). The background may be necrotic, hemodilute, inflamed (macrophages and small lymphocytes) (see Fig. 19.9), or pink and cystic-appearing (see Fig. 19.10). Well-differentiated pancreatic adenocarcinomas may result in false-negative cytological interpretations.

In one study, well-differentiated adenocarcinomas were differentiated from high-grade adenocarcinomas by the absence of necrosis, mitoses, and macronuclei.[29] Differential diagnoses for large sheets or clusters of fairly well-differentiated pancreatic epithelial cells should include normal pancreas, adenoma, nodular hyperplasia, or well-differentiated carcinoma (see Fig. 19.3).

Endocrine (Neuroendocrine) Tumors of the Pancreas

Neuroendocrine tumors of the pancreas (NETPs) (i.e., tumors of pancreatic islet cells, islet cell adenomas, and islet cell adenocarcinomas) include insulinomas (β-cell neoplasms), gastrinomas, somatostatinomas, glucagonomas, and carcinoid tumors.[24] In small animal patients, insulinomas are the most common NETP, followed in frequency by gastrinoma. Somatostatinoma, glucagonoma, and carcinoid tumor are

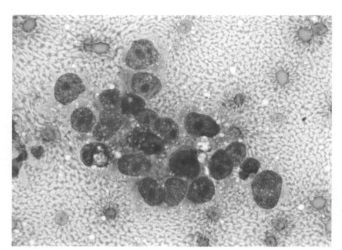

Fig. 19.10 Fine-needle aspirate of pancreatic adenocarcinoma in a cat. This cluster of cells show marked nuclear and nucleolar criteria of malignancy. Note the markedly elevated nucleus-to-cytoplasm (N:C) ratio, marked nuclear enlargement, irregular nuclear membrane contours, and prominent, deeply basophilic, single to multiple, occasionally irregular nucleoli. The dense, pink, stippled background of the slide may represent a cystic component to this neoplasm (Wright-Giemsa stain, original magnification 1000×).

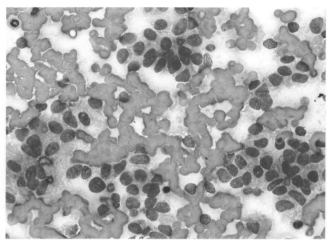

Fig. 19.11 Fine-needle aspirate of a malignant insulinoma in a dog. The sample is highly cellular, with cells found in loosely cohesive groups. Cell-to-cell borders are indistinct, and free nuclei appear scattered in a mass of shared cytoplasm. Compared with adenocarcinomas, anisokaryosis is relatively mild, although rare large nuclei are noted. Overall, the cells have a monomorphic appearance. As with other neuroendocrine tumors, individual cells are generally nondescript. Definitive tumor classification can be made only in light of imaging findings, physical examination findings, and clinicopathological data. This patient had a persistently low glucose of 23 milligrams per deciliter (mg/dL) (reference interval: 70–120 mg/dL) and a fasting insulin concentration of 138 international units per milliliter (IU/mL) (reference interval: 5–15 IU/mL). Necropsy confirmed metastases to mesenteric lymph nodes and liver (Wright-Giemsa stain, original magnification 500×).

rarely or not yet reported in small animals. Most NETPs are multihormonal; as such, they may secrete or express one or more neuroendocrine markers, including pancreatic hormones (e.g., insulin, glucagon, pancreatic polypeptide, and somatostatin) and hormones not normally expressed in mammalian pancreas (e.g., gastrin, adrenocorticotropic hormone, and calcitonin). The majority of NETPs are immunohistochemically positive for insulin (89%), and approximately 30% are positive for somatostatin, glucagon, and pancreatic polypeptide.[24,33] Amyloid deposits may be found in 17% to 32% of NETPs.[33] Superficial necrolytic dermatitis occurs most commonly with liver disease (often called "hepatocutaneous syndrome") but has also been reported secondary to glucagonoma, diabetes mellitus, and insulinoma, which all cause varying metabolic and hormonal imbalances.[34]

Tumors of the exocrine and endocrine pancreas (NETPs) (see Fig. 19.3) can usually be readily distinguished from each other on cytology. However, the biological behavior of NETPs may be difficult to predict. Pancreatic NETPs in human beings are classified as well-differentiated neuroendocrine tumors (benign, uncertain malignant potential, low-grade malignant) or poorly differentiated neuroendocrine carcinoma (high-grade malignant). This is not based on cytology; rather, differentiation is based on tumor size, the presence of vascular invasion or metastases, the number of mitoses per high power field and the Ki67 proliferation index.[35] The degree of multihormonality and growth pattern show no correlation with biological behavior.[33] In addition, cytology is often not helpful in differentiating between benign NETPs (islet cell adenomas) and their malignant counterparts (islet cell carcinomas) unless profound criteria of malignancy are met. The absence of anaplastic features does not rule out malignancy. Histological evidence of invasion by the tumor cells through the capsule and into adjacent pancreatic parenchyma or lymphatics, or metastatic disease, are the most important criteria of malignancy for NETPs.[36,37] When the cytological specimen is characterized by minimally pleomorphic neuroendocrine cells, in the absence of history or clinical findings, the cytological diagnosis of neuroendocrine tumor or islet cell tumor is most appropriate.

Insulinomas are seen most frequently in dogs ages 5 to 12 years. Grossly, they appear as single, small nodules visible from the serosal surface of the pancreas; however, malignant tumors may be larger and multilobular and show extensive invasion into the adjacent parenchyma. Malignant insulinomas are more common than benign insulinomas in dogs.[36] In one study, 45% to 55% of insulin-producing NETPs were malignant in dogs (in contrast to 10%–15% in humans).[33] There is a single case report of osseous metaplasia within a malignant insulinoma; histopathology confirmed that approximately 60% of the mass comprised mineralized compact bone.[38] Metastasis to regional lymph nodes, liver, mesentery, and omentum is noted in about 50% of cases.[39] Many breeds are affected; however, Boxers, Irish Terriers, Labrador Retrievers, and German Shepherds appear overrepresented. Both sexes appear to be affected equally.[36] Because most insulinomas are secretory, a tentative diagnosis may be made by demonstrating profound hypoglycemia and an abnormal insulin-to-glucose ratio. Surgical removal (partial pancreatectomy) may significantly increase median survival time.[39] In one study of dogs with insulinomas, it was reported that (1) dogs with higher preoperative serum insulin levels had shorter survival times, (2) dogs with tumors confined to the pancreas had longer disease-free intervals, and (3) younger dogs had significantly shorter survival time compared with older dogs.[39] Gastrinoma, although a rare tumor in veterinary medicine, frequently metastasizes to regional lymph nodes and liver. Prognosis is considered grave.[37,40]

The cytological and histological appearance of NETPs is typical of other neuroendocrine tumors. They are generally highly cellular but fragile, with many single cells, small, poorly cohesive groups, or both (Figs. 19.11 and 19.12). Aspirates frequently contain free (bare) nuclei on a background of lightly basophilic cytoplasm (see Figs. 19.11 and 19.12). Intact cells are medium to large with often poorly defined cytoplasmic borders (see Fig. 19.11) and pale blue, sometimes vacuolated cytoplasm (see Fig. 19.12). Anisokaryosis is usually mild to moderate,

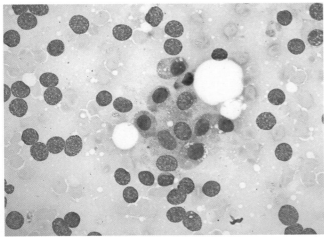

Fig. 19.12 Fine-needle aspirate of an islet-cell insulinoma in a dog. A small cluster of intact cells is noted with free nuclei in the background. Cells have distinct borders in that cluster. Anisokaryosis is mild with finely stippled chromatin, 0 to 2 small poorly defined nucleoli, and a moderate amount of lightly basophilic cytoplasm with few punctate vacuoles. The patient had persistent hypoglycemia on dextrose continuous rate infusion (CRI) and abnormal insulin level (Wright-Giemsa stain, original magnification 1000×).

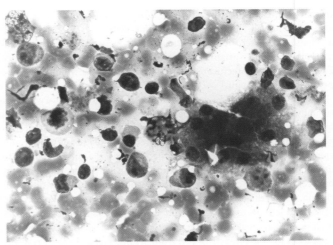

Fig. 19.13 Fine-needle aspirate of pancreatic lymphoma in a dog. The sample is moderately cellular with several clusters of benign exocrine epithelial cells and moderate numbers of large neoplastic lymphocytes showing prominent nucleoli. Mitotic figures are observed, such as on the far left. The patient had multicentric lymphoma and sample is from a hypoechoic nodule in the body of the pancreas (Wright-Giemsa stain, original magnification 1000×).

giving a monomorphic appearance to the cells (see Figs. 19.11 and 19.12). Additional nuclear features may include nuclear molding, eccentrically placed nuclei (giving a plasmacytoid appearance), and binucleation. Chromatin is generally fine and granular with a single prominent nucleolus (see Figs. 19.11 and 19.12).[13,39,41,42] Rarely, pancreatic neoplasms can contain both neuroendocrine and exocrine neoplastic epithelial cells, as reported recently in a young cat with a pancreatic neuroendocrine carcinoma with exocrine differentiation.[43]

Nonepithelial Tumors

Nonepithelial pancreatic tumors in small animals are rare (see Fig. 19.3). Fibrosarcoma and multicentric system disease, including histiocytic sarcoma, lymphoma (Fig. 19.13), hemangiosarcoma, liposarcoma, malignant nerve sheath tumor, and malignant melanoma, have been described.[13,25,44] Bloodborne metastasis from thyroid and mammary gland carcinoma and direct extension from contiguous organs in alimentary lymphoma and from carcinoma of gastric, duodenal, or common bile duct origin are reported.[23,45]

Nonneoplastic Lesions

Nonneoplastic lesions are common in the pancreas. Some initiative has been taken to develop a histopathological grading classification scheme for exocrine pancreatic diseases in the dog.[4,46] In a published case series, pancreatic hyperplastic nodules (80.2%) were found to be most common, followed by lymphocytic inflammation (52.5%), fibrosis (49.5%), atrophy (46.5%), neutrophilic inflammation (31.7%), pancreatic fat necrosis (25.7%), pancreatic necrosis (16.8%), and edema (9.9%).[46]

Nodular Hyperplasia of Acinar Cells

Nodular hyperplasia of acinar cells (i.e., pancreatic exocrine nodular hyperplasia) is a common, often incidental lesion in older dogs and cats (up to 80% of dogs may have nodular hyperplasia at necropsy).[47] In one study, the mean age of dogs with nodular hyperplasia was 9.5 years.[47] Grossly, the lesion may be a solitary nodule or, more commonly appears as multiple, small, white-to-tan, well-circumscribed nodules. Ultrasonographically, nodular hyperplasia tends to manifest

as multiple smaller lesions, compared with a single, large lesion for neoplasia; however, imaging findings for these entities overlap.[11] Histologically, nodular hyperplasia is distinguished from adenomas by their multiplicity, small size, lack of a capsule, and close resemblance to normal exocrine pancreatic tissue.[25] Fibrosis, atrophy, lymphocytic infiltration, or all of these commonly accompany nodules.[46] These lesions are not preneoplastic, and patients are generally asymptomatic. Cytologically, nodular hyperplasia consists of sheets of well-differentiated exocrine pancreatic epithelial cells and, as such, is not distinguishable from an adenoma or well-differentiated carcinoma (see Fig. 19.3). In these cases, cytology should be interpreted in light of imaging findings.

Miscellaneous

Although rarely reported in cats and dogs, ectopic splenic tissue can be found in the pancreas, and this is an incidental finding that could be mistaken for pancreatic neoplasia on imaging. These will contain splenic stromal tissue, lymphoid cells, and hemosiderin-laden macrophages.[48]

Pancreatitis

Acute pancreatitis. Pancreatitis is the most frequent disease process of the exocrine pancreas in dogs. For many canine patients, physical examination, biochemical testing, and imaging studies are adequate to diagnose acute pancreatitis in the absence of pancreatic cytological evaluation.[3,4,46] However, increasingly, FNA of the pancreas is recommended to confirm the diagnosis and rule out secondary disease processes, such as underlying neoplasia. In human medicine, a uniform classification system has been developed for pancreatitis.[49] In veterinary medicine, the classification is less clear because clinical, cytological, and histopathological findings vary (and overlap), depending on the duration/stage of disease and the location sampled within the organ. Some people use the terms "pancreatitis," "acute pancreatitis," and "acute pancreatic necrosis" and other similar terms interchangeably. Strictly speaking, there is a histopathological distinction between acute pancreatitis/acute necrotizing pancreatitis (where inflammation predominates, and any necrosis present is secondary) and acute pancreatic necrosis (where necrosis is the primary feature). The disorders have different etiologies, pathogenesis, and histological characteristics, so the distinction is not entirely academic; however, both necrosis and inflammation are often found concurrently and variably on cytology slides, and histopathological evaluation of architecture is required to determine which process is primary/predominant.[46]

Acute pancreatitis is defined as an acute inflammatory process (usually neutrophilic) of the pancreas, with variable involvement of other regional tissues or remote organ systems that does not lead to permanent changes, often with concurrent pancreatic and/or peripancreatic necrosis. Acute necrotizing pancreatitis is a more severe form of acute pancreatitis characterized by extensive pancreatic and peripancreatic necrosis, sometimes with dissolution of pancreatic parenchyma, hemorrhage, interstitial fluid accumulation, and deposition of fibrin and leukocytes.[49,50] Acute pancreatic necrosis is more common than acute pancreatitis in dogs. The initial necrosis results from the activation of trypsinogen into trypsin within acinar cells in response to an insult, such as a large fatty meal (dietary indiscretion). Idiopathic hyperlipidemia (e.g., in the Miniature Schnauzer), hyperadrenocorticism, hypothyroidism, hypercalcemia, abdominal trauma, and some drugs, such as azathioprine, may also be risk factors. Mortality rates of 27% to 42% are reported in dogs with acute pancreatic necrosis, although dogs with mild disease clinically recover within a few days. Most cases are thought to then become asymptomatic with a continuing smoldering necrosis until there is almost complete destruction of the pancreas. Samples from these will often reveal mainly necrotic material, necrotic peripancreatic fatty tissue, colorless mineralized material with minimal inflammation, and minimal exocrine pancreatic glandular epithelial cells.[51]

Acute pancreatitis appears to be both less common and more difficult to diagnose in the cat,[6,7,9] requiring a combination of clinical suspicion, appropriate physical examination findings, elevations in serum feline pancreatic lipase activity, and changes on AUS. Even when these tests are employed, diagnosis can still be problematic because clinical signs are variable, are nonspecific, and can wax and wane over time. As such, cytology may be even more useful distinguishing between pancreatic inflammation and other pancreatic disorders (especially neoplasia) in cats. In cats, pancreatitis, pancreatic necrosis, pancreatic degeneration, or all of these may also occur in association with other diseases, including toxoplasmosis, hepatic lipidosis, feline infectious peritonitis, Easter lily toxicosis, *Amphimerus pseudofelineus* infection, and virulent systemic feline calicivirus infection.[52-54] Therefore concurrent cytological evaluation of the pancreas and other organs, notably the liver, the GI system, or both, may prove useful for evaluating pancreatic manifestations of systemic disease. Histologically, acute pancreatitis consists of neutrophilic inflammation associated with interstitial edema, steatitis, and necrosis of mesenteric fat (Figs. 19.14 and 19.15).[5] However, as with dogs, some degree of pancreatic inflammation, necrosis, and fibrosis are common histopathological findings at necropsy, even with no clinical evidence of pancreatic disease. As such, the cytological diagnosis of pancreatic inflammation should not be based solely on the number of inflammatory cells present but also on concurrent abnormalities, including necrosis, hemorrhage, epithelial reactivity, or all.

Aspirates are generally highly cellular with abundant exocrine epithelial cells and inflammatory cells (see Fig. 19.3; Fig. 19.16). Neutrophils predominate in acute or acute necrotizing pancreatitis. The neutrophils are classically nondegenerate; however, they may appear mildly to moderately degenerate, likely secondary to concurrent necrosis (see Fig. 19.16; Fig. 19.17). Neutrophils are frequently noted in large aggregates, occasionally embedded in necrotic or cystic-appearing debris (see Figs. 19.14 to 19.19). The background may

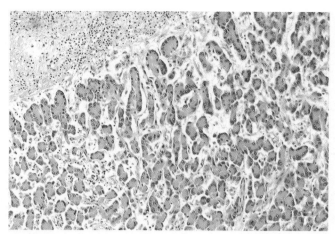

Fig. 19.14 Histopathological section of necrotizing pancreatitis in a dog. The section consists of relatively uniform tubuloacinar secretory units separated by pale-pink material consistent with edema. Infiltrating neutrophils are focally abundant *(upper left area of section)* and dissect through pancreatic acinar cells. Multifocal clusters of acinar cells are degenerate and necrotic (hematoxylin and eosin [H&E] stain, original magnification 100×).

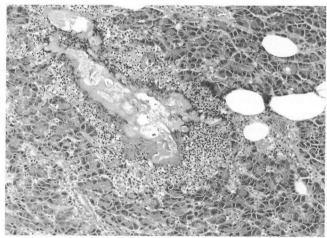

Fig. 19.15 Histopathological section of suppurative pancreatitis in a dog. The section consists of mildly atypical tubuloacinar secretory units with a large focus of suppurative inflammation surrounding an area of eosinophilic material lacking histological detail (fat necrosis, *center*). Areas of dissecting fibrosis *(upper right)* are also noted along with small areas of hemorrhage and mineralization (hematoxylin and eosin [H&E] stain, original magnification 100×).

contain amorphous blue to pink material consistent with necrosis (see Fig. 19.19) or aggregates of crystalline, clear material consistent with calcific debris (Fig. 19.18). Necrosis may be accompanied by hemorrhage, as evidenced by activated, vacuolated, and hemosiderin and hematoidin-laden macrophages (Fig. 19.19). Epithelial cells often appear atypical and reactive. They may have deeply basophilic cytoplasm (with fewer distinct pink granules), cytoplasmic vacuolation, increased N:C ratio, and even prominent or multiple small nucleoli (see Fig. 19.17). Although generally mild, the epithelial atypia can be fairly marked and may result in a false-positive diagnosis of pancreatic carcinoma if the presence of inflammatory cells or other evidence of pancreatitis is lacking (e.g., necrosis, hemorrhage, or fibrosis). Thus distinguishing between pancreatitis with marked reactivity and pancreatic carcinoma with secondary inflammation and necrosis may

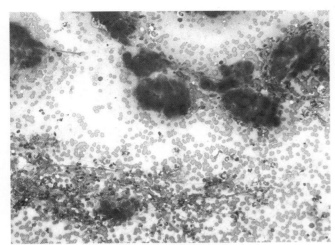

Fig. 19.16 Fine-needle aspirate of acute pancreatitis in a dog. The sample consists of multiple cell populations, including exocrine pancreatic epithelial cells and mixed, primarily neutrophilic, inflammatory cells. Epithelial cells are highly cohesive. They have abundant pink or blue cytoplasm and a low nucleus-to-cytoplasm (N:C) ratio. Inflammatory cells are present in large aggregates surrounding and adjacent to epithelial cells (Wright-Giemsa stain, original magnification 200×).

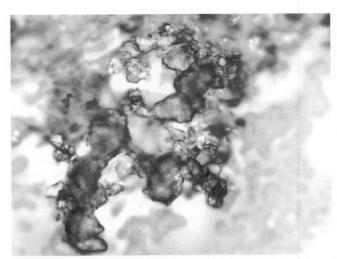

Fig. 19.18 Calcific or mineralized debris obtained from fine-needle aspirate of canine pancreas. This debris is often multidimensional and refractile. It may be noted in large chunks, as depicted, or scattered throughout the background as crystalline material. It appears to be primarily associated with necrosis; however, it is not indicative of any specific pancreatic disorder. In this case, it was associated with necrotizing pancreatitis; however, it may also be noted if the necrotic center of a pancreatic adenocarcinoma is aspirated (Wright-Giemsa stain, original magnification 500×).

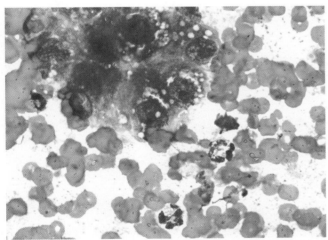

Fig. 19.17 Fine-needle aspirate of acute pancreatitis in a dog. The sample consists of multiple cell populations. Note that the neutrophils appear ragged, and one neutrophil contains clear, punctate cytoplasmic vacuoles. Epithelial cells are atypical and reactive (deeply basophilic) with some criteria of malignancy, including prominent nucleoli. In the absence of inflammation, these cellular changes could be mistaken as indicative of malignancy (Wright-Giemsa stain, original magnification 1000×).

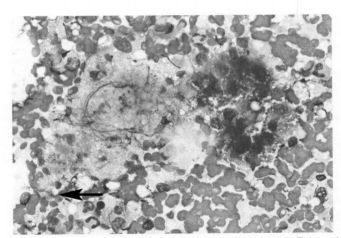

Fig. 19.19 Fine-needle aspirate of acute pancreatitis in a dog. This aspirate was characterized by reactive, deeply basophilic, and atypical epithelial cells admixed with mixed inflammatory cells in a background of amorphous pink and blue material consistent with necrotic and cystic debris. Golden heme breakdown products were also noted consistent with hemorrhage *(arrow)* (Wright-Giemsa stain, original magnification 500×).

present a challenge and should be recognized as a potential pitfall. Additionally, negative FNA and intraoperative biopsy results are insufficient to rule out pancreatitis because inflammatory lesions may be highly localized and missed on sampling.[9] In half the dogs with acute pancreatitis, and two-thirds of dogs with chronic pancreatitis, evidence of pancreatic inflammation was found in less than 25% of sections.[54]

As a final point, pancreatitis may be accompanied by ascites, usually a modified transudate or a nonseptic, purulent exudate. The effusion may have a proteinaceous background that is basophilic or "dirty" and may indicate saponified fat.

Chronic pancreatitis or lymphocytic inflammation. Chronic pancreatitis is defined as a chronic inflammatory process (usually lymphocytic) of the pancreas, with variable involvement of other regional tissues or remote organ systems that leads to permanent changes, mainly fibrosis or atrophy and adhesions.[50] Histopathologically, chronic pancreatitis is characterized by focal aggregation of ducts and endocrine cells set in fibrous tissue infiltrated by chronic inflammatory cells.[23] Pure-bred dogs are significantly overrepresented, especially those belonging to the American Kennel Club (AKC) toy and nonsporting breeds; additionally, dogs in the toy and nonsporting breeds had a significantly higher likelihood of being categorized as having clinical as opposed to incidental chronic pancreatitis.[55] Cocker Spaniels have an increased relative risk for combined acute and chronic pancreatitis,[56] and chronic pancreatitis, which has been described in

English Cocker Spaniels, is characterized by periductular distribution of fibrosis and inflammation (primarily CD3 + T-lymphocytes) with duct destruction. This duct destruction is similar to autoimmune pancreatitis in humans.[57] The histopathological lesions of chronic pancreatitis in cats are similar to chronic pancreatitis in humans, with cystic degeneration and fibrosis being more prominent than inflammatory changes.[5] On imaging, the pancreas may appear fibrotic, nodular, or atrophied. As such, FNA is rarely performed. Described features of chronic pancreatitis include low numbers of mixed acinar and ductal epithelial cells; mild epithelial reactivity or atypia (demonstrated by slight nuclear enlargement and slight nuclear contour irregularities); mixed inflammatory cells, especially small lymphocytes; calcified debris; and, possibly, wispy pink fibrous material.[58] Unfortunately, underlying carcinoma may be associated with, or surrounded by, lesions compatible with acute and chronic pancreatitis, which leads to a potential sample bias.

Occasionally, lymphocytic inflammation of the pancreas that is not associated with chronic pancreatitis may occur. Considerations for increased numbers of small, well-differentiated lymphocytes in a pancreatic aspirate include lymphocytic inflammation of pancreatic islets associated with diabetes, underlying viral disease, small cell lymphoma, or, as mentioned in a previous section, ectopic splenic tissue (see Fig. 19.3).[59] In cats, there is a high prevalence of chronic pancreatitis: 67% in healthy and ill cats and 45% in clinically healthy cats only in a survey necropsy study. Based on survey results from patients submitted for necropsy for a variety of reasons, 64% of 73 dogs[50] and 67% of 115 cats (including 45% of clinically healthy cats) had histological evidence of pancreatitis, making determination of the significance challenging.[5]

Pancreatic cysts. Pancreatic cysts may be congenital, acquired, or pseudocysts. Congenital cysts and acquired retention cysts are rarely described in small animals. Pseudocysts are also rare but are the most common pancreatic cystic lesion seen in small animals.[60,61] In humans, pseudocysts are a common sequela of acute and chronic pancreatitis. Pseudocysts are lined with granulation tissue and contain pancreatic enzymes and debris. They are suspected to result from the release of pancreatic secretions into the periductular connective tissue during an episode of acute pancreatitis. This may also hold true for dogs and cats; in one retrospective study, all six animals had a clinical diagnosis of pancreatitis.[61] Pseudocysts can be safely aspirated. In addition, preferential localization of pseudocysts to the left pancreatic limb may occur.[61,62] Their fluid contents may be measured for amylase and lipase activities, and cytology may be performed to rule out an abscess. In one retrospective study, six animals had high lipase activity in the pseudocyst fluid, and in two dogs and one cat the lipase activity in the fluid was greater than in serum.[61] Low pancreatic enzyme activity suggests a cystic neoplasm, whereas high levels of pancreatic enzyme activity suggest a pseudocyst. In humans, many pseudocysts resolve spontaneously; however, they may also hemorrhage, rupture, or become secondarily infected.

Regardless of ontogeny, the cytological appearance of cyst fluid derived from the pancreas is similar to that from cysts from any organ or structure. Cellularity is usually low, comprising rare nondegenerate neutrophils and occasional macrophages with a light-pink to deep-blue background that may contain abundant amorphous or crystalline debris (see Fig. 19.3; Figs. 19.20 and 19.21). Macrophages may be cytophagic, being erythrophagocytic or hemosiderin-laden, if hemorrhage is present (see Fig. 19.21). Pseudocyst fluid is aseptic and may have elevated total protein concentration. Cytological evaluation of cystic fluid from the pancreas is most useful to rule out other fluid-filled masses of the pancreas, including abscesses and cystic neoplasms.

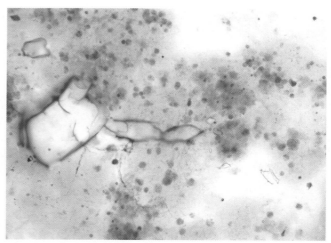

Fig. 19.20 Fine-needle aspirate of a pancreatic cyst in a dog. The sample is of low cellularity with amorphous cellular and crystalline debris in a dense, pink background. Epithelial cells are generally absent. Differential diagnoses should include a primary cyst (the type of cyst cannot be determined on cytological examination alone) or cystic neoplasm (Wright-Giemsa stain, original magnification 500×).

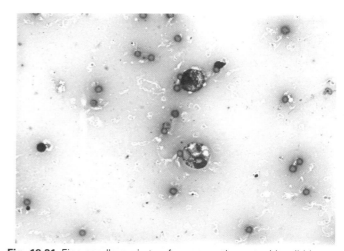

Fig. 19.21 Fine-needle aspirate of a pancreatic cyst with mild hemorrhage in a cat. Samples are characterized by low cellularity and primarily activated erythrophagocytic macrophages. The background contains rare red blood cells and pink stippling consistent with increased protein (Wright-Giemsa stain, original magnification 500×).

Pancreatic abscesses. Primary pancreatic abscesses in small animals are rare. Sources of infection for abscesses include the biliary tract, the transverse colon, or the bloodstream. Aspirates of abscesses yield abundant neutrophils (see Fig. 19.3; Fig. 19.22), often on a background filled with lysed nuclear and cellular debris. Neutrophil nuclei are swollen (degenerate) and intracellular bacteria may be seen (see Figs. 19.3 and Fig. 19.22 *[arrow]*). The absence of bacteria does not rule out an abscess; as such, if an abscess is suspected based on clinical or imaging findings, culture and sensitivity are warranted. The cytological distinction between an abscess and acute pancreatitis is not always straightforward. Occasionally, an abscess may be characterized by nondegenerate neutrophils and scattered reactive epithelial cells in the absence of bacteria. This is most likely if the patient has been, or is currently being, treated with antibiotics. As such, differential diagnoses for purulent inflammation should include an abscess or acute pancreatitis in the absence of additional cytological clues.

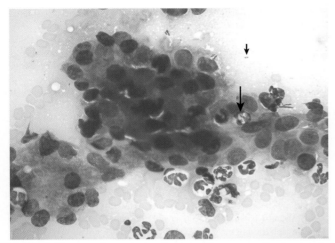

Fig. 19.22 Fine-needle aspirate of a mass-like pancreatic abscess in a cat. The sample contains exocrine pancreatic epithelial cells surrounded and infiltrated by neutrophils sometimes containing intracellular bacterial rods, which are also observed free in the background *(arrows)* (Wright-Giemsa stain, original magnification 1000×).

REFERENCES

1. Cortner AP, Armstrong PJ, Newman SJ, et al. Effect of pancreatic tissue sampling on serum pancreatic enzyme levels in clinically healthy dogs. *J Vet Diagn Invest.* 2010;22:702.
2. Pratschke KM, Ryan J, McAlinden A, McLauchlan G. Pancreatic surgical biopsy in 24 dogs and 19 cats: postoperative complications and clinical relevance of histological findings. *J Small Anim Pract.* 2015;56:60.
3. Steiner JM, Newman S, Xenoulis P, et al. Sensitivity of serum markers for pancreatitis in dogs with macroscopic evidence of pancreatitis. *Vet Ther.* 2008;9:263.
4. Trivedi S, Marks SL, Kass PH, et al. Sensitivity and specificity of canine pancreas-specific lipase (cPL) and other markers for pancreatitis in 70 dogs with and without histopathologic evidence of pancreatitis. *J Vet Intern Med.* 2011;25:1241.
5. De Cock HE, Forman MA, Farver TB, et al. Prevalence and histopathologic characteristics of pancreatitis in cats. *Vet Pathol.* 2007;44:39.
6. Ferreri JA, Hardam E, Kimmel SE, et al. Clinical differentiation of acute necrotizing from chronic nonsuppurative pancreatitis in cats: 63 cases (1996-2001). *J Am Vet Med Assoc.* 2003;223:469.
7. Saunders HM, VanWinkle TJ, Drobatz K, et al. Ultrasonographic findings in cats with clinical, gross pathologic, and histologic evidence of acute pancreatic necrosis: 20 cases (1994-2001). *J Am Vet Med Assoc.* 2002;221:1724.
8. Swift NC, Marks SL, MacLachlan NJ, et al. Evaluation of serum feline trypsin-like immunoreactivity for the diagnosis of pancreatitis in cats. *J Am Vet Med Assoc.* 2000;217:37.
9. Xenoulis PG. Diagnosis of pancreatitis in dogs and cats. *J Sm Anim Pract.* 2015;56:13.
10. Hecht S, Henry G. Sonographic evaluation of the normal and abnormal pancreas. *Clin Tech Small Anim Pract.* 2007;22:115.
11. Hecht S, Penninck DG, Keating JH. Imaging findings in pancreatic neoplasia and nodular hyperplasia in 19 cats. *Vet Radiol Ultrasound.* 2007;48:45.
12. Hess RS, Saunders HM, Van Winkle TJ, et al. Clinical, clinicopathologic, radiographic, and ultrasonographic abnormalities in dogs with fatal acute pancreatitis: 70 cases (1986-1995). *J Am Vet Med Assoc.* 1998;213:665.
13. Jones TC, Hunt RD, King NW. *Veterinary Pathology.* 6th ed. Baltimore, MD: Williams & Wilkins; 1997.
14. Bacha WJ, Bacha LM. *Color Atlas of Veterinary Histology.* 2nd ed. Baltimore, MD: Lippincott Williams & Wilkins; 2000.
15. Bjorneby JM, Kari S. Cytology of the pancreas. *Vet Clin North Am Small Anim Pract.* 2002;32:1293.
16. Iseri T, Yamada K, Chijiwa K, et al. Dynamic computed tomography of the pancreas in normal dogs and in a dog with pancreatic insulinoma. *Vet Radiol Ultrasound.* 2007;48:328.
17. Kook PH, Baloi P, Ruetten M, et al. Feasibility and safety of endoscopic ultrasound-guided fine needle aspiration of the pancreas in dogs. *J Vet Intern Med.* 2012;26:513.
18. Schweighauser A, Gaschen F, Steiner J, et al. Evaluation of endosonography as a new diagnostic tool for feline pancreatitis. *J Feline Med Surg.* 2009;11:492.
19. Bennett PF, Hahn KA, Toal RL, et al. Ultrasonographic and cytopathological diagnosis of exocrine pancreatic carcinoma in the dog and cat. *J Am Anim Hosp Assoc.* 2001;37:466.
20. Menard M, Papageorges M. Fine-needle biopsies: how to increase diagnostic yield. *Compend Contin Educ Vet.* 1997;19:738.
21. Cordner AP, Sharkey LC, Armstrong PJ, et al. Cytologic findings and diagnostic yield in 92 dogs undergoing fine-needle aspiration of the pancreas. *J Vet Diagn Invest.* 2015;27:236.
22. Crain KC, Sharkey LC, Cordner AP, et al. Safety of ultrasound fine-needle aspiration of the feline pancreas: a case-control study. *J Feline Med Surg.* 2015;17:858.
23. Head KW, Cullen J, Dubielzig RR, et al. *WHO Histological Classification of Tumors of the Alimentary System of Domestic Animals.* Washington, DC: Armed Forces Institute of Pathology; 2003.
24. Kiupel M, Capen CC, Miller M, et al. *Histological Classification of Tumors of the Endocrine System of Domestic Animals, World Health Organization International Histological Classification of Tumors of Domestic Animals.* Vol 12. Washington, DC: Armed Forces Institute of Pathology; 2008.
25. Munday JS, Lohr CV, Kiupel M. Tumors of the alimentary tract. In: Meuten DJ, ed. *Tumors in Domestic Animals.* 5th ed. Ames, IA: Wiley-Blackwell; 2016.
26. Tasker S, Griffon DJ, Nuttall TJ, et al. Resolution of paraneoplastic alopecia following surgical removal of a pancreatic carcinoma in a cat. *J Small Anim Pract.* 1999;40:16.
27. Bright JM. Pancreatic adenocarcinoma in a dog with a maldigestion syndrome. *J Am Vet Med Assoc.* 1985;187:420.
28. Fabbrini F, Anfray P, Viacava P, et al. Feline cutaneous and visceral necrotizing panniculitis and steatitis associated with a pancreatic tumour. *Vet Dermatol.* 2005;16:413.
29. Lin F, Staerkel G. Cytologic criteria for well differentiated adenocarcinoma of the pancreas in fine-needle aspiration biopsy specimens. *Cancer.* 2003;99:44.
30. Robins DB, Katz RL, Evans DB, et al. Fine needle aspiration of the pancreas: in quest of accuracy. *Acta Cytol.* 1995;39:1.
31. Eloubeidi MA, Jhala D, Chhieng DC, et al. Yield of endoscopic ultrasound-guided fine-needle aspiration biopsy in patients with suspected pancreatic carcinoma. *Cancer.* 2003;99:285.
32. Ylagan LR, Edmundowicz S, Kasal K, et al. Endoscopic ultrasound guided fine-needle aspiration cytology of pancreatic carcinoma: a 3-year experience and review of the literature. *Cancer.* 2002;96:362.
33. Minkus G, Jutting U, Aubele M, et al. Canine neuroendocrine tumors of the pancreas: a study using image analysis techniques for the discrimination of metastatic versus nonmetastatic tumors. *Vet Pathol.* 1997;34:138.
34. Isidoro-Ayza M, Lloret A, Bardagí M, et al. Superficial necrolytic dermatitis in a dog with an insulin-producing pancreatic islet cell carcinoma. *Vet Pathol.* 2014;51:805.
35. Verbeke CS. Endocrine tumours of the pancreas. *Histopathology.* 2010;56:669.
36. Rosol JR, Meuten DJ. Tumors of the endocrine gland. In: Meuten DJ, ed. *Tumors in Domestic Animals.* 5th ed. Ames, IA: Wiley-Blackwell; 2016.
37. Tobin RL, Nelson RW, Lucroy MD, et al. Outcome of surgical versus medical treatment of dogs with beta cell neoplasia: 39 cases (1990-1997). *J Am Vet Med Assoc.* 1999;215:226.
38. Pieczarka EM, Russell DS, Santangelo KS, et al. Osseous metaplasia within a canine insulinoma. *Vet Clin Pathol.* 2014;43:89.
39. Caywood D, Klausner J, O'Leary T, et al. Pancreatic insulin-secreting neoplasms: clinical, diagnostic, and prognostic features in 73 dogs. *J Am Anim Hosp Assoc.* 1988;24:577.
40. Green RA, Gartrell CL. Gastrinoma: a retrospective study of four cases (1985-1995). *J Am Anim Hosp Assoc.* 1997;33:524.

41. Ardengh JC, de Paulo GA, Ferrari AP. EUS-guided FNA in the diagnosis of pancreatic neuroendocrine tumors before surgery. *Gastrointest Endosc.* 2004;60:378.

42. Jimenez-Heffernan JA, Vicandi B, Lopez-Ferrer P, et al. Fine needle aspiration cytology of endocrine neoplasms of the pancreas. Morphologic and immunocytochemical findings in 20 cases. *Acta Cytol.* 2004;48:295.

43. Michishita M, Tagaki M, Kishimoto TE, et al. Pancreatic neuroendocrine carcinoma with exocrine differentiation in a young cat. *J Vet Diagn Invest.* 2017;29:325.

44. Hayden DW, Waters DJ, Burke BA, et al. Disseminated malignant histiocytosis in a golden retriever: clinicopathologic, ultrastructural, and immunohistochemical findings. *Vet Pathol.* 1993;30:256.

45. Swann HM, Holt DE. Canine gastric adenocarcinoma and leiomyosarcoma: a retrospective study of 21 cases (1986-1999) and literature review. *J Am Anim Hosp Assoc.* 2002;38:157.

46. Newman SJ, Steiner JM, Woosley K, et al. Histologic assessment and grading of the exocrine pancreas in the dog. *J Vet Diagn Invest.* 2006;18:115.

47. Newman SJ, Steiner JM, Woosley K, et al. Correlation of age and incidence of pancreatic exocrine nodular hyperplasia in the dog. *Vet Pathol.* 2005;42:510.

48. Ramirez GA, Altimira J, Garcia-Gonzalez B, et al. Intrapancreatic ectopic splenic tissue in dogs and cats. *J Comp Pathol.* 2013;148:361.

49. Bradley 3rd EL. A clinically based classification system for acute pancreatitis. Summary of the International Symposium on Acute Pancreatitis, Atlanta, GA, September 11 through 13, 1992. *Arch Surg.* 1993;128:586.

50. Newman S, Steiner J, Woosley K, et al. Localization of pancreatic inflammation and necrosis in dogs. *J Vet Intern Med.* 2004;18:488.

51. Jubb, Kennedy. *Palmer's Pathology of Domestic Animals.* 5th ed. Vol 2. Philadelphia, PA: Elsevier Saunders; 2007:398–401.

52. Rumbeiha WK, Francis JA, Fitzgerald SD, et al. A comprehensive study of Easter lily poisoning in cats. *J Vet Diagn Invest.* 2004;16:527.

53. Pesavento PA, MacLachlan NJ, Dillard-Telm L, et al. Pathologic, immunohistochemical, and electron microscopic findings in naturally occurring virulent systemic feline calicivirus infection in cats. *Vet Pathol.* 2004;41:257.

54. Zoran DL. Pancreatitis in cats: diagnosis and management of a challenging disease. *J Am Anim Hosp Assoc.* 2006;42:1.

55. Bostrom BM, Xenoulis PG, Newman SJ, et al. Chronic pancreatitis in dogs: a retrospective study of clinical, clinicopathological, and histopathological findings in 61 cases. *Vet J.* 2013;195:73.

56. Watson PJ, Roulois AJ, Scase T, et al. Prevalence and breed distribution of chronic pancreatitis at post-mortem examination in first-opinion dogs. *J Small Anim Pract.* 2007;48:609.

57. Watson PJ, Roulois A, Scase T, et al. Characterization of chronic pancreatitis in English Cocker Spaniels. *J Vet Intern Med.* 2011;25:797.

58. Afify AM, al-Khafaji BM, Kim B, et al. Endoscopic ultrasound-guided fine needle aspiration of the pancreas: diagnostic utility and accuracy. *Acta Cytol.* 2003;47:341.

59. Hall DG, Kelley LC, Gray ML, et al. Lymphocytic inflammation of pancreatic islets in a diabetic cat. *J Vet Diagn Invest.* 1997;9:98.

60. Coleman MG, Robson MC, Harvey C. Pancreatic cyst in a cat. *N Z Vet J.* 2005;53:157.

61. VanEnkevort BA, O'Brien RT, Young KM. Pancreatic pseudocysts in 4 dogs and 2 cats: ultrasonographic and clinicopathologic findings. *J Vet Intern Med.* 1999;13:309.

62. Hines BL, Salisbury SK, Jakovljevic S, et al. Pancreatic pseudocyst associated with chronic-active necrotizing pancreatitis in a cat. *J Am Anim Hosp Assoc.* 1996;32:147.

20

The Liver

Andrea Siegel and Michael D. Wiseman

The liver is a vital organ and the primary site for many physiological functions, including carbohydrate and lipid metabolism, synthesis of most plasma and coagulation proteins, and detoxification of many endogenous/exogenous compounds, drugs, and toxins.[1] In part because of these different functions, diseases afflicting the hepatobiliary system present clinically in various ways. Cytology of the liver and gallbladder by use of ultrasound-guided fine-needle aspiration (FNA) is a practical and less invasive tool that can help make a definitive diagnosis of certain liver diseases. It is important to note, however, that cytology has limitations, and some conditions will require architectural assessment by histopathology for their accurate diagnoses.[2-4] For instance, cytology is excellent for diagnosing feline hepatic lipidosis, for many types of neoplasia, and for identifying nonspecific hepatocellular vacuolar changes; however, it cannot always detect the inflammatory infiltrate of cholangitis, nor can it adequately assess the fibrosis, patchy nature of inflammation, and other subtle features of canine chronic hepatitis.[5] Similarly, differentiating among a regenerative hyperplastic liver nodule, hepatocellular adenoma, and well-differentiated hepatocellular carcinoma is often challenging with cytology alone. The goal of this chapter is to describe and illustrate the cytological features, limits, and clinical differentials for canine and feline hepatobiliary parenchymal, inflammatory, and neoplastic diseases. This chapter does not discuss circulatory disorders of the liver (e.g., congenital portosystemic shunts, portal vein hypoplasia/microvascular dysplasia) because the accuracy of these diagnoses cannot be improved by using FNA cytology.

SAMPLING THE LIVER

Indications for performing liver cytology or histology include any concern about liver disease or involvement, such as persistently increased liver enzymes or altered hepatic function markers on biochemistry panels; hepatic enlargement on palpation or imaging; and abnormal parenchymal echogenicity or nodules/masses observed on ultrasonography. Cytology or histology is also used for staging disease in patients with multicentric and metastatic neoplasia. It is imperative to communicate any such clinical and imaging abnormalities to the person performing the microscopic evaluation to obtain the most accurate and meaningful interpretation.

The main contraindication of liver (or any vascular organ) sampling is abnormal hemostasis and a high risk for hemorrhage. There is no clear consensus as to what magnitude of thrombocytopenia or abnormal coagulation test result poses a risk too severe for a sampling procedure; furthermore, hemorrhage can occur even if screening results are normal.[6] A reduced platelet count less than 50,000/μL is certainly most concerning, and less than 20,000/μL may warrant a platelet-rich plasma transfusion before FNA is attempted.[7] Other precautionary tests include the buccal mucosal bleeding time (BMBT),

especially in breeds with known higher prevalence of von Willebrand disease, and a standard coagulation profile with prothrombin time (PT) and activated partial thromboplastin time (aPTT). Inquiring about any prior bleeding episodes or current medications, such as aspirin or other nonsteroidal antiinflammatory drugs (NSAIDs), is prudent. If liver sampling is deemed an acceptable risk in any patient, it is advisable to perform it early in the day and have hospital staff and the owner monitor the patient for 24 hours. All that said, the overall risk for excess bleeding after liver aspiration or biopsy is very low to rare.

Another rare potential complication is seeding of neoplastic cells along needle tracts when sampling a neoplastic liver lesion; however, the relative risk usually does not outweigh the benefit of information obtained by the procedure. The exception would be a presumed hemangiosarcoma, where needle aspiration of a larger-sized cavitational mass should be avoided because of the risk for capsule rupture, hemorrhage, and tumor seeding.

Various techniques for sampling the hepatobiliary system have been described, whether it be percutaneous FNA, percutaneous needle core biopsy (Tru-Cut needle), laparoscopic collection, or surgical wedge biopsy.[8] The chosen sampling method should factor in the lesion location, characteristics, suspected abnormality, and overall risk to the patient. For the blind FNA technique, which might be considered for hepatomegaly with suspected diffuse disease or a large lobar mass, the usual entry point is caudal to the costal arch. Ultrasound guidance greatly enhances sampling precision for percutaneous collections and is generally recommended. The patient should be positioned in dorsal recumbency or right lateral side down; the use of chemical restraint depends on patient temperament. A 20- to 23-gauge needle of 1½- to 3-inch length is chosen. It can be used alone or attached to a 6- or 12-mL syringe preloaded with 2 to 3 mL of air. With a patient in dorsal recumbency, the needle is directed at a craniodorsal angle toward the diaphragm, entering subcostally to the left of midline. (The needle is generally too short to cause concern about penetration past the diaphragm). If a patient is deep chested, then the right-lateral-side-down position may be easier, whereby the needle enters from the left caudal intercostal spaces. A nonaspiration collection method (using capillary action) is often preferred for vascular organs to reduce hemodilution by taking several passes of the needle in a back-and-forth motion. The traditional syringe-suction FNA method can also be used with the air-preloaded syringe. Several glass slide smears should be promptly made (see Chapter 1). If the procedure is tolerated by and safe for the patient, multiple aspirates obtained from the relevant liver locations will help gain better representation of the lesion(s) in question, with each glass slide labeled appropriately. Once fully dried, some slides can be stained for in-house microscope viewing and to verify sufficient cellularity; otherwise, they should be placed in a protective slide case and kept away from any possible formalin fumes.

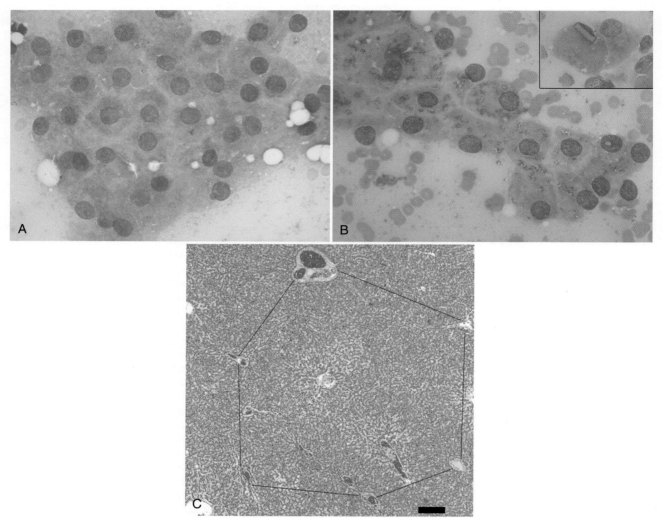

Fig. 20.1 Normal hepatocytes. (A) Fine-needle aspiration (FNA) cytology showing a cluster of normal hepatocytes from a dog (Wright-Giemsa, 100× objective). (B) This aspirate from a different dog displays hepatocytes with cytoplasmic lipofuscin pigment granules, a product of normal cellular aging. The inset image shows a rectangular intranuclear "brick" inclusion that can be incidentally found in sporadic hepatocytes and has no known significance (Wright-Giemsa, 100× objective). (C) Normal canine liver histological section. Lines are shown connecting the portal regions, which depict a classic hexagonal lobule, the basic structural and functional unit of the liver. Blood flows from the peripheral portal triads toward a central vein, and bile flows in the opposite direction (hematoxylin and eosin [H&E], 4× objective; bar is 200 μm). (C, Courtesy Dr. Taryn A. Donovan.)

NORMAL CYTOLOGY AND LIVER PIGMENTS

Normal Liver

Recognition of normal liver cytology is necessary before any pathological features can be interpreted. Hepatocytes exfoliate readily in sheets, clusters, and few stray individual cells on a background of variable hemodilution. They are large, fairly uniform cells approximately 25 to 30 μm in size, usually with distinct cell borders and polygonal to slightly oval shape (Fig. 20.1). Hepatocytes have a centrally placed, round nucleus of coarsely granular to stippled chromatin and a single prominent nucleolus, surrounded by abundant bluish and faint pink, grainy cytoplasm. The cytoplasmic tincture reflects the different organelles of these metabolically active cells. Hepatocytes often contain some lipofuscin pigment granules (see "Pigments" section below), and few binucleate cells may be seen. Rarely, a rectangular crystalline intranuclear "brick" inclusion is identified in sporadic hepatocytes, which are of no known significance (see Fig. 20.1, B).

Bile duct epithelial cells are infrequently observed in normal liver cytology; instead, they are encountered most often when biliary hyperplasia exists. Biliary epithelium consists of columnar to cuboidal shaped cells with relatively uniform round nuclei of densely granular to smooth chromatin and a minimal, small, or moderate volume of pale blue cytoplasm (Fig. 20.2). Biliary epithelial cells can be found as clusters with high nucleus-to-cytoplasm (N:C) ratio, in ductal tubular formation or as flattened sheets.

Other resident cell types found in liver cytology but seen in low numbers, if at all, are hepatic macrophages (Kupffer cells), hepatic stellate cells (Ito cells), and mast cells. Macrophages may be interspersed within hepatocyte clusters or in the background of peripheral blood. Hepatic stellate cells are not usually appreciated in cytology but can be observed as lipid-laden cells in histological samples, especially from older cats and less so in older dogs.[9,10] They are a major storage site of vitamin A and have the capacity to transform into myofibroblasts, which lay down extracellular matrix material (fibrosis) during chronic

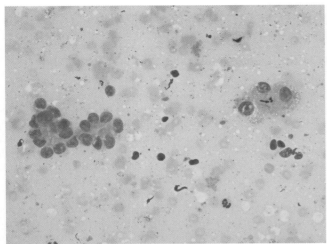

Fig. 20.2 Biliary epithelium. Bile duct epithelial cells are most frequently encountered when biliary hyperplasia exists, as shown in this canine case. On the left side, two small clusters of biliary epithelial cells display a tubular ring formation, and three hepatocytes are on the right side. In cytology, biliary epithelium is observed as either columnar-shaped cells with basilar-located nuclei or cuboidal clusters *(not depicted here)* with minimally visible cytoplasm (Wright-Giemsa, 50× objective).

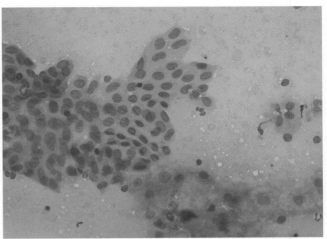

Fig. 20.3 Mesothelial lining cells. A large, partially folded sheet of mesothelial cells has been inadvertently collected during liver fine-needle aspiration (FNA) from a dog. The mesothelial cells are shown on the left, adjacent to a lower right cluster of hepatocytes. Nonreactive, normal mesothelial cells can have a "fish scale–like" sheet appearance, with slightly angular shape and relatively uniform nuclei. A characteristic pink colored outer glycocalyx fringe can be appreciated along the edges of the top right mesothelial cells (Wright-Giemsa, 50× objective).

disease states. Mast cells are a common and normal finding in the liver when present in low numbers and individually placed. They can be mildly increased in various inflammatory conditions and may even promote fibrous matrix production by transformed hepatic stellate cells.[11-13] It is important to distinguish these inflammatory mast cells from a neoplastic mast cell population, which would be expected in groupings and in significantly increased numbers.

Miscellaneous background cells and material that are also commonly observed in liver aspirates include a variable but proportional quantity of peripheral blood neutrophils and other leukocytes, usually evenly distributed among the erythrocytes, platelets, and tissue cells. Intact adipocytes and free lipid vacuoles may reflect inadvertently sampled mesenteric fat. Mesothelial lining cells can also be inadvertently collected and are displayed as flat or folded sheets with a characteristic slightly angular shape and a "fish scale–like" pattern (Fig. 20.3). Their outer pink glycocalyx fringe can sometimes be appreciated. Care should be taken not to mistake mesothelial cells for the slightly smaller biliary epithelial or neoplastic cells. Ultrasound gel contamination is a common artifact seen as extracellular, magenta-colored, chucky granular debris (Fig. 20.4).

Pigments

Several pigments can be observed within hepatocytes either as a normal finding or increased quantity in disease states. Lipofuscin is the most commonly observed cytoplasmic pigment versus pigments granules of bile, hemosiderin, or copper.[14] A fifth liver pigment named *ceroid* is not found within hepatocytes but, rather, accumulates in hepatic macrophages; it is a lipid breakdown product resulting from increased hepatocellular turnover or injury.[10] Ceroid is a golden brown, granular to globular pigment and can resemble hemosiderin. Differentiating the pigments within hepatocytes (and macrophages, as applicable) solely on the basis of routine Romanowsky-type cytochemical staining or standard hematoxylin and eosin (H&E) histochemical staining is sometimes difficult, so special stains may have to be employed, when necessary.

Lipofuscin

Lipofuscin is a "wear and tear" pigment frequently observed in hepatocytes and represents indigestible cellular residue within lysosomes; a

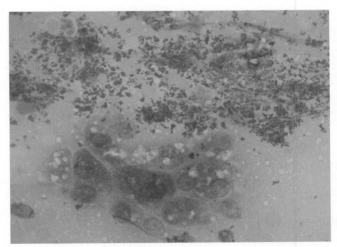

Fig. 20.4 Ultrasound gel artifact. Canine liver. A pool of extracellular, bright pink– to magenta-colored granular debris reflects ultrasound gel contamination, resting above a cluster of hepatocytes (Wright-Giemsa, 100× objective).

product of normal cellular aging (see Fig. 20.1, B). Larger amounts may be seen in older cats and dogs. Lipofuscin cytologically appears as small, blue to blue-green granules, whereas on H&E histological sections, they are yellow-brown in color.

Bile Pigment

Bile retention within hepatocytes is recognized as variably sized, dark green to black clumpy granules on cytology. It reflects cholestasis and may precede hyperbilirubinemia. Bile cholestasis can occur with prehepatic hemolysis, hepatic, or posthepatic diseases and is most easily recognized when it accumulates around hepatocytes within canaliculi, showing linear inspissated bile plugs (Fig. 20.5). On standard H&E histological sections, bile pigment has a brownish yellow color and will appear green with the special Hall stain.

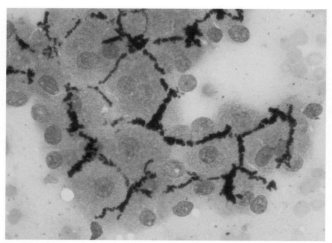

Fig. 20.5 Bile retention and cholestasis. Surrounding hepatocytes in this canine liver aspirate are inspissated plugs of bile. The dark green to black bile pigment is retained within the canaliculi and indicative of cholestasis (Wright-Giemsa, 100× objective).

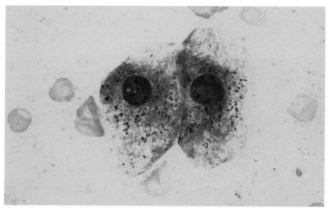

Fig. 20.6 Hemosiderin pigment. The golden-brown granules within these two hepatocytes are consistent with hemosiderin (Wright, 40× objective). (Courtesy Dr. Tara P. Arndt and Dr. Sonjia M. Shelly.)

Hemosiderin

Hemosiderin is a granular, iron-containing pigment resulting from the phagocytic breakdown of heme protein (Fig. 20.6). It can accumulate not only within hepatocytes during disease states, such as hemolytic anemia and chronic inflammatory conditions, but also with repeated blood transfusions and iron injections. It is also commonly seen within macrophages with or without phagocytized erythrocytes. Hemosiderin color can range from golden-brown to blue-black in cytology stains, whereas it has a more consistent golden-brown tint on H&E histological sections. Should verification of hemosiderin pigment be needed, the special Prussian blue stain is used.

Copper

Copper accumulation within hepatocytes has a subtle staining character as pale blue, coarse, crystalline granules on routine cytochemical stains (Fig. 20.7, A), whereas the coloration ranges from gray-yellow to gray-brown or gray-blue on standard H&E staining. Special stains are applied most often in histological samples to better visualize and semi-quantify the copper amount; rubeanic acid stains copper a green-black color, and rhodanine dye turns it red (see Fig. 20.7, B). More precise copper quantification is analyzed on fresh, frozen, or paraffin-embedded tissue samples to confirm copper-associated hepatopathy, which is discussed later in the "Chronic Hepatitis" section.

NONNEOPLASTIC CONDITIONS AND INFLAMMATORY DISEASES

Hepatocellular Vacuolar Changes and Associated Conditions

Hepatocellular vacuolar change is a common yet often nonspecific finding associated with metabolic disease or occurs secondary to cellular injury. The cytoplasmic swelling is usually reversible; it results from the intracellular accumulation of lipid, glycogen, or water. Although usually not necessary, the vacuolar contents can be confirmed with special stains for lipid (Sudan black, Oil Red O) or glycogen/glycoproteins (periodic acid–Schiff [PAS] stain with or without diastase).

Lipid vacuolation within hepatocytes reflects increased accumulation of triglycerides. The discrete clear lipid vacuoles can appear either *microvesicular* (relatively uniform vacuoles smaller than the centrally placed nucleus) or *macrovesicular* (variably sized vacuoles larger than the often-displaced nucleus). Feline hepatic lipidosis syndrome (fatty liver, steatosis) is the most commonly encountered condition where fatty change is evident (Fig. 20.8). The magnitude of cellular lipidosis is usually marked, typically affecting greater than 80% of hepatocytes, and shows a mixture of both macrovesicular and microvesicular change.[15] This condition is either primary (and idiopathic) or secondary to underlying diseases, such as chronic pancreatitis, diabetes mellitus, cholangitis, inflammatory bowel disease, lymphoma, or other neoplasia. Cats with primary hepatic lipidosis syndrome may classically present with hepatomegaly, clinical icterus, significantly increased serum alkaline phosphatase (ALP) activity and hyperbilirubinemia combined with a normal or minimally increased γ-glutamyltransferase activity (GGT). The patient history may reveal a period of anorexia, environmental changes, and stress; overweight/obese cats are predisposed. It is crucial to investigate for a possible underlying cause before making a diagnosis of primary idiopathic hepatic lipidosis. Secondary hepatic lipidosis is also common, and cats with this condition may not necessarily have the same extreme clinical presentation.

In contrast to cats, dogs do not usually have liver pathology showing diffuse lipid vacuolation, although it has been rarely reported as cases of aflatoxicosis caused by eating fungal-contaminated dog food.[16] Both dogs and cats, however, will show some degree of lipid vacuolation that variably affects hepatocytes in metabolic disorders, such as diabetes mellitus. In the rare congenital lysosomal storage diseases, juvenile animals will typically develop hepatomegaly with diffuse microvesicular vacuolation, reflecting glycolipid/glycoprotein accumulation because of their specific lysosomal enzyme deficiency.[10] Similarly, microvesicular steatosis (lipidosis) has been documented in very young toy-breed puppies associated with hypoglycemia and anorexia.[9]

Nonlipid hepatocellular vacuolar swelling is referred to as *rarefaction*, cytoplasm that is of thinner density than normal. It is the most common type of hepatocellular vacuolation in canine pathology. This cytoplasmic swelling appears feathery, without obvious discrete vacuoles; instead, it shows distended cytoplasmic clearings that are caused by accumulation of glycogen or water, the latter of which is termed *hydropic degeneration* and caused by nonspecific cellular injury (Figs. 20.9 and 20.10). The nucleus usually remains centrally located. The cytological appearance of glycogen accumulation versus water accumulation is very similar and often cannot be distinguished. Glycogen deposition within hepatocytes is induced by exogenous or endogenously derived glucocorticoids. Common in dogs and only rarely observed/reported in cats[17] is the so-called "steroid hepatopathy," in which exposure to high/exaggerated plasma concentrations of glucocorticoid hormone causes a relatively diffuse, moderate to marked cytoplasmic swelling of most hepatocytes (see Fig. 20.9, B). Hyperadrenocorticism (HAC; Cushing disease) or exogenous

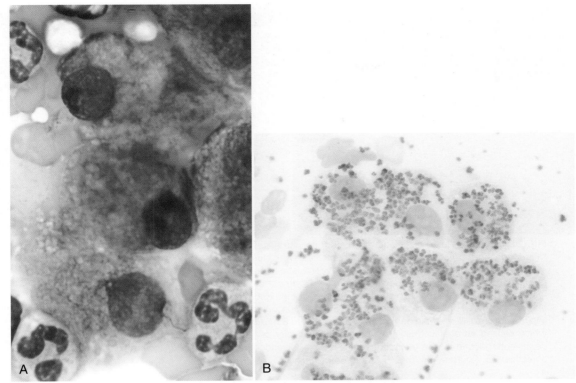

Fig. 20.7 Copper pigment and accumulation. (A) Liver aspirate from a 3-year-old Bedlington Terrier with a copper storage hepatopathy. The copper stains as pale-blue crystalline granules (Wright, 100× objective). (B) Rhodanine dye turns the copper granules red, providing better visibility of the pigment within these hepatocytes from a different dog (Rhodanine, 40× objective). (A, Courtesy Dr. Michael Scott, 1991, ASVCP slide review session.)

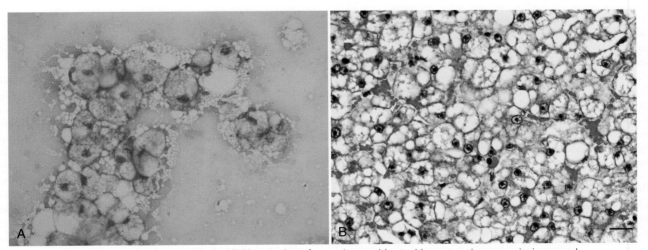

Fig. 20.8 Feline hepatic lipidosis. (A) Liver aspirate from a 4-year-old cat with progressive anorexia, increased serum liver enzyme activity (especially alkaline phosphatase [ALP]), and hyperbilirubinemia. Hepatocytes demonstrate marked fatty change with mixture of microvesicular (relatively uniform discrete vacuoles smaller than the centrally placed nucleus) and macrovesicular lipid vacuolation (variably sized discrete vacuoles larger than the often-displaced nucleus). Few of the hepatocytes contain a small amount of black bile pigment (Wright-Giemsa, 50× objective). (B) Histology correlate from a different cat also with an advanced stage of hepatic lipidosis (hematoxylin and eosin [H&E], 50× objective; bar is 20 μm). (B, Courtesy Dr. Taryn A. Donovan.)

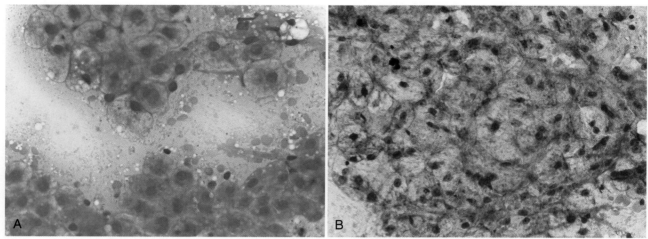

Fig. 20.9 Hepatocellular vacuolation in dogs (nonlipid). (A) The top cluster of hepatocytes demonstrates moderate nonlipid vacuolar change, whereas the lower clusters show relatively mild vacuolation in this 11-year-old dog, sampled from one of many hyperplastic nodules in its liver (same case as Fig. 20.10A). This rarefaction, a thinner density cytoplasm compared with normal, is the result of either glycogen deposition or water. Compared with the discrete lipid vacuoles of Fig. 20.8, glycogen and water cytoplasmic vacuolation shows indistinct, feathery clearings (Wright-Giemsa, 50× objective). (B) This thick cluster of hepatocytes was aspirated from a 12-year-old dog that had been treated 8 months with glucocorticoids for a persistent cough, which caused iatrogenic Cushing syndrome. A vacuolar or "steroid" hepatopathy results from glycogen deposition induced by the exogenous (in this case) or endogenously derived glucocorticoids (Wright, 50× objective). (B, Courtesy Dr. Tara P. Arndt and Dr. Sonjia M. Shelly.)

glucocorticoid therapy become top differentials, particularly if the dog shows expected clinicopathological signs of polyuria, polydipsia, polyphagia, hepatomegaly, hypercholesterolemia, and significantly increased serum ALP without hyperbilirubinemia. An interesting "atypical HAC" scenario is the breed-specific, progressive vacuolar hepatopathy of Scottish Terriers.[18] Their atypical adrenal hyperactivity and associated hepatopathy appear as a result of excessive production of the sex hormones (progesterone and androstenedione) in addition to cortisol. Unfortunately, these affected Scotties do not usually respond to conventional medical treatment (and even experience serious adverse reactions) and frequently go on to develop hepatocellular carcinoma (as was seen in 34% of the 114 dogs in a study).[18] Further investigation for the cause of nonlipid hepatocellular vacuolation is warranted if HAC and exogenous glucocorticoid differentials have been ruled out.[19] Nonlipid vacuolar change, whether it be from glycogen accumulation or water accumulation, is frequently observed in nonspecific conditions, such as low-level stress with acute and chronic illness, tissue hypoxia, drug/toxin exposure, inflammation, neoplasia, and nodular hyperplasia.

Nodular Hyperplasia and Regenerative Nodules

Nodular hyperplasia is a spontaneous, age-related, very common proliferation of hepatocytes found in older dogs and rarely observed in other domestic species. The etiology is unknown and has no clinical consequence. It is usually encountered incidentally on ultrasound evaluation. Nodular hyperplasia typically first arises at ages 6 to 8 years, and most dogs are likely to develop them in their geriatric years.[20] The nodules can appear as single or, more often, multiple (even numerous) lesions, randomly distributed and well-circumscribed, and ranging from 0.2 to 3 cm in diameter. Cytologically, the hepatocytes within the nodules will have normal morphology with or without a mixture of nonlipid and/or lipid vacuolation focally distributed or diffused within a given nodule (see Fig. 20.10). Subtle cytological changes that may be found in hyperplastic nodules include mild variation in cellular and nuclear sizes (mild anisocytosis and anisokaryosis, respectively),

increased cytoplasmic basophilia, and increased numbers of binucleate hepatocytes. Focal inflammatory infiltrates are often present, to a variable extent, as macrophages or pigment-laden macrophages and sometimes are mixed with neutrophils and lymphocytes. Extramedullary hematopoiesis can also rarely be observed. The combination of cellular hypertrophy, vacuolation, and hyperplasia is responsible for the mass effect.[20] Nodular hyperplasia may be accompanied by a mild to moderate increase in serum liver enzyme activity, especially ALP, together with a normal bilirubin level. A key feature of nodular hyperplasia when histologically evaluated is that hepatocyte lobular architecture is retained and the adjacent hepatic parenchyma is normal, albeit mildly compressed in some areas.

Regenerative hyperplastic nodules also occur most commonly in dogs but are not age related. The nodules are usually multiple and appear identical to nodular hyperplasia when sampled with cytology; however, they have a significantly different pathogenesis and appearance on histology. Regenerative nodules reflect a compensatory hepatocyte hyperplastic outgrowth from surrounding diseased liver tissue, and the original insult may not always be determined. It is commonly seen in canine chronic hepatitis. On histological sections, there will *always* be loss of lobular architecture within the nodule and significantly abnormal lesions in the surrounding parenchyma, usually with fibrosis.[20] Extramedullary hematopoiesis is not a feature. Some regenerative nodules may even be difficult to distinguish from benign neoplastic hepatocellular adenoma on histology, particularly if insufficient tissue quantity is submitted for evaluation.

The cytological appearance of both hyperplastic and regenerative liver nodules is not specific. If correlated with its multinodular ultrasonographic appearance, relative sizes of 0.2 to 3 cm diameter, and patient history, however, a tentative diagnosis of hyperplasia is reasonable. All such lesions should be carefully monitored with ultrasonography. If there are any changes, growth, or clinical suspicion of neoplasia, then biopsy and histopathology should be further pursued to rule out the possibility of hepatocellular adenoma or even well-differentiated hepatocellular carcinoma.

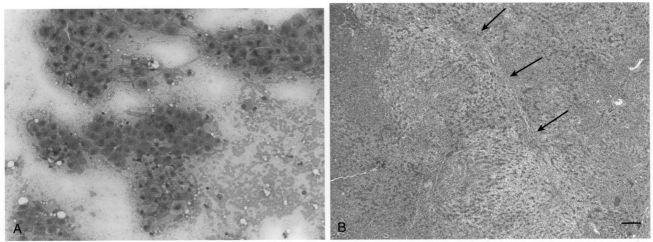

Fig. 20.10 Hepatocellular nodular hyperplasia. (A) Liver aspirate from an 11-year-old Siberian Husky with diffuse liver nodules and progressively increased serum alkaline phosphatase (ALP) and mild alanine amino-transferase (ALT) activity. The top and bottom of the photograph show hepatocytes with moderate nonlipid vacuolar change, and the central hepatocytes demonstrate minimal to mild vacuolation. A single, incidental mast cell is present at the center of the photograph. Overall, these findings are nonspecific; thus, only a tentative diagnosis of nodular hyperplasia can be reached when combined with imaging results and cytological and clinical information (Wright-Giemsa, 20× objective). (B) Histological section, low-power magnification from a different dog with confirmed canine nodular hyperplasia. The nodule is represented in the region left of the arrows and shows a mixture of hepatocytes without and with significant vacuolation (shown by areas with white cytoplasmic clearings), as well as mild regional compression. Lobular architecture is retained (hematoxylin and eosin [H&E], 4× objective; bar is 200 μm). (B, Courtesy Dr. A. Taryn Donovan.)

Inflammatory Diseases

Acute and chronic inflammatory diseases affecting the liver and its biliary system are common in dogs and cats; they are related to a multitude of causes that can be primary to the liver, multisystemic, or secondary to inflammation elsewhere (pancreatitis, gastroenteritis, etc.).[21-24] Confirming the true presence of hepatobiliary inflammatory disease with cytology alone is challenging. For instance, the magnitude of infiltrate may be mild and its distribution patchy such that the inflammation may not even be detected. Observing degenerative neutrophils, infectious agents, or necrotic cellular debris, however, may provide supportive evidence. Other helpful clues are the presence of aggregates of neutrophils and/or lymphocytes, particularly if they are intimately associated with or embedded within hepatocyte sheets and mixed with cells not found in blood (i.e., increased macrophages and/or plasma cells, mixed inflammation with chronic disease). The recognition of inflammation is blurred when peripheral blood contamination (inevitably present) has neutrophilia or lymphocytosis; it is even more ambiguous if the complete blood count (CBC) data are not known or not specified. Furthermore, cytology does not have the benefit of assessing tissue architecture, so it cannot determine to what extent or location the inflammation is directed; specifically, whether it is general hepatic parenchyma (hepatitis), bile ducts in the portal region (cholangitis), or extension from the portal region into surrounding parenchyma (cholangiohepatitis). Last, the absence of inflammation on cytology does not necessarily rule out an inflammatory differential.[3]

Guided by the classification scheme and terminology set forth by the Liver Standardization Group of the World Small Animal Veterinary Association (WSAVA), the following section highlights the expected patterns and etiopathogenesis for the most frequently encountered canine and feline inflammatory liver diseases.[5,9,10,25]

Neutrophilic Inflammation

Neutrophilic or suppurative inflammation is present when increased neutrophils are the predominant cell type, where they may exceed 85% of the inflammatory infiltrate. A variable number of macrophages will be admixed; their relative proportion increases with chronicity, as may lesser number of lymphocytes and plasma cells (i.e., the inflammation becomes a mixed cell appearance) (Fig. 20.11). A careful search for bacteria or other infectious agents should be made, but the findings are usually negative.

Neutrophilic cholangitis is the leading cause of inflammatory liver disease in both dogs and cats.[21,23,26] This reflects inflammation centered around the portal region, and it can extend into the surrounding hepatic parenchyma (cholangiohepatitis). Remember, the specific anatomical location of the inflammation cannot be determined with cytology and requires histopathology for characterization, whereby some degree of biliary hyperplasia and fibrosis (chronic changes) is usually documented. Correlation with ultrasonography findings should influence the suspicion for cholangitis; the liver may show a dilated or tortuous route of the biliary tree, sludgy appearance to the bile fluid, and/or a distended gallbladder. Clinical signs are nonspecific and sometimes include fever. Most cases have increased serum liver enzyme activity and bilirubin, whereas CBC may sometimes show a left shift neutrophilia.[22,23]

Neutrophilic cholangitis can be a sterile inflammatory process, but a bacterial etiology is usually suspected and occasionally confirmed by culture.[22,23,27,28] *Escherichia coli* and *Enterococcus* spp. are the most commonly cultured organisms from either gallbladder fluid or liver tissue biopsy specimens. There is frequent gallbladder involvement (cholecystitis and/or bactibilia) in both dogs and cats (Fig. 20.12). Furthermore, concurrent inflammatory disease within the adjacent pancreas and/or gastrointestinal (GI) tract is common in cats (i.e., so-called "triaditis") and increasingly recognized in dogs.[22,23,27] Both gallbladder fluid

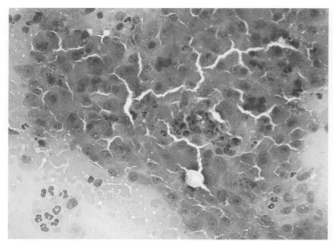

Fig. 20.11 Marked neutrophilic to mixed inflammation. There is marked infiltrate of predominantly neutrophils and fewer macrophages and lymphocytes in this liver aspirate from a 13-year-old Chihuahua with fever. The inflammatory cells are seen grouped together and embedded within the smudged hepatocyte tissue. A Tru-Cut biopsy sample from this dog confirmed a neutrophilic necrotizing hepatitis. An underlying bacterial etiology was suspected despite negative culture results from histology of the liver biopsy specimen (Wright-Giemsa, 50× objective).

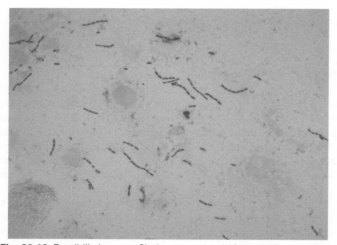

Fig. 20.12 Bactibilia in a cat. Cholecystocentesis from a 16-year-old cat confirms bactibilia with numerous rod bacteria forming chains on a stippled mucoproteinaceous background of gallbladder fluid. *Escherichia coli* bacteria were cultured. Concurrent liver cytology showed moderate to marked hepatic lipidosis and neutrophilic to mixed inflammation (Wright-Giemsa, 100× objective).

cytology and bacterial culture are recommended in most cases of suspected cholangitis, when safe and appropriate for the patient.[22,23] If there is any question regarding the structural integrity of the gallbladder wall, then FNA sampling should not be attempted. A bile duct obstruction (dogs/cats) and gallbladder mucocele (dogs) are additional contraindications for cholecystocentesis because they pose a risk for gallbladder rupture and consequent bile peritonitis. The cytological characteristics of bile peritonitis are described in Chapter 15, regarding effusions.

Lymphocytic Inflammation

The presence of a lymphocytic-predominant inflammatory infiltrate in the liver is relatively common in cats but rare in dogs. In fact, some healthy cats may have low-level infiltrate of small mature lymphocytes

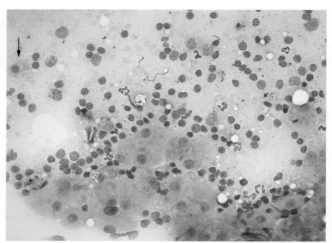

Fig. 20.13 Lymphocytic inflammation in a cat. Marked quantities of small mature lymphocytes are admixed with hepatocytes, along with rare plasma cells *(arrow)* and low numbers of neutrophils and macrophages. This hepatic lymphocyte population is consistent with an inflammatory infiltrate (probable lymphocytic cholangitis–cholangiohepatitis) in this 13-year-old cat; however, distinction from a small cell lymphoma is challenging for both cytological and histological evaluations. Ideally, a subsequent tissue biopsy and molecular test for neoplastic clonality (polymerase chain reaction for antigen receptor rearrangement [PARR] assay) can further characterize the lymphocyte population to more confidently rule in or rule out a neoplastic differential (Wright-Giemsa, 50× objective).

and plasma cells restricted to the portal tract regions, but this is a nonspecific finding.[29] More clinically important is the inflammatory condition of lymphocytic or nonsuppurative cholangitis/cholangiohepatitis (older term *lymphocytic portal hepatitis*). Lymphocytic cholangitis and cholangiohepatitis will have moderate to potentially marked infiltrate of small mature lymphocytes, along with lower number of plasma cells, potentially few intermediate sized lymphocytes, and minority of neutrophils and macrophages (Fig. 20.13). These affected cats typically have slowly progressive illness over weeks/months with nonspecific clinical signs. Patient presentation ranges from clinically silent to jaundice, hepatomegaly, and ascites.[23,24] Compared to cats with neutrophilic cholangitis, the magnitude of increased liver enzyme activity and bilirubin may be less pronounced in cats with lymphocytic cholangitis, not to mention a less clear association with comorbidities, such as bactibilia, pancreatic disease, and/or intestinal disease. Lymphocytic cholangitis/cholangiohepatitis is thought to be an immune-mediated process that targets the bile ducts, usually consisting of a T-lymphocyte population.[30] Biliary hyperplasia, peribiliary fibrosis, and portal lipogranulomas (aggregates of ceroid and lipid-containing macrophages) are other features consistently found on histological tissue sections. Histology is necessary to confirm the extent and cause of any significant lymphocytic infiltrate, particularly because it closely resembles some forms of lymphoma. Accurate distinction between lymphocytic cholangitis and small- to intermediate-size lymphoma is challenging for both cytological and histological evaluations, such that immunohistochemistry and PARR (polymerase chain reaction [PCR] for antigen receptor rearrangement) assay are also recommended. The PARR assay is an ancillary molecular test that can sometimes help distinguish a reactive lymphocyte population (usually polyclonal) from a neoplastic one (usually clonal). It can be performed on previously stained cytology slides. Full integration of *all* clinicopathological findings is important because a minority subset of cats with lymphocytic cholangitis can have an unexpected clonal PARR assay result.[30] Lymphoma and its various morphologies and subtypes are discussed in the section on neoplastic diseases.

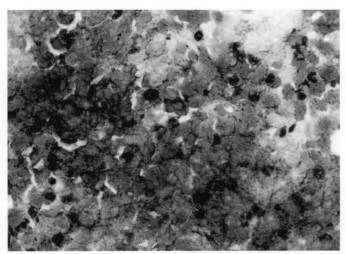

Fig. 20.14 Acute liver injury and necrosis. Fine-needle aspiration (FNA) liver cytology from a young dog known to have ingested poisonous wild mushrooms. Tissue necrosis is depicted as large amounts of amorphous blue/purple to gray-colored cellular material. Hepatocytes are no longer recognizable, but increased and poorly preserved neutrophils are evident. These findings are not specific to mycotoxin or any other noxious insult. In many cases of acute liver injury, the cause will not be known or microscopically evident (Wright, 100× objective). (Courtesy Dr. Tara P. Arndt and Dr. Sonjia M. Shelly.)

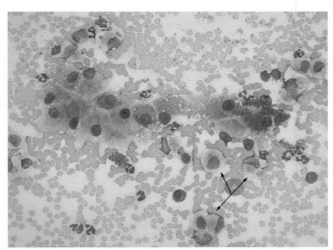

Fig. 20.15 Mixed inflammation with feline infectious peritonitis (FIP). There is moderate to marked mixed inflammation with mostly macrophages *(arrows)*, increased but fewer neutrophils, and a sole plasma cell to the left of the triple arrow. They surround a small raft of hepatocytes. These findings could represent mixed inflammation associated with any disease process, but because this 1-year-old cat also had hyperglobulinemia and large-volume and high-protein (6.6 g/dL and relative low cellularity) exudative peritoneal effusion, the observed liver inflammation was proposedly related to FIP infection (Wright-Giemsa, 50× objective).

Acute Liver Injury, Toxins, and Infectious Liver Diseases

Various liver insults can cause reversible hepatocellular injury, but if sustained or severe enough, then irreversible damage will result in hepatocyte necrosis or apoptosis and usually observed concomitant inflammation. Neutrophilic inflammation may predominate in acute/peracute liver injuries, but with chronicity, most cases will show mixed cell or macrophage-predominant inflammation. The various noxious stimuli include ischemia and tissue hypoxia; toxins (plant/mycotoxins, xylitol); dose-dependent and idiosyncratic drug reactions (acetaminophen/paracetamol, phenobarbital, sulfonamide antibiotics, carprofen, oral benzodiazepine, etc.); severe metabolic disturbances; and microorganisms.[31] In many cases of acute liver injury, the patient is too rapidly ill or unstable for liver sampling, whereas other cases deemed safe for liver FNA may show necrosis and/or inflammation but not identify the cause (Fig. 20.14). Similarly, histological assessment of a liver biopsy may localize the pattern of inflammation (centrilobular, periportal, midzonal, or massive), but the findings are usually nonspecific.[5] Coordinated testing with serology, PCR tests, toxicology screening assays, and sample cultures may help rule in or rule out a specific etiology, as tailored to the patient's history and exposure risk. For example, leptospirosis has a characteristic multisystemic clinical presentation, but its hepatic histopathology is nonspecific; thus, serology and/or PCR tests are needed for its specific diagnosis. In cats with feline infectious peritonitis (FIP) virus, the liver may have randomly dispersed areas of mixed inflammation (+/− observed necrosis), but only a coordinated effort with body fluid effusion analysis, serology, or PCR will yield a conclusion of probable/consistent with FIP (Fig. 20.15). Other instances where an infectious agent may be microscopically identified or at least highly suspected are infectious canine hepatitis (canine adenovirus 1) revealing round intranuclear viral inclusions within hepatocytes; granulomatous/pyogranulomatous infiltrate (often including multinucleated giant macrophages) associated with mycobacterial, fungal, or protozoal infections in dogs and cats; and marked eosinophilic cholangitis/cholangiohepatitis and liver fluke infestation in cats from a tropical climate, as in Florida, the Caribbean

islands, or Hawaii. Last, caution is strongly advised in sampling a solitary hypoechoic hepatic mass in a febrile dog or cat with peripheral blood neutrophilia because of the risk for potentially rupturing a bacterial abscess.

Chronic Hepatitis

In chronic inflammatory liver diseases, there is ongoing hepatocellular damage and loss, with the liver's response being regeneration and fibrosis. The following discussion pertains to canine chronic hepatitis, which affects the hepatic parenchyma and can involve the portal regions. Advanced cases lead to cirrhosis and end-stage liver failure. Cytology has inherent limitations that prevent it from establishing a diagnosis of canine chronic hepatitis. On rare occasion, cytology might suggest the presence of fibrosis (Fig. 20.16), but histopathology is necessary to characterize its extent and significance.[12] The four histological criteria for a chronic hepatitis diagnosis are hepatocellular apoptosis or necrosis; a variable mononuclear or mixed inflammatory infiltrate; hepatocyte regeneration (often including regenerative nodules and biliary ductal proliferation); and fibrosis (Fig. 20.17).[5] The magnitude, distribution, and relative proportions among these criteria vary widely in affected dogs.

Canine chronic hepatitis is a slowly progressive disease, and its underlying cause remains undetermined in most cases. Even the breed-specific and copper-associated hepatopathies have unanswered questions. On the basis of the most current research, however, the breeds deemed likely to have an immune-mediated cause of chronic hepatitis are, in decreasing levels of evidence, Doberman Pinchers, English Springer Spaniels, and Cocker Spaniels.[32] Copper accumulation can be a primary cause or a secondary consequence of chronic hepatitis. Copper is an essential trace mineral required for many body functions, but it is potentially toxic and leads to oxidative cell damage if not properly stored in the liver or excreted via the biliary system.[33] The dog breeds most likely to have a primary (hereditary) copper-storage disease are, in decreasing levels of evidence, Bedlington Terriers, Dalmatians, Labrador Retrievers, Doberman Pinchers, and West

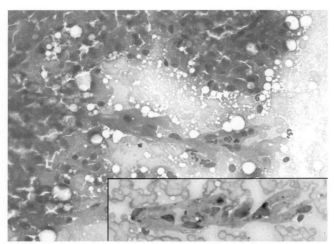

Fig. 20.16 Fibrosis in liver cytology. Pink fibrillar extracellular matrix material and its associated spindled mesenchymal cells are consistent with fibrous tissue in this liver aspirate from a 14-year-old Border Collie. The fibrous tissue is associated with few neutrophils and lymphocytes. The lower inset of spindle cells is from the same liver cytology and shows cytoplasmic granules of no known significance. Although fibrosis may be cytologically recognized on rare occasion, histopathology is necessary to characterize its extent and significance (Wright-Giemsa, 50× objective. *Inset:* 50× objective).

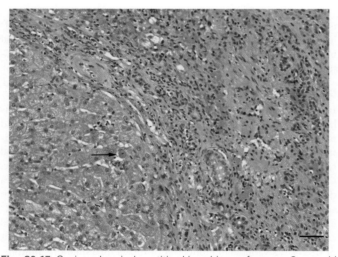

Fig. 20.17 Canine chronic hepatitis. Liver biopsy from an 8-year-old Boxer. The central, vertical portion of the photograph depicts linear, portal-to-portal bridging with fibrosis, biliary hyperplasia, and a mixed mononuclear inflammatory infiltrate. The left side of the photograph shows a regenerative nodule with focal individual hepatocyte necrosis *(arrow)* (hematoxylin and eosin [H&E], 20× objective; bar is 50 μm). (Courtesy Dr. Taryn A. Donovan.)

Highland White Terriers.[32,33] Only the Bedlington Terrier and the Labrador Retriever breeds have proven genetic mutations in their copper metabolism/transport. There are case reports of other dog breeds with suspected hereditary copper-associated hepatitis, such as the Skye Terrier breed, but the evidence is ambiguous. Dietary composition of food likely plays a role in both primary and secondary copper-associated hepatopathies. It is recommended that excess copper accumulation be ruled out in all cases of canine chronic hepatitis. Similarly, recent studies in cats with chronic biliary disease have shown that hepatic copper accumulation occurs more frequently than previously reported.[34,35]

Gallbladder and Biliary Tract Disorders

Gallbladder and biliary tract disorders are often a component of some inflammatory liver diseases, as discussed in the preceding section. Cholecystitis is most commonly observed with bacterial or sterile cholangitis, biliary tract obstruction (including choleliths), gallbladder mucocele (progressive, cystic mucinous hyperplasia in dogs), or a combination therein. Correlation with ultrasonography findings is essential for diagnosing biliary and gallbladder conditions.

A benign biliary cystic proliferation worth clarifying is adult polycystic disease, a form of congenital cystic liver disease caused by malformation of the primitive biliary ductal plate during embryological/fetal development.[20,25] Although these ductal plate anomalies are present at birth, the most recognized type is the adult-onset formation of multiple (even numerous) cysts, which in the past and recent veterinary literature have been misclassified as "neoplastic biliary cystadenomas." A true biliary cystadenoma (cholangiocellular adenoma) is extremely rare in dogs and cats and would be a solitary lesion. In both species, adult polycystic disease is characterized by slowly progressive biliary dilatations that can range in diameter from 1 mm to 12 cm, lined by a single layer of cuboidal to low columnar epithelium. The resultant single- and multiple-chambered cysts contain clear, colorless fluid, separated by fibrosis of variable thickness that can compress adjacent hepatic parenchyma (Fig. 20.18). Adult polycystic disease frequently and concurrently involves similar cyst formations in the kidneys. The "poster child" Persian cat and Persian crossbreeds with dual liver and kidney polycystic disease may have juvenile- and/or adult-onset congenital ductal plate anomalies.[25]

Amyloidosis

Amyloid A (AA) is an insoluble extracellular fibrillar protein that can pathologically accumulate in various organs as a consequence of long-standing inflammation, infection, or tissue destruction. It is derived from the circulating acute phase reactant protein, serum amyloid A (SAA), which is produced mainly in the liver. Hepatic amyloidosis in dogs and cats is a relatively uncommon occurrence and results in amyloid fibrils adhering along blood vessel walls and in the perisinusoidal space of Disse, where blood plasma interacts with hepatocytes.[9] With excessive amyloid deposition, the liver will become markedly enlarged and fragile with increased susceptibility to vessel rupture. Hepatic AA amyloidosis is also hereditary in the Chinese Shar Pei dogs and in Abyssinian, Siamese, and Oriental cat breeds.[9,36] In both reactive and familial cases, amyloidosis can be localized to the liver or other organs (kidney, heart, pancreas, etc.) or be systemic. Cytologically, hepatic amyloid appears as extracellular bright pink amorphous to fibrillar material intimately associated with hepatocytes (Fig. 20.19). A variable degree of mixed inflammation is often present in the surrounding tissue. Congo red stain will confirm the presence of amyloid on cytology and histology; the amyloid will be red/orange and show green birefringence under polarized light. Immunohistochemistry staining can also be performed.

Extramedullary Hematopoiesis

The liver is able to bolster the bone marrow's hematopoietic efforts in response to a pronounced anemia or inflammatory stimulus. Perhaps not as frequently encountered as splenic extramedullary hematopoiesis (EMH), the liver can produce foci of hematopoietic activity that may tend to favor the cell lineage needed most. In cases of immune-mediated hemolytic anemia and thrombocytopenia, there would be an expected predominance of erythroid precursors along with some megakaryocytes, whereas in chronic purulent inflammatory diseases, granulopoiesis should be favored in its production of neutrophils.

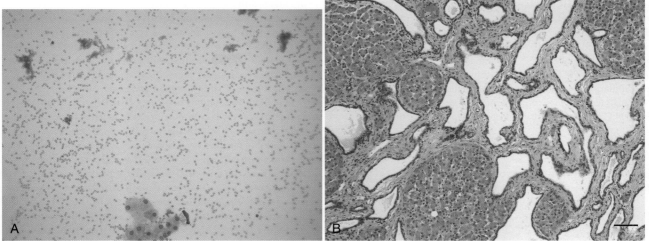

Fig. 20.18 Adult polycystic disease in the liver. (A) Cytological evaluation of fluid obtained from one of several, variably sized cysts within the liver of a 14-year-old Domestic Shorthair cat. The minimally cellular cyst fluid contains some amorphous light-blue mucoproteinaceous fluid material mixed with mild peripheral blood erythrocyte contamination. A raft hepatocyte (from hepatic parenchyma adjacent to the cyst) is present at the bottom of the photograph (Wright-Giemsa, 20× objective). (B) Histological correlate showing the multiple cystic dilated bile duct malformations that are lined by a single layer of biliary epithelium and separated by fibrous stroma and islands of hepatic parenchyma. Adult polycystic disease is the most common type of congenital ductal plate anomaly in both dogs and cats. Past and recent veterinary literature has frequently misclassified this polycystic disease as biliary cystadenoma (hematoxylin and eosin [H&E], 10× objective; bar is 100 μm). (B, Courtesy Dr. Taryn A. Donovan.)

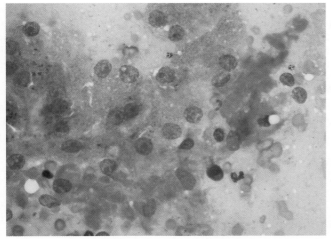

Fig. 20.19 Hepatic amyloid deposition in a cat. The fibrillar to amorphous bright-pink extracellular material is consistent with reactive amyloid protein deposition in the liver. A nearby plasma cell and neutrophil are seen. This 7-year-old cat had chronic inflammatory disease. Although amyloid material resembles other pink extracellular matrix, such as collagen, chondroid, and osteoid, one might expect to see associated spindle cells with those differentials. Congo red stain can help distinguish amyloid in both cytology and histology (Wright-Giemsa, 100× objective).

Regardless of which lineage is in highest demand, EMH usually shows orderly, complete, and synchronous maturation of hematopoietic cells, where late-stage precursors are more numerous than earlier ones. EMH is also rarely observed in canine nodular hyperplasia. Myelolipoma is a rare benign tumor seen in older cats and dogs. It is an incidental tumor in liver or spleen and will appear identical to EMH or normal bone marrow elements, except that it is intermixed with a variable quantity of mature adipose tissue.

Neoplasia

The following section describes and illustrates the most commonly encountered primary and secondary (metastatic and multicentric) neoplasms involving the liver. Primary tumors are mostly epithelial and can be classified as hepatocellular adenoma, hepatocellular carcinoma (HCC), cholangiocellular (bile duct) carcinoma, and carcinoid; hemangiosarcoma is the main mesenchymal neoplasm that can originate within the liver.[20] Furthermore, hepatoblastoma is a rare primary neoplasm in dogs and cats and is derived from pluripotential stem cells; only single case reports exist.[37,38] Tumors that metastasize to the liver most commonly originate from the GI tract, pancreas, or spleen; they spread hematogenously or through the lymphatics.[39] Secondary tumors of hemolymphatic origin, notably lymphoma, are often multicentric in presentation.

Hepatocellular Neoplasia

Hepatocellular adenoma is a benign tumor of hepatocytes and is referred to as a *hepatoma*. It is reported to occur less frequently compared with HCC in dogs, in part because there is morphological overlap with well-differentiated hepatocellular carcinoma and even a hyperplastic nodule.[20,40] Hepatocellular adenoma presents as a single mass, 2 to 12 cm in diameter, composed of well differentiated hepatocytes that are histologically well demarcated by compression of the adjacent parenchyma (nonencapsulated) and lack of normal lobular architecture.[20] Cytologically, the hepatocytes of a hepatocellular adenoma display only subtle changes, such as mild anisocytosis and increased cytoplasmic basophilia (Fig. 20.20).[20] Histological evaluation is necessary for a definitive diagnosis.

Hepatocellular carcinoma accounts for about half of the primary hepatic neoplasia in dogs and occurs less frequently in cats.[41-44] Morphologically, they can be classified as massive (single large tumor), nodular (multiple tumors in several lobes), and diffuse.[41] The massive form of canine HCC most commonly involves the left lateral liver lobe and has a reported low rate of metastasis after lobectomy.[45]

Nodular and diffuse HCCs occur less often but have a higher potential for metastasis to the regional lymph nodes, peritoneum, and lungs.[20] Cytologically, the neoplastic hepatocytes of HCC can appear either well differentiated (difficult to distinguish from a benign process) or look highly pleomorphic.[20] Cytological features used to identify well-differentiated HCCs include the presence of lysed cells and free nuclei; capillary vessels coursing through sheets/clusters; individualized hepatocytes and loss of cell cohesion; significant anisokaryosis, increased N:C ratio; and multinucleated cells with three or more nuclei (Fig. 20.21).[46]

Bile Duct Neoplasia

Cholangiocellular neoplasms arise from the epithelial lining of the biliary tract. Contrary to reports in the past and recent veterinary literature,

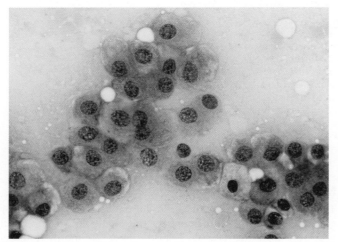

Fig. 20.20 Hepatocellular adenoma. Fine-needle aspiration (FNA) cytology from a single liver mass in a dog. Clusters of well-differentiated hepatocytes display only subtle changes characterized by mild anisocytosis and increased cytoplasmic basophilia. A diagnosis of hepatocellular adenoma requires histopathology, as was confirmed in this case (Wright-Giemsa, 50× objective). (Courtesy Dr. Andrew G. Burton.)

cholangiocellular adenoma (biliary adenoma) is extremely rare in dogs and cats.[25] Feline congenital polycystic disease has been historically confused with biliary adenomas (cystadenomas) accounting for the discrepancy.[20] (See "Gallbladder and Biliary Tract Disorders" in the "Nonneoplastic Conditions and Inflammatory Diseases" section). True biliary adenomas are solitary and well circumscribed, with a solid/fibrous stromal component and small-caliber cysts.[20]

Malignant bile duct neoplasia, namely cholangiocellular carcinoma, is the most common primary hepatic tumor in cats. It frequently originates within the intrahepatic biliary tract and presents with multiple nodules involving all of the liver lobes.[25,39,47] There can be variable proportions of cystic areas.[20,25] Cytologically, cholangiocellular carcinoma is characterized by relatively uniform cuboidal epithelial cells, with a scant amount of cytoplasm arranged in densely packed sheets and tubular cluster formations (Fig. 20.22). Despite an often well-differentiated cytomorphology, bile duct carcinoma has an aggressive biological behavior and a high rate of metastasis.[48]

Hepatic Carcinoid

Hepatic carcinoid is a rare aggressive neoplasm arising from the neuroendocrine cells found in the biliary system and frequently metastasizes throughout the liver and to the regional lymph nodes and the peritoneum.[43,48] The typical presentation in dogs is characterized by multiple and diffuse, small, distinct intrahepatic nodules without hepatomegaly.[20] In cats, carcinoids may be of either intrahepatic or extrahepatic bile duct origin.[20] As with any neuroendocrine neoplasm, aspirates from hepatic carcinoid(s) yield high numbers of cells, most of which are lysed (bare nuclei) or partially disrupted, in sheets with indistinct cell borders and overlapping nuclei (Fig. 20.23). The nuclei are often relatively uniform in appearance with only mild anisokaryosis despite the high-grade behavior. Cytological distinction of hepatic carcinoids from metastatic neuroendocrine tumors, such as islet cell tumors, pheochromocytoma, and intestinal carcinoid, is not possible.

Metastatic Carcinoma

Pancreatic carcinoma is the most frequent epithelial malignancy to spread to the liver.[40] Although cytological assessment of these lesions

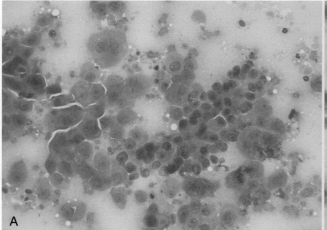
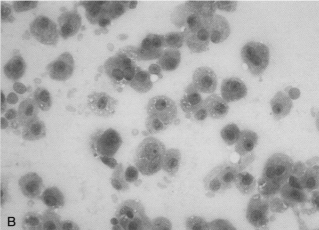

Fig. 20.21 Hepatocellular carcinoma. (A) Sheets and clusters of neoplastic hepatocytes display significant pleomorphism in this aspirate from a dog with a large left-sided liver mass. There is moderate to marked variation is cell size, nuclear size, variable nucleus-to-cytoplasm (N:C) ratio, and multinucleation (Wright-Giemsa, 50× objective). (B) Same canine case showing the neoplastic hepatocytes with loss of cellular cohesion—frequent individualized hepatocytes—an abnormal cytological feature. Some cases of well-differentiated hepatocellular carcinoma show less pronounced cytological criteria of malignancy; thus, all hepatocellular tumors require histology for a definitive diagnosis (Wright-Giemsa, 50× objective).

readily identifies a carcinoma, determination of the primary site of origin is not possible on the basis of cytomorphology and requires histopathology (Fig. 20.24). Furthermore, distinguishing metastatic carcinoma (especially of pancreatic origin) from primary cholangiocellular carcinoma is challenging on both cytology and histology.[49]

Primary and Metastatic Sarcomas

Primary sarcomas of the liver are rare, whereas metastatic mesenchymal tumors occur more frequently. Hemangiosarcoma is the most encountered spindle cell tumor in the liver, whether it be primary or, more often, originating in the spleen.[20] Perhaps more so than other spindle cell tumor types, hemangiosarcoma is usually poorly

exfoliating by FNA and typically only yields hemodilution from the tumor's blood-filled channels. If neoplastic cells are present, they will be spindle-shaped to polygonal cells, with tapering tails and variable degrees of anisocytosis and anisokaryosis. As stated at the beginning of this chapter, FNA of larger cavitational liver masses should be avoided because of the risk for capsule rupture, hemorrhage, and potential tumor seeding. Other sarcoma types to infiltrate the liver can include fibrosarcoma and leiomyosarcoma, among others. Histopathology is usually necessary to determine the specific sarcoma type (Fig. 20.25).

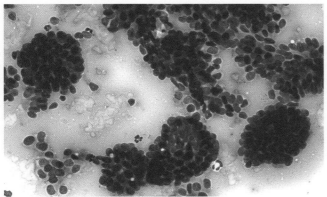

Fig. 20.22 Cholangiocellular carcinoma (biliary carcinoma). Liver aspirate from a cat with multiple liver masses/nodules. Note the densely packed clusters of relatively uniform cuboidal epithelial cells, sometimes in palisading arrangements. The cells have round to oval nuclei with a stippled chromatin pattern, mild anisokaryosis, and scant volume of cytoplasm. This highly cellular neoplastic epithelial population is characteristic of a cholangiocellular carcinoma (Wright-Giemsa, 50× objective). (Courtesy Dr. Emily Walters.)

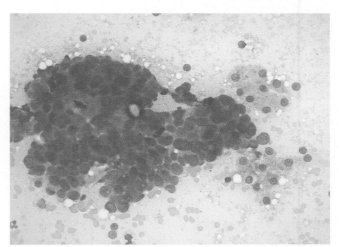

Fig. 20.24 Metastatic carcinoma. This liver aspirate is taken from a cat with a known pancreatic mass and multinodular liver appearance on ultrasonography. The criteria of malignancy in this large densely cellular cluster of epithelial cells include large nuclear size with moderate anisokaryosis and variably prominent large nucleoli. For size comparison, two clusters of hepatocytes are present on the right side of the photograph. Histopathology is required to determine the carcinoma type (Wright-Giemsa, 50× objective).

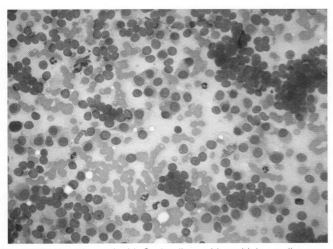

Fig. 20.23 Hepatic carcinoid. Canine liver with multiple small masses. This highly cellular aspirate contains numerous lysed cells (bare nuclei) and fewer intact cells, all of which are arranged individually and in disorganized sheets/clusters with indistinct borders. Intact cells are oval shaped, with moderate amount of pale basophilic cytoplasm surrounding a round nucleus of finely stippled chromatin and sometimes a visible single, variably prominent nucleolus. Anisocytosis and anisokaryosis are mild. This epithelial neoplasm displays features of neuroendocrine origin, and with multiple masses throughout the liver, it is consistent with hepatic carcinoid (Wright-Giemsa, 50× objective).

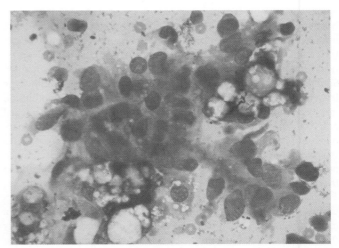

Fig. 20.25 Sarcoma in the liver. Ultrasound-guided aspirate from an 8-year-old dog with a large liver mass and history of progressive anorexia. The spleen had normal echogenicity. Atypical spindled mesenchymal cells are intimately associated with extracellular pink matrix material and flanked by two small clusters of hepatocytes on the lower left and upper right sides (note that the hepatocytes show cytoplasmic lipid vacuolation). The spindle cells have large ovoid nuclei of finely stippled chromatin with multiple, variably sized nucleoli and moderate amounts of basophilic tapered cytoplasm. Many medium-size spindle cell aggregates were identified in the liver mass aspirate, sufficiently to conclude a sarcoma but unknown as to which type and whether primary or metastatic (Wright-Giemsa, 100× objective).

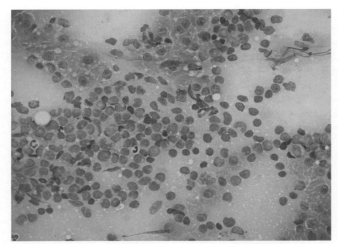

Fig. 20.26 Large cell lymphoma. This liver aspirate from a dog with hepatosplenomegaly and generalized peripheral and mesenteric lymphadenopathy shows a relatively monomorphic population of large immature lymphocytes. The lymphocytes have rounded to indented nuclei that are equal and just larger than a neutrophil diameter. The cytological findings and clinical presentation are indicative of a multicentric large cell lymphoma (Wright-Giemsa, 50× objective).

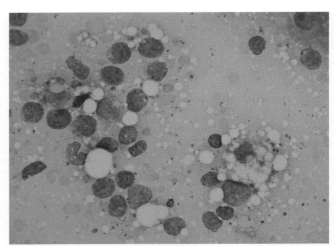

Fig. 20.27 Large granular lymphoma (LGL). Liver aspirate from an icteric and anorexic 15-year-old cat. There are significantly expanded numbers of large granular lymphocytes with characteristic pink/magenta cytoplasmic granules, usually seen packeted together near the nucleus. Note the numerous LGL granules free in the background and a single hepatocyte on the right side with lipid vacuolation. Hepatic lipidosis was evident elsewhere on the sample slides, secondary to this LGL (Wright-Giemsa, 100× objective).

Hemolymphatic Neoplasia

The following is a brief summary of the features of "round cell tumors" as they involve the liver and include the diverse group of lymphoma, histiocytic sarcoma, mast cell tumor, and plasma cell neoplasia.

In dogs, the large cell lymphoma involving the liver is usually the classic multicentric lymphoma, whereas hepatic lymphoma in cats is usually derived from the GI tract.[40] The liver is usually diffusely enlarged and exfoliates high numbers of cells on FNA. Lymphocytes of large cell lymphoma have rounded nuclei that are larger than a neutrophil in diameter, are immature in appearance, and have a modest amount of variably basophilic cytoplasm (Fig. 20.26). Large granular lymphoma (LGL) is often an aggressive neoplasm derived from the intraepithelial enteric lymphocytes and occurs most frequently in cats (i.e., feline intestinal LGL lymphoma). It can have circulating neoplastic cells in blood and disseminate to the liver as well as other organs.[50] Similarly, neoplastic lymphocytes of a large granular lymphocytic leukemia can also be observed in liver cytology (with hemodilution inevitably present), but these neoplastic cells originate from splenic red pulp.[50] Compared with cats, canine large granular lymphocytic leukemia and some LGLs may have a more indolent disease course. LGLs typically have an intermediate- to large-sized nucleus and clumped or smooth chromatin. They have characteristic fine or coarse pink/magenta cytoplasmic granules that are often grouped near the nucleus. The packeted nature of LGL granules is a helpful comparative distinction from the wide and random dispersal of cytoplasmic granules of a mast cell (Fig. 20.27). A diagnosis of lymphoma on FNA is generally straightforward for both the LGL and large cell lymphoma types. If a markedly expanded small- to intermediate-size lymphocyte population is present, then differential diagnoses must include small- to intermediate-size lymphoma, chronic lymphocytic leukemia (CLL; only if concurrent lymphocytosis), and severe lymphocytic inflammation (i.e., severe feline cholangitis). This represents a conundrum—lymphoma or leukemia (or neither). The recommended diagnostic approach and appropriate ancillary tests have been discussed earlier in the "Lymphocytic Inflammation" section under "Inflammatory Diseases."

Hepatosplenic and hepatocytotropic lymphomas are two rare specific types of T-cell lymphoma (HS-TCL and HC-TCL, respectively), which infiltrate the hepatic sinusoids (and hepatic cords in HC-TCL) without peripheral lymphadenopathy.[51] HS-TCL is an aggressive neoplasm in dogs, suspected to originate in the spleen and characterized by erythrophagocytic lymphocytes, along with a variable number of nonneoplastic hemophagocytic macrophages.[51] Erythrophagocytic lymphoma resembling HS-TCL has been reported in a cat; however, the indolent clinical course of the disease and the paucity of hemophagocytic macrophages in that case differed from the HS-TCL reported in dogs (Fig. 20.28).[52] In contrast, HC-TCL in both dogs and cats likely originates in the liver and invades the hepatocyte cords.[51] Ultrastructurally, neoplastic lymphocytes cause cytoplasmic invaginations of hepatocyte cell membranes; a phenomenon that has been referred to as *emperipolesis-like invasion*.[53] On light microscopy, this gives the impression of lymphocytes being present within hepatocytes (Fig. 20.29). Even with these unique cytological features, both HS-TCL and HC-TCL require histological confirmation, immunophenotyping, and clonality testing.

Histiocytic sarcoma (HS) is an aggressive neoplasm of dendritic cell origin that can quickly and widely disseminate throughout the body, often involving the spleen, liver, lung, lymph nodes, and beyond.[54,55] Disseminated HS is most frequently observed in dogs but is also rarely recognized as a malignant and progressive disease in cats.[55] Malignant histiocytes have a pleomorphic morphology and typically yield high numbers of cells. They are large in size and are round, oval, or irregularly shaped, with large round/irregular nuclei, fine to stippled chromatin, and single to multiple, variably sized, prominent nucleoli. Their abundant light-blue cytoplasm often contains clear vacuoles (Fig. 20.30). Another histiocytic malignancy is hemophagocytic histiocytic sarcoma, which is derived from splenic red pulp or bone marrow macrophages, rather than being of dendritic cell origin.[56] As its name implies, exuberant and marked erythrophagia by neoplastic histiocytes is a characteristic feature. Neoplastic cells of hemophagocytic histiocytic sarcoma vary from a well-differentiated "typical" macrophage appearance (especially when observed in bone marrow) to moderate

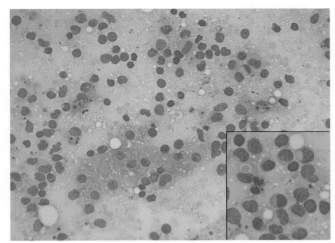

Fig. 20.28 Lymphoma resembling hepatosplenic lymphoma. There is marked infiltration of lymphocytes in this liver aspirate from a 6-year-old cat with hepatosplenomegaly and a severe nonregenerative anemia. The lymphocyte population consists of mostly intermediate- and larger-sized lymphocytes, whose nuclei are approximately 1.5× to 2.5× an erythrocyte diameter along with a modest volume of cytoplasm. Low numbers of small lymphocytes are also seen. A striking feature is the unusual erythrophagocytic behavior of the lymphocyte population *(see inset)*. This case of lymphoma resembles the expected cytological presentation for a hepatosplenic lymphoma, but definitive classification would require further characterization and immunophenotyping (Wright-Giemsa, 50× objective).

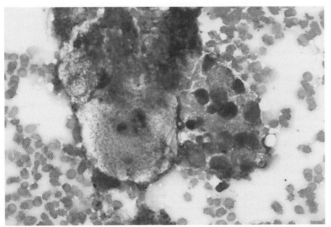

Fig. 20.29 Hepatocytotropic lymphoma. FNA liver cytology from an 11-year-old cat that presented for progressive icterus and elevated liver enzymes. This cluster of hepatocytes is markedly swollen with microvesicular lipid vacuolation. Two hepatocytes on the right side show multiple intermediate- to large-size lymphocytes that appear to be in the cytoplasm (emperipolesis-like appearance). Unfortunately, the disease was advanced and the cat humanely euthanized. The lymphoma diagnosis was achieved on postmortem tissue evaluation, special staining, immunophenotyping, and a molecular clonality assay. With coordinated assistance from Dr. Peter Moore and the Leukocyte Antigen Biology Laboratory at UC Davis, CA, the neoplastic lymphocytes were positive for CD3 and Granzyme B, negative for CD11d and suspected to be gamma-delta T-cell lineage, representing a case of hepatocytotropic lymphoma (Wright-Giemsa, 100× objective). (Histology and ancillary testing courtesy Dr. Taryn A. Donovan.)

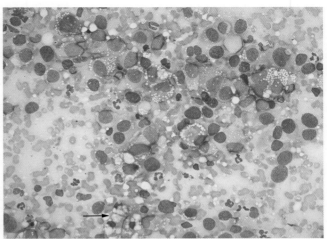

Fig. 20.30 Histiocytic sarcoma. A 12-year-old Basset Hound with severe intraabdominal lymphadenopathy and large hypoechoic masses in the liver and spleen. This highly cellular liver aspirate contains many intact (and some ruptured) large discrete cells with an atypical morphology characteristic of disseminated histiocytic sarcoma. The neoplastic cells have large, round-to-irregular-shaped nuclei with fine chromatin, multiple large prominent nucleoli, and light blue cytoplasm containing punctate clear vacuoles. Moderate to marked variation in nuclear and cell size is seen, along with bizarre mitotic figures and multinucleation observed elsewhere in the aspirate sample. Compare the size of these malignant histiocytes to the neutrophils and rare cluster of lipid-vacuolated hepatocytes *(arrow)* (Wright-Giemsa, 50× objective).

pleomorphism, although not as wild as their dendritic cell counterpart.[56] A clinical syndrome of dogs with hemophagocytic histiocytic sarcoma often includes a severe (Coombs-negative) regenerative anemia, thrombocytopenia, hypoalbuminemia, and hypocholesterolemia.[56] Any dog of any breed can potentially be afflicted by histiocytic sarcoma, but the disease complex in Bernese Mountain Dogs is familial, and the Rottweiler, Golden Retriever, and Flat-Coated Retriever breeds are also predisposed.[55]

Mast cell neoplasia involving the liver typically reflects visceral (splenic) mast cell disease in cats, whereas metastasis from cutaneous mast cell tumor(s) is more common in dogs.[57] Significantly increased numbers of mast cells grouped together or in large sheets within the liver are diagnostic for metastatic mast cell neoplasia (Fig. 20.31, A). If their cell morphology is atypical, with pleomorphism and decreased/variable cytoplasmic granulation, then the diagnosis is even more convincing (see Fig. 20.31, B).

Plasma cell neoplasia is the least common of the round cell tumor group to infiltrate the liver, and it falls under the umbrella term *myeloma-related disorders* (MRDs).[58] In dogs, the classic myeloma disease follows a similar presentation as that seen in humans, namely, bone marrow origin of the plasma cell neoplasia, with or without extramedullary involvement.[58] Although some cats may also have bone marrow involvement, plasma cell infiltration of the liver and spleen (primary extramedullary development without bone marrow disease) is more frequent in this species.[59] Monoclonal gammopathy is a common feature in both canine and feline MRDs. Cytologically, if MRD neoplasia involves the liver, there will be a marked infiltration of well-differentiated plasma cells. These round-to-ovoid cells have a characteristic eccentrically placed round nucleus, clumped to granular chromatin; perinuclear clear zone (Golgi body apparatus); and deep-blue cytoplasm (Fig. 20.32). Despite the well-differentiated cytological appearance, MRDs display an aggressive biological behavior.

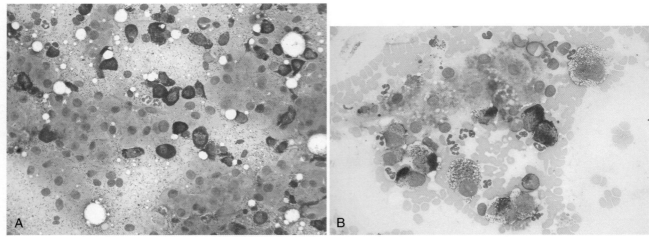

Fig. 20.31 Metastatic mast cell neoplasia in a cat and dog. (A) Markedly increased numbers of mast cells, including those seen grouped together, have infiltrated the liver of this 18-year-old cat. The neoplastic mast cells are highly granulated with many free mast cell granules in the background (Wright-Giemsa, 50× objective). (B) Staging disease with liver (and splenic) ultrasonography and cytology in a dog with a large cutaneous mast cell tumor on the right shoulder. Both liver and spleen are infiltrated with high number of atypical-appearing mast cells. The mast cells in this liver aspirate are pleomorphic; they have large, round to irregular–shaped nuclei, fine chromatin, faint nucleoli, and variable degree of cytoplasmic granulation. The adjacent hepatocytes contain blue lipofuscin granules, a normal cellular pigment (Wright-Giemsa, 50× objective).

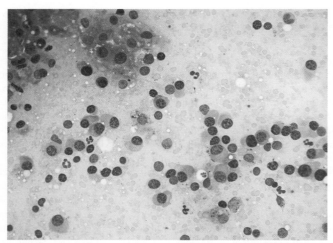

Fig. 20.32 Plasma cell neoplasia (myeloma-related disorder [MRD]) in a 14-year-old cat with hepatosplenomegaly and a monoclonal gammopathy. The liver is markedly infiltrated by a well-differentiated neoplastic population of plasma cells. The (intact) plasma cells show characteristic eccentrically placed nuclei with clumped chromatin, often a perinuclear clearing and moderate volume of deep-blue cytoplasm. Hepatocytes are depicted in the upper left of the photograph. A complete workup in this cat revealed splenic infiltration but no bone marrow involvement, which is different from dogs and the most common presentation for cats (MRD without bone marrow involvement) (Wright-Giemsa, 50× objective).

REFERENCES

1. Stockham SL, Scott MA. *Fundamentals of Veterinary Clinical Pathology*. 2nd ed. Ames: Blackwell Publishing; 2008:676–677.
2. Bahr KL, Sharkey LC, Murakami T, et al. Accuracy of US-guided FNA of focal liver lesions in dogs: 140 cases (2005-2008). *J Am Anim Hosp Assoc*. 2013;49(3):190–196.
3. Roth L. Comparison of liver cytology and biopsy diagnoses in dogs and cats: 56 cases. *Vet Clin Pathol*. 2001;30(1):35–38.
4. Wang KJ, Panciera DL, Al-Rukibat RK, et al. Accuracy of ultrasound-guided fine-needle aspiration of the liver and cytologic findings in dogs and cats: 97 cases (1990-2000). *J Am Vet Med Assoc*. 2004;224(1):75–78.
5. Van den Ingh TSGAM, Van Winkle T, Cullen JM, et al. Morphological classification of parenchymal disorders of the canine and feline liver: 2. Hepatocellular death, hepatitis and cirrhosis. In: Rothuizen J, Bunch SE, Charles JA, et al., eds. *WSAVA Standards for Clinical and Histological Diagnosis of Canine and Feline Liver Disease*. 1st ed. Philadelphia: Saunders Elsevier; 2006:85–101.
6. Webster CR. Hemostatic disorders associated with hepatobiliary disease. In: Lidbury JA, ed. Hepatology, *Vet Clin North Am Small Anim Pract*. Philadelphia: Elsevier; 2017:47(3): 601–615.
7. Meyer DJ. The liver. In: Raskin RE, Meyer DJ, eds. *Canine and Feline Cytology: A Color Atlas and Interpretation Guide*. 3rd ed. St. Louis: Elsevier; 2016:259–283.
8. Rothuizen J, Twedt DC. Liver biopsy techniques. In: Armstrong PJ, Rothuizen J, eds. *Hepatology, Vet Clin North Am Small Anim Pract*. Philadelphia: Elsevier; 2009;39(3):469–480.
9. Cullen JM, Van den Ingh TSGAM, Van Winkle T, et al. Morphological classification of parenchymal disorders of the canine and feline liver: 1. Normal histology, reversible hepatocellular injury and hepatic amyloidosis. In: Rothuizen J, Bunch SE, Charles JA, et al., eds. *WSAVA Standards for Clinical and Histological Diagnosis of Canine and Feline Liver Disease*. Philadelphia: Saunders Elsevier; 2006:77–84.
10. Van Winkle T, Cullen JM, Van den Ingh TSGAM, et al. Morphological classification of parenchymal disorders of the canine and feline liver: 3. Hepatic abscesses and granulomas, hepatic metabolic storage disorders and miscellaneous conditions. In: Rothuizen J, Bunch SE, Charles JA, et al., eds. *WSAVA Standards for Clinical and Histological Diagnosis of Canine and Feline Liver Disease*. Philadelphia: Saunders Elsevier; 2006:103–116.
11. Stockhaus C, Van den Ingh T, Rothuizen J, et al. A multistep approach in the cytologic evaluation of liver biopsy samples of dogs with hepatic diseases. *Vet Pathol*. 2004;41:461–470.
12. Masserdotti C, Bertazzolo W. Cytologic features of hepatic fibrosis in dogs: a retrospective study on 22 cases. *Vet Clin Pathol*. 2016;45(2):361–367.
13. Jeong DH, Lee GP, Jeong WI, et al. Alterations of mast cells and TGF-beta1 on the silymarin treatment of CCl₄-induced hepatic fibrosis. *World J Gastrenterol*. 2005;11(8):1141–1148.
14. Scott M, Buriko K. Characterization of the pigmented cytoplasmic granules common in canine hepatocytes. *Vet Clin Pathol*. 2005;34 (suppl):281–282.

15. Valtolina C, Favier RP. Feline hepatic lipidosis. In: Lidbury JA, ed. *Hepatology, Vet Clin North Am Small Anim Pract*. Philadelphia: Elsevier; 2017:47(3): 683–702.

16. Newman SJ, Smith JR, Stenske KA, et al. Aflatoxicosis in nine dogs after exposure to contaminated commercial dog food. *J Vet Diagn Invest*. 2007;19(2):168–175.

17. Lowe AD, Campbell KL, Barger A, et al. Clinical, clinicopathological and histological changes observed in 14 cats treated with glucocorticoids. *Vet Rec*. 2008;162(24):777–783.

18. Cortright CC, Center SA, Randolph JF, et al. Clinical features of progressive vacuolar hepatopathy in Scottish Terriers with and without hepatocellular carcinoma: 114 cases (1980-2013). *J Am Vet Med Assoc*. 2014;245(7):797–808.

19. Sepesy LM, Center SA, Randolph JF, et al. Vacuolar hepatopathy in dogs: 336 cases (1993-2005). *J Am Vet Med Assoc*. 2006;229(2):246–252.

20. Cullen JM. Tumors of the liver and gallbladder. In: Meuten DJ, ed. *Tumors in Domestic Animals*. 5th ed. Ames: Wiley Blackwell; 2017:602–631.

21. Hirose N, Uchida K, Kanemoto H, et al. A retrospective histopathological survey on canine and feline liver diseases at the University of Tokyo between 2006 and 2012. *J Vet Med Sci*. 2014;76(7):1015–1020.

22. Harrison JL, Turek BJ, Brown DC, et al. Cholangitis and cholangiohepatitis in dogs: a descriptive study of 54 cases based on histopathologic diagnosis (2004-2014). *J Vet Intern Med*. 2018;32(1):172–180.

23. Boland L, Beatty J. Feline cholangitis. In: Lidbury JA, editor. *Hepatology, Vet Clin North Am Small Anim Pract*. Philadelphia: Elsevier, 2017:47(3):703–724.

24. Gagne JM, Weiss DJ, Armstrong PJ. Histopathologic evaluation of feline inflammatory liver disease. *Vet Pathol*. 1996;33(5):521–526.

25. Van den Ingh TSGAM, Cullen JM, Twedt DC, et al. Morphological classification of biliary disorders of the canine and feline liver. In: Rothuizen J, Bunch SE, Charles JA, et al., eds. *WSAVA Standards for Clinical and Histological Diagnosis of Canine and Feline Liver Disease*. Philadelphia: Saunders Elsevier; 2006:103–116.

26. Callahan Clark JE, Haddad JL, Brown DC, et al. Feline cholangitis: a necropsy study of 44 cats (1986-2008). *J Feline Med Surg*. 2011;13(8): 570–576.

27. Peters LM, Glanemann B, Garden OA, et al. Cytological findings of 140 bile samples from dogs and cats and associated clinical pathological data. *J Vet Intern Med*. 2016;30(1):123–131.

28. Wagner KA, Hartmann FA, Trepanier LA. Bacterial culture results from liver, gallbladder, or bile in 248 dogs and cats evaluated for hepatobiliary disease: 1998-2003. *J Vet Intern Med*. 2007;21(3):417–424.

29. Weiss DJ, Gagne JM, Armstrong PJ. Characterization of portal lymphocytic infiltrates in feline liver. *Vet Clin Pathol*. 1995;24(3):91–95.

30. Warren A, Center S, McDonough S, et al. Histopathologic features, immunophenotyping, clonality, and eubacterial fluorescence in situ hybridization in cats with lymphocytic cholangitis/cholangiohepatitis. *Vet Pathol*. 2011;48(3):627–641.

31. Thawley V. Acute liver injury and failure. In: Lidbury JA, ed. *Hepatology, Vet Clin North Am Small Anim Pract*. Philadelphia: Elsevier; 2017:47(3):617–630.

32. Watson P. Canine breed-specific hepatopathies. In: Lidbury JA, ed. *Hepatology, Vet Clin North Am Small Anim Pract*. Philadelphia: Elsevier, 2017; 47(3): 665-682.

33. Dirksen K, Fieten H. Canine copper-associated hepatitis. In: Lidbury JA, ed. Hepatology, *Vet Clin North Am Small Anim Pract*. Philadelphia: Elsevier, 2017; 47(3): 631-644.

34. Whittemore JC, Newkirk KM, Reel DM, et al. Hepatic copper and iron accumulation and histologic findings in 104 feline liver biopsies. *J Vet Diagn Invest*. 2012;24(2):656–661.

35. Hurwitz BM, Center SA, Randolph JF, et al. Presumed primary and secondary hepatic copper accumulation in cats. *J Am Vet Med Assoc*. 2014;244(1):68–77.

36. Flatland B, Moore RR, Wolf CM, et al. Liver aspirate from a Shar Pei dog. *Vet Clin Pathol*. 2007;36(1):105–108.

37. Shiga A, Shirota K, Shida T, et al. Hepatoblastoma in a dog. *J Vet Med Sci*. 1997;59(12):1167–1170.

38. Ano N, Ozaki K, Nomura, et al. Hepatoblastoma in a cat. *Vet Pathol*. 2011;48(5):1020–1023.

39. Patnaik AK. A morphologic and immunocytochemical study of hepatic neoplasms in cats. *Vet Pathol*. 1992;29:405–412.

40. Trigo FJ, Thompson H, Breeze RG, et al. The pathology of liver tumors in the dog. *J Comp Path*. 1982;92:21–39.

41. Patnaik AK, Hurvitz AI, Lieberman PH, et al. Canine hepatocellular carcinoma. *Vet Pathol*. 1981;18:427–438.

42. Lawrence HJ, Erb HN, Harvey HJ. Nonlymphomatous hepatobiliary masses in cats: 41 cases (1972 to 1991). *Vet Surg*. 1994;23:365–368.

43. Van Sprundel RGHM, Van den Ingh TSGAM, Guscetti F. Classification of primary hepatic tumors in the dog. *Vet J*. 2013;197:596–606.

44. Goussev SA, Center SA, Randolph JF, et al. Clinical characteristics of hepatocellular carcinoma in 19 cats from a single institution (1980-2013). *J Am Anim Hosp Assoc*. 2016;52(1):36–41.

45. Liptak JM, Dernell WS, Monnet E, et al. Massive hepatocellular carcinoma in dogs: 48 cases (1992-2002). *J Am Vet Med Assoc*. 2004;225(8):1225–1230.

46. Masserdotti C, Drigo M. Retrospective study of cytologic features of well-differentiated hepatocellular carcinomas in dogs. *Vet Clin Pathol*. 2012;41(3):382–390.

47. Post GP, Patkaik AK. Nonhematopoietic hepatic neoplasms in cats: 21 cases (1983-1988). *J Am Vet Med Assoc*. 1992;201(7):1080–1082.

48. Selmic LE. Hepatobiliary neoplasia. In: Lidbury JA, ed. *Hepatology, Vet Clin North Am Small Anim Pract*. Philadelphia: Elsevier, 2017;47(3):725–736.

49. Stalker MJ, Hayes MA. In: Grant Maxie M, ed. *Liver and Biliary System, Jubb, Kennedy and Palmer's Pathology of Domestic Animals*. 5th ed. Edinburgh: Elsevier; 2007:297–388.

50. Valli VE, Bienzle D, Meuton DJ. Tumors of the hemolymphatic system. In: Meuten DJ, editor. *Tumors in Domestic Animals*. 5th ed. Ames, IA: Wiley Blackwell; 2017:203–321.

51. Keller SM, Vernau W, Hodges J, et al. Hepatosplenic and hepatocytotropic T-cell lymphoma: two distinct types of T-cell lymphoma in dogs. *Vet Pathol*. 2012;50(2):281–290.

52. Carter JE, Tarigo JL, Vernau W, et al. Erythrophagocytic low-grade extranodal T-cell lymphoma in a cat. *Vet Clin Pathol*. 2008;37(4):416–421.

53. Suzuki M, Kanae Y, Kagawa Y, et al. all. Emperipolesis-like invasion of neoplastic lymphocytes into hepatocytes in feline T-cell lymphoma. *J Comp Path*. 2011;44:312–316.

54. Affolter VK, Moore PF. Localized and disseminated histiocytic sarcoma of dendritic cell origin in dogs. *Vet Pathol*. 2002;39:74–83.

55. Moore PF. A review of histiocytic diseases of dogs and cats. *Vet Pathol*. 2014;51:167–184.

56. Moore PF, Affolter VK, Vernau W. Canine hemophagocytic histiocytic sarcoma: a proliferative disorder of CD11+ macrophages. *Vet Pathol*. 2006;43(5):636–645.

57. Takahashi T, Kadosawa T, Nagase M, et al. Visceral mast cell tumors in dogs:10 cases (1982-1997). *J Am Vet Med Assoc*. 2000;216(2):222–226.

58. Mellor PJ, Haugland S, Murphy S, et al. Myeloma-related disorders in cats commonly present as extramedullary neoplasms in contrast to myeloma in human patients: 24 cases with clinical follow up. *J Vet Intern Med*. 2006;20(1):1376–1383.

59. Mellor PJ, Haugland S, Smith KC, et al. Histopathologic, immunocytochemical, and cytologic analysis of feline myeloma-related disorders: further evidence for primary extramedullary development in the cat. *Vet Pathol*. 2008;45:159–173.

21

The Spleen

Janice Cruz Cardona, Jocelyn D. Johnsrude, Patricia M. McManus, and Peter S. MacWilliams

The spleen is a large organ with various functions ranging from immune reactions to storage of platelets and mature red blood cells (RBCs) to filtering of senescent erythrocytes and other cells. It is generally composed of three parts: the splenic capsule and connective tissue trabeculae,[1] white pulp, and red pulp. The high number of elastic fibers and smooth musculature allow for storage of blood. Contraction can lead to release of stored blood into circulation. Species with a high storage spleen have an increased number of these tissues to allow for greater release into circulation. The red pulp acts as a filter of foreign material and senescent or damaged erythrocytes. It also plays a role in iron metabolism. The white pulp is composed of macrophages, antigen presenting cells, and B and T lymphocytes. It functions to initiate immune responses to bloodborne antigens.[2]

Depending on the cause, splenomegaly may be accompanied by hematological abnormalities such as anemia, thrombocytopenia, neutropenia, and leukemia. Concurrent evaluation of a complete blood count (CBC) and careful examination of morphologies of RBCs, white blood cells (WBCs), and platelets in a peripheral blood film may aid in the diagnosis of causative factors. Causes of splenomegaly in dogs and cats include hyperplasia, extramedullary hematopoiesis, neoplasia (hemolymphatic, primary, or metastatic), and circulatory disturbances (Table 21.1).[2-8] Careful palpation and radiographic imaging should reveal the severity of splenomegaly and whether enlargement is diffuse or localized. Ultrasonography provides a more detailed assessment of architectural abnormalities. By visualizing small nodules, target lesions, or changes in echogenicity in the spleen, ultrasonography can detect suspect areas of neoplasia, hyperplasia, inflammation, or extramedullary hematopoiesis and enables precise localization for fine-needle aspiration (FNA) or fine-needle biopsy (FNB).[9-11]

Indications for sampling of spleen include diffuse or symmetrical enlargement, abnormal architecture or echogenicity, nodular or focal lesions, for diagnosis of neoplasia or tumor staging.[6] Hypercalcemia or a monoclonal gammopathy are other indications for cytological assessment. These are summarized in Box 21.1, but invasive collection of splenic tissue is not always required if the underlying cause is revealed by other means.[12,13] For example, splenomegaly is likely linked to immune-mediated disease if a patient tests positive for erythrocytic antiglobulins (Coombs test), antinuclear antibodies, or rheumatoid factor. Serological tests may suggest fungal or protozoal infections. Detection of hemoparasites, such as *Mycoplasma*, *Cytauxzoon*, or *Babesia* spp., in a peripheral blood film also supports an infectious cause for splenomegaly. Reevaluation of the patient for splenomegaly after resolution of an underlying infectious or immune mediated process negates the need for cytology of the spleen. Cytological examination of bone marrow or peripheral lymph nodes may also be diagnostic for hematopoietic and lymphocytic neoplasia or systemic infections.

When splenomegaly is accompanied by peritoneal effusion, collection and cytological evaluation of abdominal fluid are indicated before direct sampling of the spleen.

SAMPLING METHODS

Needle collections of splenic tissue are indicated when the cause of splenomegaly cannot be determined by other means. Specimens for cytological assessment of the spleen may be collected by using needle and syringe or by using material collected at the time of a surgical biopsy or at necropsy.

Needle Methods

Collection of splenic samples by needle puncture should be carefully considered. An enlarged spleen may be turgid, friable, and engorged with blood. Profuse intraabdominal hemorrhage and tumor metastasis within the abdominal cavity are possible complications; however, several studies in dogs and humans concluded that thrombocytopenia, number of needle passes during collection, repeat collections, and core biopsies were not associated with an increase in the number or severity of complications.[14-16]

FNA of splenic specimens can usually be done without general anesthesia. The size and location of the spleen within the abdominal cavity determine the actual site for penetration, which should be at the site where the spleen is most easily apposed to the abdominal wall. The site is prepared as if for surgery by clipping, washing, and applying an antiseptic. If the collection is aided by ultrasonography, care must be taken to not contaminate the skin, the slides, and the needles with lubricant because this material stains a rich purple to magenta on slides and will interfere with microscopic evaluation (Fig. 21.1). Infiltration of the abdominal wall with local anesthetic is usually unnecessary. A 22-gauge needle may be either directly attached to a 12-mL (milliliter) syringe for aspiration (FNA) or attached via an intravenous extension set for the nonaspiration method (FNB), which may reduce hemodilution of the sample, yield more highly cellular tissue fragments, and produce superior preparations.[17,18] Needle length is determined by the size of the animal, but usually a 1- or 1{1/2}-inch needle is adequate.

The spleen is gently pressed against the abdominal wall at the prepared site. The needle is inserted through the skin and muscle layer into the spleen. For the FNA method, the syringe plunger produces negative pressure, while the needle is moved within the spleen along several axes. Maintaining suction while redirecting the needle in the parenchyma collects cells and tissue fragments from several areas. To minimize hemorrhage and dilution of the sample, negative pressure on the plunger should be released immediately if bloody fluid appears in the syringe tip. It is very important to release the syringe plunger before the needle is withdrawn from the spleen. Immediately after

TABLE 21.1 Causes and Characteristics of Splenomegaly in Dogs and Cats With Supportive Findings

Cause	Type of Enlargement	Possible Concurrent Findings	Supportive Diagnostic Tests
Hyperplasia	Symmetrical or nodular		
Infection		Hyperglobulinemia Inflammatory leukogram, presence of infectious agent	CBC, serum biochemistry panel, culture, serology, PCR
Immunological disease		Hyper-/hypoglobulinemia, current drug therapy	Coomb test, ANA titers, rheumatoid factor; immunoglobulin quantification
Extramedullary Hematopoiesis	Symmetrical or nodular	Anemia, other cytopenias, or inflammation seen on leukogram	CBC
Hemolymphatic Neoplasia	Symmetrical		
Lymphoma or lymphocytic leukemia		Leukocytosis/lymphocytosis, atypical cells or blasts in circulation	CBC, bone marrow FNA and core biopsy, lymph node cytology/histology
Myeloid neoplasms		Circulating blasts, increased NCC +/− dysplastic changes +/− cytopenias (of nonneoplastic lineages)	CBC, bone marrow FNA and core biopsies
Systemic mastocytosis		Circulating mast cells, eosinophilia, basophilia (rare)	CBC, diagnostic imaging or microscopic evaluation of other affected tissue
Plasma cell tumor or multiple myeloma		Hyperglobulinemia, monoclonal gammopathy, paraproteinuria	serum globulins, serum/urine protein electrophoresis; immunofixation
Other Neoplasia	Symmetrical or nodular		
Hemangioma or hemangiosarcoma	Nodular	Regenerative anemia; schistocytes, acanthocytes, thrombocytopenia (hemangiosarcoma); may be subclinical in hemangioma	CBC
Fibrosarcoma or undifferentiated sarcoma	Nodular	Nonspecific	Variable
Histiocytic sarcoma	Nodular	Other lesions	Variable
Hemophagocytic histiocytic sarcoma	Symmetrical	anemia +/− other cytopenias	CBC
Leiomyoma or leiomyosarcoma	Nodular	May be primary or secondary; look for intestinal mass +/− anemia (chronic blood loss anemia)	CBC
Metastatic neoplasms	Asymmetrical or nodular	Variable	Variable
Other	Symmetrical or nodular		
Systemic histiocytosis		Nonspecific	Variable
Hemophagocytic syndrome		Anemia, other cytopenias	CBC
Fibrohistiocytic nodules		Nonspecific	Variable
Hypereosinophilic syndrome		Eosinophilia	CBC +/− bone marrow aspirate and core
Inflammation		Inflammatory leukogram, hyperglobulinemia	CBC
Circulatory Disturbances			
Hematoma	Asymmetrical/ Symmetrical	Regenerative anemia, hemoabdomen, if ruptured	CBC
Portal hypertension with splenic congestion	Symmetrical	Abnormal liver values	Serum biochemistry
Torsion	Symmetrical	Inflammation seen on leukogram	CBC

ANA, antinuclear antibody; *CBC,* complete blood count (includes blood smear review); *FNA,* fine-needle aspiration; *PCR,* polymerase chain reaction.

Adapted from Spangler WL, Culbertson MR: Prevalence and type of splenic diseases in cats: 455 cases (1985–1991). *J Am Vet Med Assoc.* 1992;201:773–776.

withdrawing the needle from the animal, small drops of the aspirate are applied to glass slides and prepared as described below.

For the FNB method, the needle is attached to an intravenous extension set, which is attached to the syringe.[17] The syringe is filled with air

before penetration of the skin and does not need to be handled during the actual collection of specimen, unlike with the FNA method. After the spleen is penetrated, the needle tip is rapidly moved in and out 8 to 10 times without changing its path and without allowing the tip of the needle to leave the spleen. This will dislodge a small sample that will be retained within the bore of the needle. The needle is then withdrawn, and the specimen contained within the needle is immediately expelled onto a glass slide by using the air-filled syringe. Preparation of the smear is described below. This method usually results in only a single slide per penetration; therefore, three to five collections are suggested, each time targeting different areas of the spleen or splenic nodule.

The consistency of the specimen determines the method of smear preparation. Most specimens collected by the aspiration method have the consistency of blood, and slides are prepared in the same manner as blood films. Specimens that are thick or contain tissue fragments, for example, specimens collected by FNB, are prepared by using the squash technique, with the material gently compressed between two slides. Too much material on the slide can result in slides that are too thick to evaluate (Fig. 21.2). Chapter 1 contains a detailed description of slide preparation techniques.

Impression, Scraping, and Squash Preparations

Impression, scraping, and squash preparations of splenic tissue may be made from biopsy samples taken during surgical exploration and often complement histological assessment. In some situations, an immediate diagnosis may be obtained. For example, a homogeneous population of large lymphoblasts (Fig. 21.3) or a pure population of mast cells (Fig. 21.4) confirms a diagnosis of lymphoma and mast cell neoplasia, respectively. Cytological preparations of splenic tissue reveal nuclear and cytoplasmic details not visible in tissue sections. The different tinctorial characteristics of hematological stains allow for more accurate identification of erythroid precursors versus lymphocytes, basophils versus histiocytes, and mast cells versus other round cells. Although tissue architecture is lost in collection, recognition of individual cell types, fungi, protozoa, RBC parasites, and neoplastic cells is sometimes easier on Wright-stained slides. Cytological preparations are particularly valuable in identifying subtle dysplastic morphologies. However, changes attributable to circulatory disturbances as causes of splenomegaly, for example, congestion, hemorrhage, torsion, or infarction, are better assessed by histological evaluation.

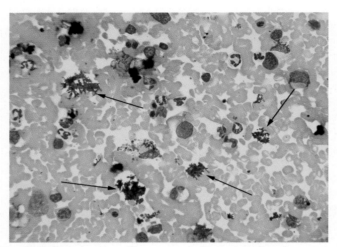

Fig. 21.1 Canine spleen. The arrows indicate deposits of magenta-stained material, typical for aqueous lubricant used for ultrasound-guided fine-needle methods. Heavy contamination can prevent evaluation of a slide (Wright-Giemsa, original magnification 50× oil objective).

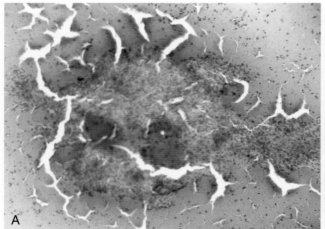

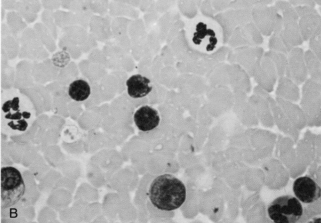

Fig. 21.2 Canine spleen. (A) This preparation is very thick and cracked because of slow drying of the thick areas. The splenic tissue fragment cannot be evaluated, and most of the dispersed nucleated cells are difficult to identify. In this type of preparation, it is difficult to distinguish small lymphocytes from larger, potentially neoplastic cells. However, detection of these fragments confirms successful aspiration of spleen (Wright-Giemsa, original magnification 10× objective). (B) In some cases, the smear cannot be evaluated at all, but, as this image demonstrates, patient examination of thinner areas between fragments will be rewarded by finding cells spread thin enough to identify and evaluate (Wright-Giemsa, original magnification 100× oil).

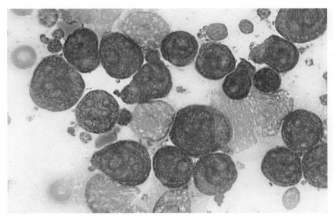

Fig. 21.3 Canine spleen. Impression smear prepared from a splenic biopsy specimen from a dog with lymphoma contains a homogeneous population of large lymphocytes characterized by multiple prominent nucleoli (Wright stain, original magnification 100× oil objective).

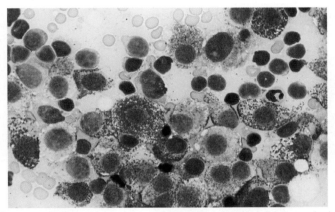

Fig. 21.4 Feline spleen. Impression smear prepared from a splenic biopsy specimen from a cat with systemic mastocytosis and marked symmetrical splenomegaly. The spleen is diffusely infiltrated with neoplastic mast cells that have round nuclei and numerous intracytoplasmic purple granules. Numerous small lymphocytes, plus a single neutrophil in the upper right corner, are also present (Wright stain, original magnification 100× oil objective).

Preliminary to making impression and scraping smears from whole-tissue specimens, the tissue should be blotted on a paper towel to remove excess blood and fluid. If feasible, the tissue is trimmed with a scalpel blade to expose a fresh-cut surface. Then, tissue imprints are made on the slides or the surface scraped with the scalpel blade and the scrapings spread on the slide. Also, making squash preparations from tissue fragments should be considered. Using a variety of techniques increases the likelihood of getting smears that contain adequate specimen with good preservation of cell morphology. Further details are provided in Chapter 1.

Staining

Wright-Giemsa stain or a similar Romanowsky stain is the ideal stain for splenic cytology because it provides excellent definition of cytoplasmic features, facilitates identification of cytoplasmic granulation, and allows for evaluation of hematopoietic cells. If using "quick" or "rapid" modified Wright stains, fixation and staining times will need to be increased for preparations that are thicker than blood films. Cytoplasmic granulation (e.g., granular lymphocytes, mast cells, myeloid precursors) may not be preserved with quick

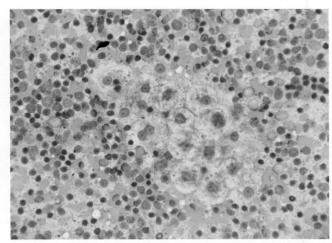

Fig. 21.5 Canine spleen. Occasionally, hepatic tissue may be inadvertently included in an aspirate and should not be mistaken for metastatic carcinoma (Wright stain, original magnification 50× objective).

stains, although longer fixation times may ameliorate that problem to some extent. Chapter 1 contains specific information on staining techniques.

MICROSCOPIC EXAMINATION

Low-power objectives (4× and 10×) are used to assess cellularity and stain quality, locate cellular clusters and tissue fragments, and select slides and microscopic fields for further examination under higher magnification. Occasionally, miscellaneous structures that have no clinical significance, for example, fragments of mechanically exfoliated mesothelial tissue or hepatic tissue that was inadvertently included will be found (Fig. 21.5). The 40× (or 50× oil to allow examination without a coverslip), and 100× oil objectives are used to assess the general composition of the cell population and study the nuclear and cytoplasmic details of individual cells. At these magnifications, it is helpful to find a small lymphocyte or segmented neutrophil for size and color comparisons (Fig. 21.6; also see Fig. 21.2). Small lymphocytes are smaller than segmented neutrophils and have round, slightly indented, or narrowly cleaved nuclei; dark condensed chromatin; no visible nucleoli; and scant light-blue cytoplasm.

Table 21.1 lists five general causes of splenic enlargement, but more than one mechanism may be responsible in any given animal. Examples of supportive findings and potential diagnostic tests are included. For example, a dog with immune-mediated hemolytic anemia may have splenomegaly caused by both lymphoid hyperplasia and extramedullary hematopoiesis. Animals with infections, such as *Histoplasma*, *Cytauxzoon*, and *Babesia* spp. infections (Figs. 21.7 and 21.8), may have splenomegaly from both lymphoid hyperplasia and granulomatous inflammation. Figure 21.9 presents an algorithm for classification of splenic cytological findings.

Normal Cytological Features

Smears of normal splenic tissue can have microscopic features similar to those of normal lymph nodes. Often, aspirates are of low cellularity, containing mostly blood and splenic stromal cells, especially if there are no hyperplastic responses or neoplastic lesions. Aspirates may contain a heterogeneous population of cells, including lymphoid, hematopoietic, macrophages and stromal elements.[2,3,13]

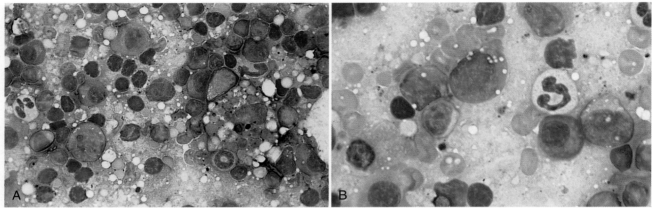

Fig. 21.6 Canine spleen. Fine-needle aspirate of hyperplastic splenic tissue from a dog with immune-mediated hemolytic anemia. (A) Small lymphocytes predominate, but increased numbers of large lymphocytes *(lower left)* and plasma cells *(upper left)* indicate hyperplasia. A large macrophage *(lower right)* contains many phagocytized erythrocytes (Wright stain, original magnification 48× objective). (B) Higher magnification reveals two lymphoblasts *(left)* adjacent to a small lymphocyte. A neutrophil, a plasma cell, and a lymphoblast are located to the right of center. The plasma cell is recognized by its round, eccentric nucleus; smooth blue cytoplasm; and prominent Golgi zone. Compare the sizes of the neutrophil, plasma cell, lymphoblast, and lymphocyte (Wright stain, original magnification 100× oil objective).

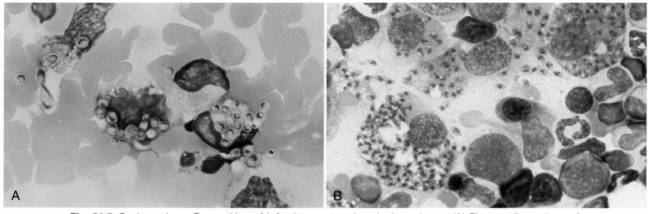

Fig. 21.7 Canine spleen. Recognition of infectious agents in splenic aspirates. (A) Fine-needle aspirate of spleen from a dog infected with the fungus *Histoplasma capsulatum*. Macrophages contain phagocytized *Histoplasma* organisms; one organism in the upper left appears to be budding (Wright stain, original magnification 100× oil objective). (B) Impression smear of spleen from a dog infected with the protozoan parasite of the genus *Leishmania*, most likely of the *L. donovani* complex, the cause of visceral leishmaniasis. Numerous *Leishmania* amastigotes are present in macrophages and in the background. The image also contains several plasma cells, neutrophils, and immature granulocytes (Wright stain, original magnification 100× oil objective).

Lymphoid cells are a mixture of small lymphocytes, few to moderate numbers of larger lymphocytes, and occasional plasma cells. Hematopoietic cells may include both erythroid and myeloid precursors. Macrophages and few mast cells may also accompany them.[2,12] A representative sample contains variably sized fragments of splenic tissue, which consist of reticular fibers, stroma cells (also called *myofibroblasts* and *fibrohistiocytes*), endothelial cells, macrophages, and plasma cells (Fig. 21.10). Small lymphocytes predominate in most fields; however, because the spleen contains numerous lymphoid follicles with germinal centers, large lymphocytes may predominate in other areas (Fig. 21.11). The larger lymphocytes may display loosely clumped to vesicular chromatin, and nucleoli may be visible, similar to neoplastic lymphocytes. Because of the possibility of lymphoid hyperplasia with expansion of intermediate- to large-size lymphocytes, context is needed to rule out a neoplastic proliferation. Finding areas of the smears that contain a heterogeneous

collection of lymphocytes and plasma cells precludes definitive designation of immature-appearing cells as neoplastic (Fig. 21.12). Macrophages may contain small to moderate amounts of intracytoplasmic pigment, consistent with hemosiderin (iron), particularly in dogs.

Nonneoplastic Lesions
Hyperplasia and Inflammation
Splenomegaly secondary to lymphocytic hyperplasia results from a variety of inflammatory diseases, both septic and nonseptic. Mild to moderate degrees of splenomegaly are found in immune-mediated disorders and in systemic infectious diseases caused by bacteria, rickettsiae, protozoa, and fungi. Cytological findings in hyperplastic splenomegaly depend on the causative agent, the mechanism of disease, and the host's immune response. In general, splenic hyperplasia is characterized by increased numbers of macrophages, plasma

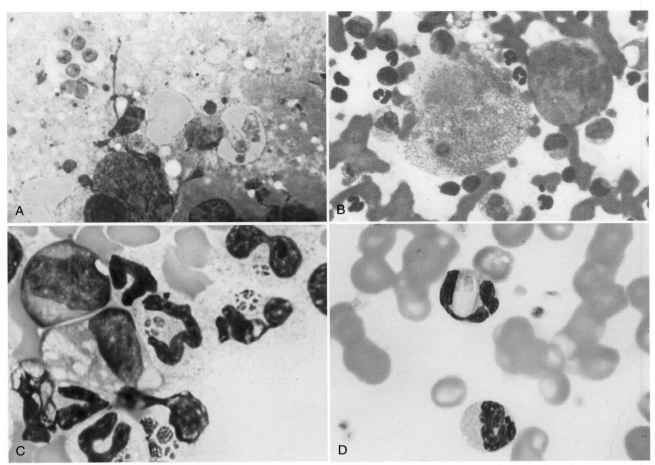

Fig. 21.8 Hemotropic parasites that are seen in peripheral blood erythrocytes or leukocytes that also may be seen in splenic aspirates include *Babesia canis* (A), *Cytauxzoon* (B), *Anaplasma phagocytophilum* (C), and *Hepatozoan* spp. (D). A, Canine spleen. Impression smear of the spleen from a dog infected with the protozoa *B. canis*; organisms are present in an erythrocyte and in the background (Wright stain, original magnification 100× oil objective). (B) Feline spleen. The two huge mononuclear cells with abundant cytoplasm, eccentric nuclei, and prominent nucleoli are macrophages that contain many developing *Cytauxzoon* merozoites. The organisms appear as small, dark-staining bodies in one cell and as larger, irregularly defined clusters in the other (Wright stain, original magnification 100× oil objective). (C) Canine spleen. Morulae of the bacterial pathogen *A. phagocytophilum* are present in the cytoplasm of several neutrophils (Wright stain, original magnification 100× oil objective). (D) Canine spleen. A protozoal *Hepatozoon* organism is present in the cytoplasm of a neutrophil. Infected leukocytes may be seen in peripheral blood and may become entrapped in splenic sinusoids. Fine-needle aspirates of spleen are often diluted with peripheral blood. Red blood cells and platelets are present, indicating that some hemodilution has occurred (Wright stain, original magnification 100× oil objective).

cells, and larger lymphocytes (see Fig. 21.6). A relative decrease in numbers of small lymphocytes occurs; however, these cells remain the predominant cell type. A slight to occasional increase in neutrophil numbers may be seen, but marked predominance of neutrophils is uncommon and suggests splenitis, necrosis, abscessation, or inflammation secondary to a neoplastic cell infiltrate. Presence of degenerate neutrophils would also support an inflammatory focus. As in other cytological preparations, interpretation of inflammation is dependent on the degree of blood contamination and peripheral cell counts. For example, a severe peripheral neutrophilia could potentially lead to misinterpretation as splenitis, when the inflammation causing the neutrophilia may be elsewhere.

A marked increase in eosinophils may correlate with enteric parasites, severe allergies, some neoplasms, or idiopathic eosinophilic infiltrative disease. With some infections and immune responses, increases in macrophages and plasma cells are pronounced. Flame cells, plasma cells with a pink cytoplasmic appearance, and Mott cells, which are plasma cells with cytoplasmic inclusions of immunoglobulin, may be part of the plasma cell population. When macrophages are increased, it is important to examine their cytoplasm for cellular debris, pigment, phagocytized erythrocytes (see Fig. 21.6), bacteria, and organisms, such as *Histoplasma* (see Fig. 21.7, A) and *Leishmania* spp. (see Fig. 21.7, B). Erythrocytes in background blood can be examined for *Babesia* (see Fig. 21.8, A), *Cytauxzoon*, *Mycoplasma haemofelis*, or morphological changes to erythrocytes, such as Heinz bodies and eccentrocytes[12]; however, peripheral blood smears are preferable for evaluation of red blood cell morphology. Although neoplasia is a common cause

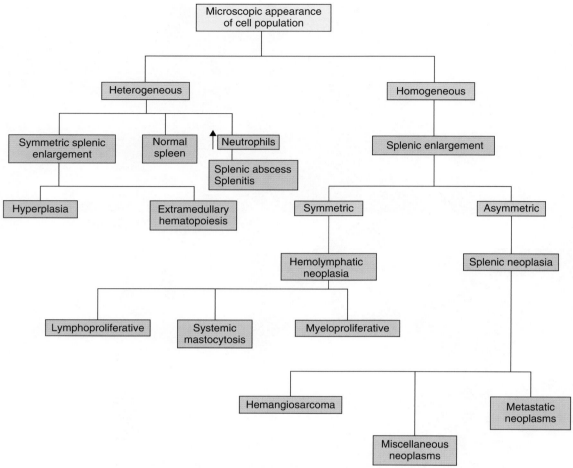

Fig. 21.9 Cytological classification of fine-needle aspirates and impression smears from the spleens of dogs and cats.

of concurrent splenomegaly and peripheral lymphadenopathy, one must always consider hyperplasia as a differential and pursue additional diagnostics, as needed, to achieve a definitive diagnosis. Antigenic stimulation from inflammation and even drug therapy may be an underlying cause.[19] Cytological evaluation may help distinguish the cause of splenomegaly in these two clinically similar processes.

Leukocytes should be scrutinized for inclusions, such as morulae of *Anaplasma phagocytophilum* (see Fig. 21.8, C) and *Hepatozoon* organisms (see Fig. 21.8, D) or other infectious agents. Mast cells can also increase in a stimulated spleen; therefore few to moderate numbers are not sufficient to diagnose neoplastic systemic mastocytosis or mast cell tumor metastasis (Figs. 21.13 and 21.14). A marked increase in hemosiderin deposits within macrophages is often best assessed by examination of tissue fragments (see Fig. 21.13). The change may be incidental, as quantity will increase with age, but increases may also correlate with chronic congestion (e.g., with chronic liver or heart disease), hemorrhage, or hemolysis. Gamna-Gandy bodies, which are deposits composed of calcium and iron, have been documented in the spleen of a cat with neoplasia as a result of intratumoral hemorrhage and formation of iron–calcium complexes.[20] Care must be taken to not confuse these with fungal hyphae (Fig. 21.15 A–D).

Extramedullary Hematopoiesis

Extramedullary hematopoiesis (EMH) is the development of sites of hematopoiesis outside of bone marrow. Hematopoietic cells include precursors of erythroid, myeloid, and platelet (megakaryocytes) origin. They are often detected at a low frequency in splenic tissue from healthy cats and dogs, but disorders that markedly increase their numbers are numerous and diverse. Responses of the hematopoietic cells are similar to those of bone marrow, with increases reflective of the current demand. For example, with inflammatory disease, there may be an increase in granulopoietic cells, whereas with immune-mediated hemolytic anemia or hemorrhage, erythroid precursors may predominate among the hematopoietic precursors seen. Rare to occasional megakaryocytes are often found in the spleen of healthy animals but may be increased with thrombocytopenia. Most commonly, clinically significant EMH is found secondary to inflammatory disease, immune-mediated hemolytic anemia and/or thrombocytopenia, and hemorrhage. A combination of the three lineages may be seen with representation of both mature cells and precursors found in orderly maturation. Less common causes of splenic EMH include recovery from chemotherapy or cytotoxins, bone marrow disorders, and association with certain tumors (e.g., disseminated histiocytic sarcoma, hemangiosarcoma, myelolipoma). Splenomegaly and/or hypoechoic splenic foci are common progressing to blue-gray to "polychromatophilic" with maturation as ribosomes decrease and hemoglobin increases. The less mature forms often display a small clear zone adjacent to the nucleus (see Fig. 21.18). EMH involving the myeloid series will show precursors, including progranulocytes, myelocytes, metamyelocytes, bands, and segmented cells, in an orderly progression of maturation.

Neoplasia
Round Cell Neoplasms
Round cell tumors seen in spleen may be derived from myeloid (granulocytes, monocytes, erythroid, megakaryocytic), lymphoid (including plasma cells; Fig. 21.19), mast cells (see Fig. 21.4), cells of uncertain lineage (Fig. 21.20), or primitive, undifferentiated cells (Fig. 21.21). A monotonous population of the involved cell type usually replaces normal lymphocytes and hematopoietic cells, although inflammatory cell infiltrates may be seen. Some of these neoplasms are described in more detail in Chapter 27.

The cells obtained from normal spleen are heterogeneous in terms of morphology and lineage, whereas with a lymphocytic or myeloid neoplasm, the slides contain a more homogeneous population of neoplastic cells. For cytological diagnosis of lymphoma or myeloid neoplasms, replacement of parenchyma with these cells is nearly complete, leaving few normal lymphocytes, plasma cells, and macrophages.

In most dogs and cats with high-grade lymphoma and acute lymphocytic leukemia, normal cells are replaced by a homogeneous population of large to very large lymphocytes characterized by dark blue cytoplasm, round or indented nuclei, and multiple distinct nucleoli (see Fig. 21.3). If only small fields are examined and the smears are thick, lymphoid hyperplasia may be mistaken for lymphoma (see Fig. 21.11). Disrupted cells, yielding free nuclei, can be misinterpreted as blasts because of enhancement of nuclear detail upon cellular lysis. Chronic lymphocytic leukemia and small cell lymphoma (indolent lymphoma) are more difficult to identify cytologically because the neoplastic cells are small and are difficult to differentiate from nonneoplastic lymphocytes. Because the cells are not overtly neoplastic, surgical biopsy with histopathology is the preferred method of diagnosis. Other diagnostic methods, such as, immunocytochemistry (see Chapter 29), flow cytometric immunophenotyping (see Chapter 30), or polymerase chain reaction for antigen receptor rearrangement (PARR) (see Chapter 31), may help support a diagnosis of neoplasia over atypical hyperplasia. Other clues that the cells are neoplastic may include a lack heterogeneity of the sample, lack of a plasmacytic component, extreme cellularity of the specimen, detection of consistently atypical granules in the cytoplasm (as in lymphoma of granular lymphocytes), and clinical history—for example, the finding of severe splenomegaly, peripheral blood lymphocytosis (persistent, moderate to marked), or hypercalcemia. As previously mentioned, concurrent evaluation of a peripheral blood smear is advised to detect possible lymphocytosis, blast cells, or a marked leukocytosis.

Splenic impression smears from cats with erythroid leukemia have a cellular profile similar to their marrow; that is, numerous large round cells with round nuclei, fine granular chromatin, single nucleoli, and dark-blue cytoplasm are present. In some cells, the cytoplasm contains a small, localized clear zone (Fig. 21.22). The relatively few late-stage erythroid precursors often display nuclear-to-cytoplasmic asynchronous maturation.

Mesenchymal Neoplasms
Primary malignant mesenchymal neoplasms of the spleen include disseminated histiocytic sarcoma, hemophagocytic histiocytic sarcoma, hemangiosarcoma, leiomyosarcoma, fibrosarcoma, and undifferentiated sarcoma.

Hemangiosarcoma may be recognized on impression smears and aspirates, but slides made from scrapings of fresh-cut surfaces of

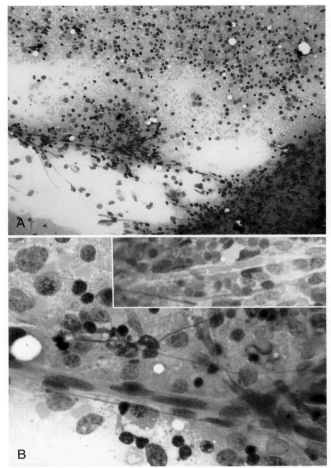

Fig. 21.10 Canine spleen. (A) Note the capillary fragment emerging from the thick splenic tissue fragment. A smaller fragment of splenic tissue is still adherent to it. The large fragment is too thick to evaluate, but the thinner areas between fragments contain nicely spread cells, amenable to evaluation (Wright-Giemsa, original magnification 20× objective). (B) This is a higher magnification of that same blood vessel. Note the small, narrow oval nuclei. Cytoplasm of endothelial cells is often almost invisible, as it stains a very light gray (Wright-Giemsa, original magnification 100× objective). *Inset,* Note the capillary that still has erythrocytes within it (Wright-Giemsa, original magnification 100× objective).

manifestations in animals with extramedullary hematopoiesis, which may be encountered as the primary change or in combination with lymphocytic hyperplasia and neoplasia.

Erythrophagocytosis (Fig. 21.6) is increased with immune-mediated hemolytic anemia and intralesional hemorrhage; the peripheral blood smear is desired for identification of spherocytes. In hemolytic anemia caused by immunological disease or infectious agents, the cytological appearance is dominated by erythroid precursors, which sometimes exfoliate as clusters around central macrophages (see Fig. 21.16). These clusters are referred to as erythroblastic islets. The central macrophages are considered intrinsic to the regulation of erythropoiesis, and they also phagocytize nuclei from maturing cells. Macrophages containing hemosiderin and phagocytized RBCs are typically found (Fig. 21.17). Late-stage erythroid precursors are numerous and recognized easily, but the more immature erythroid cells could be confused with lymphocytes (Fig. 21.18). Features of immature RBCs that differentiate them from lymphocytes include an evenly round nucleus with irregularly clumped chromatin imparting a "wheel spoke" or "checkerboard" appearance (see Fig. 21.18). The cytoplasm is dark-blue in coloration,

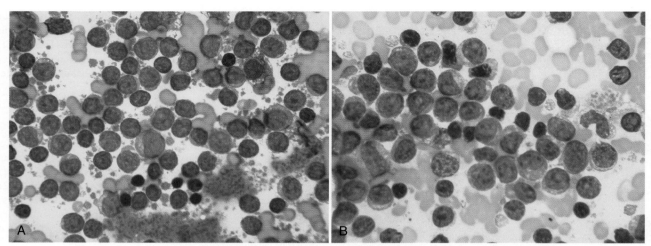

Fig. 21.11 (A) Feline spleen. Ultrasonographic evaluation of this 14-year-old cat showed liver and spleen enlargement and diffusely thickened intestines. Lymphoma was diagnosed based on detection of a diffuse and homogeneous infiltrate of these moderately large lymphocytes within the splenic fine-needle biopsy specimen. No evidence of a plasmacytosis in any area of the aspirates was present, and very few small lymphocytes were seen (Wright-Giemsa, original magnification 100× objective). (B) Canine spleen. This is an area of a splenic aspirate from a dog with lymphocytic hyperplasia. It also contains a homogeneous collection of moderately large lymphocytes; however, a broader evaluation of several areas of the spleen revealed a heterogeneous population of smaller lymphocytes, plasma cells, and extramedullary hematopoiesis (see Fig. 21.12) (Wright-Giemsa, original magnification 100× objective).

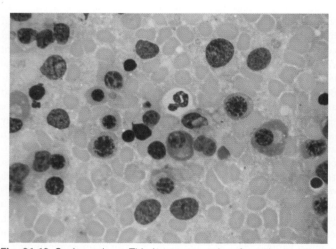

Fig. 21.12 Canine spleen. This image was taken from the same aspirate as seen in Fig. 21.11, B. Detection of significant numbers of plasma cells precludes designating the cells seen in Fig. 21.11B as neoplastic. This image also contains numerous mid- to late-stage erythroid precursors (Wright-Giemsa, original magnification 100× objective).

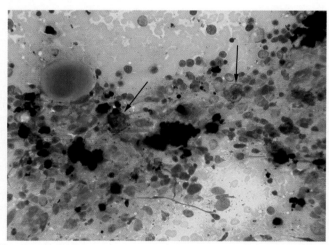

Fig. 21.13 Canine spleen. This 13-year-old Labrador Retriever has splenic lymphocytic hyperplasia. The fragment of splenic tissue demonstrates increased hemosiderin deposits that may be seen not only in older animals but also in animals with hemolytic anemia, hemorrhage, and chronic congestion. Note that this dog also had a high frequency of mast cells *(arrows)* throughout its spleen, but frequency was not diagnostic for systemic mastocytosis or mast cell tumor metastasis. Note the megakaryocyte in the upper left. The area is too thick to clearly see its nucleus (Wright-Giemsa, original magnification 50× objective).

tissue are often superior. The microscopic appearance of hemangiosarcoma in a cytological preparation (Fig. 21.23) may be typical of other high-grade sarcomas, but in histological sections the cells characteristically line blood-filled sinuses (see Fig. 21.23). In cytology, cells may exfoliate individually or in loose aggregates. Tumor cells are highly pleomorphic, with marked anisokaryosis and marked anisocytosis. Giant forms are not unusual. Some cells are fusiform, with indistinct borders, and others are irregularly shaped, with angular margins. Nuclei are round to oval, with variable chromatin patterns and many large, pleomorphic nucleoli. Cytoplasm is light blue and variably abundant (see Fig. 21.23). Erythroid precursors are often present, indicating extramedullary hematopoiesis. Because of associated hemorrhage, macrophages may contain abundant hemosiderin and numerous phagocytized erythrocytes.

Histiocytic sarcomas can be diagnosed by using FNA and FNB because the cells usually exfoliate readily, unlike hemangiosarcoma, and the cells may be embedded within highly cellular splenic tissue rather than being associated with cavernous areas of hemorrhage. Splenic disseminated histiocytic sarcoma may contain many neoplastic cells and few lymphoid and hematopoietic elements (Fig. 21.24), but this may also be reversed; that is, the neoplastic cells may be noted at a low frequency within highly cellular aspirates containing lymphocytes, plasma cells, nonneoplastic macrophages, neutrophils, and hematopoietic cells. When giant sized, they may be as large as or

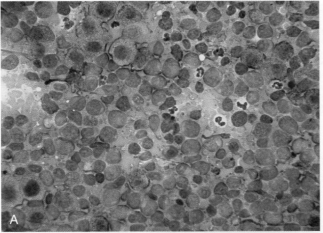

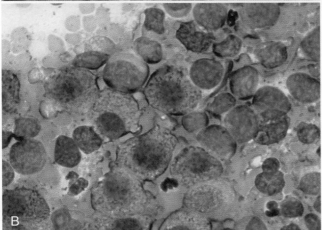

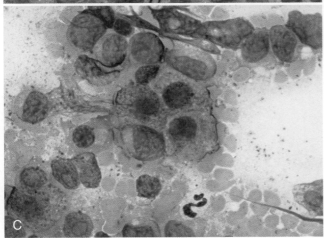

Fig. 21.14 Canine spleen. This 11-year-old mixed-breed dog had a confusing smear that included both large immature round cells and approximately equivalent numbers of mast cells. No morphological progression connected the two cell types. The neoplastic round cells are most likely of lymphocytic lineage, although immunophenotyping is needed for confirmation. The mastocytosis may indicate concurrent mast cell neoplasia or the mastocytosis may be a reactive infiltrate secondary to lymphoma (considered more likely). The opinion was that whether or not the mast cells were neoplastic, they were likely of lesser importance in terms of long-term prognosis for this dog compared with high-grade lymphoma (*all images,* Wright-Giemsa stained. A, Original magnification 50× objective; B and C, original magnification 100× objective).

larger than megakaryocytes (Fig. 21.25). They are rarely diagnosed in cats (Figs. 21.26 and 21.27) and more widely reported in dogs.[21] Histiocytosis involving the spleen may be part of a complex of histiocytic disorders, including feline progressive histiocytosis, which is a disease of cats, or systemic histiocytosis (see Chapter 4). Although cytology supports the diagnosis, immunophenotyping and histopathology may be required to distinguish between these diseases when the cells lack features of malignancy.

Fibrosarcoma and leiomyosarcoma occur less frequently compared with hemangiosarcoma and histiocytic sarcoma and have the cytological appearance of low- to intermediate-grade spindle cell tumors. The diagnostic criteria discussed in Chapter 2 may be used to identify these tumors. Fibrosarcoma is discussed in more detail in Chapter 5. Rarely, primary extraskeletal chondrosarcomas and osteosarcomas can occur in the spleen.[22,23] Metastatic splenic infiltrates of the spleen are seen with some frequency in cytology, and they may arise from various organs and tissues. Well-differentiated neoplasms can be more fully characterized cytologically, but anaplastic or poorly differentiated cells may pose a challenge. Unless a primary mass has been documented and diagnosed, specific identification of the neoplastic cell type may require additional tests, such as immunostaining or histopathology.

Myelolipomas are benign nodular lesions that are observed incidentally in the spleen in dogs and occasionally in cats. Their cytological appearance is characterized by marked EMH with small groups of normal adipocytes. The key difference between myelolipomas and EMH is the presence of embedded fat tissue in the former.

CONCLUSIONS

Cytological evaluation of splenic tissue may be key to achieving an accurate, clinically relevant diagnosis, but success hinges on the experience of the pathologist, the skill of the person collecting the specimen, and the quality of the slides.

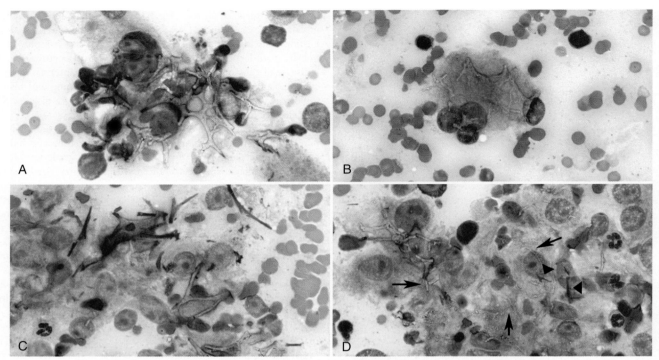

Fig. 21.15 Gamma-Gandy bodies, cat spleen. Gamma-Gandy bodies are calcium–iron complexes that may form with intralesional chronic hemorrhage along collagenous fibers. Note the angular branching, septal-like divisions of these crystalline linear structures that may display uniform thickness, resembling fungal hyphae. (Image courtesy Ryseff JK, Duncan C. Sfiligoi G et al. Gamna-Gandy bodies: a case of mistaken identity in the spleen of a cat. *Vet Clin Pathol*, 43:94–100.)

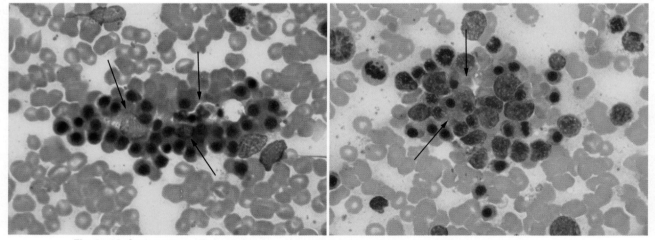

Fig. 21.16 Canine spleen. These images were from the spleen of an 8-year-old Rottweiler with hemophago-cytic histiocytic sarcoma (also see Fig. 21.24). This dog has marked erythropoiesis. These images demonstrate the small islands of maturing erythroid precursors (erythroblastic islets) that are seen adherent to central macrophages *(arrows)* (Wright-Giemsa, original magnification 100× objective).

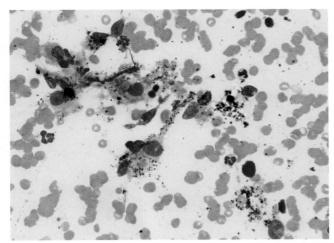

Fig. 21.17 Canine spleen. This was an 8-year-old Cain Terrier with severe nonregenerative anemia and ineffective erythroid hyperplasia in the marrow. Destruction of red blood cells and their precursors was thought to be immune mediated. The spleen contained many macrophages that demonstrated phagocytosis of erythrocytes, their precursors, and apoptotic nuclear debris. Similar cells were seen in bone marrow (Wright-Giemsa, original magnification 50× objective).

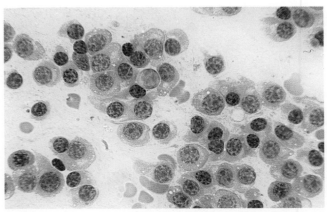

Fig. 21.19 Canine spleen. Impression smear of splenic tissue from a dog with multiple myeloma. The spleen is effaced by a homogeneous population of neoplastic plasma cells (Wright stain, original magnification 48× objective).

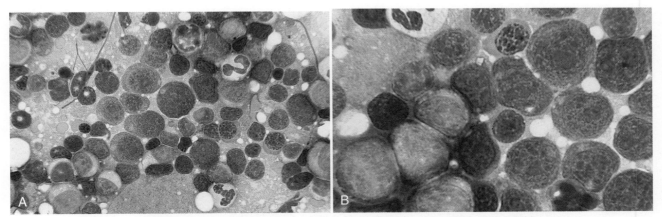

Fig. 21.18 Feline spleen, with extramedullary hematopoiesis. (A) Most of the cells are erythroid precursors at various stages of development, with a few neutrophils and several lymphocytes (lower right). The large round cells in the center are early to intermediate stage erythroid precursors (Wright stain, original magnification 48× objective). (B) Large lymphocytes are in the lower left, whereas erythroid precursors are on the right. These may be difficult to distinguish. Immunophenotypic analysis that demonstrates a lack of lymphocytic markers may be needed when the lineage of a round cell population is uncertain. Immature erythroid precursors at the rubriblast and prorubricyte stages have round nuclei, dark basophilic cytoplasm, coarse granular or loosely clumped chromatin, and, when visible, singular nucleoli. The metarubricyte at the top of the field has an immature nucleus but well-differentiated cytoplasm (nucleus–cytoplasm asynchrony) (Wright stain, original magnification 100× objective).

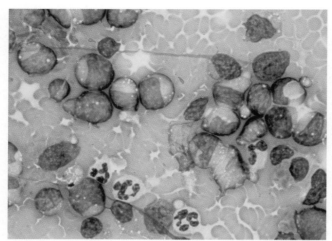

Fig. 21.20 Canine spleen. Round cell tumor of uncertain lineage. This dog had hepatosplenomegaly and 10,900 per microliter (μL) unclassifiable cells in peripheral blood. The spleen contains many large, vacuolated cells of uncertain lineage; one cell in the upper left contains a phagocytized erythrocyte. Note the irregular shape of the nuclei and size relative to neutrophils and small lymphocytes. The chief differentials are high-grade lymphoma and acute monocytic leukemia (Wright-Giemsa, original magnification 100×).

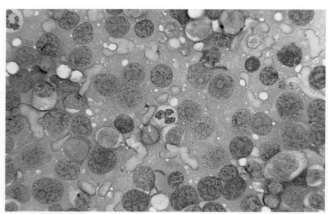

Fig. 21.21 Feline spleen. Impression smear of splenic tissue from a cat with an undifferentiated round cell neoplasm. A neutrophil and several small lymphocytes in the center are surrounded by primitive cells with indistinct cell margins, round nuclei, vesicular chromatin, and singular prominent nucleoli (Wright stain, original magnification 48× objective).

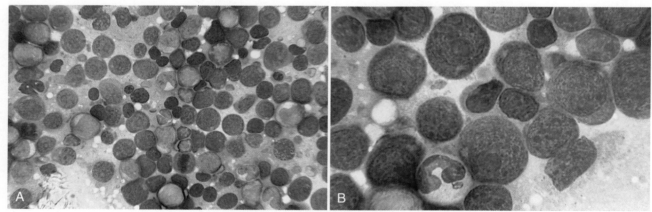

Fig. 21.22 Feline spleen. Impression smear of splenic tissue from a cat with erythroid leukemia. (A) Many large round cells have replaced the normal cell population. No differentiation toward more mature forms in the erythroid series is evident (Wright stain, original magnification 48× objective). (B) The neoplastic cells are similar to very early erythroid precursors. Morphological features include a round nucleus, coarse granular chromatin, a single large nucleolus, and a small clear zone within dark blue cytoplasm (Wright stain, original magnification 100× oil objective).

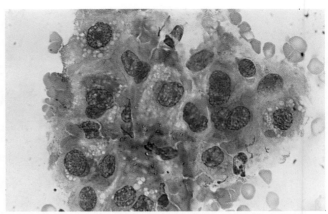

Fig. 21.24 Canine spleen. Fine-needle aspirate of spleen from a dog with histiocytic sarcoma. Lymphoid cells normally present in the spleen have been replaced by pleomorphic cells characterized by marked anisocytosis, indistinct cell margins, cytoplasmic vacuolation, marked anisokaryosis, and irregular chromatin clumping (Wright stain, original magnification 100× oil objective).

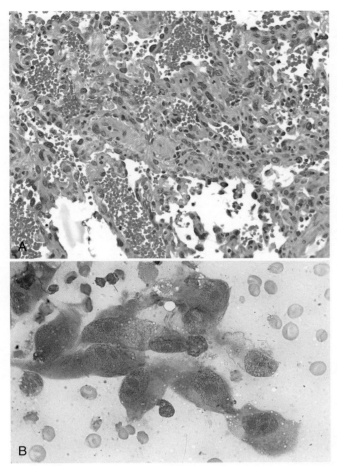

Fig. 21.23 Canine spleen. (A) Surgical biopsy of hemangiosarcoma in the spleen of a dog. Note the large blood-filled sinuses lined by neoplastic cells (hematoxylin and eosin [H&E], original magnification 20× objective). (B) Impression smear of splenic tissue from a dog with hemangiosarcoma. The neoplastic cells have features of a mesenchymal malignancy, such as marked anisocytosis, indistinct cell margins, marked anisokaryosis, and variable nucleolar size, shape, and number (Wright stain, original magnification 100× oil objective). (A, Contributed by Dr. Michael Goldschmidt, University of Pennsylvania, School of Veterinary Medicine, Department of Pathobiology, Philadelphia, PA.)

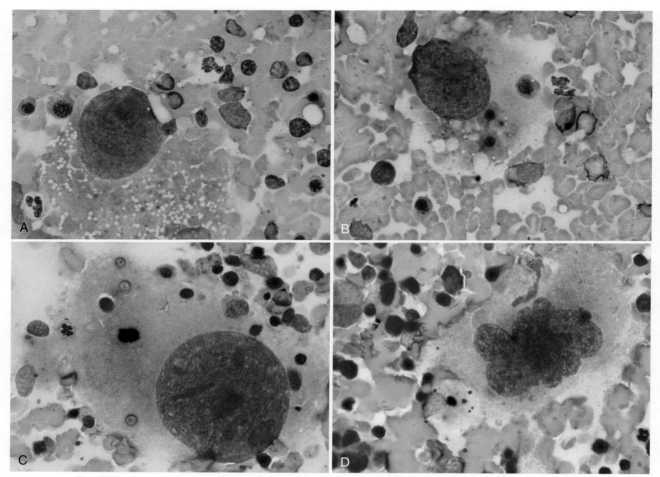

Fig. 21.25 Canine spleen. Hemophagocytic histiocytic sarcoma. This was an 8-year-old female spayed Rottweiler with lethargy, decreased appetite, pale mucous membranes, splenomegaly, severe regenerative anemia (packed cell volume [PCV] 18%), and leukopenia. The splenic aspirate indicated marked extramedullary hematopoiesis (predominantly erythroid precursors) and lymphocytic hyperplasia. A low frequency of giant hemophagocytic cells, characterized by giant round nuclei, macronucleoli, and fine granular to lacey chromatin, was seen. (A) This neoplastic macrophage (phagocytic histiocyte) displays a macronucleolus and phagocytosis of erythrocytes (Wright-Giemsa stain, original magnification 100× oil objective). (B) The neoplastic cell has phagocytized both erythrocytes and late-stage erythrocytic precursors. The nucleolus is giant sized and misshapen. Compare the size of the cell and its nucleus to the neutrophil next to it (Wright-Giemsa stain. 100× oil objective). (C) The neoplastic cell displays multiple misshapen nucleoli and a particle of hemosiderin in its cytoplasm (Wright-Giemsa stain, original magnification 100× oil objective). (D) Compare the neoplastic cells in images (A), (B), and (C) to this normal megakaryocyte found in the same aspirate and to a more typical macrophage to the left of the megakaryocyte. The megakaryocyte has a lobulated nucleus, moderately coarse chromatin, indistinct small nucleoli, and finely granular light purple stained cytoplasm. It is possible to occasionally detect cells within the cytoplasm of megakaryocytes (emperipolesis), but only a few should be present, and they are usually mature neutrophils rather than erythrocytes (Wright-Giemsa stain, original magnification 100× oil objective).

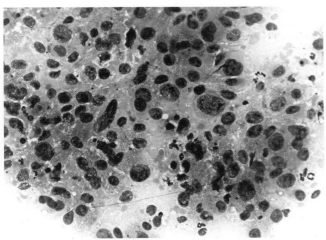

Fig. 21.26 Cat spleen. Histiocytic sarcoma in spleen of a cat with a nodular appearance on ultrasonography. There is marked atypia and evidence of phagocytosis along with scant extramedullary hematopoiesis (EMH), Diff-Quik stain, original magnification 50× oil. (Image courtesy Dr. Jess-Sebastien Latouche, IDEXX Laboratories, USA.)

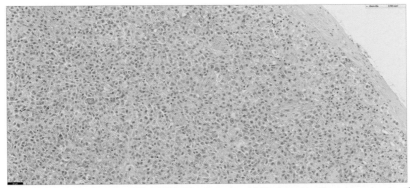

Fig. 21.27 Cat spleen. Same case as Fig 21.26. The splenic architecture is effaced by sheets of neoplastic cells with similar features as those observed on cytology (hematoxylin and eosin [H&E] stain). (Image courtesy Dr. Catherine Lamm, IDEXX Laboratories, USA.)

REFERENCES

1. Valli VE, Kiupel M, Bienzle D. Hematopoietic system. In: Maxie MG, ed. *Pathology of Domestic Animals*. 6th ed. St. Louis: Elsevier; 2016:158–196.
2. Cesta MF. Normal structure, function, and histology of the spleen. *Toxicol Pathol*. 2006;34:455–465.
3. Valli VE. *Veterinary Comparative Hematopathology*. Ames, IA: Blackwell Publishing; 2007:47–77.
4. Spangler WL, Culbertson MR. Prevalence type and importance of splenic diseases in dogs: 1,480 cases (1985-1989). *J Am Vet Med Assoc*. 1992;200:829–834.
5. Spangler WL, Culbertson MR. Prevalence and type of splenic diseases in cats: 455 cases (1985-1991). *J Am Vet Med Assoc*. 1992;201:773–776.
6. Spangler WL, Kass PH. Pathologic and prognostic characteristics of splenomegaly in dogs due to fibrohistiocytic nodules: 98 cases. *Vet Pathol*. 1998;35:488–498.
7. Spangler WL, Kass PH. Splenic myeloid metaplasia, histiocytosis, and hypersplenism in the dog (65 cases). *Vet Pathol*. 1999;36:583–593.
8. Sykes JE, et al. Idiopathic hypereosinophilic syndrome in 3 Rottweilers. *J Vet Int Med*. 2001;15:162–166.
9. Hanson JA, Papageorges M, Girard E, et al. Ultrasonographic appearance of splenic disease in 101 cats. *Vet Radiol Ultrasound*. 2001;42:441–445.
10. Ballegeer EA, Forrest LJ, Dickinson RM, et al. Correlation of ultrasonographic appearance of lesions and cytologic and histologic diagnoses in splenic aspirates from dogs and cats: 32 cases (2002-2005). *J Am Vet Med Assoc*. 2007;230:690–696.
11. Crabtree AC, et al. Diagnostic accuracy of gray-scale ultrasonography for the detection of hepatic and splenic lymphoma in dogs. *Vet Radiol Ultrasound*. 2010;51:661–664.
12. O'Keefe DA, Couto CG. Fine-needle aspiration of the spleen as an aid in the diagnosis of splenomegaly. *J Vet Int Med*. 1987;1:102–109.
13. Christopher MM. Cytology of the spleen. *Vet Clin North Am Small Anim Pract*. 2003;33:135–152.
14. Lal A, et al. Splenic fine needle aspiration and core biopsy: a review of 49 cases. *Acta Cytol*. 2003;47:951–959.
15. Watson AT, Penninck D, Knoll JS, et al. Safety and correlation of test results of combined ultrasound-guided fine-needle aspiration and needle core biopsy of the canine spleen. *Vet Radiol Ultrasound*. 2011;52:317–322.
16. McInnes MD, Kielar AZ, Macdonald DB. Percutaneous image-guided biopsy of the spleen: systematic review and meta-analysis of the complication rate and diagnostic accuracy. *Radiology*. 2011;260:699–708.
17. Papageorges M, et al. Ultrasound-guided fine-needle aspiration: an inexpensive modification of the technique. *Vet Radiol*. 1988;29:269–271.
18. Leblanc CJ, Head LL, Fry MM. Comparison of aspiration and nonaspiration techniques for obtaining cytologic samples from the canine and feline spleen. *Vet Clin Pathol*. 2009;38:242–246.
19. Lampe R, Manens J, Sharp N. Suspected phenobarbital-induced pseudolymphoma in a dog. *J Vet Intern Med*. 2017;31:1858–1859.
20. Ryseff JK, Duncan C. Sfiligoi G et al. Gamna-Gandy bodies: a case of mistaken identity in the spleen of a cat. *Vet Clin Pathol*. 43:94–100.
21. Friedrichs KR, Young K. Histiocytic sarcoma of macrophage origin in a cat: case report with a literature review of feline histiocytoic malignancies and comparison with canine hemophagocytic histiocytic sarcoma. *Vet Clin Pathol*. 2008;37:121–127.
22. Kawabata A, Husnik R, Le Donne V. Pathology in practice. *J Am Vet Med Assoc*. 2017;250:1113–1116.
23. Carr AH, Brumitt J, Sellon RK. What is your diagnosis? *J Am Vet Med Assoc*. 2010;236:513–514.

The Kidneys

Patty J. Ewing, James H. Meinkoth, Rick L. Cowell, and Ronald D. Tyler

Cytological evaluation (e.g., fine-needle aspiration [FNA]) of the kidney, in correlation with history, clinical data, and imaging findings, is a useful tool in diagnosing certain renal lesions, especially neoplasms, in dogs and cats. The advantages and disadvantages of FNA (cytology) compared with incisional biopsy (histopathology) of the kidney are presented in Table 22.1. Although the examination of cytological specimens does not provide the cellular architecture necessary to characterize many lesions in which structural relationships are important, it may provide sufficient diagnostic information to aid in the clinical management of cases and is less invasive and associated with fewer complications compared with full-tissue biopsy. Major complications resulting from FNA of the kidney are relatively uncommon if appropriate procedures are followed.[1]

Disease conditions that are most likely and least likely to yield diagnostic cytological results are presented in Boxes 22.1 and 22.2. Renal cytology is especially useful for rapid confirmation of neoplasia but is not helpful for diagnosis of chronic kidney disease. Ultrasonography (US) is a valuable tool for approximating the likelihood of acquiring a diagnostic renal FNA sample and for selecting optimal sites of collection. Ultrasonographic findings most likely and least likely to yield diagnostic samples in dogs and cats are shown in Boxes 22.3 and 22.4. Kidneys with infiltrative or nodular appearance and unclear corticomedullary interface are most likely to yield diagnostic cytological results.[2] Although positive cytological findings are useful in establishing

a diagnosis, differential diagnoses cannot always be excluded on the basis of negative findings because representative material may not have been recovered during collection attempts. The diagnostic yield of renal FNA cytology is reported as 68% for cats and 72% for dogs, which is comparable with other soft tissue FNA samples, including aspirates of cutaneous/subcutaneous masses and lymph nodes.[2,3]

Percutaneous FNA of the kidney without image-guiding was performed in cats with diffuse renomegaly in the past because their kidneys are easily palpated and can be immobilized against the body wall,

TABLE 22.1 Advantages and Disadvantages of Renal Cytology Compared With Incisional Biopsy

Advantages	Disadvantages
Less invasive, fewer complications	Does not allow for assessment of tissue architecture
Less expensive	Does not allow for evaluation of glomeruli
Rapid diagnosis of some conditions, such as feline lymphoma	Blood contamination and low cell yield may limit usefulness

BOX 22.1 Disease Conditions Most Likely to Yield Diagnostic Renal Aspirates

- Neoplasms
- Abscesses
- Fungal granulomas
- Renal tubular hyperplasia

BOX 22.2 Disease Conditions Least Likely to Yield Diagnostic Renal Aspirates

- Chronic kidney disease or end-stage kidney disease (small or shrunken fibrotic kidneys)
- Renal tubular degeneration
- Interstitial nephritis
- Glomerulonephritis

BOX 22.3 Ultrasonographic Findings Most Likely to Yield Diagnostic Renal Aspirates

Cats
- Subcapsular infiltrate
- Diffuse renal enlargement (any echogenicity) without pelvic dilation
- Normal or enlarged kidneys with infiltrative/nodular appearance
- Hypoechoic kidney (less echogenic than liver)
- Unclear corticomedullary interface

Dogs
- Infiltrative nodular appearance
- Pelvic dilation
- Unclear corticomedullary interface

BOX 22.4 Ultrasonographic Findings Least Likely to Yield Diagnostic Renal Aspirates

Cats
- Presence of a mass
- Pelvic dilation

Dogs
- Iso- or hyperechoic medulla, compared with cortex
- Hyperechoic kidney (iso- or hyperechoic to spleen), normal or enlarged
- Bilateral isoechoic/mixed echogenicity mass

BOX 22.5 Contraindications for Renal Aspiration Cytology

- Marked thrombocytopenia (platelet count <50,000/μL)
- Platelet function disorder (increased buccal mucosal bleeding time)
- Coagulopathy, acquired (including patients receiving anticoagulation medications) or hereditary (one-stage prothrombin time or activated partial thromboplastin time prolonged >20%)
- Patients at high risk for anesthesia or sedation complications
- Obstructive uropathy (severe hydronephrosis or septic pyonephrosis) if risk for abdominal cavity contamination is high
- Mass lesions that are suspected to be septic abscesses at risk for rupturing and highly vascularized masses at risk for hemorrhage

but this modality is no longer recommended given the widespread availability of US. Using US or computed tomography (CT) to detect optimal sites to collect specimens, avoid highly vascular lesions, and obtain additional information about the nature and extent of lesions increases safety and diagnostic yield. US-guided percutaneous renal FNA, the current modality of choice, readily identifies cortical tissue, large renal vessels, and focal lesions; guides correct needle placement; and allows for monitoring for postaspiration hemorrhage. Because of the highly vascular nature of the kidneys, blood contamination is a significant problem during sample collection. Use of a nonaspiration (i.e., capillary action) technique (see Chapter 1) facilitates the collection of cellular specimens that are not heavily contaminated with blood. Highly cellular, solid lesions (e.g., neoplasms) are also more likely to yield cellular samples compared with many degenerative or inflammatory diseases.

SAMPLING TECHNIQUE

FNA is associated with less tissue trauma compared with core needle biopsies, and there are only a few contraindications for collecting cytological specimens from the kidneys. Contraindications for renal FNA are listed in Box 22.5. As with other renal biopsy procedures, the main complication is excessive hemorrhage.[1,4] The risk for hemorrhage is increased in masses that are highly vascularized. Patients should be evaluated for the presence of hemostatic derangements, severe anemia, and hypertension before the procedure. The concurrent use of US and CT for sample collection is preferred, and tranquilization, sedation, or anesthesia (required for CT) is used, as necessary, to adequately restrain the patient, thus preventing unexpected movement during the procedure.

Seeding of the needle tract with neoplastic cells during fine-needle sampling of malignant lesions has been suggested as a complication; however, clinical experience and results of retrospective studies in humans show such seeding to be uncommon.[5,6]

After complete bilateral renal US, the patient's skin and the transducer are prepped aseptically. The patient may be restrained in dorsal or lateral recumbency. A 22-gauge 1.5-inch needle attached to a 10- to 12-milliliter (mL) syringe that has been prefilled with air is held at the base of the needle with the thumb and forefinger. Real-time guidance of the needle through the path of least tissue resistance is executed, followed by rapid forward and reverse thrusts of the needle through the region of interest, ideally without negative pressure (nonaspiration technique) and avoiding the arcuate blood vessels near the corticomedullary junction.[3,7] Depending on the type of lesion, the needle is directed either into the lesion (focal lesions) or tangentially into the cortex of the kidney (diffuse lesions). Care should be taken to avoid the renal hilus, which contains large vascular structures. The needle is

passed through approximately two-thirds the thickness of the lesion about five to seven times with a stabbing motion. Samples may be collected from different portions of the lesion in multiple (two or three) collection attempts or by redirecting the needle. Collection of several slides (at least five) from different areas of the lesion helps increase the chances of obtaining a diagnostic specimen. Whenever blood is visible in the hub of the needle or syringe, collection should be stopped and the material spread onto a glass slide, because continued collection attempts usually result in gross blood contamination, rendering the sample worthless. Color Doppler US may be used to assess for hemorrhage after the aspiration procedure.

After collection, the material in the needle (none is usually visible in the syringe) should be carefully dispersed on one end of a glass slide and gently spread out using a slide-over-slide technique (see Chapter 1). If fluid is obtained, direct and line smears should be made and the remainder of the fluid put into an ethylenetetraacetic acid (EDTA) tube. Fluid or exudate collected for culture should be placed in a red-top tube or sterile plastic tube. If the fluid is clear (suggesting low cellularity) and sufficient sample has been obtained, concentrated sediment smears, which are similar to urine sediments, are prepared and air-dried.

Impression smears may be made from renal biopsy specimens or kidneys removed at surgery or necropsy before the specimen is fixed in formalin for histological analysis. Before the impression smears are made, excess blood should be gently blotted from the tissue to increase the number of cells that transfer to the glass slides. Whenever sufficient tissue has been obtained for histological analysis, the specimen should be submitted in case the cytological preparations are nondiagnostic. Samples for histological and cytological examinations must be mailed in separate packages because formalin fumes (even from sealed containers) will partially fix the cells on unstained smears, making evaluation impossible.

CYTOLOGICAL EVALUATION

Normal and Abnormal Cell Types Encountered

The normal histological anatomies of the canine and feline renal cortices are shown in Fig. 22.1. The renal parenchyma consists of glomeruli, tubules, interstitium, and blood vessels. Renal tubules make up the bulk of the parenchyma. Findings in normal renal aspirates are listed in Table 22.2. Renal tubular epithelial cells are the predominant cell type seen in fine-needle aspirates from normal kidneys. They are rather large, round-to-polygonal cells that occur singly and in clusters (Fig. 22.2, A). They have a round, eccentrically placed nucleus and moderately abundant pale basophilic cytoplasm, which, in cats, often contains several distinct, clear vacuoles from the presence of lipid droplets (see Fig. 22.2, B). Clear cytoplasmic vacuoles may also be present in dogs with diabetes mellitus, long-term exposure to corticosteroids, or lysosomal storage disease (Box 22.6). Cells of the distal convoluted tubules and ascending limb of the loop of Henle may contain dark intracytoplasmic granules (see Fig. 22.2, C).[6]

Differentiation of the various epithelial cell types is not practical or of diagnostic importance. The cells and their nuclei should be relatively uniform in size and shape; however, the different types of epithelial cells differ slightly in size. The nucleus-to-cytoplasm (N:C) ratio of normal tubular cells is low, except for feline lipid-laden proximal tubular epithelial cells, and tubular cells that are well spread out often have a single, visible nucleolus (see Fig. 22.2, A–C). When present, nucleoli should be small and round. Renal tubular hyperplasia, observed in feline infectious peritonitis (FIP) and chronic renal disease, features disorganized clusters of epithelial cells exhibiting mild to moderate anisocytosis, anisokaryosis, increased N:C ratios, binucleation, and

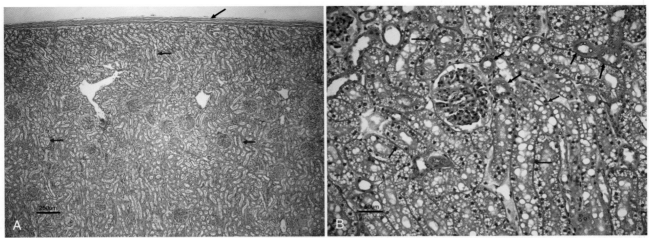

Fig. 22.1 (A) Histological section of normal canine kidney. Renal tubules comprise the majority of the normal renal parenchyma. Note absence of vacuoles in the proximal tubular epithelial cells *(blue arrows)* in contrast to the cat kidney shown in image (B). Glomeruli *(green arrows)* are prominent structures in the renal cortex and consist of a tuft of interconnected capillaries enclosed in the Bowman capsule. Orange arrows identify dilated intralobular veins. The black arrow identifies the thick fibrous capsule through which the needle penetrates during the fine-needle aspiration procedure (hematoxylin and eosin [H&E] stain). (B) Histological section of normal feline kidney. Note prominent lipid vacuolation of proximal tubular epithelial cells *(blue arrows)*. The lipid vacuolation is what accounts for the grossly pale tan–yellow appearance of a normal feline kidney. Note cuboidal cells without vacuoles that line the distal tubules *(black arrows)* and low cuboidal, nonvacuolated epithelial cells of the collecting duct *(orange arrows)*. The *green arrow* identifies a glomerulus (H&E stain). (A and B, Courtesy Dr. Pam Mouser.)

TABLE 22.2   Findings in Normal Renal Aspirates

Cell Types or Structures	Appearance	Comments
Renal tubular epithelial cells (see Fig. 22.2)	Medium to large, round-to-polygonal cells that occur singly and in clusters; slightly eccentric round nucleus with single visible nucleolus, pale basophilic cytoplasm, which may have clear vacuoles (especially in cats)	Predominant cell type seen
Intact renal tubules (see Figs. 22.3 and 22.4)	Densely packed cells, as described above, arranged in linear structures	Variably present
Glomeruli (see Fig. 22.5)	Lobulated dense clusters of slender, oval to spindle-shaped cells	Infrequently seen
Collagen matrix	Strands of homogeneous, acellular eosinophilic material	Absent or present in only small amounts; collagen obtained from renal capsule or interstitium
Peripheral blood	Many erythrocytes with platelet aggregates and leukocytes (neutrophils, lymphocytes, and monocytes)	Marked blood contamination is common; subjective assessment of types and number of leukocytes present is only way to differentiate blood contamination versus inflammation

atypical vacuolar pattern (see Fig. 22.2, D).[2] Renal tubular hyperplasia can be difficult to differentiate from renal cell neoplasia in some cases. Renal tubular cells often remain together as recognizable tubule fragments of various sizes (Fig. 22.3). Tubular casts may also be seen in renal aspirates from some animals (Fig. 22.4). Their significance depends on the amount and type of cast present, similar to those in urine sediments. Glomeruli may be seen in cellular samples and appear as somewhat lobulated clusters of slender, spindloid cells (Fig. 22.5).[6,8] Individual cells are difficult to see because they are tightly clustered. Abnormalities of the glomeruli (e.g., glomerulonephritis) are not readily discernible cytologically and require histological analysis. A few homogeneous strands of acellular eosinophilic matrix (collagen) may be seen in normal renal aspirates. The matrix is typically obtained as the needle passes through the fibrous capsule of the kidney (see Fig. 22.1, A).

Some degree (often marked) of peripheral blood contamination is always present in renal aspirates. Various peripheral blood leukocytes (i.e., neutrophils, small mature lymphocytes, monocytes, and possibly eosinophils) and platelets, often in aggregates, will be present as a result of peripheral blood contamination. A subjective assessment of the number and type of leukocytes present, compared with the amount of peripheral blood on the slide, is the only way to assess whether the leukocytes most likely represent blood contamination or renal inflammation. Inflammation is suggested by a disproportionate number of leukocytes relative to red blood cells (RBCs) or the presence of cells not associated with peripheral blood (e.g., overt plasma cells, vacuolated or phagocytologically active macrophages). Plasma cells are lymphoid cells with eccentric nuclei, increased amounts of deeply basophilic cytoplasm (compared with small lymphocytes), and a perinuclear clear area (Fig. 22.6). Macrophages, which must be differentiated from

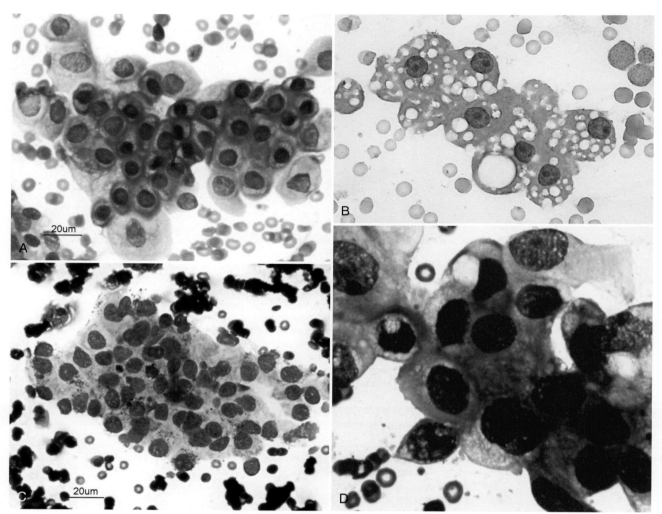

Fig. 22.2 (A) Renal fine-needle aspiration (FNA) sample from a dog. Numerous renal tubular cells showing mature, uniform nuclei with dark, mature chromatin (Wright-Giemsa stain). (B) Renal FNA sample from a cat. Note the cluster of renal tubular epithelial cells with some blood contamination; feline renal tubular cells are often vacuolated. Nucleoli are visible but are small and round (Wright stain, original magnification 330×). (C) Cluster of renal tubular cells from a renal FNA sample from a cat. The cells are mature and uniform and show cytoplasmic granules (Wright-Giemsa stain). (D) Cluster of renal tubular epithelial cells exhibiting hyperplasia from a renal FNA from a cat. Note disorganized clusters of epithelial cells exhibiting mild to moderate anisocytosis, anisokaryosis, increased nuclear-to-cytoplasmic (N:C) ratios, binucleation, and atypical vacuolar pattern (Diff-Quik stain, original magnification 1250×).

BOX 22.6 Causes of Clear Vacuoles in Renal Tubular Epithelial Cells

- Normal cat renal proximal tubular cells (lipid)
- Diabetes mellitus in dogs (lipid)
- Long-term exposure to corticosteroids in dogs (glycogen)
- Nephrotoxicity
- Lysosomal storage disorders—congenital or drug induced (lipid or glycogen)

peripheral blood monocytes, have more abundant cytoplasm that may have phagocytized cellular debris or many small vacuoles (see Figs. 22.18 and 22.25 later in the chapter). Macrophage nuclei are usually round, unlike irregular, pleomorphic monocyte nuclei. Additionally, finding neutrophils with degenerate changes (e.g., swelling of the nuclear lobes) and phagocytized bacteria (see Fig. 22.18 later in the chapter) is abnormal and indicates septic inflammation.

Small mature lymphocytes, which are approximately 10 micrometers (μm) in diameter (slightly smaller than neutrophils) and have only scant amounts of basophilic cytoplasm, are often present as the result of blood contamination. Their deep purple nuclei are round and slightly indented (see Fig. 22.6). The presence of reactive lymphocytes (Fig. 22.7) or prolymphocytes, which are slightly larger than small mature lymphocytes, suggests inflammatory infiltrates. Their nuclei are larger, stain a less dense color, and do not have prominent nucleoli. These cells also have moderately increased amounts of basophilic cytoplasm. Large atypical lymphoid cells are usually seen in cases of renal lymphoma. These cells are distinctly larger than inflammatory lymphocytes (equal to or larger than the diameter of a neutrophil) and have prominent nucleoli and less dense nuclear chromatin. Their cytoplasm is more abundant, is deeply basophilic, and often completely encircles the nucleus (Fig. 22.8).

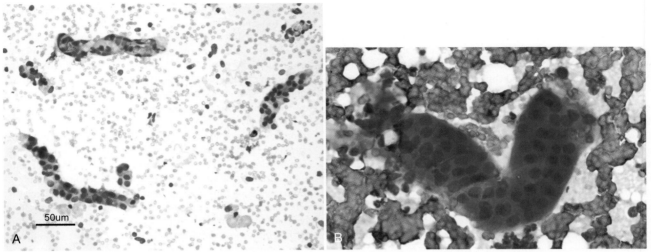

Fig. 22.3 (A) Small tubular fragments in a renal fine-needle aspiration (FNA) sample from a dog (Wright stain, original magnification 50×). (B) Higher magnification of tubular fragment in a renal FNA from a cat. Dark nuclei of individual tubular cells are visible, but cell margins are difficult to discern (Wright stain, original magnification 500×).

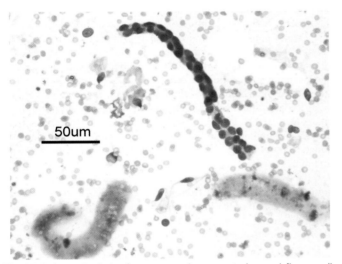

Fig. 22.4 A renal tubular fragment and two casts in renal fine-needle aspirate from a dog (Wright stain, original magnification 50×).

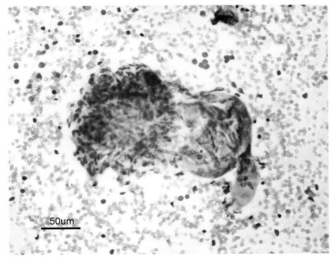

Fig. 22.5 A glomerulus present in renal fine-needle aspirate from a dog (Wright stain, original magnification 50×).

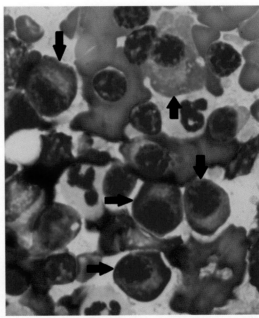

Fig. 22.6 Plasma cells *(arrows)* characterized by an eccentric round nucleus with abundant, deep-blue cytoplasm and a prominent, clear Golgi apparatus, and small lymphocytes and neutrophils (Diff-Quik stain, original magnification 1500×).

Cytological Characteristics of Solid Lesions

Cytological preparations from enlarged or abnormally shaped kidneys or discrete, solid kidney masses are evaluated for the presence of neoplasia or inflammatory responses (Fig. 22.9).

Neoplasia

Renal cytology is especially diagnostically useful for the rapid confirmation of lymphoma and carcinoma in cats, with sensitivity, specificity, positive predictive value, and negative predictive value all reported as 100%.[2] A similar high degree of sensitivity for detecting lymphoma (100%) and moderate sensitivity for all types of renal neoplasia (78%) has been shown in dogs.[3] Renal lymphoma is the most common neoplastic disease affecting feline kidneys and may occur as a single, discrete nodule but more often causes diffuse bilateral renomegaly, enlarged infiltrative/nodular kidneys, unclear corticomedullary interface, perinephric fluid, and/or subcapsular renal infiltrate noted ultrasonographically.[2,9] The lymphoma is not usually limited to the kidneys. Aspirates are of high cellularity and consist almost entirely of lymphoid cells. In most cases, most of these cells (>80%) are large atypical lymphoid cells (see Fig. 22.8). Lymphoid cells are fragile, and slides may contain many ruptured cells. Nearly all cells may be ruptured if downward pressure is applied to the spreader slide during slide preparation. Depending on the degree to which the tumor has replaced normal tissue in the area sampled, renal tubular cells may be present. Slides made from animals with lymphoma are often very thick, and in many areas the cells are not well spread out. In such areas, it is difficult to accurately classify the lymphoid cells. Neoplastic lymphoid cells that are not well spread out appear smaller; their nucleoli are indistinct, and it is difficult to determine the amount of cytoplasm present. Thus it is imperative to find thin areas of the smear where the cells have assumed their normal morphology. Forms of lymphoma in which the neoplastic cell

populations cytologically appear as small or intermediate lymphocytes occur, but these forms are much less common. In such cases, it may be difficult to differentiate these lesions from severe lymphocytic infiltrates resulting from chronic inflammatory conditions. Inflammatory lesions typically result in lower numbers of lymphoid cells admixed with normal renal tubular cells. A mixture of small lymphocytes, prolymphocytes, intermediate lymphocytes, and some plasma cells may be present. Lymphoma is suggested if a dense, monotonous population of lymphoid cells exist in an extremely cellular smear from an enlarged kidney, but histological confirmation or immunophenotyping (flow cytometry, polymerase chain reaction [PCR] for B-cell and T-cell receptor clonality on FNA specimens, or both) is often warranted.

In retrospective studies of primary renal neoplasia, excluding lymphoma, 94% or greater of primary canine and feline renal tumors were malignant.[10,11] Carcinomas (e.g., tubular adenocarcinomas or renal cell carcinomas, transitional cell carcinomas, and squamous cell carcinomas of the renal pelvis) are the most common primary renal neoplasms of dogs and cats, but the overall incidence of renal cancer is fairly low (approximately 1% of all canine neoplasms and 1.5%–2.5% of all feline neoplasms).[9] A diagnosis of carcinoma is made from smears containing a population of epithelial cells that demonstrate adequate criteria of malignancy (see Chapter 2). Aspirates from renal carcinomas are often of much higher cellularity compared with aspirates from normal kidneys or renal inflammatory diseases and yield a dense population of renal epithelial cells (Fig. 22.10, A). Well-differentiated renal cell carcinomas may yield a majority of cells that are somewhat uniform, and cells demonstrating criteria of malignancy must be found among uniform cells (see Fig. 22.10, B; see Fig. 22.25, C, later in the chapter). The high cellularity of the aspirates correlates with the histological finding of densely packed epithelial cells arranged in lobules (Fig. 22.11). Poorly differentiated renal cell carcinomas, transitional cell carcinomas, and squamous cell carcinomas typically show moderate to marked cytological atypia (Figs. 22.12 and 22.13). Adrenal carcinomas may be encountered in animals with masses in the kidney area. If a blind aspirate is performed, these carcinomas are difficult or impossible to differentiate from renal carcinomas. Adrenal cortical cells are larger and have more abundant cytoplasm that often contains many fine vacuoles (Fig. 22.14).[8,12] Adrenal carcinomas should be considered if the patient shows clinical evidence of hyperadrenocorticism;

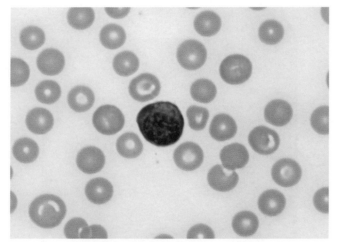

Fig. 22.7 A reactive lymphocyte (Wright-Giemsa stain, original magnification 1000×).

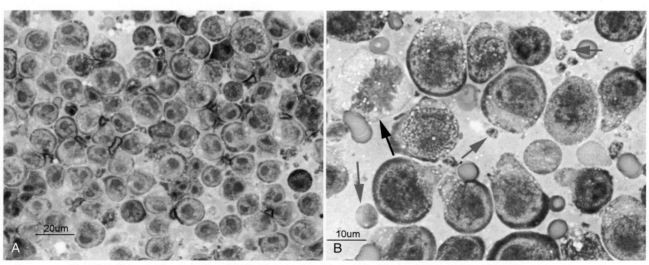

Fig. 22.8 Fine-needle aspiration samples from a cat with renal lymphoma presenting as bilateral renomegaly. (A) The specimen is densely cellular with a population of discrete cells (Wright-Giemsa stain). (B) Greater than 90% of the cells present are atypical medium to large lymphoid cells. Numerous lymphoglandular bodies are present *(red arrows)*, and one mitotic figure is seen *(black arrow)* (Wright-Giemsa stain).

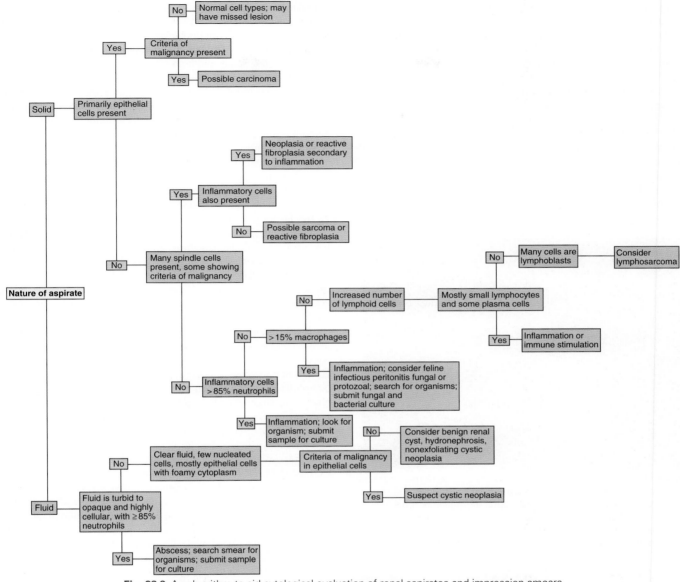

Fig. 22.9 An algorithm to aid cytological evaluation of renal aspirates and impression smears.

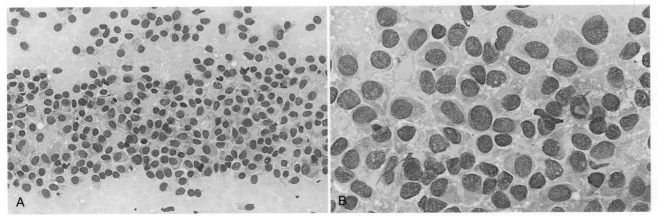

Fig. 22.10 Fine-needle aspirates from a mass involving the right kidney of a dog. (A) The samples are highly cellular, consisting of a single population of epithelial cells (Wright stain, original magnification 100×). (B) The epithelial cells present show criteria of malignancy, allowing for a diagnosis of carcinoma. Histopathological examination confirmed a diagnosis of renal cell carcinoma (Wright stain, original magnification 250×).

diagnostic imaging studies may help identify the location of the tumor in such cases.

Nephroblastoma is an uncommon embryonal tumor that occurs primarily in the kidney and thoracolumbar region of young dogs but has also been reported to occur as a primary renal tumor of cats.[10,11,13,14] Nephroblastomas typically present as a solitary unilateral mass at one pole of the kidney located primarily in the cortex with possible extension through the capsule or as a solitary mass in the spinal cord (T3–L3). Aspirates or impression smears of nephroblastomas are highly cellular and composed of numerous large (12–30 μm in diameter), epithelioid mononuclear, round-to-oval cells arranged individually and in clusters, often in combination with a mesenchymal cell population (Fig. 22.15, A). They exhibit mild to moderate anisocytosis and anisokaryosis and a variable but high N:C ratio. The cells have eccentrically located round, oval, or pleomorphic nuclei with a finely

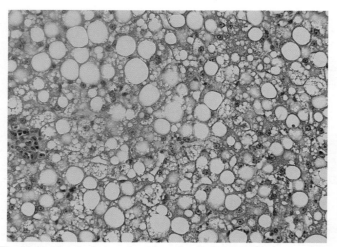

Fig. 22.11 Histological section of renal cell carcinoma from a dog. Note the densely packed large polygonal epithelial cells divided into distinct lobules by fibrous connective tissue septa. Individual cells have abundant clear to granular eosinophilic cytoplasm and a centrally located round nucleus with vesicular chromatin and a single prominent nucleolus (hematoxylin and eosin [H&E] stain, original magnification 200×).

granular to smudged chromatin, single to multiple small nucleoli, and a scant rim of basophilic and occasionally vacuolated cytoplasm. They may be mistaken for lymphoma, given their high N:C ratio and finely granular chromatin. Nuclear molding and pseudorosette formation may be evident. Small spindloid cells with dark nuclei are frequently admixed with the round-to-oval mononuclear cells.[13,14] Confirmation of diagnosis via histological evaluation is warranted (see Fig. 22.15, B). The mesenchymal component exhibits immunopositivity for vimentin, and the epithelial component exhibits immunopositivity for cytokeratin. Immunohistochemical expression for marker WT-1 may also be useful in confirming a diagnosis of nephroblastoma.[14]

Mesenchymal tumors are less common than epithelial tumors, accounting for approximately 5% of feline and 34% of canine renal neoplasms.[10,11] Types of mesenchymal tumors that may be found in the canine or feline kidney include malignant fibrous histiocytoma (Fig. 22.16), histiocytic sarcoma (Fig. 22.17), plasma cell tumor (or multiple myeloma), neurofibroma, fibroleiomyosarcoma, leiomyosarcoma, hemangiosarcoma, hemangioma, angiomyolipoma, cortical fibroma, congenital mesoblastic nephroma, oncocytoma, chondrosarcoma, and extramedullary osteosarcoma.[2,9-11,15,16] Mesenchymal tumors of the kidney may be primary, disseminated, or metastatic.[9,10,14,17] An example of a disseminated mesenchymal neoplasm that may occur in the kidney, especially in dogs, is histiocytic sarcoma. Histiocytic sarcoma is a tumor of neoplastic dendritic cells.[16] More common sites of involvement include the periarticular regions, lungs, spleen, liver, and lymph nodes. The neoplastic cells are large, round cells occurring singly and in noncohesive aggregates. The round cells contain abundant basophilic cytoplasm, which may exhibit vacuolation or phagocytosis. Nuclei are large, round to indented, and eccentrically located with vesicular to coarse chromatin and one or more prominent nucleoli. Neoplastic cells frequently exhibit moderate to marked anisocytosis and anisokaryosis (see Fig. 22.17). Neoplastic cells typically exhibit immunopositivity for the following markers: CD45, CD18, CD1, CD11c, and MHCII. An example of a disseminated round cell neoplasm other than lymphoma, reported in cats, is plasma cell tumor or multiple myeloma.[2] Neoplastic plasma cells are large, atypical round cells that occur singly and have abundant amphophilic to basophilic cytoplasm with eosinophilic margins. Single or multiple, round-to-oval, eccentrically placed nuclei have coarsely stippled chromatin and

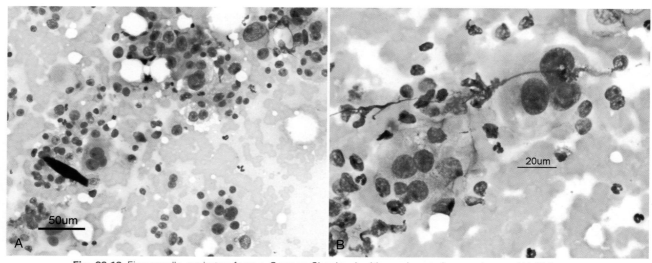

Fig. 22.12 Fine-needle aspirates from a German Shepherd with renal cystadenocarcinoma. (A) Slides are highly cellular and display marked atypia, including marked anisocytosis, marked anisokaryosis, multinucleation, and large prominent nuclei (Wright-Giemsa stain). (B) Higher magnification shows multiple large, irregularly shaped nucleoli (Wright-Giemsa stain).

inapparent variably prominent round nucleoli. Neoplastic cells exhibit minimal to moderate anisocytosis and anisokaryosis. Monoclonal or biclonal gammopathy may be present concurrently in affected cats.

Inflammation

Most inflammatory diseases affecting the kidney (e.g., chronic interstitial nephritis, pyelonephritis, glomerulonephritis) are diagnosed on the basis of history, physical examination findings, and ancillary diagnostic procedure results. Cytological examination is not usually indicated in such conditions; however, inflammatory responses are occasionally encountered in aspirates from clinical cases or impression smears taken at necropsy. Because kidneys are highly vascular, nearly all renal aspirates contain some leukocytes secondary to peripheral blood contamination. A diagnosis of inflammation depends on the presence of cells not typically found in blood (e.g., plasma cells, macrophages) or of greater numbers of leukocytes than expected from the degree of blood contamination.

Purulent inflammation is denoted by a marked predominance of neutrophils (usually >80%) with only scattered macrophages and suggests inflammation produced by pyogenic bacteria (Fig. 22.18) but may also result from noninfectious causes. Many species of pyogenic bacteria, which are usually the result of ascending infection from the lower urinary tract but may also be of hematogenous origin, have been cultured from dogs with acute pyelonephritis. Increased percentages of

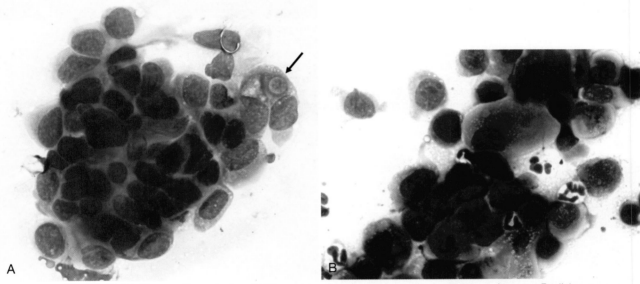

Fig. 22.13 (A) Fine-needle aspiration (FNA) sample of renal transitional cell carcinoma from an English Springer Spaniel. Note cohesive aggregate of medium polygonal cells typical of an epithelial neoplasm. Cells exhibit increased nuclear-to-cytoplasmic (N:C) ratio, moderate anisocytosis and anisokaryosis, and a distinctive intracytoplasmic eosinophilic inclusion *(black arrow)*. Histopathological examination confirmed a diagnosis of transitional cell carcinoma arising from the renal pelvis (Wright-Giemsa stain, original magnification 500×). (B) FNA sample of renal squamous cell carcinoma from a dog. Note large polygonal, angular, and oval cells that exhibit marked anisocytosis, anisokaryosis, vesicular cytoplasm, and large, oval-to-irregular, multiple nucleoli (Diff-Quik stain, original magnification 1000×).

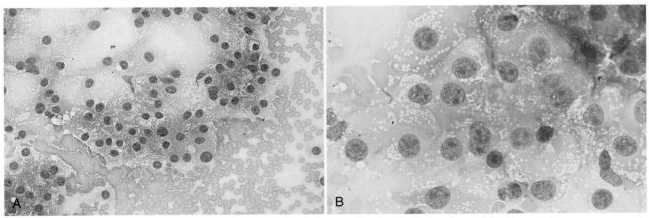

Fig. 22.14 Fine-needle aspirates from an abdominal mass of a dog displaying signs of Cushing syndrome. Ultrasonography revealed an extremely large right adrenal gland mass. The left adrenal gland could not be seen. (A) Samples are highly cellular and consist of finely vacuolated epithelial cells (DipStat, original magnification 100×). (B) Cells show moderate variability and prominent nucleoli. Some extremely large cells displaying macronuclei were present in other fields (DipStat, original magnification 250×).

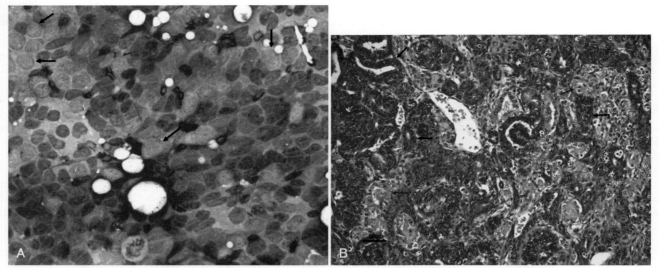

Fig. 22.15 (A) Fine-needle aspiration (FNA) sample of canine nephroblastoma. Note predominance of round-to-oval epithelial cells in dense aggregates. The cells have a high nuclear-to-cytoplasmic (N:C) ratio, dispersed chromatin, and inapparent to indistinct nucleoli *(black arrows)*. Fewer spindle (mesenchymal) cells with oblong nuclei are observed *(red arrows)*. A bizarre mitotic figure is present *(green arrow)* (Wright-Giemsa stain, original magnification 500×). (B) Histological section of canine nephroblastoma. Densely packed epithelial cells form aggregates, primitive tubules *(black arrows)* and tuft-like invaginations *(green arrow)*. Paler eosinophilic areas *(blue arrows)* represent stroma containing mesenchymal cells (hematoxylin and eosin [H&E] stain). (Courtesy Dr. Pam Mouser.)

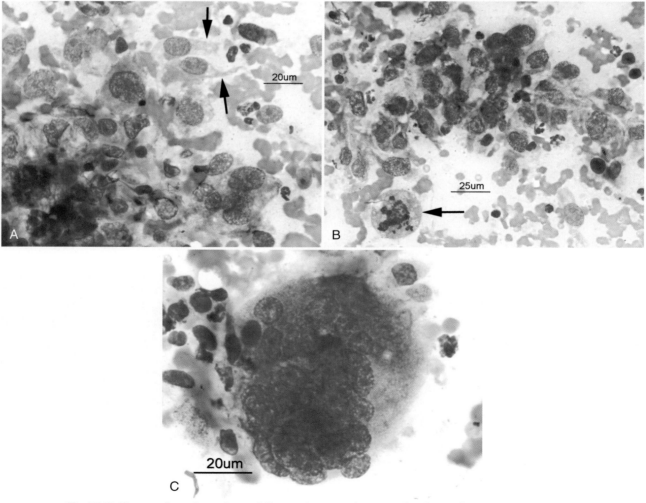

Fig. 22.16 Fine-needle aspirates from a feline renal sarcoma (suspected malignant fibrous histiocytoma). (A) Aspirates are highly cellular and show a pleomorphic population of mesenchymal cells. Tapered cytoplasm is evident in some cells *(arrows)*. Most cells have large, prominent nucleoli (Wright-Giemsa stain). (B) Image showing pleomorphic mesenchymal cells and a bizarre mitotic figure *(arrow)* (Wright-Giemsa stain). (C) Large multinucleated giant cells containing greater than 20 nuclei are common, suggesting malignant fibrous histiocytoma. Further diagnostics were not performed. (Courtesy Dr. Robin Allison.)

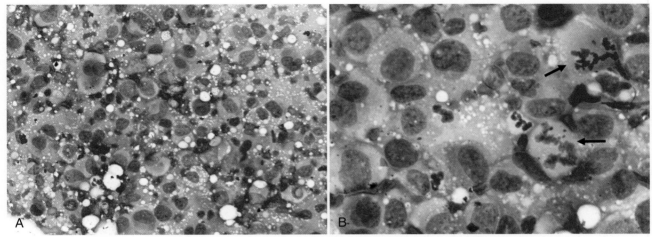

Fig. 22.17 Fine-needle aspirates from a dog with disseminated histiocytic sarcoma involving the kidney. (A) Aspirates are highly cellular and consist of singly occurring round cells of variable size. Some are binucleate or have vacuolated cytoplasm (Wright-Giemsa stain, original magnification 500×). (B) Higher-magnification view showing neoplastic round cells with variable amounts (often abundant) of pale blue-to-gray cytoplasm and an eccentric large, oval–to–irregularly round nucleus with smudged chromatin and multiple irregular nucleoli. Cells exhibit moderate anisocytosis and anisokaryosis. Two bizarre mitotic figures are present *(black arrows)* (Wright-Giemsa stain, original magnification 1000×).

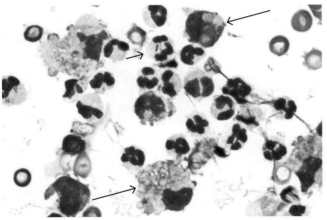

Fig. 22.18 Fine-needle aspirates from the kidney of a dog with septic pyelonephritis. The smears are highly cellular and contain degenerate neutrophils, some of which contain phagocytized bacterial rods *(short arrow)*. Macrophages containing cytoplasmic vacuoles or phagocytized cellular debris are present in lesser numbers *(long arrows)* (Diff-Quik, original magnification 1000×).

macrophages (>15%) are seen in cases of pyogranulomatous and granulomatous inflammation. FIP is one cause of such lesions that should be considered in cats with appropriate clinical features (Figs. 22.19 and 22.20). Slides should also be searched for the presence of atypical bacteria (e.g., *Mycobacterium* spp.), protozoal (e.g., *Leishmania* spp.), amoebic (e.g., *Balamuthia* spp.), systemic algae (e.g., *Prototheca zopfii*; refer to Chapter 3), and fungal organisms. Yeast phases of *Blastomyces dermatitidis*, *Cryptococcus neoformans*, *Coccidioides immitis*, *Histoplasma capsulatum*, and pseudohyphal forms of *Candida* spp. (Fig. 22.21) have all been found in the kidneys of animals with disseminated disease, although such organisms are more commonly encountered in other tissues. The yeast phase of *Cryptococcus* spp. is typically characterized by a thick nonstaining capsule; however, nonencapsulated or poorly encapsulated forms of *Cryptococcus* spp. have been observed in the feline kidney (Fig. 22.22). Nonencapsulated forms of *Cryptococcus* spp. may be difficult to differentiate morphologically from other fungal

yeast and protozoal organisms. Fungal hyphae (Fig. 22.23) may occasionally be found in imprints or aspirates, but culture is necessary to further identify the fungus. Special stains, such as Gomori-Grocott methenamine silver (GMS) and periodic acid–Schiff (PAS), are often required to highlight the presence of fungal organisms in tissue specimens (Fig. 22.24), whereas routinely used Romanowsky-type stains, such as Diff-Quik, are typically sufficient to identify fungal organisms in cytological specimens.

Inflammatory infiltrates characterized by a predominance of small, mature lymphocytes and plasma cells are typical of chronic inflammatory lesions and must be differentiated from cases of renal lymphoma, as previously discussed.

Degeneration/Necrosis

FNA of chronic renal infarcts and regions of tubular degeneration may be nondiagnostic in many cases because of poor cell yield. On US, acute infarcts usually present as mass-like lesions with decreased or mixed echogenicity within 24 hours of blood vessel occlusion. They become more hyperechoic with increasing fibrosis.[18] FNA of acute or subacute renal infarcts may yield aspirates of decreased cellularity with indicators of hemorrhage (erythrophagocytosis, hemosiderin and hematoidin pigmentation), variable inflammation (mostly neutrophils and macrophages), and amorphous basophilic debris consistent with necrosis (Fig. 22.25). These cytological findings together with US features described above may be useful in making a presumptive diagnosis of an infarct.

Cytological Characteristics of Fluid Lesions

FNA may be performed to collect samples for cytological examination and bacterial culture from animals with fluid lesions (e.g., hydronephrosis, abscesses).

Cysts

In humans, renal cysts are a commonly reported cause of space-occupying kidney lesions and have also been reported in domestic animals. Renal cysts may be single or multiple, congenital or acquired, and they frequently do not cause symptomatic disease. They may enlarge and induce local tissue hypoxia, however, resulting in

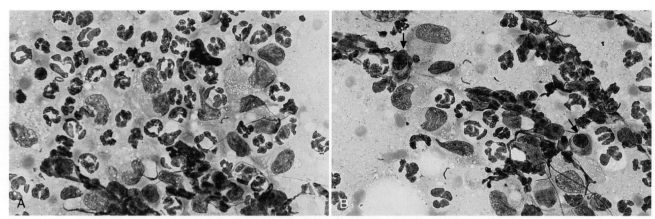

Fig. 22.19 Fine-needle aspirates from the kidney of a cat with feline infectious peritonitis. The smears are highly cellular and contain a pyogranulomatous inflammatory response. (A) Nondegenerate neutrophils and numerous macrophages are shown. In other areas of the smear, macrophages predominate (Diff-Quik, original magnification 250×). (B) Same slide as image (A) and similar cell population as image (A). Note the presence of two mature plasma cells *(arrows)* (Diff-Quik, original magnification 250×).

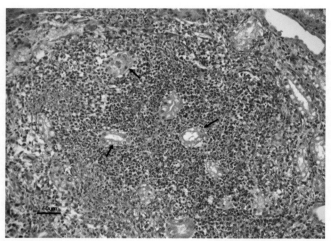

Fig. 22.20 Histological section of kidney from cat with feline infectious peritonitis. Renal parenchyma is largely replaced by sheets of inflammatory cells including lysed neutrophils and fewer macrophages, lymphocytes, and plasma cells. Renal tubules *(black arrows)* are widely separated by the interstitial inflammatory cell infiltrate (hematoxylin and eosin [H&E]). (Courtesy Dr. Pam Mouser.)

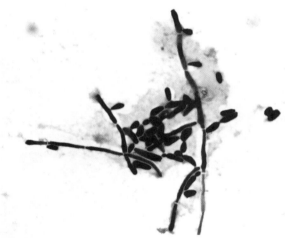

Fig. 22.21 Urine sediment from dog with renal candidiasis. Basophilic pseudohyphae and blastospores of *Candida* spp. (Diff-Quik stain, original magnification 1000×).

overproduction of erythropoietin with resultant polycythemia, or causing sufficient loss of parenchyma from pressure atrophy that eventually results in renal failure. Aspiration of renal cysts may be performed to rule out other causes of renal enlargement and evaluate for secondary bacterial infection. Benign cysts contain a clear, colorless or straw-colored fluid that is of low cellularity but may contain a few cuboidal, epithelial lining cells. These cells occur singly and generally have foamy cytoplasm and a low N:C ratio with absent or small nucleoli. Neutrophils, macrophages, including hemosiderophages or debris-laden macrophages, and cellular debris may also be present (Fig. 22.26, A and B).

Some renal carcinomas are cystic and must be differentiated from benign cysts (see Fig. 22.26, C). Exfoliated cells should be evaluated for malignant changes (see Chapter 2), but not all cystic neoplasms exfoliate recognizably malignant cells into the fluid. Histopathology may be required to differentiate between a benign cyst and cystic renal carcinoma (see Fig. 22.26, B and C).

Hydronephrosis

Hydronephrosis is the dilation of the renal pelvis and the associated parenchymal atrophy and cystic enlargement of the kidney that results from an obstruction of urine flow. The obstruction may be complete or partial, arise suddenly or progressively, and occur at any level of the urinary tract. A variable amount of clear fluid is recovered from aspiration, and smears of this fluid contain few cells; a few inflammatory cells and epithelial lining cells may be present. High numbers of inflammatory cells are seen with secondary infections. The causes of hydronephrosis, which may be distinguished from renal cysts via US, include ectopic ureters, chronic ureteritis, renal calculi, neoplasia, benign prostatic hyperplasia, pregnancy, and inadvertent surgical ligation of the ureter.[18]

Abscesses

Renal abscesses occur infrequently in dogs and cats but may occur secondary to a septic process, such as pyelonephritis or septicemia. The physical appearance of the aspirated material is like that of any other purulent exudate. Cytologically, the smears are highly cellular and typically consist of greater than 80% neutrophils with varying numbers of macrophages (see Fig. 22.18). A search should be made for infectious agents, and material should be submitted for culture and sensitivity (C&S). Identifying bacterial rods or cocci

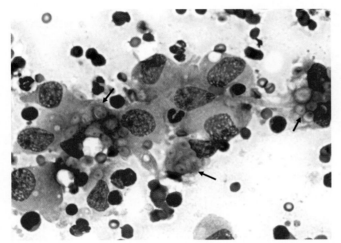

Fig. 22.22 Fine-needle aspirates from the kidney of a cat with cryptococcosis. The very cellular smears contain macrophages, neutrophils, and lymphocytes consistent with pyogranulomatous inflammation. Macrophages contain several phagocytized *Cryptococcus* spp., organisms *(black arrows)* that lack a thick nonstaining capsule that this organism typically displays. Poorly encapsulated forms of *Cryptococcus* spp. must be differentiated from other fungal yeast and protozoal organisms (Diff-Quik stain, original magnification 1000×).

helps in choosing antibiotic therapy while awaiting culture and sensitivity results. With Romanowsky-type stains, bacteria (both gram-positive and gram-negative) stain blue-black (see Fig. 22.18). If bacterial rods (especially bipolar rods) are seen cytologically, an antimicrobial effective against gram-negative bacteria should be used while C&S results are awaited. The pathological bacterial cocci are generally *Staphylococcus* and *Streptococcus* spp.; therefore, when bacterial cocci are seen cytologically, an antimicrobial effective against gram-positive bacteria should be used while C&S results are awaited.

Cytological Characteristics of Crystals

Crystals are rarely encountered in FNA of normal or diseased kidneys but, when present, may provide important diagnostic clues in nephrotoxicosis cases. Calcium oxalate monohydrate crystals may be seen in FNA or impression smears of kidneys from dogs or cats with oxalate nephrosis, which occurs most commonly in ethylene glycol poisoning cases. The calcium oxalate monohydrate crystals may appear as flat, elongated structures with pointed ends that resemble a picket fence or as groupings of crystals that resemble sheaves of wheat (Fig. 22.27). The crystals exhibit birefringence when viewed under polarized light (see Fig. 22.27, B). It is important to differentiate oxalate crystals from another important crystal type found in dogs and cats with nephrotoxicosis because of ingestion of contaminated pet food. Such crystals are thought to result from precipitation of melamine and cyanuric acid. They are pale yellow to golden, round to oval, polarizable crystals with distinctive radiating striations or globular dense green aggregates found in distal tubules and collecting ducts (Fig. 22.28).[19]

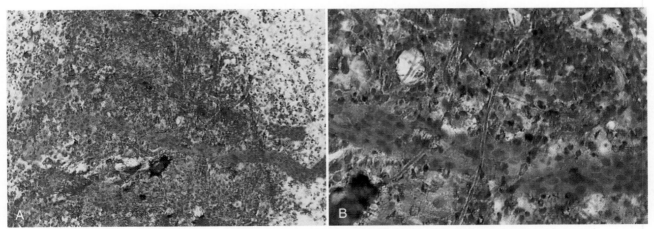

Fig. 22.23 Impression smears taken at necropsy from the kidney of a dog. (A) Highly cellular smear with recognizable tubules and fungal hyphae (Wright stain, original magnification 33×). (B) Higher magnification of the same area (Wright stain, original magnification 200×).

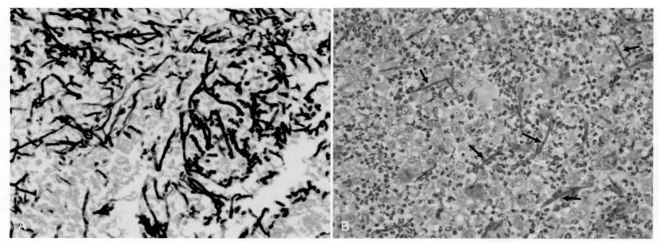

Fig. 22.24 (A) Histological section of fungal nephritis in a Newfoundland dog. Gomori-Grocott methenamine silver (GMS) stain highlights fungal hyphae in tissue as black branching structures against a pale-green background. *Aspergillus terreus* was cultured from the patient (GMS stain, original magnification 400×). (B) Histological section of fungal nephritis in a cat. Periodic acid–Schiff (PAS) stain highlights fungal hyphae in tissue as pink branching structures *(black arrows)* in a background of pyogranulomatous inflammation. *Phialophora verrucosa* was cultured from the patient (PAS stain, original magnification 400×). (Courtesy Dr. Pam Mouser.)

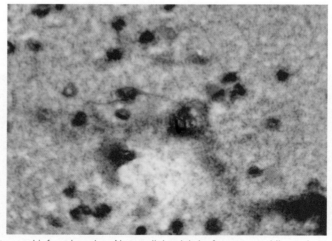

Fig. 22.25 Fine-needle aspirate of acute renal infarct in a dog. Note cellular debris, few neutrophils, and macrophage containing hematoidin *(arrow)* in amorphous basophilic background (Diff-Quik stain, original magnification 1000×).

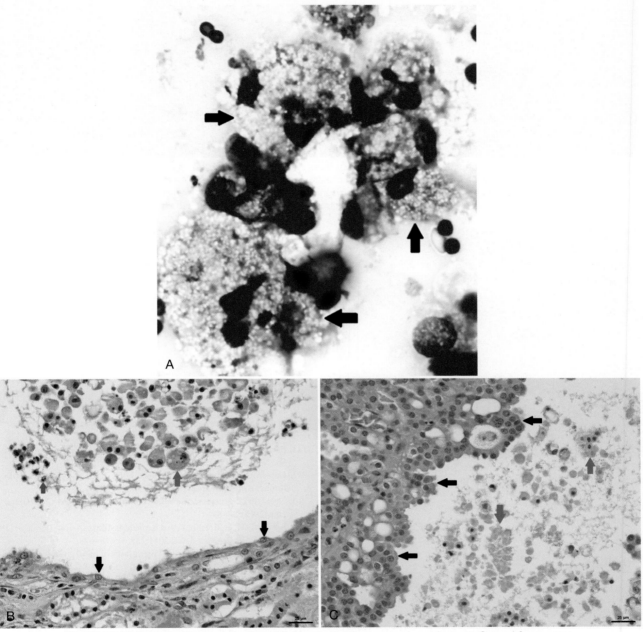

Fig. 22.26 (A) Cytocentrifuge preparation of fluid collected from a renal cyst in a cat. Several foamy macrophages, some containing phagocytized amorphous blue debris *(black arrows)*, are found in the fluid. The findings in cystic fluid are relatively nonspecific (Diff-Quik stain, original magnification 1000×). (B) Histological section of feline benign renal cyst showing cyst lined by low cuboidal tubular epithelial cells *(black arrows)*, and macrophages *(green arrow)* and neutrophils *(blue arrow)* within cyst lumen (hematoxylin and eosin [H&E] stain). (C) Histological section of canine cystic renal carcinoma showing cyst lined by multiple disorderly layers of neoplastic renal tubular epithelial cells *(black arrows)*, and macrophages, sloughed degenerate epithelial cells, and necrotic debris *(green arrows)* in cyst lumen (H&E stain). (B and C, Courtesy Dr. Pam Mouser.)

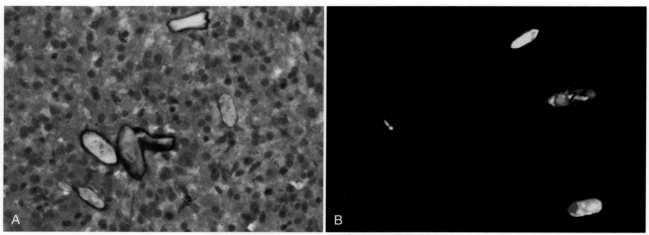

Fig. 22.27 Impression smears taken at necropsy from the kidney of a dog. (A) Highly cellular smear with degenerate tubular epithelial cells and calcium oxalate monohydrate crystals. Crystals resemble a picket fence with pointed ends (Wright stain, original magnification 500×). (B) Lower magnification of crystals as viewed under polarized light demonstrating birefringence (Wright stain, original magnification 250×).

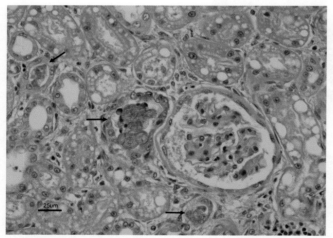

Fig. 22.28 Histological section of kidney from a cat that ingested pet food contaminated with melamine and cyanuric acid. Pale tan-to-golden, round-to-oval crystals with distinctive radiating striations or globular dense aggregates are found in lumens of distal tubules and collecting ducts (hematoxylin and eosin [H&E] stain). (Courtesy Dr. Pam Mouser.)

REFERENCES

1. Borjesson DL. Renal cytology. *Vet Clin North Am Small Anim Pract.* 2003;33:119–134.
2. McAloney CA, et al. Diagnostic utility of renal fine-needle aspirate cytology and ultrasound in the cat. *J Fel Med Surg.* 2017:1–10. Epub ahead of print.
3. McAloney CA, et al. Diagnostic utility of renal fine needle aspirate cytology, ultrasound, and combined finding in the dog. *J Am Vet Med Assoc.* 2017. [In press].
4. Zatelli A, et al. Echo-assisted percutaneous renal biopsy in dogs. A retrospective study of 229 cases. *Vet J1.* 2003;266:257–264.
5. Leiman G. Audit of fine needle aspiration cytology of 120 renal lesions. *Cytopathology.* 1990;1:65–72.
6. Nguyen GK. Percutaneous fine-needle aspiration biopsy cytology of the kidney and adrenal. *Pathol Annu.* 1987;1:163–197.
7. Menard M, Papageorges M. Technique for ultrasound-guided fine needle biopsies. *Vet Radiol Ultrasound.* 1995;36:137–138.
8. DeMay RM. *The Art and Science of Cytopathology.* Chicago, IL: ASCP Press; 1996:1083–1134.
9. Maxie MG, Newman SJ. Urinary system. In: Maxie MG, ed. *Jubb, Kennedy, and Palmer's Pathology of Domestic Animals.* Vol 2. Philadelphia, PA: Saunders; 2007:498–503.
10. Henry CJ, et al. Primary renal tumors in cats: 19 cases (1992-1998). *J Feline Med Surg.* 1999;1(3):165–170.
11. Bryan JN, et al. Primary renal neoplasia of dogs. *J Vet Intern Med.* 2006;20:1155–1160.
11a. Barton. Cytology of the endocrine and neuroendocrine tumors. *Vet Can Soc Newslett.* 1993;17:5–9.
12. Gasser AM, et al. Extradural spinal, bone marrow, and renal nephroblastoma. *J Am Anim Hosp Assoc.* 2003;39(1):80–85.
13. Neel J, et al. A mass in the spinal column of a dog. *Vet Clin Pathol.* 2000;29(3):87–89.
14. Brewer DM, et al. Spinal cord nephroblastoma in dogs: 11 cases (1985-2007). *J Am Vet Med Assoc.* 2011;238(5):618–624.
15. Hahn KA, et al. Bilateral renal metastases of nasal chondrosarcoma in a dog. *Vet Pathol.* 1997;34(4):326–352.
16. Affolter VK, Moore PF. Localized and disseminated histiocytic sarcoma of dendritic cell origin in the dog. *Vet Pathol.* 2002;39:74–83.
17. Munday JS, et al. Renal osteosarcoma in a dog. *J Small Anim Pract.* 2004;45(12):618–622.
18. Debruyn K, et al. Ultrasonography of the feline kidney—technique, anatomy and changes associated with disease. *J Fel Med Surg.* 2012;14:794–803.
19. Brown CA, et al. Outbreaks of renal failure associated with melamine and cyanuric acid in dogs and cats in 2004 and 2007. *J Vet Diagn Invest.* 2007;19:525–531.

23

Examination of the Urine Sediment

Heather L. Wamsley

SPECIMEN COLLECTION

Urinalysis results are influenced by the biological variability of patients, the urine collection method, the timing of urine collection, the administration of therapeutic or diagnostic agents before collection, and the method of handling the sample before analysis.[1] Ideally, at least 6 milliliters (mL) of urine should be collected before the administration of therapeutic or diagnostic agents to establish baseline information; however, in patients with cystitis and urge incontinence, this may be challenging. In urinalysis, 5 mL of urine may be used; 1 mL may be used for urine culture, if necessary. When choosing the urine collection method and the timing of urine collection, it is useful to consider the patient's clinical status, the logistics of the collection method, and the intended use of the sample (Tables 23.1 and 23.2).

First-morning, preprandial urine samples, which are inherently collected after a period of nil per os (NPO, nothing by mouth), will have the highest urine specific gravity and the highest concentration of sediment; however, the cytomorphology of the sediment contents and the viability of fastidious microorganisms may be reduced because of the relatively prolonged retention of urine within the bladder. If sediment examination and urine culture are primary goals, cystocentesis of a randomly timed urine sample may be preferred in patients without contraindications for cystocentesis (e.g., thrombocytopenia, urethral obstruction). Cystocentesis samples are also useful to localize urinalysis findings (e.g., sediment abnormalities, proteinuria) to the bladder or proximal urinary tract because samples obtained via cystocentesis will lack contributions from the lower genitourinary tract.

Samples collected during midstream micturition or by transurethral catheterization are also suitable for sediment examination and quantitative urine culture, which should be interpreted by using guidelines based on collection method and colony-forming units per milliliter (CFU/mL) (Table 23.3). Manual compression of the bladder to induce micturition should be avoided because doing so may cause reflux of potentially infectious urine, traumatic hematuria, or, rarely, uroabdomen. Voided urine samples rescued from the examination room tabletop have limited utility; but, if the sediment is examined without delay, some components can still be assessed, specifically cells that might come from the patient (e.g., leukocytes, erythrocytes, atypical cells). Such a sample should not be used for biochemical analysis or to screen for infectious organisms.

In addition to routine urine sediment evaluation, urine samples may be converted to a dry-mount cytology sample[2,3]; this allows for more sensitive detection of bacteria and more accurate assessment of bacterial morphology and greatly facilitates evaluation of atypical cells in-house or by a reference laboratory. The method is described in Box 23.1. If available, cytocentrifugation of the urine sediment is equally useful. When possible, obtaining cells directly from a mass (i.e., ultrasound-guided fine-needle biopsy [FNB] or surgical biopsy imprint) usually produces a sample with the best morphology for cytological examination. However, seeding carcinoma cells in the abdominal wall is an uncommon, but grave, complication of cystotomy and percutaneous FNB.[4]

SPECIMEN HANDLING BEFORE URINALYSIS

With proper sample handling and testing, complete urinalysis may rapidly provide information about the genitourinary tract and screen for diseases of other body systems (e.g., endocrine, hepatic). Urine should be collected into a sterile, single-use vessel to avoid potential contamination by cleanser residues and microorganisms. The body of the container, not just the lid, should be labeled, and the container should be sealed to avoid leakage of the sample and evaporation of volatile compounds (e.g., ketones). Urine specimen cups often leak during transport. If urine will be sent to a reference laboratory, it should be transferred to a labeled, plain, white-top tube. To minimize postcollection artifacts and to obtain results that are most representative of urine in vivo, urine samples should be evaluated within 30 minutes of collection.[5] If urinalysis will be delayed, the sample should be refrigerated and protected from light to prevent overgrowth of microorganisms and photodegradation of bilirubin, respectively. If necessary, samples may be stored for approximately 12 to 24 hours (i.e., overnight). However, depending on the initial sample composition (e.g., pH and concentration of crystallogenic substances), the sediment content may be modified from what was initially present immediately ex vivo—crystals may form with refrigerated storage (i.e., struvite, calcium oxalate dihydrate), renal tubular casts may degrade, and cytomorphology may be detrimentally altered.[6] Freezing or routine use of chemical preservatives should be avoided. Refrigeration is preferred for preservation of urine samples. Because cold urine may influence urinalysis results (e.g., falsely increase specific gravity, inhibit enzymatic urine dipstick reactions, and promote crystal formation), a sample that has been refrigerated should be permitted to warm to room temperature before urinalysis. If crystalluria is a medically important problem that is being diagnosed or monitored, then the finding should be confirmed in a freshly obtained sample collected into a single-use container and analyzed within 30 to 60 minutes without interim refrigeration.[5,6]

PREPARATION OF URINE SEDIMENT WET MOUNT

Evaluation of the urine sediment for the presence of increased concentrations of cells, casts, microorganisms, or crystals is useful for the detection of underlying urinary tract disease or diseases of other organs. Gross clarity of the urine sample should not be used as the sole means to determine potentially normal sediment findings because even nonturbid samples may be abnormal on

TABLE 23.1   Methods of Urine Collection With Their Advantages and Disadvantages or Precautions

Collection Method	Advantages	Disadvantages / Precautions
Midstream, naturally voided	• Noninvasive, relatively easy technique in dogs • May be performed by clients and is useful to collect first-morning, maximally concentrated urine samples from outpatients • Unlike cystocentesis or catheterization, is not associated with iatrogenic hematuria • Although not ideal, a freshly voided sample may be used for urine culture, as long as a quantitative urine culture is performed	• Likely contaminated by a variable amount of material from the lower genitourinary tract (e.g., bacteria, epithelial cells, blood, sperm, debris), perineum, or environment (e.g., pollen), which may be observed in the urine sediment • Cleanser residues or microorganisms within the collection vessel may affect results • Urine should be collected into a sterile, single-use urine collection cup, rather than into a reusable container • Avoid manual bladder compression to induce micturition, which may cause reflux of urine into other organs (e.g., kidneys, prostate) or iatrogenic hematuria
Transurethral catheterization	• Useful collection method when an indwelling urinary catheter is already present for another reason • Although not ideal, sample may be used for urine culture, as long as a quantitative urine culture is performed	• Risk of traumatic catheterization, which may injure the patient and contaminate the sample with blood • Risk of iatrogenic infection, especially in patients predisposed to urinary tract infection (e.g., lower urinary tract disease, renal failure, diabetes mellitus, hyperadrenocorticism) • Should be performed aseptically and atraumatically by a trained, experienced individual • Urine sample may be contaminated by variable numbers of epithelial cells, bacteria, and debris from the lower genitourinary tract, which may be observed in the urine sediment • Catheters that are chemically sterilized may contain residue of the antiseptic solution, which may irritate mucosal linings and affect results of urinalysis and urine culture • Catheterization may be technically challenging in female patients • May require use of a vaginal endoscope
Antepubic cystocentesis	• Avoids lower genitourinary tract contamination of urine sample • Ideal sample for urine culture • Less risk of iatrogenic infection compared with transurethral catheterization • Easier than collection of voided samples from cats • Better tolerated than catheterization	• Contraindicated in patients with urethral obstruction or bleeding diathesis (e.g., thrombocytopenia), may be performed with caution after cystotomy • An adequate volume of urine within the bladder is required • Blind cystocentesis without at least manual localization and immobilization of the bladder is not recommended • Ultrasound-guided needle placement is helpful, though not mandatory • Misdirection of the needle may lead to a nondiagnostic or contaminated sample (e.g., enterocentesis) • A variable degree of iatrogenic microscopic hematuria, which cannot be readily distinguished from pathological, disease-induced hematuria, may be caused by this collection method • This type of contamination may be particularly pronounced when the bladder wall is inflamed or congested • Iatrogenic hematuria may limit the utility of this collection method when monitoring the progression of disease in a patient that has pathological hematuria

TABLE 23.2   Timing of Urine Sample Collection, Indications, and Potential Effects on Urinalysis Results

Collection Time	Advantages	Disadvantages
First-morning urine—urine is formed after a several-hour period of nil per os (NPO)	• Represents the patient's maximally concentrated urine and is therefore ideal for assessing renal tubular ability to concentrate urine • Microscopic sediment will be more concentrated • Postprandial alterations unlikely • Urine more likely to be acidic, so casts may be better preserved (proteinaceous structures dissolve in alkaline urine)	• Urine present within bladder for a relatively prolonged period • May alter cellular morphology observed during microscopic examination • May decrease viability of fastidious microorganisms, causing false-negative culture results
Postprandially	• Useful to assess the effect of diets intended to modulate urinary pH when collected 3–6 hours postprandially • More likely to detect hyperglycemic glucosuria when collected 3–4 hours postprandially	• pH may be elevated by postprandial alkaline tide when collected within 1 hour postprandially
Randomly timed urine sample—represents urine that has accumulated within the bladder for minutes to hours or urine that has been diluted by recent ingestion of water	• Cytomorphology and viability of fastidious microorganisms may be better preserved because urine is stored within the bladder for relatively less time	• If the urine is isosthenuric or minimally concentrated, no conclusion can be drawn about renal tubular concentrating ability

TABLE 23.3 Guidelines for Interpretation of Quantitative Urine Cultures

Collection Method	SIGNIFICANT (CFU/ML)		QUESTIONABLE (CFU/ML)		CONTAMINATION (CFU/ML)	
	Dog	Cat	Dog	Cat	Dog	Cat
Cystocentesis	>1000	>1000	100–1000	>1000	<100	>1000
Catheterization	>10,000	>1000	1000–10,000	100–1000	<1000	<100
Voided	>100,000	>10,000	10,000–100,000	1000–10,000	<10,000	<1000

CFU/mL, colony-forming units per milliliter.

BOX 23.1 Method to Prepare Urine Sediment Dry-Mount for Routine Cytological Examination

- Centrifuge the urine at 400× to 500× gravity (*g*) (≈1000–1500 revolutions per minute [rpm]) in a conical centrifuge tube for 5 minutes.
- Remove the supernatant fluid by either gently decanting or using a transfer pipette to aspirate it.
- Use a transfer pipette to aspirate the sediment pellet from the bottom of the centrifuge tube.
- Place a small drop of the aspirated material onto a clean, glass microscope slide.
- Use a second clean, glass microscope slide to spread the material in a monolayer as is done for tissue aspirate cytology.
- Allow the slide to air-dry. Heat fixation is not necessary and will alter cell morphology.
- Stain as a routine cytology using quick Romanowsky-type stain. Alternatively, the slide may be stored in a covered container at room temperature and sent to a reference diagnostic laboratory for evaluation.

BOX 23.2 Guidelines for Urine Sediment Preparation and Evaluation

- Because cells, crystals, casts, and so on will spontaneously form a sediment because of gravity, mix the whole urine sample well before removing an aliquot for centrifugation to ensure that the urine sediment wet mount is representative of the whole sample.
- Use a standard volume aliquot of urine for centrifugation (e.g., 5 milliliters [mL]).
- Use a standard volume of urine supernatant to gently resuspend the sediment pellet (i.e., 10% of the original aliquot volume).
  - If 5 mL of urine is centrifuged, remove 4.5 mL of supernatant and resuspend the pellet in the remaining 0.5 mL.
  - If 4 mL of urine is centrifuged, remove 3.6 mL of supernatant and resuspend the pellet in the remaining 0.4 mL.
  - If 3 mL of urine is centrifuged, remove 2.7 mL of supernatant and resuspend the pellet in the remaining 0.3 mL.
  - If 2 mL of urine is centrifuged, remove 1.8 mL of supernatant and resuspend the pellet in the remaining 0.2 mL.
- Examine the whole coverslip and a standard number of microscopic fields (i.e., 10 fields) using both the 10× and 40× objectives and reduced illumination.
- Use the unstained wet mount to determine the concentration of materials within the sediment, because the addition of stain dilutes the sediment.
- Staining (e.g., with NMB stain) is helpful for identification of nucleated structures but may form crystals or may be contaminated with microorganisms. If crystals or microorganisms are observed in a stained sediment wet mount, confirm their presence in an unstained wet mount of the sediment.

---

microscopy. The urine sample should be mixed well before removing an aliquot for centrifugation. Most urine sediment findings are reported semiquantitatively, although the coefficient of variation is high for microsopy.[7] For result interpretation and intersample result comparisons, laboratories should use a standardized technique for urine sediment preparation and evaluation (Box 23.2). The starting volume of urine used to prepare the sediment, the speed and duration of centrifugation, and the volume in which the sediment pellet is resuspended after centrifugation affect the concentration of the urine sediment. Ideally, both a standard starting volume of urine and a standard volume to resuspend the sediment pellet should be used. When possible, 5 mL of well-mixed urine should be centrifuged at 400 to 500 times gravity (*g*) (approximately 1000–1500 revolutions per minute [rpm]) in a conical centrifuge tube for 5 minutes; 4.5 mL of supernatant should be removed and either discarded or saved for subsequent biochemical testing (e.g., urine specific gravity, sulfosalicylic acid precipitation of protein). The sediment pellet should be gently resuspended in 0.5 mL of supernatant, which represents 10% of the original starting volume. When restricted by a lower volume of urine sample, the volume of supernatant used to resuspend the pellet for wet mounting should be accordingly reduced to 10% of the initial volume of urine centrifuged (see Box 23.2). Commercial systems for urine sediment preparation (e.g., Stat-Spin, IRIS International, Inc., Chatsworth, CA; Kova, HYCOR Biomedical, Indianapolis, IN) are available. Adherence to the manufacturer's guidelines will ensure standardized results. The urine sediment pellet may be gently resuspended either by using a disposable transfer pipet to gently aspirate and

expel the contents of the centrifuge tube to form a suspension or by holding the conical centrifuge tube between an index finger and thumb to form a fulcrum and gently flicking the tube with the contralateral index finger to create a weak vortex. Aggressive mixing or mechanical vortexing may degrade fragile structures, such as casts.

To prepare an unstained wet mount, a single drop of the well-mixed pellet suspension should be transferred to a clean glass microscope slide and a coverslip applied. A stained wet mount prepared by using a drop of 0.5% new methylene blue (NMB) or Sternheimer-Malbin stain (Sedi-Stain, Becton Dickinson, Rutherford, NJ) added to the pellet suspension may aid in the identification of nucleated cells, but it is typically not necessary. Addition of stain will dilute the concentration of the sediment or may contaminate the sample with crystals or microorganisms. Semiquantitative results should be determined by using an unstained wet mount, and any crystals or microorganisms that are identified in a stained wet mount should be confirmed in an unstained wet mount. It may be useful to mount a stained wet mount and an unstained wet mount side by side on a single slide. In general, wet mounts should be examined without delay. However, a humidified chamber prepared from a Petri dish, a thin layer of dampened absorbent material, and a halved cotton-tip applicator stick (Fig. 23.1) may be used to temporarily preserve a wet mount in instances when consultation with an in-house colleague is desired.

MICROSCOPIC EXAMINATION OF THE URINE SEDIMENT

To enhance visualization of materials in wet mounts, samples are observed with modified illumination to increase the refraction of formed elements relative to the surrounding liquid. Proper illumination while using a light microscope is achieved either by lowering the substage condenser a few centimeters or by partial closure of the iris diaphragm of the condenser; the latter is considered optically superior. In addition to scanning the entire coverslip, 10 microscopic fields at

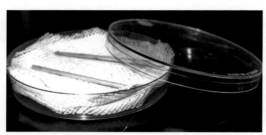

Fig. 23.1 Wet mounts may be temporarily preserved in a humidified Petri dish created by placing dampened material in the bottom of the dish with struts formed from the broken wooden handle of a cotton-tipped applicator.

both 10× and 40× should be examined to determine the concentration of formed elements. Box 23.3 details the steps for systematic microscopic urine sediment evaluation and reporting.

URINE SEDIMENT FINDINGS

Cells (Table 23.4), microorganisms (see Table 23.4), casts (Table 23.5), crystals (Tables 23.6 and 23.7), lipid, and contaminating substances may be found in the urine sediment. Urine obtained from healthy dogs and cats forms little sediment. Small numbers of epithelial cells, mucous threads, erythrocytes, leukocytes, hyaline casts, and various types of crystals may be found in the urine of most healthy animals. Bacteria and squamous epithelial cells derived from external genital surfaces may be present in voided and catheterized urine. When interpreting the urine sediment, it is also necessary to keep in mind the biochemical findings that may influence the sediment content; for example, in dilute urine (specific gravity <1.008) erythrocytes will likely be lysed; highly alkaline urine may reduce the numbers of cells and casts; bacteria influence urine pH (up or down), and urine pH influences crystal formation.

Epithelial Cells

Epithelial cells in urine vary in size, depending on the origin. They are larger in the lower urinary tract versus in the ureters, renal pelves, and renal tubules. It is routine to see fewer than 5 epithelial cells/10× low-power field (lpf) in normal urine samples. At times, it may be challenging to distinguish the different types of epithelial cells. Transitional epithelial cells are highly pleomorphic, and, within the urine fluid, all nucleated cells will become rounded and degrade. When evaluation

---

BOX 23.3 Detailed Steps for Microscopic Urine Sediment Evaluation

- Reduce the illumination of the microscope slide by either lowering the microscope's condenser to a couple centimeters below the stage or by partially closing the aperture of the iris diaphragm within the condenser.
- Scan the entire area of the wet-mount using the 10× objective to find the plane of focus in which material has settled and to detect larger structures, for example, casts, which tend to flow to the edges of the coverslip.
- Examine 10 microscopic fields of the slide from low power using the 10× objective for the presence of the following, and provide an assessment of their amounts in the unstained wet mount:
  - Crystals
    1. Record type(s) present.
    2. Record qualitative impression of the amount of each type of crystal (i.e., none, few, moderate, or many).
  - Casts
    1. May be better visualized at the margins of the coverslip.
    2. Record type(s) present (e.g., hyaline, cellular, granular, waxy).
    3. Record the number of each cast type per 10× low-power field (lpf) as a range (e.g., 0–2/lpf).
  - Epithelial cells
    1. Record type(s) present.
    2. Record the number of each type of epithelial cell per 10× lpf as a range (e.g., 0–4/lpf).
    3. Observe cytomorphology for the presence of dysplastic or neoplastic changes.
  - Mucous threads
    1. Record qualitative impression of the number of mucous threads (none, few, moderate, or many).
  - Helminth ova, larva, adult worms, or other parasites
    1. Record qualitative impression of the number of parasite structures (none, few, moderate, or many).
- Examine 10 microscopic fields of the slide from higher power using the 40× objective.
  - Scrutinize the morphology of structures observed at low power.
    1. Confirm the identification of the structures observed at low power.
    2. Again, inspect epithelial cells for dysplastic or neoplastic cytomorphology.
  - Inspect the slide for the presence of the following things and provide an assessment of their amounts in the unstained wet mount:
    1. Erythrocytes: Record the number of erythrocytes per 40× high-power field (hpf) as a range (e.g., 2–4/hpf).
    2. Leukocytes: Record the number of leukocytes per 40× hpf as a range (e.g., 0–3/hpf).
    3. Microorganisms (e.g., bacteria, yeast, fungi, algae)
       a. Record morphology of bacteria (e.g., cocci, bacilli, filamentous, spore-forming).
       b. Record qualitative impression of the number of each type of microorganism (none, few, moderate, or many).
    4. Lipid droplets
       a. Lipid droplets need to be distinguished from erythrocytes.
       b. Lipid droplets are variably sized, are refractive, and often float above the focal plane.
       c. Record qualitative impression of the number of lipid droplets (none, few, moderate, or many).
    5. Sperm
       a. Record qualitative impression of the number of sperm (none, few, moderate, or many).
    6. Other structures or unidentified structures
       a. Identify the structures or describe their morphology.
       b. Record qualitative impression of the number of these structures (none, few, moderate, or many).

TABLE 23.4 Routine Microscopic Urine Examination: Cells, Cell-like Structures, Microorganisms, Parasites, and Confusing Artifacts

Finding	Normal	Interpretation If Increased	Follow-up
Erythrocytes	<5/hpf	Bleeding—if voided, urethra, prepuce, and vagina (e.g., proestrus, estrus, postpartum) must be considered as well as bladder	Imaging, ultrasonography
			Culture if white blood cells (WBCs) are present
Leukocytes	<3/hpf, by cystocentesis <8/hpf, by catheterization or micturition	Inflammation—if voided, urethra, prepuce, and vagina (e.g., proestrus, estrus, postpartum) must be considered as well as proximal urinary tract	Culture, imaging, ultrasonography
Epithelial cells: Squamous	Rare in samples collected by cystocentesis	Presence of squamous epithelial cells in cystocentesis urine samples suggests squamous metaplasia of urinary bladder transitional cells; consider chronic irritation and/or neoplasia	Imaging, ultrasonography
	Variable by catheterization or micturition	None unless cellular abnormalities are noted	None, unless neoplasia is suspected, then cytology, imaging, and ultrasonography should be considered
Transitional	<5/lpf	Catheterization, inflammation (WBCs should also be present), chronic irritation, neoplasia, chemotherapy	Cytology, imaging, and ultrasonography
Spermatozoa	Occasional in males	None in males; after coitus in females	None
Microorganisms	Depends on collection method	Strongly suggestive of infection if sample collected by cystocentesis or catheterization (usually accompanied by WBCs). Voided samples may be contaminated with organisms from the prepuce, vagina, or vulva	Culture, look for WBCs in urine, check urine protein and glucose, consider possibility of diabetes mellitus, dry-mount cytology
Parasites	None	Fecal contamination, blood contamination, or *Capillaria plica* (bladder worm of dogs and cats) or *Dioctophyma renale* (kidney worm of dogs)	Imaging or ultrasonography if bladder or kidney worm suspected
Fat droplets	cats—frequent	Increased numbers of fat droplets may be seen with lubricants used for catheterization, obesity, diabetes mellitus, and hypothyroidism	Physical examination for evidence of hypothyroidism and obesity, urine and serum glucose for diabetes mellitus
	Dogs—occasional		
Artifacts—air bubbles, glass chips, oil droplets, starch granules, pollen, fungal conidia, feces, yeast, bacteria, parasitical ova	Variable, depending on method of collection	Associated with contamination or slide preparation	Beware of contamination

hpf, high-power field (40× objective); *lpf,* low-power field (10× objective).

TABLE 23.5 Routine Microscopic Urine Examination: Casts and Confusing Artifacts

Cast Type	Normal	Interpretation If Increased	Follow-Up
Hyaline	≤2/lpf in moderately concentrated urine	Diuresis of dehydrated animals or proteinuria of preglomerular (e.g., fever, strenuous exercise, seizures) or renal etiology	Urine and serum protein concentration, physical examination, history
Granular	≤2/lpf in moderately concentrated urine	Acute to subacute renal tubular injury	Physical examination, history, CBC, serum chemistries
Cellular	None	Acute renal tubular injury	Physical examination, history, CBC, serum chemistries
Waxy	None	Chronic renal tubular injury	Physical examination, history, CBC, serum chemistries
Fatty	≤1/lpf	Excessive numbers suggest renal tubule necrosis or degeneration; more commonly seen in cats than dogs; occasionally seen in dogs with diabetes mellitus	Physical examination, history, CBC, serum chemistries (especially glucose)

continued

TABLE 23.5 Routine Microscopic Urine Examination: Casts and Confusing Artifacts—cont'd

Cast Type	Normal	Interpretation If Increased	Follow-Up
Bilirubin	None	Indicate moderate to marked bilirubinuria	Check for hemolysis or hepatobiliary dysfunction
Hemoglobin or myoglobin (red-brown casts)	None	Hemoglobin casts and myoglobin casts both orange to red-brown and cannot be differentiated microscopically; hemoglobin casts occur with intravascular hemolysis, whereas myoglobin casts occur with severe myolysis	Check for intravascular hemolysis (CBC) and muscle injury (serum chemistries, especially LDH, CK, and AST)
Castlike artifacts (mucus threads, fibers)	Occasional	Urethral irritation or contamination with genital secretions	None
Other confusing artifacts: Hair, fecal material, fungal hyphae	None	Associated with contamination or slide preparation	Beware of contamination

AST, aspartate aminotransferase; *CBC,* complete blood count; *CK,* creatine kinase; *LDH,* lactate dehydrogenase; *lpf,* low-power field (10× objective).

TABLE 23.6 Routine Microscopic Urine Examination: Crystals and Confusing Artifacts

Crystal	Causes
Struvite (magnesium ammonium phosphate)	• Refrigerated storage for >1 hour • Commonly seen in clinically normal animals • Urinary tract infection by urease-producing bacteria • Alkaline urine for reasons other than infection (e.g., diet, recent meal, renal tubular ammoniagenesis in cats, postcollection artifact) • Sterile or infection-associated uroliths of potentially mixed mineral composition
Calcium oxalate dihydrate	• Storage for >1 hour with or without refrigeration • Acidic urine (e.g., diet, postcollection artifact) • May be seen in clinically normal animals • Calcium oxalate urolithiasis • Hypercalciuria (e.g., from hypercalcemia or hypercortisolemia) • Hyperoxaluria (e.g., ingestion of oxalate-containing vegetables, ethylene glycol, or chocolate)
Calcium oxalate monohydrate	• Hyperoxaluria (e.g., ingestion of ethylene glycol or uncommonly chocolate)
Calcium carbonate	• Anecdotally reported rarely in dogs and cats • Sulfonamide crystals with similar morphology may be mistaken for calcium carbonate
Bilirubin	• A low number commonly found in concentrated canine urine, especially males • Altered bilirubin metabolism (e.g., hemolytic or hepatobiliary diseases)
Amorphous phosphates	• Insignificant finding in clinically normal animals
Amorphous urates—uric acid, ammonium biurate	• Portovascular malformation • Severe hepatic disease • Ammonium biurate urolithiasis • Breed-associated: Dalmatians, English Bulldogs, Weimaraners, others; may represent risk factor for urolithiasis, especially in males
Cystine	• Defect in proximal renal tubular transport of amino acids; represents risk factor for urolithiasis
Iatrogenic	• Antibiotic administration (e.g., sulfonamides, ciprofloxacin) • Other drugs: anticonvulsants (particularly with polytherapy, alkaline urine, and certain drugs), xanthine crystals with allopurinol administration • Radiocontrast medium crystals
Artifacts from contamination or slide preparation	• Starch granules • Glass chips • Fecal material and microorganisms • Pollen • Fungal microconidia or macroconidia

TABLE 23.7 pH Influence on Crystalluria

Crystal	Acidic Urine	Neutral Urine	Alkaline Urine
Ammonium biurate	✓	✓	
Amorphous phosphates			✓
Amorphous urates	✓		
Bilirubin	✓		
Calcium carbonate			✓
Calcium oxalate dihydrate	✓	✓	✓ (in stored samples)
Calcium oxalate monohydrate	✓	✓	
Cystine	✓	✓	
Drug metabolites	✓	✓	✓
Struvite		✓	✓
Uric acid	✓		

of cell morphology is critical, urine sediment dry-mount cytology is useful for examination in-house or in a reference laboratory. A greater number of epithelial cells are seen in urine samples collected by transurethral catheterization or in patients with inflamed, hyperplastic, or neoplastic mucosa. Methods to diagnose structural lesions within the urinary tract (e.g., ultrasonography, traumatic catheter biopsy, FNB, surgical biopsy imprint, *braf* mutation detection assay[8]) are often more conclusive than urinalysis alone.

Squamous Epithelial Cells

Squamous epithelial cells line the distal third of the urethra, the vagina, and the prepuce and are usually not considered significant. It is useful to note that squamous epithelial cells are the largest cell from the patient found in the urine sediment. They are flat or rolled cells that have at least one angular border and either a single small, condensed nucleus or no nucleus (Figs. 23.2, Fig. 23.3; see Figs. 23.16, 23.17, and 23.18 later in the chapter).

Squamous epithelial cells are most commonly observed with lower genitourinary tract contamination of voided or catheterized samples. Squamous epithelial cells are typically not present in samples collected

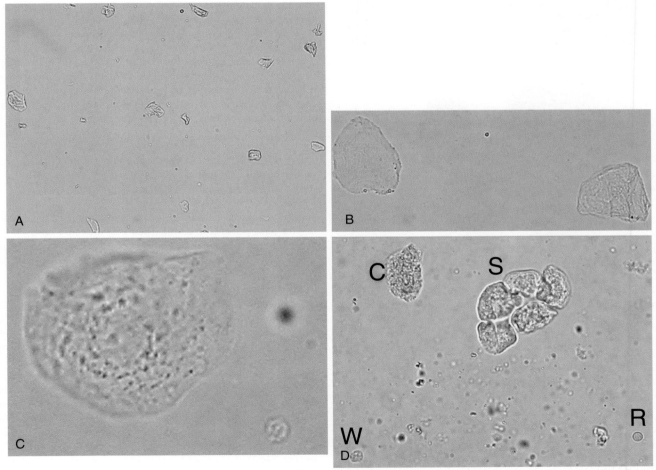

Fig. 23.2 A, Voided urine sediment with squamous epithelial cells, which are lying flat or partially twisted (unstained, original magnification 100×). B, Two anucleate squamous epithelial cells with one of more angular borders. A small lipid droplet is in the center (unstained, original magnification 400×). C, Nucleated squamous epithelial cell with granular cytoplasm with a crenated erythrocyte *(lower right)*. Note the relative size of these cells (unstained, original magnification 400×). D, A sheet of squamous epithelial cells (*S*), a leukocyte (*W*), an erythrocyte (*R*), and a granular cast fragment (*C*) (same dog as in Fig. 23.40). The erythrocyte is biconcave and more translucent than the epithelial cells and the leukocyte. Small, refractive amorphous crystals are scattered in the background (unstained, original magnification 400×).

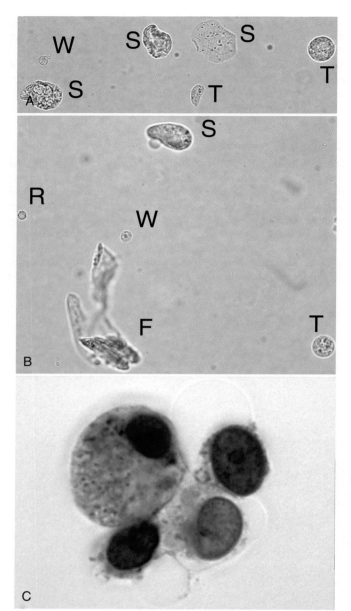

Fig. 23.3 (A) Two transitional epithelial cells (*T*), three squamous epithelial cells (*S*), and one leukocyte (*W*). Note the relative size and varied appearance of these cells (unstained, original magnification 400×). (B) Note the relative size and appearance of a rounded squamous epithelial cell (*S*), a transitional epithelial cell (*T*), a leukocyte (*W*), and an erythrocyte (*R*). A segmented nucleus is visible in the leukocyte, and the erythrocyte is a ghost. A contaminating fiber (*F*) is present in several focal planes (unstained, original magnification 400×). C, Four variably sized transitional epithelial cells (NMB stain, original magnification 1000×).

through cystocentesis. A high number of squamous epithelial cells are rarely seen in cystocentesis samples because of the presence of squamous cell carcinoma of the bladder or squamous metaplasia of the bladder—which may occur with transitional cell carcinoma or chronic bladder irritation—or because of misdirection of the needle into the uterus. Squamous metaplasia of the prostate is another uncommon source of squamous cells in the urine sediment.

Transitional Epithelial Cells

Transitional epithelial cells line the proximal two thirds of the urethra, bladder, ureters, and renal pelves. They are highly pleomorphic,

variably sized cells that are smaller than squamous epithelial cells and two to four times larger than leukocytes. Those originating in the proximal urethra and bladder are the largest. They may be round, oval, pear-shaped, polygonal, or caudate and often have granular cytoplasm with a single nucleus that is larger than that of squamous epithelial cells (see Fig. 23.3; see Figs. 23.22 and Fig. 23.51 later in the chapter).

There should be fewer than five transitional epithelial cells/10× lpf in the normal urine sediment. Higher numbers are seen in urine samples collected via catheterization or from patients with inflamed (Fig. 23.4), hyperplastic, or neoplastic mucosa. Urolithiasis and some chemotherapeutic agents (e.g., cyclophosphamide) may induce epithelial hyperplasia with mild to moderate atypia (Fig. 23.5). Variable numbers of epithelial cells and leukocytes are found in the urine sediment from animals with transitional cell carcinomas. Neoplastic epithelial cells may be present individually, in small aggregates, or in variably sized, cohesive sheets. They are usually larger than normal and exhibit darker blue cytoplasm, increased nucleus-to-cytoplasm (N:C) ratio, and other malignant features (Figs. 23.6 to 23.8). Eccentric eosinophilic cytoplasmic inclusions (i.e., Melamed-Wolinska bodies) are commonly seen but are not specific for transitional cell carcinoma. Knowledge of clinical context is important when determining the significance of atypical epithelial cells in the urine sediment, for example, the presence of uroliths, the presence of urinary tract mass, or medication administration.

If a large number of atypical epithelial cells are found, then dry-mount sediment cytology should be prepared and evaluated (see Box 23.1). Dry-mount cytology (see Fig. 23.7) is the best means to avoid degraded cytomorphology caused by transport delay. Slides prepared in this manner may be shipped either stained or unstained to a reference laboratory. Concurrent inflammation, infection, and poor preservation of atypical cells often confounds diagnosis of neoplasia from the urine sediment alone (see Fig. 23.8, A). Evaluation of cells obtained directly from a mass by traumatic catheterization (see Fig. 23.8, B), ultrasound-guided FNB (Fig. 23.9), or surgical biopsy imprint (see Fig. 23.7, B) is often helpful for diagnosis.

Caudate Transitional Epithelial Cells

Smaller transitional epithelial cells with caudate morphology specifically line the renal pelves (Fig. 23.10). These cells are rarely observed in the urine sediment. They are an abnormal finding that may be seen in patients with renal pelves disease, for example, pyelonephritis, renal pelvic calculi.

Renal Tubular Epithelial Cells

Renal tubular epithelial cells are cuboidal to low columnar, with a moderate amount of cytoplasm and a single eccentric, round nucleus (Fig. 23.11, A). Once exfoliated, these cells often become small and rounded within urine (see Fig. 23.11, B and C). This makes it very challenging to distinguish them from leukocytes and small transitional epithelial cells. Great caution is often needed in their identification. Observation of a large number of these rounded cells with consistently eccentric nucleus or with their cuboidal–to–low columnar morphology intact would indicate active renal tubular disease (see Fig. 23.11). Renal tubular epithelial cells may contain variably sized, refractive lipid vacuoles; cells with this morphology are sometimes referred to as *oval fat bodies* (Fig. 23.12). A few lipid-laden renal tubular cells may be a normal finding in feline urine. They are also sometimes present in urine from animals with nephrotic syndrome or other causes of lipiduria.

Spermatozoa

Spermatozoa are occasionally seen in the urine sediment of intact or recently castrated males, and rarely in intact females after coitus. They are easily recognized and typically have no clinical significance (see Figs. 23.19, 23.21, and 23.47, B, later in the chapter).

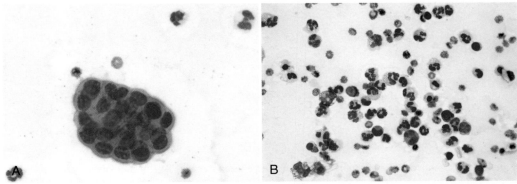

Fig. 23.4 Urine sediment dry-mount cytology from a Labrador Retriever with chronic cystitis. (A) A tightly cohesive, mildly atypical, small sheet of transitional epithelial cells with high nuclear-to-cytoplasmic ratio, but minimal size and shape variation is present with three mildly degenerate neutrophils. (B) Another microscopic field from the same sample that demonstrates mixed inflammation. A few of the neutrophils are pyknotic (Wright-Giemsa stain, original magnification of both images 500×).

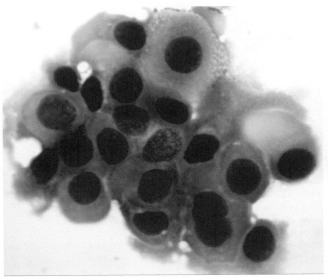

Fig. 23.5 Urine sediment dry-mount cytology from a cat with urolithiasis. Sheet of moderately atypical transitional epithelial cells, as evidenced by increased nuclear-to-cytoplasmic ratio, anisocytosis, anisokaryosis, pleomorphism, binucleation, coarse chromatin, and single prominent nucleoli. Case presentation is important when determining the significance of atypia in transitional epithelial cells (Wright-Giemsa stain, original magnification 500×).

Erythrocytes and Lipid Droplets

Erythrocytes are translucent and may be pale orange in color because of their hemoglobin content. The shape of erythrocytes varies with urine tonicity. They may maintain their biconcave disk morphology; shrivel, becoming crenated in concentrated urine; or swell, becoming rounded in dilute urine (see Fig. 23.12, A; Fig. 23.13; see Figs. 23.16 through 23.20, 23.50, and 23.51 later in the chapter). Erythrocytes may lyse in very dilute or highly alkaline urine. Generally, there should be less than 5 erythrocytes/40× high-power field (hpf). However, the number observed is influenced by collection method (e.g., cystocentesis, catheterization). Hematuria is nonspecific and may be seen with infection, inflammation, necrosis, neoplasia, hemorrhagic diathesis, toxicity (e.g., cyclophosphamide), trauma, and glomerular disease. Voided samples from females in proestrus, in estrus, or after parturition often contain erythrocytes from the genital tract.

Lipid droplets are variably sized, refractive, flat disks that are usually smaller than erythrocytes, often float above the focal plane

in which the cells settle, and never exhibit the biconcave appearance of erythrocytes (Figs. 23.14 and 23.15; see Figs. 23.21 and 23.24 later in the chapter). Beyond their potential to be misidentified as erythrocytes, lipid droplets typically are of little significance. They are common in normal feline urine and may be increased with obesity, diabetes mellitus, hypothyroidism, and other causes of lipiduria.

Erythrocytes are the smallest cell that may come from the patient, and squamous epithelial cells are the largest (Fig. 23.16). Confident identification of erythrocytes and squamous epithelial cells may be useful when trying to identify intermediate-size cells, such as leukocytes or transitional epithelial cells (Fig. 23.17; see Fig. 23.3, B). Erythrocytes are more translucent than leukocytes and transitional epithelial cells, both of which contain nuclei and often a stippled cytoplasm.

Leukocytes

In animals without genitourinary disease, few leukocytes are observed in the urine sediment. In samples collected by cystocentesis, less than three leukocytes/40× hpf should be present. In samples collected by catheterization or midstream voiding, less than 8 leukocytes/40× hpf should be present. Leukocytes are intermediate in size compared with other cells from the patient that may be present in the sediment (Fig. 23.18; see Figs. 23.2, 23.3, and 23.17). They are usually round and stippled that transmits less light compared with erythrocytes (see Fig. 23.14; Fig. 23.19, A). Segmented nuclei are sometimes visible in unstained wet mounts (Fig. 23.20; see Fig. 23.55 later in the chapter); nuclei are more easily identified in stained wet mounts (Fig. 23.21) or in the dry-mount cytology of the urine sediment pellet (see Figs. 23.18, B; 23.19, B; and 23.26 later in the chapter). Some leukocytes contain granules that are occasionally visible as refractive structures within the cytoplasm exhibiting Brownian motion. These cells are sometimes referred to as *glitter cells* (see Fig. 23.21).

When neutrophils are present in increased number, even if bacteria are not detected in the sediment wet mount, the urine sample should be cultured because microscopic examination is much less sensitive than culture for detecting bacteria. At least 10,000 bacilli/mL or 100,000 cocci/mL are required for detection by light microscopy. When leukocytes are increased but bacteria are not visible in the wet mount, it is useful to prepare a dry-mount cytology of the urine sediment pellet (see Box 23.1). This technique is a more sensitive microscopic method to detect bacteria compared with wet

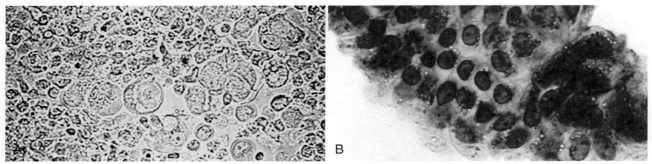

Fig. 23.6 Urine sediment wet mounts from a dog with a bladder mass. (A) The large atypical epithelial cells are so abundant that most cellular detail is obscured. A few very large individualized cells are visible *(center)* (unstained, original magnification 100×). (B) Stained wet-mount from the same case showing a large, cohesive sheet of atypical epithelial cells (NMB stain, original magnification 400×).

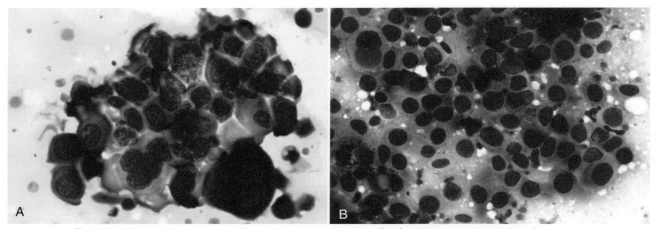

Fig. 23.7 Urine sediment dry-mount cytology and postmortem Tru-Cut biopsy imprint cytology from a toy poodle with transitional cell carcinoma of the bladder. (A) Urine sediment dry-mount cytology has indefinitely preserved the markedly abnormal cytomorphology of these sloughed cells. The concurrent observation of a bladder trigone mass, abundant epithelial cells bearing numerous malignant criteria, and the absence of concurrent inflammation permitted confident cytodiagnosis of transitional cell carcinoma in this case. (B) Imprint of postmortem Tru-Cut biopsy of the mass from the same dog reveals similar atypia and lack of inflammation (Wright-Giemsa stain, original magnification of both images 500×).

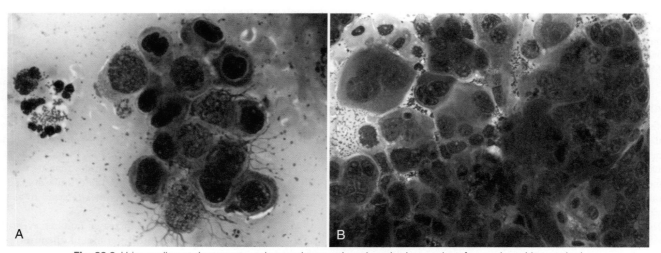

Fig. 23.8 Urine sediment dry-mount cytology and traumatic catheterization cytology from a dog with a urethral transitional cell carcinoma. (A) Poor cellular preservation and concurrent inflammation or infection may confound definitive diagnosis of neoplasia based on urine sediment alone. Neutrophils with phagocytized bacteria are present along with a cohesive sheet of partially degraded, moderately atypical epithelial cells. Purple nucleoproteinaceous material is streaming from lysed cells. (B) The urethral mass traumatic catheterization cytology yielded cells with intact cytomorphology, including a papillary projection *(top right)*, and dramatic malignant features (e.g., cellular disorganization, size variation, multinucleation, nuclear molding, pleomorphism, coarse chromatin, prominent and multiple nucleoli) (Wright-Giemsa stain, original magnification of both images 1000×).

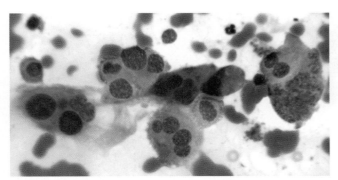

Fig. 23.9 Fine-needle biopsy (FNB) of a renal mass from a dog. Many large cells with several malignant features (e.g., multinucleation, abnormal mitosis, size variation, pleomorphism, karyomegaly) were obtained by FNB from this renal carcinoma (Wright-Giemsa stain, original magnification 500×).

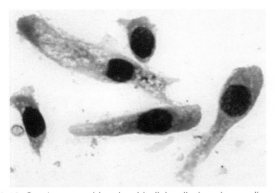

Fig. 23.10 Caudate transitional epithelial cells in urine sediment dry-mount cytology from a cat with chronic renal failure. The cells are elongated-pyriform with a unipolar round or oval nucleus (Wright-Giemsa stain, original magnification 1000×).

mounting, and bacterial morphology is accurately identified more often with this method.[2,3]

The absence of pyuria does not exclude urinary tract infection. Immunosuppressed animals may develop infection without detectable leukocytes (i.e., "silent urinary tract infection," which may be seen with hypercortisolemia, diabetes mellitus, and other immunosuppressed states) (Fig. 23.22). Also, with polyuric conditions (e.g., pyelonephritis), which are associated with production of large volumes of dilute urine, leukocytes and bacteria may be diluted below the detection limit of light microscopy. Urine culture is considered a more definitive test for detecting infection.

Observation of pyuria with concurrent bacteriuria indicates active urinary tract inflammation with either primary or secondary bacterial infection (Fig. 23.23; see Figs. 23.26 and 23.55 later in the chapter). Urine culture is useful to characterize microorganisms and to determine their antimicrobial sensitivities. Pyuria can also be seen with urolithiasis, neoplasms (see Fig. 23.8, A), prostatitis, and pyometra and with less common infections caused by viruses, mycoplasmas, or ureaplasmas. Cystocentesis may avoid contamination of the urine sample by leukocytes from the genital tract and aid in localizing the source of pyuria.

Bacteria and Other Infectious Organisms

Normal urine is free of microorganisms, but organisms in the vagina, vulva, or prepuce may contaminate urine during micturition. Bacteria are the most common microorganisms in urine (see

Fig. 23.23; Fig. 23.24). In voided samples analyzed after a delay in transport to a reference laboratory, yeast consistent with *Candida* (see Fig. 23.28 later in the chapter) and environmental fungi with pigmented macroconidia are common. In cystocentesis samples, observation of fungal hyphae is abnormal (see Fig. 23.29 later in the chapter). Bacteria proliferate in urine that has been standing at room temperature, it is important to either perform microscopic examination immediately or refrigerate the sample until microscopic examination can be performed, regardless of the urine collection method. Bacteria are very small and can be identified only at high magnifications. They may be round (cocci), rod shaped (bacilli) (see Figs. 23.22 through 23.24), filamentous (Fig. 23.25), or spore forming and usually refract light and quiver because of Brownian motion. When examining wet mounts for definitive identification of cocci, it is helpful to identify structures that are very uniformly spherical in short chains or doublets (see Fig. 23.24; see Fig. 23.62 later in the chapter). If doubt exists, dry-mount sediment cytology is beneficial (Fig. 23.26). The presence of a high number of bacteria accompanied by a high number of leukocytes indicates infection accompanied by inflammation of the urinary tract, genital tract, or both, depending on how the sample was obtained (see Figs. 23.23 and 23.26). Usually, when bacteria are observed without accompanying increase in leukocytes, it is likely that the sample has been contaminated (e.g., by external genitalia or nonsterile collection materials) (Fig. 23.27), bacteria in the sample have overgrown because of delayed urinalysis and lack of refrigeration, the observer is mistaking amorphous mineral precipitates for bacteria, or, less commonly, there is silent urinary tract infection (see Fig. 23.22). When bacteria or other microorganisms are observed in a stained wet mount, it is useful to distinguish them from stain contaminants by confirming their presence in an unstained wet mount or by sediment dry-mount cytology.

Although bacteria may be confidently identified during urinalysis, urine cultures may occasionally be negative. Reasons for this disparity, for example, antimicrobial administration before sample collection, are listed in Box 23.4. Uncommon infections by viruses or highly fastidious microorganisms (e.g., *Mycoplasma*, *Ureaplasma*) may yield negative urine culture results, even when infection is truly present.

Dependent on geographical distribution, other infectious organisms, such as fungi (e.g., *Candida* [Fig. 23.28], *Aspergillus* [Figs. 23.29 to 23.31], *Blastomyces dermatitidis*, *Cryptococcus*); algae (e.g., *Prototheca* [Figs. 23.32 and 23.33]); and nematode ova, larvae, or adults (e.g., *Capillaria* [Fig. 23.34], *Dirofilaria immitis* [Fig. 23.35], *Dioctophyma renale*) are occasionally identified in urine sediment.

Yeast organisms may be confused with red blood cells (RBCs) or lipid droplets, but yeast organisms usually display characteristic budding, often have double refractive walls, and do not dissolve in acetic acid (see Fig. 23.28). They can result from lower urinary tract contamination, secondary to long-term antibiotic administration, or diabetes mellitus–associated infection.

Fungal hyphae (see Fig. 23.29) are larger than bacteria and are long, branched structures with parallel walls and perpendicular septa. Primary fungal infections of the urinary tract are uncommon. Systemic mycosis in German Shepherds or immunosuppressed patients may affect the kidneys (see Figs. 23.30 and 23.31) and the lower urinary tract. Urine sediment evaluation is also useful when evaluating suspected discospondylitis cases.

Trichuris (whipworm) ova may be present in samples contaminated by feces or enteric contents. These ova are similar to *Capillaria plica* ova (see Fig. 23.34) but have important distinguishing features. The bipolar opercula of *Capillaria* ova are slightly askew, rather than being perfectly bipolar as they are in *Trichuris* ova. The shells of *Capillaria* ova are knobby (i.e., mammillated), rather than perfectly smooth as they are

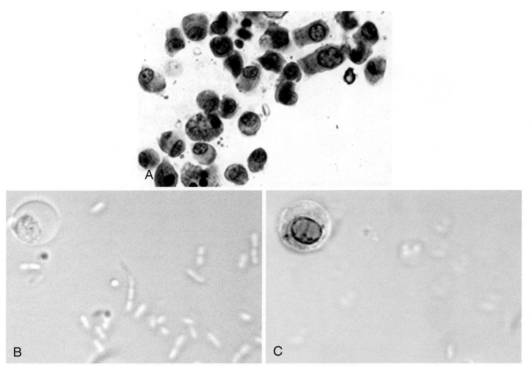

Fig. 23.11 Urine sediment wet mounts with renal tubular epithelial cells. (A) Several individualized cells that can be confidently identified as renal tubular epithelial cells based on their cuboidal or oval shape with eccentric nuclei (NMB stain, original magnification 400×). (B) Renal tubular epithelial cells *(upper left)* tend to become rounded once sloughed, which makes distinction from small transitional epithelial cells challenging. Several bacilli are also in the background (unstained, original magnification 1000×). (C) Same specimen as shown in image B (NMB stain, original magnification 1000×).

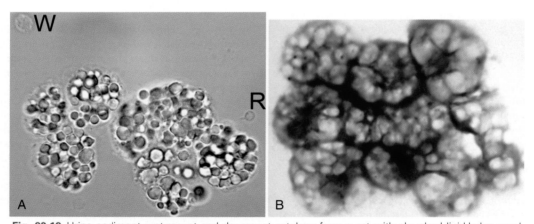

Fig. 23.12 Urine sediment wet-mount and dry-mount cytology from a cat with sloughed lipid-laden renal tubular epithelial cells, sometimes referred to as *oval fat bodies*. (A) A small group of round cells contain several refractive lipid vacuoles that project three-dimensionally from the focal plane. A leukocyte (*W*) and an erythrocyte ghost (*R*) are also present (unstained, original magnification 500×). (B) Dry-mount sediment cytology of the same specimen shown in image A exhibits an aggregate of partially degraded, lipid-laden renal tubular epithelial cells (Wright-Giemsa stain, original magnification 500×).

in *Trichuris* ova. *Capillaria* may be an incidental finding in the urine of asymptomatic cats. However, *Capillaria* ova are rarely identified in cats with lower urinary tract signs, which resolve after appropriate treatment.

When evaluating the importance of potentially infectious organisms in urine, it is important to consider whether clinical and microscopic evidence of urinary tract irritation or inflammation exists or if the animal has a condition that might inhibit such an inflammatory reaction (e.g., diabetes mellitus, hypercortisolemia). To assess the

likelihood of contamination, consideration should also be given to the method of collection and the subsequent handling of the urine sample.

Casts and Castlike Artifacts

Casts (see Table 23.5) are formed in the lumen of the distal nephron (i.e., Henle loop, distal tubule, collecting duct). The increased concentration and acidity of the urine in the tubules promotes

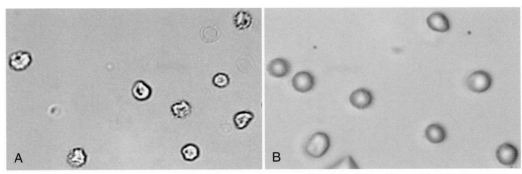

Fig. 23.13 Urine sediment wet mounts showing the effects of urine tonicity on erythrocyte appearance. Erythrocytes usually are pale orange-red because of the presence of hemoglobin and may maintain their biconcave shape. (A) Shriveled, crenated, and ghost erythrocytes are present in highly concentrated urine. (B) Swollen, round erythrocytes are present in dilute urine (unstained, original magnification both images 500×).

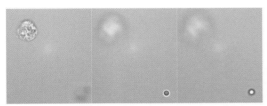

Fig. 23.14 Three images of the same urine sediment wet-mount field showing a flat, round, refractive lipid droplet *(lower right)* that is floating above the focal plane of a leukocyte *(upper left)* with granular cytoplasm and visible nuclear lobule (unstained, original magnification all images 1000×).

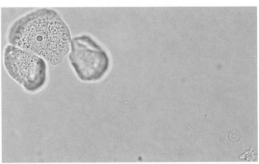

Fig. 23.16 Urine sediment wet mount with three large angular squamous epithelial cells *(upper left)* and a crenated erythrocyte *(lower right)*. The squamous epithelial cell in the center has a small, round, condensed nucleus. Note the relative size of the cells (unstained, original magnification 400×).

Fig. 23.15 Urine sediment wet mount with multiple variably sized, flat, round, refractive lipid droplets (unstained, original magnification 400×).

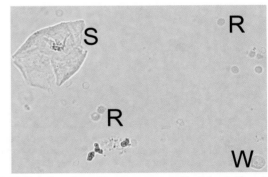

Fig. 23.17 Relative sizes of a squamous epithelial cell (*S*), a leukocyte (*W*), and several erythrocytes that are often crenated (*R*) and a few erythrocytes ghosts in a urine sediment wet mount. A few amorphous crystals are also in the background (unstained, original magnification 400×).

precipitation of protein present in the tubules. Because casts are formed in the renal tubules, they are cylindrical with parallel sides. When the cells in the tubules die and exfoliate, they are often incorporated into the precipitated meshlike mucoprotein matrix (i.e., Tamm-Horsfall mucoprotein). During microscopic evaluation of the urine sediment, cellular casts are further classified as epithelial, leukocyte, or erythrocyte casts, if the constituent cells can be discerned, which is rare. Once locked within the proteinaceous matrix, cells continue to degrade, progressing from intact cells, to granular cellular remnants, and finally to a waxy, cholesterol-rich end product. A renal tubular cast may dislodge at any time during this degenerative process and may be observed in the urine sediment.

Other materials, such as lipid from degenerated renal tubular epithelial cells, hemoglobin during hemolytic disease, and bilirubin, may be trapped within the proteinaceous matrix. Casts are fragile and prone to degeneration, particularly in alkaline urine; therefore, fresh urine and proper technique should be used when preparing specimens for evaluation. In most instances, cylindruria—casts in the urine sediment— is an insensitive, but specific, indicator of renal tubular disease. The number of casts present does not predict the severity or reversibility of disease.

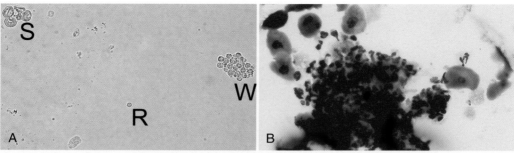

Fig. 23.18 (A) Aggregates of squamous epithelial cells (*S*) and leukocytes (*W*) with an erythrocyte (*R*). Note the relative sizes of the cells (unstained, original magnification 400×). (B) Urine sediment dry-mount cytology of the same case with epithelial cells and a large clump of neutrophils (Wright-Giemsa stain, original magnification 500×).

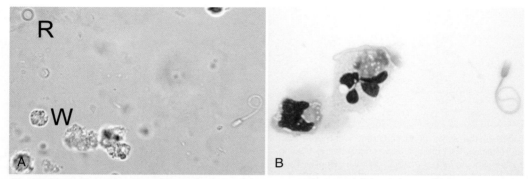

Fig. 23.19 (A) The leukocytes (*W*) are stippled and do not transmit as much light as the smaller erythrocyte (*R*). A sperm is present on the right (unstained, original magnification 1000×). (B) Urine sediment dry-mount cytology of the same case with two leukocytes and two sperm (Wright-Giemsa stain, original magnification 1000×).

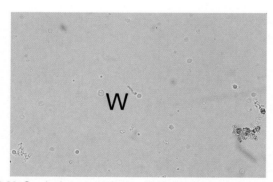

Fig. 23.20 One leukocyte (*W*) with a U-shaped nucleus is present along with several erythrocytes and variably sized aggregates of amorphous crystals (unstained, original magnification 400×).

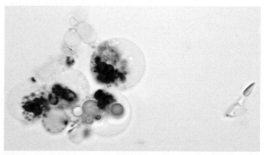

Fig. 23.21 A group of neutrophils in which the granules are visible and refractive. In the wet mount, the neutrophil granules may exhibit Brownian movement; these cells may be referred to as *glitter cells* by some. Lipid droplets overlay and surround the leukocytes, and a sperm is present *(right)* (NMB stain, original magnification 1000×).

Very low numbers (i.e., 0–2/10× lpf) of hyaline or granular casts may be seen in normal urine, but higher numbers of casts suggest a renal tubular lesion. The number of casts observed in the sediment does not correlate with the severity of renal disease or its reversibility; and the absence of casts from the urine sediment cannot be used to exclude the possibility of renal disease. When hyaline or granular casts are present in increased numbers or when other cast types are observed, the only conclusion is that the renal tubules are diseased, but the severity and reversibility remain indeterminate. The type of cast observed may provide additional information. Leukocyte casts indicate active renal tubulointerstitial inflammation. Waxy casts reflect a chronic tubular lesion. To recognize the onset of nephrotoxicity in patients receiving aminoglycoside antibiotic therapy, it is useful to

monitor the urine sediment for the appearance of tubular casts, which should prompt withdrawal of the antibiotic. Other abnormalities seen with aminoglycoside-induced nephrotoxicity include isosthenuria, proteinuria, glucosuria, and aminoaciduria, all of which may precede the onset of azotemia.

Mucous threads or fibers, which are much more common than cylindruria, should not be mistaken for casts during evaluation of the urine sediment. Mucus threads are distinguished by their variable width, curvilinear shape, and tapered ends (Fig. 23.36). Mucous threads are an expected finding in horses and may also be seen with urethral irritation or contamination by genital secretions. Fibers are typically larger than the surrounding cells and may contain a repetitive

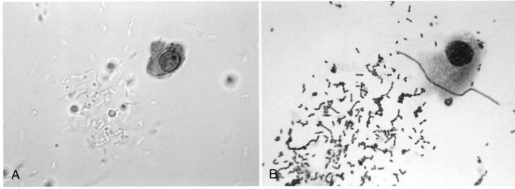

Fig. 23.22 Diabetic canine cystocentesis urine sediment. (A) Many bacilli and chains of cocci are present with a transitional epithelial cell. Note the lack of inflammatory response (NMB stain, original magnification 1000×). (B) Urine sediment dry-mount cytology of the same case permits reliable identification of bacterial morphology. A lysed transitional epithelial cell is also present (Wright-Giemsa stain, original magnification 1000×).

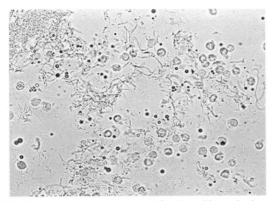

Fig. 23.23 Evidence of a urinary tract infection with marked pyuria and numerous bacilli in mats and long chains. Small, refractive lipid droplets are dispersed throughout the field (unstained, original magnification 400×).

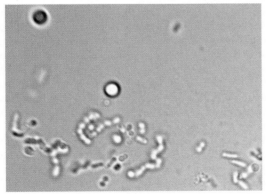

Fig. 23.24 Urine sediment with bacilli and chains of cocci with two refractive lipid droplets (unstained, original magnification 1000×).

internal geometric structure (Figs. 23.37 and 23.38; see Fig. 23.57, A, later in the chapter).

Hyaline Casts

A few (i.e., 0–2/10× lpf) hyaline casts, which are clear, colorless, and refractive, may be seen in moderately concentrated urine from animals without renal disease (Fig. 23.39). Similar to all casts, hyaline casts are cylindrical, with parallel sides and rounded termini. Diuresis of dehydrated animals or proteinuria of preglomerular (e.g., fever, strenuous exercise, seizures) or renal etiology may cause an increased number of hyaline casts in urine.

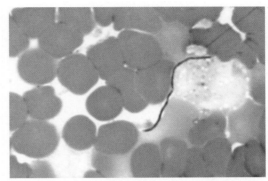

Fig. 23.25 Urine sediment dry-mount cytology with a filamentous bacterium and hematuria (Wright-Giemsa stain, original magnification 1000×).

Hyaline casts may also be increased with renal tubular disease, which should typically be accompanied by an abnormally low urine specific gravity.

Granular Casts

Granular casts are commonly seen in urine sediment (see Fig. 23.38; Figs. 23.40 and 23.41). A few (i.e., 0–2/10× lpf) granular casts may be seen in moderately concentrated urine from animals without renal disease. Granular casts may be increased with renal tubular injury and are more specific than hyaline casts.

Cellular Casts

Cellular casts may contain epithelial cells, leukocytes, or erythrocytes (see Figs. 23.38; Fig. 23.42). Epithelial cell casts are formed when dead epithelial cells are sloughed intact from the renal tubules and the cast is passed into the urine before the cells degenerate to granular material. Leukocyte casts are uncommon but indicate active tubulointerstitial inflammation. Erythrocyte casts are also uncommon but may form with renal hemorrhage. Granular casts usually accompany cellular casts, and mixed casts may occur (see Fig. 23.38; Fig. 23.43).

Waxy Casts

Waxy casts (see Fig. 23.38; Fig. 23.44), which indicate chronic tubular injury, look somewhat like hyaline casts but usually are wider, have blunt, square ends instead of round, and are dull, homogenous, and waxy (see Fig. 23.44; Fig. 23.45). They are more opaque than hyaline casts and may appear to have fissures. Broad waxy casts are sloughed from distal tubules and indicate chronic renal tubular disease (see Fig. 23.43)

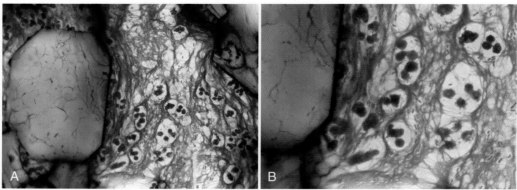

Fig. 23.26 Canine urinary tract infection with struvite crystalluria. (A) Urine sediment dry-mount cytology with struvite crystalluria, many degenerate neutrophils, abundant bacteria, and streaming, purple nucleoprotein (Wright-Giemsa stain, original magnification 500×). (B) Close examination facilitates accurate characterization of bacterial morphology, in this case bacilli (Wright-Giemsa stain, original magnification 1000×).

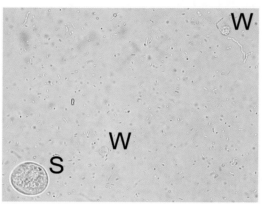

Fig. 23.27 Voided urine sediment with abundant bacteria that are present individually and in chains. Although two leukocytes (*W*) are present in the field, their overall concentration is not increased. A squamous epithelial cell (*S*) is also present (unstained, original magnification 400×).

BOX 23.4 Causes of a Negative Urine Culture Despite Identification of Bacteria in the Urine Sediment

- Observed bacteria represent contaminants of the urine sample incurred during collection or processing.
- Observed bacteria may actually be nonbacterial structures in the sediment that were mistakenly identified as bacteria during urinalysis.
- Observed bacteria may be not viable or may be "viable, but nonculturable" by routine method as a result of:
  - Prior antimicrobial administration.
  - Prolonged urine storage.
  - Fastidious nutritional and culture requirements.
  - Exposure to chemical or environmental stress (e.g., nutrient deficiency, oxygen lack, pH, temperature extreme, salinity, others).
- Observed bacteria may not grow because of improper culture technique.

Fatty Casts

Fatty casts contain many small fat droplets, which are round, highly refractive structures (Fig. 23.46). They are frequently seen in cats because cats have fat in their renal tubular epithelial cells and are occasionally seen in dogs with diabetes mellitus. A high number of fatty casts suggest renal tubule degeneration.

Other Casts

Casts are occasionally mixed with other materials, such as bilirubin, hemoglobin, myoglobin, or crystalline precipitates (i.e., calcium oxalate monohydrate).[9] Bilirubin-stained casts indicate the presence of moderate to marked bilirubinuria (see Fig. 23.45). Hemoglobin and myoglobin both impart a red to red-brown tint. The presence of hemoglobin casts and precipitates suggests intravascular hemolysis (Fig. 23.47, A and B). Myoglobin-stained casts or precipitates may be seen with severe myolysis (see Fig. 23.47, C and D).

Crystals

Crystals are identified and reported semiquantitatively per 10× lpf. When urine is saturated with dissolved minerals or other crystallogenic substances that precipitate, crystalluria occurs. Crystals may form in vivo for either pathological or nonpathological reasons, or crystals may precipitate ex vivo because of cold temperature, prolonged storage, postcollection alterations of urine pH, or evaporation of water from the sample (Tables 23.6 and 23.7). To increase the likelihood of crystals present in urine sediment being representative of those in vivo, fresh, nonrefrigerated urine specimens that have been collected into a single-use container should be analyzed within 30 to 60 minutes of sampling.[5,6]

Decisions about when crystalluria may be clinically significant are based on other urine sediment findings and case presentations. Detection of crystalluria may be diagnostically useful when abnormal crystal types are identified (e.g., ammonium biurate, calcium oxalate monohydrate, cystine); when struvite or calcium oxalate dihydrate crystals are found along with pyuria or hematuria; or when crystalluria is observed in a patient that has confirmed urolithiasis. In most instances, crystalluria does not necessarily indicate the presence of uroliths or even a predisposition to form uroliths. For individuals with urolithiasis confirmed on diagnostic imaging or bladder palpation, determination of crystalluria type may be useful to estimate the mineral content of the urolith(s) while results of complete urolith analysis are pending. Uroliths are often heterogeneous; therefore crystalluria type cannot be used as the sole indicator of urolith mineral content. Sequential evaluation of crystalluria may aid in monitoring a patient's response to urolith dissolution therapy.

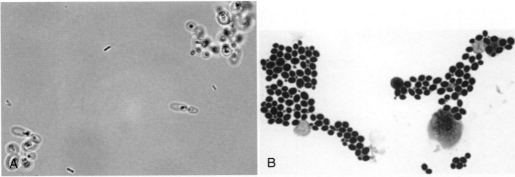

Fig. 23.28 Yeast in feline cystocentesis urine sediment after chronic antibiotic administration. (A) Small, budding yeast are present individually and in two aggregates with scant amorphous crystals (unstained, original magnification 1000×). (B) Urine sediment dry-mount cytology of the same case with numerous small, budding yeast, consistent with *Candida*. A few erythrocytes and a degraded epithelial cell are also present (Wright-Giemsa stain, original magnification 1000×).

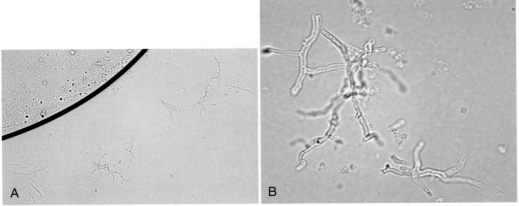

Fig. 23.29 Canine systemic fungal infection after chronic immunosuppressant administration. (A) Urine sediment with three mats of fungal hyphae, pyuria, hematuria, and an air bubble artifact *(top left)* (unstained, original magnification 200×). (B) Perpendicular septa are visible in the branching fungal hyphae; pyuria is also present. Compare with bacilli growing in chains in Fig. 23.23 (unstained, original magnification 500×). Fig. 23.30 shows renal fine-needle biopsy (FNB) specimen of the same case.

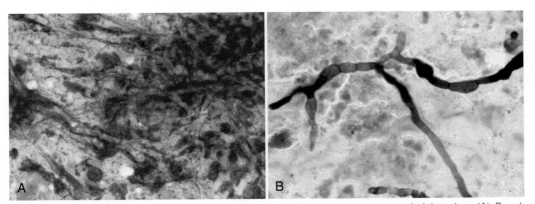

Fig. 23.30 Canine systemic fungal infection after chronic immunosuppressant administration. (A) Renal fine-needle biopsy (FNB) specimen with a dense mat of negatively stained, branched fungal hyphae, which is outlined by purple nucleoproteinaceous material and highly karyolytic cells. A single golden hematoidin crystal *(top middle)* indicates chronic hemorrhage (Wright-Giemsa stain, original magnification 1000×). (B) Renal FNB with branching, septate fungal hyphae stained black by silver stain (Gomori methenamine silver [GMS] stain, original magnification 1000×). Fig. 23.29 shows urine sediment of the same case.

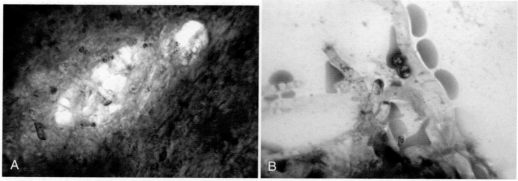

Fig. 23.31 Renal pelvis fine-needle biopsy (FNB) specimen. (A) A three-dimensional mat of partially stained fungal hyphae is present with several partially stained microconidia and golden, rhomboid hematoidin crystals (Wright-Giemsa stain, original magnification 500×). (B) Closer view with two thinly encapsulated microconidia, partially stained hyphal termini, and hematoidin (Wright-Giemsa stain, original magnification 1000×).

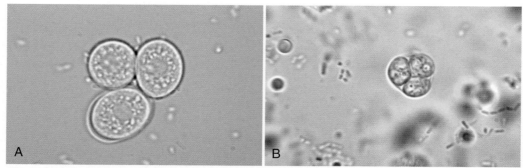

Fig. 23.32 Urine sediment from a dog with cystic lesions in the kidneys and brain. (A) Three algal sporangiospores and bacteria in a different focal plane (unstained, original magnification 1000×). (B) An endosporulated sporangiospore with bacteria and lipid droplets (NMB stain, original magnification 1000×). Fig. 23.33 shows fine-needle biopsy (FNB) specimen of a cystic renal mass from same case.

Struvite

Struvite crystals are also referred to as *magnesium ammonium phosphate crystals*, *triple phosphate crystals* (technically a misnomer), or *infection crystals* (an older term). They are colorless and frequently form variably sized prisms or casket cover–shaped crystals. They also form three- to eight-sided needles, flat crystals with oblique ends, or three-dimensional square or rectangular crystals sometimes with an internal "X." Uncommonly, X-shaped crystals or X-shaped fern leaves form when the urine ammonia concentration is high (Figs. 23.48 and 23.49; see Fig. 23.54 later in the chapter).

Struvite crystals are nonspecific. They are very commonly seen in dogs and occasionally in cats with neutral to alkaline urine. When found in high number in fresh specimens, they are often associated with bacterial infection by urease-producing bacteria, such as *Staphylococcus* or *Proteus*, which would typically be accompanied by pyuria, hematuria, and bacteriuria (see Fig. 23.26). In cats, struvite crystalluria may occur in the absence of infection, likely as a result of ammonia excretion by the renal tubules. Struvite crystals may also be found in clinically normal animals that have alkaline urine for reasons other than infection (e.g., diet, recent meal with postprandial alkaline tide), in animals that have sterile or infection-associated uroliths of potentially mixed mineral composition, or in patients with urinary tract disease in the absence of urolithiasis. Concurrent hematuria or pyuria is expected with urolithiasis.

Struvite crystals may develop after collection in refrigerated, stored urine samples.[6] They may also develop in samples that become alkaline during storage, for example, from bacterial overgrowth or contamination with ammonium-containing cleanser residues. When struvite crystalluria is detected in a stored urine sample and is considered a potentially medically significant observation, the finding should be verified in a freshly obtained specimen collected into a single-use container and examined promptly without interim refrigeration.

Calcium Oxalate

There are two forms of calcium oxalate crystals. One is considered pathological and the other is not. Calcium oxalate dihydrate crystals are observed more commonly. They are colorless, variably sized, octahedrons with three-dimensional intersecting lines that resemble a small envelope or a Maltese cross and form in neutral to acidic urine (Fig. 23.50). Calcium oxalate dihydrate crystalluria is nonspecific. It occurs in normal animals and in animals with urolithiasis, with which concurrent pyuria or hematuria would be expected; increased calciuresis, as seen with hypercalcemia or hypercortisolemia; or hyperoxaluria, as seen with ingestion of vegetables high in oxalates (e.g., *Brassica* family), ethylene glycol, or chocolate. Acidification treatments instituted to mitigate struvite crystalluria may cause secondary calcium oxalate dihydrate crystalluria. Calcium oxalate dihydrate crystals may develop ex vivo in stored urine specimens with or without refrigeration.[6] They may also develop in those that become acidic during storage from overgrowth of bacteria that produce lactic acid. When calcium oxalate dihydrate crystals are detected in a stored urine sample

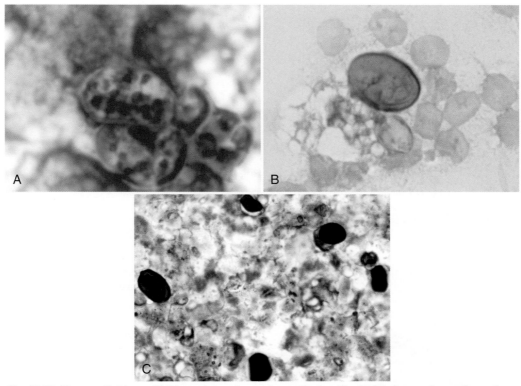

Fig. 23.33 Fine-needle biopsy (FNB) specimen of a cystic renal lesion; Fig. 23.32 shows urine sediment from the same case. (A) Two sporangiospores are adjacent to a neutrophil with free purple nucleoproteins in the background (Wright-Giemsa stain, original magnification 1000×). (B) A sporangiospore and an empty theca within a degraded macrophage. The staining pattern distinguishes *Prototheca* from *Chlorella;* in the former, only the wall is periodic acid–Schiff (PAS) positive, the latter contains starch granules that are strongly PAS positive (PAS stain, original magnification 1000×). (C) Several Gomori methenamine silver [GMS]–positive sporangiospores (GMS stain, original magnification 1000×).

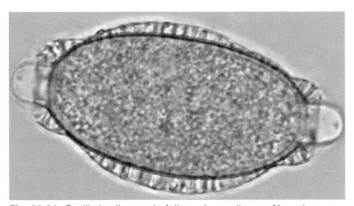

Fig. 23.34 *Capillaria plica* ova in feline urine sediment. Note the mammillated shell and askew polar opercula (unstained, original magnification 500×).

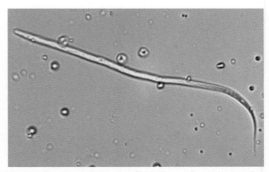

Fig. 23.35 *Dirofilaria immitis* microfilaria in canine urine sediment with hematuria (unstained, original magnification 200×).

and are considered potentially medically significant, the finding should be verified in freshly obtained urine that is examined within 30 to 60 minutes of collection without refrigeration.

Calcium oxalate monohydrate crystalluria is considered pathological and is an early feature of ethylene glycol intoxication. Crystalluria may be observed within 3 hours of ingestion in cats or within 6 hours in dogs and may persist for 18 hours after ingestion. This crystal is colorless, variably sized, birefringent with polarized light, and somewhat pleomorphic with two morphologies commonly observed. They may

be flat with pointed ends and resemble picket fence boards or may form spindles or dumbbell-shaped crystals (Fig. 23.51). Other calcium-containing crystals, for example, the nonpathological calcium carbonate, may also form spindles, dumbbell shapes, and plump fusiform shapes that are very similar to calcium oxalate monohydrate. Because calcium oxalate monohydrate crystals are a medically significant finding, one should rely on observation of the more specific flat, picket fence board–like morphology when making this diagnosis. Calcium oxalate dihydrate crystalluria often accompanies monohydrate crystalluria during ethylene glycol intoxication. Calcium oxalate monohydrate crystals with spindle- or dumbbell-shaped morphology are uncommonly observed with other causes of hyperoxaluria (e.g., chocolate ingestion).

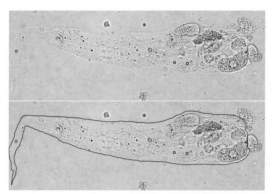

Fig. 23.36 A translucent mucous thread of varied width with a fine, curvilinear, wispy terminus on the left has adherent granular material and cells on the right terminus. The lower panel is a digital duplicate of the mucous thread outlined to aid visualization. Several small, refractive, flat, round lipid droplets are also present (unstained, original magnification 400×).

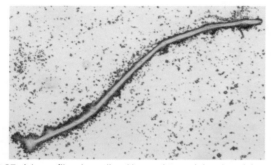

Fig. 23.37 A large fiber is outlined by copious miniscule calcium oxalate dihydrate crystals (unstained, original magnification 40×).

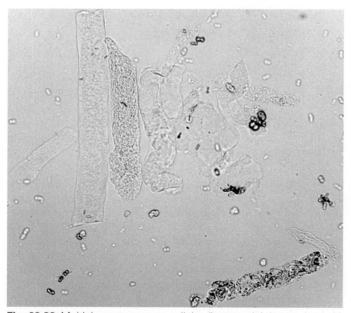

Fig. 23.38 Multiple casts—waxy, cellular *(bottom right)*, granular *(middle left)* (unstained, original magnification 200×).

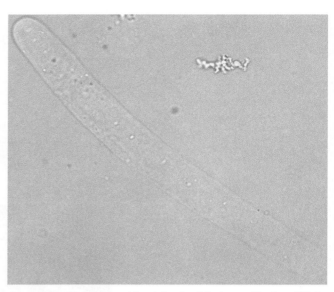

Fig. 23.39 A hyaline cast (unstained, original magnification 400×).

Calcium Carbonate

Calcium carbonate crystals are variably sized, yellow-brown or colorless, pleomorphic crystals that are found individually or in clusters usually within alkaline urine. The crystals may be elongated oval–shaped, dumbbell-shaped, clover leaf–like, or large spheres with radiating striations (Fig. 23.52). Calcium carbonate crystals are an expected finding in clinically normal horses, elephants, goats, rabbits, and guinea pigs. Anecdotally, they are uncommonly seen in dogs. Sulfonamide crystals, which may be seen in dogs and cats after sulfa-containing antibiotic ingestion, may form globules with radiant striations that could be mistaken for calcium carbonate crystals.

Bilirubin

Bilirubin precipitates as orange to copper granules or acicular crystals that are typically present in small bundles (Fig. 23.53). Low numbers of bilirubin crystals are routinely observed in highly concentrated canine urine, particularly samples from male dogs. When bilirubin crystals are found in other species or in large quantity in a canine patient, hemolytic or hepatobiliary diseases associated with icterus may be present.

Amorphous Crystals

Two types of amorphous crystals, amorphous phosphates and urates, are similar in shape and may form amorphous debris or small spheroids that could be misidentified as bacteria—bacteria are less pleomorphic and not as refractive (Figs. 23.54 and 23.55). Amorphous phosphates are distinguished from amorphous urates in two ways: (1) phosphates are colorless or light yellow and form in alkaline urine; (2) urates are yellow-brown to black and form in acidic urine. Amorphous phosphates are commonly observed in alkaline urine of clinically normal animals, and they are not clinically significant. Conversely, amorphous urates are an uncommon abnormal finding in most breeds. They may be seen in animals with portovascular malformation, severe hepatic disease, or ammonium biurate urolithiasis. In Dalmatians and English Bulldogs, amorphous urates may represent a predisposition for urate urolithiasis.

Uric Acid

Uric acid crystals are colorless, flat, variably shaped, six-sided crystals that occur as blunt ovals, triangles, or diamonds (Fig. 23.56). These crystals are expected in avian and reptile urine but are rarely seen in cats and in most dog breeds. In cats and most

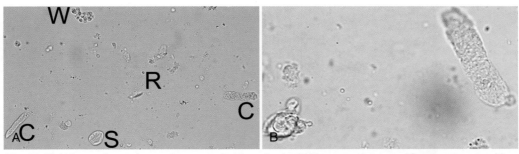

Fig. 23.40 Urine sediment from a dog treated with amikacin. (A) Two granular casts (*C*), a squamous epithelial cell (*S*), an aggregate of leukocytes (*W*), and an erythrocyte (*R*) are present with refractive lipid droplets and amorphous crystals dispersed throughout the field (unstained, original magnification 100×). (B) A granular cast *(right)* and epithelial cells *(left)* are shown (unstained, original magnification 400×).

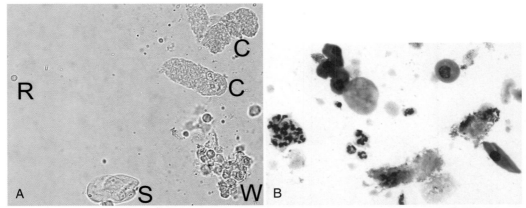

Fig. 23.41 Urine sediment from a dog treated with amikacin. (A) Two granular casts (*C*), a squamous epithelial cell (*S*), an aggregate of leukocytes (*W*), and an erythrocyte (*R*) (unstained, original magnification 400×). (B) Urine sediment dry-mount cytology of the same case with a fragmented cast *(lower right)*—homogeneous purple material with granular terminus, epithelial cells, and clumped neutrophils (Wright-Giemsa stain, original magnification 500×).

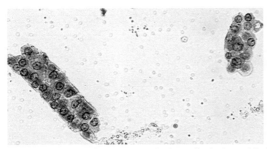

Fig. 23.42 Two cellular casts composed of renal tubular epithelial cells (NMB stain, original magnification 400×).

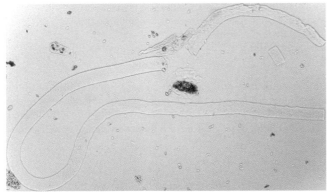

Fig. 23.43 A broad waxy cast *(top)* with a mixed cellular cast *(bottom)* (unstained, original magnification 200×).

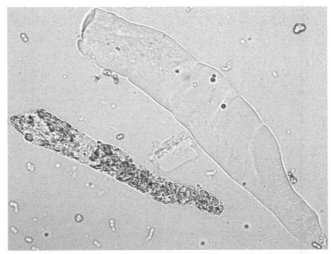

Fig. 23.44 Waxy casts (unstained, original magnification 200×).

dogs, these crystals have the same significance as amorphous urate or ammonium biurate crystals. Some canine breeds (e.g., Dalmatian, English Bulldog, Black Russian Terrier, Weimaraner, and others) have an autosomal recessive trait that causes hyperuricosuria, which is a risk factor for urate urolithiasis.[10] Males are more likely than females to develop urate urolithiasis, which may be an important consideration when selecting long-term preventive therapy.[11]

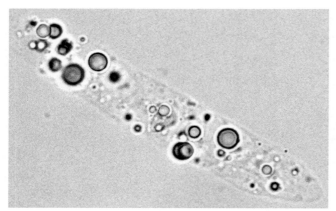

Fig. 23.45 Bilirubin-stained, mixed granular and waxy cast (unstained, original magnification 400×).

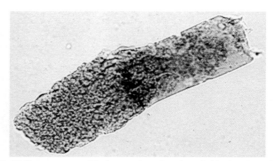

Fig. 23.46 Fatty cast with internal, refractive lipid droplets (original magnification 400×).

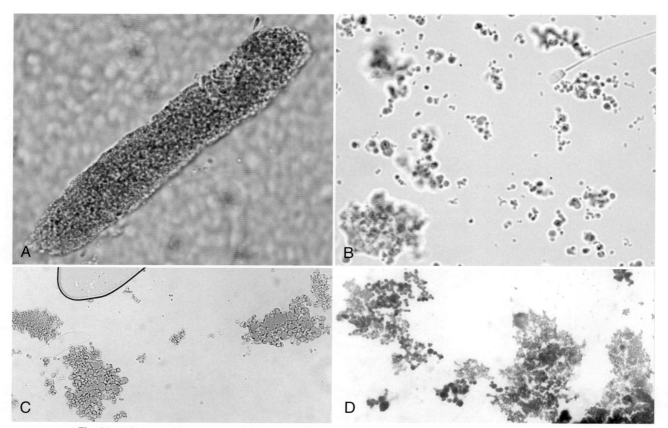

Fig. 23.47 Urine sediment from a dog with autoimmune hemolytic anemia. (A) A hemoglobin cast is present on a dense background of hemoglobin precipitate in a different focal plane (unstained, original magnification 500×). (B) Globular hemoglobin precipitates and a sperm *(upper right)*. (C) Globular myoglobin precipitates from a dog with high serum kinase (unstained, original magnification 500×). (D) Same dog with myoglobin precipitates (Wright-Giemsa, original magnification 500×).

Ammonium Biurate

Ammonium biurate (sometimes called *ammonium urate*) are golden-brown in color and spherical shaped, with irregular protrusions that render a thorn apple–like or a sarcoptic mange–like appearance (Fig. 23.57). They may occur as aggregates of smooth spheroids in cats. In most instances, ammonium biurate crystals are considered a pathological crystal observed in animals with acquired or congenital causes of hepatic failure and hyperammonemia. They are commonly seen in animals with portovascular malformation or, less commonly, in those

with hepatotoxicity, other acquired causes of liver failure, or ammonium biurate urolithiasis. Ammonium biurate crystals may uncommonly be found in very low numbers in the urine of Dalmatians, English Bulldogs, and Schnauzers and may represent a predisposition for urate urolithiasis.

Cystine

Cystine crystals are pathological and occur as colorless, flat hexagonal plates that may have unequal sides. Daughter crystals form

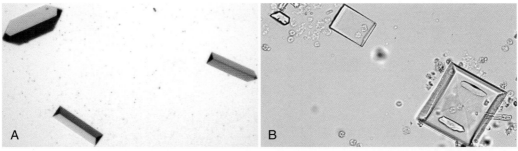

Fig. 23.48 (A) Struvite crystals as five- to eight-sided prisms and a casket cover *(bottom)* (unstained, original magnification 100×). (B) Struvite crystals as three-dimensional squares with an internal "X" *(lower right)*. Degraded leukocytes and bacteria are in the background (unstained, original magnification 200×).

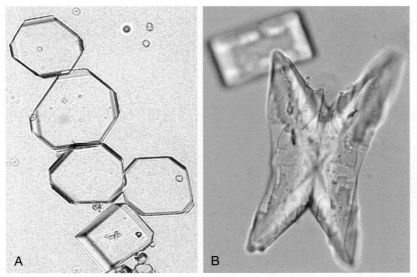

Fig. 23.49 (A) Atypical struvite crystals in feline urine as six- to eight-sided, three-dimensional irregular shapes that have a central spine *(not shown)* (unstained, original magnification 200×). (B) Struvite crystal with uncommon X-shaped, fern leaf–like morphology. A three-dimensional rectangle is in a different focal plane (unstained, original magnification 1000×).

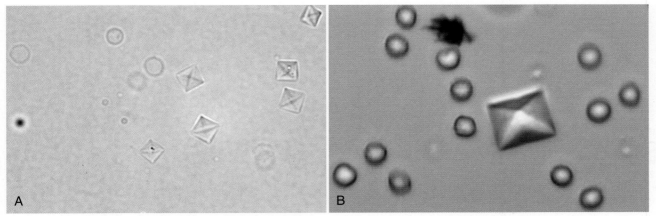

Fig. 23.50 (A) Calcium oxalate dihydrate as small, colorless, three-dimensional, Maltese cross–like crystals in a dog with hematuria (unstained, original magnification 1000×). (B) An oblique calcium oxalate dihydrate crystal that demonstrates the three-dimensional projection, where the lines crossing through the crystal intersect. Erythrocytes and a contaminating stain crystal are also present (NMB stain, original magnification 1000×).

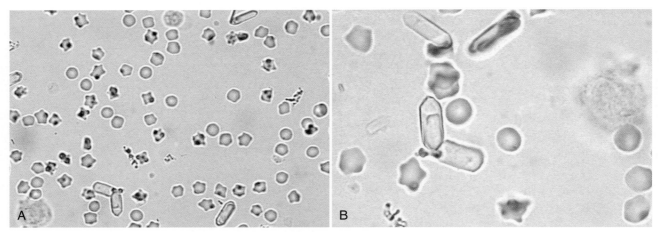

Fig. 23.51 (A) Calcium oxalate monohydrate as flat picket fence board–like crystals in a cat with ethylene glycol intoxication and hematuria, a leukocyte *(top center)*, and a transitional epithelial cell *(lower left)* (unstained, original magnification 500×). (B) Same cat with calcium oxalate monohydrate crystalluria, hematuria, and a transitional epithelial cell *(right)* (unstained, original magnification 1000×).

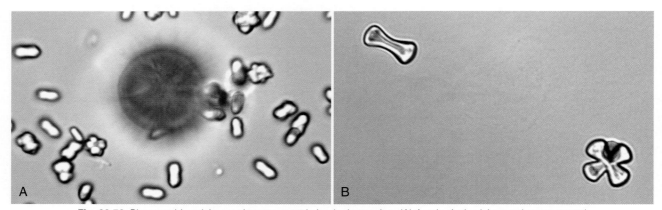

Fig. 23.52 Pleomorphic calcium carbonate crystals in elephant urine. (A) A spherical calcium carbonate crystal with radiating striations is present with smaller elongated oval forms (unstained, original magnification 500×). (B) Dumbbell-shaped and clover leaf–like calcium carbonate crystals (unstained, original magnification 500×).

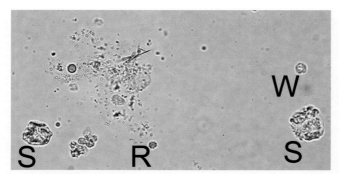

Fig. 23.53 Bilirubin as small bundle of copper, acicular crystals in canine urine with squamous epithelial cells (*S*), a leukocyte (*W*), and an erythrocyte (*R*) (unstained, original magnification 400×).

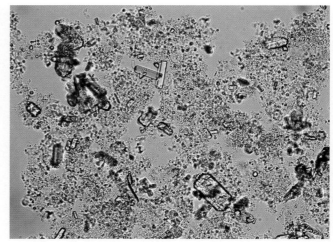

Fig. 23.54 Colorless, amorphous phosphates and struvite crystals in alkaline canine urine (unstained, original magnification 200×).

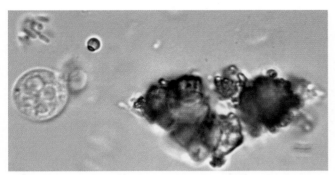

Fig. 23.55 Yellow-brown amorphous urates in acidic urine in a Dalmatian with a neutrophil (*left*) and bacilli *(top left)* that are less refractive than the crystals (unstained, original magnification 1000×).

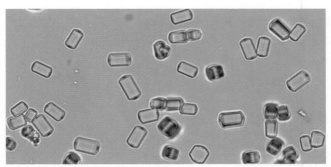

Fig. 23.56 Colorless, flat, pleomorphic, six-sided uric acid crystals forming blunt ovals (unstained, original magnification 400×).

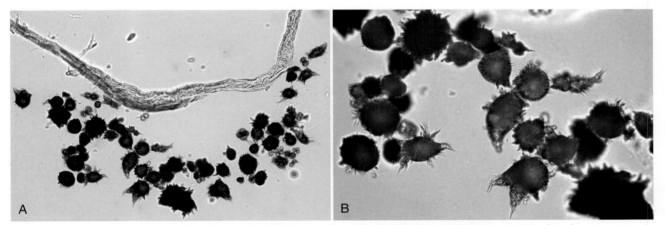

Fig. 23.57 (A) Ammonium biurate crystalluria in a dog with acquired hepatic failure caused by intoxication with the glycoside cycasin after sago palm ingestion. A large contaminating fiber is also present *(top)* (unstained, original magnification 200×). (B) Dark amber to brown ammonium biurate crystals with thorn apple–like or sarcoptic mange–like appearance (unstained, original magnification 500×).

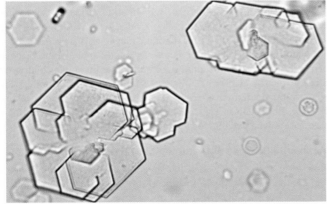

Fig. 23.58 Cystine crystalluria in a dog with hematuria. Cystine crystals form colorless, flat hexagonal plates that bud in three-dimensions (unstained, original magnification 500×).

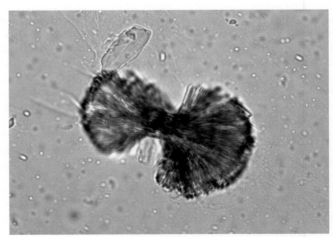

Fig. 23.59 Iatrogenic crystalluria in a dog treated with trimethoprim sulfamethoxazole. This sulfa crystal exhibits a sheaf of wheat–like appearance (unstained, original magnification 500×).

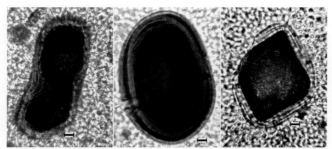

Fig. 23.60 Iatrogenic crystalluria in acidic urine from a dog receiving polytherapy that included zonisamide (a sulfonamide), levetiracetam, dexamethasone, acetylcysteine, furosemide, mannitol, and other medications. Erythrocytes and amorphous debris are abundant in a different, background focal plane (unstained; bar ≡ 10 μm; original magnification 500×).

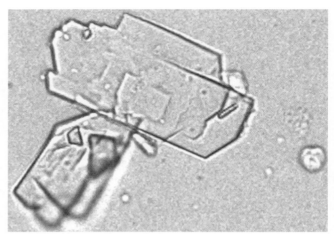

Fig. 23.61 A flat, notched cholesterol crystal (unstained, original magnification 500×).

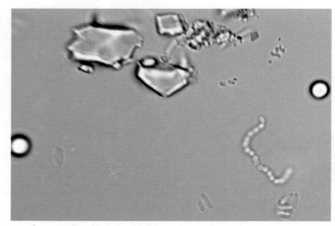

Fig. 23.62 Fragments of coverslip glass *(top)* with a chain of cocci, two small groups of bacilli, and two refractive lipid droplets (unstained, original magnification 1000×).

as hexagons that bud vertically from the seed crystal (Fig. 23.58). Crystals occur in cystinuric patients with concentrated, acidic urine. Cystinuria causes predisposition for the development of cystine urolithiasis, where the crystals often lodge at the base of the os penis and may be missed on survey radiography because the crystals are relatively radiolucent. Cystinuria may be caused by acquired proximal renal tubular disease or a congenital defect of proximal renal tubular transport of several amino acids (i.e., arginine, cystine, lysine, ornithine). Transient aminoacidurias may occur during the diuretic phase after acute renal insufficiency, or as a result of potassium deficiency. Cystinuria may be androgen dependent in some dogs. Some canine breeds are predisposed, but the nonpredisposed breeds may also be affected. Breeds predisposed include Australian Cattle Dog, Bassett Hound, Bulldog, Chihuahua, Dachshund, French Bulldog, Irish Terrier, Labrador Retriever, Mastiff, Miniature Pinscher, Newfoundland, Rottweiler, Staffordshire Bull Terrier, and Yorkshire Terrier. Female dogs and other breeds also may be affected. In cats, this disease has been recognized in male and female Siamese and American Domestic Shorthair cats.

Iatrogenic Crystals

Crystals may be seen with administration of some antibiotics (e.g., sulfonamides, ciprofloxacin); anticonvulsants (e.g., zonisamide, acetazolamide,

polytherapy); xanthine crystals with allopurinol administration, particularly when dietary protein and purine are not concurrently restricted; and radiocontrast medium administration. Sulfonamide crystals (Fig. 23.59) are more likely to be observed in acidic urine as pale-yellow crystals that may form haystack-like bundles or round globules with radiant striations. The latter morphology may be mistaken for calcium carbonate crystals. Zonisamide is a sulfonamide antiepileptic that has been reported to cause crystalluria and urolithiasis in human children on ketogenic diets; antiepileptic polytherapy is also a risk factor for crystalluria in human children. Veterinary publications are currently lacking; however, the crystals in Fig. 23.60 were observed in the urine sediment of a dog receiving polytherapy that included zonisamide.

Uncommon Crystals of Unknown Significance

Cholesterol crystals are large, flat rectangles with a notched border (Fig. 23.61). These crystals are uncommon, and their significance is unknown, but they may be found in the urine of animals with previous urinary tract hemorrhage or diseases with cellular degeneration. Leucine and tyrosine crystals are rarely observed in humans with certain hereditary diseases or severe hepatic failure, and their significance in animal urine is poorly defined. Tyrosine crystals are dark, fine acicular crystals found individually or in small clusters. Leucine crystals appear as large spheroids with concentric striations.

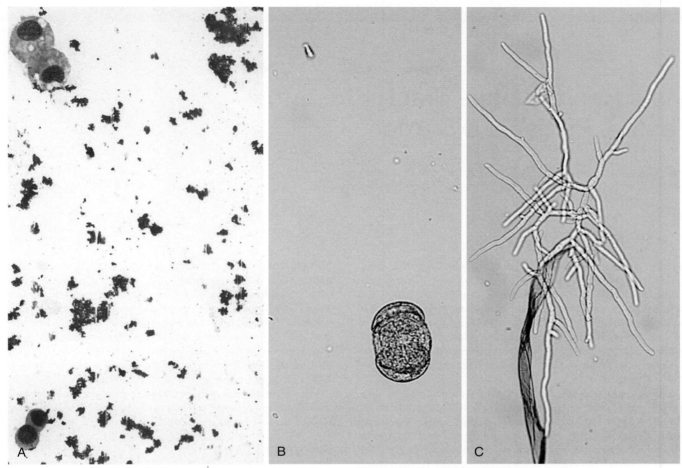

Fig. 23.63 (A) Catheter lubricant *(purple)* with few transitional epithelial cells (Wright-Giemsa, original magnification 500×). (B) Plant pollen (unstained, original magnification 200×). (C) Branching fungal hyphae and a fiber *(bottom center;* unstained, original magnification 500×).

Common Contaminants

Urine sample contaminants are common and may come from either the environment or the patient, depending on sample collection method (e.g., epithelial cells or sperm from the distal genitourinary tract [see Fig. 23.47, B]). Care should be taken to distinguish common contaminants from other relevant sediment findings. Starch granules from powdered gloves or coverslip glass chips (Fig. 23.62) may be mistaken for crystalluria; plant pollen (Fig. 23.63, B) could be mistaken for transitional epithelial cells or ova; and hair or synthetic fibers could be misconstrued as casts (see Figs. 23.37; 23.57, A; and 23.63, C). Other possible contaminants include air bubbles (see Figs. 23.29, A and 23.47, C), lubricant from catheters, bacteria, yeast, fungi (see Fig. 23.63), or feces. Abundant pleomorphic bacilli that may include spore formers, yeasts (e.g., *Cyniclomyces*), intestinal parasite ova, and digesta without pyuria may be found with fecal contamination of the urine sample.

REFERENCES

1. Osborne CA, Stevens JB. In: Osborne CA, Stevens JB, eds. *Urinalysis: a clinical guide to compassionate patient care.* Shawnee Mission, KS: Veterinary Learning Systems, Bayer Corporation; 1999.
2. Swenson CL, et al. Evaluation of modified wright-staining of urine sediment as a method for accurate detection of bacteriuria in dogs. *J Am Vet Med Assoc.* 2004;224:1282–1289.
3. Swenson CL, et al. Evaluation of modified wright-staining of dried urinary sediment as a method for accurate detection of bacteriuria in cats. *Vet Clin Pathol.* 2011;40:256–264.
4. Higuchi T, et al. Characterization and treatment of transitional cell carcinoma of the abdominal wall in dogs: 24 cases (1985-2010). *J Am Vet Med Assoc.* 2013;242:499–506.
5. Gunn-Christie RG, et al. American Society for Veterinary Clinical Pathology (ASVCP): ASVCP quality assurance guidelines: control of preanalytical, analytical, and postanalytical factors for urinalysis, cytology, and clinical chemistry in veterinary laboratories. *Vet Clin Pathol.* 2012;41:18–26.
6. Albasan H, et al. Effects of storage time and temperature on pH, specific gravity, and crystal formation in urine samples from dogs and cats. *J Am Vet Med Assoc.* 2003;222:176–179.
7. Kenyon SM, Cradic KW. Automated urinalysis in the clinical lab. *MLO Med Lab Obs.* 2017;49:22–23.
8. Mochizuki H, et al. Detection of BRAF mutation in urine DNA as a molecular diagnostic for canine urothelial and prostatic carcinoma. *PLoS One.* 2015;10(12):e0144170. https://doi.org/10.1371/journal.pone.0144170. PubMed PMID: 26649430.
9. Morfin J, Chin A. Images in clinical medicine. Urinary calcium oxalate crystals in ethylene glycol intoxication. *N Engl J Med.* 2005;353:e21.
10. Karmi N, et al. Estimated frequency of the canine hyperuricosuria mutation in different dog breeds. *J Vet Intern Med.* 2010;24:1337–1342.
11. Albasan H, et al. Evaluation of the association between sex and risk of forming urate uroliths in dalmatians. *J Am Vet Med Assoc.* 2005;227:565–569.

Male Reproductive Tract: Prostate, Testes, Penis, and Semen

Sabrina D. Clark and Mary B. Nabity

The most commonly evaluated organs of the male reproductive system are the prostate and the testes, typically because of enlargement or other abnormalities identified during a physical examination. It is important to remember, particularly in all intact males, that evaluation of the prostate should always include a digital rectal examination (DRE) as part of a full physical examination. Additionally, semen evaluation is commonly used to evaluate concerns regarding male infertility, and it can be performed in conjunction with fine-needle aspiration (FNA) of the testes.

Although prostatic disease is frequently encountered in dogs, especially older, intact dogs, it seems to be extremely rare in cats.[1-3] In dogs, breed predisposition for development of prostatic disease has been described in German Shepherds and Bernese Mountain Dogs, with conflicting reports for breed disposition in Doberman Pinschers, Scottish Terriers, Rottweilers, American Staffordshire Terriers, Berger de Beauce, Bouvier des Flandres, and German Pointers.[4-6] Regardless of etiology, clinical signs that suggest disease of the prostate include urinary abnormalities, such as hematuria, dysuria, and pollakiuria, preputial or urethral discharge, tenesmus, and ribbon or tapered stools.[1,3] Animals may be presented for abnormalities in micturition, although it is less frequent. Intact animals may also exhibit decreased fertility or loss of libido. Rectal digital palpation of the prostate is best achieved while simultaneously pushing the prostate up into the pelvic canal by caudal ventral abdominal palpation.[1] The normal prostate should be smooth, symmetrical, and nonpainful, and the dorsal sulcus or groove should be palpable.[1,3] Detection of abnormalities warrants further diagnostics, including a minimum database (complete blood count [CBC], biochemistry profile, and urinalysis), radiography, ultrasonography, and/or FNA for cytological evaluation, bacterial culture, and susceptibility testing. Ultrasonography is a particularly useful tool for evaluating the prostate because it allows for visualization of the external texture and the internal architecture.[7] Although the gold standard for the diagnosis of prostatic disease is histological examination of a prostatic biopsy specimen, it has been shown that in prostatic disease, there is a high concordance (>80%) between cytological and histological diagnoses.[8]

Unlike prostatic disease, testicular disease rarely causes clinical signs, and enlargement of the testes and/or palpation of a mass on physical examination are the most common means for identifying abnormalities, such as testicular tumors. Surgical biopsy is recommended to distinguish between testicular tumors types. However, because of the advantages of FNA compared with surgical biopsy (e.g., minimal invasiveness, speed, low cost, less pain to the animal), testicular FNA is frequently used to evaluate for pathological conditions.[9] Furthermore,

FNA allows for sampling of multiple areas within the testes, making FNA samples more representative of the testes as a whole compared with a single biopsy sample.[9] In general, testicular FNA is considered a safe procedure. It has been shown that testicular FNA, even in dogs that have multiple samples taken over a long period and with different-sized needles, does not appear to result in immediate or long-term adverse effects on male sexual performance or fertility.[10-12] Testicular FNA has also been shown to be a safe procedure in cats even with up to eight pierces performed.[13]

Although disorders of the penis and prepuce are relatively uncommon, penile and preputial cytology can be helpful if purulent discharge is identified or if a mass is present.

PROSTATE GLAND

Collecting and Preparing Samples

Material from the prostate may be obtained directly through the urethra (known as *prostatic massage*), ejaculation, or direct FNA of the gland.[1,3] For prostatic massage, the bladder must be emptied of all urine and rinsed with sterile saline, using aseptic catheterization. A small volume of saline rinse (approximately 5 mL) should be retained as a premassage sample.[1,3] Using transrectal guidance, the catheter is withdrawn so that the tip is just distal to the prostate. The prostate is then vigorously massaged either through the rectum or the abdomen, followed by infusion of 5 to 10 mL of sterile saline, making sure to occlude the urethral opening so that fluid is not lost. Continuous aspiration is performed (particularly in the area of the prostate) as the catheter is slowly advanced into the bladder (postmassage sample). A portion of the fluid should be placed in an ethylenediaminetetraacetic acid (EDTA) tube for preparation of direct and concentrated smears. Additionally, some fluid should be directed into a red-top tube in case bacterial culture and susceptibility testing are indicated.[1,3]

Semen can be an ideal sample for evaluation of prostatic disease. The first fraction of ejaculate is presperm fluid that originates from both the urethra and the prostate.[14] The second fraction is rich in sperm and is typically cloudy in appearance. The third fraction is solely prostatic fluid (>90%) and should be clear.[1,14] The sample volume of the third fraction is typically large, and it is highly specific for evaluation of the prostate.[1] However, fluid obtained via this method will contain contaminants from other parts of the reproductive tract.[15] During collection of the third fraction, the prostate can be gently massaged to increase the proportion of material originating from the prostate. Interpretation of bacteria in prostatic fluid must be done with caution because bacteria are part of the normal flora from the distal urinary tract.[1,15] Heavy growth of a pure culture is typically indicative of a true infection.[15] The main disadvantage for both prostatic massage and ejaculation is that prostatic disease located in an area that does not communicate with the urethra will not be identified with use of these methods.[3]

Fluid or tissue from the prostate can also be sampled via direct FNA by using a small-gauge needle. It should be noted that if prostatitis is the main differential diagnosis, FNA is contraindicated to prevent inadvertent seeding of bacteria along the needle tract.[1,3] However, in a study involving 13 dogs with either prostatic abscesses or cysts, treatment with percutaneous ultrasound-guided drainage did not result in any complications after drainage.[16] Aspiration of the prostate is typically performed by using ultrasound guidance. While the animal is sedated, samples may be collected either transabdominally (most common) or perineally.[1,3] Collection of any fluid from the prostate should be considered abnormal, and fluid obtained should be submitted for both cytological evaluation and bacterial culture and susceptibility testing.[1] If tissue is collected via FNA, smear preparations should be made. Disadvantages of performing FNA of the prostate include such complications as hemorrhage or peritonitis if the bladder is punctured, failure to diagnose localized disease, and potential seeding of an infection or tumor along the needle tract.[3] Ultrasound guidance should help decrease the likelihood of some of these events.

Although ultrasound-guided aspiration is preferred, the prostate in dogs can be sampled without imaging guidance when it is large enough to be palpated through the abdomen. In this scenario, the needle can be passed through the posterior abdominal wall by using digital guidance while the dog is placed in either lateral or dorsal recumbency. The prostate is immobilized with one hand while the gland is gently aspirated, directing the needle in different directions within the gland.[1,7,17]

Staining of the smear preparations is similar to that for other tissues. If fluid is obtained, such as from a prostatic cyst, preparation should include concentrating the cells by using centrifugation. The sediment can then be used to obtain slides with sufficient material for proper cytological evaluation. Some fluid should be directed into a red-top tube in case bacterial culture and susceptibility testing are needed.

Cytological Evaluation of Normal Prostate

The cytological features of the normal prostate can vary, depending on the method used to obtain the samples. Samples obtained via FNA are generally more cellular than those obtained through ejaculation or prostatic massage and typically contain less contaminating material.

Prostatic Epithelial Cells

Glandular cells of the normal prostate are found in small- to medium-size cohesive clusters and sheets and are overall uniform in appearance. Cells are cuboidal to lowly columnar with a small to moderate amount of basophilic, finely granular cytoplasm, which may contain variable numbers of vacuoles. Nuclei are round to oval, basally to centrally located, and display a finely stippled or reticular chromatin pattern with an indistinct to subtle, small nucleolus (Figs. 24.1 to 24.3). In general, bacteria should not be present in the normal canine prostate gland. If prostatic massage or ejaculation was used for sample collection, contaminating material from the urogenital tract (described below) may be identified (Fig. 24.4).

Spermatozoa

Spermatozoa are most frequently found in ejaculated material but can also be found in fluid obtained through prostatic massage. Sperm characteristically stain aqua with Romanowsky stains (see Fig. 24.4), and they often adhere to other cells, sometimes with numerous sperm adhering to a single epithelial cell.

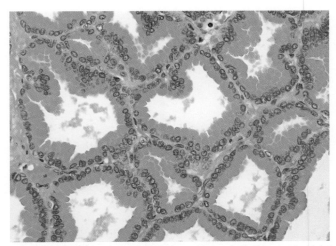

Fig. 24.1 Histology of a normal dog prostate. Uniform cuboidal to columnar epithelial cells with apical eosinophilic cytoplasm and basally located nuclei are forming single-layered tubular structures (hematoxylin and eosin [H&E] stain, original magnification 400×). (Courtesy Dr. John Edwards.)

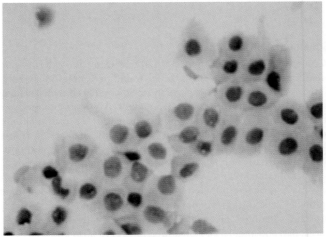

Fig. 24.2 Prostatic epithelial cells from a normal dog. The cells are in cohesive clusters and have light blue cytoplasm and relatively large nuclei. Prostatic massage concentrated by centrifugation (Wright-Giemsa stain, original magnification 400×).

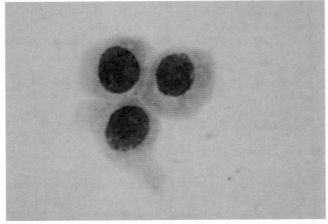

Fig. 24.3 Prostatic epithelial cells from a normal dog. The cytoplasm is light blue and finely granular. Nuclei are centrally located and display a reticular chromatin pattern. Prostatic massage concentrated by centrifugation (Wright-Giemsa stain, original magnification 1000×).

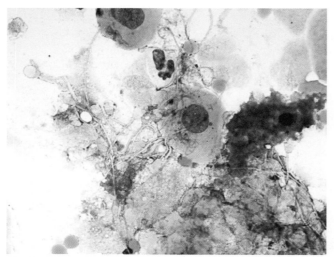

Fig. 24.4 Fluid obtained by prostatic massage from a normal dog. Many spermatozoa (characteristically stained aqua with Romanowsky stains), few epithelial cells, and a small amount of blood (few erythrocytes and rare neutrophils) are present (Wright-Giemsa stain, original magnification 1000×). (Courtesy Dr. Rick Cowell.)

Squamous Cells

Because they originate from the distal urethra or the external genitalia, squamous epithelial cells can be found in samples obtained via both prostatic massage and ejaculation. Squamous epithelial cells are large, flattened cells with round to angular cell borders and moderate to large amounts of lightly basophilic cytoplasm. More differentiated squamous cells have a pyknotic or karyorrhectic nucleus. Squamous cells can be difficult to differentiate from urothelial cells and possibly even prostatic epithelial cells, especially if they are immature. In samples obtained via prostatic massage or ejaculation, contaminating bacteria may be seen adhered to the cells. Identification of squamous epithelial cells in samples obtained via FNA is more supportive of prostatic squamous metaplasia (see Fig. 24.10 later in the chapter). Large, flat, and angular or rolled squamous cells (also known as *squames*) can represent contamination from external skin surfaces; contamination can be minimized by cleaning the skin before obtaining a sample.

Urothelial Cells

Urothelial cells (also known as *transitional epithelial cells*) originate from the proximal two-thirds of the urethra, bladder, ureters, and renal pelves and are most frequently found in samples obtained through ejaculation and prostatic massage. These cells usually appear as single cells but can also be present in small, cohesive clusters. Normal urothelial cells can be highly variable but are typically distinguishable from prostatic epithelial cells based on their larger size and lower nuclear-to-cytoplasmic (N:C) ratio (see Chapter 23 for figures and descriptions of urothelial cells).

Other Contaminant Cells

Prostatic massage samples from normal dogs may contain low numbers of erythrocytes. Samples obtained through normal prostatic ejaculation may also contain low numbers of erythrocytes in addition to leukocytes. Rarely, few bacteria may be identified in both sample types, most likely contamination from the lower urethra. Although cells of the ductus deferens and the epididymis may be present, they are difficult to distinguish from prostatic cells and may not be specifically identified.

Ultrasound Contact Gel

When ultrasound-guided aspiration is used, the ultrasound gel can contaminate the sample. On cytology, this typically appears as magenta-colored, granular, rod-shaped material scattered throughout the slide in aggregates of variable size. To minimize this artifact, excess gel should be removed by wiping the skin before aspiration.

Benign Prostatic Hyperplasia

Benign prostatic hyperplasia (BPH) is the most common prostatic disorder that occurs in older, intact male dogs but is very rare in cats. Beginning as early as age 2 years, an overproduction of the hormone dihydrotestosterone (DHT) is the primary mediator of BPH, ultimately leading to both hyperplasia and hypertrophy of the stromal and glandular components.[1,18] An alteration of the ratio of 17β-estradiol to testosterone secreted by the testes is also involved.[19] BPH is part of the normal aging process, and although most dogs will not develop clinical signs, almost all intact male dogs will develop BPH, with greater than 95% affected by age 9 years.[20] Palpation of the prostate by DRE typically reveals a symmetrically enlarged and nonpainful prostate; however, prostatitis can be a sequela of BPH. Once the prostate becomes large enough, the dog may present with clinical signs, including urethral discharge, tenesmus, hematuria, fertility abnormalities, or, rarely, a stilted gait caused by prostatic pain.[20,21] Although histopathological diagnosis is the gold standard, a presumptive diagnosis of BPH can be made on the basis of history and findings from physical examination, imaging, and FNA of the prostate.[1,8] More recently, blood measurement of canine prostate-specific arginine esterase (CPSE), a serine protease similar to the human prostate-specific antigen, has proven to be helpful as an alternative or complementary method to diagnose BPH in middle-aged dogs.[19] This test is commercially available, and samples can be submitted through Biobest Laboratories Ltd. (Penicuik, UK). Because BPH can be an underlying cause of other prostatic disorders, including prostatitis and neoplasia, treatment is important to minimize the development of pathological processes.[7] The most effective treatment for BPH is castration. The prostate begins to decrease in size approximately 7 to 14 days after surgery.[1] Overall, an approximately 70% reduction in size occurs, and it may require up to 4 months to achieve.[1] For breeding dogs, available medical options for treatment of BPH use variable mechanisms to counteract the action of hormones.

On cytology, the prostatic epithelial cells in BPH are typically uniform and appear very similar to the normal prostatic epithelium. The cellularity of the smear is generally moderate to high, with cells arranged in variably sized cohesive sheets and clusters. Occasionally, acinar-like arrangements may be seen. If exfoliated in large sheets, cells may be described as having a "honeycomb" appearance. Cells have variably distinct cytoplasmic borders with low to moderate amounts of basophilic, slightly granular cytoplasm with or without vacuoles. Nuclei are round to oval and display a finely reticulated to stippled chromatin pattern. Nucleoli are usually not observed, although few nuclei may have a small, round nucleolus. Mild anisocytosis and anisokaryosis may be seen, and overall the N:C ratio is similar to slightly increased compared with that of normal prostatic cells (Figs. 24.5 and 24.6).

Prostatitis and Prostatic Abscess

Prostatitis is defined as inflammation of the prostate gland, which can be caused by infectious agents or may be aseptic. In dogs, approximately one-third of prostatitis cases result from bacterial infection.[7] The primary route of infection is ascending (via the urethra), but bacteria can also colonize the prostate by hematogenous spread.[1,22] On

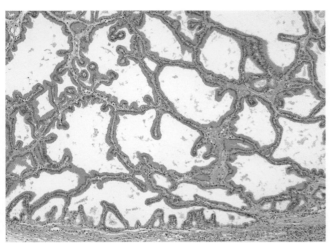

Fig. 24.5 Histology of the prostate from a dog with benign prostatic hyperplasia. Glandular lumens are dilated, and papillary projections extend into the lumen (hematoxylin and eosin [H&E] stain, original magnification 100×). (Courtesy Dr. John Edwards.)

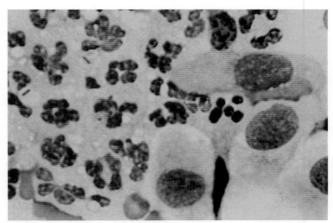

Fig. 24.7 Neutrophils and prostatic epithelial cells from a dog with acute prostatitis. Neutrophils, which are mildly degenerative, contain phagocytized, intracellular bacterial rods consistent with septic inflammation. Prostatic massage concentrated by centrifugation (Wright-Giemsa stain, original magnification 1000×).

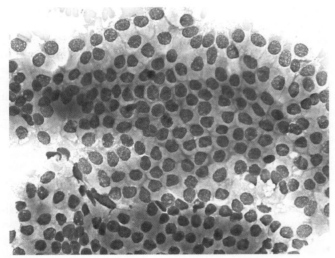

Fig. 24.6 A large cluster of uniform prostatic epithelial cells from an older dog with benign prostatic hyperplasia. When exfoliated in large sheets, cells may be described as having a "honeycomb" appearance with low to moderate amounts of blue granular cytoplasm that may contain vacuoles (fine-needle aspiration and biopsy) (Wright-Giemsa stain, original magnification 500×). (Courtesy Dr. Rick Cowell.)

DRE, the prostate may appear normal to enlarged and is typically painful. Abdominal ultrasonography often reveals changes in the echodensity of the prostate.

Prostatitis is classified as either acute or chronic, primarily depending on clinical signs.[1,7] Acute prostatitis typically occurs in mature, intact male dogs but has been reported in castrated males.[1,23] Animals will often present with signs of systemic disease, such as fever, depression, and anorexia.[1] Prostatitis frequently leads to cystitis; conversely, cystitis can extend to the prostate and cause prostatitis.[1,7] In one study, urinary symptoms were present in greater than 50% of male dogs (regardless of genital status) that were diagnosed with prostatitis.[4] In cases where clinical signs were suggestive of cystitis, results of culture performed on urine obtained via cystocentesis correlated with bacteria isolated from the prostate.[7] Chronic prostatitis can be more difficult to detect and is commonly associated with recurrent

urinary tract infections or urethral discharge.[1] Although relatively uncommon, prostatic abscessation can occur as a sequela to chronic prostatitis and is defined by cavities of purulent material within the prostatic parenchyma.[1] Bacterial prostatitis and prostatic abscessation has been reported in one intact and one castrated cat, respectively.[2,24] In both cases, the cats presented with a primary complaint of dyschezia, including straining and constipation.[2,24]

If bacterial prostatitis is suspected, ejaculation or prostatic wash may be a preferred method for sample collection to prevent complications that might occur from FNA. However, bacterial contamination from the lower urinary and genital tracts could lead to misdiagnosis. Should FNA be performed, care should be taken to maintain continual negative pressure until the needle is fully extracted from the tissue to avoid leakage of material. Cytological evaluation of samples obtained via ultrasound-guided FNA may be more sensitive than histology for the diagnosis of sepsis, because the thickness of the histological sections can impede visualization of bacteria.[8] Sample material obtained from cases of suspected prostatitis should be submitted for bacterial culture and susceptibility testing. Treatment of prostatitis involves medical management (e.g., appropriate antibiotic therapy) in conjunction with castration, which will help control the infection more quickly.

Cytological evaluation of prostatitis reveals predominantly neutrophilic inflammation. Additionally, variable numbers of macrophages, lymphocytes, and plasma cells may be present, particularly in chronic prostatitis. Bacteria may be present both extracellularly and intracellularly. If intracellular bacteria are present (i.e., septic), the neutrophils will generally have features of degenerative change, indicated by swelling of the nucleus (Fig. 24.7). If the sample was obtained via FNA, it is reasonable to assume that bacteria are the cause of prostatitis, particularly if they are intracellular. However, if the sample was obtained through the urogenital system or the rectum, it is less likely that bacteria are the cause. Culture results of urine obtained by cystocentesis may be helpful in differentiating true infection from contamination.[1,7] In dogs, the most common bacterial isolate of prostatitis is *Escherichia coli*; however, *Mycoplasma* spp., *Staphylococcus* spp., *Streptococcus* spp., *Brucella canis*, *Proteus mirabilis*, *Klebsiella* spp., and *Pseudomonas* spp. have all been reported.[25] Fungal causes of prostatitis, such as blastomycosis, coccidiomycosis, and cryptococcosis, are infrequent but have also been reported.[1,26,27] In addition, leishmaniasis has been reported as a cause of chronic prostatitis in a dog presented for infertility.[28] Along with inflammatory cells, clusters of variably

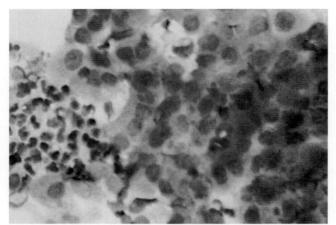

Fig. 24.8 Hyperplasia of the prostatic epithelium from a dog with acute prostatitis. Cells display mild anisocytosis and anisokaryosis and have an increased nuclear-to-cytoplasmic ratio. Prostate massage concentrated by centrifugation (Wright-Giemsa stain, original magnification 500×).

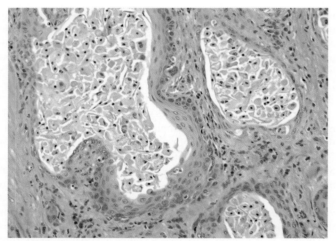

Fig. 24.9 Histology of the prostate from a dog with squamous metaplasia caused by a Sertoli cell tumor. Glandular epithelium has been replaced by a stratified squamous epithelium, and numerous sloughed squamous cells are present within the lumens. Note increased connective tissue between acini (hematoxylin and eosin [H&E] stain, original magnification 200×). (Courtesy Dr. John Edwards.)

sized, intact prostatic epithelial cells may be observed. These cells may exhibit increased cytoplasmic basophilia with mild anisocytosis and anisokaryosis and an increased N:C ratio, indicating that the prostatic epithelium is hyperplastic as a result of inflammation (Fig. 24.8). In the presence of severe inflammation, cells may display some criteria of malignancy, making cytological diagnosis of hyperplasia versus prostatic neoplasia challenging. In chronic inflammatory conditions, squamous metaplasia may be observed (see Fig. 24.10 below). Aggregates of blue-gray to purple amorphous material may also be noted, consistent with necrotic cellular debris.

Squamous Metaplasia

Metaplasia occurs when epithelial stem cells are induced to differentiate along a new developmental pathway, leading to the replacement of one differentiated somatic cell type with another in the same tissue.[29] In the prostate, this involves the replacement of normal cuboidal to low-columnar epithelial cells by squamous epithelial cells (Figs. 24.9 and 24.10). In dogs, this process is typically and most dramatically

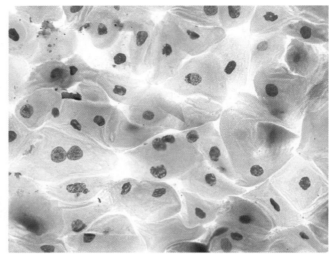

Fig. 24.10 Squamous metaplasia of the prostatic epithelium in a dog with a Sertoli cell tumor. The squamous cells are large and polygonal with pale-staining cytoplasm. Some cells have karyorrhectic nuclei. Prostatic massage concentrated by centrifugation (Wright-Giemsa stain, original magnification 500×). (Courtesy Dr. Rick Cowell.)

induced under the influence of estrogen or an estrogen-like hormone excreted from a Sertoli cell tumor, or, rarely, from an interstitial cell tumor.[7,30] One case report described prostatic squamous metaplasia associated with interstitial cell neoplasia identified in a retained testicle in a cat; however, hormone assays had not been performed in that case.[31] Squamous metaplasia may also occur secondary to chronic irritation or inflammation, as with prostatitis, or in dogs exposed to high levels of exogenous estrogen.[15]

Aspirates are moderately cellular and are composed of cells arranged singly or in small- to moderate-size aggregates. Consistent with well-differentiated squamous epithelial cells, cells are large and round to polygonal and have indistinct cell borders and abundant pale- to light-blue cytoplasm, and appear flattened or folded. Frequently, cells contain a pyknotic or karyorrhectic nucleus, thus exhibiting a low N:C ratio (see Fig. 24.10). Additionally, depending on the underlying disease process, inflammatory cells, bacteria, amorphic debris, and/or hyperplastic prostatic epithelial cells may be observed. Squamous metaplasia of the prostate is not considered a preneoplastic process.[27]

Prostatic and Paraprostatic Cysts

Prostatic cysts are formed by accumulation of fluid as a result of obstruction of prostatic canaliculi.[1] Initially, cysts are microscopic and can only be detected through histological evaluation. However, as a cyst grows and communicates with other cysts, it becomes evident macroscopically.[32] Prostatic cysts may be identified as an incidental finding without clinical signs during a routine physical examination or discovered during diagnostic workup of a dog that presents with clinical signs suggestive of prostatic disease. Prevalence of prostatic cysts was approximately 14% in one study evaluating 85 intact, adult male large-breed dogs.[32] In that same study, approximately 42% of those cysts had evidence for bacterial infection on culture.[32] Typically, cysts are found in dogs with concurrent BPH or other prostatic diseases.[1,32] Prostatic cysts can be classified as either retention cysts or paraprostatic cysts. Retention cysts form within the parenchyma of the prostate and communicate with the urethra. Paraprostatic cysts form outside the parenchyma and are generally attached to the prostate via a stalk of tissue or adhesions.[1,3] Although cysts are primarily seen in intact dogs, one case report describes a paraprostatic cyst in a neutered cat.[33]

Prostatic cysts are quite variable cytologically. Grossly, fluid obtained from cysts may appear serosanguinous to brown. Smears may be acellular or, even when concentrated, contain only a few epithelial cells, rare neutrophils and erythrocytes, and some debris. Sometimes, small numbers of normal or slightly hyperplastic epithelial cells are seen. Squamous cells resulting from metaplasia secondary to chronic inflammation are rarely observed. The protein concentration of prostatic cysts is usually similar to that of transudate fluid.

Prostatic Neoplasia

Prostatic neoplasia is relatively uncommon in the dog (prevalence of 0.2%–0.6%) and has rarely been reported in cats.[4,7,34-39] Most affected dogs tend to be medium- to large-breed, older dogs (average age 8–10 years). Although both intact and neutered dogs can develop prostatic neoplasia, studies have shown an increased incidence in castrated dogs.[4,6,40] Reports have described both intact and neutered cats being affected. In dogs, the most common clinical signs of prostatic neoplasia include stranguria and dysuria, constipation, diarrhea, pain and paresis of the hind limbs (caused by metastasis), anorexia, and severe weight loss.[1,7] On DRE, the prostate tends to be large, irregular, asymmetrical and, in some cases, painful.[1,34] Cats with prostatic neoplasia may present with similar clinical signs.[34] A palpable prostate in a castrated animal should raise suspicion of prostatic disease, particularly neoplasia.[1,34] For evaluation of prostatic neoplasia, ultrasonography is preferred, although radiography is helpful to identify pulmonary nodules, enlarged lymph nodes, and/or bone lesions caused by metastasis.[7] Mineralization of the prostate may be observed and can be identified by using either imaging modality. A study evaluating the relationship of mineralization and prostatic disease in dogs found that neutered dogs with prostatic mineralization were more likely to have neoplasia than intact dogs.[41] Intact dogs without identifiable mineralization in the prostate were unlikely to have prostatic neoplasia.[41] Retroperitoneal lymphadenopathy can be observed in both neoplastic and nonneoplastic diseases; however, if pulmonary metastasis or periosteal reactions on the vertebrae, femur, and/or pelvic bones are identified, neoplasia is highly likely. Unfortunately, in both dogs and cats, because of the aggressive nature of prostatic carcinoma, by the time it is diagnosed, metastasis has likely already occurred, making the prognosis poor.[1,34,38]

In both dogs and cats, carcinoma is the most commonly diagnosed neoplasm of the prostate. In dogs, other primary prostatic tumors have been reported, such as fibrosarcoma, leiomyoma, leiomyosarcoma, hemangiosarcoma, and lymphoma.[34,42,43] Metastasis to the prostate is rare.[44] Prostatic carcinomas can arise from the prostatic acinar epithelium, the urothelium lining the prostatic urethra (e.g., urothelial or transitional cell carcinoma), or the ductal epithelium. In dogs, adenocarcinomas of the prostate and urothelial (transitional) cell carcinomas of the prostatic urethra are most commonly diagnosed.[1,34] The type of carcinoma is difficult to distinguish cytologically and even histologically. Most tumors exhibit glandular or acinar structures and are therefore usually classified as adenocarcinomas, but many also contain patterns similar to that of urothelial cell carcinoma. A panel of antibodies for definitive diagnosis by using immunohistochemistry (IHC) has yet to be determined.[45] Although a few cases of adenocarcinomas have been reported in cats, urothelial cell carcinoma has not been reported.

Cytological samples can be obtained by using any of the methods described above. Although direct aspiration of the prostate through the skin can lead to seeding of neoplastic cells along the needle tract, many believe that the usefulness of FNA in diagnosis, and thus prognosis, outweighs the risks.[7] The cellularity of a cytological sample is typically moderate to marked, composed of round to highly pleomorphic cells

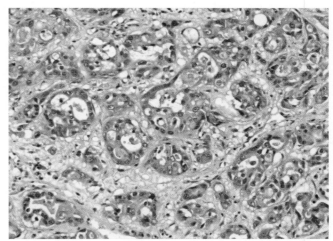

Fig. 24.11 Histology of the prostate from a dog with prostatic carcinoma. Cells display marked atypia and form nests and occasionally tubelike structures separated by a fibroblastic response (hematoxylin and eosin [H&E] stain, original magnification 200×). (Courtesy Dr. John Edwards.)

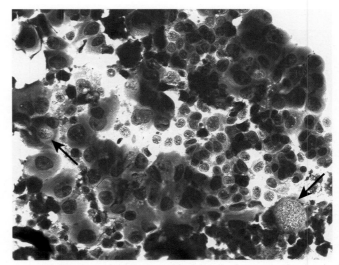

Fig. 24.12 Clusters of prostatic epithelial cells demonstrating marked criteria of malignancy. Note the occasional intracellular vacuoles containing pink granular material (arrows) (fine-needle aspiration from a dog) (Wright-Giemsa stain, original magnification 500×). (Courtesy Dr. Amy Valenciano.)

arranged in variably sized cohesive clusters and sheets and as scattered single cells (Figs. 24.11 and 24.12). Cells assembled in glandular or acinar-like structures, supporting a diagnosis of adenocarcinoma may also be observed (Fig. 24.13). Cell borders may be distinct in well-differentiated carcinomas but can be indistinct in poorly differentiated tumors. Cells contain variable amounts of basophilic cytoplasm that occasionally contains numerous round, clear vacuoles. Cells may also have cytoplasmic aggregates of eosinophilic granular material (which may represent glycosylated protein) confined within a large, single vacuole (see Fig. 24.12). Typical features of malignancy are pronounced and can include single to multiple nuclei with coarse to clumped chromatin and multiple, prominent nucleoli. Cells often display marked anisocytosis and anisokaryosis with a variable N:C ratio, along with nuclear molding, satellite nuclei, and mitotic figures (including bizarre

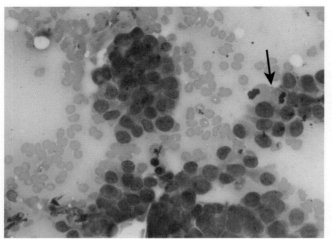

Fig. 24.13 Neoplastic epithelial cells from a prostatic adenocarcinoma in a dog. Cells are assembled in cohesive clusters, and one group displays an acinar-like arrangement, supporting a diagnosis of prostatic adenocarcinoma (confirmed on histopathology). Cells display criteria of malignancy including multiple, prominent nucleoli, moderate anisocytosis and anisokaryosis, multinucleation, and a mitotic figure *(arrow)* (modified Wright stain, original magnification 500×).

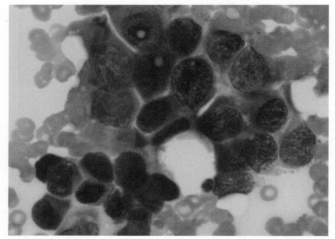

Fig. 24.14 A group of neoplastic epithelial cells from a prostatic adenocarcinoma in a dog. Cells are highly pleomorphic, demonstrating multiple prominent, variably sized nucleoli within the same nucleus (anisonucleoleosis), increased nuclear-to-cytoplasmic ratio, and marked anisocytosis and anisokaryosis (modified Wright stain, original magnification 1000×).

forms) (see Figs. 24.12 and 24.13; Fig. 24.14). However, some carcinomas may demonstrate only mild cellular atypia (Fig. 24.15). Cells obtained from a prostatic wash may be less preserved, but morphological features consistent with malignancy are usually still identifiable. In the presence of concurrent marked inflammation, caution must be taken while determining whether the cells present are truly neoplastic.

TESTES

Collecting and Preparing Samples

Enlargement of the testes, either unilateral or bilateral, and infertility are the primary indications for FNA and cytological evaluation to help differentiate inflammatory from neoplastic causes. When aspirating

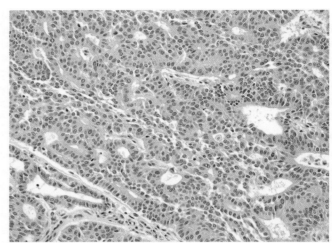

Fig. 24.15 Histology of the prostate of a dog with a prostatic carcinoma. Cellular atypia is mild, but glandular structures are disorganized, and apical eosinophilic cytoplasm is lost. The neoplasm metastasized widely (hematoxylin and eosin [H&E] stain, original magnification 200×). (Courtesy Dr. John Edwards.)

the testis, care should be taken to prevent injury to the epididymis. Although several different aspiration techniques have been described, the testis can be aspirated just as any other tissue. Once the needle is removed, pressure should be applied to the puncture site to minimize scrotal bleeding and help prevent formation of an intraparenchymatous hematoma.[11,13] An enlarged epididymis can also be sampled via FNA. Testes that are decreased in size with increased firmness suggest atrophy, and FNA does not usually yield a sample that is adequate for cytological evaluation. In this case, biopsy with histopathological evaluation may be required for an informed diagnosis.[46] Semen evaluation may also provide information on testicular lesions, although such evaluation is mainly used for determining sperm quality.

Cytological Evaluation of Normal Testes

The cellularity of a sample obtained from an aspirate or core of a normal testicle may be quite variable, depending on the aggressiveness of sampling. Cellularity is typically moderate to high, composed of a pleomorphic population of cells consisting of spermatozoa and their precursors, scattered Sertoli cells, and, rarely, Leydig (interstitial) cells, typically seen in loosely cohesive clusters or as single cells (Figs. 24.16 and 24.17). The material obtained from normal testicles is often contaminated with blood, and many bare nuclei and cytoplasmic fragments may be observed in the background.[9] Morphology of the testicular cell types is similar in dogs and cats.[47] Because multinucleate and large cells with prominent nucleoli may be apparent, care should be taken not to diagnose malignant neoplasia. In addition, some of the spermatogenic precursors may appear similar to large lymphocytes, and a misdiagnosis of lymphoma is possible (Fig. 24.18).

Spermatogenic Cells

Spermatogenic cells should be present in an orderly and complete fashion to include numerous spermatozoa with lower numbers of precursors (spermatogonia, spermatocytes, and early and late spermatids) (see Figs. 24.16 and Fig. 24.17). Spermatogonia are large- to medium-size round cells with low to moderate amounts of blue cytoplasm and an oval-shaped nucleus without a distinct nucleolus. A commonly observed distinguishing characteristic of these cells is a distinct, condensed, crescent-shaped section of chromatin in their nucleus.[9] Spermatocytes are the largest of the spermatozoa precursor cells and

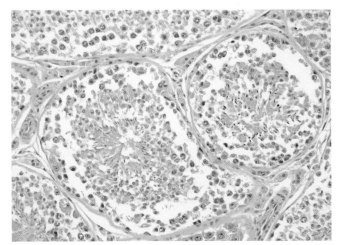

Fig. 24.16 Histology of a normal testicle from an 8-year-old dog. Cells display orderly progression through maturation within each tubule, with immature cells present along the periphery and mature spermatids and spermatozoa within the lumen (hematoxylin and eosin [H&E] stain, original magnification 200×). (Courtesy Dr. John Edwards.)

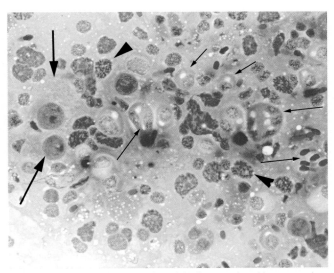

Fig. 24.17 Aspirate of a normal testicle from a dog. Numerous lysed and intact cells are present, with many cytoplasmic fragments observed in the background. Few Sertoli cells *(thick arrows)*, few spermatocytes *(arrowheads)*, and many early and late spermatids *(thin arrows)* are present (Diff-Quik stain, original magnification 500×).

are round in shape, with scant to moderate amounts of light blue cytoplasm surrounding a round nucleus that displays a coarse to clumped cordlike chromatin pattern, similar in appearance to a mitotic figure. A round prominent nucleolus is rarely observed. Occasionally, multinucleate cells are noted. Spermatids are the most common and easily identifiable cells. As the spermatids progress through maturation, four phases are visible. Early spermatids go through the following phases:

1. Golgi phase—the cells are round, are slightly smaller than spermatocytes, and contain a small to moderate amount of basophilic cytoplasm, which often has a single perinuclear vacuole or several small, dispersed, clear vacuoles. Cells have a round nucleus with an indistinct nucleolus, and are frequently multinucleated.
2. Cap phase—the cytoplasm becomes less distinct and the acrosomal cap is often visible as a lighter, crescent shape area in the nucleus, which is round to pear-shaped and darker. Late stage spermatids

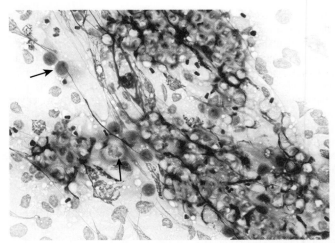

Fig. 24.18 Impression smear of a normal testicle from a dog. Nuclear streaming is present, and the majority of cells appear to be spermatids in various stages of maturation, with the earlier stages resembling lymphocytes. Few Sertoli cells *(thick arrow)* and mitotic figures *(thin arrow)* are observed (Wright-Giemsa stain, original magnification 500×). (Courtesy Dr. Amy Valenciano.)

are differentiated by their scant amount of cytoplasm and are present in the next phase.
3. Acrosomal phase—this phase is characterized by a darker, elongated nucleus
4. Maturation phase—nuclear condensation is complete, and there is scant cytoplasm around the area of tail formation. Finally, mature spermatozoa are characterized by a lack of cytoplasm with a small, dense, oval pale blue to purple nucleus and a long, thin, nonstaining tail (see Figs. 24.17 and Fig. 24.18).

Sertoli Cells

Most Sertoli cells appear as bare nuclei but, if intact, are usually intermingled with spermatogenic cells or in small groups. Sertoli cells can be identified as round to slightly oval cells, with poorly defined cell borders and abundant amounts of pale blue cytoplasm that surrounds a large round nucleus with finely stippled to reticular chromatin and a single, prominent, round nucleolus (see Fig. 24.17). Commonly, the cytoplasm contains numerous, variably sized, clear, distinct vacuoles. Multinucleation or mitotic figures are not typical characteristics of Sertoli cells.

Leydig Cells

Although rarely observed in normal testicular cytology, Leydig (interstitial) cells may be seen in small sheets or as single cells. Cells are round with abundant basophilic cytoplasm that is often microvacuolated and may occasionally contain multiple, small blue granules. The nucleus is eccentrically located, round, and displays a coarsely clumped chromatin pattern with one to two small nucleoli.

Other Cells

Rare mesenchymal cells may be observed. These appear as benign single cells with scant, light blue cytoplasm and a small, centrally located, oval nucleus that displays a stippled chromatin pattern. They are most likely part of the endothelial or peritubular cell population within the testis.

Testicular Inflammation (Orchitis and Epididymitis)

In general, orchitis is a rare occurrence in small animals, and when diagnosed clinically, it is actually a manifestation of epididymitis, which is much more common.[27] Most causes of epididymitis and orchitis are infectious in nature, although severe trauma to the scrotum can also cause testicular inflammation. In dogs, *Brucella canis* is attributed as the primary etiological agent of orchitis, but other infectious causes have been reported, including *E. coli*,[27] *Proteus vulgaris*,[27] *Blastomyces dermatitidis*,[26] *M. canis*,[48] *Leishmania infantum*,[49] and *Rickettsia rickettsia* (which causes Rocky Mountain spotted fever).[50] Distemper virus can induce testicular inflammation characterized by an infiltration of lymphocytes, and intranuclear or intracytoplasmic inclusions may be identified in epithelial cells.[27] Dual infections may also occur. In one case report of a 2-year-old Border Collie, *B. dermatitidis* was identified on histology, and bacterial culture revealed a gram-negative bacterium, *Aureimonas altamirensis*.[51] Cats may develop primary orchitis or epididymitis from feline infectious peritonitis (FIP) or scrotal trauma.[27]

The cytological findings of orchitis and epididymitis are similar to the cytological findings of inflammation in other tissues. Neutrophils with variable degrees of degenerative change are usually the predominant cell type, but other inflammatory cells, such as macrophages (including multinucleate giant cells), small lymphocytes, and/or plasma cells, may be identified, especially in fungal and/or chronic inflammatory processes. Occasionally, the cause of inflammation can be determined on cytology; however, submission of a sample of testicular material for bacterial culture and susceptibility testing is always encouraged.

Testicular Neoplasia

In male dogs, the testes are a common site for tumor development.[34] Testicular tumors may occur in both intact and neutered animals.[52] In neutered animals, tumors may be located in the scrotum or at the prescrotal incision site and are thought to arise from embryological testicular remnants, ectopic testis-like tissue (including polyorchidism), or transplanted testicular tissue from trauma to the testes during castration.[52] In dogs, testicular torsion is commonly associated with a testicular tumor, which is also typically intraabdominal.[34] Despite a report of 100% specificity in one study,[53] cytological diagnosis of testicular tumors can be challenging, and histology is often required to make a definitive diagnosis. In dogs, the three major tumors of the testes are Sertoli cell tumors, Leydig (interstitial) cell tumors, and seminomas.[34,53,54] Conflicting reports exist regarding both incidence of and breed predilection for tumor development in dogs. Testicular tumors are rare in cats, with only few isolated published case reports.[34,52,55,56] It is common for an animal to have more than one type of testicular tumor.[53] FNA can be performed on a suspected intraabdominal tumor using ultrasound guidance; inguinal cryptorchid testicles with suspected neoplasia can be easily aspirated without imaging.

Sertoli Cell Tumors

Sertoli cell tumors are a type of sex cord stromal tumor (arising from the sustentacular cells of seminiferous tubules). They frequently occur in the testicles of older dogs or the undescended testicles of cryptorchid dogs. On palpation, they are typically firm, and grossly, they appear lobulated and greasy with a white or gray surface.[22,34] Approximately 70% of these tumors are functional, releasing estrogen. This may result in the occurrence of feminization paraneoplastic syndrome.[57] In addition to various clinical signs, such as bone marrow hypoplasia, symmetrical alopecia, and mammary hypertrophy, feminization syndrome results in atrophy of the contralateral testicle.[34,58] As a result of estrogen release, squamous metaplasia of the prostate may also occur (see Fig. 24.11). To the authors' knowledge, feminization syndrome has not been reported in cats with Sertoli cell tumors.[52] Extratesticular Sertoli cell tumors, particularly in the scrotal skin or spermatic cord, have been reported in dogs.[52]

Cytologically, smears from Sertoli cell tumors are moderately to highly cellular with cells typically arranged in variably sized aggregates,

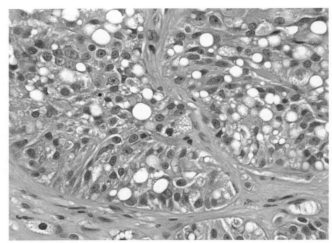

Fig. 24.19 Histology of a Sertoli cell neoplasm in a dog. Cells demonstrate the palisading arrangement and variably sized, intracytoplasmic vacuoles often seen in this tumor type (hematoxylin and eosin [H&E] stain, original magnification 400×). (Courtesy Dr. John Edwards.)

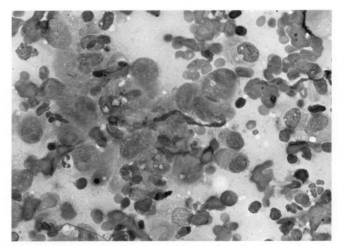

Fig. 24.20 A group of cells aspirated from a Sertoli cell tumor in a dog. The cells have a moderate amount of light blue wispy, cytoplasm. Nuclei have prominent large nucleoli often seen with these tumors (Wright-Giemsa stain, original magnification 100×).

sheets, or distinct palisades (Fig. 24.19) with occasional single cells. Cells are generally large and round to elongate, with variably distinct cell borders (Fig. 24.20). A distinct feature of these tumors is the abundant light blue cytoplasm that often contains few, large, distinct, clear vacuoles (see Fig. 24.19; Fig. 24.21). Nuclei are round to oval and display a finely stippled to reticulated chromatin pattern, with one to several prominent, round nucleoli. Moderate anisocytosis and anisokaryosis are observed, and mitotic figures are rare. Although typically associated with ovarian granulosa cell tumors, Call-Exner bodies have been reported in dogs with Sertoli cell tumors.[59] These structures are characterized by a large cluster of round to elongated cells arranged in a rosette-like pattern surrounding dark pink to magenta, hyaline material that stains intensely with Periodic acid–Schiff (PAS), toluidine blue, and Ziehl-Neelsen stains.[59] Sertoli cell tumors express vimentin, inhibin-α, and anti-Müllerian hormone, and they can be distinguished from Leydig cell tumors with nuclear staining of the transcription factor SOX9 using IHC.[60-62]

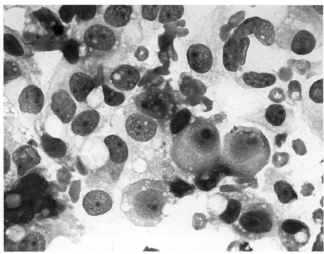

Fig. 24.21 Aspirate of a Sertoli cell tumor from a dog. The cells have abundant blue cytoplasm that contains variably sized, clear vacuoles. Nuclei display a finely stippled chromatin pattern with a single, round, prominent nucleolus (Wright-Giemsa stain, original magnification 1000×).

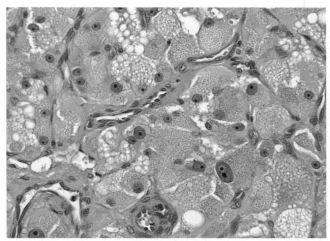

Fig. 24.22 Histology of a Leydig (interstitial) cell tumor from a dog. The cytoplasm contains numerous fine to moderately sized vacuoles, and cells display moderate anisocytosis and anisokaryosis. Frequent capillaries are observed throughout the tumor (hematoxylin and eosin [H&E] stain, original magnification 400×). (Courtesy Dr. John Edwards.)

Leydig (Interstitial) Cell Tumors

Leydig (interstitial) cell tumors, another type of sex cord stromal tumor, arise from Leydig cells between the seminiferous tubules in the testes. Clinical signs are typically uncommon in dogs; thus, these tumors are often an incidental finding. On palpation, these tumors are soft and bulging. On cut surface, they are well circumscribed and noninvasive and may appear tan to bright yellow or orange in color, with many vascular channels.[22,34] These tumors have been associated with increased testosterone production, leading to a high prevalence of prostatic disease and perianal gland neoplasms.[34] In some studies, cats with interstitial cell tumors, although castrated (or presumed so), were observed to display some form of secondary male sexual characteristics, such as aggressive behavior, inappropriate urination, and penile barbs, suggesting testosterone production.[52,55] In dogs, Leydig cell tumors have rarely been reported to produce estrogen, resulting in feminization syndrome and related clinical signs.[63] Metastasis of Leydig cell tumors is generally rare and has been reported in dogs but not in cats.[64,65]

Aspirates of interstitial cell tumors are overall highly cellular and frequently contain aggregates of cells surrounding capillaries, known as a *perivascular pattern* (Fig. 24.22), making this a distinguishing characteristic for cytological diagnosis (Fig. 24.23).[52] Cells are round to columnar to spindle shaped, with indistinct cell borders and moderate to abundant amounts of dark blue cytoplasm. As opposed to Sertoli cell tumors, the cytoplasm of interstitial cell tumors tends to contain numerous fine, punctate, clear vacuoles (microvacuoles), which can also be observed in the background as a result of cell rupture (Figs. 24.24 and 24.25).[53] Occasionally, fine, blue-to-black cytoplasmic granules are seen, and this is not a common finding in other testicular tumors (see Fig. 24.24).[53] Nuclei are round and display a finely stippled to reticular chromatin pattern with a prominent, round nucleolus. Nuclear pseudoinclusions, appearing as small vacuoles embedded within the nucleus, may also be identified and used as a distinguishing cytological characteristic of Leydig cell tumors because they, too, have not been observed in other testicular tumors.[53] Overall, cells display mild to moderate (and rarely marked) anisocytosis and anisokaryosis with a low to moderate N:C ratio. Mitotic figures are rare. On IHC, Leydig cell tumors intensely stain with inhibin-α and calretinin. In

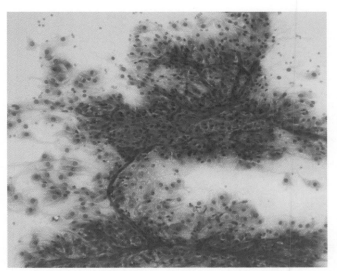

Fig. 24.23 An aspirate of a Leydig (interstitial) cell tumor from a dog. The smear is highly cellular, composed of cells surrounding capillaries, which is a distinguishing characteristic for cytological diagnosis (Wright-Giemsa stain, original magnification 200×).

dogs, calretinin is consistently positive and can be used to distinguish Leydig cell tumors from other testicular tumors.[64,66]

Seminomas

Seminomas are derived from germ cells in the testes. Although not routinely subdivided in veterinary medicine, two types of seminomas have been recognized in dogs that are morphologically consistent with human spermatocytic seminomas and classic seminomas.[67,68] Seminomas are commonly associated with cryptorchidism, and undescended testicles have an increased risk of seminoma occurrence.[67] There is also an increased incidence of seminoma occurring within the right testicle in dogs.[67] Seminomas commonly occur along with other testicular tumors, particularly Sertoli cell tumors. Seminomas are soft on palpation, bulge on cut surface, and grossly appear as a well-circumscribed, homogenous, white mass.[22,34] A major feature of seminomas is testicular enlargement, which is usually unilateral but

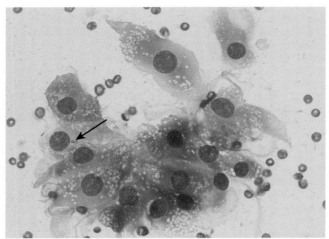

Fig. 24.24 Cells from an aspirate of a Leydig (interstitial) cell tumor from a dog. In addition to cytoplasmic vacuoles, one cell contains blue-black cytoplasmic vacuoles *(arrow)*, which are occasionally identified in cells from this tumor. Cells demonstrate mild to moderate anisocytosis and mild anisokaryosis (Wright-Giemsa stain, original magnification 500×).

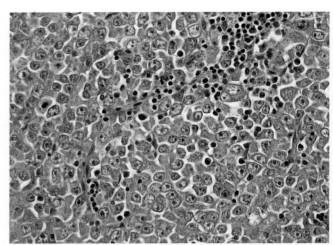

Fig. 24.26 Histology of a seminoma from a dog, solid variant. Cells are arranged in a solid sheet and have a mild infiltrate of small lymphocytes. Neoplastic cells have a large, round nucleus with vesicular chromatin and typically a single prominent nucleolus (hematoxylin and eosin [H&E] stain, original magnification 400×). (Courtesy Dr. John Edwards.)

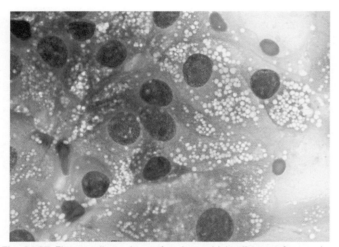

Fig. 24.25 Fine-needle aspirate of an interstitial cell tumor from a dog. Cells have numerous, fine, punctate, clear vacuoles that are characteristic of this tumor. Mild to moderate anisocytosis and mild anisokaryosis is observed (Wright-Giemsa stain, original magnification 1000×).

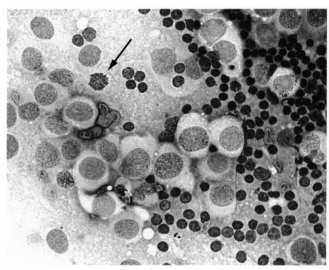

Fig. 24.27 Impression smear of a seminoma from a dog. Large numbers of characteristic discrete, round cells with nuclei that display a reticular chromatin pattern and a prominent nucleolus are present. In addition, a large number of small lymphocytes that infiltrate the tumor can be identified. A mitotic figure is also observed *(arrow)* (Diff-Quik stain, original magnification 500×).

occasionally can be bilateral.[34] Typically, few clinical signs are seen in dogs with seminomas, although they have been reported to result in feminization syndrome alone or, more commonly, in cases where a concurrent Sertoli cell tumor is present.[34] Although relatively uncommon, metastasis is more likely with seminomas than other testicular tumors.[34] Seminoma occurring in a cat with bilateral cryptorchidism with metastasis to the sublumbar lymph nodes has been reported.[34]

Aspiration usually yields moderate to large numbers of large, discrete round cells (Fig. 24.26) that contain a sparse to moderate amount of homogeneous, medium to deep blue cytoplasm with low numbers of large, round, clear vacuoles. Nuclei are large in size and round to oval in shape and display characteristic coarsely reticular to irregularly clumped chromatin with a large, round, prominent nucleolus (Fig. 24.27). Multinucleation is common (Fig. 24.28), and mitotic figures are frequently identified (see Figs. 24.27 and 24.28; Fig. 24.29). The presence of a granular, lacey eosinophilic background (tigroid background), lymphocytic infiltrate (see Figs. 24.26 and 24.27), and atypical mitoses (see Fig. 24.29) are diagnostic

features commonly observed with seminomas.[53] In canine seminomas, c-KIT is potently expressed, as shown by IHC, and is potentially helpful for differentiating seminomas from other testicular tumors.[69]

Other Testicular Neoplasms

Although the tumors listed above are the most prevalent, other testicular tumors, including mixed germ cell sex cord stromal tumor (described below), leiomyoma, schwannoma, and hemangioma, have been reported.[34,70,71] Metastases to the testes is rare but has been reported in dogs.[72]

Mixed Germ Cell Sex Cord Stromal Tumors

Although rarely reported, mixed germ cell sex cord stromal tumors are a distinct and separate group of testicular neoplasms in the dog

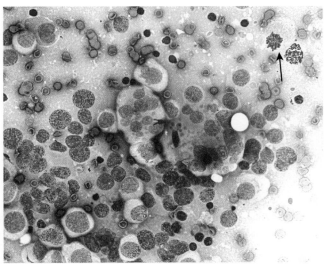

Fig. 24.28 Impression smear of a seminoma from a dog. Large multinucleated cells containing numerous nuclei, including satellite nuclei, are seen, along with several other intact and lysed neoplastic cells and few small lymphocytes. Mitotic figures are present *(arrow)* (Diff-Quik stain, original magnification 400×).

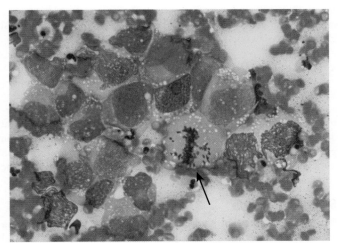

Fig. 24.29 Aspirate from a seminoma in a dog. Frequent mitotic figures, including atypical mitotic figures *(arrow)*, are commonly observed with seminomas (Diff-Quik stain, original magnification 500×).

and are characterized by a mixture of atypical germ cells and sex cord stromal derivatives (either Sertoli cells or Leydig cells).[70,71,73] In dogs, they are typically unilateral, but a bilateral case has been reported.[71] Grossly, these tumors are difficult to distinguish from other testicular tumors, appearing as firm, gray-white to tan, single to multilobed masses.[71]

On cytology, a mixed germ cell stromal tumor should be suspected when two populations of neoplastic cells are observed. Most commonly this includes a mixture of neoplastic germ cells, as seen in seminomas, in conjunction with Sertoli cells; however, Leydig cells can also be present. Histologically, mixed gonadal tumors are differentiated from collision tumors (two individual tumors that have grown into one another) on the basis of the degree of intermingling of the two cell populations. To help differentiate this tumor type, an antibody panel, including E-cadherin, GATA-4, inhibin-α, c-KIT, neuron specific enolase (NSE), and protein gene product 9.5 (PGP 9.5), may be useful.[70]

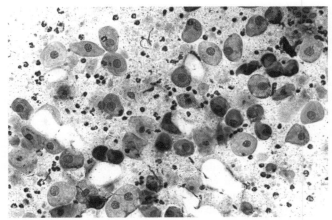

Fig. 24.30 Impression smear of the tip of the penis from an intact dog. Many nucleated squamous epithelial cells, neutrophils, and bacteria are present. Mild variation in cell appearance is evident among the epithelial cells (Diff-Quik stain, original magnification 200×).

Teratomas

A teratoma is a complex tumor that is composed of multiple germ layers in various stages of maturation and, as a result, may consist of tissue that is foreign to the area in which it arises. Testicular teratomas have been described in various textbooks to occur in both dogs and cats. However, the only currently available published case reports have described teratomas in the cryptorchid testicles of cats, including one that metastasized to the omentum.[56,74]

Sperm Granulomas

Sperm granulomas develop because of a chronic inflammatory response elicited by extravasation of spermatozoa from the reproductive tract. The occurrence of granuloma has been associated with congenital alterations of the epididymal duct, trauma, infection, and surgical procedures.[75,76] On physical examination of the scrotum, sperm granulomas are palpated as variably sized, firm nodules in the epididymis. Abnormalities on semen evaluation (described below) may also be noted.[75] FNA of the nodule(s) and histopathology reveals numerous spermatozoa in conjunction with a marked inflammatory response characterized predominantly by macrophages and lymphocytes.

PENIS AND PREPUCE

Cytological Evaluation of the Normal Penis

Cytological evaluation of the penis can be helpful in assessing for inflammatory and neoplastic conditions. The most prevalent cell observed on normal penile cytology (obtained by impression smear) is the nucleated squamous epithelial cell. In addition, variable numbers of nondegenerate to slightly degenerate neutrophils are present, and bacteria may be found, both extracellularly and intracellularly (Fig. 24.30). *Simonsiella* spp. from oral contamination (licking) may also be identified. Because the preputial covering is an extension of the skin, criteria used for cytological evaluation of the skin should be applied.

Balanitis and Posthitis

It is not uncommon for male dogs to have a small amount of greenish-yellow, purulent discharge (smegma) extruding at the tip of the penis and preputial opening. Copious amounts of this material, however, may be an indication of an underlying infection. The penis should be gently extruded from the preputial sheath and examined closely for any abnormalities, such as the presence of a foreign body, discoloration, injury, and/or masses. Excessive licking for any reason can lead to hyperemia of the penis. Cytological evaluation of the purulent material may reveal a nonspecific inflammatory response characterized by variably degenerate neutrophils, macrophages, and intracellular and/or extracellular bacteria with exfoliated mature squamous epithelial cells. Bacterial culture and susceptibility testing are typically not helpful but can be considered if there is suspicion of a bacterial infection that does not resolve with antibiotic therapy.

Penile and Preputial Neoplasia

Although not common, neoplasia of the penis has been reported in dogs, and cytological evaluation can be done by making impression smears of the mass or via FNA. Not having knowledge of normal canine anatomy, some owners may mistake the swelling of the bulbus glandus of the penis for an abnormal "mass."

Penile Squamous Papilloma

Dogs with a penile squamous papilloma may present for preputial swelling, genital masses, and urinary abnormalities.[77] Evaluation of the penis reveals a variably sized, single, pedunculated, soft, pinkish red, cauliflower-like mass, which may also have ulceration and bleeding.[77] Smears are composed of a homogeneous population of squamous epithelial cells that display minimal atypia, in conjunction with a secondary inflammatory response that is characterized predominantly by neutrophils. Bacteria may be identified if the sample was obtained from an area of ulceration and there is infection secondary to continuous licking of the mass. Although papillomas are mostly associated with papillomavirus infection, they can also be nonviral (induced by trauma or idiopathic).[77]

Canine Transmissible Venereal Tumors

The most common penile neoplasm in dogs is the transmissible venereal tumor (TVT).[34] This is rare in the United States but is endemic in areas where there are large populations of stray dogs, especially in tropical and subtropical environments. The tumors usually occur on the external genitalia but can also be found on the nasal and oral mucosae (especially near the tonsils) and on nongenital skin.

On cytology, smears reveal high cellularity and are composed of cells that are round to slightly oval, with discrete cell borders and moderate amounts of light to dark blue cytoplasm. Frequently, the cytoplasm contains small, punctate vacuoles, giving these tumor cells a distinct cytological characteristic (Fig. 24.31). Nuclei are round to oval and display an immature, finely reticulated chromatin pattern that occasionally contains a large, round nucleolus. Overall, cells display mild to moderate anisocytosis and mild anisokaryosis with a moderate to high N:C ratio. Mitotic figures are frequently observed. As the tumor regresses, increased numbers of lymphocytes are seen, along with a few neutrophils and macrophages. If impression smears are made from the surface of an ulcerated tumor, bacteria, neutrophils, and epithelial cells can also be present. Recent reports in the literature have suggested that it may be beneficial to classify TVTs into three cytomorphological subtypes—plasmacytoid, lymphocytoid, and mixed—because each type may exhibit different biological behavior and thus may influence treatment options.[78]

Other Neoplasms

In dogs, the second most common penile neoplasm is squamous cell carcinoma, which is cytologically identical to squamous cell carcinomas from other locations.[34,79] A number of other penile neoplasms have been reported in dogs, including lymphoma, fibrosarcoma,

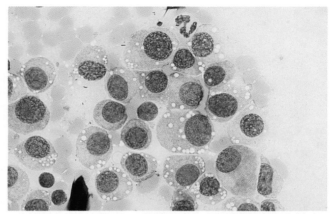

Fig. 24.31 Fine-needle aspirate of a transmissible venereal tumor from a dog. Numerous, discrete, round cells are present and contain medium blue cytoplasm with multiple punctate vacuoles. Nuclei display a reticulated chromatin pattern with indistinct nucleoli (Wright-Giemsa stain, original magnification 500×).

sebaceous gland adenoma, ossifying fibroma, osteosarcoma, hemangiosarcoma, and chondrosarcoma.[34,80-84]

As mentioned previously, because the prepuce is a continuation of the skin, any cutaneous neoplasm may be encountered, such as lipomas, melanomas, or mast cell tumors.[34] The skin of the prepuce contains perianal gland cells (modified sebaceous glands); thus perianal gland tumors can occur.

SEMEN

Evaluation of semen quality is performed as part of a routine breeding soundness examination or to investigate causes of subfertility or infertility in both male dogs and cats.[85-87] Because semen contains material derived from the testes and the entire reproductive tract, including the prostate gland, examination of semen can also provide information on lesions in the genital tract, including inflammatory or neoplastic conditions.

Semen Collection

Semen collection can be performed on most dogs in a clinical setting without the need for special equipment. Likelihood of successful sample collection is increased by proper preparation of the collection room and the presence of a teaser bitch.[88] Before collection, the male should have at least 4 to 5 days of sexual rest. Evaluation of semen collected after more than 10 days of sexual rest may result in increased morphological abnormalities, decreased motility caused by spermatozoal aging, and an increased amount of cellular debris.[88] Collection should not occur more frequently than every 2 to 5 days for purposes of evaluation.[88] The procedure itself involves collecting semen into an artificial latex vagina while the penis is manually manipulated in the presence of a teaser female that is, ideally, in proestrus or estrus. However, vaginal swabs obtained from a bitch in estrus can also be used. For further details on sample collection techniques, the reader is referred to other resources.[88,89] In cats, collection of semen via electroejaculation has become the method of choice, as it produces higher ejaculate volumes; however, collection can also be done with the use of an artificial vagina and a teaser queen.[87] In dogs, FNA of the testicle can be used as a tool for semen evaluation to provide information on procession of spermatogenesis.[10] Identification of cells is described in the discussion on normal testicle cytology above.

Semen Evaluation

The gross characteristics of the fluid, including volume, color, and consistency, should be determined immediately after collection. Dogs ejaculate in three fractions.[86,88] The first fraction, known as the *presperm fraction*, comes from the prostate gland. Its volume is typically 0.5 to 20 milliliters (mL), and it contains little to no sperm. The second fraction, the *sperm-rich fraction*, comes from the epididymis and testes and is normally opaque, milky-white, and approximately 0.5 to 2.0 mL in volume.[88] The third fraction, or *prostatic fraction*, is normally clear and should not be collected with the sperm-rich portion, especially for semen evaluation, as it can cause decreased motility after 2 hours.[88] Cats produce a much lower volume of sperm ejaculate, ranging from 0.03 to 0.7 mL, depending on the method used.[87] In cats, the second fraction should normally be homogeneous and cream-white in color. In either animal, yellow coloration can indicate that semen is contaminated by urine. Red, pink, or brown coloration indicates that fresh or hemolyzed blood is present in the sample. Serous, green, or gray coloration of semen indicates inflammation, especially when small flecks of material are present.

Sperm motility should be evaluated immediately after collection. The sample should be maintained at body temperature. A drop of semen is placed on a warmed microscope slide, which is immediately covered with a warm coverslip. Samples with a high concentration of spermatozoa may be diluted 1:1 with warm physiological saline to aid in evaluation.[88] Microscopic evaluation should be performed at 20× and 40×, with the condenser lowered. Normal motility is described as rapid, progressive, forward motion, with at least 70% of sperm showing this movement.[88] Motility is thought to reflect viability and thus ability to fertilize an ovum. Abnormal motility may include side-to-side motion without forward progression, movement in small circles, rolling, hypomotility, or nonmotile sperm. Decreased motility may be seen in semen contaminated by urine or exposed to blood or inflammation. After a long period of sexual inactivity, sperm motility may be decreased significantly as a result of aging, and many sperm may be dead. The percentage of progressive motility increases after 5 days of sexual rest compared with only 1 day of rest.[88]

Sperm concentration is determined by using a Neubauer hemocytometer after appropriate dilution. The procedure should be performed according the manufacturer's protocol. Although there are several protocols, one method is to draw semen into the 0.02 mL Unopette (Becton-Dickinson, Rutherford, NJ) capillary tube, which is then dispensed into the 1.98 mL Unopette chamber and mixed. The diluted sample is dispensed into both sides of the hemocytometer chambers and allowed to settle. The total number of sperm in the central primary square is counted on each side and averaged. The numbers should be within 10% of each other. This represents the number of spermatozoa (in millions) per milliliter of semen. This number is then multiplied by the total volume of the ejaculate (in milliliters) to determine the total sperm count. An average-sized dog should produce approximately 250 to 300 million sperm per ejaculate, whereas the average cat should produce 6 to 13 million sperm per ejaculate. Sperm count can be affected by a variety of factors including age of the animal, time of year, animal disposition, and frequency of ejaculation.[88]

For evaluation of sperm morphology, phase-contrast microscopy of an unstained smear is considered the gold standard, because alteration in osmolality or pH caused by the addition of stain may increase the abnormalities observed.[86] There are several ways to prepare the smear, although a "squash prep" (i.e., placing a drop of semen on a glass slide,

TABLE 24.1	Abnormalities of Spermatozoa
Primary	**Secondary**
Head	**Head**
• Tapered	• Detached
• Narrow	**Midpiece**
• Small	• Retained distal droplet
• Giant	**Tail**
• Round	• Bent
• Deformed	• Hairpin
• Double	**Other**
Midpiece	• Detached acrosome
• Double	
• Swollen	
• Retained proximal droplet	
Tail	
• Tightly coiled	
• Double	

laying another slide directly on top of it, and pulling the two slides apart) or a "blood smear prep" (putting a drop of semen on a slide and using a "pusher" slide at a 45-degree angle) is recommended.[86] For bright-field light microscopy, the eosin-nigrosin stain and Romanowsky-type stains (e.g., Wright-Giemsa, Diff-Quik) are most commonly used, although others have been described.[86,88,90] Sperm should be evaluated under 100× (immersion oil) with a minimum of 200 sperm examined. Abnormalities can be classified as either primary or secondary (Table 24.1). Primary abnormalities occur during spermatogenesis and are thus of higher concern. Secondary abnormalities may occur either by passage through the epididymis, during collection, and/or during slide preparation. Examples of some of these defects are shown in Fig. 24.32. Normal semen should have less than 10% primary abnormalities and less than 20% secondary abnormalities with a total of less than 20% to 30% abnormalities overall.[88] Although an increased percentage of abnormalities may indicate poor quality and breeding potential, a recent study involving 39 male Labrador Retrievers found that there was no significant association between sperm abnormalities and declining fertility rate.[91] This indicates that many factors influence fertility, and a discussion of all of them is beyond the scope of this chapter. Although not sensitive enough for identifying subtle infertility problems, the use of testicular FNA and cytological analysis has shown to be helpful in identifying azoospermia as a cause of infertility in dogs.[10]

Cytological evaluation of the sperm-rich fraction can be performed if inflammation or neoplasia of the reproductive tract is suspected. A concentrated smear or cytocentrifuge preparation is most useful, but evaluation of a direct smear can also be performed. In addition to spermatozoa, normal sperm-rich fluid can contain approximately two to four white blood cells per high-power field along with rare to few epithelial cells, bacteria, and erythrocytes. If increased numbers and/or abnormal cells are noted, additional diagnostics to evaluate the entirety of the reproductive tract should be pursued. Semen is not sterile, so extra precautions should be taken to minimize as much contamination as possible if a sample for bacterial culture is submitted. Infection is indicated if greater than 10,000 colony-forming units per milliliter of semen is grown on culture.[92]

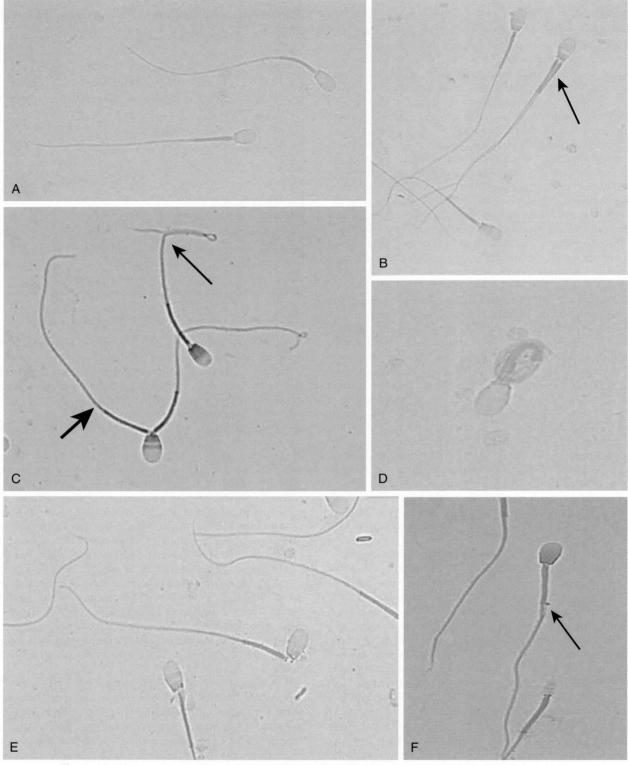

Fig. 24.32 (A) Normal spermatozoa. (B) Spermatozoa with a double midpiece and tail *(arrow)*. (C) Spermatozoa with a double tail *(thick arrow)* and spermatozoa with a hairpin tail *(thin arrow)*. (D) Spermatozoa with a tightly coiled tail. E, Spermatozoa with a detached head. F, Spermatozoa with a retained distal droplet (new methylene blue stain, original magnification 1000×).

REFERENCES

1. Smith J. Canine prostatic disease: a review of anatomy, pathology, diagnosis, and treatment. *Theriogenology*. 2008;70:375–383.
2. Mordecai A, Liptak JM, Hofstede T, et al. Prostatic abscess in a neutered cat. *J Am Anim Hosp Assoc*. 2008;44:90–94.
3. Williams J, Niles J. Prostatic disease in the dog. *In Practice*. 1999;21:558–575.
4. Polisca A, Troisi A, Fontaine E, et al. A retrospective study of canine prostatic diseases from 2002 to 2009 at the Alfort Veterinary College in France. *Theriogenology*. 2016;85:835–840.
5. Krawiec DR, Heflin D. Study of prostatic disease in dogs—177 cases (1981-1986). *J Am Vet Med Assoc*. 1992;200:1119–1122.
6. Teske E, Naan EC, van Dijk EM, et al. Canine prostate carcinoma: epidemiological evidence of an increased risk in castrated dogs. *Mol Cell Endocrinol*. 2002;197:251–255.
7. Levy X, Nizanski W, Heimendahl A, et al. Diagnosis of common prostatic conditions in dogs: an update. *Reprod Domest Anim*. 2014;49:50–57.
8. Powe JR, Canfield PJ, Martin PA. Evaluation of the cytologic diagnosis of canine prostatic disorders. *Vet Clin Pathol*. 2004;33:150–154.
9. Santos M, Marcos R, Caniatti M. Cytologic study of normal canine testis. *Theriogenology*. 2010;73:208–214.
10. Dahlbom M, Makinen A, Suominen J. Testicular fine needle aspiration cytology as a diagnostic tool in dog infertility. *J Small Anim Pract*. 1997;38:506–512.
11. Gouletsou PG, Galatos AD, Leontides LS, et al. Impact of fine- or large-needle aspiration on canine testes: clinical, in vivo ultrasonographic and seminological assessment. *Reprod Domest Anim*. 2011;46:712–719.
12. James RW, Heywood R, Fowler DJ. Serial percutaneous testicular biopsy in the Beagle dog. *J Small Anim Pract*. 1979;20:219–228.
13. Gouletsou PG, Galatos AD, Sideri AI, et al. Impact of fine needle aspiration (FNA) and of the number of punctures on the feline testis: clinical, gross anatomy and histological assessment. *Theriogenology*. 2012;78:172–181.
14. Kustritz MVR. Collection of tissue and culture samples from the canine reproductive tract. *Theriogenology*. 2006;66:567–574.
15. Ling GV, Branam JE, Ruby AL, et al. Canine prostatic fluid: techniques of collection, quantitative bacterial culture, and interpretation of results. *J Am Vet Med Assoc*. 1983;183:201–206.
16. Boland LE, Hardie RJ, Gregory SP, et al. Ultrasound-guided percutaneous drainage as the primary treatment for prostatic abscesses and cysts in dogs. *J Am Anim Hosp Assoc*. 2003;39:151–159.
17. Ling GV. *Lower Urinary Tract Diseases of Dogs and Cats: Diagnosis, Medical Management, Prevention*. St. Louis: Mosby; 1995.
18. Berry SJ, Strandberg JD, Saunders WJ, et al. Development of canine benign prostatic hyperplasia with age. *Prostate*. 1986;9:363–373.
19. Pinheiro D, Machado J, Viegas C, et al. Evaluation of biomarker canine-prostate specific arginine esterase (CPSE) for the diagnosis of benign prostatic hyperplasia. *BMC Vet Res*. 2017;13:76.
20. Gobello C, Corrada Y. Noninfectious prostatic diseases in dogs. *Compend Contin Educ*. 2002;24:99–107.
21. Krawiec DR. Canine prostate disease. *J Am Vet Med Assoc*. 1994;204:1561–1564.
22. Foster RA. Common lesions in the male reproductive tract of cats and dogs. *Vet Clin North Am Small Anim Pract*. 2012;42:527–545.
23. Duque J, Macias-Garcia B, Tapia PR, et al. Two unusual cases of canine prostatitis: prostatitis in a castrated dog and preputial oedema in an intact male. *Reprod Domest Anim*. 2010;45:e199–e200.
24. Roura X, Camps-Palau MA, Lloret A, et al. Bacterial prostatitis in a cat. *J Vet Intern Med*. 2002;16:593–597.
25. Dorfman M, Barsanti J. Diseases of the canine prostate-gland. *Compend Contin Educ*. 1995;17:791.
26. Totten AK, Ridgway MD, Sauerli DS. Blastomyces dermatitidis prostatic and testicular infection in eight dogs (1992-2005). *J Am Anim Hosp Assoc*. 2011;47:413–418.
27. Foster RA. Male genital system In: Maxie MG. In: Jubb Kennedy, ed. *Palmer's Pathology of Domestic Animals*. 6th ed. St. Louis, Missouri: Elsevier; 2016:465–510.
28. Mir F, Fontaine E, Reyes-Gomez E, et al. Subclinical leishmaniasis associated with infertility and chronic prostatitis in a dog. *J Small Anim Pract*. 2012;53:419–422.
29. Giroux V, Rustgi AK. Metaplasia: tissue injury adaptation and a precursor to the dysplasia-cancer sequence. *Nat Rev Cancer*. 2017;17:594–604.
30. Palmieri C, Lean FZ, Akter SH, et al. A retrospective analysis of 111 canine prostatic samples: histopathological findings and classification. *Res Vet Sci*. 2014;97:568–573.
31. Tucker AR, Smith JR. Prostatic squamous metaplasia in a cat with interstitial cell neoplasia in a retained testis. *Vet Pathol*. 2008;45:905–909.
32. Black GM, Ling GV, Nyland TG, et al. Prevalence of prostatic cysts in adult, large-breed dogs. *J Am Anim Hosp Assoc*. 1998;34:177–180.
33. Newell SM, Mahaffey MB, Binhazim A, et al. Paraprostatic cyst in a cat. *J Small Anim Pract*. 1992;33:399–401.
34. McEntee MC. Reproductive oncology. *Top Companion Anim Med*. 2002;17:133–149.
35. Weaver AD. Fifteen cases of prostatic carcinoma in the dog. *Vet Rec*. 1981;109:71–75.
36. LeRoy BE, Lech ME. Prostatic carcinoma causing urethral obstruction and obstipation in a cat. *J Feline Med Surg*. 2004;6:397–400.
37. Tursi M, Costa T, Valenza F, et al. Adenocarcinoma of the disseminated prostate in a cat. *J Feline Med Surg*. 2008;10:600–602.
38. Caney SMA, Holt PE, Day MJ, et al. Prostatic carcinoma in two cats. *J Small Anim Pract*. 1998;39:140–143.
39. Hubbard BS, Vulgamott JC, Liska WD. Prostatic adenocarcinoma in a cat. *J Am Vet Med Assoc*. 1990;197:1493–1494.
40. Bryan JN, Keeler MR, Henry CJ, et al. A population study of neutering status as a risk factor for canine prostate cancer. *Prostate*. 2007;67:1174–1181.
41. Bradbury CA, Westropp JL, Pollard RE. Relationship between Prostatomegaly, Prostatic Mineralization, and Cytologic Diagnosis. *Vet Radiol Ultrasound*. 2009;50:167–171.
42. Winter MD, Locke JE, Penninck DG. Imaging diagnosis—urinary obstruction secondary to prostatic lymphoma in a young dog. *Vet Radiol Ultrasound*. 2006;47:597–601.
43. Hayden DW, Klausner JS, Waters DJ. Prostatic leiomyosarcoma in a dog. *J Vet Diagn Invest*. 1999;11:283–286.
44. Harmelin A, Nyska A, Aroch I, et al. Canine medullary thyroid carcinoma with unusual distant metastases. *J Vet Diagn Invest*. 1993;5:284–288.
45. Leroy BE, Northrup N. Prostate cancer in dogs: comparative and clinical aspects. *Vet J*. 2009;180:149–162.
46. Larsen RE. Testicular biopsy in dog. *Vet Clin North Am Small Anim Pract*. 1977;7:747–755.
47. Diagone KV, Feliciano MAR, Pacheco MR, et al. Histology and morphometry of the testes of adult domestic cats (*Felis catus*). *J Feline Med Surg*. 2012;14:124–130.
48. Rosendal S. Canine mycoplasmas—their ecologic niche and role in disease. *J Am Vet Med Assoc*. 1982;180:1212–1214.
49. Manna L, Paciello O, Della Morte R, et al. Detection of Leishmania parasites in the testis of a dog affected by orchitis: case report. *Parasit Vectors*. 2012;5.
50. Ober CP, Spaulding K, Breitschwerdt EB, et al. Orchitis in two dogs with rocky mountain spotted fever. *Vet Radiol Ultrasound*. 2004;45:458–465.
51. Reilly TJ, Calcutt MJ, Wennerdahl LA, et al. Isolation of *Aureimonas altamirensis*, a *Brucella canis*-like bacterium, from an edematous canine testicle. *J Vet Diagn Invest*. 2014;26:795–798.
52. Doxsee AL, Yager JA, Best SJ, et al. Extratesticular interstitial and Sertoli cell tumors in previously neutered dogs and cats: a report of 17 cases. *Can Vet*. 2006;47:763–766.
53. Masserdotti C, Bonfanti U, De Lorenzi D, et al. Cytologic features of testicular tumours in dog. *J Vet Med A Physiol Pathol Clin Med*. 2005;52:339–346.
54. Grieco V, Riccardi E, Greppi GF, et al. Canine testicular tumours: a study on 232 dogs. *J Comp Pathol*. 2008;138:86–89.
55. Miller MA, Hartnett SE, Ramos-Vara JA. Interstitial cell tumor and sertoli cell tumor in the testis of a cat. *Vet Pathol*. 2007;44:394–397.
56. Miyoshi N, Yasuda N, Kamimura Y, et al. Teratoma in a feline unilateral cryptorchid testis. *Vet Pathol*. 2001;38:729–730.
57. Quartuccio M, Marino G, Garufi G, et al. Sertoli cell tumors associated with feminizing syndrome and spermatic cord torsion in two cryptorchid dogs. *J Vet Med Sci*. 2012;13:207–209.
58. Sherding RG, Wilson 3rd GP, Kociba GJ. Bone marrow hypoplasia in eight dogs with Sertoli cell tumor. *J Am Vet Med Assoc*. 1981;178:497–501.

59. Masserdotti C, De Lorenzi D, Gasparotto L. Cytologic detection of Call-Exner bodies in Sertoli cell tumors from 2 dogs. *Vet Clin Pathol.* 2008;37:112–114.

60. Banco B, Giudice C, Veronesi MC, et al. An immunohistochemical study of normal and neoplastic canine sertoli cells. *J Comp Pathol.* 2010;143:239–247.

61. Banco B, Palmieri C, Sironi G, et al. Immunohistochemical expression of SOX9 protein in immature, mature, and neoplastic canine sertoli cells. *Theriogenology.* 2016;85:1408–1414.

62. Banco B, Veronesi MC, Giudice C, et al. Immunohistochemical evaluation of the expression of anti-mullerian hormone in mature, immature and neoplastic canine sertoli cells. *J Comp Pathol.* 2012;146:18–23.

63. Suess RP, Barr SC, Sacre BJ, et al. Bone-marrow hypoplasia in a feminized dog with an interstitial cell tumor. *J Am Vet Med Assoc.* 1992;200:1346–1348.

64. Canadas A, Romao P, Gartner F. Multiple cutaneous metastasis of a malignant leydig cell tumour in a dog. *J Comp Pathol.* 2016;155:181–184.

65. Togni A, Rutten M, Bley CR, et al. Metastasized leydig cell tumor in a dog. *Schweiz Arch Tierheilkd.* 2015;157:111–115.

66. Radi ZA, Miller DL. Immunohistochemical expression of calretinin in canine testicular tumours and normal canine testicular tissue. *Res Vet Sci.* 2005;79:125–129.

67. Bush JM, Gardiner DW, Palmer JS, et al. Testicular germ cell tumours in dogs are predominantly of spermatocytic seminoma type and are frequently associated with somatic cell tumours. *Int J Andro.* 2011;34:E288–E295.

68. Hohsteter M, Artukovic B, Severin K, et al. Canine testicular tumors: two types of seminomas can be differentiated by immunohistochemistry. *BMC Vet Res.* 2014;10:169.

69. Yu CH, Hwang DN, Yhee JY, et al. Comparative immunohistochemical characterization of canine seminomas and Sertoli cell tumors. *J Vet Sci.* 2009;10:1–7.

70. Owston MA, Ramos-Vara JA. Histologic and immunohistochemical characterization of a testicular mixed germ cell sex cord-stromal tumor and a leydig cell tumor in a dog. *Vet Pathol.* 2007;44:936–943.

71. Patnaik AK, Mostofi FK. A clinicopathological, histologic, and immunohistochemical study of mixed germ-cell stromal tumors of the testis in 16 dogs. *Vet Pathol.* 1993;30:287–295.

72. Esplin DG, Wilson SR. Gastrointestinal adenocarcinomas metastatic to the testes and associated structures in three dogs. *J Am Anim Hosp Assoc.* 1998;34:287–290.

73. Bolen JW. Mixed germ-cell sex cord stromal tumor - a gonadal tumor distinct from gonadoblastoma. *Am J Clin Pathol.* 1981;75:565–573.

74. Ferreira da Silva J. Tertoma in a feline unilateral cryptorchid testis. *Vet Pathol.* 2002;39:516.

75. Kawakami E, Koga H, Hori T, et al. Sperm granuloma and sperm agglutination in a dog with asthenozoospermia. *J Vet Med Sci.* 2003;65:409–412.

76. Batista-Arteaga M, Santana M, Lozano O, et al. Bilateral epididymal sperm granulomas following urethrostomy in a german shepherd dog. *Reprod Domest Anim.* 2011;46:731–733.

77. Cornegliani L, Vercelli A, Abramo F. Idiopathic mucosal penile squamous papillomas in dogs. *Vet Dermatol.* 2007;18:439–443.

78. Florez MM, Pedraza F, Grandi F, et al. Cytologic subtypes of canine transmissible venereal tumor. *Vet Clin Pathol.* 2012;41:4–5.

79. Wakui S, Furusato M, Nomura Y, et al. Testicular epidermoid cyst and penile squamous-cell carcinoma in a dog. *Vet Pathol.* 1992;29:543–545.

80. Michels GM, Knapp DW, David M, et al. Penile prolapse and urethral obstruction secondary to lymphosarcoma of the penis in a dog. *J Am Anim Hosp Assoc.* 2001;37:474–477.

81. Peppler C, Weissert D, Kappe E, et al. Osteosarcoma of the penile bone (os penis) in a dog. *Aust Vet J.* 2009;87:52–55.

82. Davis GJ, Holt D. Two chondrosarcomas in the urethra of a German shepherd dog. *J Small Anim Pract.* 2003;44:169–171.

83. Burchell RK, Kirberger RM, Janse van Rensberg DD. Haemangiosarcoma of the os penis in a dog: the most common neoplasm of the canine penis. *J S Afr Vet Assoc.* 2014;85:1092.

84. Mirkovic TK, Shmon CL, Allen AL. Urinary obstruction secondary to an ossifying fibroma of the os penis in a dog. *J Am Anim Hosp Assoc.* 2004;40:152–156.

85. England G, Bright L, Pritchard B, et al. Canine reproductive ultrasound examination for predicting future sperm quality. *Reprod Domest Anim.* 2017;52(suppl 2):202–207.

86. Kustritz MVR. The value of canine semen evaluation for practitioners. *Theriogenology.* 2007;68:329–337.

87. Zambelli D, Cunto M. Semen collection in cats: techniques and analysis. *Theriogenology.* 2006;66:159–165.

88. Freshman JL. Semen collection and evaluation. *Top Companion Anim Med.* 2002;17:104–107.

89. England GCW, Russo M, Freeman SL. Artificial insemination in dogs and cats 1. Collection and preservation of canine semen. *Practice.* 2014;36:77–81.

90. Prochowska S, Nizanski W, Ochota M, et al. Characteristics of urethral and epididymal semen collected from domestic cats—A retrospective study of 214 cases. *Theriogenology.* 2015;84:1565–1571.

91. Hesser A, Darr C, Gonzales K, et al. Semen evaluation and fertility assessment in a purebred dog breeding facility. *Theriogenology.* 2017;87:115–123.

92. Kustritz MVR, Johnston SD, Olson PN, et al. Relationship between inflammatory cytology of canine seminal fluid and significant aerobic bacterial, anaerobic bacterial or mycoplasma cultures of canine seminal fluid: 95 cases (1987-2000). *Theriogenology.* 2005;64:1333–1339.

25

Female Reproductive Tract

Melinda S. Camus, Robin W. Allison, and Doris Miller

Examination of exfoliated cells from the vagina is a simple technique and is useful to monitor the progression of proestrus and estrus in dogs and cats.[1-3] The vaginal epithelium undergoes a predictable hyperplastic response to increasing plasma estrogen concentrations during proestrus. Starting as only a few cell layers, the epithelium becomes 20 to 30 cell layers thick, eventually exfoliating large numbers of superficial epithelial cells during estrus. Vaginal cytology, often in tandem with hormone analysis, may provide valuable information about the stage of the ovarian cycle.[4] In addition, vaginal cytology has proven useful in detecting inflammatory and neoplastic conditions in the female reproductive tract.[5]

VAGINA

Collecting Vaginal Samples

Cells are obtained by passing a cotton-tipped swab into the caudal vagina (Figs. 25.1 and 25.2). A narrow spreading speculum may be used to allow unimpeded swab passage. If no vaginal discharge is present, the swab may be moistened with sterile saline to avoid discomfort. The swab should be directed craniodorsad when entering the vaginal vault to avoid the clitoral fossa. Keratinized epithelium normally present in the fossa could lead to an inappropriate cytological interpretation.[3] Once the swab is directed cranial to the urethral orifice, the vaginal wall is gently swabbed. The cells are then transferred to a glass slide by gently rolling the swab with minimal pressure to avoid rupturing cells. The smear is allowed to air-dry thoroughly before staining. Romanowsky-type stains typically used for blood smears (Wright or modified Wright-Giemsa stains, including quick-type stains) provide good morphological detail.

Classifying Vaginal Cells

Vaginal epithelial cells are described beginning with the deepest, most immature layer near the basement membrane and progressing superficially to the most mature layer nearest the vaginal lumen (Fig. 25.3).

Basal Cells

Basal cells give rise to all epithelial cell types observed in a vaginal smear. They are small cells with round nuclei and a high nucleus-to-cytoplasm (N:C) ratio and are rarely observed in vaginal smears (Fig. 25.4, A).

Parabasal Cells

Parabasal cells are small round cells with round vesiculated nuclei and a small amount of cytoplasm and are usually uniform in size and shape (see Fig. 25.4, B). Large numbers of parabasal cells may exfoliate when the vagina of a prepubertal animal is swabbed.

Intermediate Cells

Intermediate cells vary in size, depending on the amount of cytoplasm present. Although the nuclei of both small and large intermediate cells are similar in size to parabasal cell nuclei, intermediate cells are larger than parabasal cells because of an increased amount of cytoplasm (see Fig. 25.4, C and D). Intermediate cells still have vesiculated nuclei, but as they increase in size, their cytoplasm becomes irregular, folded, and angular, similar to the cytoplasm of superficial cells. Large intermediate cells are sometimes called *superficial intermediate cells* or *transitional intermediate cells*.

Superficial Cells

Superficial cells are the largest epithelial cells seen in vaginal smears (see Fig. 25.4, E). These are dead cells, whose nuclei become pyknotic and then faded, often progressing to anucleate forms (see Fig. 25.4, F). Their cytoplasm is abundant, angular, and folded. As cells degenerate, their cytoplasm may develop small vacuoles (Fig. 25.5). The degeneration process of stratified squamous epithelial cells into large, flat, dead cells is called *cornification*. Superficial epithelial cells are commonly called *cornified cells*.

Other Normal Cytological Findings

Metestrum cells have been described as vaginal epithelial cells containing neutrophils in their cytoplasm (Fig. 25.6).[3,6] They are not specific for any stage of the cycle and may be seen whenever neutrophils are present for any reason.

In dogs and cats, the vagina contains normal bacterial flora, and bacteria are frequently observed on vaginal cytology slides.[7,8] Unless the bacteria are accompanied by large numbers of neutrophils, they are generally considered normal flora.

Spermatozoa are sometimes observed in vaginal cytological preparations from mated females (Fig. 25.7), but the period during which they are present varies. The presence of spermatozoa confirms mating, but their absence does not preclude breeding. Intact spermatozoa or sperm heads have been observed in about 65% of vaginal smears made 24 hours after natural mating in dogs and in 50% of smears made 48 hours after mating (R. Allison, personal observation).

Cells that appear to be placental trophoblast-like syncytia may be occasionally observed in vaginal cytological preparations, particularly several weeks after whelping in dogs with suspected subinvolution of placental sites (Fig. 25.8).[5]

STAGING THE CANINE ESTROUS CYCLE

Fig. 25.9 provides an overview of the changes in vaginal cytology related to plasma estrogen levels during the normal canine estrous cycle.

Proestrus

As ovarian follicles mature and serum concentrations of estrogen (estradiol) increase, the vaginal epithelium proliferates, and erythrocytes pass through uterine capillaries. These changes result in the typical appearance of vaginal cytological preparations made during proestrus (Fig. 25.10). Cytological specimens obtained in early and midproestrus are characterized by a mixture of epithelial cells, including parabasal, small and large intermediate cells, and superficial cells, along with variable numbers of neutrophils and erythrocytes. Basophilic mucous may be present in the background. As proestrus continues and the vaginal epithelium thickens, neutrophils are no longer able to traverse the vaginal wall, so their numbers decrease. Progressively higher percentages of large intermediate and superficial cells are present, with fewer parabasal and small intermediate cells. After serum estrogen levels peak in late proestrus, greater than 80% of epithelial cells are superficial, and neutrophils are absent. This is identical to the vaginal cytology during estrus.[9] Erythrocytes may be abundant or absent throughout proestrus. Bacteria, both free and on the surface of epithelial cells, are often present in large numbers. The mean duration of proestrus in mature dogs is 9 days, although a range of 2 to 17 days has been reported.[2]

Estrus

Most (80%–90%) of the epithelial cells exfoliated during estrus are superficial cells. Typically, almost all of these superficial cells contain small pyknotic nuclei (Fig. 25.11). However, occasional samples contain nearly 100% anuclear cells, whereas in others, large intermediate cells are retained. Maximal cornification follows the serum estrogen peak in late proestrus and continues throughout estrus.[1,9] Ovulation usually occurs about 2 days after the luteinizing hormone (LH) surge, following a decrease in serum estrogen and an increase in serum progesterone (Fig. 25.12).[2] Because maximal cornification may occur as much as 6 days before or 3 days after the LH surge, vaginal cytology is an imprecise predictor of ovulation. Cytological preparations made during estrus usually have a background that is clear and free of mucus and may or may not contain erythrocytes. Large numbers of bacteria are commonly observed on and around superficial epithelial cells, but neutrophils are normally absent unless inflammation is present (Fig. 25.13).[3] The average duration of estrus is 9 days for mature dogs, but a range of 3 to 21 days has been reported.[2]

Diestrus

Diestrus occurs about 8 days (range 6–10 days) after the LH peak in most cycles and is characterized cytologically by an abrupt change in the relative numbers of superficial epithelial cells. Over a 24- to 48-hour period, superficial cell numbers dramatically

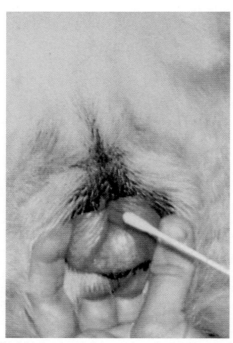

Fig. 25.1 The labia are carefully parted to allow unimpeded passage of the swab. (Courtesy Kal Kan Forum.)

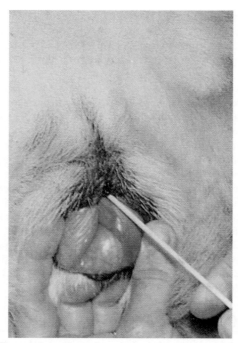

Fig. 25.2 The swab is directed craniodorsad to avoid entering the clitoral fossa. (Courtesy Kal Kan Forum.)

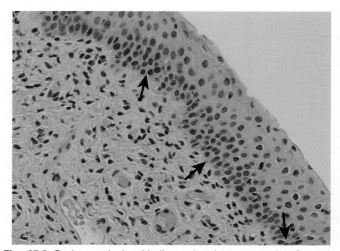

Fig. 25.3 Canine vaginal epithelium, showing progression from the basal cell layer to more superficial epithelial cells near the vaginal lumen (H&E stain, original magnification 40×).

decrease to about 20%, whereas parabasal and intermediate cell numbers increase.[6] Neutrophils appear in variable numbers, and this usually coincides with an increase in the numbers of parabasal and intermediate cells (Fig. 25.14). Some dogs have few or no neutrophils in vaginal smears made during diestrus (Fig. 25.15). Erythrocytes and bacteria may or may not be present. Bacteria engulfed by neutrophils are occasionally seen during diestrus in clinically normal dogs.[5] Behavioral diestrus is defined by the female's refusal of the male and usually lags behind cytological diestrus by several days.[3]

Individual cytological preparations made during the transition period from late estrus to early diestrus, without benefit of prior preparations, may appear very similar to smears made in early or midproestrus. At both times, a similar mixture of superficial and nonsuperficial cells may be present, as well as both erythrocytes and neutrophils. Vaginoscopy, vulvar examination, and the animal's behavior are usually helpful in making differentiations. When in doubt, repeating vaginal cytology in 3 or 4 days should provide clarity.

Anestrus

Parabasal and intermediate cells predominate during anestrus (Fig. 25.16). If present, neutrophils and bacteria are few in number.

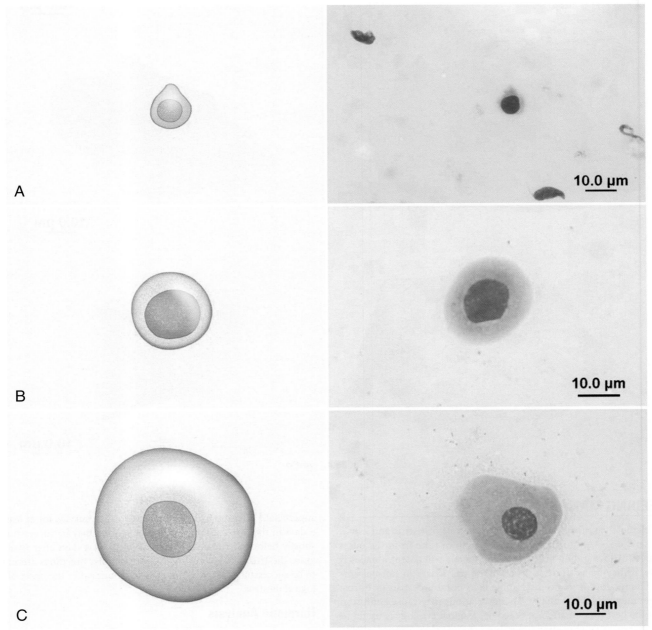

Fig. 25.4 Diagrams and corresponding images of epithelial cell types from the canine vagina. (A) Basal epithelial cells. (B) Parabasal epithelial cells. (C) Small intermediate cells. (D) Large intermediate cells. (E) Superficial cells with pyknotic nuclei (note bacteria adhered to the cell on the right). (F) Anuclear superficial cells (note bacteria adhered to the cell on the right) (all cytology images stained with Wright stain, original magnification 100× [B–F]).

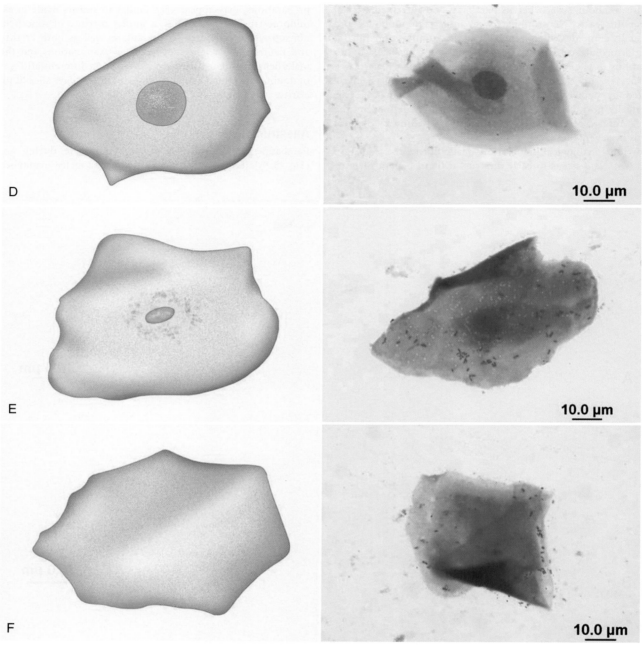

D

10.0 µm

E

10.0 µm

F

10.0 µm

Fig. 25.4, cont'd

BREEDING MANAGEMENT

Considerable variation exists in the duration of proestrus and estrus in normal dogs. Although the average length of time from the onset of proestrus to standing heat (when the female will accept a male) is 9 days, it may be as short as 2 or as long as 25 days in normal animals.[6] Some dogs have no discernible behavioral proestrus or estrus, and yet they ovulate normally. These variations may cause confusion about the best time to attempt breeding. Vaginal cytology is useful to suggest appropriate breeding times, but cytology alone cannot reliably distinguish between late proestrus and estrus and does not give specific information about the date of ovulation.

Normal, healthy dogs should be bred every 3 to 4 days throughout the period when greater than 90% of vaginal epithelial cells are superficial.[3,9] Because canine spermatozoa can survive for at least 4 to 6 days in the uterus of dogs in estrus, mating may be successful from shortly before the time of ovulation to about 4 days after ovulation. Once diestrus occurs, fertility declines rapidly. Breedings are unlikely to be successful if delayed more than 24 hours after the onset of cytological diestrus.

Hormone Analysis

Ovulation occurs about 48 hours (range 24–72 hours) after the LH surge.[9,10] Serum LH concentrations may be measured but stay elevated only 12 to 24 hours, making them inconvenient as a marker of ovulation for routine breedings. However, measuring LH levels may be justified in animals experiencing reproductive difficulties or when frozen

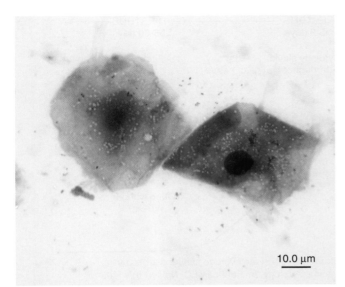

Fig. 25.5 Degenerating superficial vaginal epithelial cells with vacuolated cytoplasm in a canine vaginal smear (Wright stain, original magnification 100×).

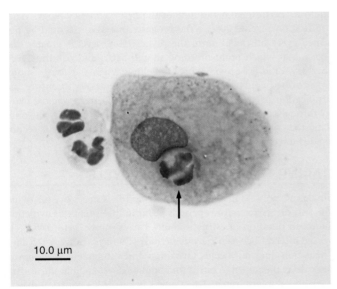

Fig. 25.6 Neutrophil *(arrow)* within the cytoplasm of an epithelial cell. These cells have been termed *metestrum cells* but may be seen any time neutrophils are present (Wright stain, original magnification 100×).

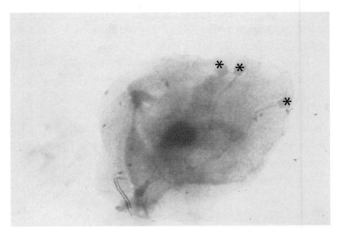

Fig. 25.7 Spermatozoa (*) and a superficial epithelial cell in a vaginal smear from a female dog several hours after mating (Wright stain, original magnification 40×).

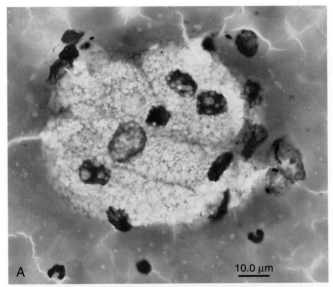

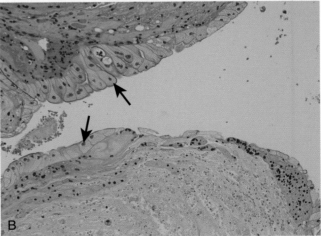

Fig. 25.8 (A) Vaginal smear from a dog with subinvolution of placental sites after whelping containing cells consistent with placental trophoblasts (Wright stain, original magnification 100×). (B) Corresponding histological section of the canine vagina where the uterine lumen is lined by finely vacuolated cells, often called "progesterone cells" (H&E stain, original magnification 40×).

semen is used for artificial insemination. By contrast, serum progesterone levels rise from basal levels of less than 0.5 nanogram per milliliter (ng/mL) to greater than 1 ng/mL shortly before the LH surge, 2 to 4 ng/mL during the LH surge, and typically reach greater than 4 ng/mL by the time ovulation occurs.[4,9,11] Commercial laboratories offer rapid turnaround time on serum progesterone assays, making them a convenient adjunct to vaginal cytology, with the benefit of more precise estimation of the fertile period.

Combining Vaginal Cytology and Hormone Analysis

Evaluation of serial progesterone levels and vaginal cytologies during proestrus and estrus helps obtain the most information about the fertile period and have proven useful in the management of animals with variable estrus cycles.[4] A protocol proposed by Goodman recommends beginning vaginal cytology at the first clinical sign of proestrus (vaginal

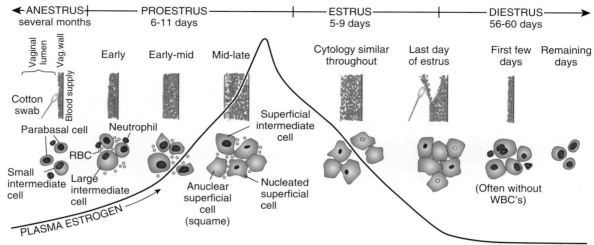

Fig. 25.9 Changes in vaginal cytology related to plasma estrogen levels in the average canine estrous cycle. (Image from Feldman EC, Nelson RW. Ovarian cycle and vaginal cytology. In: Feldman EC, Nelson RW, editors. *Canine and Feline Endocrinology and Reproduction.* 3rd ed. Philadelphia: Saunders; 200:755.)

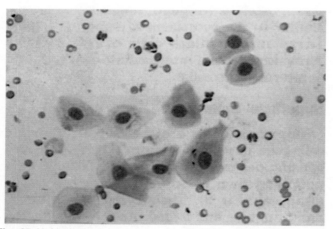

Fig. 25.10 Vaginal smear from a dog in proestrus. Intermediate epithelial cells predominate. Note the erythrocytes and a few neutrophils (Wright stain, original magnification 100×).

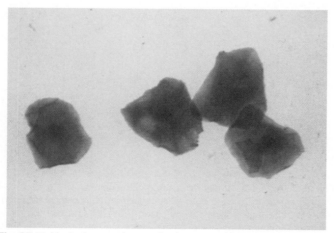

Fig. 25.11 Vaginal smear from a dog in estrus. Note superficial epithelial cells with pyknotic nuclei (Wright stain, original magnification 100×).

discharge or vulvar swelling) and following with cytology every few days until cornification reaches 70%.[9] A baseline progesterone level should be performed at the time of the first vaginal cytology. When cornification reaches 70%, serial progesterone assays should be performed every other day until the progesterone level is greater than 2 ng/mL, at which point breeding should begin and continue every other day for at least two or three breedings. Vaginal cytology should be performed concurrently with progesterone assays to ensure that cornification progresses to 80% to 100%. Performing vaginal cytology throughout the breeding period is suggested to identify the onset of diestrus, and at least one additional progesterone assay is recommended to verify that concentrations continue to rise.

STAGING THE FELINE ESTROUS CYCLE

Female cats are seasonally polyestrous. Coitus is necessary for ovulation, and successive estrous periods occur in the absence of ovulation. The mean duration of estrus is about 8 days (range 3–16 days). The average interval between estrous periods is 9 days (range 4–22 days) if ovulation does not occur. Ovulation and subsequent pseudopregnancy delay the return to estrus for about 45 days. Vaginal smears may be examined to accurately detect estrus in cats.[12-16] Ovulation may be induced while obtaining cells for vaginal cytological preparations.

The vaginal cytological characteristics of the cat are similar to those of the dog. The differences are outlined below.

Proestrus

Proestrus is usually difficult to detect because, unlike dogs, cats do not typically have vaginal discharge.[2] Duration of proestrus is short (0.5–2 days).[17] Erythrocytes and leukocytes are not usually present on cytological samples, but clearing of the background mucus is seen on vaginal smears because of increasing estrogen levels before the onset of estrus. Epithelial cells consist of a mixture of intermediate and nucleated superficial cells, with low numbers of parabasal cells and anuclear superficial cells.[16]

Estrus

Epithelial cells become progressively cornified as serum estrogen levels rise above 20 picograms per milliliter (pg/mL) during estrus.[16] The proportion of anuclear superficial cells increases to greater than 10% on the first day of estrus. By the fourth day of estrus, about 40% of the cells are anuclear superficial cells, whereas intermediate cell

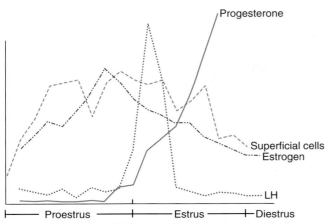

Fig. 25.12 Illustration of hormone fluctuations and vaginal cytology during the average canine estrous cycle. (Image adapted from Feldman EC, Nelson RW. Ovarian cycle and vaginal cytology. In: Feldman EC, Nelson RW, editors. *Canine and Feline Endocrinology and Reproduction.* 3rd ed. Philadelphia: Saunders; 200:755.)

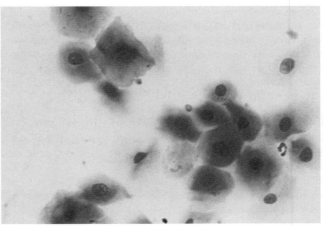

Fig. 25.15 Vaginal smear from a dog in diestrus that contains very few neutrophils (Wright stain, original magnification 100×).

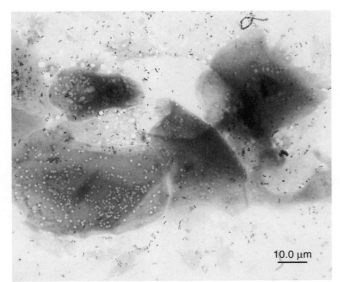

Fig. 25.13 Vaginal smear from a dog in estrus. Superficial cells predominate, and many bacteria are present in the background and adhered to the epithelial cells (Wright stain, original magnification 100×).

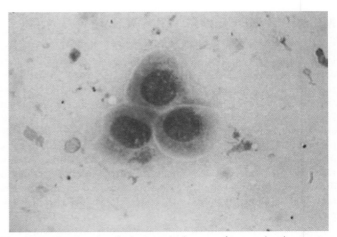

Fig. 25.16 Parabasal cells in a vaginal smear from a dog in anestrus (Wright stain, original magnification 400×).

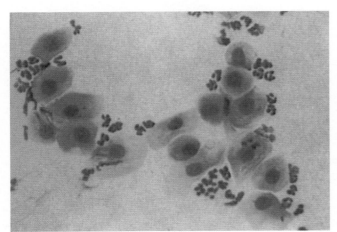

Fig. 25.14 Vaginal smear from a dog in diestrus. Note the numerous neutrophils and intermediate cells (Wright stain, original magnification 100×).

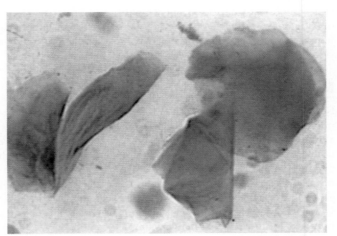

Fig. 25.17 Vaginal smear from a cat in estrus. Note the anuclear superficial epithelial cells with folded angular cytoplasm (Wright stain, original magnification 400×).

numbers decrease to less than 10% (Fig. 25.17).[16] The number of anuclear superficial cells stays relatively constant during the remainder of estrus, ranging from 40% to 60% of the total. Neutrophils and parabasal cells are absent during estrus. It has been suggested that the pronounced clearing of the background mucus and debris on vaginal smears obtained during estrus may be the most sensitive indicator of estrogen activity in cats.[16]

Interestrous Period and Diestrus

Estrus is followed by the interestrous period (if no ovulation occurs) or diestrus (if ovulation occurs). As estrus ends, background debris and parabasal cells reappear on vaginal smears. Anuclear superficial cell numbers decrease, and the majority of cells are a mixture of intermediate and nucleated superficial cells. Low numbers of neutrophils are occasionally present.[16]

Anestrus

Vaginal cytology during anestrus is similar to that of the interestrous period. Epithelial cells are predominantly intermediate, with up to 40% nucleated superficial cells and about 10% parabasal cells.[17]

MICROSCOPIC CHARACTERISTICS OF VAGINITIS

Samples obtained from animals with inflammation of the vagina or in the upper reproductive tract are characterized by large numbers of neutrophils (Fig. 25.18, A and B; canine vaginitis 40×). If a bacterial infection is the cause, neutrophils often show degenerate changes (swollen, pale nuclei with loss of segmentation) and may contain phagocytized bacteria. Cytological samples from dogs in early diestrus also contain many neutrophils and may contain bacteria, occasionally phagocytized by neutrophils.[5] Thus vaginal smears from early diestrus may resemble those from dogs with vaginal or uterine inflammation. However, the number of neutrophils in smears from normal dogs in diestrus markedly decreases by postestrus week 1. Mucus and a few macrophages and lymphocytes may be seen in cases of chronic vaginitis (Fig. 25.19).[5]

Vaginitis is often caused by noninfectious factors (e.g., vaginal anomalies, clitoral hypertrophy, foreign bodies, or vaginal immaturity), in which case nondegenerate neutrophils will be present. Basophilic epithelial intracytoplasmic inclusions have been observed in dogs with vaginitis, but their significance is not known (Fig. 25.20) (R. Allison, personal observation). Vaginal smears from animals with pyometra or metritis usually contain large numbers of degenerate neutrophils, and bacteria are frequently observed (Fig. 25.21). Muscle fibers from decomposing fetuses may rarely be seen with metritis secondary to dystocia (Fig. 25.22).

MICROSCOPIC CHARACTERISTICS OF NEOPLASIA

Neoplasia of the urinary and reproductive tracts may be diagnosed occasionally by cytological examination of vaginal smears, although direct aspiration or biopsy of the mass are often more useful. The most common vaginal tumors in dogs are of smooth muscle or fibrous tissue origin (leiomyoma, fibroma, and leiomyosarcoma), which do not exfoliate cells readily and so are not generally recognized with routine vaginal cytology.[18] Histologic samples from benign tumors will contain fairly uniform cells with round to oval nuclei and relatively abundant spindled cytoplasm, present individually or in aggregates (Fig. 25.23). Aspirates from sarcomas will contain similar cells, but with prominent pleomorphism (Fig. 25.24).

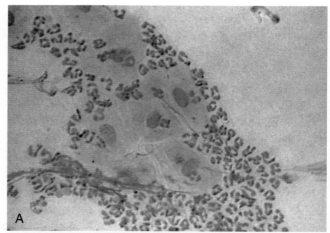

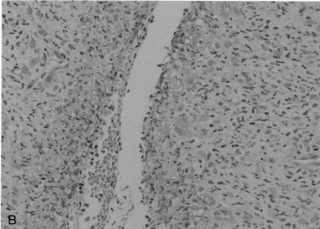

Fig. 25.18 (A) Vaginal smear from a puppy with vaginitis containing large numbers of neutrophils and intermediate epithelial cells (Wright stain, original magnification 100×). (B) Corresponding histological section showing diffuse neutrophils and edema in subepithelial region (H&E stain, original magnification 40×)

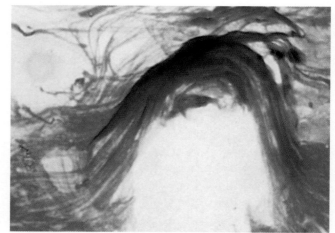

Fig. 25.19 Mucus in a vaginal smear from a bitch with a chronic vulvar discharge (Wright stain, original magnification 40×).

Canine transmissible venereal tumors (TVTs) may be diagnosed through vaginal cytology or direct mass aspiration or biopsy. These contagious tumors are transmitted by direct contact and occur not only on genitalia but also in other locations (oral and nasal cavity,

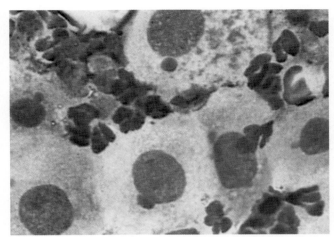

Fig. 25.20 Basophilic intracytoplasmic inclusions in epithelial cells in a vaginal smear from a dog with vaginitis (Wright stain, original magnification 40×).

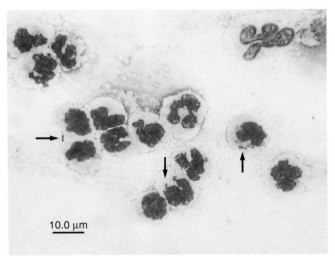

Fig. 25.21 Degenerate neutrophils exhibiting swollen, pale nuclei with loss of segmentation in a vaginal smear from a dog with metritis. Note the intracytoplasmic bacteria *(arrows)* (Wright stain, original magnification 100×).

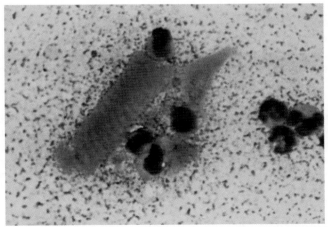

Fig. 25.22 Neutrophils and muscle fibers from decomposing puppies in a vaginal smear from a bitch with a herniated uterus and metritis (Wright stain, original magnification 40×).

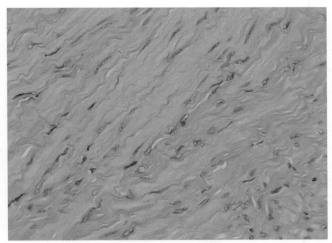

Fig. 25.23 Histological section of a leiomyoma in the canine uterine wall. The mass is composed of cells with abundant eosinophilic cytoplasm and vesicular nuclei, which are elongated/oval and have a low mitotic index (H&E stain, original magnification 40×).

rectum, skin, subcutaneous tissue).[19,20] Malignant cells are discrete and round, containing round nuclei with stippled to coarse chromatin and often prominent nucleoli. They have a moderate amount of pale basophilic cytoplasm, which usually contains multiple clear, punctate vacuoles (Fig. 25.25, A and B). Because these tumors are frequently ulcerated and inflamed, variable numbers of inflammatory cells may be present.[19]

Vaginal carcinomas are less common but sometimes result from extension of urinary tract carcinomas into the vagina or vestibule (Figs. 25.26 and 25.27) These carcinomas may be of transitional cell or squamous cell origin because the distal portion of the canine urethra is lined by modified squamous epithelium.[18] In one report of seven dogs with urinary tract carcinomas involving the vagina or the vestibule, six dogs had vaginal smears performed, and neoplastic epithelial cells were identified in all six samples.[21]

Cytological and histological features of vaginal carcinomas are the same as those occurring in carcinomas arising at other locations. See discussion of cell types and criteria of malignancy in Chapter 2 and carcinomas in Chapter 5.

UTERUS

Uterine cytology is performed infrequently in small animal patients and is done typically when investigating poor reproductive performance or when looking for evidence of inflammation or neoplasia, often in response to a vaginal discharge of unknown origin in sexually intact females.

Collecting Uterine Samples

Uterine specimens can be obtained via a uterine flush, which is accomplished typically by transcervical endoscopy.[22] This method allows for collection of relatively large sample volumes and sterile culture specimens. Additionally, impression smears of biopsy samples collected either via endoscopy or abdominal surgery can be evaluated, keeping in mind that the collection method affects overall cellularity.

As with vaginal cytologies, expected findings on uterine cytologies vary with stages of the estrous cycle. The endometrium is lined by simple cuboidal to columnar epithelial cells, depending on the stage of the estrous cycle, with columnar epithelium predominating during

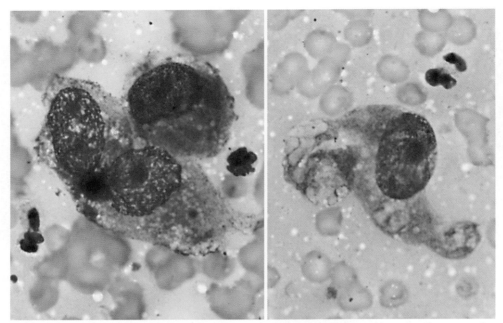

Fig. 25.24 Pleomorphic mesenchymal cells from a vaginal sarcoma in a dog. Note the plump cytoplasm, anisocytosis, anisokaryosis, and prominent nucleoli (Wright stain, original magnification 100×).

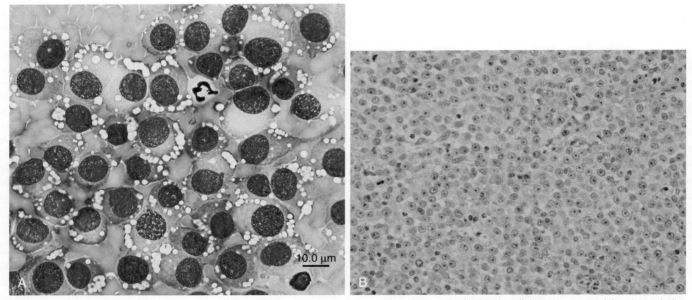

Fig. 25.25 Canine transmissible venereal tumor (TVT). (A) Direct aspiration of the vaginal mass resulted in highly cellular smears containing the typical vacuolated discrete cells of a transmissible venereal tumor (Wright stain, original magnification 100×). (B) Typical histological appearance of a canine TVT from the vagina. Note the round nuclei with prominent nucleoli and finely vacuolated cytoplasm (H&E stain, original magnification 40×).

estrogen peaks. Cells are well-preserved during proestrus, estrus, and early diestrus, with evidence for degeneration and loss of cellular detail in late diestrus through midanestrus. Although typically not appreciable with light microscopy, cell morphology, including the presence of cilia and microtubules, varies with cyclic stage.[23] The presence of erythrocytes and neutrophils parallels that seen in vaginal smears during each stage of the estrous cycle.[24]

Microscopic Characteristics of Metritis

Inflammation of the uterus appears similar to inflammation in other locations, and inflammatory cells may or may not exfoliate well into uterine flushes, depending on localization of the inflammatory cells within the uterus or uterine stump. With the presence of infectious agents, inflammatory cells are often free within the uterine lumen and typically exfoliate well through an open cervix (Fig. 25.28, A and B). Bacterial endotoxins, if present, often induce degenerate change within neutrophils. Necrotic debris is commonly observed in such specimens.

Microscopic Characteristics of Uterine Neoplasia

Uterine neoplasia is uncommon in domestic animals, with mesenchymal neoplasms occurring more frequently than epithelial

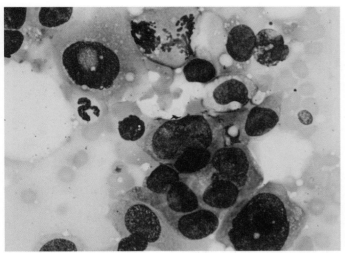

Fig. 25.26 Neoplastic epithelial cells in a vaginal smear from a dog with transitional cell carcinoma invading the vagina. Note the marked pleomorphism, prominent nucleoli, and the presence of an irregular mitotic figure (modified Wright stain, original magnification 100×).

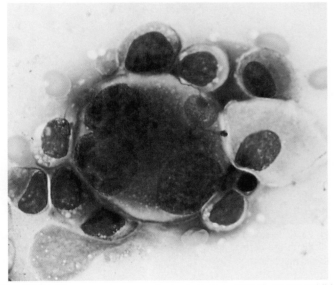

Fig. 25.27 These carcinoma cells in a canine vaginal smear exhibit criteria of malignancy, including marked anisokaryosis, anisocytosis, multinucleation with loss of contact inhibition, and multiple prominent nucleoli (Wright stain, original magnification 100×).

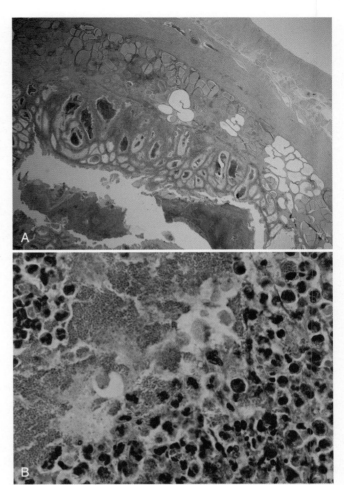

Fig. 25.28 Histological section of a canine uterus with cystic endometrial hyperplasia, pyometra, and metritis. (A) Note purulent exudate in uterine lumen, cystic endometrial glands filled with inflammatory cells, and inflammatory cells in the myometrium (H&E stain, original magnification 2×). (B) Uterine lumen showing many bacteria and degenerate neutrophils (H&E stain, original magnification 100×).

tumors, which are rarely reported. Of the mesenchymal neoplasms, benign tumors are much more common compared with their malignant counterparts. Myometrial leiomyomas are the most frequent, with fewer fibromas and leiomyofibromas reported (see Fig. 25.23). There is a reported positive association between nulliparity and frequency of tumor formation.[25] In dogs, uterine leiomyomas are accompanied frequently by concurrent vaginal smooth muscle tumors. As with all mesenchymal tissues, these neoplasms tend to exfoliate poorly and often yield very poor cellular samples for cytological evaluation.[18] Despite their rarity, uterine adenocarcinomas are reportedly the most common feline uterine neoplasm, with cytological features similar to those of other malignant epithelial neoplasms (Fig. 25.29, A and B).[25]

Mass-forming, nonneoplastic uterine lesions consist of polyps, cysts, and hyperplasia in response to excess estrogen or progesterone. Polyps are composed of both dilated glands and proliferative stromal tissue, yielding aspirates that may contain both epithelial and mesenchymal components (Fig. 25.30). Adenomyosis, which is nonneoplastic glandular proliferation within the myometrium, often forms mass lesions in dogs with endometrial hyperplasia (Fig. 25.31).[18]

OVARIES

Collecting Ovarian Samples

Cytology of ovarian tissue is performed infrequently. Such samples can be collected via ultrasound-guided fine-needle aspiration (FNA) or surgery via laparoscopy or laparotomy. Normal ovary is composed of tissue from all three embryological cell lines and, as such, can produce cytological samples containing a heterogeneous mixture of cells (Fig. 25.32). However, ovarian aspirates are typically poorly cellular and contain and abundance of adipose tissue, with individualized mesenchymal cells and luteal cells and occasional clusters of granulosa cells (Fig. 25.33, A and B). The relative proportions of these

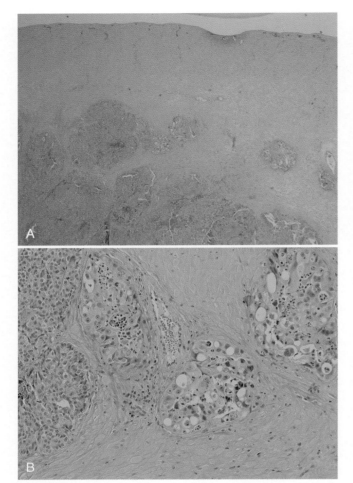

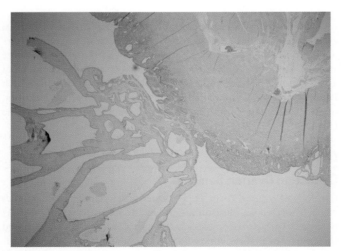

Fig. 25.29 Histological section of a feline uterine adenocarcinoma. (A) Note nests of neoplastic epithelial cells within the myometrium. Pyometra/metritis is also present (H&E stain, original magnification 4×). (B) Note the marked pleomorphism of individual cells, including multinucleation and prominent nucleoli (H&E stain, original magnification 20×).

Fig. 25.30 Histological section of a feline uterus with a cystic endometrial polyp protruding into the lumen (H&E stain, original magnification 2×).

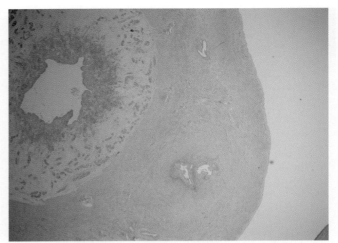

Fig. 25.31 Histological cross-section of a canine uterus with areas of adenomyosis in the myometrium. The edema and hemorrhage in the endometrium are surgically induced (H&E stain, original magnification 2×).

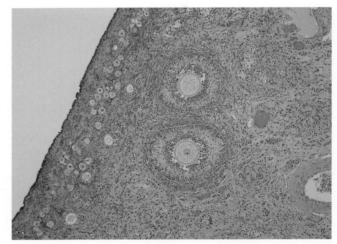

Fig. 25.32 Histological section of normal canine ovary with primordial follicles in the cortex, and granulosa cells within a follicle (H&E stain, original magnification 10×).

cells and their cytological appearance can vary with stage of estrus.[26] It is important to recognize ovarian tissue, as ovarian remnants often result in clinical signs of estrus in spayed females. Although these generally are suspected on the basis of clinical signs and presence of predominately superficial epithelial cells on a vaginal smear, the diagnosis can be strengthened through assessment of estradiol and/ or progesterone concentrations, both of which are elevated with follicular activity.[27]

Microscopic Characteristics of Ovarian Inflammation

Oophoritis occurs very uncommonly in dogs and cats. When affected ovaries are examined histologically, inflammatory cells often surround the entire organ and infiltrate the oviduct, suggesting ascension from the uterus. Inflammation of the feline ovary can occur with feline infectious peritonitis (FIP) (Fig. 25.34).[28]

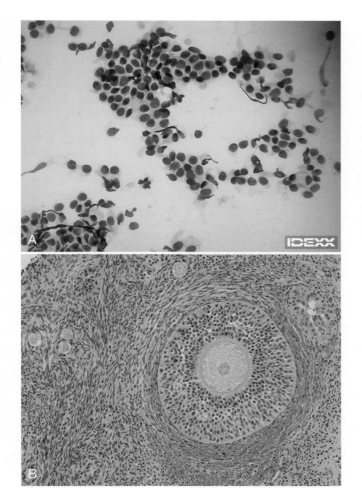

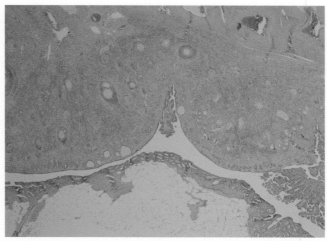

Fig. 25.35 Histological section of canine ovary with a papillary cystade-nocarcinoma on the surface and cystic subsurface epithelial structures (H&E stain, original magnification 2×).

Fig. 25.33 Normal canine ovary. (A) Impression smear with aggregates of uniform granulosa cells. (Wright stain, original magnification 100×). (B) Histological section containing a primary follicle with granulosa cells (H&E stain, original magnification 20×). (A, Courtesy Dr. Daniel Valenciano.)

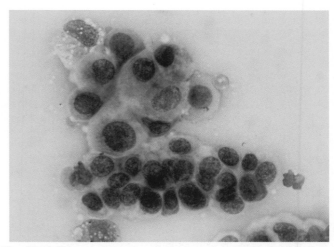

Fig. 25.36 These carcinoma cells in impression smears of a canine ovary exhibit criteria of malignancy including anisocytosis, anisokaryosis, multinucleation, nuclear crowding, and prominent nucleoli (Wright stain, original magnification 100×).

Microscopic Characteristics of Ovarian Neoplasia

Ovarian epithelial tumors are more frequent in the dog than in other domestic species. This may be attributed to the unique species difference in the canine species, which has subsurface epithelial structures not present in other species, which are prone to tumor formation (Fig. 25.35).[29] Morphologically, these tumors resemble epithelial tumors arising from other locations and have been demonstrated to invade through the capsule and into the peritoneal space, resulting in carcinomatosis with associated abdominal effusion (Fig. 25.36).[18]

Sex cord stromal tumors arise from the endocrine cells of the ovary. Formerly divided into subtypes, including granulosa cell tumor, granulosa–theca cell tumor, luteoma, thecoma, Sertoli cell tumor, and Leydig cell tumor, the term *sex cord stromal tumor* or *gonadostromal tumor* is preferred because the embryological origin of these cells is uncertain and often there are multiple cell types within the same neoplasm. Gonadostromal tumors typically exfoliate well for cytology and

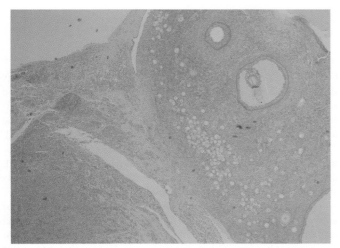

Fig. 25.34 Histological section of feline ovary with oophoritis and salpingitis. The ovarian cortex has primordial follicles adjacent to the mixed inflammatory infiltrate (H&E stain, original magnification 4×).

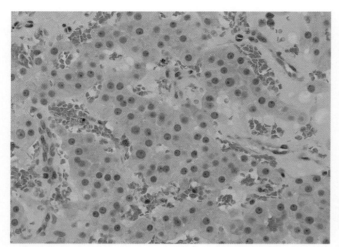

Fig. 25.37 Histological section of a canine ovarian luteoma with cells that have abundant, finely vacuolated cytoplasm and abundant supporting blood vessels (H&E stain, original magnification 40×).

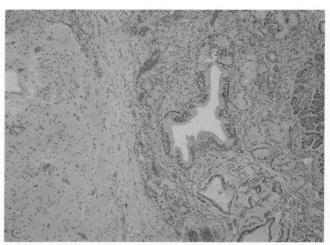

Fig. 25.39 Histological section of a canine ovarian teratoma with presence of multiple tissue types (H&E stain, original magnification 10×).

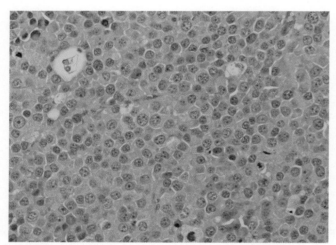

Fig. 25.38 Histological section of a canine ovarian dysgerminoma characterized by a uniform population of polyhedral cells with abundant cytoplasm. The round to irregular nuclei vary in size, with granular chromatin and one to two prominent nucleoli (H&E stain, original magnification 40×).

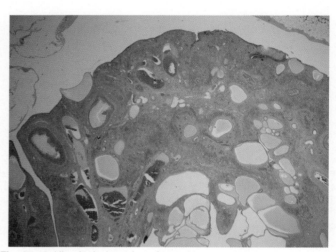

Fig. 25.40 Histological section of a canine polycystic ovary with cystic subsurface epithelial structures and multiple other cysts (H&E stain, original magnification 2×).

have a classic neuroendocrine appearance of free nuclei surrounded by abundant cytoplasm. Free nuclei occasionally form acinar-like structures, particularly within the previously classified granulosa cell tumors (Fig. 25.37). Sex cord stromal tumors may be hormonally active, although classification of tumors by their endocrine products may be challenging because of the variability in production and diurnal variation.[18]

Germ cell tumors are uncommon neoplasms arising from primordial germ cells, which migrate to the ovary from the yolk sac. These tumors include dysgerminomas and teratomas, the latter of which contain abnormal tissue from all three embryonal cell lines. Microscopic specimens from dysgerminomas are composed of pleomorphic round shaped cells with variable amounts of basophilic cytoplasm and nuclei with reticulated chromatin and large, prominent nucleoli (Fig. 25.38). They may stain positive for placental alkaline phosphatase, which could

be helpful differentiating them from other neoplasms on cytology slides.[30] Typically, aspirates of teratomas contain abundant epithelial cells and necrotic debris, with fewer other cell types, making cytological diagnosis extremely challenging. Histological examination may be required for complete characterization of these neoplasms (Fig. 25.39).

Ovarian tumors of mesenchymal origin include fibromas, leiomyomas, and hemangiomas, and share morphological characteristics with mesenchymal tumors arising elsewhere. They often exfoliate poorly and contain abundant amounts of blood or lipid.

Nonneoplastic cysts can arise from numerous tissues within or around the ovary (Fig. 25.40). They often secrete steroid hormones resulting in clinical signs, including pancytopenia secondary to bone marrow suppression. Other nonneoplastic lesions that can occur within the ovary include hematomas and choriostomas (aberrantly located tissue) of adrenal origin.[31]

REFERENCES

1. Linde C, Karlsson I. The correlation between the cytology of the vaginal smear and the time of ovulation in the bitch. *J Small Anim Pract.* 1984;25:77–82.

2. Olson PN, Hulsted PW, Allen TA, et al. Reproductive endocrinology and physiology of the bitch and queen. *Vet Clin North Am Small Anim Pract.* 1984;14(4):927–946.

3. Olson PN, Thrall MA, Wykes PM, et al. Vaginal cytology. I. A useful tool for staging the canine estrous cycle. *Comp Cont Ed Pract Vet.* 1984;6(4):288–297.

4. Wright PJ. Application of vaginal cytology and plasma progesterone determinations to the management of reproduction in the bitch. *J Small Anim Pract.* 1990;31:335–340.

5. Olson PN, Thrall MA, Wykes PM, et al. Vaginal cytology. II. Its use in diagnosing canine reproductive disorders. *Comp Cont Ed Pract Vet.* 1984;6(5):385–390.

6. Feldman EC, Nelson RW. Ovarian cycle and vaginal cytology. In: Feldman EC, Nelson RW, eds. *Canine and Feline Endocrinology and Reproduction.* 3rd ed. St. Louis: Elsevier; 2004:752–774.

7. Clemetson LL, Ward AC. Bacterial flora of the vagina and uterus of healthy cats. *J Am Vet Med Assoc.* 1990;196(6):902–906.

8. Watts JR, Wright PJ, Whithear KC. Uterine, cervical and vaginal microflora of the normal bitch throughout the reproductive cycle. *J Small Anim Pract.* 1996;37(2):54–60.

9. Goodman M. Ovulation timing: concepts and controversies. *Vet Clin North Am Small Anim Pract.* 2001;31(2):219–235.

10. Hase M, Hori T, Kawakami E, et al. Plasma LH and progesterone levels before and after ovulation and observation of ovarian follicles by ultrasonographic diagnosis system in dogs. *J Vet Med Sci.* 2000;62(3):243–248.

11. Feldman EC, Nelson RW. Breeding, pregnancy, and parturition. In: Feldman EC, Nelson RW, eds. *Canine and Feline Endocrinology and Reproduction.* 3rd ed. St. Louis: Elsevier; 2004:775–807.

12. Cline EM, Jennings LL, Sojka NJ. Analysis of the feline vaginal epithelial cycle. *Feline Pract.* 1980;10(2):47–49.

13. Herron MA. Feline vaginal cytologic examination. *Feline Pract.* 1977;7(2):36–39.

14. Mowrer RT, Conti PA, Rossow CF. Vaginal cytology an approach of improvement of cat breeding. *Vet Med Small Anim Clin.* 1975;70(6):691–696.

15. Shille VM, Lundstrom KE, Stabenfeldt GH. Follicular function in the domestic cat as determined by estradiol-17 beta concentrations in plasma: relation to estrous behavior and cornification of exfoliated vaginal epithelium. *Biol Reprod.* 1979;21(4):953–963.

16. Feldman EC, Nelson RW. Feline reproduction. In: Feldman EC, Nelson RW, eds. *Canine and Feline Endocrinology and Reproduction.* 3rd ed. St. Louis: Elsevier; 2004:1016–1045.

17. Mills JN, Valli VE, Lumsden JH. Cyclical changes of vaginal cytology in the cat. *Can Vet J.* 1979;20(4):95–101.

18. Agnew DW, MacLachlan NJ. Tumors of the genital systems. In: Meuten DJ, ed. *Tumors of Domestic Animals.* 5th ed. Ames, IA: John Wiley & Sons, Inc.; 2017:689–722.

19. Rogers KS. Transmissible venereal tumor. *Compend Cont Ed Pract Vet.* 1997;19(9):1036–1045.

20. Ibrahim AM, Porter BF. Pathology in practice. *J Am Vet Med Assoc.* 2012;241(6):707–709.

21. Magne ML, Hoopes PJ, Kainer RA, et al. Urinary tract carcinomas involving the canine vagina and vestibule. *J Am Anim Hosp Assoc.* 1985;21(6):767–772.

22. Root Kustritz MW. The value of canine semen evaluation for practitioners. *Theriogenology.* 2007;68:329–337.

23. Van Crutchen S, Van den Broeck W, Roels F, et al. Cyclic changes of the canine endometrial surface: an electron-microscopic study. *Cells Tissues Organs.* 2003;173:46–53.

24. Gropetti D, Pecile A, Arrighi S, et al. Endometrial cytology and computerized morphometric analysis of epithelial nuclei: a useful tool for reproductive diagnosis in the bitch. *Theriogenology.* 2010;73:927–941.

25. Saba CF, Lawrence JA. Tumors of the female reproductive system. In: Withrow SJ, Vail DM, eds. *Withrow & Macewen's Small Animal Clinical Oncology.* 5th ed. St. Louis: Elsevier; 2013:532–536.

26. Piseddu E, Masserdoti C, Milesi C, Solano-Gallego L. Cytologic features of normal canine ovaries in different stages of estrus with histologic comparison. *Vet Clin Pathol.* 2012;41(3):396–401.

27. Feldman EC, Nelson RW. Infertility, associated breeding disorders, and disorders of sexual development. In: Feldman EC, Nelson RW, eds. *Canine and Feline Endocrinology and Reproduction.* 3rd ed. St. Louis: Elsevier; 2004:868–900.

28. Foster RA. Female reproductive system and mammae. In: Zachary J, ed. *Pathologic Basis of Veterinary Disease.* 6th ed. St. Louis: Elsevier; 2017:1147–1193.

29. Andersen AC, Simpson ME. *The Ovary and Reproductive Cycle of the Dog (Beagle).* Los Altos, CA: Geron-X; 1973.

30. Brazzell J, Borjesson DL. Intra-abdominal mass aspirate from an alopecic dog. *Vet Clin Pathol.* 2006;35(2):259–262.

31. Altera KP, Miller LN. Recognition of feline parovarian nodules as ectopic adrenocortical tissue. *J Am Vet Med Assoc.* 1986;189(1):71–72.

26

Peripheral Blood Smears

Shanon M. Zabolotzky and Dana B. Walker

Blood smear evaluation as part of the complete hematology profile (complete blood count [CBC]) is a fundamental step in overall patient health assessment. Blood smear examination can yield a broad range of diagnostic information well beyond a differential leukocyte count. For example, altered red blood cell (RBC) morphology can suggest chronic blood loss, exposure to exogenous toxins, diseases involving select organs, or primary immune-mediated conditions. Changes in leukocyte morphology may be the earliest laboratory finding suggestive of acute inflammation, leukemia, or certain inherited conditions. In some cases, specific organisms, pathognomonic inclusions, or particular neoplastic cell types on blood films yield an immediate definitive diagnosis. In addition, monitoring cytological changes found in peripheral blood can help determine a patient's response to treatment, short- and long-term prognoses, and future treatment plan.

Blood smear evaluation should be performed as a supplement to an automated CBC, whether the latter is obtained in-house or from an outside laboratory. The evaluation provides a synopsis of essentially all other hematological parameter values and assurance of the accuracy of values obtained from other methods and sources. The greatest amount of information is generally obtained when the white blood cell (WBC) differential count is not a primary objective and when the person evaluating the smear has access to the patient's current and previous laboratory findings, current clinical condition, and medical history.

Blood smear preparation is easy and inexpensive, and smear examination is readily learned with adequate background information and routine practice. This chapter describes techniques of preparation and interpretation of canine and feline blood smears and addresses integrating findings from blood smears with other parameters in CBCs. Supplementary information on interpreting routine hematological parameter values is available in several well-written reviews and texts.[1-5]

EQUIPMENT AND SUPPLIES

The only major equipment for blood smear evaluation is a well-maintained binocular microscope with high-quality 10, 20, 40 or 50 (ideally, oil-immersion), and 100× (oil-immersion) objectives. Other items, such as Coplin jars and staining racks, are convenient for preparing smears. Standard plain or frosted glass slides can be used directly from the package without special treatment or cleaning. Slides with frosted ends facilitate labeling with patient information. Slide surfaces should be free of dust, fingerprints, and residue from detergent, alcohol, or tap water. The use of special cytological adhesives can result in background staining and is not recommended. An ample supply of slides facilitates preparation of multiple smears per sample, avoiding the frustration of interpreting any poorly made smears. Any additional smears can also

be reserved for alternative types of staining or, if indicated, a specialist's review.

SAMPLE COLLECTION

Ideally, blood samples should be collected on the first attempt from a medium to large vein of a calm patient. Ethylenetetraacetic acid (EDTA) is the preferred anticoagulant for blood used in cytological preparations. The liquid form of EDTA (usually K3EDTA) disperses more rapidly in samples compared with the powder form (usually K2EDTA) and may be preferable to prevent platelet aggregates with feline blood or for viscous or difficult-to-collect samples. However, powdered K2EDTA provides better erythrocyte preservation for automated counts and lacks dilutional effect on low-volume samples. Both forms of EDTA preserve general cellular morphology in refrigerated samples for up to 4 hours, although the fresher the sample, the more reliable is the morphology.

Alternatively (particularly if sample volume is limited), blood without an anticoagulant can be placed directly from the collection needle onto the slide. Samples collected from superficial skin-puncture wounds or clipped toenails (as a result of excessive contamination with tissue procoagulants) and blood anticoagulated with heparin (a relatively poor preservative of cellular morphology and staining characteristics) are less acceptable. Blood anticoagulated with citrate can be used to evaluate cell morphology on blood smears and may be particularly useful to avoid anticoagulant-associated pseudothrombocytopenia; however, the required 10% sample dilution interferes with cell count estimates.

Collection of blood in proper proportion to anticoagulant helps avoid certain artifacts of cell morphology and may be facilitated by the use of commercial vacutainers.

HEMATOLOGICAL REFERENCE INTERVALS

Hematological reference intervals should be established by individual diagnostic laboratories; however, published reference ranges can be used as a general guide for in-clinic laboratories, although most instruments will come with some reference interval information generated on that methodology. Typical values for dogs and cats are listed in Table 26.1. Certain physiological factors occasionally cause a healthy patient's hematological values to deviate from reference ranges. Because they are rapidly expanding their vascular space, very young animals tend to have relatively low hematocrits. Because they are also actively replacing fetal with adult RBCs, animals in early growth periods have greater RBC anisocytosis, polychromasia, and incidence of nucleated RBCs compared with mature animals.

TABLE 26.1   Reference Intervals for Hematological Values in Dogs and Cats

Erythrocytes	Canine Values	Feline Values
Hematocrit (%)	37.0–55.0	24.0–45.0
Hemoglobin (g/dL)	12.0–18.0	8.0–15.0
Erythrocyte count (×10⁶/μL)	5.5–8.5	5.0–10.0
Reticulocytes (%)	≤1.0	≤ 1.0
MCV (fl)	60.6–77.0	39.0–55.0
MCH (pg)	19.5–24.5	12.5–17.5
MCHC (g/dL)	32.0–36.0	30.0–36.0

Leukocytes

	CANINE VALUES		FELINE VALUES	
Cell Types	Distribution Range (%)	Absolute Range (cells/μL)	Distribution Range (%)	Absolute Range (cells/μL)
Total leukocytes	–	6000–17,000	–	5500–19,500
Neutrophils segmented	60–77	3000–11,000	35–75	2500–12,500
band	0–3	0–500	0–3	0–500
Lymphocytes	12–30	1000–4800	20–55	1500–7000
Monocytes	3–10	150–1350	1–4	0–850
Eosinophils	2–10	100–1250	2–12	0–1500
Basophils	Rare	Rare	Rare	Rare

Platelets	Canine Values	Feline Values
Platelets count (×10³/μL)	200–500	300–800
Mean platelet volume (fl)	5.4–9.2	12.1–15.1

Proteins	Canine Values	Feline Values
Plasma protein (refractometry; g/dL)	5.7–7.0	6.1–7.4
Albumin (g/dL)	2.4–3.6	2.5–3.3
Globulins (g/dL)	2.1–4.6	2.6–4.9

MCH, mean corpuscular hemoglobin; *MCHC*, mean corpuscular hemoglobin concentration; *MCV*, mean corpuscular volume.

Relatively high lymphocyte counts are also common in young animals, and lymphopenia is suggested if lymphocyte counts drop below 2000 cells/μL in puppies and kittens under 6 months of age.[3] Transient elevations above the reference range for lymphocyte counts and occasionally reticulocyte counts may be seen in excited or vigorously exercised patients, especially if they are immature. This epinephrine-induced response can also result in temporarily increased counts of other WBC types in the peripheral blood of healthy patients. At least one canine breed, the Greyhound, has hematological reference ranges reported to fall slightly outside of reference ranges commonly used for the species.[6-8] Greyhound crossbreed dogs may also have similar changes.[9] Although these normal physiological conditions should be considered, they generally explain less than 5% of the patient values that fall outside reference ranges for any single hematological parameter.

SMEAR PREPARATION

Well-made smears are required for reliable identification and evaluation of peripheral blood cells. Smears can be prepared on glass slides or coverslips. The glass slide technique is generally easier and more reliable than preparing smears on coverslips. Glass slides can also be processed through automatic stainers and so may be most suitable for laboratories using such equipment. The coverslip method may result in more uniform WBC distribution and less trauma to fragile blood components, such as large or neoplastic cells, within the sample. For both methods, blood samples should be fresh and well mixed at smear preparation time, and smears should be completely air-dried before staining. Checking with the reference laboratory before submitting coverslip smears may be prudent, as the laboratory may prefer the coverslips be affixed (i.e., with superglue) to a full-size slide to decrease the risk of breakage or loss in transit and to allow staining at the laboratory.

Glass Slides

Smears are prepared on glass slides by placing a drop of blood (2–3 mm in diameter) on the broad face of the slide about 1 to 1.5 cm from the frosted border (or edge of a nonfrosted slide). Another clean, dry slide (i.e., spreader slide) is held loosely against the surface of the first slide at a 30-degree angle and drawn smoothly toward the blood drop, as illustrated in Fig. 1.16 (see Chapter 1). The spreader slide should be brought to a position where it just meets, but is not drawn into, the blood drop. When the spreader slide makes contact with the blood drop, capillary action immediately distributes the blood drop between the two slides. Then, with no downward pressure, the spreader slide is quickly and smoothly swept across the remaining length of the underlying slide.

Ideally, blood smears have a smooth transition from the thick region to the feathered edge and cover an area half the length and slightly less than the width of the slide (see Fig. 1.16, D, in Chapter 1). If the edge is blunt instead of feathered, the second slide was probably raised off the first before the blood drop was spread completely. Unequal smear thickness usually results from the spreader slide being held at too obtuse an angle or placing too much pressure on the first slide while spreading the blood drop. Too much pressure on the second slide can also result in WBC clumping along the smear's feathered edge. Too little pressure can result in short, thick smears. Smear thickness can also be affected by the viscosity of the blood sample. Adjusting the angle at which the second slide is held against the first can help compensate for very viscous (e.g., hemoconcentrated) or watery (i.e., anemic) blood samples. A more obtuse, 40- to 45-degree angle between the two slides makes thicker smears for very anemic samples, and an angle less than 30 degrees may be necessary for preparing smears of severely hemoconcentrated blood. Smears need to be thoroughly air-dried before staining; those that are thick may require additional drying time. Use (at the low setting) of a heat block or a blow dryer may shorten the drying time.

Glass Coverslips

The first step in creating coverslip smears is to place a small drop of blood drawn from a capillary tube in the center of a 22- × 22-mm glass coverslip and a second coverslip on top. The corners of the two coverslips should point in opposite directions. Then, without downward pressure, the top coverslip is quickly and smoothly drawn horizontally off the underlying one. The smears created on both coverslips are air-dried, stained (see the following discussion of stains), and placed face down on a drop of immersion oil or mounting medium on the same or separate glass slide(s) for evaluation.

Coverslip smears can also be made using both sides of a single coverslip to spread blood in two separate regions of a glass slide surface, resulting in two adjacent smears with fairly uniform WBC distribution on a single slide. This method provides the benefits of coverslip smears but avoids the problems inherent to handling delicate glass coverslips during manual staining. This method also allows for processing the smears with an automatic stainer.

STAINS

As with cytological preparations, Romanowsky-type stains are good general stains for microscopically evaluating blood smears. Quick Romanowsky-type stains are advantageous because they are less sensitive to solution pH and staining time and less susceptible to precipitate formation compared with Wright stains. However, many quick stains are also less effective at demonstrating polychromasia of immature erythrocytes.

Wright staining is achieved by flooding the air-dried blood smear with, or dipping it into Coplin jars containing, filtered Wright stain. After 2 to 4 minutes of incubation with the stain, the smear is flooded with a volume of phosphate buffer solution roughly equal to the amount of stain. To mix the buffer with the stain, one should gently rock or blow on the slide or dip it into another Coplin jar containing the buffer. The slides are incubated for another 3 to 6 minutes with the buffer. A metallic sheen will begin to appear on the fluid surface of flooded smears. The slide is then rinsed with tap water (or a 50:50 mixture of tap and distilled water to achieve a pH around 7.0) and blotted with bibulous paper or placed upright on an absorptive surface to hasten drying. A blowdryer set on low power and held 8 to 10 inches from the slide also shortens drying time.

Quick stain methods vary somewhat and should be used according to manufacturer's recommendations. The two-step Prodiff is unique among quick stains in differentially staining polychromatophilic and mature RBCs. Most quick stains, such as Diff-Quik, Hemacolor, and Quick III, lack the ability to distinguish polychromatophilic erythrocytes well, but they provide particularly consistent staining between smear preparations. The quick stains generally require slowly dipping the smear first in an alcohol fixative, then in a methylene blue dye mixture, and last in an eosin-containing solution. One edge of the slide is briefly blotted between solutions. Tap or distilled water can be used to rinse the slide after the last solution and before air-drying.

TROUBLESHOOTING

Artifacts of Cell Morphology and Staining

Most artifactual changes in cell morphology and staining can be readily recognized by their appearance and/or distribution within a smear. Examining multiple smears of the same blood sample is also helpful because alterations that are inconstant from smear to smear are likely to be artifactual.

Crenated Erythrocytes

Crenated erythrocytes (see Fig. 26.36 later in the chapter), artifacts especially common in feline blood samples, have a thorn apple–like shape with many short, uniformly spaced, blunt or pointed spicules that protrude from the cell membrane. Crenated RBCs can result from drying the smear too slowly or a relative excess of anticoagulant in the sample. Prolonged storage time of the blood (e.g., more than 2 hours at 4° C or at room temperature), particularly with an EDTA anticoagulant, can also result in RBC crenation. Differences in surface tension between the cell membrane and the glass slide may be an unpredictable cause of the artifact.

In Vitro Aging Artifacts

These are common in smears made from blood samples left at room temperature for longer than 2 to 4 hours or refrigerated for longer than 12 hours. Neutrophils, monocytes, and immature and neoplastic WBCs degenerate slightly earlier compared with other cell types. The nuclei of affected cells initially become condensed and stain homogeneously, and segmentation of granulocyte nuclei becomes more prominent, with only thin strands of chromatin separating lobules (e.g., hypersegmented neutrophils). Basophilia and vacuolation may be evident in the cytoplasm of neutrophils, and nuclei later become pyknotic and fragmented. The cytoplasmic borders of degenerating cells often show blebbing (Fig. 26.1), and the cytoplasm of lymphocytes and monocytes may become vacuolated. These changes interfere with accurate identification of cell type and invalidate differential WBC counts if greater than 10% of the cells in the smear are affected. Platelet aggregation/clumping is also prevalent in aged samples. Avoiding aging artifacts is one reason to include fresh well-made smears with a sample submitted for hematology analysis to an outside laboratory.

Pale or Unstained Nuclei

Pale or unstained nuclei (Fig. 26.2) on smears suggest that there has been inadequate staining time, or the stain has aged. Of the three-step quick stain solutions, the new methylene blue (NMB) mixture is usually that which has begun to degrade and may require longer incubation time with the smear or replacement. On Wright-stained preparations, pale nuclei with bright orange-red RBCs can result from overzealous washing or low pH of the buffer. Conversely, Wright-stained smears with pale nuclei and RBCs that stain slightly brown to green may occur when preparations are thick, inadequately washed, or stained with too little or too alkaline a buffer. A neutral buffer (i.e., pH 6.4–7.0) is most effective for Wright staining. The pH of the distilled or tap water wash solution can occasionally interfere with the intensity of the nuclear staining with both Wright and quick stains. Additional causes of inadequate nuclear staining are noted in Table 1.3 in Chapter 1.

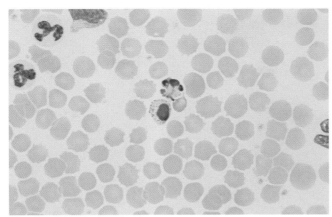

Fig. 26.1 Aging artifact in blood stored at room temperature for more than 1 hour. One cell has a densely stained, fragmented nucleus and cytoplasmic blebbing, and the adjacent cell has a condensed, rounded nucleus with a homogeneous chromatin pattern (Wright stain, original magnification 250×).

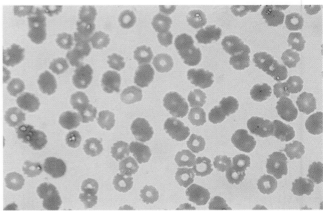

Fig. 26.3 This blood film was inadequately dried before staining. The punched-out, unstained regions in the RBCs are a result of moisture interfering with the contact between cells and stain (Diff-Quik stain, original magnification 250×).

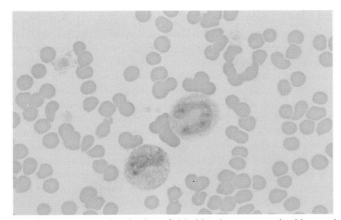

Fig. 26.2 Inadequate incubation of this blood smear resulted in poorly stained WBCs despite adequate RBC staining (Wright stain, original magnification 250×).

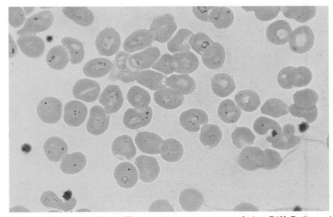

Fig. 26.4 Drying artifact. The eosin component of the Diff-Quik stain has precipitated around RBC areas that were inadequately dried. This artifact could be mistaken for erythroparasites, cytoplasmic inclusions, or basophilic stippling (Diff-Quik stain, original magnification 330×).

Drying Artifact

Drying artifact (Figs. 26.3 and 26.4) results if a smear is insufficiently air-dried before it is stained. The artifact is recognized in RBCs as round to crescent-shaped, punched-out regions or refractile vacuole-like structures. Stain condensations may border these pale cell areas or precipitate in the background between cells.

Overall Blue Tint

This may be seen on blood smears stained after prolonged storage, prepared from heparin-anticoagulated blood, or exposed to formalin or formalin fumes before staining. Even indirect exposure to formalin fumes (as may occur when slides are packaged with fixed tissues for shipment) may result in an overall pale, hazy, and often basophilic smear (Fig. 26.5).

Stain Precipitate

Stain precipitate is more often a problem with Wright stains than with quick stains. Wright stain will precipitate in storage, if incubated on a slide too long, or if insufficiently washed from a slide after incubation. Precipitate formed during storage and from insufficient washing occurs as random aggregates of spherical and dumbbell-shaped granules that appear both in and out of the

smear's plane of focus (Fig. 26.6). With prolonged incubation time, stain precipitate appears throughout the smear as uniformly dispersed, irregular globules of stain. Precipitate formed during storage can be removed by filtering the stain through Whatman filter paper into clean vials.

BLOOD SMEAR EVALUATION

Smears should be initially examined from the thickest region to the feathered edge by using the 10× or 20× objective. At this low magnification, blood films can be checked for staining, overall thickness, smooth transitions in thickness, cell distribution, and adequacy of the monolayer area. The monolayer is generally found within the distal half of the smear adjacent to the feathered edge and is luminescent when the unstained slide is held under indirect light. The monolayer represents the limited region where cell morphology is most reliably evaluated. WBCs should be fairly uniformly distributed within this region and only mildly clustered along the feathered edge. Examination of the borders and especially the feathered edge of the smear under low magnification may demonstrate the presence of platelet aggregates, microfilaria, large atypical cells, or cells with phagocytosed organisms.

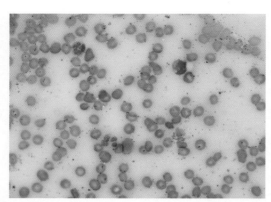

Fig. 26.5 Formalin artifact. Erythrocytes showing a pale, hazy, and often basophilic appearance characteristic of formalin fume exposure (Wright stain). (Courtesy Dr. Amy Valenciano.)

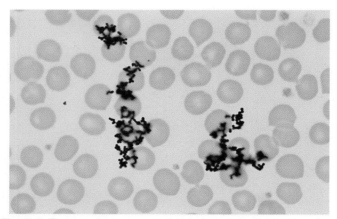

Fig. 26.6 The granular stain precipitate appears in and out of the plane of focus for the smear. This precipitate formed as a result of insufficient washing of Wright stain after buffer application. The granular precipitate that forms in the stain during storage can also be deposited on blood smears. The latter can be prevented by filtering the stain before use (Wright stain, original magnification 330×).

A patient's hematocrit can be roughly approximated by examining a blood smear at low magnification. Blood films from nonanemic animals generally have RBCs that are closely apposed in the monolayer in addition to several RBC layers at the thick end of the smear that obstruct penetrance of most condenser light. In contrast, smears from animals that are moderately to markedly anemic usually have RBCs that are widely separated from one another in the monolayer and only one or two RBC layers in the thick end of the smear that allow considerable condenser light to penetrate. Unless the angle between slides was adjusted during smear preparation of hemoconcentrated samples, the monolayer occupies a relatively reduced area. Estimates should ultimately be checked against the patient's measured hematocrit or packed cell volume (PCV).

The WBC count can also be roughly estimated or simply classified as low, normal, or high by examining the smear under low magnification. Accurate identification of the different WBC types and their relative proportions is more easily performed using the 40× or 50× objective. Cell morphology is typically evaluated under magnifications of 40× to 100×; platelet number and morphology are assessed at the highest of these magnification levels.

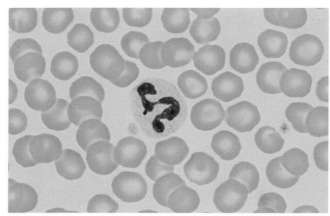

Fig. 26.7 Canine neutrophil with pale, eosinophilic cytoplasm and a lobulated nucleus containing mostly dense heterochromatin (Wright stain, original magnification 330×).

NORMAL CELL COMPONENTS OF BLOOD

Red Blood Cells

RBC morphology is primarily evaluated within the monolayer where artifactual distortion induced during preparation and differences in smear thickness are less apt to influence cell appearance. Nearly all significant morphological abnormalities of RBCs can be detected at 40× or 50× magnification, although some alterations may require additional examination at higher magnification. Initial examination of RBC morphology with the 100× objective, however, often results in overdiagnosis of aberrations.

Mature RBCs in healthy adult dogs are about 7 μm in diameter (slightly larger than the 5.5– to 6.0 μm diameter of feline RBCs). As is apparent in the monolayer of blood smears, canine RBCs are biconcave with an area of central pallor occupying about one third of the cell's diameter. Feline RBCs do not consistently have discernible central pallor and tend to vary slightly more in shape compared with canine RBCs. Both species have mild RBC anisocytosis and may show an occasional immature polychromatophilic cell on peripheral blood smears.

White Blood Cells

Neutrophils

Canine and feline neutrophils have similar appearance on blood films (Fig. 26.7). The neutrophil nucleus is elongated and separated into multiple lobules by invaginations of the nuclear border. Demarcations between lobules are seldom distinct enough to be considered filamentous. Chromatin is organized into dense clumps of dark-purple to black staining heterochromatin separated by narrow areas of less condensed euchromatin. Female animals may have a notable small, drumstick-like projection on one of the lobes of some neutrophils known as a *Barr body*. This represents the inactivated X chromosome. Cytoplasm is clear, pale eosinophilic to faintly basophilic, with a fine grainy texture, and, rarely, contains one or two small vacuoles. Neutrophil granules range from indiscernible to faintly eosinophilic but are pale and much smaller than the prominent granules of mature eosinophils.

Band Neutrophils

Band neutrophils, low numbers of which occur in the peripheral blood of healthy dogs and cats, have an elongated, U- or J-shaped to slightly twisted nucleus and less chromatin condensation compared with mature neutrophils (Fig. 26.8). Nuclear lobulation is absent or poorly defined. Constrictions of canine band neutrophil nuclei are less than half the width of the remainder (nonconstricted sections) of the nucleus; feline band neutrophils lack nuclear constrictions entirely. Cytoplasm is similar in granule content and staining to that of mature neutrophils.

Monocytes

Canine and feline monocytes are larger than neutrophils and similar in size to eosinophils and basophils. Nuclei vary greatly in morphology, ranging from elongated U shapes that resemble band neutrophils to irregular multilobulated forms. The nuclear chromatin of monocytes is generally distinct from that of both mature and immature granulocytes and is characteristically lacy to ropy with only a few small isolated clumps of heterochromatin (Fig. 26.9). The moderate to abundant gray-blue cytoplasm of monocytes has a ground-glass texture, is often sparsely dusted with minute eosinophilic granules, and occasionally contains vacuoles. Cytoplasmic borders are usually irregular, sometimes with fine, filamentous, pseudopodia-like extensions. Because of their relatively large size, monocytes may be concentrated along the feathered edge, and their proportion underestimated in blood smear differential WBC counts.

Lymphocytes

Lymphocytes vary in size in the peripheral blood of dogs and cats, with small cells predominating. Small lymphocytes have densely staining, round to oval nuclei that are sometimes slightly indented and usually have large, well-defined chromatin clumps (Fig. 26.10). Alternatively, nuclear chromatin may appear smudged, especially when stained with a quick stain. The moderately blue cytoplasm of small lymphocytes is scant, and cytoplasmic borders are partially obscured by the nuclei, particularly with feline lymphocytes. Larger lymphocytes in peripheral blood have less densely staining, but still clearly clumped, nuclear chromatin. Cytoplasm of the larger cells is more abundant and ranges from light to moderately basophilic. Some lymphocytes have a few variably sized eosinophilic cytoplasmic granules that are usually concentrated within a single perinuclear cell area (Fig. 26.11).

Eosinophils

Eosinophils, which are slightly larger than neutrophils, can usually be found in very low numbers on blood smears of healthy dogs and cats. Nuclei are less lobulated (often being divided into only two distinct lobules) with less condensed chromatin (Fig. 26.12) than those of mature neutrophils. Cytoplasm is clear to faintly basophilic and contains prominent pink granules, which are abundant, small, and rod shaped in cats (Fig. 26.13) but vary widely in number and size in dogs. Canine eosinophils occasionally contain a single, large granule that may be mistaken for an inclusion body or unusual organism (Fig. 26.14). Eosinophils

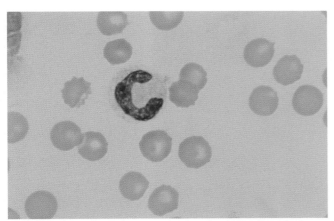

Fig. 26.8 Canine band neutrophil with pale eosinophilic cytoplasm that is similar to a mature cell and a U-shaped nucleus lacking distinct segmentation (Wright stain, original magnification 330×).

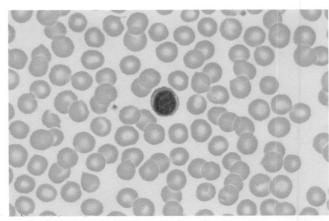

Fig. 26.10 Canine lymphocyte with densely clumped nuclear chromatin and scant basophilic cytoplasm (Wright stain, original magnification 250×).

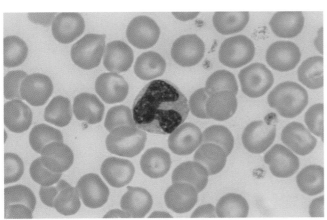

Fig. 26.9 This canine monocyte has an irregular nucleus with a ropey chromatin pattern and grainy basophilic cytoplasm (Wright stain, original magnification 330×).

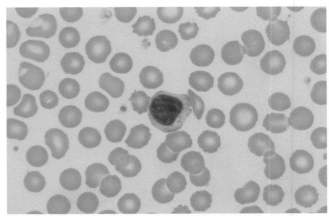

Fig. 26.11 Large granular lymphocyte in a healthy dog. Both canine and feline lymphocytes occasionally contain a few eosinophilic granules in a moderate amount of homogeneous basophilic cytoplasm (Wright stain, original magnification 250×).

of Greyhounds are peculiar in that they may appear vacuolated on smears—a breed difference that has been attributed to differential staining properties of the specific granules (Fig. 26.15).[10] Eosinophil granules that are ruptured in vitro are also sometimes freely scattered in the background of canine and feline blood smears.

Basophils

Basophils are the largest of the mature granulocytic cell types and rare in peripheral blood of healthy dogs and cats. Nuclei are less densely staining and have fewer lobulations and a more elongated, ribbonlike appearance than the nuclei of other granulocytic cell types (Fig. 26.16). Cytoplasm is moderately blue-gray to slightly purple and usually contains granules. In dogs, basophil granules are usually low in number and stain dark-blue to metachromatic. Canine basophils also occasionally lack obvious granules but are recognizable by their size, nuclear morphology, and cytoplasmic staining (Fig. 26.17). In cats, basophils contain abundant oval, pale-lavender to gray specific granules (Fig. 26.18), although immature basophils may also contain a few primary, dark purple granules.

Platelets

Canine and feline platelets appear oval, round, or rod shaped on peripheral blood smears. Their clear to pale-gray cytoplasm usually contains a central cluster of eosinophilic to metachromatic granules. Platelets

normally vary in size from about one-fourth to two-thirds of the diameter of RBCs in canine blood, and occasionally are even larger than the RBCs in feline blood. These larger platelets may be noted as macroplatelets in hematology reports (see Fig. 26.35 later in the chapter). Partially activated platelets have a spiderlike appearance with thin cytoplasmic processes extending from a small spherical cell body. Platelets may also

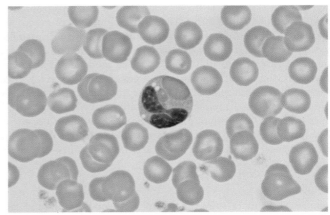

Fig. 26.14 Canine eosinophil with only two large cytoplasmic granules (Wright stain, original magnification 330×).

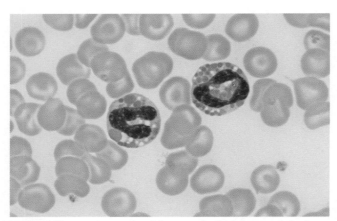

Fig. 26.12 Two canine eosinophils, one of which has partially degranulated cytoplasm. Eosinophil nuclei are less condensed and lobulated than those of neutrophils (Wright stain, original magnification 330×).

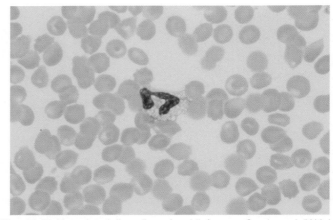

Fig. 26.15 Vacuolated "gray" eosinophil from a Greyhound (Wright stain). (From *Hematology Atlas of the Dog and Cat*; slide courtesy Dr. Theresa Rizzi at Oklahoma State; photo courtesy Dr. Amy Valenciano.)

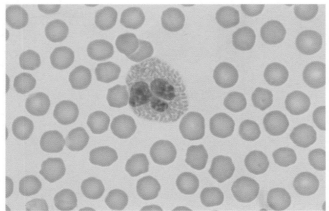

Fig. 26.13 Feline eosinophil with small, rod-shaped, eosinophilic granules filling the cytoplasm and partially obscuring the nucleus (Wright stain, original magnification 250×).

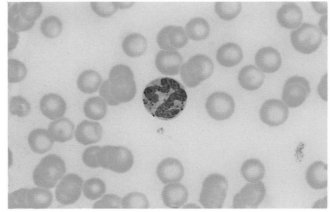

Fig. 26.16 Canine basophil with metachromatic granules scattered in the cytoplasm (Wright stain, original magnification 250×).

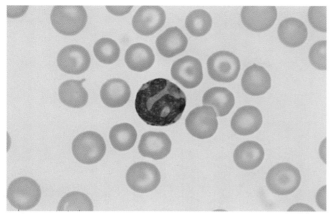

Fig. 26.17 Poorly granulated canine basophil, which can be identified as such by its size, ribbonlike nuclear shape, and cytoplasmic staining, despite the near absence of cytoplasmic granules (Wright stain, original magnification 330×).

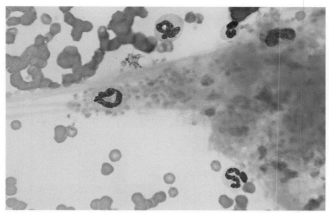

Fig. 26.19 Large mass of aggregated platelets, fibrin, and a few enmeshed leukocytes. Platelet aggregation or agglutination sometimes results in artifactually low platelet counts (Wright stain, original magnification 200×).

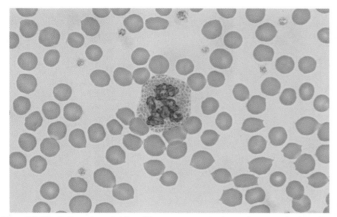

Fig. 26.18 Feline basophil with a segmented nucleus and abundant oval to polygonal, lavender-gray, cytoplasmic granules (Wright stain, original magnification 250×).

appear aggregated (Fig. 26.19) or clumped into an amorphous mass on blood smears, a finding particularly common in feline blood smears. Pale-blue fibrin strands indicating active clotting and fibrin formation may also be noted. Aggregated and clumped platelets are usually pushed to the feathered edge, and this may result in the false impression of thrombocytopenia if only the monolayer of the smear is evaluated.

ALTERATIONS OF RBCs IN DISEASE

Alterations in RBC Numbers

Alterations in RBC density on a smear may reflect erythrocytosis (polycythemia) or anemia. Erythrocytosis and polycythemia both refer to an increase in the RBC density, and some like to reserve the term *polycythemia* for a primary marrow proliferation of neoplastic RBC elements. The most common cause of erythrocytosis is hemoconcentration with dehydration, resulting in a relative increase in RBC numbers and plasma protein concentration. Alternatively, relative erythrocytosis may occur secondary to splenic contraction, a condition that is more likely to occur in dogs than in cats, and can be supported by the animal's recent history, lack of a corresponding increase in plasma proteins, and transient nature of the finding. Absolute erythrocytosis is a persistent increase in circulating erythroid elements and is less common, but when observed, it is usually the result of an appropriate erythropoietic response to chronic hypoxia. The hypoxia may be generalized, as with respiratory

or cardiovascular conditions, or localized to the kidney; both conditions can lead to low renal tissue oxygenation and increased circulating erythropoietin resulting in increased production of erythrocytes.

Absolute erythrocytosis secondary to inappropriate erythropoietin production, and primary polycythemia, or polycythemia vera, which is independent of erythropoietin levels, are both rare in dogs and cats. These two conditions are tentatively diagnosed by excluding the more common causes of erythrocytosis. Erythrocytosis associated with tumor erythropoietin production has been reported in dogs with renal and nonrenal tumor types, with the latter including cecal leiomyoma, nasal fibrosarcoma, and extradural schwannoma.[11-13] Inappropriate administration of recombinant erythropoietin or androgens may also be a cause of absolute secondary erythrocytosis in dogs or cats as in other species, although treatment with human erythropoietin can also lead to RBC aplasia in both species.[14] The algorithm shown in Fig. 26.20 may further aid in determining the cause of erythrocytosis in dogs and cats.

Anemia is an especially common finding in dogs and cats and can be secondary to almost any type of illness. Anemia is often suspected before blood samples are collected on the basis of a patient's clinical signs and physical examination. Evidence to support the condition as being acute or chronic can be derived from the clinical presentation and history. An animal with peracute to acute blood loss is often anxious and tachypneic and may have mucous membranes that are paler than expected for the degree of anemia as a result of transient peripheral vasoconstriction. With chronic blood loss, through upregulation of RBC 2,3-diphosphoglycerate in dogs and likely by an alternative mechanism in cats, oxygen is more readily released from hemoglobin to the tissues. Animals with chronic anemia are apt to be relatively inactive and show distress and dyspnea only if further stressed by physical exertion, an additional medical condition, or if the blood loss is severe. A dog or cat presenting with a PCV of 12% or less typically has some degree of chronic anemia, because acute or subacute blood loss of this magnitude is generally not life-supporting. Blood smear examination, as described in the following section and Fig. 26.21, may further aid in determining the cause of anemia in dogs and cats.

Blood Smear Examination in the Evaluation of Anemia

Cytological examination of peripheral blood is important in determining the cause, treatment, and prognosis of a patient's anemia. The procedure is also valuable in monitoring anemic conditions over time. Alterations of RBC morphology are usually most indicative of the primary cause of the anemia. For example, anisocytosis may be detected in animals with regenerative erythropoietic response or immune-mediated hemolysis with spherocytic RBC and is especially profound when the two conditions are concurrent (see Figs. 26.26

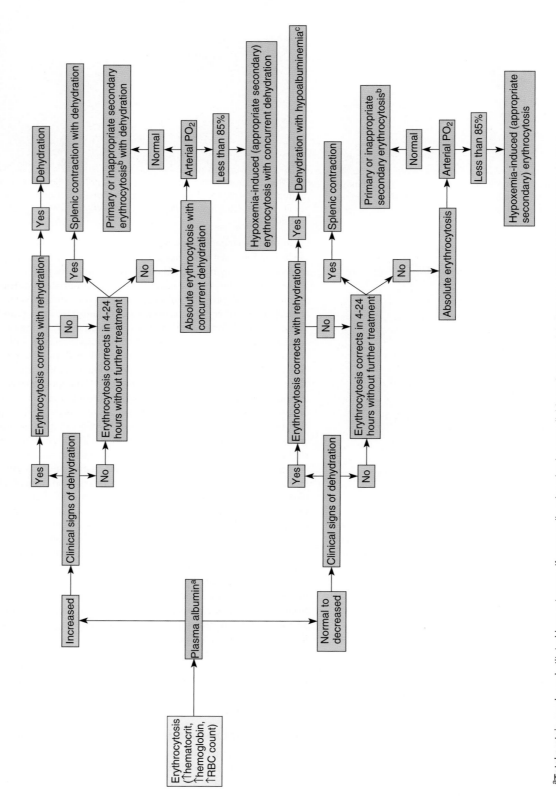

Fig. 26.20 Algorithm to aid in the diagnosis of polycythemia.

[a]Total protein can be substituted in most cases if serum albumin value is unavailable and serum globulins are unlikely to be markedly elevated.

[b]Inappropriate secondary erythrocytosis may be caused by renal lesions or selective neoplastic conditions (presumably associated with tumor production of erythropoietin-like factors) including, but not limited to, primary renal tumors (see text).

[c]Albumin loss may be due to plasma protein loss, insufficient dietary protein, hepatic protein synthesis, or a combination of these.

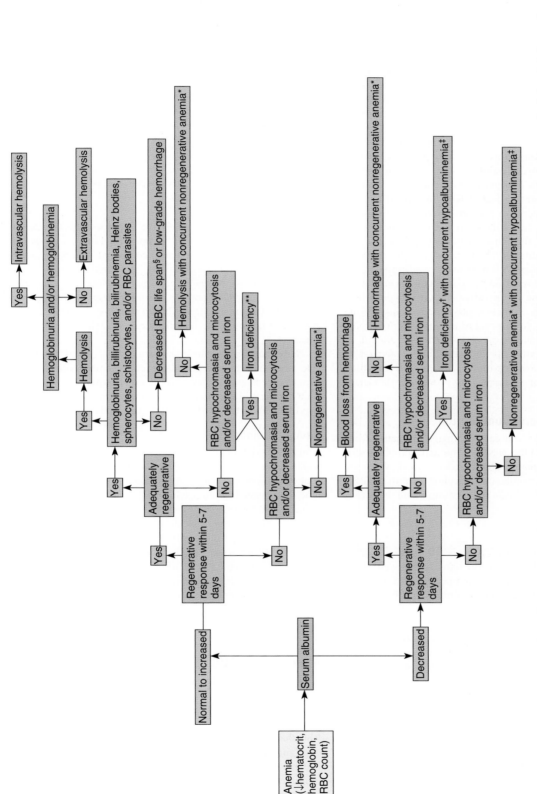

Fig. 26.21 Algorithm to aid in the diagnosis of anemia.

*Refers to anemia of chronic systemic disease or the underlying condition of the bone marrow impairing RBC production. The former includes anemia of chronic inflammation, certain endocrinopathies, and major organ (e.g., kidney, liver) diseases, neoplasia, and malnutrition. The latter includes toxin-induced and immune-mediated conditions affecting RBC precursor cells.

† Copper deficiency may also be a consideration in these cases.

‡ Hypoalbuminemia may be a result of plasma protein loss (including plasma loss through hemorrhage), insufficient hepatic synthesis, or insufficient dietary protein.

§ Includes chronic low-grade hemolysis. The presence of abnormally high polychromasia/reticulocyte count in mildly anemic or nonanemic animals suggests chronic lead toxicity or an intrinsic RBC abnormality.

**Portosystemic shunt, copper, and/or vitamin B₆ deficiency may also be considerations in these cases.

and 26.27 later in the chapter). An increasing proportion of large, immature RBCs over time without a change in absolute RBC count suggests that an animal has persistent blood loss (or hemolysis) with compensation and a responsive marrow. Other components of the smear, including leukocytes and platelets, may also provide clues about the cause of anemia. Increased numbers of normal or enlarged platelets may be seen in association with acute or persistent blood loss. Low platelet numbers support platelet consumption or destruction, with anemia secondary to hemorrhage or immune-mediated hemolysis. Leukocytosis is usually also seen with immune-mediated RBC destruction, whereas leukopenia (especially neutropenia) and thrombocytopenia occur concomitant with anemia with impaired bone marrow hematopoiesis.

Evaluating smears for the extent of erythropoietic response can provide critical information on the cause of an anemia. Responding anemia, as suggested by an orderly shift to a greater than normal proportion of large, variably basophilic, immature RBCs on an anemic patient's blood smears, indicates RBC loss from hemorrhage or hemolysis. A regenerative response may be detected in peripheral blood as early as 2 to 4 days after initial blood loss in dogs and cats, depending on the cause, magnitude of anemia, and the animal's concurrent conditions. The response is typically rapid and profound in dogs and cats with hemolytic conditions and is more variable in onset and magnitude in patients with only mild blood loss. In all cases, if the regenerative response appears less than adequate for the degree of anemia (assuming adequate time has elapsed for bone marrow to respond to the maximum extent), a reticulocyte count, which allows for classification of anemia as regenerative or nonregenerative, is indicated. Nonregenerative anemias indicate some degree of impaired erythropoiesis for which evaluation of the patient's bone marrow may provide further diagnostic information.

Reticulocyte Evaluation and Quantitation

One of a few vital stains that can be used to distinguish immature from mature erythrocytes on blood films is NMB. The stain combines with polyribosomes retained in immature RBCs (reticulocytes), which are then recognized as dark-blue granules or "reticulum" within the RBC cytoplasm. Mature RBCs lack cytoplasmic ribosomes and stain uniformly pale blue with NMB.

Method

One-part blood is mixed with 1 to 1.5 parts NMB (0.5% in saline) in either a test or capillary tube (rolling the latter to mix well). This mixture is then allowed to stand at room temperature for either 10 (canine blood) or 15 to 20 (feline blood) minutes. The blood–stain combination is mixed again, and a small drop is used to make a thin smear, which is then air-dried and examined under the 100× oil-immersion objective. For manual reticulocyte quantitation, at least 1000 total RBCs are quantified, and the number of reticulocytes is expressed as a percentage (i.e., number of reticulocytes among 1000 total RBCs ÷ 10). An eyepiece etched with a Miller disk (available through retailers of microscope accessories) may facilitate counting.

Canine reticulocytes are of the aggregate type, recognized by their dark blue, interlacing network of cytoplasmic precipitate. Feline reticulocytes are of two readily recognizable types, aggregate reticulocytes (as in dogs) and punctate reticulocytes (Fig. 26.22). Punctate reticulocytes lack the reticular pattern of cytoplasmic staining but contain a few scattered, variably sized, dark blue cytoplasmic granules. These two reticulocyte types are counted separately in feline blood because

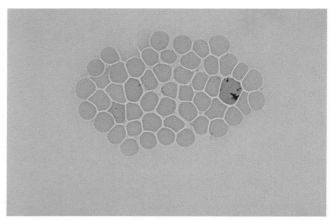

Fig. 26.22 NMB–stained blood film from a cat. Both aggregate and sparsely stippled punctate reticulocytes are seen in this field (NMB stain, original magnification 250×).

their kinetics during a regenerative response differ. Because feline punctate reticulocytes remain elevated for longer periods (up to 2 weeks after resolution of anemia) compared with aggregate reticulocytes in peripheral blood, only aggregate reticulocytes are counted to assess an active regenerative response. Note that epierythrocytic *Hemobartonella felis* organisms, basophilic stippling, and drying artifacts on RBCs can appear similar to, and thus may need to be differentiated from, punctate reticulocytes on NMB-stained feline blood smears.

Newer automated instruments are capable of performing reticulocyte counts as well and are available for assessment both at the in-clinic or reference laboratory level. These instruments use different dyes to stain nucleic acid and often enumerate a percentage and absolute numbers of reticulocytes based on large numbers of cells via flow cytometry.

Interpretation

A maximal erythropoietic response from the bone marrow is expected within 7 days of the onset of anemia. Interpretation of reticulocyte counts is often based on calculation of the absolute number of circulating reticulocytes generated by multiplying the percentage obtained on the NMB-stained smear (or generated by automated instruments) by the erythrocyte count generated by a hematology instrument. (i.e., total RBC count × reticulocyte percentage). Counts greater than 50,000 aggregate reticulocytes/μL in cats and 60,000 aggregate reticulocytes/μL in dogs are considered indicative of at least a mild regenerative response, although these interpretive ranges likely vary, depending on the reference laboratory and the method of hematology quantification (i.e., instrument type). Because feline punctate reticulocytes circulate for a prolonged period, an increase in these forms without a detectable increase in aggregates may represent a marrow response in cats with either mild acute or recently resolved anemia.

Alterations of RBC Shape or Size

Although occasional alterations of RBC shape or size can be seen on virtually all smears, such changes that occur in high proportion (i.e., >5% of RBC) or that are prominent in their appearance should be carefully evaluated for their potential diagnostic significance. Common RBC shape changes that can be detected on peripheral blood smears of dogs and cats and have diagnostic significance can be grouped into five major categories: (1) RBC fragmentation, (2) oxidative injury, (3) immune-mediated damage, (4) altered diameter, and (5) shape distortion or poikilocytosis. Table 26.2[15-28] provides a quick aid for the diagnosis of the major RBC shape changes.

TABLE 26.2 Major Changes in Peripheral Blood Smear Red Blood Cell (RBC) Morphology as Indicators of the Cause of Anemia

Prominent Morphology	Expected Associated RBC Morphological Findings	Additional Morphology/Other Findings Often Seen	Causes to Consider
Fragmented erythrocytes (schistocytes)	Keratocytes (helmet cells), blister cells, possibly occasional spherocytes	Sufficient polychromatophilic cells to indicate a regenerative erythropoietic response	Microangiopathic hemolytic anemia secondary to disseminated intravascular coagulation, inflammation of a highly vascular organ (e.g., liver, spleen, lung, renal glomeruli), turbulent blood flow (e.g., caval syndrome, hemangiosarcoma), severe burns, advanced neoplasia, lymphosarcoma[15,16]
Eccentrocytes and/or Heinz bodies	Sufficient polychromatophilic cells to indicate a regenerative erythropoietic response	Pyknocytes (small, dense, irregularly shaped RBCs), ghosted erythrocytes	Hemolytic anemia secondary to oxidative injury: consider ingestion of onion garlic, zinc, copper, or naphthalene; drug toxicity (e.g., acetaminophen, benzocaine products, propofol, d-L methionine, vitamin K3, or phenazopyridine)[17-19]
Anisocytosis	Caused by polychromatophilic macrocytes, indicative of a regenerative response	Codocytes and stomatocytes (among polychromatophilic cells) and a few nucleated red blood cells (nRBCs) may be seen with a regenerative response	If erythropoietic regenerative response is adequate relative to degree of anemia, consider blood loss from hemolysis or hemorrhage; if less than expected regenerative response, consider nonregenerative cause(s) in addition to hemolysis and/ or hemorrhage
	Or caused by combined polychromatophilic macrocytes and spherocytes or microcytes	Erythrocyte agglutination, thrombocytopenia, red cell parasites, nRBCs	Immune-mediated hemolytic anemia; infection with erythroparasites, especially hemotropic *Mycoplasma* spp.; crotalid snake or bee envenomation[20,21]; may also be seen with Heinz body formation (presumed reformed erythrocyte after removal of membrane protrusion)
	Or primarily caused by normocytic macrocytes with few/no polychromatophilic cells	nRBCs, other immature erythroid, or abnormal nucleated cells	Myelodysplastic or myeloproliferative disorder (myeloid, erythroid, or lymphoid)
Acanthocytes, echinocytes	Few to no polychromatophilic erythrocytes	If >1% fragmented cells (e.g., schistocytes, keratocytes) *(see above)*	Artifact of collection/preparation *(see text)*, disorders of lipid metabolism, liver disease, glomerulonephritis, lymphosarcoma, doxorubicin administration and elapid or crotalid snake envenomation, myeloproliferative disorders, myelofibrosis, uremia, and possibly electrolyte abnormality[16,20-28]
Hypochromic erythrocytes (increased central pallor)	Hypochromic RBCs often appear as acanthocytes, codocytes, or fragmented cells	Insufficient erythropoietic response (polychromatophilic cells) relative to degree of anemia	Iron deficiency: consider dietary deficiency or chronic blood loss (e.g., through gastrointestinal or urinary tract, repeated blood collection, chronic parasitemia); portosystemic shunt
Nucleated erythrocytes	Sufficient polychromatophilic cells to indicate a regenerative erythropoietic response	nRBCs with normal morphology; Howell-Jolly bodies	Low numbers of nRBCs sometimes accompany a robust regenerative erythropoietic response
	Few or no polychromatophilic macrocytes indicative of a nonregenerative or poorly regenerative erythropoietic response	nRBCs with normal morphology; Howell-Jolly bodies	Splenic or bone marrow dysfunction (e.g., secondary to hypoxia, neoplasia, trauma), persistent glucocorticoid treatment, hyperadrenocorticism, severe physiological stress, extramedullary hematopoiesis, hemangiosarcoma, reported as occasional in some breeds (generally without anemia)
	Few or no polychromatophilic macrocytes indicative of a nonregenerative or poorly regenerative erythropoietic response	Abnormal nRBCs (e.g., asynchronous nuclear-to-cytoplasmic ratio), other immature or abnormal nucleated cells	Dyserythropoietic, myelodysplastic, or myeloproliferative (myeloid, erythroid, or lymphoid) disorders; bone marrow dyscrasia in Poodles (with macrocytosis, and usually without anemia)

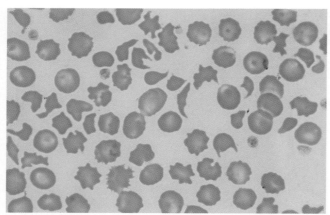

Fig. 26.23 Many fragmented RBCs are seen in this blood smear from a dog with stenosis of the pulmonic valve. Numerous schistocytes and a helmet-shaped cell can be seen (Wright stain, original magnification 250×).

Fragmentation

RBC fragmentation on blood smears represents RBCs that have lost a portion of their cell membrane generally with some associated cytoplasm. RBC fragmentation is most often a result of excessive blood turbulence from altered blood flow or extensive deposition of fibrin within microvascular lumina. The former is likely the primary mechanism of RBC fragmentation associated with cardiac valvular stenosis and caval syndrome of heartworm disease. The latter mechanism is responsible for the fragmentation hemolysis that is frequently seen in animals with disseminated intravascular coagulation or extensive inflammation of highly vascular tissues (i.e., spleen, liver, pulmonary parenchyma, bone marrow, and renal cortex). Both mechanisms may be active in cases of fragmentation hemolysis associated with large, highly vascular tumors (especially hemangiosarcoma). RBC fragmentation can also result from intrinsic abnormalities of the RBCs themselves, as with RBC oxidative injury or moderate to severe iron deficiency. Fragmented RBCs are usually recognized on blood smears as one of three morphological forms: schistocytes, keratocytes, or blister cells.

Schistocytes (or schizocytes) are irregularly shaped RBC fragments that typically have ragged asymmetrical borders and sharp, pointed projections (Fig. 26.23). Keratocytes are RBC fragments with two adjacent hornlike projections as a result of one-sided loss of cell membrane and cytoplasm. Keratocytes are sometimes referred to as *bite cells* or *helmet cells* because of their two-dimensional shape on blood smears (see Fig. 26.23). Blister cells are RBCs with a single, eccentric, vacuole-like structure thought to be created when the cell encounters fibrin strands bridging a vessel lumen. Blister cells are usually found with other forms of fragmented RBCs and probably represent the transitional form between intact erythrocytes and keratocytes (see Fig. 26.29 later). If greater than 1% of these abnormal RBCs are present in peripheral blood, significant RBC fragmentation is suggested. When 10% or greater of the RBCs on a blood film appear fragmented, clinical and other laboratory findings are likely to further support the presence of intravascular hemolytic anemia in the patient.

Increased red blood cell distribution width (RDW) with a shoulder on the left side of the RBC histogram tracing may be seen with automated analysis of blood samples with larger numbers of fragmented RBCs; this finding is supportive but not diagnostic of the condition because it can also be seen with other RBC and even platelet alterations.

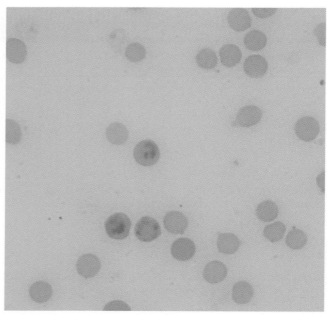

Fig. 26.24 Feline blood smear showing increased numbers of Heinz bodies and aggregate reticulocytes. Note the lysed, ghost erythrocytes with Heinz bodies at the top left, supporting some component of likely intravascular hemolysis (NMB stain, original magnification 100×).

Oxidative Injury

Oxidative injury of RBCs can lead to denaturation of the hemoglobin protein, which, when pronounced, can appear as Heinz bodies and/or eccentrocytes on patient blood films. Heinz bodies appear as single, rounded protrusions of the RBC membrane (Fig. 26.24), often with a pale-staining collar of cytoplasm around the base of the projection. They may also be seen as eccentric, round, pale-staining areas within, or refractile bodies overlying, RBCs. The presence and percentage of RBCs containing Heinz bodies can be most accurately determined by preparing wet or dry blood smears stained with 0.5% NMB, as some poikilocytes (i.e., echinocytes) can mimic Heinz bodies on Wright-stained smears. Heinz bodies occasionally fragment from the cell during sample processing and are seen as small, spherical, pink or refractile (or NMB-stained) bodies in the background of a smear. Heinz bodies vary in size, depending on the severity of oxidative injury. Cats, whose hemoglobin molecules are particularly susceptible to oxidative injury, may have very small Heinz bodies in varying percentages (generally <10%) of their circulating RBCs when healthy. Many small and, occasionally, large Heinz bodies may be found in the RBCs of cats with certain chronic conditions, such as diabetes mellitus, lymphoma, hyperthyroidism, and chronic renal disease (see Fig. 26.24). Canine Heinz bodies and numerous or large feline Heinz bodies in RBCs suggest a potential hemolytic crisis. Eccentrocytes, which may also be detected in blood smears of dogs and cats exposed to exogenous oxidative toxins, have an eccentric, ghosted region of cytoplasm with the remaining cytoplasm being slightly condensed (Fig. 26.25). Several exogenous toxins associated with oxidative RBC injury and Heinz bodies and/or eccentrocytes in dogs or cats are listed in Table 26.2.

Immune-Mediated RBC Damage

Immune-mediated RBC damage is suggested by the presence of spherocytes with minimal other poikilocytes, agglutinated RBCs, or both on smears of peripheral blood. Spherocytes are densely staining, small (less than two-thirds of the normal diameter) RBCs that lack central

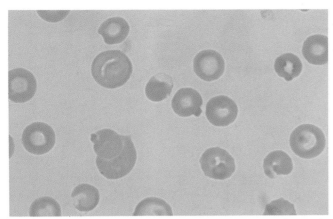

Fig. 26.25 Three canine erythrocytes with large Heinz bodies and an eccentrocyte *(center)* can be seen in this field (Wright stain, original magnification 330×).

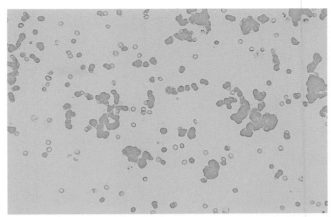

Fig. 26.27 RBC agglutination is seen in this blood film from a dog with immune-mediated hemolytic anemia. The cells remained agglutinated after saline dilution of blood (Wright stain, original magnification 100×).

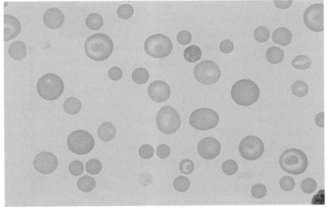

Fig. 26.26 Blood smear from a dog with immune-mediated hemolytic anemia. Note the marked anisocytosis resulting from a mixed population of small spherocytes and large, immature, and normal RBCs. The spherocytes are dense staining and lack central pallor. A few polychromatophils are in the shape of codocytes (Wright stain, original magnification 250×).

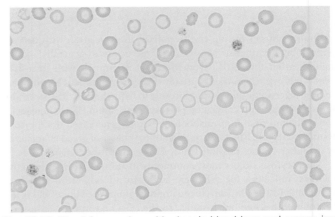

Fig. 26.28 Blood from a dog with chronic blood loss and severe iron deficiency. Iron-deficient RBCs have a broad area of central pallor and a thin rim of stained cytoplasm. Anisocytosis is also apparent (Diff-Quik stain, original magnification 132×).

pallor (Fig. 26.26). They predominantly occur as a result of immune opsonization and piecemeal removal of the RBC membrane by phagocytic cells of the vascular system. This membrane damage weakens the cell and decreases its deformability, leading to RBC loss through cell rupture. In some cases, complement may directly lyse opsonized cells. Significant spherocytosis (>1%) is usually accompanied by overt extravascular or combined extravascular and intravascular hemolytic anemia. Spherocytosis can be reliably detected only in species that have RBCs with a distinctive central pallor (e.g., dogs) and then only in the monolayer of blood smears. Both dogs and cats with immune-mediated hemolytic anemia, however, may have pronounced anisocytosis on blood films (because of a mixture of spherocytic, normal, and—in cases with regenerative responses—large immature RBCs). It should be noted that spherocyte-like particles may also be seen in a few cases of traumatic RBC injury, along with more typical morphological forms of fragmented RBCs, and may also be seen on smears from animals with recent blood transfusions. Ghost erythrocytes are cytoplasmic remnants from lysed cells (see Fig. 26.24). These are supportive of intravascular hemolysis, particularly coupled with spherocytes or agglutination, but may be seen in low numbers as a result of shearing artifact during smear preparation.

RBC agglutination (Fig. 26.27) represents a particularly severe form of immune-mediated hemolytic anemia and may be detected grossly in samples within the collection vial or on unstained blood films. A saline dilution test is suggested for all suspect samples to aid in distinguishing immune-mediated agglutination from nonspecific RBC aggregation or rouleaux. Mixing 2 or 3 to 10 to 15 drops of saline with a drop of blood on a glass slide or tube causes cells that are simply aggregated or in rouleaux to disperse. Unstained, coverslipped preparations should be evaluated under 40× magnification with the substage condenser lowered.

Alterations in RBC Diameter

RBCs with smaller or larger diameter than average can be classified as microcytes or macrocytes, respectively. Blood smear evaluation is a sensitive means of detecting these alterations if RBC diameter in peripheral blood is mixed. Uniform microcytosis or macrocytosis is not easily recognized in peripheral smears but can be indicated by the mean cell volume (MCV) value generated with automated hematology analysis of the sample. In smears containing mixed RBC diameters, or anisocytosis, determining which cells represent the abnormal population may be difficult. Adjacent leukocytes on the smear can be helpful for size comparisons. Anisocytosis with microcytosis and poorly regenerative anemia can be seen in dogs and cats with pronounced iron-deficiency anemia (Fig. 26.28). The decrease in cell diameter is a result of

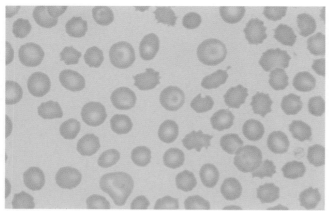

Fig. 26.29 Irregularly spiculated codocytes, echinocytes, and ovalocytes in the blood of a dog with multicentric lymphoma. The blister cell near the center of the field indicates that RBC trauma may be at least partially responsible for the acanthocytic RBCs (Wright stain, original magnification 250×).

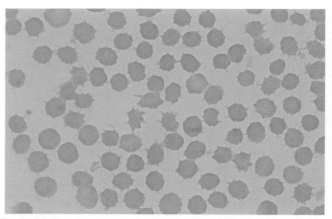

Fig. 26.30 Acanthocytes demonstrating irregularly sized spicules in a blood smear from a dog with cholestatic liver disease (Wright stain, original magnification 132×).

additional mitoses during erythropoiesis, in association with delayed hemoglobin synthesis. Measurable microcytosis generally occurs slightly earlier than RBC hypochromasia in animals with iron deficiency, but hypochromasia is usually the more prominent blood smear finding. Microcytic and normochromic to hypochromic RBCs can also be seen in dogs with congenital portosystemic shunt (likely in association with abnormal iron metabolism[29]), and generalized microcytosis of normochromic RBCs occurs as a nonpathological breed characteristic in Shibas, Akitas, possibly Chow Chows, and other Asian breeds.[30]

Macrocytosis occurs most commonly in animals with regenerative anemias, reflecting the relatively large size of immature polychromatophilic RBCs. The polychromatophilic staining of these cells is less apparent with some quick stains, so the cells may appear as normochromic macrocytes on blood films. True normochromic macrocytosis can result from impaired mitosis of RBC precursors and may be seen with myelodysplastic and myeloproliferative diseases and feline leukemia virus (FeLV) infections. Macrocytosis in association with familial bone marrow dysplasia has also been reported in some poodles, including miniature and toy poodles.[31] Macrocytosis that is attributed to these erythroid dysplastic or neoplastic conditions is usually accompanied by additional findings of increased erythrocyte anisocytosis and circulating nucleated erythroid cells (sometimes with asynchronized nucleus-to-cytoplasm development).

Macrocytosis has been rarely associated in dogs and/or cats with alterations of RBC fluid balance or cytoskeletal or membrane properties. Any of these causes may contribute to the familial macrocytosis with stomatocytosis (central fold resulting in a linear central pale region) that is uncommonly seen in Miniature or Standard Schnauzers. In the affected Schnauzers, the RBC shape change may be associated with other blood smear RBC alterations (anisocytosis, polychromasia) and increased RBC fragility and slight anemia.[32] Rare familial macrocytosis has been reported with other breeds (e.g., Giant Schnauzer, Alaskan Malamute, and Drentse Patrijshond) in association with pronounced clinical manifestations.[33-35]

Poikilocytosis

Poikilocytosis is the presence of striking shape variation in a significant number (generally 10% or greater) of peripheral blood RBCs. *Poikilocytosis* is a nonspecific term and may refer to acanthocytes, echinocytes, elliptocytes/ovalocytes, codocytes, and, less often, other RBC shape changes (Figs. 26.29 and 26.30). Poikilocytosis has been

linked to altered RBC membrane lipid content and lipid metabolism in humans; this may also be a contributing mechanism for the association of poikilocytosis in animals with hepatic disease, including cats with hepatic lipidosis, cholangiohepatitis, hepatitis/hepatopathy, systemic histoplasmosis, and portocaval shunt, and dogs with chronic hepatic or renal glomerular disease, lymphosarcoma, or hypothyroidism.[16,26-28] However, it is as likely that the poikilocytosis in these cases is also multifactorial, because abnormalities of the microvasculature and blood viscosity, hypertension, and inflammation accompany most of these conditions and can alter the physical stress on circulating erythrocytes. Poikilocytosis has also been reported in both species when treated with doxorubicin.[23,24] Poikilocytes may be the most frequent shape change seen in animals with RBC fragmentation injury as well, but the latter is generally the more diagnostic finding.

Acanthocytes are poikilocytes with one or more irregularly spaced and shaped membrane projections that may be slightly knobbed at the tip (see Fig. 26.30), whereas echinocytes have more numerous and uniformly spaced membrane projections. Acanthocytes or echinocytes can resemble, but are usually distinguishable from, in vitro crenated cells or preparation artifacts by their random distribution within blood smears (whereas the in vitro effects are generally seen in broad regions of the smear). Historically, increased numbers of acanthocytes in dogs were associated with underlying hemangiosarcoma, but a retrospective study found that acanthocytosis was noted in both neoplastic processes, including hemangiosarcoma, osteosarcoma, and lymphoma most commonly, along with nonneoplastic diseases, such as gastrointestinal, musculoskeletal, renal, and immune-mediated diseases.[25] Elliptocytes, or ovalocytes, are oval RBCs with smooth or scalloped borders that (along with acanthocytes) have been particularly reported in cats with hepatic lipidosis and myelofibrosis.

Codocytes, or target cells, are poikilocytes with three-dimensional hatlike shapes that appear on blood smears as RBCs with pale to unstained rings separating peripheral- and central-stained cytoplasmic regions. Codocytes represent RBCs with relative excess of membrane compared with volume of cytoplasm. In dogs, relatively high numbers of codocytes have been associated with the hypercholesterolemia of hypothyroidism. However, immature RBCs, which similarly have an excess of membrane to cytoplasm, can also be commonly seen as large, slightly polychromatophilic codocytes on smears (see Fig. 26.26).

With samples that show pronounced poikilocytosis on smears, increased RDW may be seen on histograms with automated analysis.

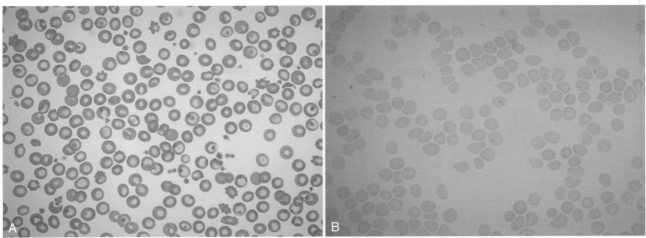

Fig. 26.31 (A) Siderocytes on Wright-stained smear from a dog. (B) Prussian Blue staining confirming iron deposits (original magnification 100×). (Courtesy Dr. Dave Fisher.)

However, this may also reflect the additional occurrence of fragmented or immature RBCs and is not specifically supportive of the morphological findings.

Alterations in RBC Staining

Polychromatophils

Polychromatophils are immature RBCs that are usually larger and more basophilic than mature cells (see Fig. 26.26). Polychromatophils occur in up to 0.5% and 1% of the circulating RBC pool of healthy cats and dogs, respectively. Higher proportions of polychromatophils suggest increased erythropoiesis.

Hypochromasia

Hypochromasia characterizes the RBCs of pronounced iron deficiency (see Fig. 26.28). These cells are recognized by their prominent central pallor and a relatively thin, peripheral ring of stained cytoplasm. Hypochromic RBCs are generally more variable in shape compared with normochromic RBCs, often occurring as poikilocytes, folded cells, and codocytes on blood smears. The hypochromic cells in iron deficiency may also appear microcytic, although this is often more subtle on blood smears than the change in tinctorial properties. Polychromatophilic RBCs are considered hypochromic in reference to their hemoglobin content but do not appear hypochromic on routinely stained blood films. Table 26.2 may further aid in determining the cause of hypochromic erythrocytes in dogs and cats.

Howell-Jolly Bodies

Howell-Jolly bodies are dark-blue to black spherical inclusions that usually occur individually within the RBC cytoplasm. These discrete structures represent nuclear remnants that are not appropriately extruded from the cell during maturation. Howell-Jolly bodies are occasionally seen as an insignificant finding in the RBCs of healthy dogs and cats. Higher numbers of cells may contain the inclusions in animals with regenerative anemia, with decreased splenic function, or in association with abnormal erythropoiesis. It is particularly important not to confuse Howell-Jolly bodies with other cellular inclusions or erythroparasites (see Fig. 26.35, B, later).

Basophilic Stippling

Basophilic stippling appears as a faint dusting of the RBC cytoplasm with fine, gray to dark-blue granules. This finding is an indication of interference with, or incomplete utilization of, polyribosomes for hemoglobin synthesis and is most often a nonspecific finding in dogs and cats with profound regenerative responses to anemia. Basophilic stippling has classically been linked to lead toxicity in dogs, but is generally limited to cases with severe lead exposure and associated with no or only mild anemia.[36]

Siderocytes

Erythrocytes containing coarse aggregates of basophilic material as a result of iron accumulation are known as *siderocytes* (Fig. 26.31, A). Confirmation of iron can be done with special staining, such as Prussian Blue (see Fig. 26.31, B). Siderocytes may be seen with myelodysplastic processes. Sideroblastic anemia is characterized by chronic hypochromic anemia with large iron deposits and can be seen with inflammatory processes such as hepatitis, pancreatitis, or glomerulonephritis as well as myelofibrosis.[37]

Nucleated RBCs

Nucleated RBCs, also known as *rubricytes* or *normoblasts*, are occasionally seen in the blood of healthy dogs and cats. Higher numbers of nucleated RBCs (but generally <5 RBCs/100 WBCs) are expected on blood smears from animals with regenerative anemias or splenic dysfunction/asplenia. Rubricytosis or normoblastemia with the latter condition can occur transiently with splenic trauma and inconsistently with splenic neoplasia, inflammation, and extramedullary hematopoiesis. Hyperadrenocorticism, severe physiological stress, and corticosteroid treatment are also associated with reduced splenic trapping of the nucleated cells and possible mild rubricytosis/normoblastosis. Variable numbers of circulating normoblasts may be seen in animals with hemangiosarcoma of the spleen or other organs and inflammatory liver conditions. Certain dog breeds (e.g., Miniature Schnauzer, Dachshund), when healthy, have also been reported to have increased numbers of nucleated RBCs.[38]

If there are greater than 5 nucleated RBCs/100 WBCs in peripheral blood, bone marrow alterations are particularly suggested. Hypoxia of the bone marrow, as occurs with hypovolemic shock, heat stroke, and marked or peracute anemia can transiently impair marrow sinusoidal integrity and result in mild to moderate rubricytosis or normoblastemia. Marrow hypoxia may be a reason that circulating, nucleated RBCs are commonly associated with—but are not an indication of—a regenerative response to anemia. In cases with 15

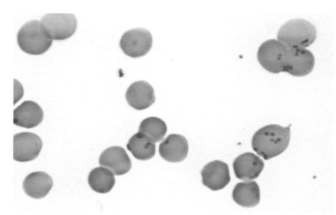

Fig. 26.32 This blood smear from a domestic cat shows a high proportion of the RBCs with single scattered or short chains of basophilic cocci or faint rings on the cell membrane that are characteristic of *Mycoplasma haemofelis* organisms (Diff-Quik stain, original magnification 400×).

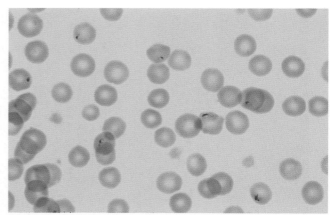

Fig. 26.33 In this smear from a domestic cat, signet ring–shaped *Cytauxzoon felis* organisms are apparent in several RBCs (Diff-Quik stain, original magnification 330×).

or more nucleated RBCs/100 WBCs on blood smears, bone marrow severe injury or disruption of architecture (i.e., fractures) or lead poisoning are more likely. Erythroid leukemias, myeloproliferative disorders predominantly occurring in cats, are characterized by severe peripheral blood rubricytosis/normoblastosis that includes erythroid progenitor cells of multiple stages (e.g., metarubricytes, rubricytes, and rubriblasts) often associated with a severe nonregenerative anemia (see Fig. 26.58 later). Table 26.2 may further aid in determining the cause of increased numbers of circulating nucleated erythrocytes in dogs and cats.

Parasitic Organisms of RBCs

Dogs and cats can be infected with several species and variants of RBC-associated parasitic organisms. A complete list of the known organisms is too large to adequately review here; hence, only those that have been reported on blood films from dogs and cats in North America are described. Notably, the taxonomy of erythrocyte-associated parasitical organisms has been evolving in recent years with advancements in molecular-based classification. For this reason and because new variants and new hosts of the organisms are increasingly being discovered in other global regions, it is prudent to keep in mind that this list may change continually.

Hemotropic Mycoplasma

Infection with *Mycoplasma haemofelis* and *Candidatus Mycoplasma haemominutum* (previously classified as *Hemobartonella felis*, large and small forms, or *H. felis* Ohio and California variants) has been reported for cats in most areas of the United States, although regional differences in prevalence and greater incidence in older, male and/or outdoor cats have been noted.[39-41] Infection with either organism can be asymptomatic or associated with a mild anemia. Infection with *M. haemofelis* can also cause a moderate to severe acute extravascular hemolytic anemia in cats. More recently, a third variant, *Candidatus Mycoplasma turicensis*, has also been detected via polymerase chain reaction (PCR) testing of anemic cats.[42]

In Wright-stained smears of peripheral blood, *M. haemofelis* appears as basophilic cocci, short rods (that may represent chains of cocci), or faint rings on the RBC membrane and are most reliably identifiable if found in chains that extend across the face of an RBC (Fig. 26.32). *Cand. M. haemominutum* organisms appear similar in staining and shape in smears, but cocci are about half the diameter and

generally not found as rings or in chains. *Cand. M. turicensis* was only detected molecularly, so cytological appearance may be small and difficult to detect. With all variants, few to a majority of RBCs can appear infected on smears. However, the number of infected RBCs seen does not necessarily correlate with the occurrence or severity of anemia. Fresh blood (without use of anticoagulants) seems to be the most reliable for detecting the bacteria; organisms are apt to detach from the RBC membrane in shaken or stored samples, especially those containing a calcium-chelating anticoagulant. Organisms also need to be differentiated on blood smears from artifacts of preparation and staining (e.g., membrane blebs in crenated RBCs or granular stain precipitate). In suspected infections, repeat sampling may be useful to detect either organism on blood smears. However, more sensitive molecular diagnostic methods are now commercially available to confirm infection. Molecular methods have also shown that cats can be infected with multiple organisms.

In dogs, two mycoplasma epierythrocytic parasites have also been reported. Distinction between these has been by molecular procedures rather than blood smear evaluation, because infections appear to be mostly occult. However, circulating infected RBCs may rarely be seen in asplenic or immunosuppressed dogs. On Wright-stained smears, these organisms appear as basophilic epierythrocytic cocci, with *Mycoplasma haemocanis* being larger than the more recently described variant. Although infection is most commonly asymptomatic, a variety of symptoms with or without anemia have been reported with acute or resurgence of latent infection in some dogs, and rare cases of severe symptoms or pronounced anemia have been described in association with *M. haemocanis*.[43,44] For suspected active cases of infection by *M. haemocanis* or *Cand. Mycoplasma hematoparvum*, a PCR-based method of detection with whole blood is also available through some university and commercial laboratories.

Cytauxzoon felis

Cytauxzoon felis has been reported in North American cats primarily from the midwestern, southeastern, and mid-Atlantic regions of the United States. Organisms occur within RBCs as signet ring and, occasionally, matchstick, safety pin, and Maltese cross forms (Fig. 26.33). Typically, less than 1% of feline RBCs appear infected unless a cat is in the terminal stages of infection. Schizogonous forms in swollen macrophages are readily detected in aspirates from the lymph nodes, spleen, liver, lungs, and bone marrow of clinically ill cats. Cytauxzoonosis is commonly acutely fatal in cats as a result of vascular obstruction from schizogony within phagocytic cells (particularly endothelial macrophages) throughout the body. The anemia that develops is usually only mild to moderate, partially masked by dehydration, and minimally regenerative at the time of the animal's death. Leukopenia and thrombocytopenia are also common during the terminal stages.[45]

Babesia spp.

Babesia spp. infection is more common in dogs. *B. canis* is the largest of these organisms that infect canine RBCs. Pyriform to amoeboid shapes of *B. canis* can extend across most of the RBC diameter (Fig. 26.34), whereas rod and fusiform shapes, which are usually present concomitantly, are much smaller and more difficult to detect. Intraerythrocytic forms of the other two species identified in dogs, *B. gibsoni* and *B. conradae*, are relatively small compared with *B. canis*, occurring within RBCs as rings, rods, and pyriform, bandlike, or coccoid forms (Fig. 26.35). Multiple organisms per RBC may be seen in acute infections with any of these species; however, only rare parasites are detected with chronic babesiosis. Detection may be facilitated by examining capillary blood smears (e.g., collected from an ear vein) and the RBCs located immediately below the buffy coat of a spun hematocrit tube. Infected cells are also most likely to be located along the periphery and feathered edge of a smear.

Additional supportive findings with acute *B. canis* infections include intravascular hemolysis with hemoglobinuria, bilirubinuria, and bilirubinemia. Extravascular hemolysis with anemia, in addition to thrombocytopenia and neutropenia, can be found in dogs with acute infections of any of these *Babesia* species. Chronic infection can result in an undulating pattern of variably regenerative anemia with clinical and laboratory evidence of chronic immune stimulation. An indirect fluorescent antibody (IFA) test can also support diagnosis, although false-negative results can occur in acutely infected animals, and antibody cross-reactivity is considerable between *Babesia* spp. Molecular methods (PCR) for detection of the different species in whole blood is offered by some university and commercial laboratories. In up to 21% of dogs with large-form babesiosis, a spurious reticulocyte profile may be noted on some automated hematology analyzers using fluorescent dye.[46,47]

ALTERATIONS IN PLATELET NUMBERS AND MORPHOLOGY

A patient's platelet count can be roughly estimated from the monolayer of a blood smear, if there are no platelet clumps along the feathered edge. Under 100× oil-immersion magnification, the platelets in each of 10 microscopic fields are counted, averaged, and multiplied by 15,000 to arrive at the estimated number per μL. Alternatively, 7 to 35 platelets per oil-immersion 100× field can be used as a reference for adequate platelet numbers (i.e., ≥100,000 platelets/μL).[3] Platelet clumps suggest that numbers are at least adequate for hemostasis (i.e., ≥50,000 platelets/μL).[3] When abnormal platelet numbers are detected on dog or cat blood smears, thrombocytopenia is found more often than thrombocytosis. A wide variety of conditions, with inflammatory states and neoplasia being the two most commonly associated with the finding in both species, have been associated with thrombocytopenia in dogs and cats.[48,49] However, marked thrombocytopenia can usually be attributed to one of the four primary causes listed with examples in Box 26.1. Conditions associated with thrombocytosis are also listed in Box 26.1.

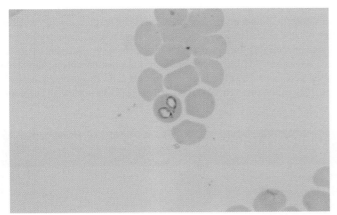

Fig. 26.34 Peripheral blood from a dog with *Babesia canis* infection. Two piroplasms are seen in a single RBC in this field (Wright stain, original magnification 330×).

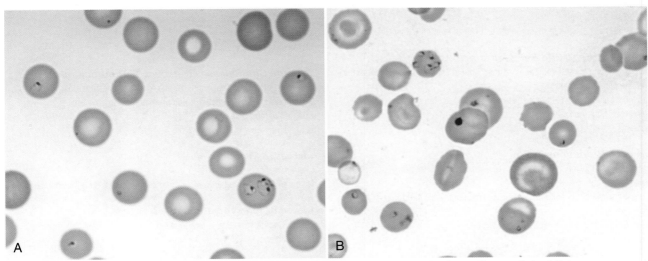

Fig. 26.35 (A) Canine erythrocytes showing the smaller, more amorphous ring forms characteristic of *Babesia gibsonii* infection. (B) More pleomorphic inclusions characteristic of *B. gibsonii*. The large, solid, more basophilic structure near the middle of the image is a Howell-Jolly body (Wright stain). (Courtesy Dr. Rick Cowell in *Hematology Atlas of the Dog and Cat*.)

The diameter of most platelets in healthy dogs range from 2 to 4 μm, or about a fourth to half the size of the erythrocytes. Platelets in cats are more variable in size, larger on average than those in dogs, and about a fourth to almost the same size of the erythrocytes. Enlarged platelets in both species are considered to be those with approximately the same diameter as RBCs. Platelets this size are uncommon in normal canine blood and constitute a minor percentage in normal feline blood. Macroplatelets (i.e., "stress platelets," "shift platelets," or megathrombocytes; Fig. 26.36) are larger than RBCs and unusual in blood smears from healthy dogs and cats. Giant or increased numbers of enlarged platelets on routinely prepared blood films suggest active thrombopoiesis or, less often, abnormal thrombopoiesis associated with myelodysplastic or myeloproliferative conditions or myelofibrosis. Irregularly shaped and/or atypically granulated platelets may also be seen in the peripheral blood of animals with bone marrow disorders, especially those animals with myeloproliferative conditions and cats with FeLV infections.

Increased incidence of small platelets has been reported as a finding on blood smears from dogs with immune-mediated thrombocytopenia or with various chronic conditions; however, because small platelets overlap into the normal range, this is a more difficult determination on the basis of blood smears alone without supportive mean platelet volume (MPV) data from automated analysis of blood. Overall, increased platelet variation in size and granulation, cytoplasmic polychromasia or vacuolation, and filamentous extensions suggestive of activation can be observed more often on smears from dogs and cats with clinical illness than those from healthy animals,[50] although these findings generally have little to no specific diagnostic value. A rare reason for abnormal platelet morphology is the appearance of a single, large granule (sometimes vacuolated) in a canine platelet, which represents the morula of *Anaplasma (Ehrlichia) platys*; infected dogs usually present with mild to moderate thrombocytopenia or cyclic thrombocytopenia (Fig. 26.37).

Familial and other genetic defects that affect platelets are usually not associated with abnormal platelet morphology that can be detected by routine blood smear evaluation. One exception, an asymptomatic familial disorder in Cavalier King Charles Spaniels, is characterized by slight thrombocytopenia and enlarged platelets that have normal ultrastructure.[51] These animals overall have a normal platelet mass and are not at risk of hemorrhage.

Platelet vacuolation may rarely be appreciated. This has been reported in a case of severe nonregenerative anemia associated with autophagy on transmission electron microscopy but also noted to occur in dogs with acute megakaryoblastic leukemia and in a dog with probable essential thrombocythemia.[52]

ALTERATIONS OF WBCs IN DISEASE

Alterations of WBC Numbers

The WBC count can be roughly classified as high, normal, or low by scanning the blood smear monolayer and the feathered edge with the 10× or 20× objective. The percentages of each WBC type can be estimated by scanning the smear or determined by a 100-differential nucleated cell count. Mature neutrophils are the most common WBC type in the peripheral blood of healthy adult cats and dogs, averaging 60% and 70% of the differential cell count, respectively, although cats have

---

BOX 26.1 Causes and Conditions Associated With Clinically Significant Alteration in Peripheral Blood Platelet Count

Thrombocytopenia

Increased Destruction
Immune-mediated thrombocytopenia
Drug induced (usually an immune-mediated process [e.g., certain antibiotics or heparin therapy])

Accelerated Utilization
Disseminated intravascular coagulation
Major vessel thrombosis
Acute severe hemorrhage (e.g., some cases of Brodifacoum toxicity)

Increased Storage Site Sequestration
Splenic disease (e.g., splenomegaly, splenic torsion, severe splenic congestion, and splenic neoplasia)
Anaphylaxis, endotoxemia (sequestration in microvasculature)
Certain drugs (e.g., barbiturates)
Addison disease

Decreased Production
Pancytopenic syndrome (e.g., chronic *Ehrlichia* spp. infection, Fanconi syndrome, estrogen toxicity)
Marrow infiltration (leukemia, myelofibrosis, myelophthisic conditions)
Cyclic hematopoiesis
Chemotherapeutic cytotoxic and cytostatic drugs
Severe nutritional deficiencies

Mixed or Idiosyncratic Causes
Certain infections, especially those involving the bone marrow (e.g., feline leukemia virus [FeLV] or histoplasmosis), acute pathological viral infections, *Babesia* spp., and rickettsial infections

Nonleukemic neoplasia
Bacterial septicemia or endotoxemia
Pronounced inflammation or necrosis (especially of highly vascular organs)
Uremia

Thrombocytosis

Reactive
Acute hemorrhage/hemolysis
Increased granulopoiesis (especially when associated with chronic inflammation)
Increased erythropoiesis

Storage Site Release (Transient Thrombocytosis)
Splenic contraction (fear, pain, trauma, physical exertion, postoperative)
Certain drugs (e.g., corticosteroids or epinephrine)
Canine Cushing disease
Postsplenectomy

Increased Production
Certain drugs (e.g., vincristine)
Myeloproliferative syndromes (e.g., myelogenous and erythroid leukemias)

Mixed or Idiosyncratic Causes
Various neoplasms (e.g., squamous cell carcinoma, mast cell sarcoma)
Iron deficiency

a slightly wider reference interval than dogs. Lymphocytes, the second most common nucleated cell type, average 20% of the differential count in adult dogs and slightly greater than 30% in cats. Monocytes constitute about 5%, and eosinophils are usually less than 5% of canine and feline peripheral blood WBCs. Interpretation of changes should be based on absolute numbers compared with appropriate reference intervals rather than on percentages of cell types. There are six major patterns of alterations in the WBC differential count commonly seen in animals; these are listed with the general mechanism of their induction in Box 26.2. Conditions associated with changes in the number of each specific WBC type have been published in several veterinary texts.[1-3]

Alterations of WBC Morphology

Neutrophilic Toxic Changes

Neutrophilic toxic changes are probably the most common morphological WBC alterations detected on blood films. These cellular changes are an outcome of aberrant granulopoiesis and indicate a systemic

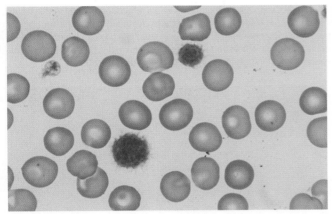

Fig. 26.36 A giant and a slightly enlarged platelet in a dog with hemorrhagic pancreatitis and a markedly inflammatory leukogram. Enlarged platelets are consistent with increased thrombopoiesis, which may be a reactive response associated with acute hemorrhage and increased granulocytopoiesis in this dog (Wright stain, original magnification 330×).

inflammatory effect on the bone marrow. The most severe changes are primarily seen in animals with sepsis, endotoxemia, or tissue necrosis. Toxic changes represent qualitative abnormalities of neutrophils, with the severity, or degree of alteration, considered at least as significant as the actual proportion of cells involved.

Döhle bodies are the mildest form of toxic neutrophilic change. These irregular gray patches in neutrophil cytoplasm (Fig. 26.38) represent aberrant aggregations of the endoplasmic reticulum. Döhle bodies always indicate a systemic effect of inflammation in dogs but are occasionally seen without significant inflammation in cats.

Cytoplasmic basophilia is a more severe form of toxic change that appears as pale, homogeneous, blue to patchy blue-purple cytoplasm in affected cells. As with Döhle bodies, cytoplasmic basophilia may occur in band neutrophils and mature neutrophils.

Foamy cytoplasmic vacuolization is an indication of severe systemic toxicity and considered a result of abnormal lysosome formation and intracellular release of the autolyzing enzymes. This toxic change appears as many vaguely defined vacuoles throughout the cytoplasm, giving it a soap bubbles–like appearance (Fig. 26.39).

Toxic granulation is an uncommon finding that occurs with severely aberrant granulopoiesis. The small, scattered, red-pink cytoplasmic granules (Fig. 26.40) represent the retained primary granule mucopolysaccharide, which is normally lost during neutrophil maturation.

Giant neutrophils represent skipped mitotic divisions of rapidly developing neutrophil precursor cells. Giant neutrophils are similar in appearance to, but about twice the size of, band or mature neutrophils and are generally found more often in cats with toxic neutropoiesis than in dogs (Fig. 26.41).

Historically, ring-shaped nuclei in neutrophils were thought to be a sign of extreme systemic toxicity and associated with sepsis (Fig. 26.42), although this has become more controversial recently. When evaluating blood smears for toxic changes, it is important not to mistake neutrophil nuclei with overlapping ends as toxic ring-shaped nuclei.

Immature Granulocytes

An increase in the number of immature granulocytes in the peripheral blood of dogs and cats usually indicates an inflammatory process. During inflammation, as in health, granulocytes exit bone marrow in an orderly manner, depending on their stage of maturation. For each

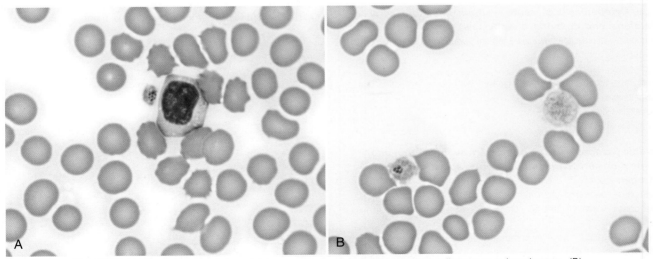

Fig. 26.37 (A) A canine platelet containing a morula of *Anaplasma platys* adjacent to a lymphocyte. (B) Left side platelet with an *A. platys* morula in the same field as an unaffected macroplatelet (Wright stain). (Courtesy Dr. Rick Cowell in *Hematology Atlas of the Dog and Cat.*)

granulocyte line, cells of the most mature stages available to an animal are found in the highest proportion in peripheral blood. Cells of sequentially less mature stages are expected to occur in blood in numbers directly proportional to their level of development. A particularly guarded prognosis is indicated when the total number of immature neutrophils, including band cells, on an inflammatory leukogram is greater than that of mature segmented neutrophils. A similar prognosis

is indicated when 10% or greater of the circulating neutrophils are immature in an animal with neutropenia. Both these conditions are called *degenerative left shifts*. In addition, accurately staging immature granulocytes may be difficult because of asynchronous cellular

---

BOX 26.2 Common Patterns of Alterations in the Leukocyte Differential Count

Leukocytosis

Physiological (Epinephrine-Mediated) Responses (e.g., with fear, excitement, pain, and trauma)
Neutrophils—mildly increased
Lymphocytes—increased
Monocytes—normal to mildly increased
Eosinophils—normal to increased
Basophils—usually absent

Stress-Related (Corticosteroid-Mediated) Responses
Neutrophils—increased
Lymphocytes—decreased
Monocytes—increased (in dogs) or variable (in cats)
Eosinophils—decreased
Basophils—absent

Acute Inflammatory Conditions
Neutrophils—increased, usually with a shift toward immature stages
Lymphocytes—normal to decreased
Monocytes—normal to increased
Eosinophils—normal to decreased
Basophils—usually absent

Chronic Inflammatory Conditions
Neutrophils—increased, with or without a shift toward immature stages
Lymphocytes—usually increased, especially with chronic infectious diseases
Monocytes—usually increased
Eosinophils—variable; may be increased
Basophils—variable; may be increased

Leukopenia

Acute Cytopenias (e.g., acute systemic infections, viral infections, endotoxemia, anaphylaxis)
Neutrophils—decreased (may have a left shift with acute inflammatory disease)
Lymphocytes—often decreased
Monocytes—variable (e.g., often increased with acute immune-mediated cytopenias)
Eosinophils—decreased
Basophils—absent

Chronic Cytopenias (e.g., bone marrow infiltration and/or infections involving bone marrow, aplastic anemia, or estrogen toxicity)
Neutrophils—decreased (often without a left shift)
Lymphocytes—usually normal to increased (increased with chronic immune stimulation)
Monocytes—usually normal to increased (may be partly compensatory to neutropenia)
Eosinophils—variable
Basophils—variable

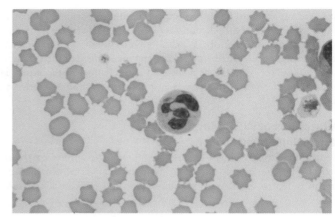

Fig. 26.38 Cytoplasmic basophilia and a large Döhle body in this neutrophil from a cat with pyothorax indicate systemic toxicity affecting marrow granulocytopoiesis. The RBCs in the background are crenated as a result of excess ethylenediaminetetraacetic acid (EDTA) in the collected blood sample (Wright stain, original magnification 250×).

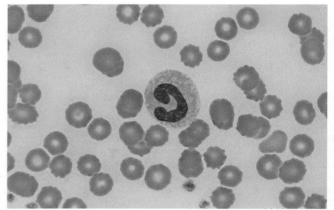

Fig. 26.39 Canine neutrophil showing changes associated with inflammation and marked systemic toxicity. The cytoplasm appears slightly basophilic and foamy (Wright stain, original magnification 250×).

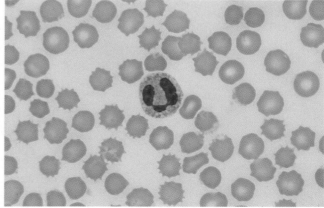

Fig. 26.40 Toxic granulation, as noted by the scattered, small, round, eosinophilic to metachromatic cytoplasmic granules, in a canine neutrophil. The cell also shows cytoplasmic basophilia and foaminess (Wright stain, original magnification 250×).

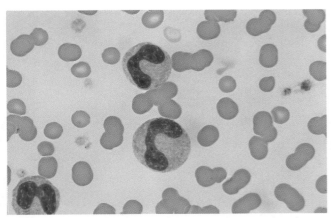

Fig. 26.41 Giant neutrophil adjacent to a normally proportioned neutrophil in a feline blood smear. The basophilic cytoplasm and Döhle bodies in both neutrophils indicate systemic toxicity (Wright stain, original magnification 250×).

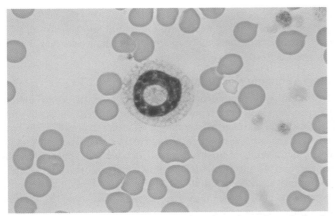

Fig. 26.42 Feline neutrophil with a ring-shaped nucleus indicating severe systemic toxicity. The cell also has highly vacuolated or foamy cytoplasm (Wright stain, original magnification 250×).

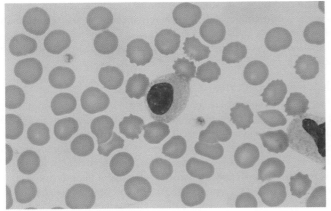

Fig. 26.43 Asynchronous development of nuclear shape (compared with cytoplasmic maturation and chromatin condensation) is seen in this canine neutrophilic myelocyte (Wright stain, original magnification 250×).

development in particularly pronounced inflammatory responses. This is often recognized as a delay in nuclear shape change relative to the degree of chromatin condensation and cytoplasmic development (Fig. 26.43).

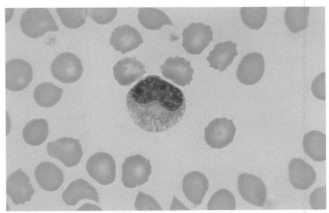

Fig. 26.44 Metamyelocyte in the blood of a dog with inflammation, as seen on a leukogram, and left shift. The cell's cytoplasm is more deeply basophilic than expected as a result of systemic toxicity (Wright stain, original magnification 330×).

Band cells of granulocytes contain cytoplasmic granules specific to cell type and nuclei generally similar to those of mature neutrophils, but they lack distinct segmentation and have less condensed chromatin.

Metamyelocytes have nuclei shaped like kidney beans or broad hourglasses, with fewer, smaller, and more widely spaced clumps of heterochromatin compared with band and segmented granulocyte nuclei (Fig. 26.44). The cytoplasm of neutrophilic metamyelocytes ranges from pale-pink to variably basophilic, depending on the degree of immaturity and toxic change. Cytoplasmic granules specific to cell type are present and are usually prominent in eosinophil and basophil metamyelocytes.

Myelocytes have round to oval, slightly eccentric nuclei that are sometimes slightly flattened on one side; they have coarse, ropy chromatin separating a few small chromatin clumps. Myelocytes are larger with a considerably higher nucleus-to-cytoplasm (N:C) ratio compared with more mature WBCs. The cytoplasm is slightly basophilic and contains granules specific to the cell type.

Pelger-Huët Anomaly

Pelger-Huët anomaly is an idiosyncratic finding reported in several dog breeds, canine mongrels, and Domestic Short-Hair cats. It is generally considered a familial disorder in which all or most granulocyte (neutrophils, eosinophils, and basophils) and monocyte nuclei fail to undergo segmentation. The defect is presumed to originate at the stem cell level because bone marrow megakaryocytes are also affected.[53] Nuclei of the affected circulating cells may be round or kidney bean shaped, whereas chromatin condensation and cytoplasmic development resemble that of normal mature cells (Fig. 26.45). The granulocytes of animals with Pelger-Huët anomaly can usually be distinguished from the immature cells of an inflammatory response on the basis of their uniform appearance and absence of toxic changes. Animals with Pelger-Huët anomaly lack overt functional immune system alterations; however, at least one study of an affected family of Foxhounds has shown impaired neutrophil and lymphocyte functions.[54] A prolonged acquired Pelger-Huët–like anomaly has also been reported in a dog as a presumed idiosyncratic reaction to chemotherapeutic treatment.[55]

Hypersegmented Neutrophils

Hypersegmented neutrophils in peripheral blood represent neutrophils that have remained in circulation for an extended period instead

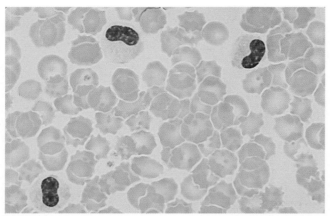

Fig. 26.45 Pelger-Huët anomaly. The nuclei of granulocyte cells retain immature shapes despite a condensed, mature, chromatin pattern (Wright stain, original magnification 250×).

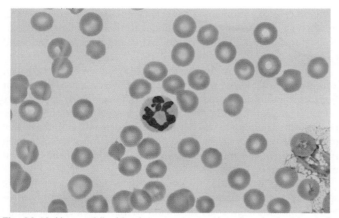

Fig. 26.46 Neutrophil with a hypersegmented nucleus in the blood of a dog 1 day after ovariohysterectomy for pyometra (Wright stain, original magnification 250×).

of migrating into the tissues. These cells, which are recognized as neutrophils with five or more distinct separations between nuclear lobes (Fig. 26.46), can be seen in peripheral blood of patients with increases in the circulating levels of exogenous or endogenous corticosteroids. Hypersegmented neutrophils are also occasionally seen in the peripheral blood of animals with marked neutrophilia associated with chronic inflammatory states and for a brief period after treatment or elimination of the source of inflammation. Hypersegmented neutrophils may be distinguished from partially pyknotic cells that have aged in vitro by evaluating other WBCs in the smear for evidence of in vitro aging changes.

Chediak-Higashi Syndrome

Chediak-Higashi syndrome is a rare genetic disorder that affects intracellular protein transport in a wide variety of tissue types and is associated with abnormally large cytoplasmic granules in peripheral blood leukocytes. The condition has been described in Persian cats with blue smoke–colored hair coats, and other species, but not in dogs. In peripheral blood smears, the abnormal granules may be seen in neutrophils, eosinophils, monocytes, and an occasional lymphocyte. With Romanowsky-type stains, the granules in affected leukocytes are usually eosinophilic and often irregular in shape. In neutrophils, the granules are considered to represent fused primary (i.e., azurophilic) granules, which have properties of lysosomes. Cats with Chediak-Higashi

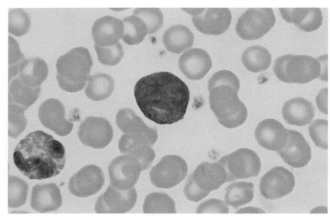

Fig. 26.47 Large, reactive lymphocyte in a cat with histoplasmosis. The cell's nuclear chromatin is less densely clumped compared with that of small mature lymphocytes. The cytoplasm is abundant, deeply basophilic, and shows a prominent, pale perinuclear Golgi region (Wright stain, original magnification 330×).

syndrome often have low neutrophil counts and functionally impaired leukocyte bacteriocidal activity and mild bleeding tendency as a result of platelet defects.[56-58]

Altered Staining of Neutrophil Granules

Neutrophils with prominent magenta granules scattered throughout the cytoplasm have been reported in peripheral blood smears of some Birman cats as an inherited condition. Granules in affected cells have similar shape and size as that of the normally barely discernible granules in neutrophils of unaffected cats. Affected cats appear clinically healthy, and no ultrastructural or functional abnormalities of their neutrophils have been found.[59] The finding is thought to reflect a benign genetic difference in neutrophil lysosomal contents, affecting the affinity for acidic dyes.

Other familial canine or feline conditions in cats or dogs can be associated with altered neutrophil granules. In mucopolysaccharidosis type VI and type VII, and GM2-gangliosidosis, reddish-purple granules may be present within the cytoplasm of circulating neutrophils and monocytes.[60,61] Eosinophil granules may be unstained or more brightly eosinophilic and abnormally shaped in affected animals. However, gross dysmorphic features and, sometimes, neurological deficits are generally far more prominent in dogs and cats with these conditions.

Reactive Lymphocytes

Reactive lymphocytes are generally regarded as immune-stimulated T or B cells with upregulated synthesis of inflammatory mediators and/or immunoglobulins (B cells). The cells may have variable morphology, ranging from intermediate size, with more abundant, pale staining cytoplasm, to large size, with abundant deeply basophilic cytoplasm and less-condensed nuclear chromatin than the more common small, mature lymphocytes. The gray to deeply basophilic cytoplasm represents an abundance of polyribosomes associated with the increased protein synthesis and often shows a contrasting pale, perinuclear Golgi region (see Fig. 26.37; Fig. 26.47). Reactive lymphocytes in peripheral blood suggest active immune stimulation but are etiologically nonspecific.

Mast Cells

Mast cells have been observed in peripheral blood of dogs and cats with systemic mastocytosis (Fig. 26.48) and in very low numbers on blood smears from dogs with pronounced inflammatory conditions,

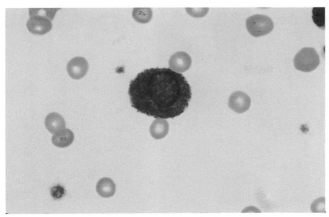

Fig. 26.48 Well-granulated mast cell in the blood of a cat with splenic mast-cell neoplasm (Wright stain, original magnification 250×).

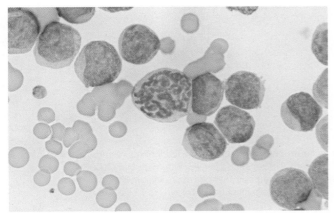

Fig. 26.49 Large, mitotic figure among other leukemic cells in the blood of a cat with large cell lymphoid leukemia (Wright stain, original magnification 250×).

regenerative anemia, trauma, or non–mast cell neoplasia.[62,63] Although rare, other neoplastic processes, such as lymphoproliferative disease and disseminated hemangiosarcoma, have been noted with circulating mast cells in cats.[64]

Mitotic Figures

Mitotic figures are rarely seen on blood films. When present, they are most often found at the feathered edges of smears and are part of a leukemic cell population (Fig. 26.49). Mitotic figures are rarely seen in the peripheral blood of nonleukemic animals, but in these cases, the most common association has been with reactive lymphocytosis or rubricytosis.

WBC Inclusions

WBC inclusions on blood smears usually represent phagocytosed material, including other cells, cell debris, and infectious organisms. Phagocytosed RBCs, hematoidin, or hemosiderin (with the last two appearing as golden or blue-black cytoplasmic material) are seen only rarely in the circulating monocytes or neutrophils of animals, generally in association with marked inflammatory responses or hemolytic anemias.

Inclusions of canine distemper virus can occur in either WBCs (i.e., lymphocytes, neutrophils, monocytes) or RBCs. The inclusions

are pathognomonic for the infection and usually appear as one or two variably sized, discrete, eosinophilic, round to oval bodies in the cytoplasm of lymphocytes and monocytes and as smaller, eosinophilic to basophilic bodies in neutrophils. In addition to, or in lieu of, their appearance in WBCs, viral inclusions may also be observed in RBCs. When seen in RBCs, the inclusions are found in a relatively high percentage of the cells and appear as pale blue, pink, or red-brown, round to irregular structures (Fig. 26.50). The occurrence of inclusions in the peripheral blood cells of infected dogs is highly variable, even within the same individual at different stages of the disease. They are reported to be found most often in the early stages of the infection but can rarely be found during the neurological phase of the disease.

Intracellular morulae of *Ehrlichia canis*, *Ehrlichia ewingii*, or *Anaplasma phagocytophilum* may be seen in canine WBCs, especially those with clinical signs of illness (e.g., fever, thrombocytopenia, leukopenia, anemia, lymphadenopathy, splenomegaly, weight loss, and/or lameness; dogs with chronic *E. canis* infections can also show severe pancytopenia). Morulae of all three species (in the bacterial order Rickettsiales) are similar in appearance as round to oval, eosinophilic to basophilic bodies in the cytoplasm of affected cells. With good microscopic resolution, morulae can be seen to be composed of varying numbers of minute cocci (Fig. 26.51). Morulae of *E. ewingii* and *A. phagocytophilum* can be readily seen in the peripheral blood neutrophils of affected dogs. In contrast, *E. canis* morulae occur in canine lymphocytes and monocytes and are detected only rarely in peripheral blood, and then only during the very early stages of infection. Diagnosis and patient monitoring of *E. canis* infection in dogs can be supplemented by testing serum with a commercial in-house or diagnostic laboratory IFA assay. However, these tests do not completely differentiate among rickettsial organisms, and false-negative results because of low IFA titers can occur. Molecular analysis (PCR) is the most reliable way to distinguish between infections with the different *Ehrlichia* or *Anaplasma* species. However, because of the low numbers of circulating organisms in cases of monocytic ehrlichiosis, false-negative results from analysis of whole blood samples from dogs with *E. canis* infection may still occur with this method.

Hepatozoon americanum gamonts are rarely found in peripheral blood leukocytes of dogs infected with the organism. The majority of infections have been in the Gulf Coast region, but the range appears to be expanding to include southeastern and south-central areas of the United States.[65,66] Despite the pronounced leukocytosis accompanying the disease (e.g., 20,000–200,000 WBCs/μL), the organism is usually found in very few circulating nucleated cells (probable monocytes). Examination of buffy coat preparations may aid detection of the intracellular parasite. *H. americanum* gamonts in Wright-stained blood films appear as aqua-staining ovoid bodies with a single eosinophilic to basophilic patch; these are large enough to displace cell nuclei and distort cytoplasmic borders (Fig. 26.52). Sometimes the ovoid structure remains unstained but is discretely outlined by the displaced host cell cytoplasm and nucleus. In addition to the high WBC count (attributed to a mostly mature neutrophilic leukocytosis), clinical infection is primarily associated with fever, muscular hyperesthesia and atrophy, and long bone and/or vertebral periosteal proliferation. Definitive diagnosis can usually be made with skeletal muscle biopsy. Serology for detection of antibodies to *H. americanum* sporozoites or PCR with whole blood are also commercially available.

Very rarely, yeast, fungal, or bacterial organisms are seen within leukocytes on blood smears from dogs or cats.[67,68] If these are seen in fresh samples, however, they are diagnostic of the systemic

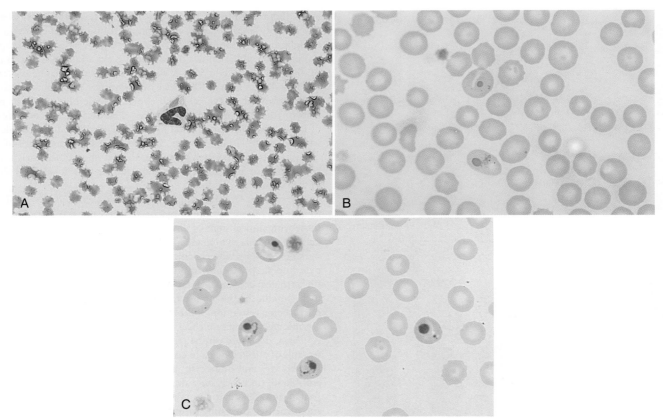

Fig. 26.50 (A) Canine distemper virus (CDV) inclusion in this neutrophil stains red-orange (Wright stain, original magnification 200×). (B) CDV inclusions in two red blood cells (RBCs) stain pale sky blue with Diff-Quik (Original magnification 330×). (C) CDV inclusions in three RBCs stained with Wright stain. Wright-stained inclusions are bright pink-purple to reddish-brown inclusions (original magnification 330×).

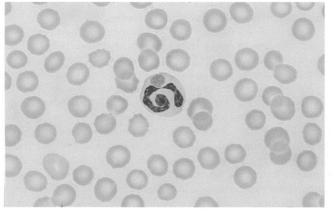

Fig. 26.51 Canine neutrophil containing an *Ehrlichia ewingii* morula (Wright stain, original magnification 250×).

infections. Special stains may aid in further characterizing the organism. Endothelial lining elements and circulating nonhemic neoplastic cells may also rarely be noted.[69,70]

Table 26.3 is presented as a quick reference to aid in the interpretation of morphological alterations in leukocytes in peripheral blood smears and conditions to consider in association with these findings.

LEUKEMIAS

Atypical or bizarre cells or a disordered collection of immature cells on peripheral blood smears suggest leukemia. A persistent, unexplained increase of a specific cell type in peripheral blood can also suggest leukemia, as exemplified by chronic lymphocytic leukemia (CLL). The majority of dogs and cats with leukemia have a moderate to marked leukocytosis (i.e., >50,000 WBCs/μL in dogs and >35,000 WBCs/μL in cats), consisting predominantly of the neoplastic cell population. Exceptions are common, however, and some patients even present with leukopenia. Peripheral blood RBC and platelet counts may be altered (i.e., most often decreased) in leukemic dogs and cats, especially with acute, rapidly progressive forms. Concomitantly, macrocytic RBCs and megathrombocytes, abnormally shaped or granulated platelets, and/or increases in nucleated RBCs may be evident on blood films, supporting bone marrow involvement. Monocytosis is also common and, in some cases, eosinophilia or basophilia are seen in addition to the neoplastic nucleated cells in peripheral blood. Numbers of neutrophils and lymphocytes in blood from dogs and cats with leukemias are highly variable, although a shift toward immature cell stages and/or toxic changes is uncommon unless secondary systemic inflammation or tissue necrosis is present. Hypersegmented neutrophils may also be seen in some cases.

Because of immaturity and anaplasia, recognition of the cell line from which the leukemic cells originated is often difficult to impossible by evaluating only routinely stained peripheral blood films. Examination of marrow aspirates may be important for confirmation and prognostication of leukemia; however, because leukemic cells

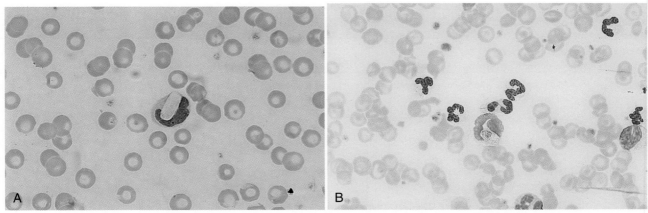

Fig. 26.52 (A) Nonstaining *Hepatozoon canis* capsule distorts this neutrophil's cytoplasmic and nuclear shape (Diff-Quik, original magnification 250×). (B) Stained with Wright-Giemsa stain, the nuclear material of the organism can be seen in the large WBC in the center of the field. Giemsa stains the organism better compared with Wright or Diff-Quik (original magnification 132×).

TABLE 26.3 **Changes in Peripheral Blood Smear Leukocyte Morphology as Indicators of the Cause of Disease**

Prominent Change	Specific Morphological Findings	Other Criteria/Considerations	Causes to Consider
Neutrophil toxic changes	Döhle bodies, cytoplasmic basophilia, cytoplasmic vacuolization, giant neutrophils, ring-shaped nuclei (listed in order of significance [see text])	Döhle bodies can be seen without significant inflammation in cats	Tissue necrosis or inflammation, septic inflammatory/infectious lesions, endotoxemia
Regenerative left shift	Increase in proportion of immature neutrophils, with orderly progression of developmental stages	Normal to increased neutrophil count, or <10% of cells are bands or more immature stages if neutropenia	Tissue necrosis, septic inflammatory/infectious lesions, endotoxemia
Degenerative left shift	Pronounced increase in proportion of immature neutrophils, with orderly progression of developmental stages; may also see asynchronous maturation (e.g., nuclear shape more immature relative to chromatin and cytoplasmic features)	Immature neutrophil stages comprise >50% of total neutrophil count with normal to increased neutrophil count, or >10% of count if neutropenia	Severe sepsis, endotoxemia
Leukocyte dysplasia	Increase in proportion of immature or bizarre leukocytes on blood smears, with discontinuous or disordered leukocyte maturation stages	Changes may involve one or multiple cell lines	Myelodysplastic or myeloproliferative disorder; Pelger-Huët anomaly; recovery from chemotherapy or severe leukocytopenia
Cytoplasmic inclusions	Morphology consistent with specific infectious organism or viral inclusion *(see text)*	Usually with inflammatory leukogram, cytopenia, and/or thrombocytopenia (depending on the organism and disease stage); consider species, cell type(s) affected, age, regional factors	*Ehrlichia* spp., *Hepatozoon* spp., canine distemper virus (CDV), *Histoplasma* spp., *Mycobacteria* spp.
	Cytoplasmic granules appear abnormally stained and/or shaped, and are often surrounded by a vacuole	If familial or genetic abnormality, multiple cell types may be similarly affected and cell counts may be unaffected or decreased	Chediak-Higashi anomaly, neutrophil granulation anomaly in Birman cats, mucopolysaccharidosis types VI and VII, or GM2-gangliosidosis
	Cytoplasmic granules appear abnormally stained and/or shaped	Transient condition	Postchemotherapy, recovery from severe leukocytopenia
	Phagocytosed cells, cell debris, red blood cells (RBCs), hematoidin, or hemosiderin	Affected cells may be neutrophils, monocytes/macrophages or neoplastic cells	May accompany marked inflammatory responses, hemolytic anemias, significant hemorrhage into tissues, blood transfusion, or neoplastic, especially myeloproliferative conditions

TABLE 26.3   Changes in Peripheral Blood Smear Leukocyte Morphology as Indicators of the Cause of Disease—cont'd

Prominent Change	Specific Morphological Findings	Other Criteria/Considerations	Causes to Consider
Neutrophil hypersegmentation	Multilobed nuclei with typically hypercondensed chromatin and mature cytoplasm staining	Rule out in vitro aging artifact	Recovery from severe chronic inflammation, corticosteroid excess (hyperadrenocorticism and iatrogenic), myelodysplastic or myeloproliferative disorder, chemotherapy, or megaloblastic anemia (e.g., Poodles)[31]
Smudged cells, or "basket cells"	Numerous ruptured cells, often found at feathered edge and periphery of smear	Repeatable and not attributable to smear technique or in vitro aging artifact	Circulating blast cells—especially leukemic lymphoblasts or myeloblasts
Basophilia and/or eosinophilia	Increased counts of eosinophils and/or basophils with normal morphology		Helminthiasis (especially with *Dirofilaria immitis*), eosinophil-associated pulmonary disease, chronic inflammation with immune stimulation (e.g., infections of epithelial surfaces), hypoadrenocorticism, snake bite toxicosis, neoplastic (especially myeloproliferative) and paraneoplastic conditions

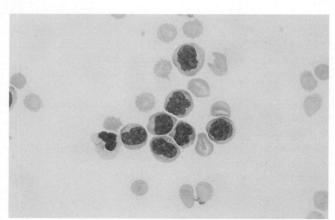

Fig. 26.53 Canine leukemic lymphocytes displaying a variety of convoluted nuclear shapes that can resemble the nuclei of monocytes or immature granulocytes. The chromatin of these cells is partially clumped into blocks of heterochromatin (Wright stain, original magnification 250×).

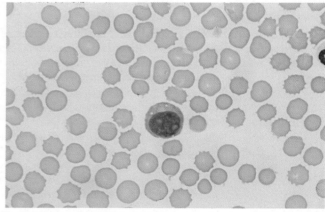

Fig. 26.54 Large lymphoblast with two prominent nucleolar rings in the peripheral blood of a cat with lymphoid leukemia (Wright stain, original magnification 250×).

within the bone marrow are typically more immature than those in peripheral blood, the procedure may not aid in specifically identifying the neoplastic cell type unless special cytochemical staining or immunophenotyping is employed. A few of the more common leukemias in dogs and cats may be suggested by a combination of leukemic cell morphology, patient history, and associated hematological abnormalities, as discussed in the following sections.

Lymphoid Leukemias

Lymphoid leukemias of two major clinical forms are recognized in dogs and cats: acute lymphoblastic leukemia (ALL) and CLL. ALL most often affects young adult to middle-aged animals, and CLL is more common in dogs over 7 years of age and cats of a wide range of ages. Circulating blast cells of ALL usually occur in high numbers and have oval or bizarre clover leaf–shaped nuclei with coarse, reticulated chromatin and moderate amounts of basophilic cytoplasm (Fig. 26.53). These cells may

also have one or more variably sized, dark, nucleolar rings (Fig. 26.54). Neoplastic cells of CLL typically occur in high numbers in peripheral blood, although more sensitive diagnostic methods, such as flow cytometry, allow for earlier detection with lower cell counts. These appear as typical mature lymphocytes, although they tend to vary more in size and have especially dark-staining cytoplasm and a few cytoplasmic vacuoles. As with other leukemic cell types, these cells may be cytophagic and erythrophagic (Fig. 26.55). About half of all canine CLL cases further exhibit monoclonal gammopathy.[71] In addition, about 10% of canine solid lymphomas, especially the multicentric forms and those in the advanced stages, have detectable neoplastic lymphoid cells in circulation, and this is termed the *leukemic phase of lymphoma*, although these cells generally occur in much lower numbers compared with the leukemic cells of dogs with ALL and CLL. Feline lymphoma is less commonly associated with circulating neoplastic cells, although a high proportion of cats with large granular cell type lymphoma were noted to have a secondary leukemia (Fig. 26.56).[72]

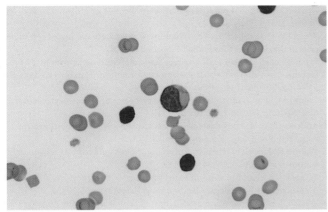

Fig. 26.55 Neoplastic lymphoid cell containing a single phagocytosed red blood cell (RBC) in this blood smear from a cat (Wright stain, original magnification 132×).

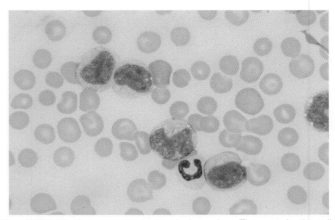

Fig. 26.57 Myelomonocytic leukemia in a dog. The neoplastic cells have irregular nuclei with minimally clumped chromatin and abundant, grainy, basophilic cytoplasm (Wright stain, original magnification 250×).

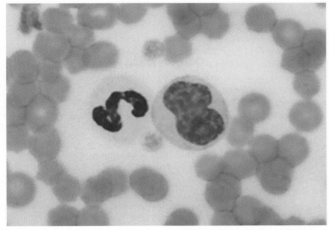

Fig. 26.56 Atypical circulating lymphocyte in the peripheral blood of a cat with high-grade, large, granular cell–type lymphoma. Note the moderately sized, faint nucleolus. Rare cells were noted with faint azurophilic cytoplasmic granules (Wright stain, original magnification 100×)

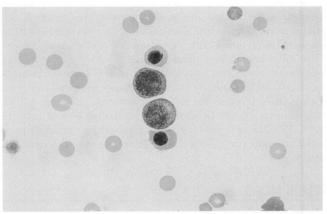

Fig. 26.58 Erythremic myelosis in a cat, characterized by rubricytes of varying maturity in peripheral blood. Note the macrocytosis of at least one of the metarubricytes on either end of this row of nucleated cells. The other two cells are basophilic rubricytes with centrally located nuclei, coarsely clumped chromatin, and deeply basophilic cytoplasm (Wright stain, original magnification 250×).

Myeloid Leukemias

In both dogs and cats, myeloid leukemia of every major lineage has been reported, including malignant (systemic) mastocytosis and eosinophilic, basophilic, and megakaryocytic leukemias. Acute myeloid and myelomonocytic leukemias (Fig. 26.57) are especially common in dogs.

Acute myelogenous (granulocytic) leukemia in dogs occurs predominantly in young animals, including dogs under age 2 years. Leukocytosis tends to be extreme and composed of a disordered mixture of immature cells that resemble myeloblasts, giant band neutrophils, and neutrophilic metamyelocytes with a separate, smaller population of seemingly normal mature to hypersegmented granulocytes. Immature myeloid cells have finely stippled, lacy or ropy chromatin and, occasionally, prominent nucleolar rings. Their cytoplasm is relatively abundant and blue-gray with a ground-glass consistency and is occasionally scattered with fine eosinophilic granules.

Acute myelomonocytic leukemia is considered if some of the more differentiated circulating neoplastic cells have a monocytoid appearance, whereas others resemble immature granulocytic cells (based on nuclear shape, chromatin pattern, and cytoplasmic features). Immunophenotyping methods have been developed to differentiate

between these two forms of myeloid leukemia,[73] although the progression of the condition in dogs is generally similar.

Chronic myelogenous leukemia (CML) is much less common in dogs and cats, and without age predilection. Cases have presented with fluctuating moderate to marked leukocytosis of predominantly mature leukocytes, with a lower proportion of immature and dysplastic cells. However, normal total leukocyte counts can also occur. Animals with this condition may survive up to 2 years; the disease is usually accompanied by persistent anemia and sometimes altered platelet counts. CMLs are differentiated from a leukemoid response, in part, by the lack of orderly progression of developmental stages among the leukocytes in peripheral blood and absence of a corresponding pyogenic condition. CML can also be associated with a subsequent showering of immature forms in peripheral blood or a blast crisis.

Erythroid Leukemias

Erythroid leukemias are more common in cats and extremely rare in dogs. Affected cats usually have severe, nonregenerative anemia and high numbers of circulating nucleated RBCs in various stages of development (Fig. 26.58). Over a few weeks to months, the leukemic

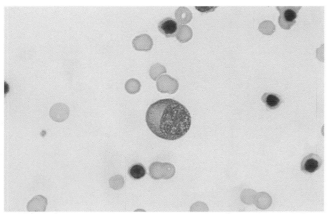

Fig. 26.59 Large plasmacytoid-like erythroblast in the blood of a cat with erythremic myelosis (Wright stain, original magnification 250×).

population usually shifts toward higher proportions of more immature stages of RBCs and sometimes to an erythroleukemic population involving both erythroid and granulocytic cell lines. There is often atypical morphology—particularly macrocytosis of the nucleated and nonnucleated erythroid cells. Very immature erythroid cells can usually be differentiated from immature cells of other blood cell lines by their centric nuclei that contain dark, coarsely clumped chromatin, and their scant to moderate amount of deeply basophilic cytoplasm. In some cases, however, the neoplastic erythroid cells have eccentric nuclei and prominent Golgi regions, resembling plasma cells (Fig. 26.59). This disease is most commonly associated with underlying retroviral infection, particularly FeLV.[73] Rare cases may be seen in FeLV negative cats.[74]

REFERENCES

1. Feldman BF, et al. *Schalm's Veterinary Hematology.* 5th ed. Philadelphia: Lea & Febiger; 2000.
2. Latimer KS, Rakich PM. Clinical interpretation of leukocyte responses. *Vet Clin North Am Small Anim Prac.* 1989;19:637–668.
3. Duncan JR, et al. Veterinary laboratory medicine. In: *Clinical Pathology.* 3rd ed. Ames, IA: Iowa State University Press; 1994.
4. Wyrick-Glatzel Gwaltney-Krause. In: *Harmening DM: Clinical Hematology and Fundamentals of Hemostasis.* 2nd ed. Philadelphia: FA Davis; 1992:523–617.
5. Shafer, et al. In: Hoffman R, ed. *Hematology Basic Principles and Practice.* 2nd ed. New York: Churchill Livingstone; 1991:1790–1801.
6. Sullivan, et al. Platelet concentration and hemoglobin function in Greyhounds. *J Am Vet Med Assoc.* 1994;205:838–841.
7. Lording. *Post-graduate Committee in Veterinary Science: Proceedings No. 122.* University of Sydney; 1989:369–392.
8. Zaldivar-Lopez S, et al. Clinical pathology of Greyhounds and other sighthounds. *Vet Clin Pathol.* 2011;40:414–425.
9. Campora, et al. Reference intervals for Greyhounds and Lurchers using the Sysmex XT-2000iV hematology analyzer. *Vet Clin Pathol.* 2011;40:467–474.
10. Iazbik MC, Couto CG. Morphologic characterization of specific granules in Greyhound eosinophils. *Vet Clin Pathol.* 2005;34:140–143.
11. Yamauchi A, et al. Secondary erythrocytosis associated with schwannoma in a dog. *J Vet Med Sci.* 2004;66:1605–1608.
12. Sato K, et al. Secondary erythrocytosis associated with high plasma erythropoietin concentrations in a dog with cecal leiomyosarcoma. *J Am Vet Med Assoc.* 2002;220:486–490.
13. Couto CG, et al. Tumor-associated erythrocytosis in a dog with nasal fibrosarcoma. *J Vet Intern Med.* 1989;3:183–185.
14. Cowgill LD, et al. Use of recombinant human erythropoietin for management of anemia in dogs and cats with renal failure. *J Am Vet Med Assoc.* 1998;212:521–528.
15. Rebar AH, et al. Red cell fragmentation in the dog: an editorial review. *Vet Pathol.* 1981;18:415–426.
16. Weiss DJ, et al. Quantitative evaluation of irregularly spiculated red-blood cells in the dog. *Vet Clin Pathol.* 1993;22:117–121.
17. Lee KW, et al. Hematologic changes associated with the appearance of eccentrocytes after intragastric administration of garlic extract to dogs. *Am J Vet Res.* 2000;61:1446–1450.
18. Caldin M, et al. A retrospective study of 60 cases of eccentrocytosis in the dog. *Vet Clin Pathol.* 2005;34:224–231.
19. Andress JL, et al. The effects of consecutive day propofol anesthesia on feline red blood cells. *Vet Surg.* 1995;24:277–282.
20. Walton RM, et al. Mechanisms of echinocytosis induced by *Crotalus atrox* venom. *Vet Pathol.* 1997;34:442–449.
21. Wysoke JM, et al. Bee sting-induced haemolysis, spherocytosis and neural dysfunction in three dogs. *J South Afr Vet Assoc.* 1990;61:29–32.
22. Weiss DJ, et al. Quantitative evaluation of echinocytes in the dog. *Vet Clin Pathol.* 1990;19:114–118.
23. Badylak SF, et al. Poikilocytosis in dogs with chronic doxorubicin toxicosis. *Am J Vet Res.* 1985;46:505–508.
24. O'Keefe DA, Schaeffer DJ. Hematologic toxicosis associated with doxorubicin administration in cats. *J Vet Intern Med.* 1992;6:276–282.
25. Warry E, et al. Disease distribution in canine patients with acanthocytosis: 123 cases. *Vet Clin Path.* 2013;42:465–470.
26. Cooper RA, et al. Red cell cholesterol enrichment and spur cell anemia in dogs fed a cholesterol-enriched atherogenic diet. *J Lipid Res.* 1980;21:1082–1089.
27. Christopher MM, Lee SE. Red cell morphologic alterations in cats with hepatic disease. *Vet Clin Pathol.* 1994;23:7–12.
28. Ogilivie GK, et al. Alterations in lipoprotein profiles in dogs with lymphoma. *J Vet Intern Med.* 1994;8. 62-22.
29. Simpson KW, et al. Iron status and erythrocyte volume in dogs with congenital portosystemic vascular anomalies. *J Vet Intern Med.* 1997;11:14–19.
30. Gookin JL. Evaluation of microcytosis in 18 Shibas. *J Am Vet Med Assoc.* 1998;212:1258–1259.
31. Canfield PJ, Watson AD. Investigations of bone marrow dyscrasia in a Poodle with macrocytosis. *J Comp Pathol.* 1989;101:269–278.
32. Bonfanti U, et al. Stomatocytosis in 7 related standard Schnauzers. *Vet Clin Pathol.* 2004;33:234–239.
33. Brown DE, et al. Erythrocyte indices and volume distribution in a dog with stomatocytosis. *Vet Pathol.* 1994;31:247–250.
34. Pinkerton PH, et al. Hereditary stomatocytosis with hemolytic anemia in the dog. *Blood.* 1974;44:557–567.
35. Slappendel RJ, et al. Familial stomatocytosis–hypertrophic gastritis (FSHG), a newly recognized disease in the dog (Drentse Patrijshond). *Vet Q.* 1991;13:30–40.
36. Berny PJ, et al. Low blood lead concentration associated with various biomarkers in household pets. *Am J Vet Res.* 1994;55:55–62.
37. Weiss DJ. Sideroblastic anemia in 7 digs (1996-2002). *J Vet Intern Med.* 2005;19:325–328.
38. Meyers, et al. *Veterinary Laboratory Medicine.* Philadelphia: Saunders; 1992:21.
39. Willi B, et al. Prevalence, risk factor analysis, and follow-up of infections caused by three feline Hemoplasma species in cats in Switzerland. *J Clin Microbiol.* 2006;44:961–969.
40. Lappin MR, et al. Prevalence of *Bartonella* species, *Haemoplasma* species, *Ehrlichia* species, *Anaplasma phagocytophilum*, and *Neorickettsia risticii* DNA in the blood of cats and their fleas in the United States. *J Feline Med Surg.* 2006;8:85–90.
41. Jensen WA, et al. Use of a polymerase chain reaction assay to detect and differentiate two strains of Haemobartonella felis in naturally infected cats. *Am J Vet Res.* 2001;62:604–608.
42. Sykes JE, et al. Prevalences of various hemoplasma species among cats in the United States with possible hemoplasmosis. *J Am Vet Med Assoc.* 2008;232:372–379.
43. Benjamin MM, Lumb WV. *Haemobartonella canis* infection in a dog. *J Am Vet Med Assoc.* 1959;135:388–390.
44. Kemming G, et al. Can we continue research in splenectomized dogs? Mycoplasma haemocanis: old problem—new insight. *Eur Surg Res.* 2004;36:198–205.
45. Hoover JP, et al. Cytauxzoonosis in domestic cats: 8 cases (1985-1992). *J Am Vet Med Assoc.* 1994;205:455–460.

46. Piane L, et al. Spurious reticulocyte profiles in a dog with babesiosis. *Vet Clin Path*. 2016;45:594–597.

47. Piane L, et al. Spurious reticulocyte profiles in dogs with large form babesiosis: a retrospective study. *Vet Clin Path*. 45:598-603.

48. Grindem CB, et al. Epidemiologic survey of thrombocytopenia in dogs: a report on 987 cases. *Vet Clin Pathol*. 1992;20:43.

49. Jordan HJ, et al. Thrombocytopenia in cats: a retrospective study of 41 cases. *J Vet Intern Med*. 1993;7:261–265.

50. Halmay D, et al. Morphological evaluation of canine platelets on Giemsa- and PAS-stained blood smears. *Acta Veterinaria Hungarica*. 2005;53:337–350.

51. Cowan SM, et al. Giant platelet disorder in the Cavalier King Charles Spaniel. *Exp Hematol*. 2004;32:344–350.

52. Pieczarka EM, et al. Platelet vacuoles in a dog with severe nonregenerative anemia: evidence of platelet autophagy. *Vet Clin Path*. 2014;43:326–329.

53. Latimer KS, et al. Nuclear segmentation, ultrastructure, and cytochemistry of blood cells from dogs with Pelger-Huët anomaly. *J Comp Pathol*. 1987;97:61–72.

54. Bowles CA, et al. Studies of the Pelger-Huët anomaly in foxhounds. *Am J Pathol*. 1979;96:237–247.

55. Shull RM, Powell D. Acquired hyposegmentation of granulocytes (pseudo-Pelger-Huët anomaly) in a dog. *Cornell Vet*. 1979;69:241–247.

56. Colgan SP, et al. Platelet aggregation and ATP secretion in whole blood of normal cats and cats homozygous and heterozygous for Chediak-Higashi syndrome. *Blood Cells*. 1989;15:585–595.

57. Colgan SP, et al. Defective in vitro motility of polymorphonuclear leukocytes of homozygote and heterozygote Chediak-Higashi cats. *Vet Immunol Immunopathol*. 1992;31:205–227.

58. Prieur DJ, Collier LL. Neutropenia in cats with the Chediak-Higashi syndrome. *Can J Vet Res*. 1987;51:407–408.

59. Hirsch VM, Cunningham TA. Hereditary anomaly of neutrophil granulation in Birman cats. *Am J Vet Res*. 1984;45:2170–2174.

60. Alroy J, et al. Morphology of leukocytes from cats affected with alpha-mannosidosis and mucopolysaccharidosis VI (MPS VI). *Vet Pathol*. 1989;26:294–302.

61. Gitzelmann R, et al. Feline mucopolysaccharidosis VII due to beta-glucuronidase deficiency. *Vet Pathol*. 1994;31:435–443.

62. Stockham SL, et al. Idiopathic mastocythemia in dogs. *Vet Clin Pathol*. 1986;15:16–21.

63. McManus PM. Frequency and severity of mastocythemia in dogs with and without mast cell tumors: 120 cases (1995-1997). *J Am Vet Med Assoc*. 1999;215:355–357.

64. Piviani M, et al. Significance of mastocythemia in cats. *Vet Clin Path*. 2013;42:4–10.

65. Ewing SA, et al. American canine hepatozoonosis: an emerging disease in the New World. *Ann NY Acad Sci*. 2000;916:81–92.

66. Cummings CA, et al. Characterization of stages of Hepatozoon americanum and of parasitized canine host cells. *Vet Pathol*. 2005;42:788–796.

67. Etienne CL, et al. A mycobacterial coinfection in a dog suspected on blood smear. *Vet Clin Path*. 2013;42:516–521.

68. Leissinger M, et al. What is your diagnosis? Blood smear from a cat. *Vet Clin Path*. 2014;43:465–466.

69. Oikonomidis IL, et al. What is your diagnosis? Unusual cells in the blood smear from a dog. *Vet Clin Path*. 2015;44:605–606.

70. Piane, et al. What is your diagnosis? Abnormal cells on a blood smear from a dog. *Vet Clin Path*. 2014;43:461–462.

71. Weiss DJ. Evaluation of proliferative disorders in canine bone marrow by use of flow cytometric scatter plots and monoclonal antibodies. *Vet Pathol*. 2001;38:512–518.

72. Roccabianca P, et al. Feline large granular lymphocyte (LGL) lymphoma with secondary leukemia: primary intestinal origin with predominance of a CD3/CD8αα phenotype. *Vet Pathol*. 2006;43:15–28.

73. McManus PM. Classification of myeloid neoplasms: a comparative review. *Vet Clin Pathol*. 2005;34:189–212.

74. Weeden AL, et al. Suspected myelodysplastic/myeloproliferative neoplasm in a feline leukemia virus-negative cat. *Vet Clin Path*. 2016;45:584–593.

27

Bone Marrow

Jamie L. Haddad, Sarah C. Roode, and Carol B. Grindem

Bone marrow is the main hematopoietic organ in the body, and bone marrow examination is a valuable tool in the identification and characterization of many hematopoietic and hematological disorders. Bone marrow is located throughout the flat and long bones of the body and is composed of hematopoietic cell populations and associated microenvironmental elements that support hematopoiesis. Basic understanding of the normal hematopoietic tissue components and familiarity with hematopoietic disorders are necessary for accurate and thorough bone marrow evaluation and interpretation. Because of the complex nature of bone marrow assessment, referral to a pathologist for review is often necessary. Knowledge of normal and potentially abnormal findings in bone marrow is crucial to comprehension of the pathology report and for correlation of the results with the accompanying clinical and clinicopathological data.[1-3]

This chapter will outline the approach to the cytological and histological evaluations of normal and abnormal bone marrow samples. The discussion will highlight key elements in this assessment, including utility of aspiration cytology versus core biopsy of bone marrow; sample collection and submission guidelines; sample quality effects; marrow cellularity evaluation; lineage assessment of erythroid, myeloid, and megakaryocytic components; and other cellular and stromal elements in bone marrow. Common infectious disorders and hematopoietic and nonhematopoietic neoplasia in bone marrow will also be discussed.

INDICATIONS AND CONTRAINDICATIONS

Bone marrow evaluation is commonly performed in patients with abnormalities in peripheral blood and has several specific indications (Box 27.1). Bone marrow assessment is most helpful in patients with unexplained or persistent cytopenias, such as neutropenia, thrombocytopenia, and/or nonregenerative or poorly regenerative anemia, or in those with immature, atypical, or dysplastic cells in circulation. Bone marrow evaluation is also indicated with unexpected or inappropriate cellular responses in peripheral blood, such as increased nucleated red blood cells (nRBCs) without reticulocytosis; unexplained persistent leukocytosis, erythrocytosis, or thrombocytosis; or other hematological abnormalities that cannot be explained by patient history, physical examination findings, and peripheral blood smear evaluation. Additional indications include staging of neoplasia that commonly involves bone marrow; investigation of lytic bone lesions; workup for serum chemistry abnormalities, including hyperglobulinemia or hypercalcemia; monitoring of treatments, such as chemotherapy; investigation for systemic infectious diseases; or assessment of iron stores.[4-9]

Bone marrow collection is typically a safe procedure with minimal complications and is generally no more of a risk than the restraint,

sedation, and/or anesthesia required for the collection procedure. Hemorrhage is rare, and infection is unlikely when using proper sampling techniques and precautions.[4] The main contraindication for bone marrow sampling is therefore evaluation being unnecessary for further characterization of a disease process. Examples of this type of unnecessary sampling include (1) an explainable hematological abnormality, such as an appropriate neutrophilia in response to inflammation; (2) unconfirmed cytopenia, such as spurious thrombocytopenia caused by traumatic venipuncture; (3) situations where bone marrow assessment would not reliably differentiate between disease states, such as between chronic myeloid leukemia and an inflammatory leukemoid reaction; or (4) cases where cytopenia is acute and could be in a pre-regenerative phase, such as acute anemia without reticulocytosis when there has not been sufficient time for an appropriate bone marrow response to develop.

BOX 27.1 Indications for Bone Marrow Evaluation

Abnormal CBC Findings
- Unexplained or persistent cytopenias (neutropenia, nonregenerative or poorly regenerative anemia, and/or thrombocytopenia)
- Immature, atypical or dysplastic cells in circulation
- Unexpected or inappropriate cellular responses in peripheral blood (i.e. increased nRBCs without reticulocytosis)
- Unexplained persistent leukocytosis, thrombocytosis, or erythrocytosis
- Other unexplained hematological abnormalities

Historical, Physical Examination, or Diagnostic Imaging Abnormalities
- Staging of neoplasia (lymphoma, mast cell tumor, histiocytic neoplasia)
- Monitoring of treatment (chemotherapy, treatment with other drugs)
- Lytic bone lesions (multiple myeloma, metastatic neoplasia, infectious disease)
- Investigation for systemic infectious disease (histoplasmosis, leishmaniasis, mycobacteriosis)
- Fever of unknown origin

Serum Chemistry Abnormalities
- Hyperproteinemia/hyperglobulinemia (lymphoid or plasma cell neoplasia, tickborne/rickettsial disease, systemic inflammatory conditions)
- Hypercalcemia (multiple myeloma, lymphoma, fungal disease, other bone neoplasia)

Assessment of Iron Status
- Suspected iron deficiency
- Differentiation of causes of anemia (chronic inflammation versus chronic blood loss)

TABLE 27.1   Aspiration Cytology versus Core Biopsy

Aspiration Cytology		Core Biopsy	
Advantages	Best for cell morphology (including evidence of dysplasia)	Advantages	Tissue architecture preserved (including cell distribution and microanatomical location)
	More precise differential count, M:E ratio, maturation assessment		Best estimate of cellularity (including megakaryocyte numbers)
	Quick and easy sample collection/preparation		Focal lesions (metastatic foci, early/occult neoplasia, granulomas)
	Best for small etiological agents		Stromal changes (bony abnormalities, myelofibrosis)
Disadvantages	Less accurate cellularity assessment	Disadvantages	Less distinct cell morphology
	May not be representative if uneven cell distribution		Differential count and calculated M:E ratio more difficult
	Less able to capture necrosis, myelofibrosis, bony remodeling		Requires laboratory for sample processing and histopathological evaluation

M:E, myeloid to erythroid ratio.

ASPIRATION CYTOLOGY VERSUS CORE BIOPSY

Bone marrow evaluation is most thorough and accurate when both cytological and histological assessments are performed together, because each modality has unique qualities to contribute to this analysis (Table 27.1). Bone marrow aspiration cytology is more commonly pursued compared with core biopsy and histopathology; however, it is recommended that both types of analysis be performed concurrently in all cases, whenever possible. Cytology of bone marrow is generally preferred for individual cell identification and morphological characterization, including assessment for maturation and evidence of dysplasia, as well as for investigation for small etiological agents, including hemoparasites. Aspiration cytology samples are quick and simple to obtain with minimal equipment needed. The quality of the sample can be assessed at the time of collection to allow for additional sampling, if necessary, either via repeated aspiration or the addition of core biopsy. Disadvantages of aspiration cytology include the risk of inaccurate representation of marrow cellularity; inadequate reflection of stromal changes within bone marrow, as with myelofibrosis or bone remodeling; and the risk of missing focal or predominantly paratrabecular lesions, as with foci of metastatic neoplasia. Core biopsy with histopathology is the preferred modality for the most accurate assessment of bone marrow cellularity, particularly in cases with suspected hypocellular marrow. Core biopsy with histopathology is also preferred for evaluation of megakaryocyte density; myelofibrosis and other stromal/vascular or bony changes, including edema, hemorrhage, necrosis, fibrin, and inflammation; occult neoplasia; and focal lesions, such as metastatic neoplasia or granulomatous inflammation. If core biopsy is not initially performed but sampling for cytology results in repeated low yield "dry taps," core biopsy with histopathology is strongly recommended to assess whether there may be hypocellular marrow, densely packed hypercellular marrow, or myelofibrosis as an explanation for the poor cytological yield.

A unique feature of core biopsy with histopathological evaluation of bone marrow is the preservation of tissue architecture, which allows for assessment of the microanatomical location of the cells present (Figs. 27.1 and 27.2).[1-3] This contrasts with cytological assessment, which more commonly represents the interstitial tissue components within the marrow and does not allow for distinct assessment of the specific localization of the hematopoietic compartments. Anatomically, the marrow environment consists of dense lamellar cortical bone along the bone surfaces with interior trabeculae of cancellous bone and an intertrabecular meshwork of thin-walled capillary–venous sinuses with accompanying extracellular matrix. It is within this intertrabecular

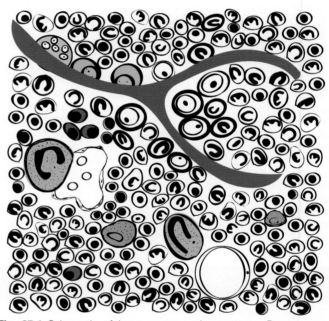

Fig. 27.1 Schematic of bone marrow microanatomy. Bone marrow comprises hematopoietic elements, including erythroid, myeloid, and megakaryocytic lineage cells, as well as a supportive network of bony trabeculae *(red)*, vascular sinuses and stromal tissue. Early myeloid cells are paratrabecular (adjacent to bone), whereas later stage myeloid cells with their more lobulated nuclei are interstitial (central). Erythroid cells are adjacent to sinuses and may be arranged in erythropoietic islands around a central macrophage *(green)*. Megakaryocytes *(pink)* are also adjacent to sinuses to allow for platelet release into the bloodstream. Plasma cells *(dark blue)* and mast cells are often perivascular, and small lymphocytes *(yellow)* are dispersed in the interstitium. With remodeling of the bone, osteoblasts *(pale blue)* and osteoclasts *(orange)* may line the bony trabeculae. (Drawing by Cari Grindem-Corbett.)

meshwork that the hematopoietic elements reside. Immature granulocytes generally are distributed along the paratrabecular zone within the marrow with maturing granulocytes located more centrally within the interstitium. Megakaryocytes and erythropoietic islands (composed of erythroid precursor cells and supportive macrophages) are located adjacent to the sinuses within the interstitial regions. Resident plasma cells and mast cells are generally perivascular in their orientation, and lymphocytes are dispersed within the interstitium or can be in perivascular aggregates.

SAMPLE COLLECTION AND PREPARATION

Bone marrow aspiration and core biopsy sites and techniques have been reviewed in the literature and will only briefly be described here.[4,10-27] Common issues with sample collection, preparation, and quality are listed in Table 27.2.

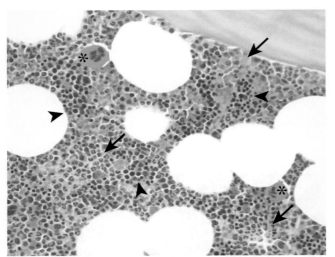

Fig. 27.2 Histological architecture of bone marrow. Microanatomical localization of the hematopoietic elements is evident with histopathology. The marrow spaces are lined by bony trabeculae *(top right corner)*, and the medullary cavity contains adipocytes *(large clear spaces)* and hematopoietic cells. As noted schematically in Fig. 27.1, early myeloid cells are paratrabecular *(arrow adjacent to bone)*, and later stage myeloid cells are interstitial *(central arrows denote groups of granulocytes with lobulated nuclei)*. Megakaryocytes *(denoted by "*")* are adjacent to sinusoids, and erythroid cells are also adjacent to sinusoids *(arrowheads denote groups of erythroid cells with dark bulleted nuclei)* (hematoxylin and eosin [H&E] stain, original magnification 400×).

Sample Site

Proper bone marrow collection and sample preparation are necessary to maximize the diagnostic yield of bone marrow sampling. Once the decision to sample bone marrow has been made and a method has been chosen (aspiration for cytology versus core biopsy for histopathology versus a combination of both), a sample site must be selected (Fig. 27.3). The most commonly used sites for both aspiration cytology and core biopsy with histopathology are the proximal humerus in dogs and cats and the trochanteric fossa of the proximal femur in cats. Additionally, the iliac crest is frequently used in large dogs and occasionally used in cats. For cytological evaluation only, sternebrae or rib sites can also be considered. Caution must be exercised to avoid puncturing the thoracic cavity with use of these sites.[15,16] Considerations regarding sample site selection, including advantages and disadvantages, can be found in Table 27.3. When considering the location for sample collection, it should be noted that in young animals, active hematopoiesis occurs throughout the flat and long bones. As growth ceases with maturity, the central/diaphyseal areas of the long bones transition to fatty tissue, with ongoing hematopoiesis being more concentrated in the metaphyseal areas of the long bones and the flat bones.

Aspiration Versus Core Biopsy

Whether performing aspiration for a cytological sample or core biopsy for histopathological sample, the overall approach is similar, and thus similar equipment is needed (Box 27.2). All equipment should be assembled and readily available for immediate use before starting the collection procedure. Sedation or anesthesia is often needed to ensure patient compliance. If the patient has an extremely calm demeanor or is critically ill, a local anesthetic without sedation may be sufficient for sample collection. For either cytology or biopsy, the sampling site is generally clipped and prepared with aseptic/sterile technique, and local anesthetic (2% lidocaine) is injected into the skin, subcutis, and periosteum. A small stab incision is made into the skin with a #11 scalpel blade. The incision can be made just adjacent to the biopsy site to avoid direct connection between the skin surface and the underlying bone tissue, and this may help prevent infection.

TABLE 27.2   Sample Collection and Quality Issues With Aspiration Cytology and Core Biopsy Samples

Aspiration Cytology		Core Biopsy	
No sample obtained	Needle plugged with skin or bone	No sample obtained	Needle not seated in marrow cavity
	Needle not seated in marrow cavity		Core not cut/retrieved from marrow cavity
	Myelofibrosis or hypercellular marrow ("dry tap")		Aspiration needle used, rather than core biopsy needle
Poor sample yield/quality	Hemodilution	Poor sample yield/quality	Sample too short (not deep enough in marrow cavity or not adequately cut/severed before removing needle)
	Hypocellular marrow		Sample damaged during collection (crushed while obtaining sample from bone, while removing core from needle, or while making touch imprints)
	Bevel of needle lodged against cortical bone		Sample taken from prior aspiration site with disruption of medullary tissue by the cytological collection procedure
	Sampling difficult site with small needle (e.g., sternum or rib)		Sample appears hypocellular due to sampling of only subcortical area (naturally hypocellular)
Good sample obtained but cannot be evaluated well microscopically	Sample too thick/not well spread	Good sample obtained but unable to evaluate well microscopically	Laboratory processing issues (chatter from microtome if not decalcified sufficiently, over-decalcification, cut too thick)
	Cells ruptured during aggressive squash preparation		Lost during processing (small sample not placed in cassette)
	Formalin exposure		
	Understained sample		

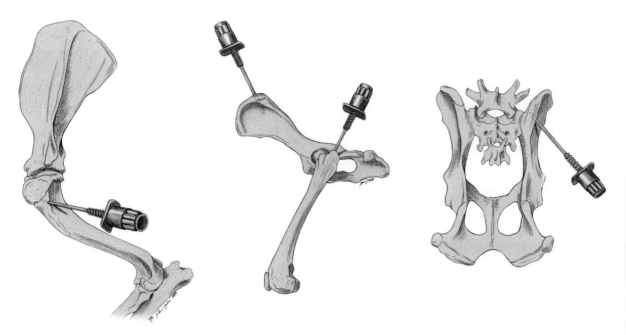

Fig. 27.3 Bone marrow sample collection sites *Left:* Proximal humerus. This is a good bone marrow collection site for dogs and cats. *Middle:* Iliac crest and proximal femur. In large dogs, a dorsal approach to the iliac crest is a good sample site. In small dogs and cats, a transilial approach can be considered *(see right image)*, or the trochanteric fossa of the proximal femur is a good option. *Right:* For small dogs and cats, the lateral approach to the wing of the ilium (transilial) is a good location for sample collection. (Reprinted with permission from Grindem CB. Bone marrow biopsy and evaluation. *Vet Clin Small Anim.* 1989;19[4]:673–674.)

TABLE 27.3 Bone Marrow Sample Site Considerations

Site	Considerations for Use	Patient Positioning	Landmarks for Sampling
Proximal humerus	Best for: • Large dogs • Small dogs • Cats Considerations: • Avoid the articular cartilage • Young growing animals should not be sampled at this location because of proximity of growth plate	Lateral recumbency	• Locate the greater tubercle by palpation. • Flex the shoulder and stabilize the limb. • Insert the biopsy needle into the flat area just distal to the greater tubercle and advance caudomedially along the long axis of the bone.
Iliac crest	Best for: • Large dogs Considerations: • May not be accessible in obese animals • Transilial approach is useful in cats, small dogs, and obese dogs	Sternal recumbency preferred; can consider sitting, standing, or lateral recumbency	• Palpate the greatest prominence of the iliac crest. • Stabilize the ilium by placing a finger on either side of the wing. • Insert the biopsy needle parallel to the ilium, and direct it ventromedially keeping it parallel to the long axis of the wing of the ilium. • Alternate approach: transilial[13]
Trochanteric fossa of the femur	Best for: • Small dogs • Cats Considerations: • May not be accessible in larger, well-muscled, or obese patients • Cortical bone may be too dense in older patients • Avoid the sciatic nerve located medial and caudal to the greater trochanter	Lateral recumbency	• Locate the greater trochanter of the proximal femur by palpation. • Stabilize the femur by grasping the stifle; slight internal rotation of the stifle may enhance exposure of the fossa. • Insert the biopsy needle medial to the trochanter with the long axis of the needle parallel to the long axis of the femur.
Sternebrae	Considerations: • Danger of penetrating thoracic cavity • Aspiration only, not core biopsy • May be more feasible in elderly or debilitated patients • May be performed with only light sedation	Sternal recumbency preferred, can consider sitting or standing or lateral recumbency for 2–4 sternebrae	• Locate the first sternebra, and stabilize with one hand. • Insert a 1-inch 20-gauge needle with attached 3-cc syringe into the cortex of the first sternebra and advance carefully until firmly embedded, then aspirate.[15] • Alternate approach: 2–4 sternebrae[14]

Continued

TABLE 27.3 Bone Marrow Sample Site Considerations—cont'd

Site	Considerations for Use	Patient Positioning	Landmarks for Sampling
Rib	Considerations: • Danger of penetrating thoracic cavity • Aspiration only, not core biopsy • May be more feasible in elderly or debilitated patients • May be performed with only light sedation • May not yield representative sample, especially in older dogs with little active hematopoiesis	Lateral recumbency	• Palpate the 10th rib and costochondral junction. • Stabilize the 10th rib. • Advance a 1-inch 22-gauge needle with attached 3-cc syringe dorsally into the medullary cavity just above the costochondral junction keeping needle parallel to the rib, and gently aspirate.[16]

BOX 27.2 Bone Marrow Sampling Equipment

- Surgical preparation supplies (gloves, scrub kit), local anesthetic (2% lidocaine) and sedative, scalpel blade (#11)
- 15- to 18-gauge, 1- to 2-inch bone marrow needles (Rosenthal, Illinois sternal, or Jamshidi) for aspiration cytology, and 11- to 15-gauge Jamshidi needles for core biopsy
  - Alternative recent option: intraosseous infusion system needles and bone injection guns (EZ-O and OnControl, Vidacare Corp)[13,21-23]
- 10- to 12-mL syringes
- 2.5%–3% ethylenediaminetetraacetic acid (EDTA) solution and EDTA tubes
  - To make EDTA solution, add 0.35 mL sterile isotonic saline to 7-mL EDTA tube to produce a 2.5%–3% EDTA solution (2.5% if EDTA tube contains liquid and 3% if tube contains powder)
- Microscope slides, coverslips, and pencil to label slides at frosted edge
- Clean Petri dish (or watch glass) and microhematocrit tubes (optional)

For aspiration sampling, a 15- to 18-gauge Jamshidi, Rosenthal, or Illinois sternal needle (preflushed with ethylenediaminetetraacetic acid [EDTA], if desired) is inserted into the stab incision with the stylet locked in place. The needle is advanced into the appropriate area of the bone (see Fig. 27.3) with a twisting/rotating motion (alternating clockwise and counterclockwise) until the needle and stylet are firmly seated in the bone. A slight decrease in resistance may be encountered upon entry into the medullary cavity. The stylet is removed and a 10- to 12-mL syringe containing a small amount (0.3 mL) of 2.5% to 3% EDTA is attached to the needle. Strong negative pressure is applied to the syringe, pulling back two-thirds to three-fourths the volume of the syringe in multiple quick successive pulls, until red marrow fluid is seen at the hub of the needle. As soon as bone marrow sample starts to enter the syringe, the negative pressure is released to avoid subsequent hemodilution. Approximately 0.2 to 0.4 mL of bone marrow fluid in the syringe is usually sufficient to prepare several smears. The needle and syringe are then withdrawn from the bone to prepare the sample. Direct pressure to the skin will aid in hemostasis, and the skin can then be sutured, if needed. The next steps in the preparation of the marrow sample are described below in the section "Sample Preparation and Staining." If marrow is not obtained, the procedure can be repeated. The needle can be repositioned at the same site by either advancing or retracting slightly or angling medially or laterally. Alternatively, the needle can be fully redirected through a different site on the same bone, or a new anatomical sampling site can be selected. Causes of aspiration failure may include poor technique, occlusion of the needle with skin or bone tissue, marrow fibrosis, hypoplasia, or a densely packed hypercellular marrow.

Core biopsy with histopathology can be performed instead of aspiration cytology, although, ideally, both sampling techniques should be performed concurrently. The core biopsy sample is preferably taken from an adjacent site slightly different from that of the aspiration sample, for example, by reangling the needle so that the aspiration procedure does not damage the area of the bone to be sampled for biopsy.[10,12,28] Jamshidi bone marrow needles (11- to 15-gauge, most often 13-gauge) are utilized for core biopsy sampling, and the placement of the needle is the same as described for cytological sampling. The needle is similarly embedded in the bone via a rotating/twisting motion of the needle, but for core biopsy sampling, the stylet is removed just after the needle is initially seated into the bone. Then, the needle is advanced at least 3 mm and to up to 1 to 2 cm deeper into bone to fully access the medullary cavity and cut a diagnostic quality sample. The needle is rotated in place completely (360 degrees) multiple times to sever the core biopsy sample from the sample site, and the needle is then removed from the bone. The sample is removed from the needle by inserting the probe into the narrow end of the needle and pushing the marrow retrograde out through the wider end. An impression smear can be made before formalin fixation of the biopsy sample via gentle rolling of the core on a glass slide, taking great care not to crush or damage the sample in the process. The core sample is then placed in 10% neutral-buffered formalin for submission to the laboratory.[24] Samples can be placed in a cassette, with or without sponge inserts, to ensure that the sample is retained and not lost during processing. Formalin-fixed samples and cytological preparations should not be shipped in the same package to avoid artifact from the formalin fumes, which can affect the cytological sample staining quality (Fig. 27.4).

Sample Preparation and Staining

Once the cytological sample is obtained and is within the syringe, the marrow material will clot very quickly (within 30 seconds) if anticoagulant is not utilized. Therefore non-anticoagulated marrow samples need to be placed on glass slides immediately. Even with EDTA, the sample should be prepared right away. This can be either via direct application of the material from the syringe onto the slides or via expulsion of the material into a Petri dish or watch glass containing EDTA solution. Bone marrow spicules can then be identified in the Petri dish and transferred to the slides with a microhematocrit tube or pipette. The spicules within a Petri dish are clear to slightly opaque, light-gray, and irregularly shaped. Once the material is on the slides, the slides are tilted 45 to 70 degrees to allow the blood to drip off the slide while the bone marrow flecks remain adhered. The sample is then spread with a squash technique or, less commonly, a smear technique, as with a blood film (Fig. 27.5). The squash technique is best performed by gently placing a second glass slide onto the sample, orienting it 90 degrees to the original slide, and then smoothly separating the slides.

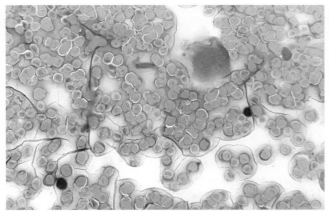

Fig. 27.4 Effects of exposure to formalin fumes on a cytological preparation. A bone cytology sample was shipped in the same container as a sealed biopsy specimen jar containing formalin. The exposure to formalin fumes, even through a sealed jar, alters the staining characteristics of the cytological sample. Formalin fumes impart a blue-green hazy quality to the cytological sample. Note the blue-green color of the red blood cells, which are typically pink to red with Wright-Giemsa stain. Smudging of the cellular features also occurs, obscuring accurate assessment of cell morphology and cellular characterization (Wright-Giemsa stain, original magnification 500×). (Courtesy Dr. Andrea Siegel.)

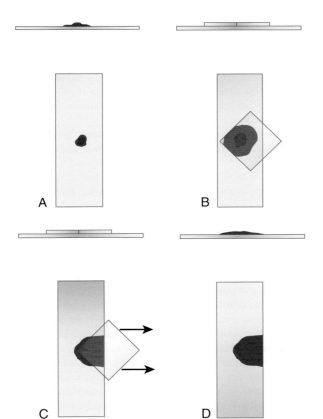

Fig. 27.5 Squash technique for bone marrow cytology samples. (A) A marrow fleck, collected from the Petri dish containing the sample, is placed on a glass microscope slide. (B) A microscope slide or a coverslip *(as pictured)* is placed over the fleck at a 45-degree angle to the slide. This spreads the fleck and accompanying fluid. (C) The coverslip or spreader slide is slid horizontally and smoothly off the glass slide. (D) Both the original glass microscope slide preparation and the coverslip or spreader slide preparation can be used for microscopic evaluation. However, a coverslip preparation is usually hard to handle during staining and is often discarded.

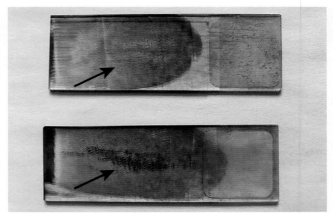

Fig. 27.6 Macroscopic appearance of two cytological preparations. *Top:* The very low number and small size of the marrow flecks *(tiny blue specks denoted by the arrow)* suggests a hypocellular marrow sample. Alternatively, this may be a poor-quality, low-diagnostic-yield sample. The number of unit particles on a slide may be more reflective of the sample adequacy than the actual marrow cellularity. *Bottom:* The dark-blue flecks of marrow represent large unit particles *(indicated by the arrow)*. This suggests a good-quality/high-yield sample, likely from a hypercellular marrow. Note the deep-blue staining quality to the marrow flecks, consistent with a well-stained preparation.

Similarly, a coverslip can be used instead of a second spreader slide for samples with very fragile cells. If flecks are not identified, the sample can be centrifuged in a small tube and additional squash preparations made from the buffy coat layer.

Once the smears are prepared and correctly labeled with pencil on the frosted edge of the slides, they are stained with a typical Romanowsky-type stain (Wright-Giemsa or Diff-Quik). Because bone marrow smears are thick, additional staining time is required, typically at least twice the length of time in each buffer and stain as would be used for a blood smear. Slides should not be blotted dry but, instead, air-dried to allow for full development of the stain color in the cells. If slides are understained, they can be restained to enhance dye penetration into the cells. Properly stained marrow has dark blue-purple spicules macroscopically (Fig. 27.6). If slides are to be submitted to a laboratory, one slide can be stained before submission to check for sample quality and then the rest submitted unstained, along with a current complete blood count (CBC) and blood smear. Any remaining bone marrow fluid can also be submitted in EDTA.

Necropsy/Postmortem Sampling

Samples can still be obtained from deceased patients for both cytological and histological evaluation. For cytology in particular, to ensure sufficient preservation of cellular morphology, samples are ideally obtained within minutes (less than 30 minutes) from the time of death to prevent introduction of autolysis and cellular degradation. This cellular degeneration can lead to misidentification of cell types and prevents accurate assessment of marrow with cytology. For histological assessment, a longer postmortem interval of several hours or even days may still preserve enough architecture to evaluate the sample, although if there is a delay in sample collection for histopathology, refrigeration of the body (not freezing) can help slow autolysis and preserve sample integrity. Postmortem sample sites typically include the metaphyseal region of the long bones, most commonly the femur. The diaphyseal region should be avoided because this is predominantly fatty tissue and may not accurately reflect hematopoietic activity. For cytological evaluation, if the sample is collected immediately after death, aspiration and smear preparation can be performed as previously described. Otherwise, a paintbrush or a gentle

BOX 27.3 Special Stains and Advanced Diagnostics in Bone Marrow Evaluation

Special Stains
Cellular Identification (Core Biopsy)
- Giemsa (highlights erythroid cells deeper blue, highlights mast cell granules)
- PAS (highlights granularity in myeloid cell cytoplasm, as well as cytoplasm of plasma cells and megakaryocytes)

Infectious Agent Investigation (Cytology or Core Biopsy)
- PAS, GMS (fungal organisms)
- Acid fast, Fites-Faraco (*Mycobacterium* spp.)
- Gram (bacteria)

Substances in Marrow (Core Biopsy)
- Iron (Perl's iron, Prussian blue)—can also be performed on cytology slides
- Myelofibrosis (reticulin, Masson's trichrome)
- Serous atrophy of fat (Alcian blue)

Advanced Diagnostics
Cytochemical Evaluation for Subtyping Leukemia (Cytology)
- Peroxidase, Sudan black B, chloroacetate esterase, nonspecific esterases, acid phosphatase

Flow Cytometry (Liquid Bone Marrow Sample)
- CD34; lymphoid, myeloid, histiocytic, and megakaryocytic markers

PARR (PCR for Antigen Receptor Rearrangement; Cytology or Core Biopsy)
- Assesses for clonality within a lymphoid population to aid in confirmation of lymphoid neoplasia

Immunocytochemistry/Immunohistochemistry
- Aids in tumor identification (cytokeratin for carcinoma, lymphoid markers for lymphoma, Mum1 for plasma cell neoplasia, etc.)

GMS, Gomori methenamine silver; *PAS,* periodic acid Schiff; *PCR,* polymerase chain reaction.

BOX 27.4 Systematic Approach to Bone Marrow Evaluation

1. Sample quality (an adequate yield, diagnostic sample)
2. Hematopoietic cellularity (relative to patient age and complete blood count [CBC] findings)
3. Iron stores (in dogs; normally absent in cats)
4. Myeloid-to-erythroid (M:E) ratio and differential count (interpreted relative to CBC findings, patient age, and marrow cellularity)
5. Assessment of each lineage (erythroid, myeloid, and megakaryocytic) for numbers, maturation, and morphology
6. Other cell types (lymphocytes, plasma cells, mast cells, macrophages/histiocytes [including phagocytic activity])
7. Stromal components (myelofibrosis, necrosis, bone changes)
8. Etiological agents (if inflammation or necrosis present)

OVERALL APPROACH TO BONE MARROW EVALUATION

Whether utilizing aspiration cytology, core biopsy with histopathology of bone marrow, or both modalities concurrently, the approach to bone marrow evaluation is similar (Box 27.4). Accurate interpretation and complete methodical assessment of marrow changes require a current CBC and blood smear assessment, ideally collected simultaneously with the bone marrow sample or within 24 hours. Additional information should include patient history (illnesses, drug administration or other therapies, travel history, diet, transfusion history, chronicity of CBC abnormalities); physical examination findings (mass lesions, organomegaly, petechiae, lymphadenopathy); additional bloodwork (chemistry or urinalysis abnormalities, testing for tickborne disease, Coomb test results); and diagnostic imaging results (hepatosplenomegaly, lung lesions, bone lesions).

Bone marrow evaluation encompasses both low- and high-magnification assessments. Features assessed at low magnification include sample quality, marrow cellularity, iron stores, and megakaryocyte numbers. Low-magnification assessment is also used to identify areas of the sample with an abnormal or distinct appearance, such as with metastatic neoplasia or focal cell aggregates, and to identify ideal areas to subsequently examine at high magnification. Components assessed at high magnification include specific cell morphology and lineage identification, maturation evaluation, and examination for etiological agents.

With cytology, the most accurate high-magnification assessment requires thin areas that contain a monolayer of intact cells with adequate staining and relatively little hemodilution. These areas are commonly identified directly adjacent to unit particles or between particles. For the most representative assessment of overall marrow findings versus a regional or focal change, evaluation should include assessment of multiple areas on multiple slides. With core biopsy, the anatomical location of the cells can aid in interpretation as to the appropriateness and nature of the population. Noting immature mitotically active cells in a paratrabecular location is an appropriate reaction for development of early myeloid precursors, but a similar immature mitotically active cell population in the interstitial area would be cause for concern about a neoplastic proliferation. Special stains can also be utilized with core biopsies to aid in classification of hematopoietic cellular elements, such as Giemsa to highlight erythroid cells and periodic acid–Schiff (PAS) to highlight granulocytes, megakaryocytes, and plasma cells. Special stains can also highlight stromal elements (reticulin, trichrome) or infectious agents (PAS, Gomori methenamine silver [GMS], acid fast, Gram stains) (see Box 27.3).

rolling technique (using a needle to roll the sample along the slide) can be used to apply a postmortem sample to a glass slide. For histological evaluation, a wedge of tissue can be collected to fix in formalin for routine processing. Marrow tissue collected postmortem for histological assessment can be placed in a cassette to keep the sample together during fixation and aid in sample processing at the laboratory. Before enclosure in a cassette, a small portion of the soft part of the marrow can be placed directly in formalin to observe whether the tissue sinks, as with a cellular marrow, or floats, as with a fatty marrow.

Sample Submission to the Laboratory

A combination of stained and unstained air-dried bone marrow cytology preparations should be submitted in break-proof containers. Include patient information, current CBC and blood smear, and any additional liquid bone marrow in EDTA. Unstained slides will then either be routinely stained at the laboratory or retained for potential special staining or advanced diagnostic testing, if warranted (Box 27.3). Bone marrow core biopsies should be mailed separately from cytology slides, even if the formalin jar containing the core biopsies is well sealed, because the formalin fumes can still escape and alter the cellular features on the cytological preparations (see Fig. 27.4).

Caution in assessment of bone marrow findings is necessary to avoid overinterpreting the changes. Bone marrow findings need to be interpreted in light of sample quality and cellularity, serial CBC results with attention to chronicity of hematological abnormalities, and patient information. It is important to understand that a single bone marrow sample captures only a "snapshot in time," reflecting a single moment in a constantly changing and evolving hematopoietic picture.

SAMPLE QUALITY

Adequate sample quality is necessary for accurate assessment of bone marrow cytology or core biopsy samples.[1] The most important factor with regard to sample quality is to avoid overinterpretation of a poor quality or inadequate sample. Artifacts within the sample or inadequate yield of cells or tissue can lead to inaccurate interpretation (see Box 27.2).

For cytology, abundant hemodilution can affect accuracy of cellularity assessment and may lead to a disproportionate percentage of erythroid lineage cells or, if there is a peripheral neutrophilia, a disproportionate component of late stage myeloid cells. A "dry tap" sample with very little yield of unit particles can be misinterpreted as a hypocellular sample. Areas too thick for evaluation cytologically can be very difficult to accurately assess for the myeloid-to-erythroid (M:E) ratio and the morphological features of the cells present. Improperly stained samples can lead to inaccurate assessment of cell morphology and, in some cases, can lead to the impression of an increased component of immature blast cells because nucleoli are often more apparent in understained samples. A more aggressive squash preparation technique can lead to excessive cell rupture, obscuring identification of the cells present. Importantly, exposure of a cytological sample to formalin fumes, even through a tightly sealed biopsy specimen jar, can impart a blue-green hazy staining quality to the sample. This can obscure accurate assessment of cell morphology and characterization (see Fig. 27.4). Therefore biopsy samples should not be shipped in the same box or container as cytological specimens.

On core biopsy with histopathology, a large amount of bone dust or crush artifact resulting from difficult sample collection, aggressive handling of the sample, or performing biopsy in a previous aspiration site can lead to an inconclusive result or can falsely mimic the appearance of myelofibrosis (Fig. 27.7). The medullary spaces in the subcortical zone (the first 2–3 trabeculae deep) are naturally hypocellular compared with the deeper medullary tissue, and therefore a shallow core biopsy or a sample taken parallel, rather than more perpendicular, to the cortical bone can lead to a falsely hypocellular appearance to the marrow (Fig. 27.8).

CELLULARITY

Cellularity of a marrow sample can be partially or initially assessed at the time of sample collection and then subsequently confirmed microscopically. At the time of collection for cytology, the sample may be of little yield without much fat (suggesting possible fibrosis), mostly fat without clear flecks of marrow (suggesting a hypocellular, fatty sample), or contain many flecks of marrow tissue (suggesting a normal to hypercellular sample). At the time of collection for core biopsy, red-gray coloration of the tissue suggests normal to hypercellular marrow, whereas white or yellow coloration of the sample suggests hypocellular, fibrotic or fatty marrow, or marked white blood cell (WBC) proliferation, as with lymphoma or leukemia. With a

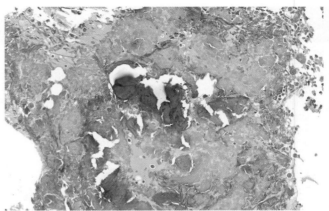

Fig. 27.7 Bone dust and crush artifact in a core biopsy. Core biopsy sample of low diagnostic yield as a result of abundant bone dust and crushed bony and medullary tissue *(blue-purple to pink smudged material)*. A small amount of yellow-brown iron pigment is identifiable, but hematopoietic cells are not intact to evaluate. The streaming pink material should not be mistaken for myelofibrosis because this streaming appearance is caused by crush artifact rather than a true change. Bone dust and crush artifact can result from aggressive handling of the core biopsy during sample collection, during removal of the biopsy sample from the needle, during preparation of touch impressions, or from collection from a prior aspiration site (H&E stain, original magnification 100×).

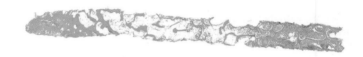

Fig. 27.8 Subgross view of a core biopsy. Excellent-quality core biopsy sample that has a superficial layer of dense cortical bone *(thick pink area at left of image)* with a subcortical region of the medullary cavity that is naturally hypocellular. The cellular marrow component is evident deeper within the sample *(middle to right of image)*. A short-core biopsy sample may only capture this naturally hypocellular area in the subcortical tissue and be misinterpreted as marrow hypoplasia. Adequate depth of penetration into the marrow cavity and complete severing of the core biopsy sample are necessary to obtain a good-quality sample of sufficient length (H&E stain, original magnification 5×).

necropsy sample, bone marrow can be tested for cellularity by placing a portion of the sample in water to see if it sinks (a cellular sample) or floats (a fatty sample).

At the time of slide preparation for cytological assessment, dark-blue aggregates of material or cleared spaces having a chatterlike effect on the slide suggest unit particles are present, whereas smooth pink to blue-gray areas suggest predominantly background blood (see Fig. 27.6). Unit particles are necessary for an estimate of marrow cellularity, so with a poor-quality sample without the presence of unit particles, accurate estimation of marrow cellularity is not possible. Taking an overall averaged estimate from multiple unit particles in multiple areas of the sample is the most accurate approach because cellularity is often not uniform throughout a sample. On microscopic evaluation of a cytological preparation, the unit particles are composed of supportive stromal and vascular

BOX 27.5 Causes of Hypocellular or Hypercellular Marrow

Hypocellular	Hypercellular
Selective or Multilineage Hypoplasia in Marrow	**Increased Hematopoiesis**
• Aplastic anemia (replacement by fatty tissue)	• Erythroid hyperplasia
	• Myeloid/granulocytic hyperplasia
• Drug-associated	
• Immune-mediated	**Nonhematopoietic Cellular**
• Toxin-induced	**Proliferation**
• Chemotherapy/radiation	• Neoplasia
• Infectious	• Inflammation
• Idiopathic	
• Selective erythroid hypoplasia (see Box 27.9)	**Hematopoietic Neoplasia**
• Selective myeloid hypoplasia (see Box 27.10)	

Stromal Changes Replacing/ Altering Marrow Tissue
- Myelofibrosis
- Myelonecrosis
- Serous atrophy of fat

"Hematopoietic hypocellularity" may be used to describe the decrease in hematopoietic cells when there is replacement of bone marrow by something other than fat (fibrosis, necrosis, tumor cells) because the marrow is still cellular, but not composed of hematopoietic cells.

elements with hematopoietic cells and adipocytes. The ratio of hematopoietic cellularity to fatty tissue within these unit particles represents the cytological assessment of cellularity within the marrow itself, whereas the number of unit particles noted on the slide may be reflective of sample adequacy more than of actual marrow cellularity.

Marrow cellularity assessment is more accurate with a core biopsy sample than with a cytology sample because tissue architecture is retained with histopathology. Core biopsy is strongly recommended when there is a cytological suspicion for hypocellular marrow to either confirm hypocellular marrow or to identify a hypercellular marrow from a "dry tap" or from myelofibrosis that may have impacted the cytological yield.

The marrow cellularity must be interpreted in light of the patient's age and the concurrent CBC data. Younger animals normally have more cellular marrow compared with older animals. Very young animals have little to no fat within the marrow, whereas juvenile animals have approximately 25% fat and 75% hematopoietic cells, young adult animals have approximately 50% fat and 50% cells, and older adult animals have approximately 75% fat and 25% cells.[4,10,12,18] General causes of hypocellular and hypercellular marrow are listed in Box 27.5. Comparison of the cytological and histological appearances of hypocellular, normocellular, and hypercellular marrow is depicted in Fig. 27.9.

Hypocellular Marrow

A hypocellular marrow (with <25% hematopoietic cells in the face of peripheral demand and taking the patient age into account; see Fig. 27.9) suggests a defect either in the marrow precursor cells themselves or in the supportive microenvironment that the cells depend on, including cytokines, hormones, and growth factors. The remaining marrow (≥75%) is composed of fatty tissue, fibrosis, necrosis, or

gelatinous transformation (serous atrophy of fat). Marrow hypocellularity can involve all cell lineages or can selectively affect one or more lines. Hypocellularity is best confirmed with core biopsy with histopathology, because there are other potential causes for hypocellular marrow with cytology, such as an inadequate sample, a "dry tap," or myelofibrosis. With hypocellular marrow, often the resident tissue cells are more prominent and account for a higher proportion of the cells present. This may include macrophages that often contain increased iron, plasma cells and lymphocytes, tissue mast cells, and possibly eosinophils. In some cases, actual hyperplasia of mast cells and plasma cells may be seen in hypocellular marrow, such as with ehrlichiosis.[29] *Aplastic anemia* refers to replacement of the marrow by fat with severely decreased hematopoiesis that leads to subsequent cytopenias. This may begin as neutropenia and thrombocytopenia with later development of anemia as a result of the longer lifespan of red blood cells (RBCs) compared with neutrophils and platelets. General causes of panhypoplasia of the bone marrow lineages (aplastic anemia) include drug-associated, immune-mediated, toxin-induced, chemotherapy/radiation–related, infectious, and idiopathic conditions[4,30,31] (see Box 27.5).

Normocellular Marrow

A normocellular marrow (approximately 50% hematopoietic cells; see Fig. 27.9) may be appropriate/normal or inappropriate/abnormal and should be interpreted in the context of the patient's age, the amount of peripheral demand for hematopoiesis, the M:E ratio, and the presence or absence of neoplasia or inflammation/infection on marrow assessment. Some marrows may appear normocellular with low magnification on cytology, but on closer inspection the cellularity within the unit particles is actually composed of increased numbers of plasma cells and macrophages with decreased numbers of hematopoietic precursors.

Hypercellular Marrow

A hypercellular marrow (>75% hematopoietic cells; see Fig. 27.9) typically indicates that one or more cell lines are increased in response to a peripheral demand for cells. This is commonly secondary to hyperplasia in one specific cell lineage (myeloid hyperplasia in response to inflammation, or erythroid hyperplasia in response to blood loss or hemolysis) but can involve multiple cell lines with a strong or combined stimulus. Hypercellularity may also be caused by the presence of other abnormal cell components, such as with effacement of the marrow by neoplasia, or with inflammation including macrophages/histiocytes, plasma cells, and/or lymphocytes. Even a markedly hypercellular marrow can have a low cytological yield in some cases, a form of "dry tap," which is why core biopsy with histopathology is often helpful to confirm cellularity, particularly in cases of cytological hypocellularity.

IRON ASSESSMENT

In dogs, marrow storage iron seen as hemosiderin in macrophages is a good indicator of total body iron stores. A few clumps of iron are expected per unit particle in a healthy adult canine patient on cytology of the bone marrow (Fig. 27.10). Depletion of marrow iron can be seen with iron deficiency, and Prussian blue or Perl's iron staining can be used to highlight any iron pigment present. In dogs, iron may be increased with old age, hemolytic anemia, anemia of chronic disease, multiple blood transfusions, dyserythropoiesis or ineffective erythropoiesis, hemochromatosis or hemosiderosis, or parenteral administration of iron. Iron may be decreased with chronic blood loss (even including as a result of repeated phlebotomy), in newborns or very young animals,

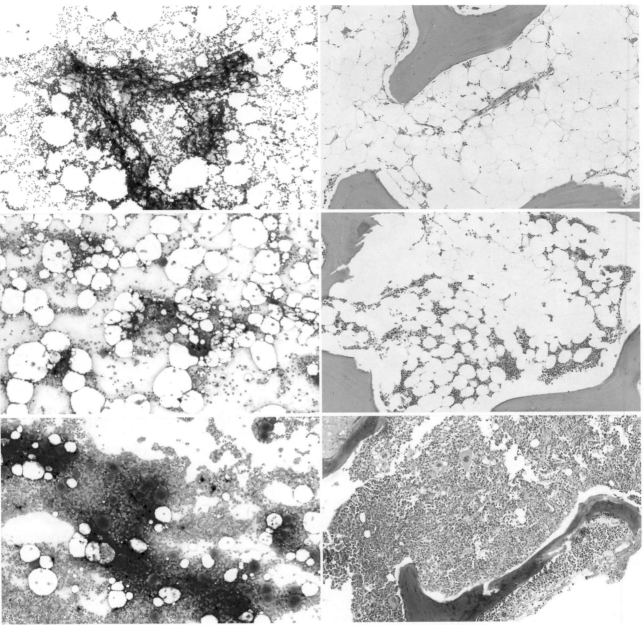

Fig. 27.9 Bone marrow cellularity with cytology and core biopsy. *Top left:* Hypocellular bone marrow cytology sample from a dog. The unit particle contains only adipose tissue and supportive stroma with little to no hematopoietic tissue (Wright-Giemsa stain, original magnification 100×). *Top right:* Hypocellular bone marrow core biopsy from a dog. The medullary spaces contain only sheets of adipocytes with rare scattered hematopoietic cells and blood-filled sinuses (H&E stain, original magnification 100×). *Middle left:* Normocellular bone marrow cytology sample from a dog. The unit particles contain approximately equal proportions of hematopoietic cells and fatty tissue. Few dark brown-black aggregates of iron are present and are expected in an adult dog (Wright-Giemsa stain, original magnification 100×). *Middle right:* Normocellular bone marrow core biopsy from a dog. The medullary tissue contains 30% to 40% hematopoietic cells and 60% to 70% fatty tissue (H&E stain, original magnification 100×). *Bottom left:* Hypercellular bone marrow cytology from a dog. The unit particles and interparticle areas have a strong predominance of hematopoietic cells with very little fat (<10%). A small amount of iron is visible, and megakaryocytes can be seen prominently within and adjacent to the unit particles (Wright-Giemsa stain, original magnification 100×). *Bottom right:* Hypercellular bone marrow core biopsy from a dog. The medullary spaces are almost entirely occupied by hematopoietic tissue with only rare adipocytes *(round clear spaces).* Note that the trabecular bone is purple rather than pink in this image. This reflects less decalcification of this sample compared with the other core biopsies pictured. The mineral component of bone is deeply basophilic with H&E stain, but as the mineral is removed with decalcification, the osteoid matrix, which stains eosinophilic, is all that remains (H&E stain, original magnification 100×).

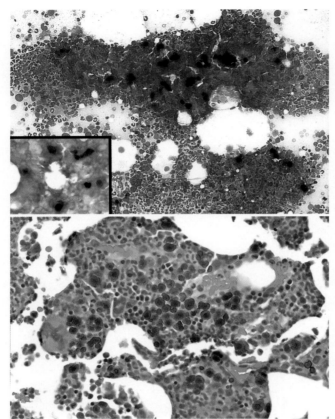

Fig. 27.10 Iron stores in bone marrow. *Top:* Hypercellular bone marrow cytology from an old dog with abundant iron stores. Iron stores with aspiration cytology stain as dark brown-black to gray-brown aggregated material, and are often superimposed on unit particles. In less darkly stained areas of a sample *(inset)*, iron stores have a yellow-brown coloration on cytological preparations (Wright-Giemsa stain, original magnification 200× and inset 500×). *Bottom:* Hypercellular bone marrow core biopsy from an adult dog with abundant iron stores. Iron stores with core biopsy stain as medium-brown to yellow-brown aggregated material. In addition to old age, given the myeloid hyperplasia and relative erythroid hypoplasia in the background, the increased iron in this patient could reflect a component of anemia of chronic/inflammatory disease (H&E stain, original magnification 400×).

or, less often, with nutritional iron deficiency (Box 27.6). Cats lack stainable iron under normal circumstances, and therefore identification of iron in marrow in cats suggests a pathological state, or it can be a sequela of multiple blood transfusions. In cats, pathological conditions that lead to visible/stainable storage iron include hemolytic anemia or dyserythropoiesis, such as with feline leukemia virus (FeLV) infection or hematopoietic neoplasia.

GENERAL LINEAGE ASSESSMENT

Complete bone marrow assessment requires evaluation of several features within each cell lineage (erythroid, myeloid, and megakaryocytic), including the total number/proportion of cells present in that lineage (hypoplasia versus normal versus hyperplasia), completeness of maturation (complete versus arrested), orderliness of maturation (orderly versus left-shifted), and assessment of cellular morphology. This requires an understanding of the normal expectations for each lineage and knowledge of the morphological differences between the various cell types present in marrow.

BOX 27.6 Interpretation of Bone Marrow Iron Stores

Increased Iron Stores
- Increasing patient age
- Hemolytic anemia
- Dyserythropoiesis or ineffective erythropoiesis
- Anemia of chronic/inflammatory disease
- Repeated blood transfusions
- Hemochromatosis or hemosiderosis (rare)
- Parenteral administration of iron

Decreased Iron Stores
- Chronic blood loss
- Newborn or very young animal
- Nutritional iron deficiency (rare in small animals)
- Repeated chronic phlebotomy

Maturation

In normal marrow, maturation within each lineage should generally be distributed in the shape of a pyramid with the least number of early/immature precursors; the greatest proportion of cells in the maturation and storage pools, which contain the later stage precursors; and middle-aged precursors in the proliferative pool making up the center of the pyramid. In the erythroid lineage, this distribution is often more of a diamond or pentagon shape with slightly fewer metarubricytes (late stage) compared with rubricytes (middle-aged cells), but early precursors (rubriblasts and prorubricytes) are still in much lower numbers (Box 27.7). If the maturation within a given lineage follows the expected pyramidal (or pentagon-shaped) distribution, then maturation is considered orderly and complete. If there are increased numbers of earlier precursors, this is considered a left shift, which is common with hyperplasia. If there is maturation up to a point in development but with a lack of later stage precursors, this is considered a maturation arrest, which is common with immune-mediated destruction of later stage precursors. Release of large numbers of band and segmented neutrophils into the peripheral circulation with an inflammatory stimulus can have the appearance of a maturation arrest in the marrow, but this can easily be ruled out by examination of peripheral blood for neutrophilia, left shift, and toxic change.

Myeloid-to-Erythroid Ratio

Overall assessment of the lineages also includes evaluation of the M:E ratio. In this ratio, "myeloid" refers to all granulocytic and monocytic precursors, including mature segmented neutrophils, and "erythroid" refers to all nucleated erythroid precursors, excluding polychromatophils/reticulocytes and mature RBCs. Lymphocytes, plasma cells, and macrophages are assessed concurrently but not included in the ratio. There are wide reported ranges for the normal M:E ratio in dogs and cats, but as a general rule, in dogs, the M:E ratio is normally 0.75:1 to 2.5:1, and in cats, the normal ratio is 1:1 to 3:1.[4,25,32] On cytology, this ratio is often calculated on the basis of a 200- to 500-cell differential count in multiple areas of multiple slides but can also be estimated by more experienced cytologists. An estimate of the M:E ratio is all that is typically performed on a core biopsy sample. The significance of the M:E ratio must be interpreted in light of the overall marrow cellularity and peripheral blood findings, which provide the context for this interpretation (Table 27.4). For example, if there is neutrophilia in the periphery and the marrow cellularity is increased with an increased M:E ratio, then this is interpreted as myeloid hyperplasia as an expected response to peripheral demand for neutrophils, as in inflammation. If there is a

BOX 27.7 Pyramidal Distribution of Cells in Marrow

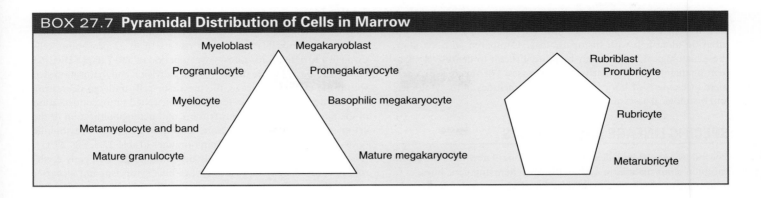

TABLE 27.4   Myeloid-to-Erythroid (M:E) Ratio Assessment

M:E Ratio	Overall Marrow Cellularity	Interpretation
Normal M:E ratio	Normocellular	Normal
	Hypercellular	Erythroid and myeloid hyperplasia
	Hypocellular	Erythroid and myeloid hypoplasia
Increased M:E ratio	Normocellular	Myeloid hyperplasia and erythroid hypoplasia
	Hypercellular	Myeloid hyperplasia
	Hypocellular	Erythroid hypoplasia
Decreased M:E ratio	Normocellular	Erythroid hyperplasia and myeloid hypoplasia
	Hypercellular	Erythroid hyperplasia
	Hypocellular	Myeloid hypoplasia

concurrent regenerative anemia caused by blood loss, then the M:E ratio may be normal because myeloid hyperplasia and erythroid hyperplasia both contribute to the increased marrow cellularity. If there is nonregenerative anemia in the periphery with decreased marrow cellularity and an increased M:E ratio, this may be interpreted as erythroid hypoplasia as an insufficient response to the peripheral demand for RBCs.

Relative Versus Absolute

Hypoplasia or hyperplasia within a given cell line can be described as an absolute change (a true increase or decrease in that marrow lineage compared with normal), or as a relative change, whether relative to the other lineages or to what would be expected given the hematopoietic stimulus. For example, if there is marrow hypercellularity with a severely increased M:E ratio but retained erythroid cells are present, then there is myeloid hyperplasia with relative erythroid hypoplasia (hypoplasia relative to the amount of myeloid present), but the absolute erythroid numbers may be normal for the patient. If the patient has a concurrent nonregenerative anemia, such as with anemia of inflammatory/chronic disease, then there may truly be concurrent absolute myeloid hyperplasia and absolute erythroid hypoplasia. Because this distinction can be difficult to confirm, interpretation may be left in relative terms.

Effective Versus Ineffective Hematopoiesis

If a lineage is identified as being hyperplastic, an important component of the assessment is whether hematopoiesis in that lineage is "effective" or "ineffective." "Effective versus ineffective" refers to the impact that the hyperplasia in the marrow has on peripheral blood in that lineage. Effective hematopoiesis leads to evidence of the regenerative bone marrow response in peripheral blood. Effective erythropoiesis leads to a subsequent regenerative anemia in peripheral blood with reticulocytosis and increasing hematocrit. Effective granulopoiesis typically leads to a developing neutrophilia in the periphery with a left shift in neutrophils with circulating bands. "Ineffective hematopoiesis" refers to hyperplasia within that lineage in bone marrow, but without evidence of that regenerative response in the periphery. Ineffective erythropoiesis indicates an attempt by bone marrow at resolution of peripheral anemia, but the anemia remains nonregenerative without an actual regenerative response seen in the periphery (without increasing hematocrit and without reticulocytosis). Ineffective granulopoiesis indicates an attempt by bone marrow at resolution of a peripheral neutropenia (with myeloid hyperplasia in bone marrow) but without an increasing neutrophil count in the periphery. Distinction between effective and ineffective hematopoiesis can aid in the differential causes to consider in a particular case. Caution is recommended with this interpretation, because a regenerative response can take 3 to 7 days to become apparent in peripheral blood. This determination is therefore best made in cases with chronic cytopenias, rather than in those with more acute anemia or neutropenia that may not have had sufficient time to respond and is still in the pre-regenerative phase.

Dysplasia

Morphological assessment is important for cellular classification, but this assessment should also include evaluation for evidence of dysplasia. *Dysplasia* refers to abnormal morphological features within a cell line caused by a pathological process. Dysplasia is not exclusively seen with hematopoietic neoplasia but is also commonly seen with severe hyperplasia within a lineage, toxic insult, nutritional deficiency (folate/cobalamin), congenital anomalies, FeLV infection, vector-borne infection, immune-mediated conditions, necrosis/inflammation/fibrosis in the marrow, nonhematopoietic neoplasia, or as an effect of certain drug administration including some chemotherapeutic agents[4,5,16,33] (Box 27.8).

Some components of the overall lineage assessment are easier and more accurate with cytological samples than with core biopsies given the relative ease of identification of individual cells with cytology compared with histopathology. Individual cells can be more difficult to specifically identify on histopathology, particularly earlier to middle-aged precursors; however, general estimations can still easily be made with histopathology. Identification of some cells may be aided by the "company they keep." In other words, earlier erythroid precursors may be more apparent when seen in the context of clear erythroid hyperplasia with many obvious late-stage erythroid precursors. Evidence of left shift, maturation arrest, or dysplasia can still often be identified with histopathology. Compared with cytology, these histological features may be more difficult to definitively confirm or quantify, particularly in subtle cases. For this reason, complete assessment of bone marrow ideally includes both cytological and histological assessments.

SPECIFIC LINEAGE ASSESSMENTS

The following sections will include descriptions of normal findings and common abnormalities in each of the main hematopoietic lineages in bone marrow (erythroid, myeloid, and megakaryocytes), following the concepts introduced by this preceding discussion.

BOX 27.8 Definition and Causes of Dysplasia

Definition of Dysplasia

Abnormal morphological features within a cell line caused by a pathological process

Causes of Dysplasia

- Neoplasia (hematopoietic neoplasia, nonhematopoietic neoplasia)
- Severe hyperplasia within a lineage
- Toxic insult; drug administration (some chemotherapy)
- Nutritional deficiency (folate, cobalamin)
- Congenital anomaly (macrocytosis in Poodle, congenital dyserythropoiesis in English Springer Spaniel)
- Infectious (FeLV, vector-borne infection)
- Necrosis/inflammation/fibrosis in bone marrow

FeLV, feline leukemia virus.

Erythroid

Normal development and maturation within the erythroid lineage begins with a rubriblast that gives rise to 16 to 32 progenitor cells through 4 to 5 divisions/mitoses over a period of 5 to 7 days.[4] Division ceases with the rubricyte stage. With each division and maturation step within the erythroid lineage, the precursor cells undergo decreasing cell size, decreasing nuclear-to-cytoplasmic (N:C) ratio, condensation of the nucleus with eventual extrusion, and hemoglobinization of the cytoplasm with a transition from deep-blue to polychromatophilic (gray-blue) to orthochromic (pink-orange) (Table 27.5; Fig. 27.11). Cytologically, compared with early myeloid lineage cells, early erythroid lineage cells generally have deeper-blue cytoplasm and a coarser chromatin pattern, whereas later-stage erythroid cells are more easily distinguished from myeloid cells by their polychromatophilic to hemoglobinized cytoplasmic coloration, condensing nucleus, and smaller cell size (Fig. 27.12). Erythroid cells may be seen in close association with a macrophage in erythropoietic islands (Fig. 27.13). On a core biopsy sample, early erythroid cells typically have a coarser chromatin pattern with smaller cytoplasmic volume compared with early myeloid cells, which have a higher volume of pale eosinophilic to clear cytoplasm with a finer chromatin pattern. Early myeloid cells are also most typically located along the paratrabecular regions within the marrow, whereas early erythroid cells are in a more interstitial location among the later stage erythroid cells (see Fig. 27.2). The later-stage erythroid cells have a very dark, round, bulleted nucleus with a small volume of eosinophilic cytoplasm.

Assessment within the erythroid lineage, as for any cell line, should include evaluation of cell numbers/proportion (hypoplasia versus normal versus hyperplasia) in absolute and/or relative terms, maturation assessment, and evaluation of morphology, including any evidence of dysplasia. The erythroid lineage development follows a pentagon-shaped distribution with only few rubriblasts and prorubricytes (approximately 2%–4%) with the highest number of rubricytes

---

TABLE 27.5 Erythroid Lineage Maturation

Name of Cell Stage	Cytological Description	Cytological Image
Rubriblast	Large-size cell; high nuclear-to-cytoplasmic ratio; small volume of deep-blue cytoplasm; large-size, round nucleus with visible nucleoli and fine to coarse granular chromatin pattern	
Prorubricyte	Medium- to large-size cell; small to moderate volume of medium- to deep-blue cytoplasm; medium- to large-size, round nucleus without nucleoli and with a coarse chromatin pattern	
Rubricyte	Small- to medium-size cell; small to moderate volume of medium-blue (basophilic) to blue-gray (polychromatophilic) to blue-pink cytoplasm; small- to medium-size, round nucleus without nucleoli and with coarse clumped chromatin pattern	
Metarubricyte	Small-size cell; small volume of blue-gray to blue-pink (polychromatophilic) to pink-orange (orthochromic) cytoplasm; small-size, round nucleus without nucleoli and with densely clumped chromatin pattern	

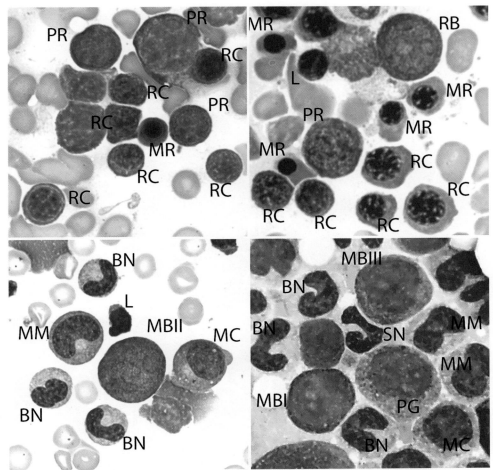

Fig. 27.11 Cellular identification in bone marrow cytology. *Top:* Erythroid lineage cell identification. Rubriblasts (*RB*), prorubricytes (*PR*), rubricytes (*RC*), and metarubricytes (*MR*) are indicated. In addition, a small lymphocyte (*L*) is present for comparison. Compared with rubricytes and metarubricytes, lymphocytes have a smaller volume of cytoplasm and a more dense and smooth chromatin pattern. Few ruptured or disrupted cells are not labeled and cannot be accurately classified. See Table 27.5 for additional description of erythroid cell characteristics (Wright-Giemsa stain, original magnification 1000×). *Bottom:* Myeloid lineage cell identification. Myeloblasts (type I, II, and III; *MBI, MBII,* and *MBIII*), progranulocytes (*PG*), neutrophilic myelocytes (*MC*), neutrophilic metamyelocytes (*MM*), band neutrophils (*BN*), and segmented neutrophils (*SN*) are indicated. In addition, a small lymphocyte is present (*L*). Few ruptured or disrupted cells are not labeled and cannot be accurately classified. See Table 27.6 for additional description of myeloid cell characteristics (Wright-Giemsa stain, original magnification 1000×).

(approximately 65%–75%) and with fewer metarubricytes (approximately 20%–35%) (see Box 27.7).[25,31] Lack or paucity of metarubricytes may suggest maturation arrest. Maturation assessment with cytology should also include evaluation for polychromasia in the background RBC population, which is not possible with core biopsy. Polychromasia is expected, particularly in dogs and to a lesser degree in cats, with normal maturation in the erythroid lineage, and lack of polychromasia with nonregenerative anemia in the periphery may indicate maturation arrest. *Dyserythropoiesis* is a general term that refers to abnormal erythroid maturation or morphology and may be used to describe either maturation arrest or other forms of ineffective erythropoiesis or to describe morphological abnormalities, as with erythroid dysplasia.

Erythroid Hyperplasia

Erythroid hyperplasia is the expected regenerative response to acute blood loss or hemolysis, and peripheral reticulocytosis would be expected in 3 to 5 days (peaking at 4 days) if the stimulus is sufficient.[4] Effective erythroid hyperplasia (effective erythropoiesis) leads to increasing hematocrit, whereas ineffective erythropoiesis does not result in resolution of the anemia with increasing hematocrit or reticulocytosis (Box 27.9). The causes of effective erythropoiesis mirror the causes of regenerative anemia, including acute blood loss or hemolysis. Effective erythropoiesis can also be seen with primary or secondary polycythemia, although marrow assessment cannot reliably distinguish between primary polycythemia vera and secondary causes of polycythemia. Effective erythroid hyperplasia typically has an accompanying left shift within the erythroid lineage with increased rubriblasts and prorubricytes, although rubricytes and metarubricytes still predominate. Polychromasia is typically seen in the background RBC population (Figs. 27.14 and 27.15).

Ineffective erythroid hyperplasia (ineffective erythropoiesis) is an increasingly more recognized pattern of hematological abnormalities and is characterized by erythroid hyperplasia in the marrow without

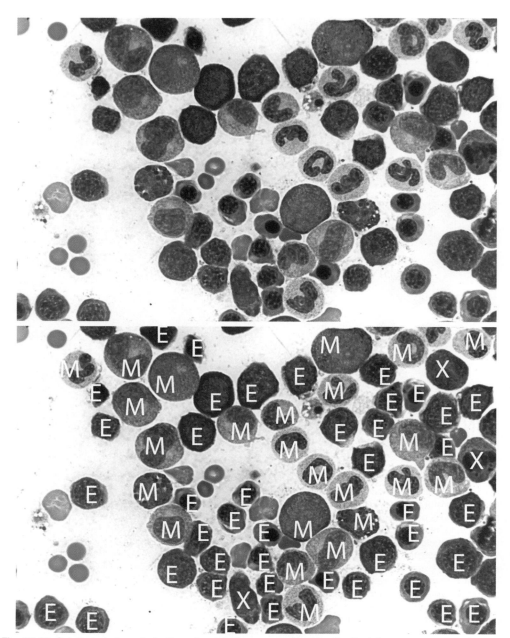

Fig. 27.12 Cytological characterization of myeloid versus erythroid cells. Both images represent the same cytological field from a dog with a hypercellular bone marrow sample. When performing a differential count to assess for an M:E ratio, each cell is identified as myeloid *(M)* or erythroid *(E)*, as denoted in the bottom image. Some cells cannot be definitively classified because of disruption or rupture, mitosis, a thicker area of the sample, or overlapping characteristics that prevent identification *(denoted with "x")*. Lymphocytes, plasma cells, and histiocytes are not included in calculating the M:E ratio (Wright-Giemsa stain, original magnification 1000×).

a regenerative response in the periphery. A common cause is precursor-targeted, immune-mediated anemia (PIMA), also referred to as nonregenerative immune-mediated hemolytic anemia (IMHA) (Figs. 27.16 and 27.17). Destruction of later-stage erythroid precursors in PIMA leads to an inability of the erythroid hyperplasia response in the marrow to effectively increase the hematocrit in the periphery. Other causes of ineffective erythroid hyperplasia include nutritional deficiency (iron deficiency, folate/cobalamin deficiency), congenital dyserythropoiesis (Poodles, English Springer Spaniels; but not usually

associated with anemia), or hematopoietic neoplasia (particularly myelodysplastic syndrome [MDS]).[4,34,35] Iron-deficiency anemia can usually be distinguished from the other differentials by the presence or absence of stainable iron in the marrow (see Fig. 27.10). Classic cases of PIMA in dogs may have evidence of phagocytosis of erythroid precursors by macrophages and often have increased marrow iron, as well as possible secondary myelofibrosis (see Figs. 27.16 and 27.17). Although maturation arrest may be identified in cases of PIMA, this finding is not specific for an immune-mediated process and can also

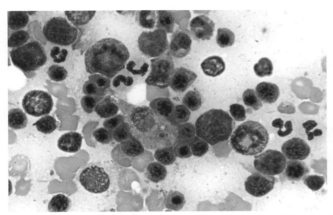

Fig. 27.13 Bone marrow cytology from a dog; erythropoietic island. Erythroid cells can be seen in erythropoietic islands, in which erythroid precursors in various stages of maturation surround a central macrophage. The macrophage supports erythropoiesis by providing nutrients, playing a role in iron metabolism, and phagocytosing extruded nuclei from metarubricytes. Erythropoietic islands may be more readily apparent with erythroid hyperplasia, as is evident in this patient (Wright-Giemsa stain, original magnification 1000×).

BOX 27.9 Causes of Erythroid Hyperplasia and Erythroid Hypoplasia

Erythroid Hyperplasia	Erythroid Hypoplasia
Effective Erythroid Hyperplasia	**Aplastic Anemia (see Box 27.5)**
• Regenerative anemia	
• Blood loss	***Selective Erythroid Hypoplasia***
• Hemolysis	• Precursor-targeting immune-mediated anemia (destruction of early-stage precursors)
• Polycythemia (absolute)	
• Primary (polycythemia vera)	• Neoplasia
• Secondary	• Drug-associated
• Appropriate (hypoxemia)	• Hyperestrogenism (dogs)
• Inappropriate (local renal hypoxia, erythropoietin-secreting tumor)	• Feline leukemia virus (FeLV) subgroup C infection (cats)
	• Recombinant human erythropoietin administration
Ineffective Erythroid Hyperplasia	• Mild causes without severe anemia
• Precursor-targeting immune-mediated anemia (destruction of late-stage precursors)	• Chronic renal disease
• Nutritional deficiency (iron, cobalamin/folate)	• Endocrinopathy
• Congenital dyserythropoiesis (Poodles, English Springer Spaniels)	• Anemia of chronic/inflammatory disease
• Hematopoietic neoplasia (particularly myelodysplastic syndrome)	

---

be seen with myeloid neoplasia, congenital dyserythropoiesis, and drug-related causes.[4] Increased erythrophagia by macrophages is also not specific for PIMA and can be seen with other causes of ineffective erythropoiesis or secondary to blood transfusion.

Erythroid Hypoplasia

Erythroid hypoplasia can occur as a selective process (affecting only the erythroid lineage) or as a component of panhypoplasia in the marrow as with causes of aplastic anemia (see Box 27.9). Causes for selective erythroid hypoplasia may include PIMA with destruction of early erythroid precursors. This is in contrast to PIMA with late stage erythroid targeting (described above), which leads to erythroid hyperplasia with persistent nonregenerative anemia.[36] Other causes include neoplasia, drug-associated causes, hyperestrogenism in dogs, FeLV infection in cats (subgroup C), or administration of recombinant human erythropoietin.[4] Chronic renal disease, endocrinopathy, and anemia of chronic/inflammatory disease can all lead to a minor degree of erythroid hypoplasia in the marrow, but most typically are not associated with as severe anemia as the other differentials.

There is variability in the literature with regard to terminology for immune-mediated precursor-targeted conditions in bone marrow in dogs and cats. Pure red cell aplasia (PRCA), which is still thought to be caused by an immune-mediated process, refers to lack or near-absence of erythropoiesis, whereas nonregenerative IMHA (PIMA) still has ongoing erythropoiesis, although erythropoiesis is incomplete and impaired. The definition of PRCA often includes an M:E ratio greater than 75:1 or less than 5% of marrow cells from the erythroid lineage, whereas PIMA often has a less severe decrease in erythropoiesis.[37-39] Lymphocytosis or lymphoid aggregates may be seen in bone marrow with these conditions, particularly in cats. Increased plasma cells and myelofibrosis may also be seen in these cases, particularly in dogs (see Fig. 27.17).[38,39] In some cases, response to immunosuppressive therapy may be very slow, often longer than 1 to 2 months.[38,39] Increased phagocytic activity by macrophages may be seen and is helpful in suggesting an immune-mediated pathogenesis, although it is not present in all cases and is not entirely specific. Myeloid hyperplasia may be seen and may even lead to severe marrow hypercellularity despite marked selective erythroid hypoplasia.

Erythroid Dysplasia

Dysplasia within the erythroid lineage may be recognized as nuclear-to-cytoplasmic asynchrony, including megaloblastic change, premature pyknosis in immature cells, nuclear fragmentation or karyolysis, multinucleation, internuclear chromatin bridging, cytoplasmic or nuclear vacuolation, or siderotic inclusions (Fig. 27.18). Possible causes for erythroid dysplasia include severe erythroid hyperplasia, ineffective erythropoiesis, myeloid neoplasia, FeLV infection, folate/cobalamin deficiency, congenital dyserythropoiesis (macrocytosis in English Springer Spaniels, Poodles), drug administration (including chemotherapy or other drugs that interfere with DNA synthesis), marrow necrosis/infection/radiation, or toxin effects.[4,31,35]

Myeloid

Myeloid lineage refers to granulocytic and monocytic precursors. Inflammatory or phagocytic macrophages will be considered in the section "Other Cell Types" below. The vast majority of the myeloid cells are granulocytic, whereas developing monocytes (discussed below) are a minority (<3%–5% of marrow cells).[4,18] Normal development and maturation within the granulocytic lineage occurs over 6 to 7 days and begins with a myeloblast that gives rise to, on average, 16 progenitor cells through 4 divisions/mitoses.[4] A division may be skipped or added, and the overall time to production of myeloid cells may be shortened, depending on peripheral demands. Division ceases with the myelocyte stage. With each division and maturation step within the granulocytic lineage, the precursor cells undergo decreasing cell size, decreasing N:C ratio, condensation and lobulation of the nucleus, and increasing pallor and alteration of granularity of the cytoplasm. Primary granules are first seen in middle-aged to late myeloblasts and are most prominent in progranulocytes and then replaced with secondary granules in myelocytes (Table 27.6; see Fig. 27.11). Cytologically, several features

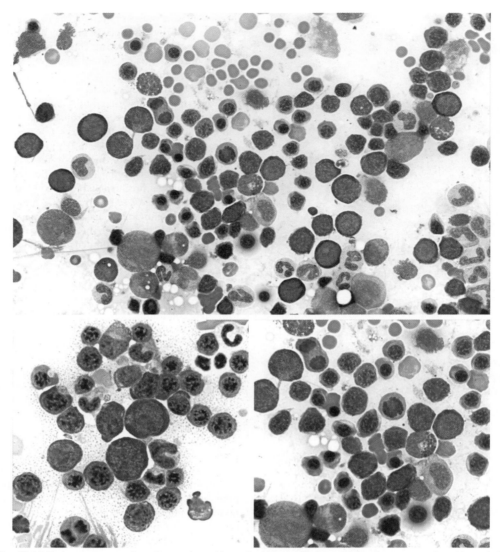

Fig. 27.14 Bone marrow cytology from a dog with erythroid hyperplasia caused by immune-mediated hemolytic anemia. Severe erythroid hyperplasia is present with a decreased M:E ratio and a left shift in erythroid cells with increased numbers of earlier stage precursors. Complete maturation is evident given the background population of polychromatophilic red blood cells with pale blue-gray cytoplasm *(top of image)*. Spherocytes among these poly- chromatophils *(top of image)* have a rounded, smaller, hyperchromic appearance. This is an example of effective erythropoiesis, because this patient has regenerative anemia (reticulocytosis) in the peripheral blood (Wright-Gi- emsa stain, original magnification 500× *[top]* and 1000× *[bottom]*).

aid in distinction of myeloid cells from erythroid lineage (see Fig. 27.12). Early myeloblasts (type I) generally have paler-blue cytoplasm and a finer chromatin pattern compared with early erythroid lineage cells. Later myeloblasts (type II and type III) and progranulocytes are distinguished from erythroid cells by their increasingly prominent and numerous pink cytoplasmic granules. Later-stage myeloid cells are easily distinguished from later-stage erythroid cells by their lobu- lated nuclear contour and cytoplasmic coloration and, in eosinophils and basophils, their brightly colored granules. Histologically, early myeloid cells typically have a more finely stippled chromatin pattern with higher cytoplasmic volume compared with early erythroid cells, with clear to granulated eosinophilic cytoplasm. Early myeloid cells are also most typically located along the paratrabecular regions within the marrow, whereas early erythroid cells are in a more interstitial location among the later-stage erythroid cells. Myelocyte stages are difficult to

specifically identify on histopathology because of lack of nuclear lob- ularity. The later-stage granulocytic cells are clearly distinguished on histopathology by their nuclear lobularity and for eosinophils in partic- ular by their prominent eosinophilic granules (see Fig. 27.2). Basophil precursors are very difficult to distinguish histologically, although are generally in low numbers.

Assessment within the granulocytic lineage, as for any cell line, should include evaluation of cell numbers/proportion (hypoplasia versus normal versus hyperplasia) in absolute and/or relative terms, maturation assessment, and evaluation of morphology, including any evidence of dysplasia. The granulocytic lineage development follows a pyramid-shaped distribution with only few myeloblasts (1%), a greater number of the proliferative pool of promyelocytes and myelo- cytes (approximately 15%) and with the largest number of the matu- ration/storage pool precursors composed of metamyelocytes, bands,

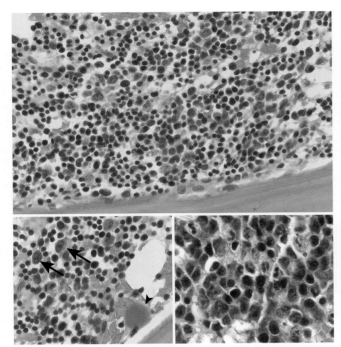

Fig. 27.15 Core biopsy from two dogs with erythroid hyperplasia. In both cases, there is severe hypercellularity with a decreased M:E ratio. On histopathology, erythroid lineage cells are identified by their darker, bulleted nuclei, particularly noticeable in later-stage precursors. Earlier erythroid precursors have a small volume of deeply eosinophilic cytoplasm with coarse chromatin (arrows), but are often most easily identified by the context of surrounding erythroid hyperplasia with many late stage precursor cells. In the top and lower left images from the same dog, there is complete maturation with many late rubricytes and metarubricytes. In contrast, in the lower right image, there are greater numbers of rubricytes with a maturation arrest and only few metarubricytes. This (lower right) is a patient with precursor-targeted immune-mediated anemia (PIMA). Also, note in the lower left image, there is a megakaryocyte (arrowhead). Portions of megakaryocyte cytoplasm may be seen without a nucleus in histological section caused by an artifact of plane of section. These anucleate brightly eosinophilic structures should be included as part of the estimate of megakaryocytic cellularity in core biopsies (H&E stain, original magnification 400× [top], 600× [bottom left], and 1000× [bottom right]).

and segmented granulocytes (approximately 85%) (see Box 27.7).[4,18,25] Relative lack of mature segmented neutrophils may be seen in cases of intense inflammation with immediate release of bands and segmented neutrophils into the periphery upon their production in the marrow, or with maturation arrest (as with an immune-mediated process). On core biopsy with histopathology, left shift may be evident as an increased thickness of the paratrabecular band of immature myeloid cells.

Monocytes

Monocytes are generally in very low numbers in bone marrow and monoblasts are not reliably distinguished from myeloblasts, even on cytology, because of overlapping morphology. Promonocytes do not contain the cytoplasmic granules noted in promyelocytes. Promonocytes and mature monocytes may be recognized as myeloid cells but are not easily distinguished from neutrophilic myelocytes or metamyelocytes. Mature monocytes are not retained in the marrow as a storage pool, unlike the abundant storage pool in the granulocytic lineages, and therefore are not generally seen in significant numbers in the marrow (generally <3%–5% of cells).[4,18] Because of their low

proportion of marrow cellularity, myeloid hyperplasia and hypoplasia are generally discussed as granulocytic hyperplasia and hypoplasia, rather than pertaining to monocytic cells.

Myeloid Hyperplasia

Myeloid/granulocytic hyperplasia, as with the discussion in the erythroid lineage above, can be effective or ineffective (Box 27.10). *Effective myeloid hyperplasia* refers to marrow granulocytic hyperplasia that leads to neutrophilia and/or left shift in the peripheral blood neutrophil population (Figs. 27.19 and 27.20). This is most common with inflammatory conditions whether they result from bacterial infection, other infectious etiologies, immune-mediated conditions, tissue necrosis, underlying neoplasia, or other causes. This type of process can also occur secondary to drug administration (granulocyte–colony stimulating factor [G-CSF]), as a paraneoplastic process (neoplasm producing G-CSF or a similar granulopoietic growth factor/stimulant), with the recovery phase of cyclic hematopoiesis in Collie dogs, with leukocyte adhesion deficiency in dogs, or with chronic myeloid leukemia (CML).[4] CML can be very difficult or even impossible to differentiate from an inflammatory process on bone marrow examination.[4] Myeloid hyperplasia is often accompanied by left shift and possibly with paucity of storage pool cells because they exit the marrow quickly upon their production. With septicemia or severe infection, this robust utilization of the storage pool with a concurrent neutropenia can mimic the marrow appearance of ineffective granulopoiesis. Mild cytoplasmic vacuolation of myeloid precursors can occur with robust myeloid hyperplasia and is considered a minor dysplastic change.

Ineffective myeloid hyperplasia (ineffective granulopoiesis) is less common than ineffective erythropoiesis but can occur with immune-mediated neutropenia with destruction of later-stage, mature, segmented neutrophils, with hematopoietic neoplasia, such as MDS or acute myeloid leukemia (AML), or with FeLV infection in cats (Fig. 27.21).[4] It should be noted that the appearance of an early myeloid hyperplasia response can overlap that of AML, given the increased proportion of myeloblasts before subsequent completion of the maturation pyramid. In cases where the neutropenia is acute, continued monitoring of CBC for an emerging regenerative response (5–7 days) is recommended before interpreting an expansion of blast cells in the marrow as a neoplastic process.

Eosinophil Hyperplasia

Eosinophil precursors are normally less than 6% of overall marrow cellularity.[4] Eosinophil hyperplasia in the marrow is the expected bone marrow finding with peripheral eosinophilia of any cause, including with parasitism, allergy/hypersensitivity, inflammatory conditions, mast cell tumor, hypereosinophilic syndrome, or hematopoietic neoplasia (CML, MDS, or AML) (Fig. 27.22). In dogs that have gray eosinophils (particularly common in greyhounds and other sighthounds), marrow eosinophil precursors also lack the typical eosinophilic coloration of the cytoplasmic secondary granules and instead contain clear cytoplasmic vacuoles (Fig. 27.23). Eosinophils in cytological and histological specimens often appear more prominent compared with other myeloid cells, likely because of their brightly colored granules, and therefore may be misinterpreted as hyperplastic even when in appropriate numbers.

Basophil Hyperplasia

Basophil precursors are normally less than 1% of overall marrow cellularity.[4] Basophil hyperplasia in the marrow typically accompanies basophilia in the periphery, and often is concurrent with eosinophilia. Basophil hyperplasia may occur with parasitism, allergy/hypersensitivity, mast cell tumor, or hematopoietic neoplasia (see Fig. 27.19).

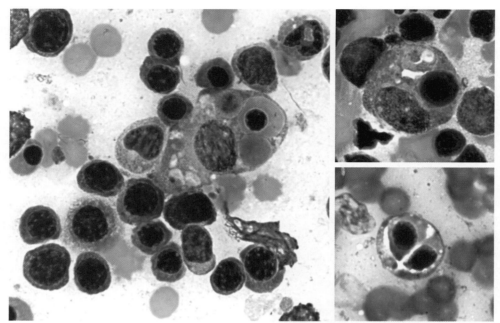

Fig. 27.16 Bone marrow cytology from a dog with ineffective erythropoiesis caused by precursor-targeted immune-mediated anemia (PIMA). Macrophages contain phagocytized red blood cells in the cytoplasm, as well as phagocytized erythroid precursors including metarubricytes *(left)* and rubricytes *(right top and bottom)*. In some cases, phagocytized erythroid cells may be seen within free cytoplasmic fragments that have artifactually broken off from phagocytic macrophages in the marrow *(lower right)*. PIMA is an example of ineffective erythropoiesis because there is severe erythroid hyperplasia in the marrow, but there is a nonregenerative anemia in peripheral blood (Wright-Giemsa stain, original magnification 1000×).

Myeloid Hypoplasia

Granulocytic hypoplasia can occur as a component of aplastic anemia with panhypoplasia in the marrow or can be selective (see Box 27.10). Granulocytic hypoplasia may also precede hypoplasia in other cell lines, as in some cases with certain drugs.[4] Selective granulocytic hypoplasia can occur with immune-mediated targeting of earlier stage myeloid precursors as a result of certain drugs, parvovirus/panleukopenia infection, FeLV infection in cats,[4,8,40] or severe inflammation/infection, such as in the early stages of septicemia (caused by depletion of the storage pool in response to high peripheral demand). Granulocytic hypoplasia can also occur transiently with inherited cyclical hematopoiesis in Collie dogs and is then followed by a restorative granulocytic hyperplasia response.

Myeloid Dysplasia

Dysgranulopoiesis, analogous to dyserythropoiesis in the erythroid lineage, refers to abnormal granulocytic maturation and/or morphology. Dysplasia within the myeloid lineage may be seen as giant neutrophils, abnormal mitotic figures, multinucleation, abnormal granulation, hyposegmentation or hypersegmentation, cytoplasmic vacuolation, or bizarre nuclear contour, including ring-form nuclei (see Fig. 27.18). These changes can be seen with MDS/AML, particularly when associated with FeLV infection, but can also be seen with severe myeloid hyperplasia, including with inflammation/infection, certain drug effects, in Giant Schnauzers with cobalamin malabsorption, and during an early recovery phase following granulocytic hypoplasia or with G-CSF administration.[4]

Megakaryocytes

Normal development and maturation within the megakaryocytic lineage begins with a megakaryoblast. Unlike in the other lineages, megakaryoblasts undergo endomitosis, rather than mitosis, to give rise to a single large polyploid megakaryocyte. *Endomitosis* refers to nuclear division without concurrent cytoplasmic division. With each division and maturation step within the megakaryocyte lineage, the cells become larger, with multiple individualized nuclei that fuse into a single large convoluted and lobular nucleus, with increasing condensation of the chromatin, decreasing N:C ratio, and transition from basophilic cytoplasm to pink granulated cytoplasm in mature megakaryocytes (Table 27.7). Cytologically, megakaryocyte precursors are clearly distinguished by their large size and multinucleation or multilobular nuclei, although megakaryoblasts are often not distinguishable from other immature or blast cells in marrow (Fig. 27.24). Megakaryocytes and their precursors are typically closely associated with the unit particles or may be in peripheral areas of the sample, in more hemodilute regions or near the edges of a smear. Megakaryocytic precursors are often not evenly distributed within a sample; therefore for assessment of cellularity within the megakaryocyte population, an estimate should be made on the basis of evaluation of multiple particles on multiple slides. Core biopsy may provide more accurate samples for assessment of megakaryocyte numbers, particularly if there is a suspicion for megakaryocytic hypoplasia on cytological evaluation. Because of the large size of megakaryocytes, an estimate of cellularity on cytology is often performed at lower magnification (10× objective) than for the other lineages (typically 40×, 50×, and/or 100× objective). In a normal marrow, several megakaryocytes are expected per unit particle on average with a strong predominance of mature megakaryocytes (>80%).[4,10,25] The literature varies with regard to specific expected numbers of megakaryocytes, but generally 5 to 10 megakaryocytes are expected per 10× low-power field (lpf) with fewer than 3 to 5 megakaryocytes suggesting megakaryocyte hypoplasia and greater than 10 to 20 megakaryocytes per 10× field suggesting megakaryocyte hyperplasia.[4,10,12,18] In more general terms, almost no megakaryocytes is considered "too few"; several per field is considered "adequate"; and

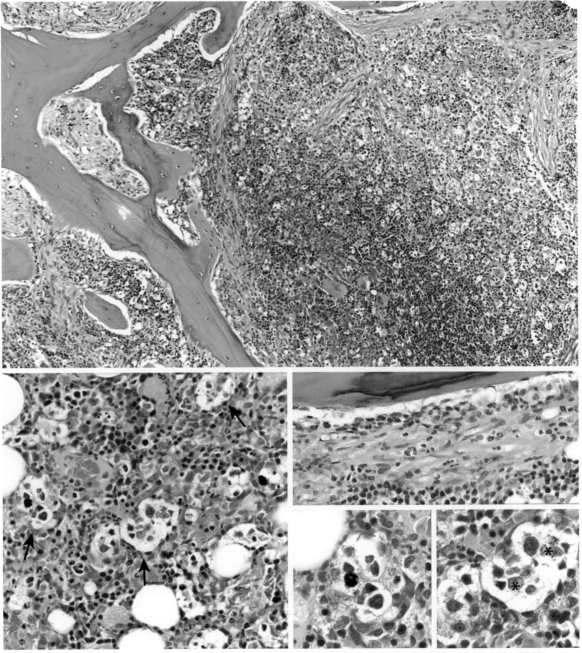

Fig. 27.17 Bone marrow core biopsy from a dog with precursor-targeted immune-mediated anemia (PIMA) and secondary myelofibrosis. Severe erythroid hyperplasia with phagocytosis of erythroid precursors by macrophages within the marrow supports a diagnosis of PIMA. Histologically, this phagocytic activity by macrophages can be seen from low magnification as areas of vacuolation within the marrow *(arrows)*. On closer inspection, macrophage nuclei *(denoted by *)* can be seen with surrounding clear cytoplasmic phagocytic vacuoles containing erythroid precursor cells. This may not be evident in all cases of PIMA, but when this feature is identified, it is a useful diagnostic aid. In this case, there is secondary myelofibrosis. The eosinophilic streaming quality within the marrow reflects the increased connective tissue *(top and right middle)*. With myelofibrosis, there is often accompanying bony remodeling with endosteal new bone formation (note the irregular contour to the less mature woven bone extending from the trabecular bone *[top]*) (H&E stain, original magnification 100× *[top]*, 400× *[lower left and right middle]*, 1000× *[bottom right]*).

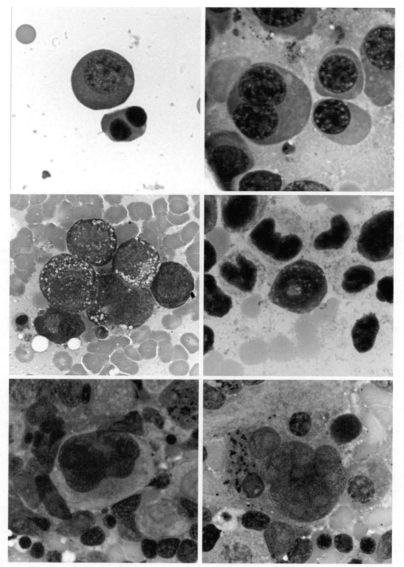

Fig. 27.18 Erythroid, myeloid, and megakaryocyte dysplasia on bone marrow cytology. *Top:* Erythroid dysplasia in two cats. *Left:* Megaloblast with nuclear to cytoplasmic asynchrony of maturation, binucleate metarubricyte (feline leukemia virus [FeLV]–associated); *Right:* Binucleate megaloblastic cell with multiple atypical rubricytes with nuclear to cytoplasmic dysmaturation (myelodysplastic syndrome with erythroid predominance [MDS-Er]). In megaloblastic cells, note the altered gray/polychromatophilic coloration to the cytoplasm with decreased N:C ratio and immature chromatin pattern. *Middle:* Myeloid dysplasia in two dogs. *Left:* Multiple myeloblasts with vacuolated cytoplasm (zonisamide toxicity). *Right:* Ring-shaped nucleus in a myeloid cell with few cytoplasmic vacuoles (mild secondary myelodysplasia accompanying severe myeloid hyperplasia). *Bottom:* Megakaryocyte dysplasia in a cat with FeLV-associated dysplastic changes. *Left:* Dwarf megakaryocyte with hypolobular nucleus and high N:C ratio. *Right:* Basophilic megakaryocyte with multiple distinct nuclei (Wright-Giemsa stain, original magnification 1000× [*top*], 1000× [*middle*], and 500× [*bottom*]).

many megakaryocytes is considered "increased." Poor-quality or low-cellularity cytological smears often have fewer megakaryocytes because these cells are typically associated with unit particles.

On core biopsies, megakaryocytes are distinguishable by their large size (Fig. 27.25). Similar to cytological evaluation, megakaryocytes are often not evenly distributed within the marrow on a core biopsy, and therefore the estimate is based on evaluation of multiple marrow spaces across the sample. Megakaryocytes may appear randomly arranged within a core biopsy but are located adjacent to sinusoids to allow for release of platelets into circulation (see Fig. 27.2). In

general, 1 to 3 megakaryocytes per 2 to 3 high-power fields (hpf; 40×) is considered to be within the reference interval.[41] It should be noted that cross-sections of megakaryocytes in histological section can lack a nuclear component, given the high cytoplasmic volume, and therefore megakaryocytes may be missed if these larger eosinophilic cytoplasmic portions are not recognized as megakaryocytes (see Fig. 27.15). In addition, care should be taken to not overinterpret the dysplastic features in megakaryocytes on histopathology, because the convoluted nuclear contour can be quite pronounced with this modality. Both cytologically and histologically, megakaryocytes must be distinguished

TABLE 27.6 Myeloid Lineage Maturation

Name of Cell Stage	Cytological Description	Cytological Image
Myeloblast	Large-size cell; high nuclear-to-cytoplasmic ratio; small volume of light to medium blue cytoplasm without granules (type I myeloblast), or with small pink-magenta primary granules in low numbers (<15 granules; type II myeloblast) or high numbers (type III myeloblast); large-size, round nucleus with visible nucleoli and fine lacy chromatin pattern	
Progranulocyte (promyelocyte)	Large-size cell; small to moderate volume of light-blue cytoplasm with numerous small pink-magenta primary granules that may also be superimposed on the nucleus; medium- to large-size, round, slightly eccentric nucleus without nucleoli and with a fine to slightly coarse chromatin pattern	
Myelocyte	Medium-size cell; small to moderate volume of clear to slightly pale-blue cytoplasm without the primary granules (but with secondary bright-pink granules in eosinophils and pale gray-lavender granules in basophils; secondary granules not visible in neutrophils); small- to medium-size, round to oval, eccentrically located nucleus without nucleoli and with coarse chromatin pattern	
Metamyelocyte	Small- to medium-size cell; small volume of clear to slightly pale-blue cytoplasm (with secondary granules visible in eosinophils and basophils but not in neutrophils); small-size, indented/reniform nucleus without nucleoli and with coarse stippled chromatin pattern	
Band granulocyte	Small-size cell; small volume of clear to slightly pale-blue cytoplasm (with secondary granules visible in eosinophils and basophils but not in neutrophils); small-size horseshoe- or S-shaped nucleus with coarse clumped chromatin pattern	
Mature granulocyte	Small-size cell; small volume of clear cytoplasm (with secondary granules visible in eosinophils and basophils but not in neutrophils); small-size, tightly segmented/lobulated nucleus (often bilobed in eosinophils and less tightly segmented in basophils) with densely clumped chromatin pattern	

from other multinucleate cells in marrow, including osteoclasts, multinucleate giant macrophages, or multinucleate tumor cells (Fig. 27.26).

Assessment within the megakaryocytic lineage, as for any cell line, should include evaluation of cell numbers/proportion (hypoplasia versus normal versus hyperplasia), maturation assessment, and evaluation of morphology, including any evidence of dysplasia.[26,42,43] The megakaryocytic lineage development follows a pyramid-shaped distribution, with only few megakaryoblasts and promegakaryocytes, a greater number of basophilic megakaryocytes, and the largest number of mature megakaryocytes (see Box 27.7). If less than 50% of the megakaryocytic cells are mature, with increased promegakaryocytes or basophilic megakaryocytes, this indicates a left shift and supports a regenerative response.

Megakaryocytic Hyperplasia

Megakaryocytic hyperplasia is the expected regenerative response to some causes of thrombocytopenia, including immune-mediated destruction of platelets; to causes of increased platelet consumption, including intravascular coagulation, hypersplenism, and vascular injury; or to an infectious etiology, such as rickettsial disease.

Megakaryocytic hyperplasia is also expected alongside thrombocytosis, as a reactive response to chronic inflammation; with iron deficiency; in response to some therapeutic drugs (vincristine)[44]; or occasionally with megakaryocytic neoplasia (megakaryocytic leukemia or essential thrombocythemia).[4,18,45] (Box 27.11). A left shift may be seen with megakaryocytic hyperplasia with increased numbers of basophilic megakaryocytes (see Fig. 27.24). This left shift may be more difficult to identify on core biopsy with histopathology compared with cytology, but a pale-gray coloration to the cytoplasm and a more open chromatin pattern can be helpful on a core biopsy (see Fig. 27.25).

Megakaryocytic Hypoplasia

Megakaryocytic hypoplasia can be seen with panhypoplasia in the marrow as with causes of aplastic anemia, but can also rarely be a selective process (see Box 27.11). Selective megakaryocytic hypoplasia may occur with immune-mediated destruction of megakaryocytes, also referred to as *amegakaryocytic thrombocytopenia*. Selective hypoplasia may also occur with drug effects or infectious etiologies. More commonly, these cause hypoplasia in multiple lineages but can affect the megakaryocytes first in some cases.[4,18,44]

BOX 27.10 Causes of Myeloid/Granulocytic Hyperplasia and Myeloid/Granulocytic Hypoplasia

Myeloid/Granulocytic Hyperplasia	Myeloid/Granulocytic Hypoplasia

Effective Granulocytic Hyperplasia
 • Inflammatory conditions
  • Bacterial or other infection
  • Immune-mediated conditions
  • Tissue necrosis
  • Neoplasia
 • G-CSF administration
 • Paraneoplastic process (neoplasm producing G-CSF or other growth factor)
 • Recovery from neutropenia with cyclical hematopoiesis in collie dogs
 • Leukocyte adhesion deficiency
 • CML
	Aplastic Anemia (see Box 27.5)
	
	 Selective Granulocytic Hypoplasia
	 • Immune-mediated neutropenia (targeting of early-stage precursors)
	 • Drug administration
	 • Infection (parvovirus/panleukopenia, FeLV in cats, early septicemia with depletion of storage pool)
	 • Cyclical hematopoiesis in collie dogs (transient)

Ineffective Granulocytic Hyperplasia • Immune-mediated neutropenia (targeting of late-stage precursors) • Hematopoietic neoplasia • FeLV infection (in cats) • Trapped neutrophil syndrome in Border Collie	
Eosinophil Hyperplasia • Parasitism • Allergy/hypersensitivity • Inflammatory conditions • Mast cell tumor; other paraneoplastic • Hypereosinophilic syndrome • Hematopoietic neoplasia (AML, MDS, CML)	

AML, acute myeloid leukemia; *CML,* chronic myelogenous leukemia; *FeLV,* feline leukemia virus; *G-CSF,* granulocyte–colony stimulating factor; *MDS,* myelodysplastic syndrome.

Bone marrow evaluation specifically regarding assessment of megakaryocytic lineage is best utilized to differentiate between various causes of thrombocytopenia and is not usually indicated in thrombocytosis unless there is suspicion for megakaryocytic or other hematopoietic neoplasia. In cases of thrombocytopenia, if there is megakaryocytic hyperplasia in the marrow, this suggests either increased consumption of platelets in the periphery or platelet destruction as with immune-mediated thrombocytopenia (IMT). If there is megakaryocytic hypoplasia in the marrow, suppression of production of megakaryocytes is the likely cause. Platelet sequestration in the spleen should not affect megakaryopoiesis.

Megakaryocyte Dysplasia

Dysmegakaryocytopoiesis, analogous to dyserythropoiesis and dysgranulopoiesis in the other lineages, refers to abnormal megakaryocyte maturation and/or morphology. Left shift with maturation arrest can be seen with immune-mediated destruction of megakaryocytes. Dysplastic features in megakaryocytes may include hypolobularity or hyperlobularity of nuclei, multiple separated nuclei in a more mature cell, prominent cytoplasmic vacuolation, or dwarf megakaryocytes (see

Fig. 27.18). Dysplasia can be seen with severe megakaryocytic hyperplasia; immune-mediated conditions; neoplasia; drugs; hereditary conditions, such as macrothrombocytopenia in Cavalier King Charles Spaniel dogs; or MDS/AML.[4] One unique feature that can occur in megakaryocytes, and can be seen on cytology or histopathology, is *emperipolesis,* which is the movement of blood cells (most commonly neutrophils) through the megakaryocyte cytoplasm (see Fig. 27.25). The significance in veterinary species is unknown, but there may be an association with inflammation.[18,33]

OTHER CELL TYPES

Additional cell types expected in bone marrow include lymphocytes, plasma cells, macrophages, mast cells, and stromal elements. These cell types are typically seen to some degree in normal bone marrow, but under certain disease states each of these cell types may become more prominent or increased in number (Box 27.12). With panhypoplasia of bone marrow, lack of hematopoietic cells often leads to apparent increased proportions of these background cellular elements (Fig. 27.27). With routine cytological bone marrow assessment, lymphocytes, plasma cells, and macrophages are typically counted as separate categories in parallel with the differential cell count of the myeloid and erythroid cells but are not included in the M:E ratio.

Lymphocytes

Lymphocytes in bone marrow are most commonly small mature lymphocytes, although a few reactive-appearing or less mature lymphocytes may be seen because a mild degree of lymphopoiesis can occur in bone marrow. Under normal circumstances, lymphocytes are expected to be less than 5% of nucleated cells in marrow in dogs and less than 10% in cats, although some reported reference intervals allow for higher numbers (10% in dogs and 20% in cats).[4,18,31] Lymphocytes on cytology appear similar to those in blood or elsewhere in the body, but on histopathology, small lymphocytes and late-stage erythroid precursor cells may be difficult to distinguish[46,47] (Fig. 27.28). Lymphoid aggregates are rare under normal circumstances but can be more frequent with chronic antigenic stimulation, such as with immune-mediated or infectious conditions. On cytology, lymphoid aggregates may be seen as a regional increase in lymphocyte numbers, whereas on histopathology their architecture is more clearly apparent (Fig. 27.29).

Increased numbers of lymphocytes can vary in significance, depending on the size and maturity of the lymphocytes in addition to their pattern and distribution in the marrow. In some cases, follow-up advanced diagnostic testing, such as immunohistochemistry (IHC; core biopsy sample), flow cytometry (liquid bone marrow sample), or polymerase chain reaction (PCR) for antigen receptor rearrangement (PARR; bone marrow smears or formalin-fixed paraffin-embedded tissue), may be necessary to further investigate for a potential neoplastic lymphoid population (see Box 27.3). Increased small lymphocytes can be seen with antigenic stimulation of any cause, including with infectious etiology (particularly tickborne disease, such as ehrlichiosis[18,31]), inflammatory conditions, or with immune-mediated disorders (including PIMA or PRCA in cats and IMHA/IMT/PIMA in dogs[38,39]), or can occur with small cell lymphoma or bone marrow involvement with chronic lymphocytic leukemia (CLL; see Box 27.12; Fig. 27.30). Classic canine and feline CLL of T-lymphocyte origin typically arises within the spleen, and therefore bone marrow involvement is often not a feature. The majority of dogs with CLL have a CD3 +, CD4− and CD8+ phenotype, whereas cats with CLL are typically CD3+,CD4+, and CD8−.[48,49] On histopathology, the pattern and distribution of lymphocytes can aid in the distinction between a reactive and neoplastic population, but if there are only subtly increased lymphocyte numbers, evenly dispersed throughout the marrow, this

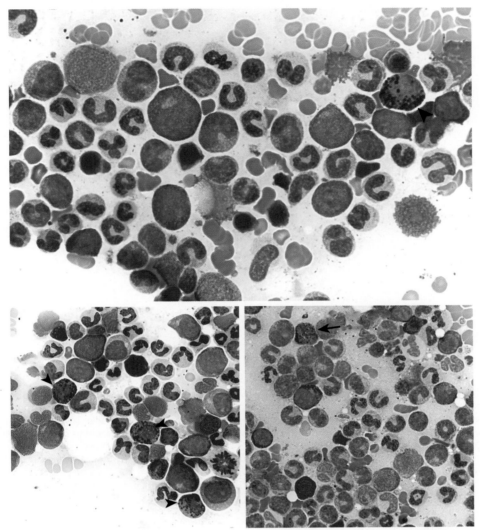

Fig. 27.19 Bone marrow cytology in three cats with myeloid hyperplasia. In each case, there is an increased M:E ratio with complete maturation that is orderly to mildly left-shifted with mildly increased immature forms. Basophil precursors can be identified by their deep purple cytoplasmic granules *(arrowheads)*, and eosinophil precursors can be identified by their bright pink cytoplasmic granules *(arrow)*. The few erythroid cells present have a more basophilic staining pattern to the cytoplasm and denser chromatin compared with the predominant myeloid population (Wright-Giemsa stain, original magnification 1000× *[top]* and 500× *[bottom]*).

distinction may not be possible without additional diagnostic testing.[12,46-48] A mixed population of lymphoid cells with IHC or clear B-lymphocyte aggregates would support a reactive process, whereas a sheetlike expansion or well-dispersed proliferation of T lymphocytes would support a neoplastic process. In some cases of lymphoma metastatic to the marrow, there may be a paratrabecular distribution of the lymphoid cells.

If significantly increased numbers of a monomorphic population of immature or large-sized lymphocytes are seen, this would support a neoplastic lymphoid population (Fig. 27.31). Distinction between lymphoid leukemia and lymphoma requires correlation to CBC findings and other potential sites of involvement (lymph nodes, internal organs), and potentially flow cytometry. With a robust lymphoid proliferation, particularly with lymphoid neoplasia, there are often background cytoplasmic fragments, referred to as *lymphoglandular bodies*. These fragments are more typical of lymphoid neoplasia than of other hematopoietic proliferations (see Fig. 27.31).

Plasma Cells

Plasma cells in bone marrow are typically in low numbers (<2%–3% of nucleated cells) in dogs and cats and have similar morphology to elsewhere in the body[4,31] (see Fig. 27.28). Occasional Mott cells may be seen, which are plasma cells that contain cytoplasmic immunoglobulin inclusions (Russell bodies), or occasional flame cells, which have a peripheral pink cytoplasmic fringe of immunoglobulin material. With cytology, plasma cells can be unevenly distributed and are often aggregated within unit particles (see Fig. 27.27). On histopathology, distinction between plasma cells and later-stage erythroid cells can be difficult, but typically plasma cells are identified by their eccentric nuclei, more abundant basophilic cytoplasm, and eosinophilic perinuclear clear zone (Fig. 27.32). Histologically, plasma cells may be in perivascular aggregates.

Increased plasma cells in bone marrow can be seen with causes of antigenic stimulation, similar to lymphocytosis. These include immune-mediated conditions; infectious etiologies, such as feline infectious peritonitis (FIP) in cats; chronic ehrlichiosis; leishmaniasis;

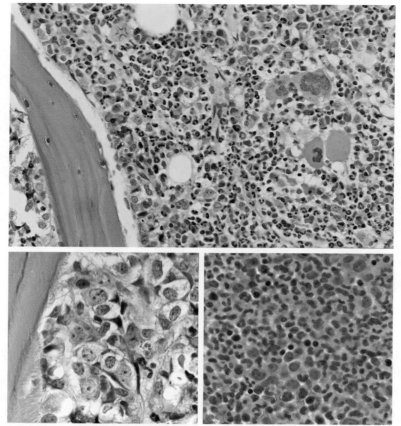

Fig. 27.20 Bone marrow core biopsy from two dogs with myeloid hyperplasia. In both cases, there is severe hypercellularity with an increased M:E ratio. On histopathology, myeloid lineage cells are identified by their convoluted lobulated nuclei, particularly in later-stage precursors *(bottom right)*. Earlier myeloid precursors arise adjacent to the bone (paratrabecular) *(top and bottom left,* note the cells adjacent to bony trabeculae*)*. Compared with early erythroid cells, early myeloid cells *(bottom left)* are larger and have increased cytoplasmic volume with eosinophilic granularity and a more open chromatin pattern (H&E stain, original magnification 400× *[top]*, 400× *[bottom right]*, and 1000× *[bottom left]*).

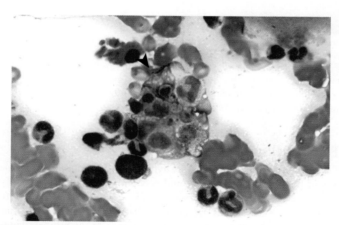

Fig. 27.21 Bone marrow cytology from a dog with immune-mediated neutropenia. Immune-mediated neutropenia may present as ineffective granulopoiesis characterized by myeloid hyperplasia in the marrow with a peripheral neutropenia. Phagocytosis of neutrophils or other myeloid cells by macrophages can aid in confirmation of precursor destruction. Note the eccentric nucleus *(arrowhead)* of this highly phagocytic macrophage with cytoplasmic neutrophils and myelocytes (Wright-Giemsa stain, original magnification 1000×).

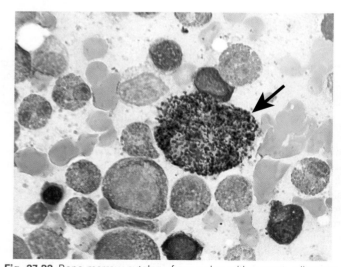

Fig. 27.22 Bone marrow cytology from a dog with a mast cell tumor. Eosinophil hyperplasia in bone marrow can be seen secondary to mast cell neoplasia. Note the brightly colored pink granules in the eosinophil myelocytes, metamyelocytes, band eosinophils, and mature eosinophils. Metastatic mast cell tumor involving bone marrow can be easily identified if there are sheets or aggregates of mast cells cytologically. However, in some cases, only low numbers of neoplastic mast cells may be seen *(arrow)*. If these cells are atypical in morphology with larger cell size *(as pictured here)*, altered granularity, or atypical nuclear features, this can aid in the interpretation of metastatic neoplasia (Wright-Giemsa stain, original magnification 250×).

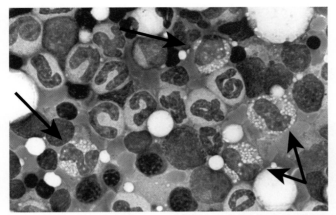

Fig. 27.23 Bone marrow cytology from a greyhound dog with gray eosinophils. This bone marrow was sampled during complete staging for a mast cell tumor. Although neoplastic mast cells were not identified, there is eosinophil hyperplasia in the bone marrow. Greyhounds, other sighthounds, and rarely other breeds of dog may have gray eosinophils *(arrows)*. These eosinophils have normal function, but have clear staining of the cytoplasmic secondary granules, rather than the typical bright pink color expected in eosinophils. These cells need to be correctly identified in peripheral blood or bone marrow as eosinophils, rather than interpreted as toxic change within neutrophils or neutrophil precursors (Wright-Giemsa stain, original magnification 1000×).

myeloid hyperplasia; multiple myeloma/plasma cell neoplasia; or aplastic anemia, although this may reflect a proportional increase resulting from lack of other hematopoietic cells, rather than a true plasmacytosis[4,31] (see Box 27.12; see Figs. 27.32; Fig. 27.33). Distinction between plasma cell neoplasia and reactive plasmacytosis can be challenging in some cases, particularly because multiple myeloma may have well-differentiated and mature plasma cell morphology. These cases may be aided by correlation with additional diagnostic testing results supporting multiple myeloma, including serum protein electrophoresis, radiography to detect lytic bone lesions, assessment for Bence Jones proteinuria, or by ruling out infectious diseases, such as rickettsial infections. Large expansive sheets of plasma cells, even if well differentiated, would suggest multiple myeloma.

Mast Cells

Mast cells can be seen in low numbers in normal bone marrow on cytology, particularly in unit particles, and are identified by their distinctive purple cytoplasmic granules. With histopathology, mast cells are often too subtle to be seen in normal marrow. Mast cells may be in increased numbers with aplastic anemia, myelofibrosis, inflammatory processes, alongside other neoplasia, such as lymphoma, with various causes of regenerative or nonregenerative anemia, or with metastatic mast cell tumor[4,31,50] (see Box 27.12; see Figs. 27.22 and 27.27). Metastatic mast cell tumor can be distinguished from hyperplasia by increased atypia within the mast cell population, dense aggregates of mast cells best seen with histopathology,

TABLE 27.7	**Megakaryocyte Lineage Maturation**	
Name of Cell Stage	**Cytological Description**	**Cytological Image**
Megakaryoblast	Large-size cell; high nuclear-to-cytoplasmic ratio; small volume of deep-blue cytoplasm with peripheral blebbing and possibly few clear vacuoles; large-size, round nucleus with visible nucleoli and fine granular chromatin pattern	
Promegakaryocyte	Very-large-size cell; moderate volume of medium- to deep-blue cytoplasm with peripheral blebbing and possibly few clear vacuoles; 2–4 medium-size, round nuclei without nucleoli and with a coarse chromatin pattern	
Basophilic megakaryocyte	Extremely large-size cell; small to moderate volume of medium-blue cytoplasm with peripheral blebbing and possibly few clear vacuoles; large multilobulated nucleus with coarse to dense chromatin pattern	
Mature (granular) megakaryocyte	Extremely large-size cell (50–200 μm diameter); high volume of pale-pink cytoplasm with numerous fine pink-magenta granules; large multilobulated nucleus with dense clumped chromatin pattern	

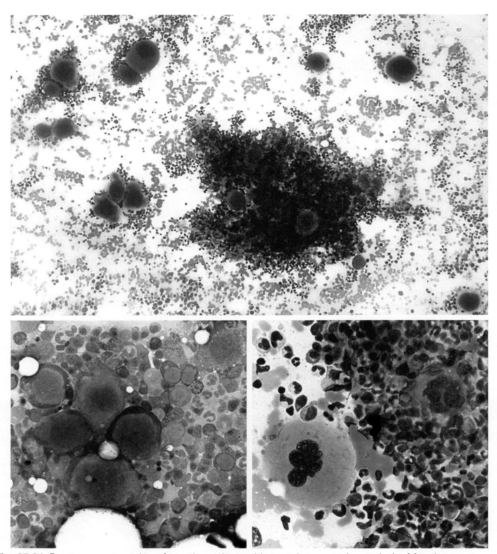

Fig. 27.24 Bone marrow cytology from three dogs with megakaryocyte hyperplasia. Megakaryocytes are identifiable from low magnification because of their large size. Megakaryocytes are often seen in close association with unit particles or can be seen in more hemodiluted areas of the slide. In each of the three cases, there is an increased number of megakaryocytes as well as a left shift with more frequent basophilic megakaryocytes (see Table 27.7 for description of mature versus basophilic megakaryocytes) (Wright-Giemsa stain, original magnification 100× *[top]* and 500× *[bottom]*).

or effacement of marrow elements by sheets of mast cells. With histopathology, if a mast cell population is suspected but is difficult to confirm, special stains, such as Giemsa or toluidine blue, can be used to highlight the metachromatic cytoplasmic granules in the mast cells.

Macrophages/Histiocytes

Macrophages are normally seen in bone marrow in low numbers (<1%–2% of nucleated cells[4]) and are morphologically typical of macrophages elsewhere in the body. Macrophages may have cytoplasmic vacuolation and phagocytized cytoplasmic debris or hemosiderin pigment, which may aid in distinction from other myeloid cells. Macrophages are normal constituents of erythropoietic islands in which a macrophage is surrounded by developing erythroid precursor cells to provide nutrients and phagocytize extruded nuclei from metarubricytes (see Fig. 27.13). Macrophages may be increased with necrosis; inflammation, including that caused by an infectious etiology; immune-mediated conditions; neoplasia; or histiocytic proliferative disorders (histiocytic sarcoma, neoplastic or non-neoplastic

hemophagocytic syndrome, or reactive histiocytosis)[4,31,51] (Figs. 27.34 and 27.35; see Box 27.13).

A minor component of phagocytosis by macrophages can be seen in normal bone marrow as a result of phagocytosis of senescent RBCs, extruded metarubricyte nuclei, and removal of apoptotic cellular debris. Increased phagocytic activity by macrophages can be seen secondary to necrosis, inflammation, infection (mycobacteriosis, leishmaniasis, histoplasmosis, cytauxzoonosis), infection by hemoparasites (*Babesia* spp., *Mycoplasma* spp.), immune-mediated destruction of precursor cells, dyserythropoiesis, severe erythroid hyperplasia, blood transfusion, neoplasia, or hemophagocytic histiocytic proliferative disorders (hemophagocytic histiocytic sarcoma or neoplastic or non-neoplastic hemophagocytic syndrome)[4] (see Box 27.13; see Figs. 27.16, 27.17, and 27.34).

Stromal Elements

Normal stromal elements that comprise bone marrow and associated bone tissue include bone trabeculae with their embedded osteocytes in lacunae and flattened surface bone-lining cells, adipocytes within the

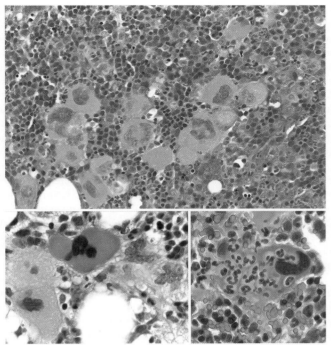

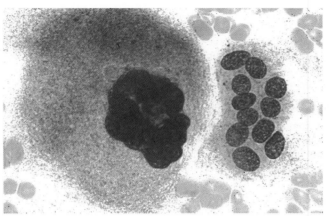

Fig. 27.26 Bone marrow cytology; megakaryocyte and osteoclast. Megakaryocytes need to be distinguished from osteoclasts cytologically. Mature megakaryocytes have a single, condensed, multilobulated nucleus and eosinophilic, granular cytoplasm *(left)*; osteoclasts have similar cytoplasmic color and granularity but have multiple separate similarly sized nuclei *(right)*; and osteoclasts are uncommonly seen in bone marrow aspirates and may be associated with bone modeling/remodeling, such as in young animals or animals with chronic renal disease, metabolic bone disease, inflammation, microfracture/trauma, or neoplasia (Wright-Giemsa stain, original magnification 240×). (Reprinted with permission from Grindem CB. Bone marrow biopsy and evaluation. *Vet Clin Small Anim.* 1989;19[4]:680.)

Fig. 27.25 Core biopsy samples from three dogs with megakaryocyte hyperplasia. In all three cases, there is an increase in megakaryocyte numbers, and left shift is also evident *(top and bottom left)*. On histopathology, megakaryocytes are easily identified by their large size. Mature megakaryocytes have eosinophilic cytoplasm and a tightly lobular nucleus with dense to clumped chromatin. Basophilic megakaryocytes have a blue-gray quality to the cytoplasm and a more open chromatin pattern of the nucleus *(several in top, right two megakaryocytes in bottom left)*. Emperipolesis is a unique feature in megakaryocytes that can be seen with cytology or core biopsy. Emperipolesis is a movement of neutrophils through the megakaryocyte cytoplasm *(bottom right)*, and is a different process than actual phagocytosis of neutrophils. There may be an association with inflammation (H&E stain, original magnification 400× *[top]*, 400× *[bottom right]*, and 1000× *[bottom left]*).

medullary spaces, and accompanying supportive interstitial stromal cells, capillaries, and larger blood vessels.

Osteoblasts and Osteoclasts

Osteoblasts can be seen in low numbers in normal marrow, but with mature quiescent bone, osteoblasts are typically not readily apparent. Osteoblasts are large rounded to elongated cells that have a perinuclear clear zone, reminiscent of plasma cells; however, osteoblasts are much larger than plasma cells and have a less condensed chromatin pattern. Osteoblasts may be increased with bone remodeling, which can accompany myelofibrosis or can be seen with inflammation, infection, or neoplasia and in young animals with active bone modeling, chronic renal disease, metabolic bone disease, or microfracture/trauma. On histopathology, osteoblasts are clearly apparent as plump, stellate-shaped cells lining up along bone trabeculae, often associated with endosteal new bone proliferation. Osteoclasts are multinucleate cells that resorb osteoid matrix with bone remodeling and therefore are often not seen in quiescent bone but can be increased with similar causes of bone reactivity/remodeling or in young animals. Osteoclasts must be differentiated from megakaryocytes, as discussed previously (see Fig. 27.26). On histopathology, osteoclasts can be seen in areas of remodeling, in scalloped areas of the bone referred to as *Howship's lacunae.* Osteosclerosis, such as that associated with pyruvate kinase deficiency, and osteopetrosis caused by a hereditary osteoclast defect are syndromes where there is expansion of the bone tissue with

narrowing of marrow spaces leading to anemia or other cytopenias. These conditions are very rare.[4]

Stromal spindle cells and capillaries are often more prominent in hypocellular marrow samples on cytology because of relative lack of hematopoietic cells superimposed on these elements. Stromal cells and associated extracellular matrix may also be increased with myelofibrosis, which most typically requires core biopsy with histopathology for confirmation, although in some cases cytological findings may be suggestive (Fig. 27.36).

Myelofibrosis

Myelofibrosis is often accompanied by hematopoietic hypocellularity. Some retained foci of persistent hematopoiesis or compensatory hyperplasia of marrow elements commonly exist, along with increased hemosiderin stores (see Fig. 27.36). Myelofibrosis is rarely a primary form of myeloproliferative neoplasia and is much more commonly secondary (Box 27.14). In dogs, causes include immune-mediated disease, especially PIMA; neoplasia; inflammation, infection, vascular injury or necrosis in the marrow; drug-associated or with irradiation; pyruvate kinase (PK) deficiency; or an idiopathic change.[4,18,31,52] Myelofibrosis is less common in cats but can occur with immune-mediated anemia, FIP, chronic renal failure, or neoplasia, such as MDS/AML.[52] Myelofibrosis is most commonly accompanied by nonregenerative anemia with normal neutrophil and platelet counts, but neutropenia and/or thrombocytopenia can be seen in more severe cases. Ovalocytes and dacryocytes can be seen in circulation in some cases but are not specific for myelofibrosis.[27,53]

Myelonecrosis

Myelonecrosis can be seen in some cases and is typically easier to confirm with histopathology than with cytology, although necrosis may be suggested with cytology on the basis of amorphous background debris and smudged cellular details. On histopathology, necrosis can be seen as regional hypereosinophilia with nuclear and cellular debris and is often accompanied by inflammation, edema, fibrin accumulation, and/or hemorrhage, and this may corroborate the suspicion and differentiate the changes from an artifact of sample collection or crush artifact (Fig. 27.37). Causes of myelonecrosis are similar to those of necrosis elsewhere in the body and include ischemia or hypoxemia, inflammation or infection, drug-related effects, neoplasia, vascular abnormality, immune-mediated processes, or severe hematopoietic cell injury[4,31,54] (Fig. 27.38).

Serous Atrophy of Fat

Gelatinous transformation or serous atrophy of fat in the marrow refers to accumulation of mucoid pink matrix (Alcian blue positive) with withered adipocytes. This change is uncommon but can be seen with chronic anorexia/starvation or cachexia.

INFLAMMATION/INFECTION IN THE MARROW

Detection of inflammation in bone marrow can be difficult in some cases because of the overlap in cell types normally in the marrow and inflammatory cells, including neutrophils, histiocytoid/monocytic

cells, lymphocytes, and plasma cells. Particularly with core biopsy with histopathology, there may be additional evidence for inflammation to corroborate a suspicion for increased inflammatory cells. For acute inflammatory conditions, this corroborative evidence may include edema, fibrin accumulation, necrosis, and/or hemorrhage. Additional evidence to support chronic inflammatory conditions may include fibrosis, granulomatous foci, or bony changes. When there is granulomatous inflammation, in particular, careful investigation for etiological agents is recommended. Common organisms causing granulomatous inflammation in the bone marrow include *Mycobacterium* spp., fungal infections and in particular systemic mycoses, or *Leishmania* spp. (see Fig. 27.32; Figs. 27.39 to 27.41). If routine staining does not identify organisms, additional special stains can be considered to further assess for *Mycobacterium* spp. (acid fast or Fites-Faraco stain) or fungal organisms (PAS or GMS stains) (see Box 27.3). Acute inflammation in the marrow can be caused by infection, including bacterial, protozoal, rickettsial, fungal, or other agents, as well as necrosis, drug-related effects, neoplasia, vascular abnormality, or immune-mediated processes.

Other infectious agents that can be discovered in bone marrow include *Cytauxzoon felis*; other hemoparasites, such as *Babesia* spp. and *Mycoplasma* spp.; rickettsial diseases; and other multisystemic protozoal infections, such as *Toxoplasma* spp.[55] In cases of hemoparasites, such as *Babesia* spp. or *Mycoplasma* spp., peripheral blood smear evaluation or PCR testing are more likely to confirm the diagnosis compared with bone marrow evaluation. *C. felis* has a blood phase of infection with merozoites in RBCs but also has a tissue phase of infection, with formation of large schizonts in macrophages, and this component may be captured with bone marrow evaluation (Fig. 27.42). Ehrlichial infection typically has an acute hypercellular phase in the marrow, but with chronic infection, dogs can develop pancytopenia with severe bone marrow hypocellularity, often with accompanying plasmacytosis and mastocytosis in the marrow.[29,31] Ehrlichial organisms are rarely seen in bone marrow myeloid cells. Some viral infections, including parvovirus and panleukopenia virus infections, can affect the marrow and are typically associated with bone marrow hypoplasia at an early stage of infection with concurrent neutropenia and subsequent marrow recovery. FeLV retroviral infection in cats commonly has hematopoietic effects, with potential for panhypoplasia/aplastic anemia, PRCA, MDS, or AML. Because of the wide range of hematopoietic disturbances that have been associated with FeLV

BOX 27.11 Causes of Megakaryocytic Hyperplasia and Megakaryocytic Hypoplasia

Megakaryocytic Hyperplasia	Megakaryocytic Hypoplasia
With Thrombocytopenia	**Aplastic Anemia**
• Immune-mediated destruction of platelets (IMT)	**(see Box 27.5)**
• Increased platelet consumption (intravascular coagulation, hypersplenism, vascular injury/abnormality)	**Selective Megakaryocytic Hypoplasia**
• Infectious etiology (rickettsial disease)	• Amegakaryocytic thrombocytopenia (immune-mediated destruction of megakaryocytes)
• Megakaryocytic leukemia	• Drug administration
With Thrombocytosis	• Infectious causes
• Drug administration (vincristine)	
• Iron deficiency	
• Chronic inflammation	
• Megakaryocytic neoplasia (megakaryocytic leukemia or essential thrombocythemia)	

BOX 27.12 Causes of Increased Lymphocytes, Plasma Cells, and Mast Cells

Increased Lymphocytes	Increased Plasma Cells	Increased Mast Cells

• Small lymphocytes
  • Antigenic stimulation (lymphoid aggregates can also be seen)
    • Immune-mediated conditions (particularly nonregenerative IMHA or PRCA in cats and IMHA/IMT, PIMA in dogs)
    • Infectious etiology (tickborne diseases, such as ehrlichiosis)
    • Inflammatory conditions
  • Small cell lymphoma or chronic lymphocytic leukemia
• Large immature lymphocytes
  • Lymphoma
  • Acute lymphoblastic leukemia
	• Antigenic stimulation
	  • Immune-mediated conditions
	  • Infectious etiology (FIP in cats, chronic ehrlichiosis, leishmaniasis)
	  • Alongside myeloid hyperplasia
	• Multiple myeloma/plasma cell neoplasia
	• Aplastic anemia
		• Aplastic anemia
		• Myelofibrosis
		• Inflammation
		• Metastatic mast cell tumor
		• Other neoplasia (lymphoma)
		• Anemia (regenerative or nonregenerative)

FIP, feline infectious peritonitis; *IMHA,* immune-mediated hemolytic anemia; *IMT,* immune-mediated thrombocytopenia; *PIMA,* precursor-targeted immune-mediated anemia; *PRCA,* pure red cell aplasia.

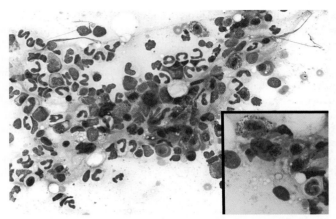

Fig. 27.27 Bone marrow cytology from a dog; prominent plasma cells and mast cells. Marrow is overall hypocellular, with only few groups of myeloid cells adjacent to unit particles. There is increased prominence of well-differentiated mast cells and plasma cells, often in aggregates or closely associated with unit particles. Few small lymphocytes are also noted. With hypocellular marrow of any cause, resident plasma cell, lymphocyte, and mast cell populations may be more prominent. In some cases, such as with chronic ehrlichiosis, there may be actual hyperplasia of the plasma cell and mast cell components (Wright-Giemsa stain, original magnification 500×, *inset:* 1000×).

infection, FeLV testing is recommended in any cat with unexplained hematological abnormalities. It should be noted that FeLV testing on bone marrow itself may reveal an infection that was not identified via testing of the peripheral blood. PCR testing on bone marrow may identify latent infection not captured with enzyme-linked immunosorbent assay (ELISA) or immunofluorescent antibody assay (IFA) testing on blood.[55]

NEOPLASIA

Neoplasia in bone marrow can be either primary or metastatic to involve the marrow[56] (Table 27.8). Primary neoplasia affecting the bone marrow may be of hematopoietic origin (myeloproliferative, lymphoid, histiocytic, or undifferentiated) or nonhematopoietic (primary bone/stromal tumors that secondarily involve the marrow spaces).[6] Bone/stromal tumors, such as osteosarcoma, chondrosarcoma, and fibrosarcoma, are not typically sampled under the guise of bone marrow evaluation because these types of neoplasia are not typically associated with cytopenias or atypical circulating cells, and therefore these are best considered with bone[57] and soft tissue tumors elsewhere in this text.

Leukemia is defined as neoplasia arising within bone marrow or blood, and most leukemias have a circulating component. Subleukemic or aleukemic leukemias are possible and affect bone marrow but are not seen in circulation. *Acute leukemia* refers to an increased immature "blast" cell component with a variable amount of maturation/

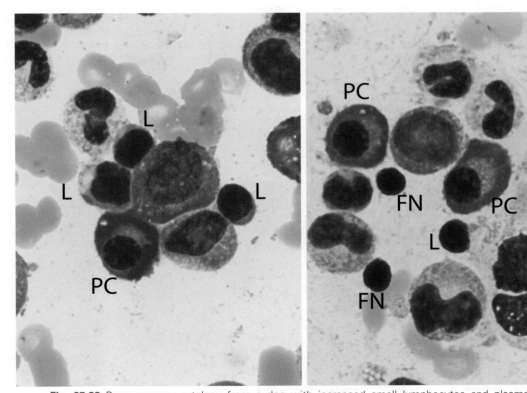

Fig. 27.28 Bone marrow cytology from a dog with increased small lymphocytes and plasma cells. Well-differentiated plasma cells (*PC*) and small lymphocytes (*L*) are indicated. Plasma cells can be distinguished from rubricytes or metarubricytes (*MR*) by their increased cytoplasmic volume, eccentric nucleus, and perinuclear clear zone. Lymphocytes can be distinguished from rubricytes and metarubricytes by their scant cytoplasm and more finely clumped chromatin pattern containing fewer clear spaces. Lymphocytes can be distinguished from free metarubricyte nuclei (*FN*) because these free nuclei have a darker, more completely filled-in chromatin pattern and lack a rim of cytoplasm (Wright-Giemsa stain, original magnification 1000×).

differentiation. Acute leukemias can be further divided into those of myeloid and lymphoid origins. Myeloid leukemias are additionally subdivided into undifferentiated; myeloblastic, with or without maturation; promyelocytic; monoblastic/monocytic; myelomonocytic; erythroblastic; and megakaryocytic variants (Figs. 27.43 and 27.44). *Chronic leukemia* refers to a neoplasm with a predominance of mature-appearing cells with a retained pyramidal distribution of cells within that lineage, and these neoplasms are now referred to as *myeloproliferative neoplasms* (MPNs).[56] In acute leukemias, typically there is rapid progression of disease, whereas chronic leukemias typically have a more slowly progressive, chronic clinical course. Primary hematopoietic neoplasia in bone marrow can be multifocal in early cases or can be diffusely effacing within the marrow, referred to as *myelophthisis*.

General accepted guidelines for an expanded cell population that would suggest a neoplasm include: greater than 20% blast cells for AML, greater than 30% lymphoid cells for lymphoma/lymphoid leukemia, and greater than 15% plasma cells for plasma cell neoplasia/multiple myeloma.[4,56] Large sheets or aggregates of other cell populations suggest neoplasia of those cell types, such as mast cells for mast cell tumor or histiocytes for histiocytic proliferative disease.

When complete marrow effacement by the neoplastic cells is absent, it can be difficult to make a definitive interpretation of neoplasia with

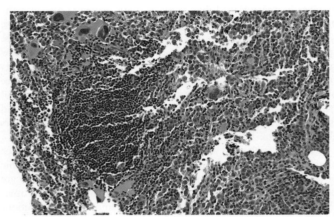

Fig. 27.29 Bone marrow core biopsy from a cat with precursor-targeted, immune-mediated anemia (PIMA). Note the large lymphoid aggregate *(dark rounded basophilic area at left aspect of image)* composed of predominantly small lymphocytes. In the background, there is evidence of erythroid hyperplasia with left shift and megakaryocyte hyperplasia. This cat had concurrent nonregenerative anemia with findings supportive of ineffective erythropoiesis associated with PIMA. Lymphoid aggregates can be seen rarely in normal animals but may be more frequent with chronic antigenic stimulation, and particularly with immune-mediated processes. On cytology, increased numbers of small lymphocytes may be noted in some areas of the sample, whereas on core biopsy the architecture of the lymphoid aggregate is apparent (H&E stain, original magnification 400×).

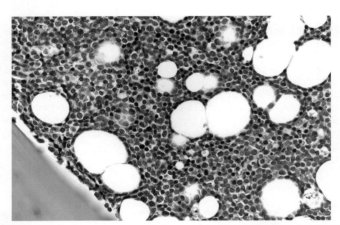

Fig. 27.30 Bone marrow core biopsy sample from a dog with lymphoid neoplasia. The hematopoietic tissue is replaced by sheets of fairly monomorphic small to intermediate-sized lymphocytes. The effacement of the tissue provides clear evidence for neoplasia. Differentials may include lymphoma or involvement with chronic lymphocytic leukemia (which usually arises from the spleen rather than the marrow). This dog had a peripheral lymphocytosis of 22,000/μL. Correlation to physical examination findings, diagnostic imaging results, and potentially flow cytometry or immunohistochemistry may help further characterize this neoplastic process (see Box 27.3) (H&E stain, original magnification 400×).

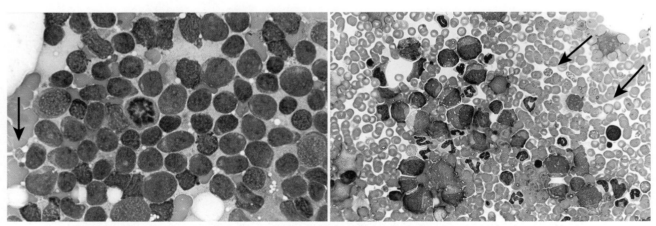

Fig. 27.31 Bone marrow cytology from two dogs with lymphoma. Both dogs have a predominance of large immature hematopoietic cells with prominent nucleoli ("blasts") in bone marrow, confirmed to be large cell lymphoma. Note the lymphoglandular bodies *(blue cytoplasmic fragments; arrows)* in the background. Lymphoma can have a somewhat variable appearance cytologically (note the cytoplasmic vacuoles in the lymphoma on the right, not evident on the left). If lymphoid origin is not clear with morphology alone, additional advanced diagnostic testing can be considered (flow cytometry, PCR for antigen receptor rearrangement (PARR), or biopsy with immunohistochemistry; see Box 27.3) (Wright-Giemsa stain, original magnification 1000× *[left]* and 500× *[right]*).

cytology or with histopathology. Early bone marrow recovery with repopulation of the marrow after a prior insult can have an increased proportion of blasts or other immature precursor cells that can mimic the appearance of neoplasia. This can also occur with a very early regenerative response to a peripheral hematopoietic stimulus, and therefore an increased immature/blast component within the marrow can be misinterpreted as potentially neoplastic. When there is an increased immature cell component, the context of historical CBC data and additional clinical information should be taken into consideration because the marrow may represent just a snapshot in time before a

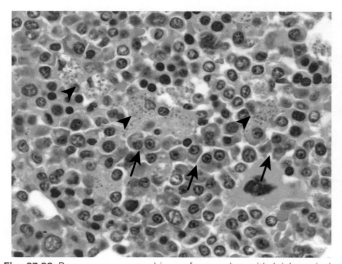

Fig. 27.32 Bone marrow core biopsy from a dog with leishmaniasis. Hypercellular-appearing marrow with numerous macrophages containing multiple small amastigotes *(arrowheads)*. Note the increased numbers of plasma cells *(arrows)*, which can be seen with antigenic stimulation or chronic inflammation. The presence of *Leishmania* spp. amastigotes clearly rules out a neoplastic plasma cell population despite the high numbers of plasma cells present. Plasma cells on histopathology may overlap in appearance with middle- to late-stage erythroid cells but are often most identifiable by their perinuclear clear zone (H&E stain, original magnification 1000×).

subsequent repopulation occurs. Reassessment of the CBC and, potentially, resampling of bone marrow in 3 to 5 or even 5 to 7 days may be necessary. With a regenerative or hyperplastic response, this would allow time for maturation of the expanded immature population and restoration of the pyramidal distribution in that lineage. A retained or further expanded immature population after 7 days would lend support for a neoplastic proliferation. The anatomical distribution within the marrow on a core biopsy sample may aid in further characterization of the cells present. When an immature mitotically active population is located along the paratrabecular area and is accompanied by maturing neutrophils with myeloid hyperplasia, this likely reflects an early hyperplastic myeloid population. When an immature cell population is present within the interstitial areas in increased numbers, there may be more concern for an emerging neoplastic component (see Fig. 27.38). Additional considerations for an interstitial expanded immature component on a core biopsy sample include a macrophage/histiocyte population, a megakaryoblast component, particularly if there is megakaryocytic hyperplasia, or a displaced expanded hyperplastic myeloid population.

If there is evidence of dysplasia within multiple cell lineages with unexplained peripheral cytopenias and accompanying marrow hypercellularity with increased immature cells in the marrow (but with <20% blasts), these features suggest MDS. MDS is a type of hematopoietic neoplasia that can eventually transition to AML (Fig. 27.45). In some cases, there can be overlapping features between other causes of ineffective hematopoiesis and MDS. In these difficult cases, response to therapy and correlation with additional clinical information may be the best differentiators.

With some types of hematopoietic neoplasia that may have a patchy distribution in the marrow or relatively low numbers of neoplastic cells present, distinction from a hyperplastic process can be very difficult. Examples include mast cell hyperplasia versus metastatic mast cell tumor, small cell lymphoma or chronic lymphocytic leukemia versus reactive lymphocytosis, or plasma cell hyperplasia versus multiple myeloma. A combination of cytology and core biopsy with histopathology, potentially with additional special stains (e.g., Giemsa for mast cell tumor) or ancillary diagnostics (IHC, flow cytometry, PARR for potential lymphoma), may be necessary for definitive diagnosis

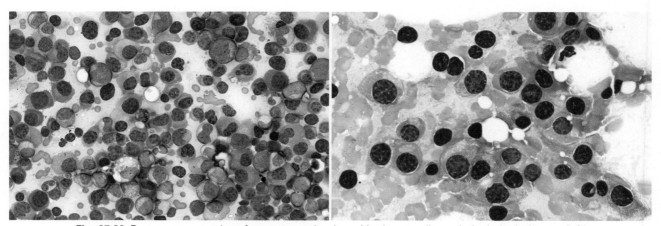

Fig. 27.33 Bone marrow cytology from a cat and a dog with plasma cell neoplasia. In both the cat *(left)* and the dog *(right)*, the vast majority of cells in the marrow are neoplastic plasma cells, with only few hematopoietic precursor cells in the background. Note the plasmacytoid morphology of the neoplastic cells, including eccentric nuclei with a coarsely clumped chromatin pattern, and characteristic blue cytoplasmic coloration with a perinuclear clear zone. Plasma cell neoplasia in bone marrow is typically a component of multiple myeloma, which is a clinical diagnosis based on certain inclusion criteria. Plasma cell neoplasia can be well differentiated, or neoplastic cells can be more pleomorphic and atypical *(left)* with binucleation, anisocytosis, and anisokaryosis (Wright-Giemsa stain, original magnification 500× left and 1000× right).

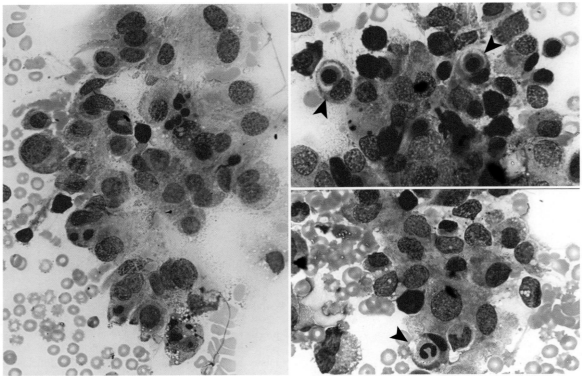

Fig. 27.34 Bone marrow cytology from a dog with histiocytosis in the marrow. Increased numbers of mildly pleomorphic histiocytes are recognized by their eccentric nuclei, high volume of medium-blue cytoplasm, and phagocytic activity with cytoplasmic iron pigment *(dark-blue intracellular pigment on left)* and occasional phagocytosis of hematopoietic precursors *(arrowheads; metarubricytes in top right, neutrophil in bottom right)*. Further characterization of a histiocytic proliferative population as neoplastic or benign/reactive can be very challenging, particularly because the hemophagocytic variant of histiocytic sarcoma often has bland morphological features. Findings need to be correlated to additional clinical information, bloodwork, and diagnostic imaging results (Wright-Giemsa, original magnification 500× left and 1000× right).

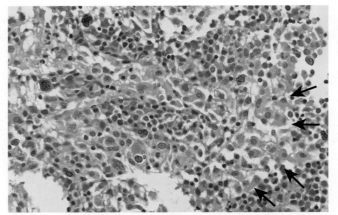

Fig. 27.35 Bone marrow core biopsy from a Bernese Mountain Dog with histiocytosis in the marrow. This marrow is hypercellular with a combination of myeloid and erythroid hyperplasia and a prominent population of histiocytes *(occupying much of the image, delineated from the surrounding marrow elements by arrows)*. There is abundant iron *(yellow-brown pigment)* in these histiocytes, but the morphological features in this population are fairly bland. Definitive distinction can be very difficult between a benign/reactive histiocytic proliferation (e.g., with an immune-mediated process, drug reaction, or benign variant of hemophagocytic syndrome) and a neoplastic proliferation (as with hemophagocytic histiocytic sarcoma). Correlation with additional clinical information, bloodwork, diagnostic imaging results, and potentially response to therapy is helpful (H&E stain, original magnification 400×).

BOX 27.13 Causes of Increased Macrophages and Increased Phagocytic Activity

Increased Macrophages/Histiocytes
- Inflammation (including infectious etiology)
- Immune-mediated conditions
- Necrosis
- Neoplasia
- Histiocytic proliferative disorders (histiocytic sarcoma, reactive histiocytosis, neoplastic or non-neoplastic hemophagocytic syndrome)

Increased Phagocytic Activity by Macrophages
- Immune-mediated conditions (particularly precursor-targeting immune-mediated anemia (PIMA) or immune-mediated neutropenia)
- Necrosis
- Inflammation
- Infection (mycobacteriosis, leishmaniasis, histoplasmosis, cytauxzoonosis), hemoparasites (*Babesia* spp., *Mycoplasma* spp.)
- Dyserythropoiesis
- Severe erythroid hyperplasia
- Blood transfusion
- Neoplasia
- Hemophagocytic histiocytic proliferative disorders (hemophagocytic histiocytic sarcoma or hemophagocytic syndrome)

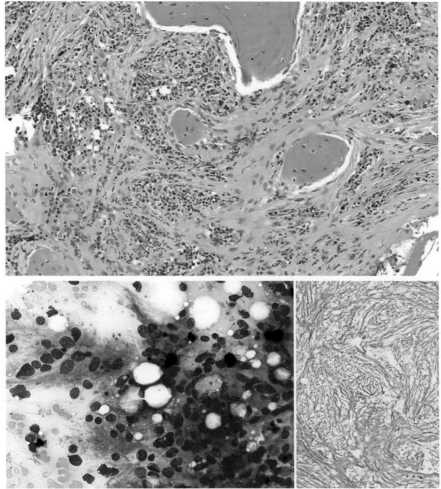

Fig. 27.36 Bone marrow core biopsy and cytology from two dogs with myelofibrosis. Myelofibrosis is often a process that can only be discerned on histopathology because there is preservation of marrow architecture with core biopsy *(top)*. In some cases, the suggestion of myelofibrosis may be evident with aspiration cytology *(bottom left; note the fibrillar pink-magenta extracellular matrix material)*. Myelofibrosis is most commonly secondary and can either be mild and multifocal within the marrow (see Fig. 27.17) or can replace most of the marrow *(top:* note the streaming eosinophilic fibrous tissue occupying the medullary space). Pockets of active hematopoiesis may be retained, though the overall hematopoietic cellularity is decreased (note groups of cells among the fibrous tissue). Reticulin stain *(bottom right:* note black-staining fibers) or trichrome stain can be utilized to highlight the fibrous tissue and is particularly useful in suspicious or borderline cases *(top:* H&E stain, original magnification 400×; *bottom left:* Wright-Giemsa stain, original magnification 500×; *bottom right:* reticulin stain, original magnification 200×).

BOX 27.14 Causes of Myelofibrosis

Primary Myelofibrosis (Rare Form of Myeloproliferative Neoplasia)

Secondary Myelofibrosis (Most Common)

- Immune-mediated disease (in particular, precursor-targeted immune-mediated anemia [PIMA])
- Neoplasia
- Inflammation, infection, vascular injury, or necrosis in bone marrow
- Drug-associated
- Irradiation
- Pyruvate kinase deficiency (in dogs)
- Feline infectious peritonitis (FIP; in cats)
- Chronic renal failure (in cats)
- Idiopathic

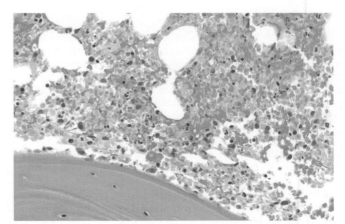

Fig. 27.37 Bone marrow core biopsy from a dog with myelonecrosis. Myelonecrosis, as with other stromal changes, is often most easily identified with core biopsy rather than with aspiration cytology. On histopathology, acute myelonecrosis is identified as areas of eosinophilic smudging of the medullary tissue with cell debris and often has accompanying hemorrhage, as in this case. Causes for myelonecrosis may include ischemia, inflammation/infection, drug effects, neoplasia, vascular abnormality, or immune-mediated processes (H&E stain, original magnification 400×).

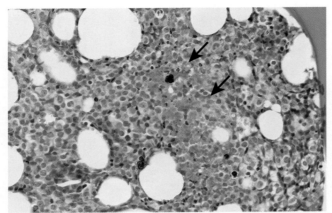

Fig. 27.38 Bone marrow core biopsy from a dog; hematopoietic neoplasia and myelonecrosis. Pancytopenia with atypical cells in circulation was observed in this dog. The marrow is replaced by sheets of monomorphic immature large round cells, consistent with hematopoietic neoplasia. There are areas of necrosis *(arrows)*, which are hypereosinophilic with amorphous/smudged debris. On the basis of the cell morphology, there is a suspicion for acute myeloid leukemia, although definitive characterization would require additional diagnostic testing, such as flow cytometry or immunohistochemistry to rule out lymphoid origin (see Box 27.3). The necrosis may be secondary to the neoplasia in this case (H&E stain, original magnification 400×).

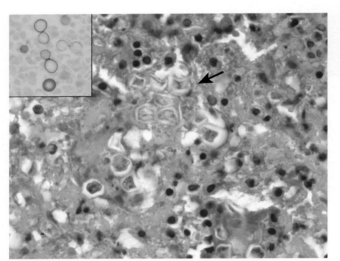

Fig. 27.39 Bone marrow core biopsy from a dog with disseminated blastomycosis. Among background hypereosinophilic necrotic debris there are groups of pale staining, degenerating round yeast organisms *(arrow)*. With Gomori methenamine silver (GMS) staining *(inset)*, the cell walls are outlined *(black)* and broad-based budding is noted, which confirms *Blastomyces dermatitidis* infection. Blastomycosis is a systemic mycotic infection that can affect bone and bone marrow in some cases, along with the skin and lungs being common sites of involvement (H&E stain, original magnification 1000×; *inset:* GMS stain, original magnification 1000×).

(see Box 27.3). With regard to lymphoma versus reactive lymphocytosis, distribution within the marrow may aid in this distinction as well because interstitial aggregates of lymphocytes are more likely to be reactive, whereas paratrabecular aggregates or diffuse distribution of lymphocytes may favor a neoplastic population.[12,46-48,58]

With immature blasts in increased numbers or entirely effacing the marrow, an interpretation of hematopoietic neoplasia may be clear, but the subtype of neoplasia may be difficult to further determine (Figs. 27.46 and 27.47). There can be morphological overlap between AML

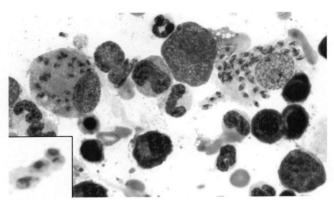

Fig. 27.40 Bone marrow cytology from a dog with disseminated leishmaniasis. Macrophages contain numerous round to oval *Leishmania* spp. amastigotes; organisms are also free in the background. There are accompanying increased plasma cells (identified by their perinuclear clear zone). *Leishmania* amastigotes have a "parachute men" appearance with a pale round nucleus and rod-shaped dark-staining kinetoplast *(inset)* (Wright-Giemsa stain, original magnification 1000×).

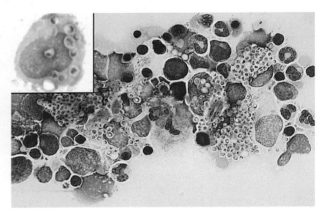

Fig. 27.41 Bone marrow from a cat with disseminated histoplasmosis. Several large macrophages are present, each containing numerous *Histoplasma capsulatum* organisms. Note the half-moon appearance of the organisms *(inset)*. Histoplasmosis is a systemic fungal infection that may affect bone marrow, in addition to the lungs, eyes, and other sites (Wright stain, original magnification 250×).

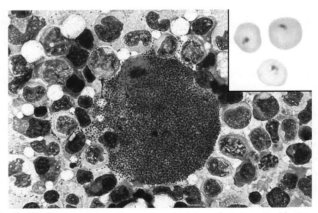

Fig. 27.42 Postmortem bone marrow cytology from a cat with cytauxzoonosis. A large macrophage containing a schizont of *Cytauxzoon felis* is surrounded by predominantly myeloid cells with occasional lymphocytes and plasma cells. *Cytauxzoon* piroplasms were seen in the peripheral blood of this cat before death *(inset)*. Scanning bone marrow smears at low magnification is helpful in identifying the large schizonts, which reflect the tissue phase of *Cytauxzoon* infection (Wright-Giemsa stain, original magnification 250×). (Case courtesy Dr. Jaime Tarigo.)

TABLE 27.8 Categories of Neoplasia in Bone Marrow

Type of Neoplasia	Subcategory of Neoplasia	Additional Subtypes
Primary hematopoietic neoplasia	Acute lymphoblastic leukemia (ALL)	T versus B cell
	Acute myeloid leukemia (AML)	Undifferentiated, myeloblastic with or without maturation, promyelocytic, monoblastic/monocytic, myelomonocytic, erythroblastic, megakaryocytic
	Chronic myeloproliferative neoplasia ("chronic leukemias")	Chronic myelogenous leukemia, polycythemia vera, essential thrombocythemia, primary myelofibrosis
	Chronic lymphocytic leukemia (CLL)	T versus B cell (but note that T cell CLL typically arises within the spleen rather than the marrow)
	Plasma cell neoplasia	Multiple myeloma
Secondary/metastatic/multicentric neoplasia	Lymphoid neoplasia	Lymphoma (various subtypes), chronic lymphocytic leukemia (if arising in the spleen and not primary to the marrow)
	Histiocytic neoplasia	Histiocytic sarcoma, hemophagocytic histiocytic sarcoma (can arise in the marrow as a primary site or involve the marrow in multicentric disease)
	Mast cell tumor	Metastatic mast cell tumor, mast cell leukemia
	Carcinoma	Transitional cell carcinoma, apocrine gland adenocarcinoma of the anal sac, etc.

*Table does not include primary bone tumors (e.g., osteosarcoma, chondrosarcoma, and fibrosarcoma) because these only affect the marrow by indirect extension/bone infiltration and are not typically associated with hematological changes.

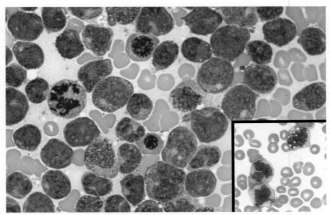

Fig. 27.43 Bone marrow cytology from a dog with acute monocytic leukemia. The marrow is largely replaced by large immature blast cells with only few background hematopoietic precursor cells noted (note a metarubricyte and a rubricyte). On the basis of morphology alone, considerations may include acute myeloid leukemia and lymphoid neoplasia (lymphoma versus acute lymphoblastic leukemia). Based on the cytoplasmic vacuoles and lobular contour of nuclei, in addition to the presence of markedly increased monocytic cells in circulation (*inset of blood smear*), the findings support an acute monocytic leukemia. Monocytic origin was confirmed with flow cytometry (Wright-Giemsa stain, original magnification 1000×).

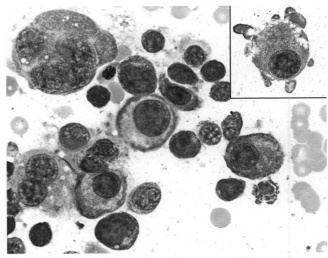

Fig. 27.44 Bone marrow cytology from a cat with megakaryocytic leukemia. Most of the cells in this image are atypical megakaryocytic precursors. Note the binucleation or multinucleation and the prominent cytoplasmic blebbing (*inset*). Megakaryocytic leukemia is rare and may be associated with either thrombocytopenia or thrombocytosis (Wright-Giemsa stain, original magnification 1000×).

(erythroid, megakaryocytic, or myeloid), acute lymphoblastic leukemia (ALL), and bone marrow involvement by lymphoma. IHC or PARR could potentially confirm lymphoid origin, but flow cytometry may be the best test for further characterization of these immature neoplasms because this test can assess for makers of lymphoid and myeloid origins in addition to CD34, which can aid in distinction between ALL and stage V lymphoma. Cytochemical stains are available in an academic setting to help distinguish among subtypes of AML, but in diagnostic practice cytochemical stains are not commonly performed, and the distinction often does not affect prognosis or treatment decisions (see Box 27.3).

Chronic myeloproliferative neoplasms ("chronic leukemias") are uncommon and include CML, polycythemia vera, and essential thrombocythemia. Bone marrow evaluation in these chronic neoplasms is often unrewarding. Bone marrow findings in chronic myeloproliferative neoplasia have a similar and indistinguishable pyramidal distribution as with a severe reactive/hyperplastic process until there is a blast crisis, as may occur at the late stage of disease. A mild degree of dysplasia can be seen in either a hyperplastic or a neoplastic process. The potential for chronic leukemia should be correlated with clinical findings, CBC data, and exclusion of inflammatory/infectious conditions (for CML), causes of secondary

polycythemia (for polycythemia vera), or reactive thrombocytosis (for essential thrombocythemia).

Some dogs may have a benign-appearing proliferative histiocytic population, which, on cytology, may be dispersed throughout the sample or in aggregates (see Fig. 27.34). On histopathology, these histiocytes may be distributed throughout the interstitium or in a more sheetlike arrangement, and cells may have increased phagocytic activity (see Fig. 27.35). Differentials for this type of benign-appearing histiocytic proliferation may include hemophagocytic syndrome, a reactive proliferation, an immune-mediated response, involvement with systemic reactive histiocytosis, or hemophagocytic histiocytic sarcoma. Typical multicentric or disseminated histiocytic sarcoma

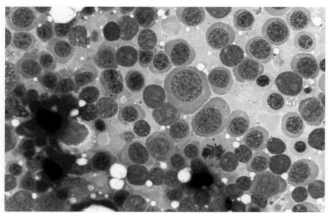

Fig. 27.45 Bone marrow cytology from a cat with myelodysplastic syndrome (MDS). The marrow contains marked erythroid hyperplasia with atypical features and prominent dysplasia within the erythroid lineage cells. Megaloblastic change, binucleation, and frequent nuclear-to-cytoplasmic asynchrony or dysmaturation are prominent. Iron pigment is noted *(dark brown-black globules in bottom left corner)*, which is abnormal in a cat and is often associated with dyserythropoiesis. Based on a blast percentage of less than 20%, erythroid dysplasia, and the marked predominance of erythroid cells, this was classified as MDS with erythroid predominance (MDS-Er). This type of hematopoietic neoplasia can progress to erythroleukemia and may be associated with feline leukemia virus (FeLV) infection (Wright-Giemsa stain, original magnification 100×).

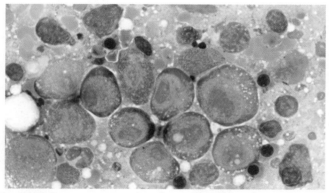

Fig. 27.46 Bone marrow cytology from a dog with poorly differentiated round cell neoplasia. The marrow contains a high number of immature large blast cells, consistent with poorly differentiated round cell neoplasia. The exceedingly large prominent nucleoli of the blast cells are not typical for myeloid, erythroid, or lymphoid cells, in particular. The basophilic background, numerous cytoplasmic fragments (lymphoglandular bodies), and scattered smaller immature lymphoid cells are suggestive of lymphoma, although additional diagnostic testing would be necessary to confirm (see Box 27.3). Increased eosinophil precursors are noted, which may be associated with lymphoma, in particular T-cell lymphoma (Wright-Giemsa stain, original magnification 1000×).

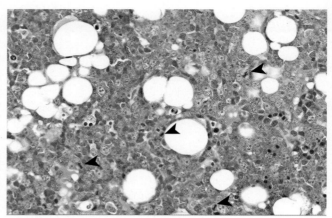

Fig. 27.47 Bone marrow core biopsy from a dog with hematopoietic neoplasia. The marrow is largely effaced by sheets of monomorphic large round cells, consistent with hematopoietic neoplasia. Note the prominent nucleoli, immature features, and increased mitotic figures *(arrowheads)*. On the basis of morphology alone, further classification is difficult, but in this case large cell lymphoma was confirmed. Advanced diagnostic testing may be necessary, in some cases, to more fully classify hematopoietic neoplasms, especially with poorly differentiated tumors (see Box 27.3) (H&E stain, original magnification 400×).

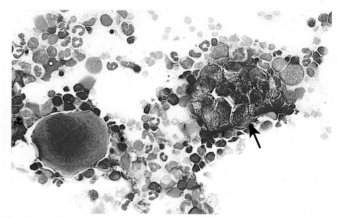

Fig. 27.48 Bone marrow cytology from a dog with metastatic carcinoma. Among the background hematopoietic cell population, there is a large cluster of cohesive, vacuolated epithelial cells *(arrow)*. This is metastasis from a pulmonary carcinoma in this dog. More common metastatic carcinomas to bone or bone marrow may include transitional cell carcinoma from the urinary bladder and apocrine gland adenocarcinoma of the anal sac. Scanning a cytological slide at low magnification to identify unusual groups of cells is an important step in assessing for foci of metastatic neoplasia. These groups are often randomly distributed within a marrow sample and therefore may be missed without careful examination (Wright stain, original magnification 250×).

cells have more prominent atypia with multinucleation and mitotic activity, whereas the hemophagocytic variant of histiocytic sarcoma can be more morphologically bland and typically affects the spleen and potentially bone marrow, liver, or other sites. The more general term *hemophagocytic syndrome* refers to a secondary process that can occur with immune-mediated, infectious, or neoplastic conditions. With hemophagocytic syndrome, there is pancytopenia or bicytopenia, with increased benign-appearing macrophages (>2% of nucleated cells) in marrow with phagocytized RBCs and/or precursors.[4] Distinction between these types of histiocytic proliferative processes is often

difficult but may be aided by correlation with CBC and chemistry data, potential additional sites of involvement (as with imaging of the spleen and the liver), and additional clinical information, as well as response to therapy. Differentiation between benign and malignant histiocytic proliferations can be very difficult in some cases.[51]

Metastatic neoplasia to bone marrow is less common than primary neoplasia. Metastatic neoplasms may include carcinomas, such as transitional cell carcinoma, apocrine gland adenocarcinoma of the anal sac, or other subtypes, as well as mast cell tumor, histiocytic sarcoma, or lymphoma (see Figs. 27.22 and 27.31; Figs. 27.48 to 27.50). Core biopsy may be necessary to best capture metastatic neoplasia

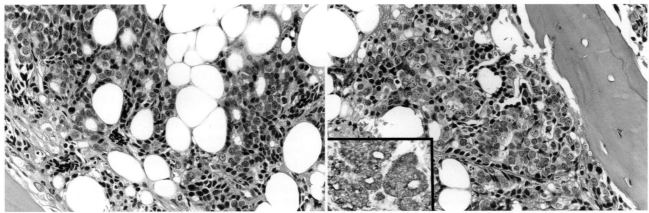

Fig. 27.49 Bone marrow core biopsy from a dog with metastatic carcinoma. In both paratrabecular and interstitial distributions, there are large rounded to polygonal cells with very few background normal hematopoietic cells. On the basis of individual cell morphology, these cells overlap with a hematopoietic population, but a cohesive aggregated pattern or acinar-type formation by these cells is noted, consistent with epithelial origin. A cytokeratin immunohistochemical stain (AE1/AE3; *inset*) confirms carcinoma in this case (note the dark brown cytoplasmic immunoreactivity). Investigation for a primary site of this carcinoma is the next step clinically (H&E stain, original magnification 400×; *inset:* cytokeratin AE1/AE3 immunohistochemical stain, original magnification 400×).

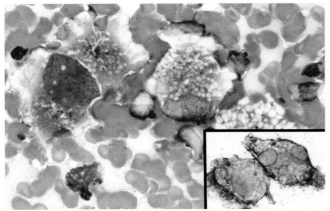

Fig. 27.50 Bone marrow cytology sample from a dog with multicentric histiocytic sarcoma. The large atypical cells are neoplastic histiocytes. They have an abundant volume of cytoplasm with cytoplasmic vacuolation and a small amount of cytoplasmic iron *(deep blue globular material in left cell)*. Cytological criteria for malignancy include the large cell size and anisokaryosis, but in other areas of the sample *(not pictured)* there was also multinucleation and karyomegaly. Immunocytochemistry for CD18 (a panleukocytic marker) highlights the cytoplasm of these cells (*inset:* note the brown cytoplasmic immunoreactivity). This CD18-positivity confirms histiocytic sarcoma versus a primary bone tumor, such as osteosarcoma (Wright-Giemsa stain, original magnification 1000×; *inset:* CD18 immunocytochemical stain, original magnification 1000×).

because this can be multifocal in the marrow and is often paratrabecular. Cytological sampling may miss these lesions because aspiration usually reflects the interstitial components of the marrow and could miss focal paratrabecular lesions (see Fig. 27.48).

CONCLUSIONS

Bone marrow evaluation and interpretation can be a diagnostic challenge even with complete CBC, blood smear analysis, aspiration cytology, and core biopsy with histopathology. A bone marrow sample provides only a single snapshot in time. Continued monitoring of CBC and potential repeat bone marrow sampling may be necessary in some cases to monitor a patient's progress and fine-tune the course of therapy. Consultation and discussion with the pathologists involved in bone marrow interpretation can be helpful and rewarding in many cases and may aid in clinical interpretation as well as inform treatment decisions.

REFERENCES

1. Riley RS, Williams D, Ross M, et al. Bone marrow aspirate and biopsy: a pathologist's perspective. II. Interpretation of the bone marrow aspirate and biopsy. *J Clin Lab Anal.* 2009;23:159–307.
2. Travlos GS. Normal structure, function, and histology of bone marrow. *Toxicol Pathol.* 2006;34:548–565.
3. Travlos GS. Histopathology of bone marrow. *Toxicol Pathol.* 2006;34:566–598.
4. Harvey JW. *Veterinary Hematology: A Diagnostic Guide and Color Atlas.* Philadelphia, PA: Saunders; 2012.
5. De Tommasi AS, Otranto D, Furlanello T, et al. Evaluation of blood and bone marrow in selected canine vector-borne disease. *Parasit Vectors.* 2014;7:534–543.
6. Bennett AI, Williams LE, Ferguson MW. Canine acute leukaemia: 50 cases (1989-2014). *Vet Comp Oncol.* 2017;15:1101–1114.
7. Frezoulis PS, Angelidou E, Karnezi D, et al. Canine pancytopenia in a Mediterranean region: a retrospective study of 119 cases (2005-2013). *J Sm Anim Pract.* 2017;58:395–402.
8. Schnelle AN, Barger AM. Neutropenia in dogs and cats: causes and consequences. *Vet Clin Sm Anim.* 2012;42:111–122.
9. Weiss DJ. A retrospective study of the incidence and classification of bone marrow disorders in the dog at a veterinary teaching hospital (1996-2004). *J Vet Intern Med.* 2006;20:955–961.
10. Stacy NI, Harvey JW. Bone marrow aspiration evaluation. *Vet Clin Small Anim.* 2017;47:31–52.
11. Harvey JW. Canine bone marrow: normal hematopoiesis, biopsy techniques and cell identification and evaluation. *Comp Cont Ed Pract Vet.* 1984;6:909–927.
12. Raskin RE, Messick JB. Bone marrow cytologic and histologic biopsies: indications, technique, and evaluation. *Vet Clin Small Anim.* 2012;42:23–42.
13. Byer CC. Diagnostic bone marrow sampling in cats: currently accepted best practices. *J Feline Med Surg.* 2017;19:759–767.
14. Paparcone R, Fiorentino E, Cappiello S, et al. Sternal aspiration of bone marrow in dogs: a practical approach for canine leishmaniasis diagnosis and monitoring. *J Vet Med.* 2013;2013:217314. https://doi.org/10.1155/2013/217314.

15. Defarges A, Abrams-Ogg A, Foster RA, et al. Comparison of sternal, iliac, and humeral bone marrow aspiration in Beagle dogs. *Vet Clin Pathol.* 2013;422:170–176.

16. Mathis JC, Yoo SH, Sullivan LA. Diagnosis of secondary dysmyelopoiesis via costochondral rib aspiration in a dog. *J Vet Emerg Crit Care.* 2014;24:739–744.

17. Grindem CB. Bone marrow biopsy and evaluation. *Vet Clin North Am Small Anim Pract.* 1989;19:669–696.

18. Grindem CB, Neel JA, Juopperi TA. Cytology of bone marrow. *Vet Clin Small Anim.* 2002;32:1313–1374.

19. Relford RL. The steps in performing a bone marrow aspiration and core biopsy. *Vet Med.* 1991;86:670–688.

20. Friedrichs KR, Young KM. How to collect diagnostic bone marrow samples. *Vet Med.* 2005100:578–588.

21. Abrams-Ogg ACG, Defarges A, Bienzle D. Comparison of feline core bone marrow biopsies from different sites using 2 techniques and needles. *Vet Clin Pathol.* 2014;43:36–42.

22. Abrams-Ogg ACG, Defarges A, Foster RA, et al. Comparison of canine core bone marrow biopsies from multiple sites using different techniques and needles. *Vet Clin Pathol.* 2012;41:235–242.

23. Tappin SW, Lorek A, Villier EJ. Use of rotary battery-powered device for the collection of bone marrow in dogs and cats. *Vet Rec.* 2014;175:173–176.

24. Weiss DJ. A review of the techniques for preparation of histopathologic sections for bone marrow. *Vet Clin Pathol.* 1987;16:90–94.

25. Jain NC. Examination of the blood and bone marrow. In: Jain NC, ed. *Essentials of Veterinary Hematology.* Philadelphia, PA: Lea & Febiger; 1993:1–18.

26. Mylonakis ME, Day MJ, Leontides LS, et al. Type of smear may influence thrombopoietic cell counts in the bone marrow of clinically healthy dogs. *Vet Clin Pathol.* 2005;34:358–361.

27. Hoff B, Lumsden JH, Valli VEO. An appraisal of bone marrow biopsy in assessment of sick dogs. *Can J Comp Med.* 1985;49:34–42.

28. Reeder JP, Hawkins EC, Cora MC, et al. Effect of a combined aspiration and core biopsy technique on quality of core bone marrow specimens. *J Am Anim Hosp Assoc.* 2013;49:16–22.

29. Walker D, Cowell RL, Clinkenbeard KD, et al. Bone marrow mast cell hyperplasia in dogs with aplastic anemia. *Vet Clin Pathol.* 1997;26:106–111.

30. Kearns SH, Ewing P. Causes of canine and feline pancytopenia. *Comp Cont Ed Pract Vet.* 2006;28:122–133.

31. Grindem CB, Haddad JL, Tyler RD, et al. The bone marrow. In: Valenciano AC, Cowell RL, eds. *Cowell and Tyler's Diagnostic Cytology and Hematology of the Dog and Cat.* 4th ed. St. Louis, MO: Elsevier; 2014:489–526.

32. Mischke R, Busse L. Reference values for the bone marrow aspirates in adult dogs. *J Vet Med Assoc.* 2002;49:499–502.

33. Manzillo VF, Restucci B, Pagano A, et al. Pathological changes in the bone marrow of dogs with leishmaniosis. *Vet Rec.* 2006;158:690–694.

34. Blue JT. Myelodysplastic syndromes and myelofibrosis. In: Feldman BF, Zinkl JG, Jain NC, eds. *Schalm's Veterinary Hematology.* 5th ed. Philadelphia, PA: Lippincott Williams & Wilkins; 2000:682–688.

35. Weiss DJ. Myelodysplastic syndromes. In: Weiss DJ, Wardrop KJ, eds. *Schalm's Veterinary Hematology.* 6th ed. Ames, IA: Wiley-Blackwell; 2010:467–474.

36. Lucidi CA, de Resende CLE, Jutkowitz LA, et al. Histologic and cytologic bone marrow findings in dogs with selected precursor-targeted immune-mediated anemia and associated phagocytosis of erythroid precursors. *Vet Clin Pathol.* 2017;46:401–415.

37. Stokol T, Blue JT, French TW. Idiopathic pure red cell aplasia and nonregenerative immune-mediated anemia in dogs: 43 cases (1988-1999). *J Am Vet Med Assoc.* 2000;216:1429–1436.

38. Day MJ. Immune-mediated anemias in the dog. In: Weiss DJ, Wardrop KJ, eds. *Schalm's Veterinary Hematology.* 6th ed. Ames, IA: Wiley-Blackwell; 2010:216–225.

39. Stokol T. Immune-mediated anemias in the cat. In: Weiss DJ, Wardrop KJ, eds. *Schalm's Veterinary Hematology.* 6th ed. Ames, IA: Wiley-Blackwell; 2010:226–232.

40. Devine L, Armstrong PJ, Whittemore JC, et al. Presumed primary immune-mediated neutropenia in 35 dogs: a retrospective study. *J Sm Anim Pract.* 2017;58:307–313.

41. Krause JR. *Bone Marrow Biopsy.* New York, NY: Churchill Livingstone; 1981.

42. Mischke R, Busse L, Bartels D, et al. Quantification of thrombopoietic activity in bone marrow aspirates of dogs. *Vet J.* 2002;164:269–274.

43. Silva LFN, Colim MA, Takahira RK. Measurement of thrombopoietic activity through the quantification of megakaryocytes in bone marrow cytology and reticulated platelets. *Res Vet Sci.* 2012;93:313–317.

44. Neel JA, Birkenheuer AJ, Grindem CB. Infectious and immune-mediated thrombocytopenia. In: Bonagura JD, Twedt DC, eds. *Kirk's Current Veterinary Therapy XIV.* St Louis, MO: Saunders Elsevier; 2009:281–287.

45. Comazzi S, Gelain ME, Bonfanti U, et al. Acute megakaryoblastic leukemia in dogs: a report of three cases and review of the literature. *J Am Anim Hosp Assoc.* 2010;46:327–335.

46. Weiss DJ. Differentiating benign and malignant causes of lymphocytosis in feline bone marrow. *J Vet Intern Med.* 2005;19:855–859.

47. Valli VE, Bienzle D, Meuten DJ. Tumors of the hemolymphatic system. In: Meuten DJ, ed. *Tumors in Domestic Animal.* 5th ed. Ames, IA: John Wiley and Sons, Inc; 2017:322–356.

48. Rout ED, Avery PA. Lymphoid neoplasia. Correlations between morphology and flow cytometry. *Vet Clin Small Anim.* 2017;47:53–70.

49. Campbell MW, Hess PR, Williams LE. Chronic lymphocytic leukaemia in the cat: 18 cases (2000-2010). *Vet Comp Oncol.* 2012;11:256–264.

50. Endicott MM, Charney SC, McKnight JA, et al. Clinicopathological findings and results of bone marrow aspiration in dogs with cutaneous mast cell tumours: 157 cases (1999-2002). *Vet Comp Oncol.* 2007;5:31–37.

51. Moore PF. Canine and feline histiocytic diseases. In: Meuten DJ, ed. *Tumors in Domestic Animal.* 5th ed. Ames, IA: John Wiley and Sons, Inc; 2017:322–356.

52. Weiss DJ. Chronic inflammation and secondary myelofibrosis. In: Weiss DJ, Wardrop KJ, eds. *Schalm's Veterinary Hematology.* 6th ed. Ames, IA: Wiley-Blackwell; 2010:112–117.

53. Regan WJ. A review of myelofibrosis in dogs. *Toxicol Pathol.* 1993;21:164–169.

54. Weiss DJ. Myelonecrosis and acute inflammation. In: Weiss DJ, Wardrop KJ, eds. *Schalm's Veterinary Hematology.* 5th ed. Ames, IA: Wiley-Blackwell; 2010:106–111.

55. Greene CE. *Infectious Diseases of the Dog and Cat.* 4th ed. St. Louis, MO: Saunders; 2011.

56. Juopperi TA, Bienzle D, Bernreuter DC, et al. Prognostic markers for myeloid neoplasms: a comparative review of the literature and goals for future investigation. *Vet Pathol.* 2011;48:182–197.

57. Barger AM. Cytology of bone. *Vet Clin Small Anim.* 2017;47:71–84.

58. Raskin RE, Krehbiel JD. Histopathology of canine bone marrow in malignant lymphoproliferative disorders. *Vet Pathol.* 1988;25:83–88.

28

The Adrenal Gland

Elizabeth K. Little, Tamara B. Wills, and Gary J. Haldorson

The increased availability and use of modern imaging techniques, such as ultrasonography, computed tomography (CT), and magnetic resonance imaging (MRI), have resulted in increased detection of adrenal masses and adrenomegaly. Although some of these lesions may be incidental findings, some cases may require a definitive diagnosis, and cytology may be a valuable tool for initial evaluation. However, caution should be exercised when considering adrenal fine-needle aspiration (FNA), especially in canine patients, because aspiration of pheochromocytomas may result in significant patient morbidity or possibly mortality from hypertensive or hypotensive emergencies and cardiac arrhythmias.[1]

NORMAL CELLULAR COMPONENTS

The adrenal glands are composed of two parts: (1) the cortex and (2) the medulla. The cortex is derived from the mesoderm and is divided into three zones functionally and histologically. Adjacent to the capsule is the zona glomerulosa, followed by the zona fasciculata and the zona reticularis, which is closest to the medulla. The cells in the zona glomerulosa (Fig. 28.1) produce and secrete aldosterone and are arranged in irregular columns histologically.[2] The middle zone, the zona fasciculata (see Fig. 28.1), is the thickest layer of the cortex and functions with the thinner inner layer, the zona reticularis, to produce

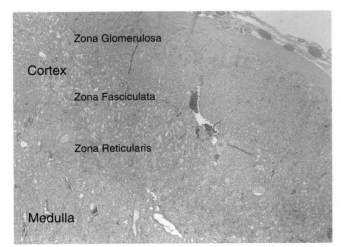

Fig. 28.1 In this histological section of normal canine adrenal gland, the cortex and medulla may be differentiated and the layers of the cortex may be observed (hematoxylin and eosin [H&E] stain, original magnification 100×).

cortisol and androgens, respectively.[2] Histologically, these two layers may be difficult to differentiate.

In the human medical literature, the cells from the zona fasciculata and glomerulosa are described as being similar cytologically and oval to polygonal in shape, with abundant, foamy to vacuolated cytoplasm because of intracytoplasmic lipids; cytological descriptions in dogs and cats are similar.[3,4] Cells from the zona reticularis are lipid poor, containing eosinophilic granular cytoplasm with no vacuoles, but some cells from this zone may contain lipofuscin granules.[3,4] The medulla, derived from neuroectoderm, secretes catecholamines. Cytologically, these cells appear different from adrenocortical cells and are sometimes described as resembling small-size hepatocytes, with centrally to eccentrically located nuclei and finely granular cytoplasm.[4]

ABNORMALITIES OF THE ADRENAL GLAND

Adrenal nodules, masses, or diffuse adrenomegaly are common reasons for the cytological evaluation of the adrenal gland in small animals. In addition to fine-needle aspirates, impression smears of surgically removed adrenal glands may also be obtained. Enlargement of the adrenal glands may occur with hyperplasia, primary or metastatic neoplasia, and, less commonly, inflammation.

Nonneoplastic Conditions
Adrenalitis
Primary adrenalitis is uncommonly reported in the literature, but when observed, canine and feline adrenalitis is often seen with septicemia or disseminated disease. Adrenalitis may occur with bacterial septicemia; disseminated fungal infections, such as with *Coccidioides immitis*, *Histoplasma capsulatum*, and *Cryptococcus neoformans*; and some protozoal infections, such as with *Toxoplasma gondii* and *Babesia* spp.[4] Granulomatous inflammation may be seen with fungal organisms, whereas some protozoal infections elicit mild histiocytic infiltration and necrosis.[4,5] Depending on the inciting cause, edema and hemorrhage may also cause adrenomegaly with systemic infections.[5]

Adrenocortical Hyperplasia
Adrenocortical nodular hyperplasia is most common in older cats and dogs. Diffuse cortical hyperplasia may also result in adrenomegaly, typically caused by oversecretion of adrenocorticotrophic hormone (ACTH) by a pituitary neoplasm.[2] Histologically, hyperplasia of the adrenal cortex results in increased width of the cortex, often because of multiple nodules of hyperplasia, consisting primarily of the zona reticularis and the zona fasciculata (Fig. 28.2).[2,5] Fine-needle aspirates of these areas contain cells resembling those described from the normal zona fasciculata. Cytological preparations are often cellular, and

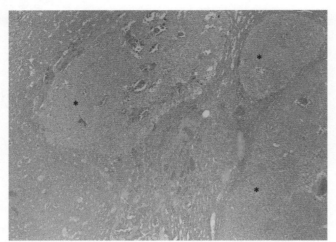

Fig. 28.2 Histopathology of a canine nodular adrenal gland reveals three nonencapsulated, poorly demarcated nodules of cortical cells (*) that have slightly different staining characteristics relative to the adjacent normal cells (adrenocortical nodular hyperplasia) (H&E stain, original magnification 100×).

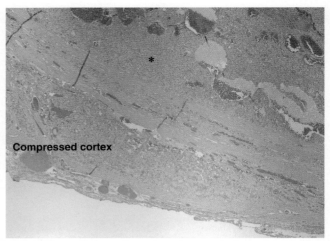

Fig. 28.3 Histopathology of a canine adrenocortical adenoma reveals an expansile, densely cellular, encapsulated mass (*) compressing normal cortex (labeled). Cells are arranged in packets supported by thin wisps of fibrovascular stroma; on higher power, individual cells were large, polygonal, with prominently vacuolated eosinophilic cytoplasm and clearly defined cellular borders (H&E stain, original magnification 100×).

cells may be more tightly arranged compared with typical adrenocortical cells. Binucleate cells are commonly reported in aspirates from human adrenocortical hyperplasia.[3] Differentiation of adrenocortical nodular hyperplasia from well-differentiated adrenal neoplasms may be challenging cytologically and will be further discussed in the next section.

Primary Tumors of the Adrenal Cortex

Functional adrenal cortical neoplasms are reported to be the underlying cause of approximately 10% to 15% cases of canine hyperadrenocorticism.[4] Rare cases of feline hyperaldosteronism are associated with adrenal neoplasms.[6,7] Neither cytology nor histopathology can determine whether a tumor is functional and serum adrenal function tests are necessary.

FNA cytology of adrenal nodules cannot be used to assess encapsulation or invasiveness, which may make cytology a difficult tool for definitive classification of adrenocortical nodules.[3] Even histological classification of adrenal lesions, including differentiation of normal from hyperplastic tissue, hyperplastic nodules from adenomas, and, in some cases, adenomas from carcinomas, may be challenging. Distinguishing adrenocortical carcinomas from pheochromocytomas may also be problematic in some cases.[2] In general, with increased malignancy of adrenocortical neoplasms, decreased lipid and nuclear atypia are encountered.[3] Necrosis is reportedly a common feature in human adrenal tumors.[3] Overlapping features of benign versus malignant adrenocortical nodules exist; however, cellular features at opposite ends of the spectrum (e.g., benign adrenal cortical nodules) may often be differentiated from a poorly differentiated adrenal cortical carcinoma.[3] Regardless, limitations of cytology should be recognized and cytological findings should be used in conjunction with the patient history, clinical signs, blood work abnormalities, and imaging, if available.

Adrenocortical Adenomas and Carcinomas

Adrenal adenomas are common in older dogs and found only rarely in cats.[2] Histologically, adrenal adenomas are surrounded by a capsule and compress adjacent normal cortex (Fig. 28.3). Cells within adrenocortical adenomas resemble the zona fasciculata or

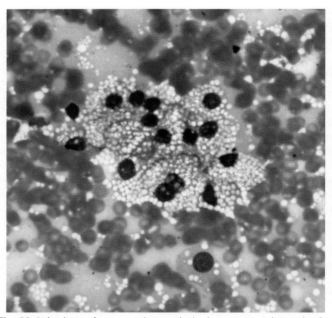

Fig. 28.4 Aspirates from a canine cortical adenoma contain a cohesive cluster of polygonal cells with abundant, highly vacuolated cytoplasm. Mild anisocytosis and anisokaryosis are observed (Wright stain, original magnification 500×).

reticularis.[4] Cytologically, adenomas are composed of cells similar to the normal zona fasciculata or reticularis and are round to polygonal, often containing several discrete vacuoles within moderate to abundant amounts of eosinophilic cytoplasm (Fig. 28.4). Nuclei are typically round, and indistinct nucleoli are occasionally observed. Cells may exhibit mild anisocytosis and anisokaryosis.[5] In humans, adrenal adenomas may sometimes exhibit more cellular pleomorphism.[3] Some adenomas will also contain extramedullary hematopoiesis (Fig. 28.5).[8]

Adrenocortical carcinomas occur less frequently compared with adenomas in dogs and rarely in cats.[8] These tumors are larger than

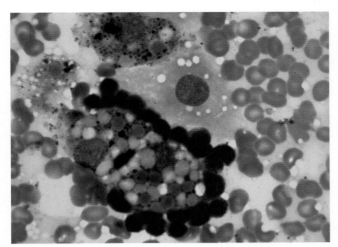

Fig. 28.5 Aspirates from a canine cortical nodule, diagnosed histopathologically as an adrenal cortical adenoma, contain macrophages containing numerous erythrocytes and dark pigment (hemosiderin) surrounded by erythroid precursors. Adjacent is one polygonal cell with abundant eosinophilic cytoplasm with few discrete vacuoles, compatible with adrenocortical origin (Wright stain, original magnification 1000×).

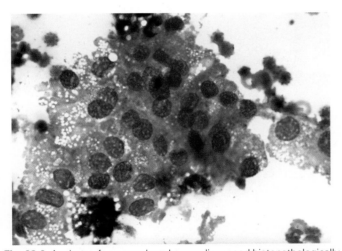

Fig. 28.6 Aspirates from an adrenal mass diagnosed histopathologically as an adrenal cortical carcinoma contain disorganized clusters of oval to polygonal cells with moderate to abundant amounts of vacuolated basophilic cytoplasm. The neoplastic cells exhibit mild to moderate pleomorphism (Wright stain, original magnification 1000×).

adenomas and may invade into surrounding tissue, including the caudal vena cava.[8] Neoplastic cells in carcinomas are typically more pleomorphic compared with neoplastic cells from adenomas, although an overlap in cellular pleomorphism exists in these two entities. Tumor cells are often large, oval to polygonal, with basophilic cytoplasm containing several discrete vacuoles, although some may contain dense eosinophilic cytoplasm (Figs. 28.6 and 28.7).[7] Nucleoli are often prominent.[8]

Myelolipoma

Myelolipomas are very uncommon in dogs but have been reported.[9] These tumors are benign and often originate in the cortex but may extend into the medulla. Expected cytological findings would include lipid and mature adipocytes admixed with hematopoietic cells and macrophages containing hemosiderin.[9]

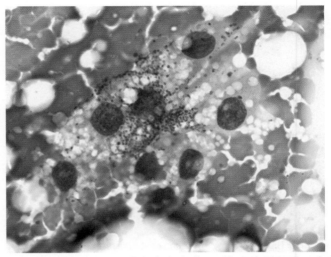

Fig. 28.7 Aspirates of a histopathologically confirmed adrenal cortical carcinoma in a dog contain cells that appear more similar to those aspirated from the adrenal cortical adenoma in Figs. 28.4 and 28.5 (Wright stain, original magnification 1000×). (Courtesy Dr. Andrea Bohn, Fort Collins, CO.)

Primary Tumors of the Adrenal Medulla

Pheochromocytomas are the most common adrenal medulla tumors in dogs and cats; however, they are quite rare in cats.[8,10] Other tumors, such as neuroblastomas and ganglioneuromas, may develop from the neuroectodermal cells within the adrenal medulla.[8]

Pheochromocytoma

Pheochromocytomas are more common in dogs than in cats and are frequently found in middle-aged and older dogs.[8] Pheochromocytomas are often locally invasive and may metastasize to the lung, liver, kidney, spleen, and pancreas.[11] Serum and urine tests measuring the levels of catecholamines and metabolites may be used to diagnose pheochromocytomas, but these tests are not widely available for dogs and cats.[12] Cytology and histopathology are often necessary for diagnosis. Because manipulation of pheochromocytomas may result in cardiac and blood pressure instability, greatly increasing risk of morbidity and mortality, FNA should be avoided. Histopathologically, the cells are arranged in nests, packets, and small lobules, separated by fine fibrovascular stroma (Fig. 28.8). Cytological specimens are often highly cellular, with occasional papillary formations described[13]; and the cells may range from small and round, to polyhedral (Fig. 28.9 through 28.11), to large, pleomorphic cells with eosinophilic to slightly basophilic, granular cytoplasm.[8,13] If a surgical specimen is obtained, application of Zenker solution (potassium dichromate) to a freshly cut surface should result in formation of a dark-brown pigment within 5 to 20 minutes because of oxidation of catecholamines.[8] This may help distinguish a pheochromocytoma from an adrenocortical tumor, which would not turn brown.

Neuroblastoma

Neuroblastomas are uncommon tumors in young dogs, typically younger than 3 years of age, and may occur in several anatomical sites, including the adrenal gland.[14] Cytologically, neuroblastomas contain round cells with scant amounts of basophilic cytoplasm containing a round hyperchromatic nucleus, mimicking the appearance of lymphocytes.[4,14] Clustered cells may also appear similar to these round cells. In one report, the epithelioid cells were described as round to polygonal in shape, with scant to moderate amounts of basophilic cytoplasm

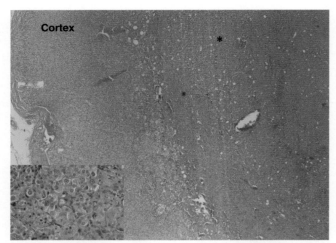

Fig. 28.8 Histopathology of a canine pheochromocytoma reveals a poorly demarcated, unencapsulated, highly cellular, nodular mass expanding the medulla (*). Cells are arranged in sheets, nests, and packets separated by a delicate fibrovascular stroma. Morphological features of the cells are better appreciated in the *inset.* Cells have indistinct margins with moderate to abundant, finely granular, and eosinophilic cytoplasm. Nuclei are round to oval, are vesicular, and have a small nucleolus (H&E stain, original magnification 100×; *inset:* H&E stain, original magnification 400×).

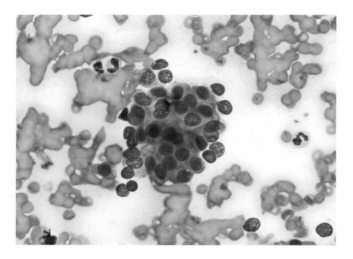

Fig. 28.9 Aspirate from a canine pheochromocytoma contains sheets of polygonal cells containing moderate amounts of eosinophilic granular cytoplasm. The nuclei are round with a stippled chromatin pattern, occasionally containing a nucleolus (Wright stain, original magnification 1000×). (Courtesy Dr. Amy Valenciano, Dallas, TX.)

exhibiting mild pleomorphism.[14] Pseudorosette formation may also be seen with cells surrounding eosinophilic fibrillar material.[3]

Ganglioneuroma

Ganglioneuromas in the adrenal gland are infrequently reported in dogs and cats. Cytology on aspirates of human ganglioneuromas has revealed ganglion cells admixed with spindle cells.[3] Cytologically, ganglion cells are large (up to 40 micrometers [μm] in diameter), round to polygonal cells containing abundant basophilic to eosinophilic cytoplasm, occasionally with cytoplasmic processes. The nuclei are large (up to 18 μm) and round with a prominent nucleolus.[15] Histopathology of human and veterinary ganglioneuromas are similarly described.[8] Cytology from aspirates of dogs and cats with ganglioneuromas would appear similar.

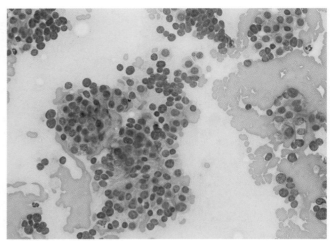

Fig. 28.10 Cells from an aspirate of a dog with a pheochromocytoma contain individual and cohesive polygonal cells with moderate amounts of eosinophilic, granular cytoplasm. Mild to moderate pleomorphism is observed (Wright stain, original magnification 500×). (Courtesy Dr. Amy Valenciano, Dallas, TX.)

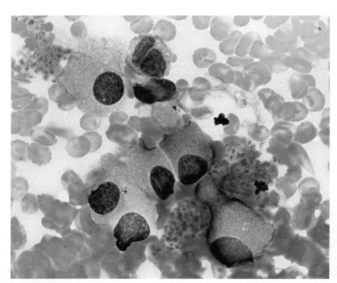

Fig. 28.11 Aspirate from a canine pheochromocytoma contains individual polygonal cells with moderate amounts of eosinophilic, granular cytoplasm. Mild to moderate pleomorphism is observed (Wright stain, original magnification 1000×). (Courtesy Dr. Andrea Bohn, Fort Collins, CO.)

REFERENCES

1. Reusch CE, Schellenberg S, Wenger M. Endocrine hypertension in small animals. *Vet Clin North Am Small Anim Pract.* 2010;40(2):335–352.
2. Feldman EC, Nelson RW. *The Adrenal Gland. Canine and Feline Endocrinology and Reproduction.* 3rd ed. St. Louis, MO: Saunders; 2004.
3. Hsu GCH, Tao LC. Primary lesions of the adrenal gland. In: Frable WJ, ed. *Transabdominal Fine-Needle Aspiration Biopsy.* 2nd ed. Hackensack, NJ: World Scientific Publishing; 2007:206–233.
4. La Perle KMD, Capen CC. Endocrine system. In: McGavin MD, Zachary JF, eds. *Pathological Bases of Veterinary Disease.* 4th ed. St. Louis, MO: Mosby Elsevier; 2007:693–741.
5. Maxie MG, ed. *Jubb, Kennedy, & Palmer's Pathology of Domestic Animals.* 5th ed. St. Louis, MO: Elsevier Saunders; 2007:413–423.
6. Renschler JS, Dean GA. What is your diagnosis? Abdominal mass aspirate in a cat with an increased Nark ratio. *Vet Clin Pathol.* 2009;38(1):69–72.

7. Ash RA, Harvey AM, Tasker S. Primary hyperaldosteronism in the cat: a series of 13 cases. *J Feline Med Surg.* 2005;7(3):173–182.

8. Capen CC. Tumors of the endocrine glands. In: Meuten DJ, ed. *Tumors in Domestic Animals.* 4th ed. Ames, IA: Iowa State Press; 2002:629–636.

9. Tursi M, et al. Adrenal myelolipoma in a dog. *Vet Pathol.* 2005;42(2):232–235.

10. Calsyn JD, et al. Adrenal pheochromocytoma with contralateral adrenocortical adenoma in a cat. *J Am Anim Hosp Assoc.* 2010;46(1):36–42.

11. Boari A, Aste G. Diagnosis and management of geriatric canine endocrine disorders. *Vet Res Commun.* 2003;27(suppl 1):543–554.

12. Kook PH, Grest P, Quante S, et al. Urinary catecholamine and metadrenaline to creatinine ratios in dogs with a phaeochromocytoma. *Vet Rec.* 2010;166(6):169–174.

13. Rosenstein DS. Diagnostic imaging in canine pheochromocytoma. *Vet Radiol Ultrasound.* 2000;41(6):499–506.

14. Marcotte L, McConkey SE, Hanna P, et al. Malignant adrenal neuroblastoma in a young dog. *Can Vet J.* 2004;45(9):773–776.

15. Koss LG, Rodriguez CA. The central nervous system. In: Koss LG, ed. *Koss' Diagnostic Cytology and Its Histopathologic Bases.* 5th ed. Philadelphia, PA: Lippincott, Williams, and Wilkins; 2005:1524.

29

Immunocytochemistry

Melinda S. Camus, Lisa S. Kelly, and Anne M. Barger

Immunohistochemistry is a diagnostic and research tool that exploits the precision of antibody–antigen binding to identify a particular cell or molecule in formalin-fixed tissue. The terms *immunohistochemistry* (IHC) and *immunocytochemistry* (ICC) are often used interchangeably. However, for the purpose of this text, ICC will be used specifically for cytological specimens that are devoid of complex architecture, including air-dried slides and cell blocks prepared from fine-needle aspirates, effusions, blood smears, urine sediments, and cell cultures. IHC is used in veterinary medicine for multiple purposes, but it predominantly aids in diagnosis to identify a cell population, to clarify or confirm a diagnosis, to gain prognostic information regarding cellular proliferation, and to identify causative agents. Currently, ICC is employed less extensively, primarily to assist in the specific identification of cell types, as in immunophenotyping of lymphoma and leukemia. Interest in ICC continues to grow, and its popularity will likely expand with increased commercial availability of validated antibodies.

GENERAL PRINCIPLES

ICC depends on the specific binding of exogenous antibody to cellular antigens, which may be lipoproteins, glycoproteins, or peptides.[1] Cells incubate with antibodies developed to recognize a particular antigen located on the cell membrane, inside the cytoplasm, or within the nucleus.[2] A basic understanding of antibody structure is required to fully comprehend and use this technique. Detailed aspects of immunology are beyond the scope of this chapter, and readers should consult a veterinary immunology text or other references for additional information.[1,3-6]

Antibodies are "Y" shaped and are composed of four polypeptides—two identical pairs of light and heavy chains, which fold into constant and variable regions (Fig. 29.1). The arms of the "Y" (Fab regions) include the variable regions of the light and heavy chains and dictate the specificity of antigen binding.[5] Four different types of bonds contribute to the noncovalent antibody binding to antigen: (1) hydrophobic bonds, (2) hydrogen bonds, (3) electrostatic bonds, and (4) van der Waals forces.[4] The parameters and reagents used in ICC are aimed at enhancing binding strength. For example, increases in temperature strengthen van der Waals forces, whereas neutral pH, low ionic buffer strength, and low incubation temperature may enhance electrostatic bonds.[5] The stem of the "Y" (Fc region), composed of constant regions of the heavy chains, contains sequences unique to the animal species from which the antibody was generated.[4] These sequences in the Fc region will serve as antigens when injected into an animal of a different species and allow for the generation of broadly useful secondary antibodies.

Production of antibodies directed against a particular antigen initiates with injection of purified antigen into an animal, commonly a mouse or rabbit. Different types of antibodies are available for many types of antigens. Monoclonal antibodies recognize one particular epitope on an antigen, imparting high specificity with minimal background staining. Polyclonal antibodies recognize multiple epitopes on a particular antigen. For this reason, they are less specific but more sensitive.[4] Most of the antibodies available for purchase are produced for use in human and murine tissues, which typically exhibit related but distinct antigens to domestic species. Therefore in veterinary medicine, polyclonal antibodies are often used because of the increased likelihood of cross-reactivity. Generally, monoclonal antibodies are produced in mice, and polyclonal antibodies are produced in rabbits, although monoclonal antibodies produced in rabbits are available for use in IHC and flow cytometry. Some proposed advantages for rabbit monoclonal antibodies include higher binding affinity, larger volume, and production of antibodies against antigens that are not immunogenic in mice.[6] This technology is still fairly new relative to mouse monoclonals, and the antibodies available are limited, so these antibodies may become more popular for ICC as more reagents become available. Because of multiple problems, including reproducibility and animal welfare associated with animal-derived antibodies, recombinant monoclonal antibody development is increasing.[7] However, the general principles for determining use of these antibodies remain the same.

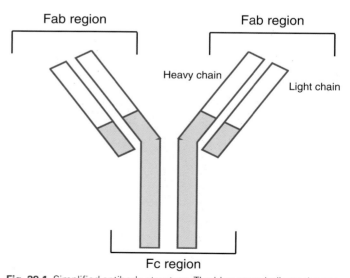

Fig. 29.1 Simplified antibody structure. The blue areas indicate the constant regions, and the white areas represent the variable regions of the paired heavy and light chains of the antibody. The Fab regions contain unique antigen binding sites at their tips. The Fc region serves as the conjugation site for detection systems or the binding site for secondary antibodies.

IMMUNOCYTOCHEMISTRY TECHNIQUE

The components of an ICC reaction include the cells (on air-dried or fixed slides, in cell blocks, or in transport media), primary antibody, secondary antibody (if necessary), labeling mechanism, and buffers.[2] Use of a general nuclear counterstain, such as hematoxylin, is not mandatory, but it improves visualization and provides context for interpreting the cells. Antibodies are classified into primary or secondary antibodies based on their target antigen and intended use. A primary antibody recognizes the cellular antigen of interest. The preferred isotype is immunoglobulin G (IgG) because of its consistent generation and binding to antigen.[1] For example, a primary IgG antibody targeting the molecule CD20 could be developed in a mouse to investigate B lymphocytes. A separate primary IgG antibody targeting the molecule CD3 could be developed in another mouse to investigate T lymphocytes. Secondary antibodies are directed against the constant, species-specific Fc region of the primary antibodies. For example, the mouse-derived primary antibodies recognizing CD20 and CD3 could each be probed with the same antimouse IgG secondary antibody developed in a rabbit.

For detection, the primary antibody, or more commonly the secondary antibody, must be conjugated to a labeling mechanism, such as a fluorochrome, an enzyme, or particulate matter (Fig. 29.2). Fluorescence was the first type of label used for immunocytochemistry described in 1942.[8] Each fluorescent label absorbs a characteristic wavelength of light and then emits a characteristic higher wavelength of light. Detection of fluorochromes requires a fluorescent microscope capable of producing and filtering these defined wavelengths, which may not be available in all diagnostic laboratories.[4] Fluorescent staining fades over time, complicating archiving of slides. However, the advent of digital slide archives eliminates this disadvantage.[9] Enzymatic labels predominate in ICC because they merely require a standard light microscope for evaluation. With this technique, an enzyme, such as horseradish peroxidase or alkaline phosphatase, labels the antibody and converts its substrate into a colored reaction product for detection.[4] The reaction is permanent, so slides may be stored for several years. Particulate labels are used rarely, with gold comprising the most frequently conjugated metal. Metal particulates are used primarily for electron microscopy.

Use of a secondary antibody has advantages and disadvantages. Secondary antibodies increase the intensity of staining because multiple labeled secondary antibodies can bind to a single primary antibody, amplifying the signal. The main disadvantage is increased background staining because of an increased chance of nonspecific binding.[4]

The literature abounds in reports of numerous manual and automated techniques for performing ICC. Sawa et al. described a rapid (45-minute) procedure for manual ICC, which can be adapted for use at individual laboratories.[10] Optimal primary antibody dilution must be determined separately within each laboratory performing the test.[7] Although technically challenging, manual ICC allows for optimization of limited samples by allowing for "splitting" of individual samples, with multiple (typically two) antibodies used per slide. Extreme care must be taken in the use of this technique to prevent antibody crossover.

Antigen Retrieval

One advantage of ICC is that it can be performed on air-dried slides acquired through minimally invasive aspiration procedures. However, the limited shelf-life of air-dried slides is a major limitation of ICC, particularly when banking positive control slides (see the section "Controls"). As a solution to the temporary nature of cytology slides, 10% neutral buffered formalin can fix slides indefinitely.[11] However, formalin cross-links deoxyribonucleic acid (DNA) and alters the structure of proteins, thereby limiting the ability of antibody recognition of a particular antigen.[12] To address this same problem in IHC, the process of antigen retrieval was identified in the early 1990s.[13] Paraffin-embedded, formalin-fixed tissues are boiled to reverse the chemical reactions between formalin and protein.[5] Antigen retrieval for cytological specimens has been evaluated by Valli et al.[11] Heating the sample in normal saline or citrate buffer allows for antigen retrieval in cytological specimens.[11] The samples may be heated by using something as common as a microwave or as specialized as a decloaking chamber (Biocare Medical, Walnut Creek, CA). If the samples are processed and stained within 24 hours, cell fixation and antigen retrieval may not be necessary, but for delayed evaluation, formalin fixation with subsequent antigen retrieval may provide excellent results (Fig. 29.3). Some antibodies (e.g., CD11d) will not recognize antigen after formalin exposure despite antigen retrieval. Antigen retrieval may also be needed in the absence of formalin fixation for certain antigens, particularly nuclear antigens.[14]

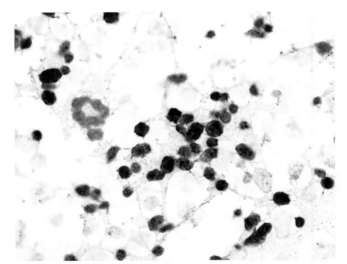

Fig. 29.3 Antigen retrieval performed on formalin-fixed cells permits delayed examination and preserves recognition by many antibodies. Buffy coat smear of blood from a cat. The specimen was fixed in formalin, followed by antigen retrieval in saline before antibody incubation. With this method, B lymphocytes exhibit strong binding of antibodies recognizing CD79a (original magnification 40× objective). Some antibodies (e.g., against some histiocytic markers) will not recognize formalin-fixed cells. (Courtesy Dr. V. E. Valli.)

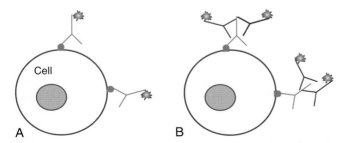

Fig. 29.2 Detection of antibody binding to cellular antigen. Detection systems frequently include fluorochromes or enzymes with chromogenic substrates. (A) Direct detection. Primary antibody *(light blue Y)* that recognizes a cellular antigen *(green circle)* with detection marker *(red starburst)* conjugated to the Fc region of the antibody. (B) Indirect detection. Unlabeled primary antibody recognized by species-specific secondary antibody *(dark blue Y)* with detection marker conjugated to the secondary antibody.

TABLE 29.1   Examples of Antibodies Used in Immunocytochemistry[a]

Cell Type	Antibody
Leukocytes (strongest for histiocytic/granulocytic lineage)	CD18
Lymphoid lineage	
T lymphocytes	CD3
Pan-T-cell marker	CD4
T-helper lymphocytes	CD8
Cytotoxic T lymphocytes	
B lymphocytes	CD79a
Pan-B-cell marker	CD20
Mature B cells	MUM-1, CD20
Plasma cells	
Megakaryocytes	CD41
Stem cells	CD34, CD117 (c-KIT)
Mast cells	CD 117 (c-KIT)
Endothelial cells	CD31
Epithelial cells	Cytokeratin
Mesenchymal cells	Vimentin
Melanocytes	Melan-A

[a]Antibodies may also bind cells not listed (e.g., CD4 is expressed on canine neutrophils).

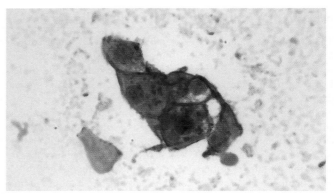

Fig. 29.4 Long-term frozen storage of positive control slides. After more than 1 year of storage at −15°C, the air-dried fine-needle aspirate smear of nonneoplastic canine liver strongly binds an anticytokeratin antibody. The immunocytochemistry protocol included brief acetone fixation and heat-induced antigen retrieval (original magnification 50× objective).

Controls

The majority of antibodies available for purchase have undergone extensive validation to ensure that the antibody is specific for the antigen being analyzed. At minimum, Western blot analysis should be performed to show that the antibody recognizes an antigen of an appropriate molecular weight. Additionally, two different antibodies recognizing different epitopes of the same antigen may be used to show that the antibodies colocalize on the same antigen.[8,15] These tests do not need to be done on each sample but should be done by each individual laboratory for each species and antibody of interest as part of the initial antibody validation process.[16] Once validated, the antibodies may be used diagnostically with appropriate positive and negative controls. These controls must be run for each antibody, and it is important that the controls match the sample type.[17] For example, it is inappropriate to use paraffin-embedded, formalin-fixed tissues as a positive or negative control for unfixed, air-dried cytological specimens. If the patient's specimen has undergone formalin fixation with antigen retrieval, so should the controls. A positive control appropriate for diagnostic use is cells that express the antigen of interest, acquired from tissue of an individual of the same species as the patient. Slides prepared from a lymph node could serve as a positive control for CD79a, CD20, CD3, CD4, and CD8 (Table 29.1). Positive control slides should contain both positive and negative areas.[2]

The negative control is performed on patient specimens, and when submitting slides for ICC, adequate numbers of slides must be provided for appropriate negative controls for each antibody. The negative control demonstrates that the secondary antibody is binding purposefully to the primary antibody without nonspecific binding to unrelated structures. There are several options, including the use of isotype matched IgG or an irrelevant monoclonal antibody, but commonly the primary antibody is omitted on this slide and replaced with serum from the same species as the secondary antibody source.[4,8,16]

Keeping banked positive control material on hand is helpful but can be challenging and time consuming in laboratories where ICC is done infrequently and control materials may expire before utilization. The American Society for Veterinary Clinical Pathology (ASVCP) guidelines for immunocytochemistry recommends that ICC control slides should be used within 2 weeks if stored at 4°C. The use of controls may be extended if control slides are placed in a freezer at or below −20°C or if antigen retrieval is utilized (Fig. 29.4).[16] Control slides placed in the freezer should be stored in a plastic container within a zip-lock bag and should be brought to room temperature before use.[2]

If external verification of results is desired, ICC reactivity may be compared against IHC results of the same tissue, as long as the same antibody clone has been validated for performance in paraffin-embedded tissues. Similarly, flow cytometry may be used for comparison of results to ICC. However, neither is a substitute for in-run cytological control samples.[2]

SAMPLE SUBMISSION

Air-dried slides submitted for cytology are acceptable for use for ICC, but cell viability and antibody binding decreases if the sample is left at room temperature. The viability of unstained slides may be prolonged by freezing the slides at or below −20°C. Slides should be placed in an airtight plastic container and sealed in a zip-lock bag.[18] Alternatively, the slides may be dipped in 10% formalin. However, as mentioned above, antigen retrieval will need to be performed with these slides.[11] Because patient slides are often limited, prestained specimens may be the only sample available, but investigations into the applicability of ICC to these samples suggest results may be antibody dependent.[19] Samples may also be submitted in transport media. Some laboratories that perform ICC will provide prepared tubes containing their preferred transport media. At a minimum, the media should consist of saline buffer with a protein source, such as bovine serum albumin, fetal calf serum, or autologous serum, and several recipes exist.[6] Acetone may be added to the sample to limit bacterial growth. However, acetone permeabilizes the cell membrane and therefore may result in cell lysis.[4] If the sample is processed quickly, the acetone will have minimal effect on the quality of the sample, but after 2 to 3 days, the cellular lysis is considerable (Fig. 29.5). The ASVCP guidelines recommend processing samples mixed with acetone to completion within 24 hours. Samples should be transported to the laboratory in a manner that prevents both freezing and overheating.[2] When sending samples to an outside laboratory for ICC, communication with the performing laboratory is paramount for proper sample selection, transport media, storage, and shipping requirements. How the specimen was handled before submission, such as storage length and condition or fixatives used, must be communicated to the performing laboratory to allow appropriate interpretation.

Multiple cytospin preparations may be made from the transport media, ideally at a concentration of 250 to 300 cells per microliter, allowing the cells to spread out and have adequate space.[20] Cells spread too thickly, whether from cytocentrifuge or direct preparations, lead to high background and poor cellular staining (Fig. 29.6). Cells from

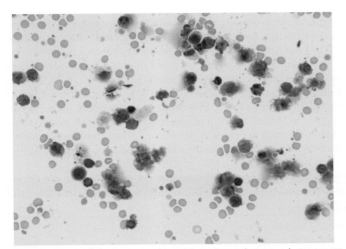

Fig. 29.5 Poor cellular preservation with prolonged storage in transport media containing acetone. The sample remained in transport media containing acetone for 72 hours before receipt by the laboratory. Many of the cells lysed, resulting in bare nuclei, swollen nuclei, and overall poor cellular morphology. Only mature erythrocytes are definitively intact and identifiable (Wright-Giemsa stain, original magnification 50× objective).

transport media may also be embedded into cell blocks, a process that converts fluid-based specimens into solid blocks that can be processed and investigated as standard histology sections. Multiple techniques are available for formation of cell blocks, and kits are available for the process.[17,21] Cell blocks permit multiple sections to be cut, allowing for panels of antibodies on limited cytological specimens.[16] The main limitation of cell blocks is the use of formalin, which necessitates the use of antigen retrieval and precludes the use of some antibodies.[17,22] The use of gel foam cell blocks has been reported in veterinary medicine and may become more widely used because of its technical ease.[23] Cytospin preparations from effusions and urine may also be prepared in a similar manner to that for cytospins from the transport media. As with cell blocks, one of the main advantages of submitting transport media or an effusion for ICC is the ability to make multiple slides from one sample, allowing for a panel of antibodies to be used, rather than just one antibody. Using a combination of possible negative and positive antibodies will result in higher diagnostic yield than the use of one antibody.[17,24] Each of these methods of sample preparation has advantages and disadvantages (Table 29.2).

CLINICAL APPLICATIONS OF IMMUNOCYTOCHEMISTRY

One of the advantages of cytology over biopsy is the relatively low cost and rapid turnaround time, both of which will increase with the use of ICC. Therefore ICC is not necessary for every sample but should be reserved for very specific purposes. Transformed cells do not elaborate a distinct "neoplastic" marker, so the diagnosis of malignancy needs to be made on standard cytology specimens before ICC.[17] Only after a diagnosis of neoplasia is made from the Romanowsky-stained cytology specimen, ICC may be able to illuminate a more specific diagnosis. Ideally, the slides used for ICC originate from the same aspirate or at least from the same location as the original cytology. In addition to increasing the specificity of a neoplasia diagnosis, ICC may allow for identification of small numbers of cells within a tissue

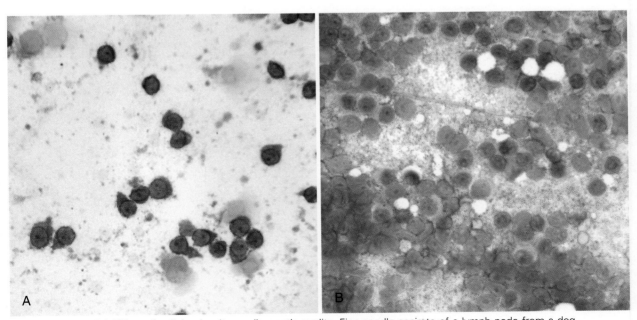

Fig. 29.6 Effect of cellular density on diagnostic quality. Fine-needle aspirate of a lymph node from a dog diagnosed with B-cell lymphoma. Images are from different areas of the same slide probed with anti-CD20. (A) Appropriate density. Cells are individualized and widely spaced, demonstrating strong antibody binding readily distinguished from the background. (B) Excessively high density. Crowded cells demonstrate poor antibody binding with high background (original magnification 50× objective).

(e.g., identification of epithelial cells in a thymoma or micrometastasis within a lymph node) or for immunophenotyping of neoplasms for prognostic information or assistance with therapeutic decisions. Results of ICC, with any associated interpretation, should be linked to the original cytology report and provided to the client for complete characterization. [2]

Diagnosis

Cytology has limits in diagnoses, especially in identifying the tissue of origin in poorly differentiated malignant tumors. Many antibodies have been validated for use in cytology to assist with the identification of tissue type (see Table 29.1). Antibodies targeting the intracytoplasmic intermediate filaments vimentin and cytokeratin are used to identify the broad tissue types of mesenchymal and epithelial tissues, respectively. Cells that express cytokeratin and do not express vimentin are considered epithelial in origin (e.g., carcinoma). A tumor that expresses vimentin, not cytokeratin, is a mesenchymal tumor (e.g., sarcoma, lymphoma). Pancytokeratin antibodies, and more specific antibodies directed against single cytokeratins (e.g., cytokeratin 7), have been evaluated for cytology, and vimentin has been validated for use in cytology of imprints and fine-needle aspirates.[25-27] A small group of neoplasms and benign tissues are known to express both cytokeratin and vimentin. These include synovial cell sarcoma,

mesothelioma, benign mesothelium, papillary renal cell carcinoma, non–small cell lung carcinoma, carcinosarcoma, and melanoma, among others.[20-24] For this reason, the expression of cytokeratin and vimentin should be probed in conjunction. Additional antibodies, such as Melan-A for melanoma (Fig. 29.7), CD31 for endothelial cells, and CD18 (Fig. 29.8) for histiocytic and granulocytic origin, are available when tumors expressing these antigens are among the differential diagnoses. Many of these antibodies have been specifically evaluated for cytology.[11,26-29] The Oncology-Pathology Working Group of the Veterinary Cancer Society has collated a list of antibodies, including manufacturer and clone, used in the veterinary literature.[16]

Neoplastic lymphocytes can be phenotyped with ICC.[30,31] Lymphomas are initially evaluated for expression of CD3 or CD79 (Fig. 29.9) to determine T- or B-cell origin, respectively. If they are of T-cell origin, they may then be further evaluated for expression of CD4 or CD8.[32] Because of the similar morphology of hematopoietic cells of different lineages, a panel of antibodies is necessary to evaluate leukemias. Lymphoid markers, such as CD3 and CD79, are valuable, but myeloperoxidase, CD18, CD45, and granzyme B should be included in the panel to identify tumors of myeloid, dendritic cell, and natural killer (NK) cell origin, respectively.[33] It should be noted that flow cytometry imparts the ability to easily and quantitatively probe with more antibodies on a small liquid sample compared with

TABLE 29.2   Advantages and Disadvantages of Sample Types

	Advantages	Disadvantages
Direct smear	• Slides from the original sample may be used, if multiple slides submitted	• Increased background artifact • Prior staining may affect results • Variability of cellularity between slides • Use of panels limited because of limited numbers of slides
Cytocentrifuge preparations	• Useful with limited material • Panels possible because multiple slides can be prepared • May control cellularity • May be used for fluids or transport media	• Background artifact • Added time, expense, equipment, and expertise to prepare transport media and cytocentrifuge specimen
Cell block	• Histology laboratory can handle like routine material • Materials, including controls, may be stored long term	• Low-cellularity samples cannot be used • Antigen retrieval necessary • Added expense, expertise, equipment, and time of cell block preparation

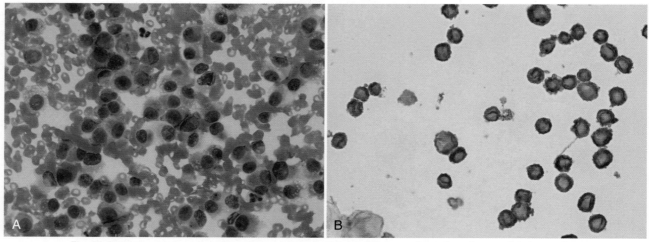

Fig. 29.7 Diagnosis of amelanotic melanoma by using Melan-A fine-needle aspirate from a digital mass in a dog. (A) In this location, a population of round neoplastic cells with prominent nucleoli but no pigmentation suggests amelanotic melanoma (Wright-Giemsa stain, original magnification 50× objective). (B) Neoplastic cells are strongly positive for Melan-A expression, supporting the diagnosis (original magnification 50× objective.)

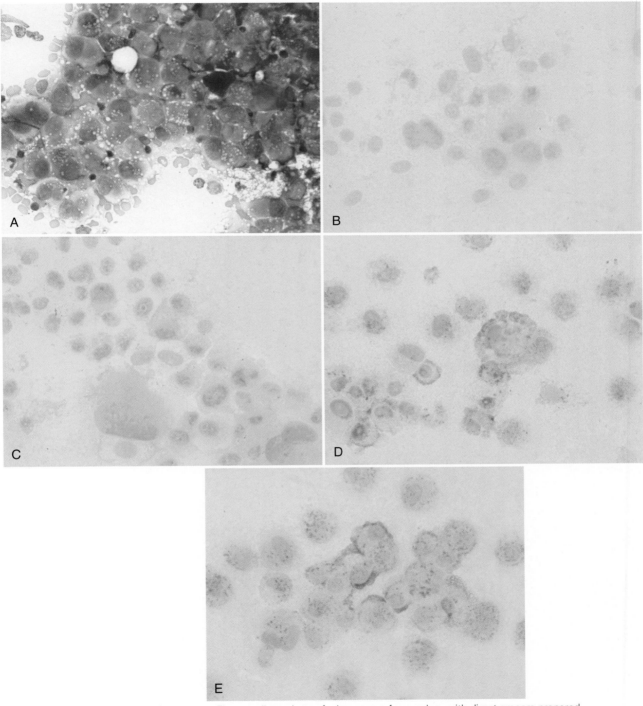

Fig. 29.8 Histiocytic sarcoma. Fine-needle aspirate of a lung mass from a dog, with direct smears prepared from sample submitted in transport media. Population of neoplastic cells. (A) cells vary from round to spindle-shaped with a moderate rim of cytoplasm (Wright-Giemsa stain). Cells do not express CD3, a T lymphocyte marker (B), or CD79a, a B lymphocyte marker (C), but do express CD18, a histiocytic/granulocytic marker (D), and vimentin, a broad mesenchymal marker (E). The immunostaining pattern combined with cellular morphology is consistent with histiocytic sarcoma (*all images:* original magnification 50× objective).

ICC, and this technique is typically the method of choice for leukemias or high-cellularity lymphoma aspirates in transport media.[34] Some acute leukemias exhibit few immunological markers (e.g., CD34+) but can be further characterized cytochemically by their expression of enzymes, such as alkaline phosphatase or α-naphthyl butyrate esterase.[35]

ICC may also be useful in identifying low numbers of cells in a tissue. In a study of dogs, the sensitivity of diagnosis of metastatic carcinoma increased from 88% to 99% with the addition of cytokeratin ICC.[36] Identification of neoplastic cells within a draining lymph node may assist in the prediction of tumor behavior and may alter the therapeutic plan for the patient.

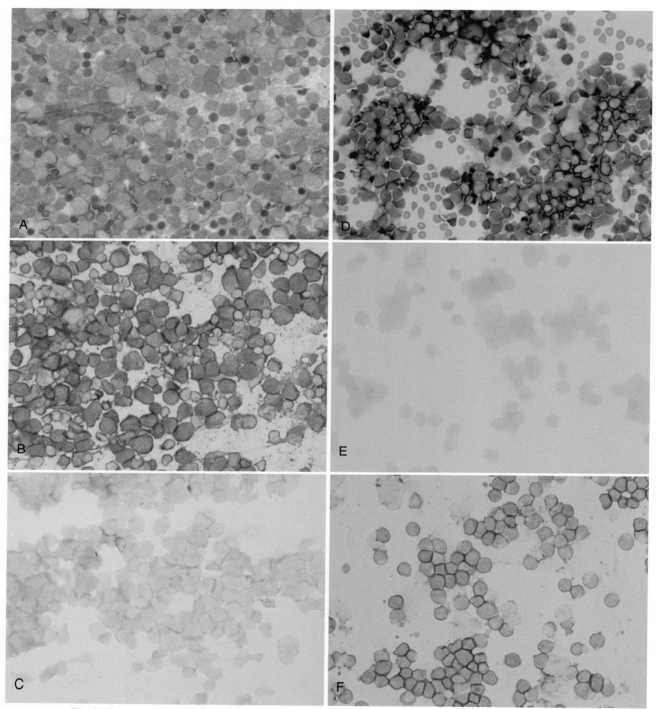

Fig. 29.9 Immunophenotyping of lymphoma. (A–C; left column). B-cell lymphoma in a lymph node. (A) Mixed lymphoid population predominated by large lymphocytes (Wright-Giemsa stain). (B) Large cells express CD79a, a B-cell marker. (C) Large cells are negative for CD3, a T-cell marker. (D–F; right column). T-cell lymphoma diagnosed from cytocentrifuge preparation of urine. (D) A population of neoplastic round cells (Wright-Giemsa stain). (E) Cells do not express CD79a. (F) Cells express CD3 (*all images:* original magnification 50× objective.)

Prognostic Information

Different groups of antibodies have been evaluated in an attempt to predict the biological behavior or assist with grading of neoplasms. Most of these studies have been done with IHC and are often used in conjunction with concurrent architectural changes. Two such examples are antibodies directed against proliferating nuclear cell antigen (PCNA) and Ki67. PCNA is a highly conserved protein found in all eukaryotic cells. PCNA is an accessory protein to DNA polymerase δ and acts as a clamp to lock the enzyme on the leading strand.[37] It has been evaluated in several different tumors, including mast cell tumors, testicular neoplasms, mammary tumors, and soft tissue sarcomas.[38-41] Ki67 is a nuclear antigen expressed in the G1, S, G2, and M phases of the cell cycle and is used to evaluate the proliferative activity of neoplasms.[37] An anti-Ki67 murine monoclonal antibody has been evaluated in mast cell tumors, melanomas, gastrointestinal stromal tumors, meningiomas, and lymphoma, among others.[40,42-46] These proliferative markers are probably most useful with histopathology because they may be interpreted with the architecture and used as part of a grading scheme. A panel of proliferative markers, including Ki67, PCNA, and agyrophilic nucleolar organizer region (AgNOR), may be used in the evaluation of canine mast cell tumors. In addition to the proliferative markers, localization of the tyrosine kinase (KIT) receptor and identification of c-KIT mutations are also used to evaluate behavior of mast cell tumors.[39,47] The combination of Ki67, AgNOR, and KIT localization have been shown to be prognostic for mast cell tumor behavior and may potentially be used in cytology for prognostic information.[47]

When used appropriately, in conjunction with routine cytological examination, ICC is a useful diagnostic tool, and its use is increasing in popularity. Currently, ICC is used primarily to assist in tumor phenotyping. Cellularity and sample type greatly affect result quality. Use of transport media allows for greater standardization of slide cellularity and the ability to produce multiple fairly uniform slides, which, in turn, allows for evaluation of an antibody panel, rather than just one or two antibodies. Communication with the laboratory and pathologist performing ICC is critical for appropriate interpretation of the sample, which should be evaluated and reported holistically for complete characterization.

REFERENCES

1. Montero C. The antigen-antibody reaction in immunohistochemistry. *J Histochem and Cytochem.* 2003;51:1–4.
2. Barger A, Raskin R, Flatland B, et al. ASVCP quality assurance guidelines: veterinary immunocytochemistry (ICC): approved guideline. [In press].
3. Tizard IR. *Veterinary Immunology.* 9th ed. St. Louis, MO: Elsevier; 2013.
4. Burry RW. *Immunocytochemistry: a Practical Guide for Biomedical Research.* New York: Springer; 2010.
5. Ramos-Vara JA. Technical aspects of immunohistochemistry. *Vet Pathol.* 2005;42:405–426.
6. Spieker-Polet H, Sethupathi P, Yam PC, et al. Rabbit monoclonal antibodies: generating a fusion partner to produce rabbit-rabbit hybridomas. *Proc Natl Acad Sci.* 1995;92:9348–9352.
7. Groff K, Brown J, Clippinger A. Modern affinity reagents: recombinant antibodies and aptamers. *Biotech Adv.* 2015;33(8):1787–1798.
8. Burry RW. Controls for immunocytochemistry: an update. *J Histochem and Cytochem.* 2011;59:6–12.
9. Al-Janabi S, Huisman A, Van Diest PJ. Digital pathology: current status and future perspectives. *Histopathology.* 2012;61(1):1–9.
10. Sawa M, Yabuki A, Miyoshi N, et al. A simple and rapid immunocytochemical technique for detection of cytokeratin, vimentin, and S-100 protein in veterinary diagnostic cytology. *Res Vet Sci.* 2012;93:1341–1345.
11. Valli V, Peters E, Williams C, et al. Optimizing methods in immunocytochemistry one laboratory's experience. *Vet Clin Pathol.* 2009;38:261–269.
12. Shi S, Shi Y, Taylor C. Antigen retrieval immunohistochemistry: review and future prospects in research and diagnosis over two decades. *J Histochem and Cytochem.* 2011;59:13–32.
13. Shi S, Key ME, Kalra KL. Antigen retrieval in formalin-fixed, paraffin-embedded tissues: an enhancement method for immunohistochemical staining based on microwave oven heating of tissue sections. *J Histochem and Cytochem.* 1991;39:741–748.
14. Skoog L, Tani E. Immunocytochemistry: an indispensable technique in routine cytology. *Cytopathol.* 2011;22:215–229.
15. Bordeaux J, Welsh AW, Agarwal S, et al. Antibody validation. *Biotechniques.* 2010;48:197–209.
16. Priest HL, Hume KR, Killick D, et al. The use, publication and future directions of immunocytochemistry in veterinary medicine: a consensus of the Oncology-Pathology Working Group. *Vet Comp Oncol.* 2016;15(3):868–880.
17. Fowler LJ, Lachar WA. Application of immunohistochemistry to cytology. *Arch Pathol Lab Med.* 2008;132:373–383.
18. Ramos-Vara JA, Avery AC, Avery PR. Advanced diagnostic techniques. In: Raskin RE, Meyer DJ, eds. *Canine and Feline Cytology: A Color Atlas and Interpretation Guide.* 3rd ed. St. Louis, MO: Elsevier; 2016:453–494.
19. Hernandez D, Priest H, Stokol T. Comparison of immunocytochemical staining for CD3, CD20, cytokeratin and vimentin in unstained and previously Wright-stained cytologic smears of canine tumors. Daniela Hernandez, Heather Priest, Tracy Stokol. Abstract presented at the ACVP Annual Meeting in New Orleans, LA, 2016.
20. Barger AM, Fan TM, de Lorimier L, et al. Expression of receptor activator of nuclear factor κB ligand (RANK-L) in canine and feline neoplasms. *J Vet Intern Med.* 2007;21:133–140.
21. Bueno A, Viero RM, Soares CT. Fine needle aspirate cell blocks are reliable for detection of hormone receptors and HER-2 by immunohistochemistry in breast carcinoma. *Cytopathol.* 2012;24(1):26–32.
22. Yung RC, Otell S, Illei P, et al. Improvement of cellularity on cell block preparations using the so-called tissue coagulum clot method during endobronchial ultrasound-guided transbronchial fine-needle aspiration. *Cancer Cytopathol.* 2011;120(3):185–195.
23. Wallace KA, Goldschmidt MH, Patel RT. Converting fluid-based cytologic specimens to histologic specimens for immunohistochemistry. *Vet Clin Pathol.* 2015;44:303–309.
24. Fetsch PA, Abati A. Immunocytochemistry in effusion cytology. *Cancer Cytopathol.* 2001;93:293–308.
25. Höinghaus R, Hewicker-Trautwien M, Mischke R. Immunocytochemical differentiation of neoplastic and hyperplastic canine epithelial lesions in cytologic imprint preparations. *Vet J.* 2007;173:79–90.
26. Höinghaus R, Hewicker-Trautwein, Mischke R. Immunocytochemical differentiation of canine mesenchymal tumors in cytologic imprint preparations. *Vet Clin Pathol.* 2008;37:104–111.
27. Barger A, Graca R, Bailey K, et al. Utilization of alkaline phosphatase staining to differentiate osteosarcoma from other vimentin positive tumors. *Vet Pathol.* 2005;42:161–165.
28. Avallone G, da Cunha NP, Palmieri C, et al. Subcutaneous embryonal rhabdomyosarcoma in a dog: cytologic, immunocytochemical, histologic and, ultrastructural features. *Vet Clin Pathol.* 2010;39:499–504.
29. Cornegliani L, Gracis M, Ferro S, et al. Sublingual reactive histiocytosis in a dog. *J Vet Dent.* 2011;28:164–170.
30. Fang J, Hussong JW, Perkins SL, et al. Diagnosis and classification of lymphoma based on cytospin preparations: a comparison of hematopathologists and cytopathologists. *Diag Cytopath.* 1999;22:336–341.
31. Caniatti M, Roccabianca P, Scanziani E, et al. Canine lymphoma: immunocytochemical analysis of fine-needle aspiration biopsy. *Vet Pathol.* 1996;33:204–212.
32. Roccabianca P, Vernau W, Caniatti M. Feline large granular lymphocyte (LGL) lymphoma with secondary leukemia: primary intestinal origin with predominance of a CD3/CD8αα phenotype. *Vet Pathol.* 2006;43:15–28.
33. Lane LV, Allison RW, Rizzi TR, et al. Canine intravascular lymphoma with overt leukemia. *Vet Clin Pathol.* 2012;41(1):84–91.
34. Seelig DM, Avery AC, Ehrhart EJ, et al. The comparative diagnostic features of canine and human lymphoma. *Vet Sci.* 2016;3(2):11–40.
35. Stokol T, Schaefer D, Shuman DM, et al. Alkaline phosphatase is a useful cytochemical marker for the diagnosis of acute myelomonocytic and monocytic leukemia in the dog. *Vet Clin Pathol.* 2015;44:79–93.
36. Höinghaus R, von Wasielewski R, Hewicker-Trauwein M, et al. Immunocytological detection of lymph node metastases in dogs with malignant epithelial tumours. *J Comp Path.* 2007;137:1–8.
37. Madewell BR. Cellular proliferation in tumors: a review of methods, interpretation, and clinical applications. *J Vet Intern Med.* 2001;15:334–340.
38. Ettinger SN, Scase TJ, Oberthaler KT, et al. Association of argyrophilic nucleolar organizing regions, Ki-67 and proliferation cell nuclear antigen scores with histologic grade and survival in dogs with soft tissue sarcomas: 60 cases (1996-2002). *J Am Vet Med Assoc.* 2006;228:1053–1062.

39. Webster JD, Yuzbasiyan-Gurkan V, Miller RA, et al. Cellular proliferation in canine cutaneous mast cell tumors: associations with c-KIT and its role in prognostication. *Vet Pathol.* 2007;44:298–308.

40. Scase TJ, Edwards D, Miller J, et al. Canine mast cell tumors: correlation of apoptosis and proliferation markers with prognosis. *J Vet Intern Med.* 2006;20:151–158.

41. Kang SK, Park NY, Cho HS, et al. Relationship between DNA ploidy and proliferative cell nuclear antigen index in canine hemangiopericytoma. *J Vet Diagn Invest.* 2006;18:211–214.

42. Vinothini G, Balachandran C, Nagini S. Evaluation of molecular markers in canine mammary tumors: correlation with histological grading. *Onco Res.* 2009;18:193–201.

43. Gillespie V, Baer K, Farrelly J, et al. Canine gastrointestinal stromal tumors: immunohistochemical expression of CD34 and examination of prognostic indicators including proliferation markers Ki67 and AgNOR. *Vet Pathol.* 2001;48:283–291.

44. Matiasek LA, Platt SR, Adams V, et al. Ki-67 and vascular endothelial growth factor expression in intracranial meningiomas in dogs. *J Vet Intern Med.* 2009;23:146–151.

45. Bergin IL, Smedley RC, Esplin DG, et al. Prognostic evaluation of Ki67 threshold value in canine oral melanoma. *Vet Pathol.* 2011;48:41–53.

46. Bauer NB, Zervos D, Moritz A. Argyrophilic nucleolar organizing regions and Ki67 equally reflect proliferation in fine needle aspirates of normal, hyperplastic inflamed and neoplastic canine lymph nodes. *J Vet Intern Med.* 2007;21:928–935.

47. Thompson JJ, Yager JA, Best SJ, et al. Canine subcutaneous mast cell tumors: cellular proliferation and KIT expression as prognostic indices. *Vet Pathol.* 2011;48:169–181.

30

Special Tests: Flow Cytometry

Deanna M. W. Schaefer and Stephanie C. Corn

Flow cytometry is commonly used to diagnose, monitor, and immuno-phenotype (identify the cell lineage) hematopoietic neoplasia, such as lymphoma and leukemia.[1] It can help differentiate between lymphoid neoplasia, such as chronic lymphocytic leukemia (CLL), and nonneoplastic lymphoid proliferation, such as reactive lymphocytosis. Flow cytometry is also used to differentiate between T-cell and B-cell lymphomas, to determine the cell line of blasts in acute leukemia, and to aid in the diagnosis of immune-mediated anemia and thrombocytopenia.

Other special tests are also available to aid in diagnosis and phenotyping of hematopoietic neoplasia, including polymerase chain reaction (PCR) for antigen receptor rearrangements (PARR), immunohistochemistry (IHC), and immunocytochemistry (ICC) (Table 30.1).[2-4] There is no consensus, to date, about comparing the sensitivity and specificity of flow cytometry, PARR, IHC, and ICC for the diagnosis of leukemia and lymphoma in dogs and cats, and false-positive and false-negative results can occur with any of these methods. Histopathology/IHC or flow cytometry are generally considered the preferred tests for diagnosis and immunophenotyping of hematopoietic neoplasia. Flow cytometry has the advantage of providing a larger panel of markers compared with IHC or ICC. Some cases of lymphoma may have concurrent clonal rearrangements in both B-cell and T-cell genes on PARR, and acute myeloid leukemia may have clonal PARR results, reducing the usefulness of PARR for immunophenotyping.[2-5] The main reasons to perform PARR would be if flow cytometry results are equivocal or if the only samples available are cytology slides.[2-4]

PRINCIPLES OF FLOW CYTOMETRY

Flow cytometry measures multiple characteristics of cells and particles in fluid as they pass through a laser beam. In its simplest form, flow cytometry is used in many hematology analyzers as part of a complete blood count (CBC). As a cell passes in front of a laser within the analyzer, light scatters at a low angle depending on the size of the cell and at a high angle with increasing cytoplasmic granularity or nuclear lobulation.[6] The analyzer uses these properties when reporting multiple measures on the CBC, including the automated leukocyte differential.[7] More complex flow cytometers can also evaluate expression of specific cell surface proteins (cluster of differentiation molecules or CD [cluster of differentiation] molecules) by using fluorescent markers. The pattern of markers expressed on cells can be used to identify cell type or lineage.

TABLE 30.1 Comparison of Flow Cytometry, PARR, IHC, and ICC for Diagnosis of Hematopoietic Neoplasia[4,14]

	Flow Cytometry	PARR	IHC and Histopathology	ICC and Cytology
Sample	Freshly collected liquid sample with intact cells	Fluid; unstained or stained cytology slides Results from formalin-fixed tissue may not be as reliable	Formalin-fixed tissue	Usually one unstained cytology slide with intact cells for each marker
Typical size of results panel[a]	Largest	Smallest	Variable	Variable
Advantages in diagnosis of hematopoietic neoplasia	Typically has the shortest turnaround time Results can sometimes provide prognostic information	Can be used if other tests are equivocal (e.g., to detect a smaller number of neoplastic cells within a mixed lymphoid population)	Allows for evaluation of tissue architecture and cytoplasmic marker expression	Allows for evaluation of cytoplasmic marker expression
Limitations in diagnosis of hematopoietic neoplasia	May not be able to confirm neoplasia within a mixed cell population or if there is no aberrant marker expression	May not be as reliable as other methods for discerning B-cell neoplasia from T-cell neoplasia Some inflammatory and infectious diseases can have clonal PARR results	May have the longest turn-around time Some markers do not work well on formalin-fixed tissue	May have a long turnaround time May be difficult to interpret because of nonspecific staining or decreased marker expression

[a]Number of markers for flow cytometry, IHC, and ICC; number of PCR products for PARR.
ICC, immunocytochemistry; *IHC,* immunohistochemistry; *PARR,* polymerase chain reaction for antigen receptor rearrangements.

Antibodies to Surface Proteins

Commercially available antibodies to cell surface proteins are available for tests in dogs and cats, and many are prelabeled with fluorescent dyes. When cells bound by these antibodies pass through the laser in the instrument, the fluorescent molecules are excited to a higher energy state and emit light at a specific wavelength that is measured by the instrument. Therefore cells that express a given surface marker are detected as a fluorescent signal. The use of different fluorescent dyes allows measurement of multiple surface proteins simultaneously within a cell population.

Sample Collection and Shipping

Flow cytometry requires viable intact cells in fluid suspension and cannot be performed on blood smears, cytology or histopathology slides, or formalin-fixed tissues. Peripheral blood or bone marrow samples can be collected into an ethylenediaminetetraacetic acid (EDTA) tube. If other tissues are sampled, these are collected in the same manner as a fine-needle aspirate and then placed in fluid suspension for transport. Laboratories may suggest using cell culture media with 10% fetal bovine serum. If media is not available, fine-needle aspiration (FNA) samples can be added to 0.9 mL saline and 0.1 mL patient serum in a red-top or clear-top no-additive tube. It is important to prepare cytology slides at the same time to ensure that the neoplastic cell population is represented in the sample.[8] Occasionally, neoplastic cells may be particularly fragile and lyse, leaving predominantly small lymphocytes from a residual normal lymphoid population. In patients with lymphoma, lymph nodes tend to exfoliate well in flow cytometry, but samples from the spleen, liver, intestinal masses, or cutaneous lesions may exfoliate poorly or be nondiagnostic because of cell disruption.[8]

The sample must be adequately cellular to obtain conclusive results. The cells to be analyzed (e.g., circulating atypical lymphocytes for blood samples, large lymphocytes from node aspirates) ideally should be present in a concentration of greater than 3000/μL. For patients with lymphadenopathy, sampling of multiple lymph nodes is recommended. Typically, two to three aspirates provide adequate numbers of cells for analysis.[8] Cell preservation is critical to preserve cell surface proteins for analysis, so care should be used when collecting samples. The sample should be promptly shipped with a cold pack to the testing facility. Ideally, samples should be analyzed within 2 to 3 days, but blood samples and those in tubes with preservatives may be viable for up to 5 days. Collecting samples early in the week is preferred to prevent delays over the weekend in shipping or sample analysis. It is also important to collect samples before initiation of chemotherapy or treatment with corticosteroids, particularly in patients with lymphoma.

In cases where atypical cells are present in both tissue and peripheral blood, a blood sample should only be submitted if the atypical cells are present in sufficient numbers. For example, if a dog with large cell lymphoma has greater than 90% large, immature lymphocytes on cytology of the lymph node but only low numbers (<3000/μL) of neoplastic cells in peripheral blood, an FNA sample of the lymph node would be the ideal sample for submission.

Sample Processing and Data Analysis

At the laboratory, red blood cells (RBCs) in the sample are lysed using a hypotonic solution and the cells are incubated with fluorescently labeled antibodies.[9] A negative isotype control is used for each fluorescent dye to identify nonspecific background fluorescence. Antibody panels are not standardized and may differ between laboratories. Some of the most commonly used commercially available surface antibodies

TABLE 30.2 Common Commercially Available Surface Markers in Dogs and Cats

Marker	Canine Cellular Expression	Feline Cellular Expression
CD21	B cells	B cells
CD5	T cells	T cells
CD4	Helper T cells and neutrophils	Helper T cells
CD8	Cytotoxic T cells	Cytotoxic T cells
CD11b	Neutrophils, monocytes	Not available
CD11c	Neutrophils, monocytes	Not available
CD11d	Some T cells, some macrophages	Not available
CD14	Monocytes	Monocytes
CD18	All leukocytes, more strongly in monocytes and granulocytes	All leukocytes, more strongly in monocytes and granulocytes
CD45	All leukocytes	Not available
CD34	Stem cells (acute leukemia)	Not available
MHC class II	Monocytes, B cells, T cells	Not available

MHC, major histocompatibility complex.

for dogs and cats are listed in Table 30.2, but other antibodies are also available. Selection of markers for cats is more limited compared with those for dogs.

INDICATIONS FOR IMMUNOPHENOTYPING BY FLOW CYTOMETRY

In veterinary medicine, flow cytometry is often used to aid in the diagnosis of leukemia or lymphoma in dogs and cats—that is, to evaluate those with peripheral blood lymphocytosis or with abnormal cells identified in blood, lymph nodes, spleen, or other tissues if the cells are present in sufficient numbers. In these cases, flow cytometry can help establish cell lineage (e.g., B cells or T cells), determine the likelihood that the cells are neoplastic, and may, in some cases, provide prognostic information. Tables 30.3 and 30.4 summarize expected results of flow cytometry and clinical behavior of common types of leukemia and multicentric lymphoma in dogs.

Flow cytometry is not typically used for diagnosis of other types of neoplasia, such as plasma cell tumor, mast cell tumor, carcinoma, sarcoma, or melanoma.[10] These are usually classified by using IHC or ICC, when necessary.

SMALL CELL LYMPHOCYTOSIS IN DOGS

The light microscopic cell morphology can be similar in cases of lymphocytosis as a result of reactive lymphocytosis, CLL, and the leukemic phase of small cell lymphoma, with the majority of circulating lymphocytes being small, morphologically well-differentiated cells. Flow cytometry may be helpful in determining whether the lymphocytes are neoplastic or nonneoplastic in these cases. The lymphocyte population in blood from healthy dogs and cats is a mixture of helper T cells, cytotoxic T cells, and B cells. If the lymphocyte population is heterogeneous on flow cytometry, the patient should be evaluated for nonneoplastic reactive lymphocytosis. Reported differential diagnoses for reactive lymphocytosis in dogs include infections (e.g., with *Ehrlichia canis, Leishmania infantum,* and *Spirocerca lupi*) and hypoadrenocorticism.[3] If immunophenotyping reveals a homogeneous population of a T-cell subset or B cells, then neoplastic lymphocytosis is most likely,

TABLE 30.3   Flow Cytometry[a] for Select Common Types of Leukemia and Multicentric Lymphoma in Dogs[14,18,26,39]

	CD45	CD34	MHC Class II	CD3	CD5	CD4	CD8	CD21	CD14	CD11	Cell Size[b]
B-cell CLL	+	–	+	–	–	–	–	+	–		Small
T-cell CLL, CD8+	+	–	+	+	+	–	+	–	–		Small to medium
T-cell ALL	+	V	–	+	+	V[a]	V[a]	–	–	V[b]	Medium to large
AML-M4 and AML-M5	+	+	–	–	–	V	–	–	+	V[c]	Medium to large
Diffuse large B-cell lymphoma	+	V[d]	V[e]	–	V[d]	–	–	+	–		Medium to large
T zone lymphoma	–	–	+	+	+	V[a]	V[a]	V			Small to medium
T-cell large cell lymphoma, CD4+	+	–	Low	+	V	+	–	–	–		Medium to large

[a]This chart summarizes the commonly reported results for flow cytometry in these types of canine neoplasia, but results may vary for individual cases.

[b]Relative cell size can be estimated on flow cytometry based on the median forward light scatter of gated neoplastic cells, with higher forward scatter correlating to increasing cell size.

V = Variable.

V[a] = May be CD4+/CD8-, CD4-/CD8+, CD4-/CD8-, or (rarely) CD4+/CD8+.

V[b] = Occasionally positive for CD11b, CD11c, and/or CD11d.

V[c] = Commonly positive for CD11b, CD11c, and/or CD11d.

V[d] = Most are negative.

V[e] = Most are positive.

ALL, acute lymphoid leukemia; AML, acute myeloid leukemia; CLL, chronic lymphocytic leukemia.

although there are exceptions. Identification of lymphocytes that have lost expression of normal surface markers or that express an abnormal combination of markers (aberrant phenotype) can also support a diagnosis of neoplasia. For example, T cells in peripheral blood and lymph nodes normally express either CD4 (helper T cells) or CD8 (cytotoxic T cells). Lack of CD4 or CD8 expression in T cells is one of the more prevalent aberrant immunophenotypes in dogs with neoplastic lymphocytosis.[11] The majority of adult dogs with persistent small cell lymphocytosis have a homogeneous lymphocyte population (>80% of the lymphocytes have the same immunophenotype) and/or aberrant antigen expression indicating neoplastic lymphocytosis.[3,12,13]

B-Cell Lymphocytosis of Small Cells

Dogs with significant B-cell small cell lymphocytosis typically have neoplastic disease—that is, B-cell CLL or the leukemic phase of a small cell B-cell lymphoma. Distinction between these two neoplastic diseases may be difficult, and they are sometimes collectively referred to as B-cell CLL/small cell lymphoma.[14] These are usually indolent diseases, although one study found a poorer prognosis in dogs diagnosed at less than 8 years of age.[11,14]

Cytotoxic T-Cell Lymphocytosis of Small Cells

Lymphocytes with this phenotype express CD8 and pan-T-cell markers CD3 and CD5. They are typically of medium size, with oval nuclei, lightly clumped chromatin, no nucleoli, and a scant to moderate amount of lightly basophilic cytoplasm. These cells may contain multiple, fine, pink cytoplasmic granules, and such cells are referred to as granular lymphocytes (Fig. 30.1). An expansion of cytotoxic T cells can occur either with neoplastic diseases, such as CLL, or with certain nonneoplastic diseases.

Chronic Ehrlichiosis

A homogeneous cytotoxic (CD8+) T-cell population occasionally can be seen in nonneoplastic diseases, particularly in dogs with E. canis infection.[15] Generally, dogs with E. canis (or any other cause of nonneoplastic lymphocytosis) have lymphocyte counts less than 30,000/μL.[3] Serology and PCR testing are helpful in excluding ehrlichiosis as a cause of persistent lymphocytosis with this phenotype.

Neoplastic Cytotoxic T-Cell Lymphocytosis of Small Cells

Cytotoxic T-cell CLL is the most commonly reported type of canine CLL.[16] It often has an indolent course and originates in the spleen. Bone marrow may be spared until late in the disease, so bone marrow cytology often is not helpful for diagnosis.[17] In a study of 33 dogs with cytotoxic T-cell CLL, those with greater than 30,000 lymphocytes/μL had shorter median survival,[11] but another study documented a long median survival time independent of cell count.[13]

Dogs with one type of indolent lymphoma, T-zone lymphoma, often have neoplastic lymphocytosis that is morphologically indistinguishable from CLL.[18] Expression of CD4 and CD8 is variable in T-zone lymphoma, and in some cases the neoplastic cells are positive for CD8 as in T-cell CLL.[18] In contrast, however, T-zone lymphoma cells are negative for the pan-leukocyte marker CD45.[14] More information on T-zone lymphoma is provided later in this chapter.

SMALL CELL LYMPHOCYTOSIS IN CATS

Nonneoplastic Lymphocytosis

There is limited published information for the incidence of neoplastic lymphocytosis versus nonneoplastic lymphocytosis in cats. Physiological lymphocytosis caused by stress or excitement is common in cats, but this

TABLE 30.4 Breed Predisposition and Clinical Behavior of Select Common Types of Leukemia and Multicentric Lymphoma in Dogs[14,18,39]

	Reported Breed Predispositions	Clinical Behavior
B-cell CLL	Small breeds	Indolent May have poorer prognosis if diagnosed at <8 years of age
T-cell CLL, CD8+	Large breeds	Indolent Dogs with lymphocytosis of >30 × 10⁶/L may have shorter survival time
T-cell ALL	Golden Retrievers	Aggressive
AML-M4 and AML-M5	German Shepherds	Aggressive
Diffuse large B-cell lymphoma		Poorer prognosis for MHC-II– compared with MHCII+, and for large cell size compared with medium cell size Similar prognosis for CD34 + and CD34–
T zone lymphoma	Golden Retrievers	Indolent Commonly have T-zone cells in peripheral blood, which does not have prognostic significance
T-cell large cell lymphoma, CD4+	Boxers and Golden Retrievers	Aggressive Those positive for CD5 may have modestly shortened survival

ALL, acute lymphoid leukemia; *AML*, acute myeloid leukemia; *CLL*, chronic lymphocytic leukemia.

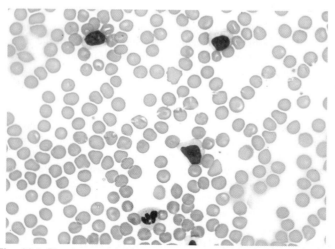

Fig. 30.1 Blood smear (1000×) from a 10-year-old Golden Retriever with persistent lymphocytosis and a lymphocyte count of 27,784/μL. On flow cytometry, greater than 90% of the lymphocytes coexpressed CD3 and CD8 in addition to CD5 and CD45, indicating cytotoxic T-cell lymphocytosis consistent with chronic lymphocytic leukemia.

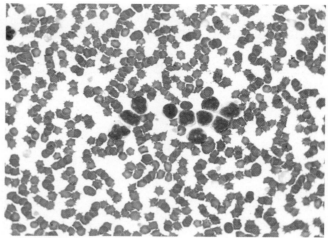

Fig. 30.2 Blood smear (1000×) from a 4-year-old Domestic Shorthair (DSH) cat with persistent mild-to-moderate lymphocytosis and a lymphocyte count of 8568/μL.

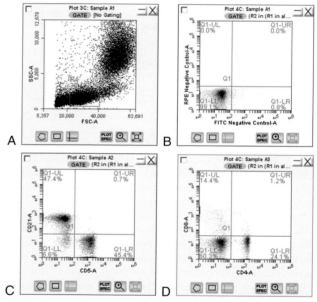

Fig. 30.3 Flow cytometry of the sample from Fig. 30.2 revealed a heterogeneous lymphoid population consistent with reactive lymphocytosis. (A) The lymphocytes are gated based on forward and light scatter and are small to intermediate in size. (B) Negative isotype control for two fluorochromes, FITC and RPE, to exclude nonspecific binding. (C) Forty-five percent of the cells express CD5 (T-cell marker, *x*-axis), and 47% of the cells express CD21 (B-cell marker, *y*-axis). (D) Twenty-four percent of the cells are CD4+ helper T cells, and 14% are CD8+ cytotoxic T cells.

is typically transient and not identified on repeat samplings. Potential causes of persistent nonneoplastic or reactive lymphocytosis in cats include infectious agents, such as hemotropic *Mycoplasma*, *Cytauxzoon felis*, *Toxoplasma gondii*, feline leukemia virus (FeLV), or feline immunodeficiency virus (FIV), and immune-mediated disease, hypoadrenocorticism, hyperthyroidism, and methimazole therapy.[3,19,20] The lymphocytes in cats with reactive lymphocytosis are typically small, have normal morphology (Fig. 30.2), and are heterogeneous on flow cytometry (Fig. 30.3). These cats may have shifts in the ratio of helper T cells and cytotoxic T cells or increased numbers of B cells compared with healthy cats.

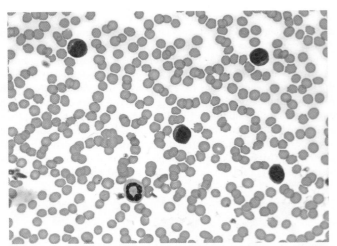

Fig. 30.4 Blood smear (1000×) from a 15-year-old Domestic Shorthair (DSH) cat with persistent moderate-to-marked lymphocytosis and a lymphocyte count of 24,745/μL.

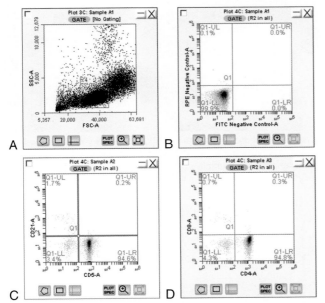

Fig. 30.5 Flow cytometry of the sample from Fig. 30.4 demonstrated a monomorphic lymphocyte population consistent with helper T-cell CLL. (A) The lymphocytes are gated, based on forward and light scatter, and are small to intermediate in size (slightly larger than the cat with reactive lymphocytosis in Fig. 30.3). (B) Negative isotype control for two fluorochromes, FITC and RPE, to exclude nonspecific binding. (C) Ninety-five percent of the cells express CD5 (T-cell marker) on the x-axis, and less than 2% express CD21 (B-cell marker). (D) Ninety-five percent of the cells are CD4+ helper T cells and less than 1% are CD8+ cytotoxic T cells.

Chronic Lymphocytic Leukemia in Cats

As in dogs, cats with CLL typically have a homogeneous expansion of a single lymphocyte subtype. Unlike in dogs, however, the most common CLL type in cats is CD4+ T-helper cells.[3,21,22] The lymphocytes may be small or intermediate in size, with less densely clumped chromatin and slightly more abundant cytoplasm (Figs. 30.4 and 30.5). Limited prognostic information is available for subtypes of CLL in cats, so the main application of flow cytometry is to differentiate neoplastic lymphocytosis from nonneoplastic lymphocytosis. In two

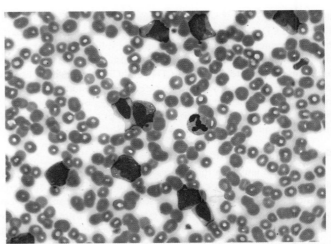

Fig. 30.6 Blood smear (1000×) from a 6-year-old spaniel dog with extreme leukocytosis, 116,278/μL circulating blasts, neutropenia, thrombocytopenia, and nonregenerative anemia. The blasts are large, round cells with irregular to lobulated nuclei, fine chromatin, indistinct nucleoli, and scant-to-moderate basophilic cytoplasm. This morphology can be seen in lymphoblasts, myeloblasts, and undifferentiated blasts. On flow cytometry, the blasts expressed only CD34 and CD45, consistent with an acute undifferentiated leukemia or acute myeloblastic leukemia with minimal differentiation. Additional testing was not pursued to further classify the cells.

studies, cats with CLL treated with chemotherapy were found to have median survival times of greater than 1 year.[22,23]

ACUTE LEUKEMIA

Flow cytometry can be performed in cases where acute leukemia is suspected on the basis of identification of blasts in blood or marrow. Blasts are intermediate- to large-size immature hematopoietic cells with a high nuclear to cytoplasmic ratio and fine chromatin. Immunophenotyping is often required to classify neoplastic blasts as lymphoid (acute lymphoblastic leukemia [ALL]) or myeloid (acute myeloid leukemia [AML]) because the microscopic appearance of blasts can be similar regardless of lineage.

Acute leukemia has traditionally been diagnosed in animals with greater than 30% blasts in peripheral blood or bone marrow.[24] More recently, this has been reduced to 20% in humans, and adopting a similar cutoff point has been proposed for veterinary medicine.[25] Flow cytometry allows blast enumeration that is objectively based on expression of the stem cell marker CD34, commonly present on acute leukemia cells.[10,16,26] Blasts may also express markers of lymphoid, granulocytic, or monocytic differentiation, allowing for more specific identification of cell lineage (Table 30.3).

Acute Undifferentiated Leukemia and Acute Myeloid Leukemia

Acute leukemia in which the neoplastic cells express only CD34 and CD45 with no lineage-specific markers is termed either *acute undifferentiated leukemia* (AUL) or *acute myeloid leukemia without differentiation* (AML-M0) (Fig. 30.6). This type of acute leukemia generally has a poor prognosis and short survival time, even with multiagent chemotherapy.[11,27]

Other types of AML that are common in dogs include acute myelomonocytic leukemia (AML-M4) and acute monocytic leukemia (AML-M5). In addition to CD34 and CD45, these types of leukemia typically express one or more lineage-specific myeloid markers, such as CD14 or CD11.[26-28] Some cases of acute leukemia expressing only CD34 and CD45 have been classified as AML-M4 or AML-M5 based on cytochemical staining with alkaline phosphatase.[26] Several cases of acute megakaryoblastic leukemia have also been reported in dogs, and markers of platelet lineage (CD41 and CD61) have been used to confirm the diagnosis by flow cytometry.[29-32] In a study of dogs with confirmed AML, median survival time was 7 days, but this was skewed by the number of dogs euthanized as a result of severe clinical signs at presentation and perceived poor prognosis.[33]

Acute Lymphoblastic Leukemia

Cases of acute leukemia that express lymphoid markers can be classified as T-cell ALL or B-cell ALL. Expression of CD34 is considered a hallmark of acute leukemia, but cases of ALL fairly commonly can be negative for this marker on flow cytometry.[26] This makes the distinction between ALL and advanced-stage V lymphoma subjective in some cases, based on the degree of involvement of lymphoid tissue versus marrow.[14] Occasionally, the neoplastic cells may only express lineage-specific markers (e.g., CD3 for T cells and CD79a for B cells) within the cytoplasm rather than on the cell surface.[10,27] Cytoplasmic expression can be evaluated with IHC, ICC, or flow cytometry by using permeabilization reagents. Nonspecific nuclear staining may occur with use of these techniques (particularly with CD79a), which is recognizable with IHC or ICC on microscopy but can be difficult to differentiate from cytoplasmic staining on flow cytometry.

IMMUNOPHENOTYPING OF LYMPHOMA IN DOGS

Flow cytometry is commonly used in dogs to either support a diagnosis of lymphoma or provide prognostic information based on the immunophenotype. Cytology is often sufficient by itself to diagnose large cell lymphoma.[4] However, small cell lymphoma can be difficult to differentiate from lymphoid hyperplasia on cytology, and definitive diagnosis often requires additional testing, such as histopathology, PARR, or flow cytometry.[4] In

these cases, flow cytometry would favor hyperplasia if the lymphoid population were heterogeneous, whereas a homogeneous lymphoid population with aberrant marker expression would support neoplasia.

Flow cytometry is also useful when the diagnosis of lymphoma has already been confirmed with cytology or histopathology because the immunophenotype may have prognostic implications. Dogs with B-cell lymphoma typically have longer survival times compared with dogs with T-cell lymphoma.[34-37] However, there are exceptions, such as T-zone lymphoma, which can have the longest median survival of any type of lymphoma.[38] Expression of major histocompatibility complex class II (MHC-II) in B-cell lymphoma may also provide prognostic information (Table 30.4).[39] Figs. 30.7 and 30.8 provide examples of

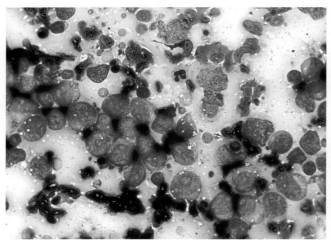

Fig. 30.7 Lymph node aspirate (1000×) from an 8-year-old mixed breed dog. There is homogeneous population of large lymphocytes with finely stippled chromatin, multiple nucleoli, and deeply basophilic cytoplasm. The cytological diagnosis was large cell lymphoma.

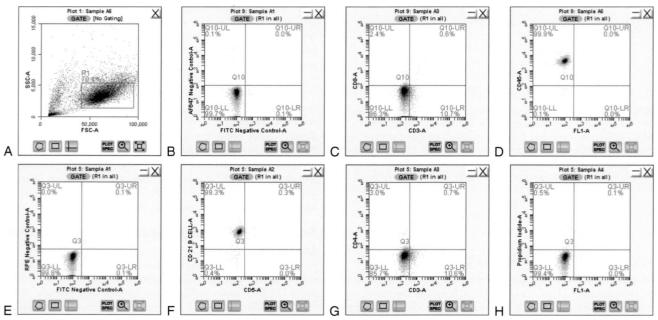

Fig. 30.8 Flow cytometry of the lymph node sample from Fig. 30.7 is consistent with large cell B-cell lymphoma. (A) The cells of interest are gated based on forward and light scatter and are large. (B) Negative isotype control for two fluorochromes, FITC and AF647, to exclude nonspecific fluorescence. (C) Expression of surface CD3 and CD8 is minimal. (D) Positive expression of CD45 in 99.9% of the cells on the y-axis with no antibody added for the x-axis. (E) Negative isotype control for two fluorochromes, FITC and RPE. (F) Strong expression of CD21 in greater than 99% of the cells indicating B-cell lineage, negative expression of CD5. (G) Expression of surface CD3 and CD4 is minimal. (H) Less than 1% of the cells in the gated population stain with propidium iodide and are not intact.

cytology and immunophenotyping results from a dog with intermediate to high-grade B-cell canine lymphoma. Figs. 30.9 and 30.10 provide examples from a dog with high-grade helper T-cell lymphoma, which often has an aggressive clinical course.[40]

Aberrant Immunophenotypes in Canine Lymphoma

Some cases of canine lymphoma, for example T-zone lymphoma and diffuse large B-cell lymphoma, can have aberrant surface marker

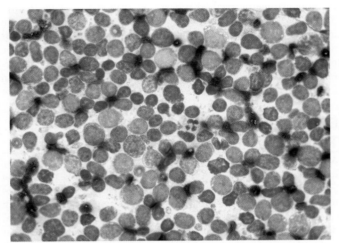

Fig. 30.9 Lymph node aspirate (1000×) from a 6-year-old Boxer dog. Most of the lymphocytes are intermediate to large with oval nuclei with fine to finely stippled chromatin and occasional indistinct nucleoli.

expression—that is, patterns not observed on normal or reactive lymphocytes or markers not commonly expressed by cells from the anatomical site that was sampled.[18,37,39]

T-Zone Lymphoma

T-zone lymphoma has a distinctive pattern on flow cytometry, with small- to intermediate-size lymphocytes that express T-cell markers (CD5 and CD3) but have lost expression of CD45. The cells also have high MHC-II expression, may express the B-cell marker CD21, and have variable expression of CD4 and CD8 (see Table 30.3).[14,18] This pattern can be readily differentiated from a reactive lymph node, where the lymphocytes retain expression of CD45 and are a mixed population of T cells and B cells. T-zone lymphoma often has an indolent course and slowly progressive lymphadenopathy.[18,41] Approximately half the dogs with this type of lymphoma have lymphocytosis, with the lymphocytes in the peripheral blood having the same immunophenotype as the cells in the lymph node.[18] This lymphocytosis is distinguished from T-cell CLL by the lack of expression of CD45. Cytologically, T-zone lymphoma is composed of a homogeneous population of small- to intermediate-size lymphocytes with smooth chromatin and a scant to moderate amount of lightly basophilic cytoplasm. The cytoplasmic borders are often distorted, giving the cells a "hand mirror" appearance, and there are only very rare mitotic figures (Fig. 30.11).[4,14,42]

B-Cell Large Cell Lymphoma

Decreased MHC-II expression in canine B-cell lymphoma may be associated with a poorer prognosis.[39] Some cases of canine B-cell large cell lymphoma express CD34 (typically expressed by acute leukemia cells), but this does not appear to have prognostic significance.[37,39]

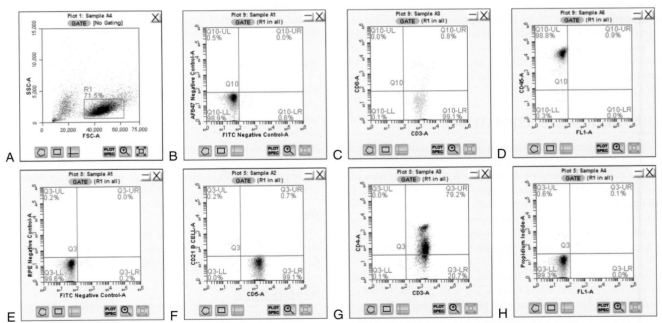

Fig. 30.10 Flow cytometry of the lymph node sample from Fig. 30.9 is consistent with large cell helper T-cell lymphoma. (A) The cells of interest are gated, based on forward and light scatter, and are intermediate to large in size (smaller than the B-cells in Fig. 30.8). (B) Negative isotype control for FITC and AF647 to exclude nonspecific fluorescence. (C) Greater than 99% of the cells express CD3, but less than 1% express CD8. (D) Positive expression of CD45 by greater than 98% of the cells on the y-axis with no antibody added for the x-axis. (E) Negative isotype control for two fluorochromes, FITC and RPE. (F) Greater than 99% of the cells express CD5, but less than 1% express CD21. (G) The neoplastic cells coexpress CD3 and CD4, indicating helper T-cell lineage. Many cells have dim CD4 expression, weaker than normal helper T cells. (F) Less than 1% of the cells in the gated population stain with propidium iodide and are not intact.

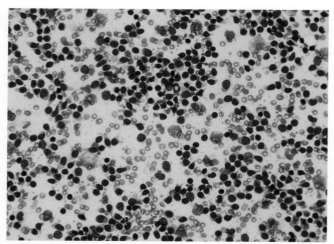

Fig. 30.11 Lymph node aspirate (500×) from a 9-year-old male Golden Retriever with a homogeneous population of intermediate-sized lymphocytes with distorted cytoplasmic borders and "hand mirror" morphology typical for T-zone lymphoma. On flow cytometry, the lymphocytes expressed T-cell markers CD3 and CD5 but did not express CD4, CD8, or CD45.

IMMUNOPHENOTYPING OF LYMPHOMA IN CATS

Immunophenotyping by flow cytometry is used less commonly in cats than in dogs because the immunophenotype of lymphoma in cats has not been strongly associated with the prognosis.[34] Also, feline lymphoma often involves the alimentary tract or other internal organs that may be difficult to sample for flow cytometry.[43] Lymphoma of granular lymphocytes is a subtype of lymphoma with a poor prognosis in cats.[44] The immunophenotype of this disorder has been described, but neoplastic granular lymphocytes are typically easily recognized on Wright-Giemsa–stained cytology slides, and immunophenotyping is generally not necessary for diagnosis. The granules in these cells may dissolve with rapid aqueous stains, such as Diff-Quick.

MEDIASTINAL MASS ASPIRATES

Flow cytometry, in conjunction with cytological evaluation, can help differentiate lymphocyte-rich thymoma from thymic lymphoma. This distinction is important because thymoma is usually treated with surgery or radiation, whereas chemotherapy is the typical treatment for lymphoma. Thymic lymphocytes are T cells that express both CD4 and CD8, whereas most T-cell lymphomas express only CD4, CD8, or neither marker. A diagnosis of thymoma is supported if greater than 10% of small lymphocytes from a canine mediastinal mass coexpress CD4 and CD8.[45]

Interestingly, there is a case report in which flow cytometry was performed on peripheral blood from a dog with lymphocytosis; the dog had a mediastinal mass that had been diagnosed as thymoma. Greater than 90% of blood lymphocytes were CD3+ T cells, with about half being double-negative for CD4 and CD8. There was no detectable increase in cells double-positive for CD4 and CD8 in blood. The blood lymphocytes were polyclonal, as shown by PARR, and were thought to represent a nonneoplastic expansion of γδ T cells secondary to altered lymphopoiesis caused by humoral influences of thymic hormones, rather than by spillover of thymocytes from the thymoma.[46]

EVALUATION OF IMMUNE-MEDIATED HEMOLYTIC ANEMIA

The Coombs test is commonly used to support a diagnosis of immune-mediated hemolytic anemia (IMHA) in dogs. This test detects increased binding of immunoglobulin G (IgG), immunoglobulin M (IgM), and/or complement to RBCs, but sensitivity can be low.[47] Erythrocyte-bound IgG, IgM, and complement (C3) can also be detected by using flow cytometry. In two studies, the sensitivity of the flow cytometric method was greater than 90%, compared with 53% to 58% for the Coombs test, so flow cytometry may be helpful in patients with equivocal results on Coombs testing.[48,49] Patients without evidence of hemolytic anemia may occasionally have positive results on the Coombs test or flow cytometry, so it is important to correlate the results with the RBC parameters, morphology, and clinical findings.[47,50]

EVALUATION OF IMMUNE-MEDIATED THROMBOCYTOPENIA

A flow cytometry assay has been developed to measure IgG binding to platelets in dogs.[51] Increased platelet surface IgG is reported in approximately 70% to 80% of dogs with primary immune-mediated thrombocytopenia (IMT) and is also usually present in dogs with secondary IMT caused by infectious agents (e.g., *Babesia gibsoni*, *Anaplasma*, *Ehrlichia*, *Leptospira*, *Leishmania*), neoplasia (lymphoma and histiocytic sarcoma), drug-induced thrombocytopenia, and other inflammatory conditions.[52-54] Additionally, one study reported that some dogs with thrombocytopenia caused by consumption or wasting disease (vasculitis, disseminated intravascular coagulation [DIC]) or decreased bone marrow production may also have detectable antibody bound to platelets.[55] Nonspecific binding of IgG occurs over time, so blood samples should be analyzed within 24 hours of collection to avoid false-positive results.[53,56]

SUMMARY

Flow cytometry is becoming more widely available to practicing veterinarians through university and private reference laboratories. In addition to its common applications, such as in CBC, flow cytometry can be used to support a diagnosis of lymphoma and leukemia and can provide important prognostic information. Flow cytometry can also be helpful in supporting a diagnosis of IMHA or idiopathic thrombocytopenic purpura (ITP). Additional applications will likely develop from current research.

Acknowledgment

The authors wish to acknowledge the contributions of the authors of the flow cytometry chapter in the fourth edition of this text: Stephanie C. Corn, Seth E. Chapman, and Emily M. Pieczarka.

REFERENCES

1. Craig FE, Foon KA. Flow cytometric immunophenotyping for hematologic neoplasms. *Blood*. 2008;111:3941–3967.
2. Avery AC. Molecular diagnostics of hematologic malignancies in small animals. *Vet Clin North Am Small Anim Pract*. 2012;42:97–110.
3. Avery AC, Avery PR. Determining the significance of persistent lymphocytosis. *Vet Clin North Am Small Anim Pract*. 2007;37:267–282. vi.
4. Burkhard MJ, Bienzle D. Making sense of lymphoma diagnostics in small animal patients. *Vet Clin North Am Small Anim Pract*. 2013;43:1331–1347. vii.

5. Stokol T, Nickerson GA, Shuman M, et al. Dogs with Acute Myeloid Leukemia Have Clonal Rearrangements in T and B Cell Receptors. *Front Vet Sci.* 2017;4:76.

6. Moritz A, Becker M. Automated hematology systems. In: Weiss DJ, Waldrop KJ, eds. *Schalm's Veterinary Hematology.* 6th ed. Ames, IA: Wiley-Blackwell; 2010.

7. Weiss DJ, Wilkerson MJ. Flow cytometry. In: Weiss DJ, Waldrop KJ, eds. *Schalm's Veterinary Hematology.* 6th ed. Ames, IA: Wiley-Blackwell; 2010.

8. Comazzi S, Gelain ME. Use of flow cytometric immunophenotyping to refine the cytological diagnosis of canine lymphoma. *Vet J.* 2011;188:149–155.

9. Nguyen D, Diamond LW, Braylan RC. *Flow Cytometry in Hematopathology.* 2nd ed. Totowa, NJ: Humana Press; 2007.

10. Avery A. Immunophenotyping and determination of clonality. In: Weiss DJ, Waldrop KJ, eds. *Schalm's Veterinary Hematology.* 6th ed. Ames, IA: Wiley-Blackwell; 2010.

11. Williams MJ, Avery AC, Lana SE, et al. Canine lymphoproliferative disease characterized by lymphocytosis: immunophenotypic markers of prognosis. *J Vet Intern Med.* 2008;22:596–601.

12. Yagihara H, Uematsu Y, Koike A, et al. Immunophenotyping and gene rearrangement analysis in dogs with lymphoproliferative disorders characterized by small-cell lymphocytosis. *J Vet Diagn Invest.* 2009;21:197–202.

13. Comazzi S, Gelain ME, Martini V, et al. Immunophenotype predicts survival time in dogs with chronic lymphocytic leukemia. *J Vet Intern Med.* 2011;25:100–106.

14. Rout ED, Avery PR. Lymphoid Neoplasia: Correlations Between Morphology and Flow Cytometry. *Vet Clin North Am Small Anim Pract.* 2017;47:53–70.

15. Heeb HL, Wilkerson MJ, Chun R, et al. Large granular lymphocytosis, lymphocyte subset inversion, thrombocytopenia, dysproteinemia, and positive Ehrlichia serology in a dog. *J Am Anim Hosp Assoc.* 2003;39:379–384.

16. Vernau W, Moore PF. An immunophenotypic study of canine leukemias and preliminary assessment of clonality by polymerase chain reaction. *Vet Immunol Immunopathol.* 1999;69:145–164.

17. McDonough SP, Moore PF. Clinical, hematologic, and immunophenotypic characterization of canine large granular lymphocytosis. *Vet Pathol.* 2000;37:637–646.

18. Seelig DM, Avery P, Webb T, et al. Canine T-zone lymphoma: unique immunophenotypic features, outcome, and population characteristics. *J Vet Intern Med.* 2014;28:878–886.

19. Gleich S, Hartmann K. Hematology and serum biochemistry of feline immunodeficiency virus-infected and feline leukemia virus-infected cats. *J Vet Intern Med.* 2009;23:552–558.

20. Reichard MV, Meinkoth JH, Edwards AC, et al. Transmission of Cytauxzoon felis to a domestic cat by Amblyomma americanum. *Vet Parasitol.* 2009;161:110–115.

21. Workman HC, Vernau W. Chronic lymphocytic leukemia in dogs and cats: the veterinary perspective. *Vet Clin North Am Small Anim Pract.* 2003;33:1379–1399. viii.

22. Campbell MW, Hess PR, Williams LE. Chronic lymphocytic leukaemia in the cat: 18 cases (2000–2010). *Vet Comp Oncol.* 2013;11:256–264.

23. Workman HC, Vernau W, Schmidt PS. Chronic lymphocytic leukemia in cats is primarily a T helper cell disease. In: *Proceedings.* 55th Annual Meeting of the American College of Veterinary Pathologists; 2004.

24. Jain NC, Blue JT, Grindem CB, et al. Proposed criteria for classification of acute myeloid leukemia in dogs and cats. *Vet Clin Pathol.* 1991;20:63–82.

25. McManus PM. Classification of myeloid neoplasms: a comparative review. *Vet Clin Pathol.* 2005;34:189–212.

26. Stokol T, Schaefer DM, Shuman M, et al. Alkaline phosphatase is a useful cytochemical marker for the diagnosis of acute myelomonocytic and monocytic leukemia in the dog. *Vet Clin Pathol.* 2015;44:79–93.

27. Tasca S, Carli E, Caldin M, et al. Hematologic abnormalities and flow cytometric immunophenotyping results in dogs with hematopoietic neoplasia: 210 cases (2002–2006). *Vet Clin Pathol.* 2009;38:2–12.

28. Adam F, Villiers E, Watson S, et al. Clinical pathological and epidemiological assessment of morphologically and immunologically confirmed canine leukaemia. *Vet Comp Oncol.* 2009;7:181–195.

29. Comazzi S, Gelain ME, Bonfanti U, et al. Acute megakaryoblastic leukemia in dogs: a report of three cases and review of the literature. *J Am Anim Hosp Assoc.* 2010;46:327–335.

30. Willmann M, Mullauer L, Schwendenwein I, et al. Chemotherapy in canine acute megakaryoblastic leukemia: a case report and review of the literature. *In Vivo.* ;23; 2009:911–918.

31. Suter SE, Vernau W, Fry MM, et al. CD34 +, CD41 + acute megakaryoblastic leukemia in a dog. *Vet Clin Pathol.* 2007;36:288–292.

32. Ameri M, Wilkerson MJ, Stockham SL, et al. Acute megakaryoblastic leukemia in a German Shepherd dog. *Vet Clin Pathol.* 2010;39:39–45.

33. Juopperi TA, Bienzle D, Bernreuter DC, et al. Prognostic markers for myeloid neoplasms: a comparative review of the literature and goals for future investigation. *Vet Pathol.* 2011;48:182–197.

34. Kisseberth WC, Helfand SC. General features of leukemia and lymphoma. In: Weiss DJ, Waldrop KJ, eds. *Schalm's Veterinary Hematology.* 6th ed. Ames, IA: Wiley-Blackwell; 2010.

35. Teske E, van Heerde P, Rutteman GR, et al. Prognostic factors for treatment of malignant lymphoma in dogs. *J Am Vet Med Assoc.* 1994;205:1722–1728.

36. Kiupel M, Teske E, Bostock D. Prognostic factors for treated canine malignant lymphoma. *Vet Pathol.* 1999;36:292–300.

37. Wilkerson MJ, Dolce K, Koopman T, et al. Lineage differentiation of canine lymphoma/leukemias and aberrant expression of CD molecules. *Vet Immunol Immunopathol.* 2005;106:179–196.

38. Valli VE, Kass PH, San Myint M, et al. Canine lymphomas: association of classification type, disease stage, tumor subtype, mitotic rate, and treatment with survival. *Vet Pathol.* 2013;50:738–748.

39. Rao S, Lana S, Eickhoff J, et al. Class II major histocompatibility complex expression and cell size independently predict survival in canine B-cell lymphoma. *J Vet Intern Med.* 2011;25:1097–1105.

40. Avery PR, Burton J, Bromberek JL, et al. Flow cytometric characterization and clinical outcome of CD4+ T-cell lymphoma in dogs: 67 cases. *J Vet Intern Med.* 2014;28:538–546.

41. Flood-Knapik KE, Durham AC, Gregor TP, et al. Clinical, histopathological and immunohistochemical characterization of canine indolent lymphoma. *Vet Comp Oncol.* 2013;11:272–286.

42. Mizutani N, Goto-Koshino Y, Takahashi M, et al. Clinical and histopathological evaluation of 16 dogs with T-zone lymphoma. *J Vet Med Sci.* 2016;78:1237–1244.

43. Milner RJ, Peyton J, Cooke K, et al. Response rates and survival times for cats with lymphoma treated with the University of Wisconsin–Madison chemotherapy protocol: 38 cases (1996–2003). *J Am Vet Med Assoc.* 2005;227:1118–1122.

44. Roccabianca P, Vernau W, Caniatti M, et al. Feline large granular lymphocyte (LGL) lymphoma with secondary leukemia: primary intestinal origin with predominance of a CD3/CD8αα phenotype. *Vet Pathol.* 2006;43:15–28.

45. Lana S, Plaza S, Hampe K, et al. Diagnosis of mediastinal masses in dogs by flow cytometry. *J Vet Intern Med.* 2006;20:1161–1165.

46. Burton AG, Borjesson DL, Vernau W. Thymoma-associated lymphocytosis in a dog. *Vet Clin Pathol.* 2014;43:584–588.

47. Wardrop KJ. The Coombs' test in veterinary medicine: past, present, future. *Vet Clin Pathol.* 2005;34:325–334.

48. Wilkerson MJ, Davis E, Shuman W, et al. Isotype-specific antibodies in horses and dogs with immune-mediated hemolytic anemia. *J Vet Intern Med.* 2000;14:190–196.

49. Quigley KA, Chelack BJ, Haines DM, et al. Application of a direct flow cytometric erythrocyte immunofluorescence assay in dogs with immune-mediated hemolytic anemia and comparison to the direct antiglobulin test. *J Vet Diagn Invest.* 2001;13:297–300.

50. Morley P, Mathes M, Guth A, et al. Anti-erythrocyte antibodies and disease associations in anemic and nonanemic dogs. *J Vet Intern Med.* 2008;22:886–892.

51. Lewis DC, McVey DS, Shuman WS, et al. Development and characterization of a flow cytometric assay for detection of platelet-bound immunoglobulin G in dogs. *Am J Vet Res.* 1995;56:1555–1558.

52. Wilkerson MJ. Principles and applications of flow cytometry and cell sorting in companion animal medicine. *Vet Clin North Am Small Anim Pract.* 2012;42:53–71.

53. Wilkerson MJ, Shuman W, Swist S, et al. Platelet size, platelet surface-associated IgG, and reticulated platelets in dogs with immune-mediated thrombocytopenia. *Vet Clin Pathol.* 2001;30:141–149.

54. Dircks BH, Schuberth HJ, Mischke R. Underlying diseases and clinico-pathologic variables of thrombocytopenic dogs with and without platelet-bound antibodies detected by use of a flow cytometric assay: 83 cases (2004–2006). *J Am Vet Med Assoc.* 2009;235:960–966.

55. Bachman DE, Forman MA, Hostutler RA, et al. Prospective diagnostic accuracy evaluation and clinical utilization of a modified assay for platelet-associated immunoglobulin in thrombocytopenic and nonthrombocytopenic dogs. *Vet Clin Pathol.* 2015;44:355–368.

56. Wilkerson MJ, Shuman W. Alterations in normal canine platelets during storage in EDTA anticoagulated blood. *Vet Clin Pathol.* 2001;30:107–113.

31

Molecular Methods in Lymphoid Malignancies

Peter F. Moore, William Vernau, Christian M. Leutenegger, and Dean Cornwell

A diagnosis of lymphoma is currently made on the basis of clinical, morphological, and immunophenotypic criteria. Morphological evidence of lymphoma includes the presence of dense cellular infiltration, a monomorphic appearance of infiltrating lymphocytes, cytological immaturity of the lymphoid infiltrate, and disruption, effacement, and replacement of the normal structures of the involved tissue by infiltrating cells. Immunophenotypic assessment is a useful aid in lymphoma diagnosis and may increase the index of suspicion of lymphoma when the majority of cells express the same or an aberrant phenotype. Diagnostic dilemmas arise with small, mature cell lymphomas, with emerging or incipient lymphomas that have not yet effaced the lymph node (and hence are "mixed" cytologically), with mixed cell lymphomas, such as T-cell and histiocyte-rich B-cell lymphoma, as well as lymphomas that occur in sites of chronic inflammation, especially in the skin and gut. In this latter instance, it may be difficult to identify lymphoma in a background of inflammation. Molecular clonality assessment is used to demonstrate clonal expansion of lymphocytes, consistent with lymphoma, in these situations.

MOLECULAR CLONALITY ASSESSMENT IN LYMPHOPROLIFERATIVE DISEASE

Lymphocyte antigen receptor gene rearrangement analysis is a methodology used to detect clonality in B-cell and T-cell populations. Although it is generally accepted that clonality is a property of neoplasia, it is not synonymous with malignancy. Benign clonal expansion occurs most often in T-cell infiltrates in a variety of clinical settings ranging from the response to infection to the response to neoplasia.[1,2] The detection of a clonal population in an equivocal lymphoproliferative lesion can be used as an important adjunctive diagnostic tool to determine the likelihood of neoplasia if interpreted in conjunction with clinical, morphological, and immunophenotypic findings.[3] Polymerase chain reaction (PCR)–based methods are most frequently used for molecular clonality assessment (commonly referred to as "PARR"—PCR for antigen receptor gene rearrangement). This methodology provides the advantage of allowing the detection of B-cell and T-cell clonality, not only in fresh samples (including smears and fluids) and frozen samples but also in formalin-fixed, paraffin-embedded (FFPE) tissues, which are routinely used for diagnosis.[3,4]

Specific antigen recognition is essential for adaptive immunity. Lymphocytes of B-cell and T-cell lineage have antigen receptors, which consist of multiple protein subunits/chains. T cells have either α-and β-chains (αβ T cells) or γ- and δ-chains (γδ T cells). B cells have immunoglobulin heavy chains (IGH) and light chains, either κ- (IGK) or λ-chains (IGL). Antigen receptor proteins have variable (V) and constant (C) domains, which are encoded by antigen receptor genes. Antigen binding occurs in the V domain.

The V domain is encoded by two or three genes—the variable (V), diversity (D), and joining (J) genes. Although multiple V, D, and J genes exist in antigen receptor loci, they are relatively limited in number and diversity (Fig. 31.1). Gene rearrangement during lymphocyte development leads to random joining of V, D (optional), and J genes, and this results in the formation of a complete V domain exon (Fig. 31.2). The diversification of the antigen receptor repertoire is markedly enhanced by modification of the junctions among the V, D, and J segments. For instance, random nucleotides (N or non–template encoded) are added by the enzyme terminal transferase. This creates the highly diverse third hypervariable region of the V domain, also known as the *complementarity determining region 3* (CDR3) (see Fig. 31.2). The CDR3 region is at the center of the antigen-binding site and hence is the major contributor to antigen specificity. The CDR3 is unique for each antigen receptor subunit and creates a "molecular fingerprint" unique to each lymphocyte.[5]

During T-cell development in the thymus, T cells rearrange their antigen receptor genes in the following order: TRD (δ), TRG (γ), TRB (β), and TRA (α). This process creates two lineages of T cells, α and γδ T cells. Rearrangement of TRA results in deletion of TRD on at least one chromosome because the TRD locus occurs within the TRA locus. A TRG gene rearrangement remains in the majority of T cells regardless of the surface T-cell receptor (TCR) phenotype, and hence TRG is the target of choice for T-cell clonality.[6]

B-cell development occurs in bone marrow. B cells first rearrange IGH followed by IGK. The B cell either expresses a κ light chain or subsequently rearranges IGL and expresses a λ light chain. If IGL is rearranged, IGK is inactivated by the rearrangement of the κ-deleting element (KDE). The IGH locus is rearranged in all B cells and is the preferred target for molecular clonality assessment. Unlike T cells, B cells can modify the sequence of IGH (and IGK or IGL) by somatic hypermutation in germinal centers of secondary lymphoid tissues (spleen, lymph nodes, and Peyer patches). This is an important property of humoral immunity and is responsible for affinity maturation of the immunoglobulin response to antigen, which occurs in germinal centers. Somatic hypermutation is a necessary, albeit dangerous, process, and targeting of genes other than immunoglobulin V, D, and J genes can precipitate lymphoma. In this regard, most B-cell lymphomas have follicular origins. Another consideration is that the sensitivity of IGH clonality assays is reduced as a result of somatic hypermutation of primer-binding sequences in the affected V and J genes. λ light chains are dominant (>90% usage) in cats, dogs, and horses. Hence IGK is frequently inactivated by rearrangement of KDE. This occurs during B-cell development in bone marrow before antigen encounter in germinal centers. Therefore KDE rearrangements are not subject to somatic hypermutation and are a useful supplemental target for molecular clonality.

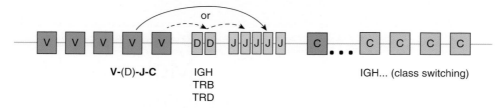

Antigen receptor locus topology

V-(D)-J-C

IGH
TRB
TRD

IGH... (class switching)

1 rearrangement per chromosome

TRG dog cat horse

V-J-C₁ ... V-J-Cₙ   TRG$_{dog}$ n=8   TRG$_{cat}$ n=6   TRG$_{horse}$ n=17   **Tandem cassettes**

> 1 rearrangement per chromosome—Oligoclonality is not demonstrable!

©pfmoore

Fig. 31.1 Antigen receptor locus topology. Most antigen receptor loci conform to the top structure with minor exceptions such as duplication of some elements (e.g., D-J-C in TRB and duplication of J-C in human TRG). Only some loci have D genes (IGH, TRB, TRD). IGH has multiple C genes, which are involved in class switching (e.g., immunoglobulin M [IgM] to IgG, IgA, or IgE). Variant TRG locus structure (bottom) consists of multiple V-J-C cassettes, which can independently rearrange resulting in more than one rearrangement per chromosome. This TRG locus structure is found in dogs, cats, and horses, but not in humans, in which only one rearrangement per chromosome is possible. Knowledge of antigen receptor locus structure is important for the design and interpretation of molecular clonality assays. (Copyright pfmoore. Used with permission.)

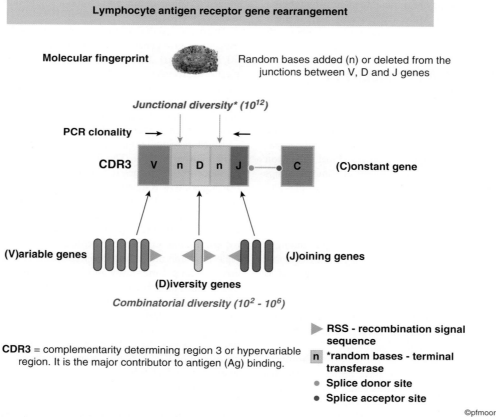

Lymphocyte antigen receptor gene rearrangement

Molecular fingerprint   Random bases added (n) or deleted from the junctions between V, D and J genes

Junctional diversity* (10^{12})

PCR clonality →

CDR3   V n D n J   C   **(C)onstant gene**

(V)ariable genes   **(D)iversity genes**   **(J)oining genes**

Combinatorial diversity (10^2 - 10^6)

▶ **RSS - recombination signal sequence**

n **random bases - terminal transferase*

● **Splice donor site**
● **Splice acceptor site**

CDR3 = complementarity determining region 3 or hypervariable region. It is the major contributor to antigen (Ag) binding.

©pfmoore

Fig. 31.2 Lymphocyte antigen receptor gene rearrangement creates a unique junctional region (CDR3) when variable (V), diversity (D), and joining (J) genes in each antigen receptor locus assemble to form the complete variable domain exon. *Combinatorial diversity* is the product of the number of V × D × J genes in an antigen receptor locus. *Junctional diversity* is created by random base addition (n) among V, D, and J genes by the enzyme terminal transferase. Junctional diversity is largely responsible for the almost limitless specificity of lymphocyte antigen receptors, and the CDR3 regions are essentially molecular fingerprints for each lymphocyte. (Copyright pfmoore. Used with permission.)

Lymphocyte antigen receptor gene rearrangements of necessity are lineage associated, but cross-lineage rearrangements are possible. In these instances, B cells rearrange T-cell loci and T cells rearrange B-cell loci. Also, rearrangement of B-cell or T-cell loci has been observed in myeloid leukemia. Because of these events, it is not recommended to assign cell lineage solely on the basis of molecular clonality results. Cell lineage assignment by immunophenotyping is more accurate.[4]

Clonality assays in veterinary medicine use heterogeneous primer sets that differ by institutions conducting the assays. Ideally, these assays should cover all appreciably rearranged gene segments in a locus. The reality is markedly different and the sensitivities of clonality assays are quite variable.[3] Antigen receptor genes can be identified within high-quality genome assemblies of species of interest (dog, cat, and horse); these are available but are not annotated to indicate the location (topology) of the genes on a chromosome (see Fig. 31.1). Antigen receptor genes can also be identified by high-throughput sequencing of the expressed V/J repertoire in messenger ribonucleic acid (mRNA) extracted from lymphoid tissues. This approach indicates V/J usage but not locus topology. By using both approaches, the primer design process can be optimized to obtain the best sensitivity.[3] Initial primer sets used for IGH and TRG clonality assessment were based on limited sequence data derived from mRNA before the genome era.[7-10] Modifications have occurred through limited genomic search or expanded mRNA sequence data.[11-18] The release of genome assemblies for dogs, cats, and horses has facilitated detailed description of antigen receptor loci and design of clonality assays that cover all genes in a locus. For instance, a complete description of the canine

TRG locus revealed a more complicated topology than was previously anticipated. The canine TRG locus consists of seven complete V-J-C clusters/cassettes, compared with only one in humans (see Fig. 31.1).[19] By using a new multiplex assay that covered all potentially rearranged genes, Keller and Moore demonstrated that canine T cells rearrange multiple V-J-C cassettes, resulting in more than one rearrangement per chromosome.[20] This novel finding changed the premise that more than two clonal rearrangements in a sample indicated oligoclonality. Indeed, knowledge of the locus topology is important in the design and interpretation of clonality assays. Preliminary indications are that cats and horses also possess multicassette TRG loci. So, in the future, existing clonality assays in veterinary medicine, which are currently prone to false-negative results, will be modified to consider locus topology and use of high-resolution V/J.

In principle, clonality assays assess the diversity of antigen receptor gene rearrangements within a population of lesional lymphocytes by PCR-based amplification of CDR3. The products (amplicons) are separated by size by using gel (or capillary) electrophoresis. To amplify CDR3 in rearranged genes, forward primers are designed for V genes, and reverse primers are designed for J genes of a given locus. Hence, the primers flank the CDR3 (see Fig. 31.2; Fig. 31.3). For T-cell clonality, TRG is the most informative locus. For B-cell clonality, IGH is the most informative locus. Other loci may be utilized (see Fig. 31.3) and may add value to the molecular clonality assessment. KDE is particularly informative in the assessment of B-cell clonality (see Fig. 31.3). In reactive/inflammatory lesions, amplicons are derived from multiple unique cells and differ in size and sequence; this is a polyclonal result

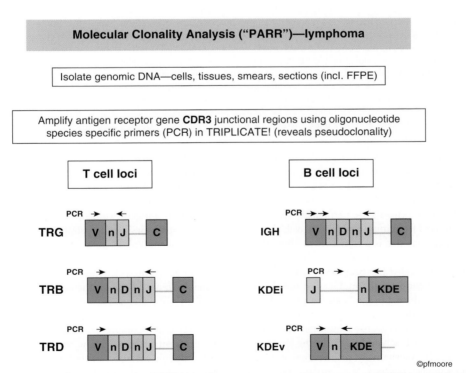

Fig. 31.3 Polymerase chain reaction (PCR) for antigen receptor gene rearrangement (PARR) is used in molecular clonality analysis for lymphoma. Molecular clonality analysis can be conducted on genomic DNA isolated from cells, cell smears (even stained), fluids, tissues, and tissue sections (including formalin-fixed, paraffin-embedded [FFPE] sections). PCR amplification of CDR3 junctional regions of T-cell (TRG) and B-cell (IGH) loci is routinely performed in molecular clonality analyses in most institutions that perform clonality testing. Additional loci are used at University of California, Davis, for molecular clonality analysis in special circumstances. κ-deleting element (KDE) rearrangement analysis (KDEi for intron and KDEv for variable gene) is also used for B-cell clonality determination to alleviate the pitfalls of somatic hypermutation of IGH. TRD (dog, cat) is also used for T-cell clonality determination, especially when a γδ T-cell lymphoma is likely and TRG analysis is uninformative. TRB (cat) is an adjunctive locus for T-cell clonality. (Copyright pfmoore. Used with permission.)

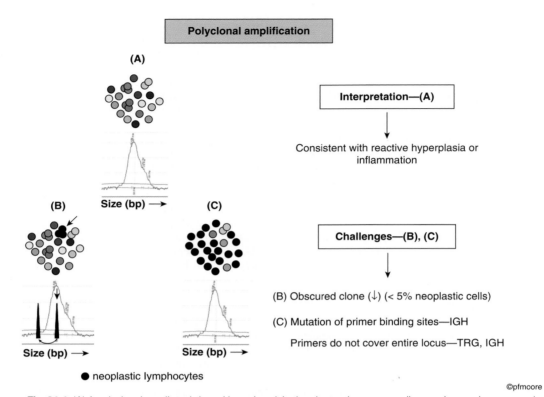

Fig. 31.4 (A) A polyclonal amplicon (a broad-based peak in the electropherogram—diverse sizes and sequences) is the product of many unique lymphocytes (represented by colors) in a lesion. A polyclonal result most commonly indicates reactive hyperplasia or inflammation. There are, however, some challenges. Sometimes a polyclonal result is a false-negative result. (B) For instance, in an inflamed lymphoma with a minor clonal population (arguably < 5%–10%), the clone (solid black peak) would not resolve from the polyclonal background if it was close to the modal size, but it would be detectable if it was markedly smaller or larger than the modal size. (C) Somatic hypermutation of IGH could result in no amplification of rearrangements in neoplastic lymphocytes, and the amplicon could be generated by residual reactive lymphocytes (polyclonal result). Last, if utilization of a V or J gene is not covered by the primers occurs, then there is a failure to detect clonality (polyclonal result or no amplification). Concurrent morphological and immunophenotypic assessments greatly assist in the resolution of these circumstances, and hence are mandatory. (Copyright pfmoore. Used with permission.)

(Fig. 31.4). False-negative results can occur if the neoplastic lymphocytes are a minor component of the lesion, the primers used do not cover the entire antigen receptor gene locus, or there is somatic hypermutation of primer-binding sites when IGH is assessed (see Fig. 31.4). In the latter instance, KDE rearrangements are particularly useful. In lymphoma, amplicons are derived from multiple identical cells and are homogeneous in size and sequence; this is a clonal result (Fig. 31.5). Not all clonal lymphoid expansions are lymphomas. Benign clonal expansion (most commonly of T cells) has been observed in several circumstances (see Fig. 31.5). Pseudoclonal amplification is only discovered if clonality assays are conducted in duplicate (or preferably in triplicate) (Fig. 31.6). Pseudoclonality, or no amplification, results if the target DNA (for the antigen receptor locus) is limiting. The reason could simply be that there are very few lymphocytes in the lesion relative to other nonlymphoid cells. Alternatively, primers may not bind to target DNA if the target sequence is altered (e.g., somatic hypermutation of IGH) or if a V or J gene not covered by the primers has been utilized (see Fig. 31.6).

IMMUNOPHENOTYPIC ASSESSMENT OF LYMPHOPROLIFERATIVE DISEASE

Immunophenotyping is a critical adjunct in the characterization of lymphoid malignancies. The diagnosis of neoplasia should first be established by morphological assessment of tumor samples, with or without molecular clonality analysis, as required. Immunophenotyping is usually necessary to classify lymphomas by the World Health Organization (WHO) system and can provide useful prognostic information in addition to further confirmation of neoplasia.[21-24] Unusual or aberrant antigen expression by an expanded population of lymphocytes provides further support for a neoplastic etiology.[21,22,24] Immunophenotyping can be done on cytology samples (immunocytochemistry), FFPE tissues (immunohistochemistry), or liquid samples (flow cytometry). Flow cytometry has become relatively widely available to aid in the characterization of lymphoid malignancies in small animal patients. Flow cytometric assessment has the advantages of increased sensitivity, precise quantitation of antigen expression, and more rapid and comprehensive assessment with larger arrays or panels of reagents. However, flow cytometry lacks morphological context, and although cell size can be assessed with flow cytometry, the key discriminator in classification schemes, such as the WHO system, is nuclear size, not overall cell size. Immunophenotyping is not a stand-alone test, but is used in conjunction with clinical, morphological, and, sometimes, molecular clonality findings. Table 31.1 lists the markers of value for determining cell lineages in leukocytic proliferations in dogs and cats. Some of these markers can also be assessed in FFPE tissues with appropriate antigen retrieval protocols. Markers are available for the detection of B and T cells. However, markers for the unequivocal detection of natural killer (NK) cells are not routinely available, so the existence of NK-cell lymphomas in dogs and cats is not easily

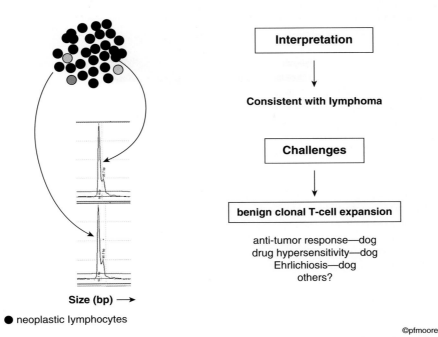

Fig. 31.5 A clonal amplicon (a narrow based peak in the electropherogram—single size and sequence) is the product of a unique lymphocyte, which is expanded in a lesion. A clonal result most commonly indicates lymphoma. There are challenges. Lymphocytes can clonally expand in a reactive/inflammatory process—benign clonal expansion. This most commonly occurs in T-cell populations in certain infectious diseases (e.g., lymphocytosis associated with ehrlichiosis), in drug hypersensitivity, and in antitumor responses (e.g., regressing histiocytoma). Clinical data and morphological and immunophenotypic assessments greatly assist in the resolution of these issues and hence are mandatory. (Copyright pfmoore. Used with permission.)

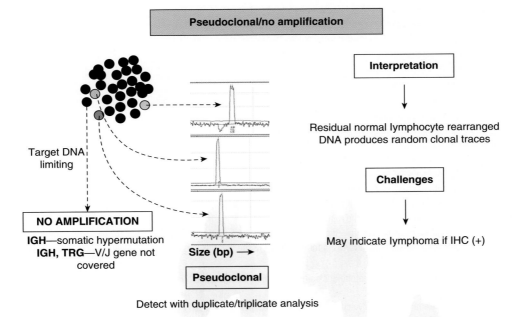

Fig. 31.6 A pseudoclonal amplicon is only demonstrable in duplicate or triplicate analysis. A pseudoclonal result indicates that target deoxyribonucleic acid (DNA) is a limiting factor. The clonal amplicons, which originate from the multiple different analysis tubes, differ in size (and sequence) and are contributed by rearrangements from residual reactive lymphocytes in a lymphoma in this example. There are no amplicons from the lymphoma cells (for a variety of reasons listed in the text). Hence, the target DNA is limited to that provided by the few residual normal lymphocytes. If the rearranged DNA from the normal lymphocytes is amplified by the primers in the early cycles of the polymerase chain reaction (PCR), then different pseudoclonal peaks are seen in the multiple analyses. Otherwise, there would be no amplification. These issues are resolvable with concurrent morphological and immunophenotypic assessments, which are, therefore, mandatory. (Copyright pfmoore. Used with permission.)

TABLE 31.1   Markers of Diagnostic Importance to Leukocytic Disease Investigation

CD1[a]	• Antigen-presenting molecule (related to major histocompatibility complex (MHC) class I molecules) that presents peptide, lipid and glycolipid antigens to T cells • The best marker of dendritic antigen-presenting cells (APCs) and hence of histiocytic sarcomas, which are most often tumors of dendritic APCs • Also expressed by cortical thymocytes (T cells) but not mature T cells • Subpopulations of B cells and monocytes can present antigen and therefore may also express CD1 • Frequently expressed in canine B-cell chronic lymphocytic leukemia (CLL)
CD3	• Signaling component of the T-cell antigen receptor complex • Expressed by $\alpha\beta$ T cells and $\gamma\delta$ T cells • Cytoplasmic expression by NK cells is possible—especially if activated
CD4[a]	• T-cell antigen receptor (TCR) associated coreceptor for MHC class II in T-helper cells • T-helper cell marker • Monocytes, macrophages, and dendritic APCs can also express or upregulate CD4 expression • Canine neutrophils constitutively express CD4 (unique to dogs)
CD8[a]	• TCR-associated coreceptor for MHC class I in cytotoxic T cells • A dimeric molecule • TCR $\alpha\beta$ T cells usually express CD8 $\alpha\beta$ heterodimers although a subset can express CD8$\alpha\alpha$ homodimers • Subsets of TCR $\gamma\delta$ T cells and natural killer (NK) cells may also express CD8 $\alpha\alpha$ homodimers
CD21[a]	• A complement receptor (CR2) that is part of the B-cell receptor–coreceptor complex • Expressed on mature B cells and follicular dendritic cells of the germinal center • Useful marker for B-cell lymphoma and B-cell CLL • Not completely lineage specific • Also variably expressed in canine T-zone lymphoma
CD79a	• Signaling component of the B-cell antigen receptor complex • Expressed by all stages of B-cell differentiation • Expression is less in plasma cells, which may even be negative
CD20	• Surface molecule expressed at all stages of B-cell differentiation • Plasma cells have diminished expression of CD20; canine plasma cells mostly lack expression of CD20, whereas feline plasma cells retain strong expression • CD20 plays a role in regulation of B-cell activation and proliferation • CD20 is not lineage specific and has been observed uncommonly in T-cell lymphomas • Caution is advised in interpretation of diffuse cytoplasmic expression, which can occur in several cell types
Pax5	• Transcription factor essential for maintenance of B-cell differentiation • Useful B-cell marker
MUM1 / IRF4	• Transcription factor essential for plasma cell differentiation • Useful plasma cell marker but not completely plasma cell specific (also expressed in some B-cell lymphomas and few T-cell malignancies)
CD11d	• αD subunit of β_2 integrin (CD18) family • Expressed by macrophages and T cells in specific hematopoietic environments, especially splenic red pulp, bone marrow, and lymph node medullary sinuses • CD11d is consistently expressed in diseases emanating from splenic red pulp (large granular lymphocyte [LGL] form of CLL, hepatosplenic lymphoma, and hemophagocytic histiocytic sarcoma)
CD18	• β subunit of the β_2 integrin family of leukocyte adhesion molecules • Expressed as a heterodimer of CD11a, CD11b, CD11c, or CD11d with CD18 • Leukocytes express at least one form of the heterodimer • Hence CD18 is expressed on all leukocytes—the expression level on myeloid cells is especially high compared to normal lymphocytes • CD18 has been used as a marker of histiocytes in formalin fixed tissue, but this is dependent on exclusion of lymphocyte differentiation by the use of other markers (CD3 and CD79a)
CD34	• Surface glycoprotein expressed on hematopoietic stem and progenitor cells, small-vessel endothelial cells, embryonic fibroblasts, and bone marrow stromal cells • Expressed in acute leukemias, especially acute myeloid leukemia (AML) and B-cell acute lymphoblastic leukemia (B-ALL) • Not (usually) expressed in lymphoma or CLL
CD45	• Surface molecule expressed by most leukocytes—formerly known as "leukocyte common antigen" • Pan-CD45 antibodies bind to the extracellular domain outside of three variably spliced exons (A, B, and C) • A useful marker of leukocytic origin • A subset of peripheral T-cell lymphomas lack expression of CD45—this is encountered in T-zone lymphomas of lymph nodes (a lymphoma type that exhibits indolent behavior)
CD204	• Class A scavenger receptor • Expressed by macrophages in tissues • Not expressed by dendritic cells in lymphoid tissues or Langerhans cells (LCs) in the epidermis • Variably expressed by neoplastic cells in canine histiocytic sarcomas, but not in histiocytomas (LC origin)

TABLE 31.1 Markers of Diagnostic Importance to Leukocytic Disease Investigation—cont'd

c-Kit	• Surface molecule and member of the receptor tyrosine kinase family (type III) • Expressed by most hematopoietic progenitor cells and by mast cells • Intense expression in high-grade mast cell tumors • Also expressed in AMLs, some ALLs, and some lymphomas
Granzyme B (GrB)	• Serine protease located in the granules of cytotoxic (CD8+) T cells and NK cells • GrB is expressed at high levels in activated cells and helps mediate rapid target cell death by apoptosis • Mast cells may also express GrB
Myeloperoxidase	• Myeloperoxidase (MPO) is a lysosomal protein stored in the azurophilic granules of neutrophils (and monocytes) • MPO is a definitive marker of myeloid differentiation • Very useful for confirming AML
Ki-67	• Cell proliferation marker (nuclear)—expressed in all phases of the cell cycle except G0 and early G1 • Excellent marker for determining the proliferative fraction of a cell population • Indolent lymphomas, such as marginal zone B-cell lymphoma and T-zone lymphoma, have proliferative fractions < 5%–10%

aNot assessable in formalin-fixed, paraffin-embedded (FFPE) tissue.

assessable. Determination of T-cell receptor use and major subsets of T cells (CD4 or CD8), as well as dissecting the lineages of histiocytes (macrophages, interstitial-type DC and Langerhans cells) is best done in unfixed cell smears or snap-frozen tissues, or by flow cytometry.

Antigen loss in lymphoma is an important occurrence because it increases diagnostic difficulty, especially if it involves a key marker. However, antigen loss (aberrant immunophenotype) also further substantiates the likelihood of neoplasia.[21,22] Partial or complete loss of CD3 expression in T-cell lymphomas has been recognized for decades.[22] A similar phenomenon may occur in high-grade B-cell lymphomas with altered expression of CD20, CD79a, and Pax-5. This necessitates the assessment of more than one of these markers in many instances. Coexpression of CD20 and CD3 occurs in some T-cell lymphomas; this underscores the importance of recognizing the limitations of lineage-*associated* molecules (CD20), which may be expressed more broadly compared with lineage-*specific* molecules (CD3 and CD79a). High-grade large granular T-cell lymphomas (T-LGL lymphomas) are readily recognized in aspirates with Wright-Giemsa staining, but the recognition of cytoplasmic granules in routine hematoxylin and eosin (H&E) sections is often difficult. Granzyme B (GrB) is a frequent component of these granules, and staining for this molecule facilitates the recognition of T-LGL lymphoma.[25]

The β_2 integrin CD11d is dominantly expressed in splenic red pulp. It is also expressed in the neoplastic counterparts of normal CD11d expressing red pulp inhabitants. For instance, CD11d+ $\gamma\delta$ T cells are rich in splenic red pulp compared with peripheral blood. Hepatosplenic T-cell lymphoma is a high-grade lymphoma of (usually) $\gamma\delta$ T cells in which CD11d and GrB are consistently expressed.[26] Knowledge of this immunophenotype is useful in establishing the diagnosis.

High-grade lymphomas have an elevated mitotic index, which correlates well with the proliferative fraction assessed by using Ki67 staining. There is marked interobserver variability in determining the mitotic index, and mitotic figures can be difficult to discern in some lesions. Ki67 staining adds cost but avoids some of these problems.

REFERENCES

1. Malik UR, Oleksowicz L, Dutcher JP, et al. Atypical clonal T-cell proliferation in infectious mononucleosis. *Med Oncol.* 1996;13:207–213.
2. Wedderburn LR, Patel A, Varsani H, et al. The developing human immune system: T-cell receptor repertoire of children and young adults shows a wide discrepancy in the frequency of persistent oligoclonal T-cell expansions. *Immunology.* 2001;102:301–309.
3. Keller SM, Vernau W, Moore PF. Clonality testing in veterinary medicine: a review with diagnostic guidelines. *Vet Pathol.* 2016;53:711–725.
4. van Dongen JJ, Langerak AW, Bruggemann M, et al. Design and standardization of PCR primers and protocols for detection of clonal immunoglobulin and T-cell receptor gene recombinations in suspect lymphoproliferations: report of the BIOMED-2 Concerted Action BMH4-CT98-3936. *Leukemia.* 2003;17:2257–2317.
5. Murphy K. *Janeway's Immunobiology.* New York: Garland Science; 2012.
6. Theodorou I, Raphael M, Bigorgne C, et al. Recombination pattern of the TCR gamma locus in human peripheral T-cell lymphomas. *J Pathol.* 1994;174:233–242.
7. Burnett RC, Vernau W, Modiano JF, et al. Diagnosis of canine lymphoid neoplasia using clonal rearrangements of antigen receptor genes. *Vet Pathol.* 2003;40:32–41.
8. Moore PF, Woo JC, Vernau W, et al. Characterization of feline T cell receptor gamma (TCRG) variable region genes for the molecular diagnosis of feline intestinal T cell lymphoma. *Vet Immunol Immunopathol.* 2005;106:167–178.
9. Valli VE, Vernau W, de Lorimier LP, et al. Canine indolent nodular lymphoma. *Vet Pathol.* 2006;43:241–256.
10. Werner JA, Woo JC, Vernau W, et al. Characterization of feline immunoglobulin heavy chain variable region genes for the molecular diagnosis of B-cell neoplasia. *Vet Pathol.* 2005;42:596–607.
11. Gentilini F, Calzolari C, Turba ME, et al. GeneScanning analysis of Ig/TCR gene rearrangements to detect clonality in canine lymphomas. *Vet Immunol Immunopathol.* 2009;127:47–56.
12. Henrich M, Hecht W, Weiss AT, et al. A new subgroup of immunoglobulin heavy chain variable region genes for the assessment of clonality in feline B-cell lymphomas. *Vet Immunol Immunopathol.* 2009;130:59–69.
13. Mochizuki H, Nakamura K, Sato H, et al. Multiplex PCR and GeneScan analysis to detect immunoglobulin heavy chain gene rearrangement in feline B-cell neoplasms. *Vet Immunol Immunopathol.* 2011;143:38–45.
14. Mochizuki H, Nakamura K, Sato H, et al. GeneScan analysis to detect clonality of T-cell receptor gamma gene rearrangement in feline lymphoid neoplasms. *Vet Immunol Immunopathol.* 2012;145:402–409.
15. Weiss AT, Hecht W, Henrich M, et al. Characterization of C-, J- and V-region-genes of the feline T-cell receptor gamma. *Vet Immunol Immunopathol.* 2008;124:63–74.
16. Weiss AT, Hecht W, Reinacher M. Feline T-cell receptor gamma V- and J-region sequences retrieved from the trace archive and from transcriptome analysis of cats. *Vet Med Int.* 2010;2010:953272.
17. Weiss AT, Klopfleisch R, Gruber AD. T-cell receptor gamma chain variable and joining region genes of subgroup 1 are clonally rearranged in feline B- and T-cell lymphoma. *J Comp Pathol.* 2011;144:123–134.
18. Yagihara H, Tamura K, Isotani M, et al. Genomic organization of the T-cell receptor gamma gene and PCR detection of its clonal rearrangement in canine T-cell lymphoma/leukemia. *Vet Immunol Immunopathol.* 2007;115:375–382.

19. Massari S, Bellahcene F, Vaccarelli G, et al. The deduced structure of the T cell receptor gamma locus in Canis lupus familiaris. *Mol Immunol.* 2009;46:2728–2736.

20. Keller SM, Moore PF. A novel clonality assay for the assessment of canine T cell proliferations. *Vet Immunol Immunopathol.* 2012;145:410–419.

21. Jamal S, Picker LJ, Aquino DB, et al. Immunophenotypic analysis of peripheral T-cell neoplasms. A multiparameter flow cytometric approach. *Am J Clin Pathol.* 2001;116:512–526.

22. Knowles DM. Immunophenotypic and antigen receptor gene rearrangement analysis in T cell neoplasia. *Am J Pathol.* 1989;134:761–785.

23. Rao S, Lana S, Eickhoff J, et al. Class II major histocompatibility complex expression and cell size independently predict survival in canine B-cell lymphoma. *J Vet Intern Med.* 2011;25:1097–1105.

24. Seelig DM, Avery P, Webb T, et al. Canine T-zone lymphoma: unique immunophenotypic features, outcome, and population characteristics. *J Vet Intern Med.* 2014;28:878–886.

25. Moore PF, Rodriguez-Bertos A, Kass PH. Feline gastrointestinal lymphoma: mucosal architecture, immunophenotype, and molecular clonality. *Vet Pathol.* 2012;49:658–668.

26. Keller SM, Vernau W, Hodges J, et al. Hepatosplenic and hepatocytotropic T-cell lymphoma two distinct types of T-cell lymphoma in dogs. *Vet Pathol.* 2013;50:281–290.

INDEX